Walter and Miller's Textbook of Radiotherapy

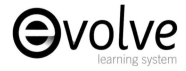

Commissioning Editor: Claire Wilson
Development Editor: Catherine Jackson
Project Manager: Mahalakshmi Nithyanand
Designer: Stewart Larking
Illustration Manager: Bruce Hogarth/Jennifer Rose
Illustrator: Antbits Ltd

Walter and Miller's Textbook of Radiotherapy

Radiation Physics, Therapy and Oncology

Seventh Edition

Edited by

Paul Symonds MD FRCP FRCR

Professor of Clinical Oncology, University of Leicester;
Consultant Oncologist to the University Hospitals of Leicester NHS Trust, UK

Charles Deehan BSc(Hons) MSc(Med Sci) PhD MInstP MIPEM CSci

Head of Radiotherapy Physics, Department of Medical Physics,
Guy's and St Thomas' NHS Foundation Trust, London;
Honorary Senior Lecturer, Imaging Sciences Division, School of Medicine, King's College, London, UK

John A. Mills PhD MinstP MIPEM CPhys

Physicist, Ariane Medical Systems Ltd, Derby, UK

Cathy Meredith MPH BA DCR(T) TQFE Cert CT Cert Couns

Senior Lecturer, School of Health, Glasgow Caledonian University, Glasgow, UK

ELSEVIER
CHURCHILL
LIVINGSTONE

ELSEVIER
CHURCHILL
LIVINGSTONE

First edition 1950
Second edition 1959
Third edition 1969
Fourth Edition 1979
Fifth Edition 1993
Sixth Edition 2003
Seventh Edition 2012

ISBN 978 0 443 07486 8

British Library Cataloguing in Publication Data
A catalogue record for this book is available from the British Library

Library of Congress Cataloging in Publication Data
A catalog record for this book is available from the Library of Congress

Notices
Knowledge and best practice in this field are constantly changing. As new research and experience broaden our understanding, changes in research methods, professional practices, or medical treatment may become necessary.

Practitioners and researchers must always rely on their own experience and knowledge in evaluating and using any information, methods, compounds, or experiments described herein. In using such information or methods they should be mindful of their own safety and the safety of others, including parties for whom they have a professional responsibility.

With respect to any drug or pharmaceutical products identified, readers are advised to check the most current information provided (i) on procedures featured or (ii) by the manufacturer of each product to be administered, to verify the recommended dose or formula, the method and duration of administration, and contraindications. It is the responsibility of practitioners, relying on their own experience and knowledge of their patients, to make diagnoses, to determine dosages and the best treatment for each individual patient, and to take all appropriate safety precautions.

To the fullest extent of the law, neither the Publisher nor the authors, contributors, or editors, assume any liability for any injury and/or damage to persons or property as a matter of products liability, negligence or otherwise, or from any use or operation of any methods, products, instructions, or ideas contained in the material herein.

ELSEVIER your source for books, journals and multimedia in the health sciences
www.elsevierhealth.com

Working together to grow libraries in developing countries

www.elsevier.com | www.bookaid.org | www.sabre.org

ELSEVIER   BOOK AID International   Sabre Foundation

The Publisher's policy is to use **paper manufactured from sustainable forests**

Printed in China

Contents

v

Contents

Contributors

Alison Armour, MB ChB BSc MSc MD MRCP FRCR
Vice-President Oncology Global Business,
GlaxoSmithKline, Philadelphia,
USA

Matthew Ahearne, MBChB MRCP
Clinical Research Fellow,
University Hospitals of Leicester,
Leicester, UK

Colin Baker, PhD MIPEM MInstP
Physics Department,
Clatterbridge Centre for Oncology,
UK

Margaret Bidmead, MSc FIPEM
Head of Physics,
Royal Marsden NHS Trust,
Fulham Road,
London, UK

Ramesh Bulusu, MD MRCP MSc FRCR (Onc)
Consultant Clinical Oncologist,
Primrose Oncology Unit,
Bedford Hospital & Oncology Centre,
Addenbrookes Hospital,
Cambridge, UK

Neil G. Burnet, FRCS FRCR MD
University Reader and Honorary Consultant Oncologist,
Department of Oncology,
Oncology Centre,
Addenbrooke's Hospital,
University of Cambridge,
Cambridge, UK

Kate E. Burton, MSc DCRT
Consultant Radiographer in Neuro-Oncology,
Oncology Centre,
Addenbrooke's Hospital,
Cambridge, UK

Peter J. Childs, MSc MIPEM
Radiotherapy Physicist,
Royal Marsden Hospital,
Sutton, Surrey, UK

Julie Clark, DCR[T] BA
Quality Assurance Superintendent,
Department of Radiotherapy,
Leicester Royal Infirmary,
University Hospitals of Leicester NHS Trust,
Leicester, UK

Robert Coleman, MD FRCP FRCPE
Yorkshire Cancer Research Professor of Medical Oncology and
Associate Director of the National Cancer Research Network
(NCRN), Academic Unit of Clinical Oncology,
Weston Park Hospital, Sheffield, UK

John Conway, PhD MIPEM CSi
Radiotherapy Research Governance Manager
Cancer Clinical Trials Centre,
Weston Park Hospital,
Sheffield, UK

Charles Deehan, BSc(Hons) MSc(Med Sci) PhD MInstP MIPEM CSci
Head of Radiotherapy Physics,
Department of Medical Physics,
Guy's and St Thomas' NHS Foundation Trust,
London; Honorary Senior Lecturer, Imaging Sciences Division,
School of Medicine, King's College, London, UK

Mike Dunn, MSc MIPEM
Head of Radiation Protection,
Leicester Royal Infirmary,
Leicester, UK

Martin J.S. Dyer, MA DPhil FRCP FRCPath
Professor of Haemato-Oncology,
University of Leicester,
Leicester, UK

Jill Emmerson, DCR[T]
Quality Radiographer,
University Hospital Coventry and Warwickshire,
Coventry, UK

David Gill, BSc
Radiotherapy Physics Technician,
University Hospital Coventry and Warwickshire,
Coventry, UK

John R. Goepel, MB ChB FRCPath
Consultant Histopathologist,
Royal Hallamshire Hospital,
Sheffield Teaching Hospitals NHS Foundation Trust;
Honorary Clinical Senior Lecturer,
University of Sheffield,
Sheffield, UK

Adrian Harnett, MBBS MRCP FRCR
Consultant Clinical Oncologist,
Department of Oncology,
Norfolk and Norwich University Hospital,
Norwich, UK

David Hastings, PhD MIPEM
Consultant Physicist,
Nuclear Medicine Group,
North Western Medical Physics,
The Christie NHS Foundation Trust,
Manchester, UK

David Hole (deceased), PhD
Professor of Epidemiology and Biostatistics,
University of Glasgow,
Glasgow, UK

Sarah J. Jeffries, PhD FRCR
Consultant Clinical Oncologist,
Oncology Centre,
Addenbrooke's Hospital,
Cambridge, UK

Janet Johnson DCR(T) BSc(Hons) MSc
Superintendent Radiographer,
Sheffield Teaching Hospitals NHS Foundation Trust,
Weston Park Hospital,
Sheffield, UK

George D.D. Jones, PhD
Reader & Deputy Head of Department,
Department of Cancer Studies & Molecular Medicine Biocentre,
University of Leicester,
Leicester, UK

Charles Kelly, MB ChB MSc FRCP FRCR FBIR DMRT
Consultant Clinical Oncologist,
Northern Centre for Cancer Care,
Newcastle upon Tyne, UK

Ian Kunkler, MA MB B Chir DMRT FRCP Ed FRCR FRSA
Honorary Professor of Clinical Oncology,
Western General Hospital,
Edinburgh, UK

Cliff Lawrence, MD FRCP
Consultant Dermatologist,
Royal Victoria Infirmary,
Newcastle upon Tyne, UK

Geoffrey P. Lawrence, PhD MIPEM
Consultant Physicist,
Clatterbridge Radiotherapy and
Oncology Centre,
Clatterbridge, UK

Duncan B. McLaren, MBBS BSc(Hons) FRCP (Ed) FRCR
Consultant Clinical Oncologist,
Edinburgh Cancer Centre,
Western General Hospital,
Edinburgh, UK

Ujjal Mallick, MS FRCP(Hon) FRCR
Consultant Clinical Oncologist,
Northern Centre for Cancer Care,
Freeman Hospital,
Newcastle upon Tyne, UK

Caroline Mansell, DCR[T]
Radiotherapy Service Manager,
The Royal Shrewsbury Hospital,
Shrewsbury, UK

Cathy Meredith, MPH BA DCR(T) TQFE Cert CT Cert Couns
Senior Lecturer,
School of Health,
Glasgow Caledonian University,
Glasgow, UK

John A. Mills, PhD MinstP MIPEM CPhys
Physicist,
Ariane Medical Systems Ltd,
Derby, UK

Sue Owens, MSc
Physicist,
Nuclear Medicine Group,
North Western Medical Physics,
The Christie NHS Foundation Trust,
Manchester, UK

Hamish Porter, PhD CPhys CChem
Radiation Physics Adviser,
London International Hospital,
Animal Health Trust,
Newmarket and Edinburgh University, UK

Trevor Roberts, FRCP FRCR
Consultant Oncologist,
Northern Centre for Cancer Care,
Newcastle upon Tyne, UK

Martin Robinson, MB BChir, MD, FRCR, FRCP
Consultant Oncologist,
Weston Park Hospital,
Whitham Road,
Sheffield, UK

Marjorie Rose, MSc MIPEM
Consultant Physicist,
Nuclear Medicine Group,
North Western Medical Physics,
The Christie NHS Foundation Trust,
Manchester, UK

John Sage, MSc PhD MIPEM
Head of Radiotherapy Physics,
University Hospitals of Leicester,
Leicester, UK

Christopher D. Scrase, MA MB CertMedEd MRCP FRCR
Macmillan Consultant Clinical Oncologist,
The Ipswich Hospital NHS Trust,
Suffolk, UK

James E. Shaw, BSc PhD
Lecturer, University of Liverpool (retired);
Director of Research and Development, Clatterbridge
Centre for Oncology (retired);
Former Head of Physics, Addenbrooke's Hospital Cambridge, UK

Michael Sokal, MB ChB FRCP FRCR
Consultant Clinical Oncologist,
Nottingham University Hospitals NHS Trust,
Nottingham City Hospital,
Hucknall Rd,
Nottingham, UK

Paul Symonds, MD FRCP FRCR
Professor of Clinical Oncology,
University of Leicester;
Consultant Oncologist to the University Hospitals of Leicester
NHS Trust

Roger E. Taylor MA FRCP (Edin) FRCP (Lond) FRCR
Professor of Clinical Oncology,
School of Medicine, Swansea University, Swansea UK;
Honorary Consultant Clinical Oncologist,
South West Wales Cancer Centre,
Singleton Hospital, Swansea, UK

Anne L. Thomas, PhD FRCP
Reader and Consultant in Medical Oncology,
University of Leicester,
Leicester, UK

Gillian D. Thomas, MD FRCR
Consultant Clinical Oncologist,
Department of Oncology,
Leicester Royal Infirmary,
Leicester, UK

Carl Tivas, MSc MIPEM
Physicist in Ultrasound,
University Hospital Coventry and Warwickshire,
Coventry, UK

Sarah Wayte, PhD MIPEM
Clinical Scientist,
Clinical Physics Department,
University Hospital,
Coventry, UK

Lorraine Webster, BSc(Hons) DCR(T) DipCouns
Macmillan Information Support Radiographer and Counsellor,
The Beatson West of Scotland Cancer Centre,
Glasgow, UK

Joyce Wilkinson, DCR(T) HDCR
Superintendent Radiographer,
Northern Centre for Cancer Care,
Newcastle upon Tyne, UK

Nigel R. Williams, PhD MIPEM
Head of Nuclear Medicine,
Department of Clinical Physics and Bioengineering,
University Hospital Coventry and Warwickshire,
Coventry, UK

Section | 1 |

Atoms, nuclei and radioactivity

Colin Baker

INTRODUCTION

The smallest identifiable amount of an element is an atom, consisting of a central nucleus composed of protons and neutrons which is orbited by electrons. The diameter of an atom and nucleus are typically 10^{-10} m and 10^{-14} m, respectively. To put these dimensions into a more accessible perspective, if the atomic nucleus is represented by the point of a pencil (diameter approximately 0.5 mm) held in the centre of a medium-sized room (say, 5 m × 5 m), then the electron cloud surrounding the nucleus would extend to the walls of the room. Most of the volume the atom occupies therefore consists of empty space, which makes it relatively easy for uncharged particles, such as photons, to pass through an atom without undergoing any interaction. An atom of carbon has six protons and six neutrons in the nucleus, surrounded by six electrons. Protons and neutrons have almost the same mass, while electrons have a mass roughly 2000 times smaller (shown in Table 1.1). The atomic nucleus therefore occupies a minute fraction (10^{-10} %) of the atomic volume, yet contains more than 99.9% of the atom's mass. Electrons and protons each carry the same magnitude of electric charge (1.602×10^{-19} Coulombs), but of opposite sign. The difference in the observed interactions of electrons and protons is therefore mostly due to their different masses: Electrons are relatively light, so scatter easily in a material while protons are less easily scattered.

Table 1.1 lists properties of *subatomic* particles of relevance to radiotherapy. Strictly, only the electron, positron and neutrinos (ν and $\bar{\nu}$) are *fundamental* particles, while protons, neutrons and pions are composed of *quarks*. Atoms are composed of just electrons, protons and neutrons. The positron is the anti-particle of the electron (having the same mass but opposite charge) and is emitted during beta decay (β^+) and in interactions of high energy photons with matter (see *pair-production*, Chapter 2). The annihilation of a positron with an electron provides the mechanism for positron emission tomography (PET). Neutrinos are uncharged particles of very small mass emitted during beta decay, sharing the energy released from the decay with the emitted beta particle (β^+ or β^-). Negative pions (π^-), one of the triplet of pions (π^0, π^+, π^-) are found in cosmic rays and are thought to be carriers of the strong force between nucleons. Despite their short life time (2.6×10^{-8} s), beams of these particles generated in physics

Table 1.1 Properties of subatomic particles of interest to radiotherapy

PARTICLE	SYMBOL	MASS* (kg)	ENERGY** (MeV)	CHARGE ($\times$ 1.6 $\times$ 10^{-19}C)
Electron	e^-	9.109×10^{-31}	0.511	-1
Positron (anti-electron)	e^+	9.109×10^{-31}	0.511	$+1$
Proton	p	1.673×10^{-27}	938	$+1$
Neutron	n	1.675×10^{-27}	940	0
Photon	γ	0	0	0
Neutrino	ν_e	>0	>0	0
Anti-neutrino	$\bar{\nu}_e$	>0	>0	0
Negative pion	π^-	2.488×10^{-28}	139.6	-1

*Rest mass
**Rest energy, see text for an explanation of these terms. From [1]

laboratories have been used for radiotherapy treatment, due to their favourable energy-deposition characteristics. This is discussed briefly in Chapter 2.

When referring to subatomic particles, it is common practice to interchange *mass* and *energy* through Einstein's famous expression:

$$E = mc^2 \qquad \boxed{1.1}$$

Where c is the speed of light, 2.998×10^8 ms^{-1}. Taking the electron as an example, the energy, E, associated with a mass, m of 9.109×10^{-31} kg is 8.187×10^{-14} Joules (J). It is more convenient to represent this very small magnitude of energy in units of the electron-volt (eV), where:

$$1 \text{ eV} = 1.602 \times 10^{-19} \text{ J} \qquad \boxed{1.2}$$

The electron mass's energy-equivalence of 8.187×10^{-14} J therefore equals 511 000 eV or 0.511 MeV, as shown in Table 1.1. Mass, m, in equation 1.1 is strictly relativistic mass, which increases as a particle's speed approaches the speed of light according to Einstein's theory of special relativity. The notation, m_0, generally refers to the concept of constant mass that we are more familiar with, corresponding to that of a particle at rest (rest mass) and the quantity m_0c^2 is then the corresponding energy associated with the particle (rest energy). The terms rest-energy and rest-mass are commonly interchangeable and both quoted in terms of energy.

The conversion of mass to energy and vice versa is demonstrated in pair-production and annihilation (Chapter 2), where the energy of an incident, mass-less photon is converted into the mass and kinetic energy of an electron and positron pair. The positron eventually annihilates with an electron (its anti-particle), releasing the combined rest mass of both particles, and any remaining kinetic energy, in the form of photons.

ATOMIC STRUCTURE

Atoms and nuclei are identified by both the number of protons or electrons (atomic number, Z) and the combined number of protons and neutrons present in the nucleus (mass number, A). An element may therefore be represented as:

$$^A_Z X \qquad \boxed{1.3}$$

The symbol, X, can be replaced by a unique identifier (chemical symbol) to remove the need for Z to be stated, e.g. ^{12}C to represent carbon (A=12, Z=6). An isotope of an element contains the same number of protons (Z), but a different number of neutrons (A–Z). Many elements appear naturally in the form of more than one isotope, some of which may be radioactive. As it is the atomic number that largely governs the chemical behaviour of elements (due to the arrangement of electrons discussed below), a stable element and its radioactive isotope will behave identically chemically. This feature can be made use of for clinical investigations, such as monitoring the uptake of iodine in the thyroid using radioactive ^{131}I as opposed to the stable isotope of ^{127}I.

Electromagnetic force

Electric and magnetic fields exert a force, F, on particles carrying a charge, q, which may be represented by:

$$F = q(E + vB) \qquad \boxed{1.4}$$

Where E is the strength of the electric field, v the velocity of the charged particle (which may be zero) and B the strength of the magnetic field perpendicular (or normal) to the particle velocity. An atomic electron is held in orbit by the electric (or electrostatic) component of this force due to the electric field of protons in the nucleus. This force of attraction (the electrostatic or Coulomb force), F_e, between electron and nucleus is proportional to the product of their charge and inversely proportional to the square of the distance, r, between them:

$$F_e = qE = k\frac{Ze^2}{r^2}$$

1.**5**

Where k is a constant, e is the electronic charge and Z the atomic number (number of protons) of the atom concerned. This *inverse-square* relationship is analogous to the gravitational force between two massive bodies (masses replace charges in equation 1.5). We can derive classical orbits (analogous to those of planets orbiting the sun) by equating this electrostatic force, F_e, with the centripetal force, F_c, due to an electron's circular motion around the nucleus:

$$F_c = \frac{mv^2}{r}$$

1.**6**

In the classical model of the atom, any value of r is possible, with a corresponding value of v. Observation of the radiation emitted by excited atoms shows that this continuous distribution of allowed orbits is not true of atoms and that only a discrete set of orbits, or *electron shells*, are allowed. This is discussed further below.

Electromagnetic waves and wave-particle duality

Energy, in the form light, heat or sound, may be transmitted from place to place by waves. These may be either transverse (as in the case of electromagnetic waves transporting light and heat) or longitudinal (sound waves). Electromagnetic waves are composed of oscillating *transverse* electric and magnetic fields, illustrated in Figure 1.1. In transverse waves, the direction of oscillation is normal to the direction of propagation, whereas longitudinal waves contain oscillations in the direction of propagation in the form of compressions and rarefactions. For radiotherapy applications, we are mostly concerned with the very high frequency end of the *electromagnetic spectrum*, shown in Figure 1.2. We can consider an x-ray photon to behave either as a particle or a wave, expressing *wave-particle duality*. The frequency, in cycles per second or Hertz (Hz), v of the radiation relates to its energy per particle, or *quantum*, through:

$$E = hv$$

1.**7**

Where h is Planck's constant (6.626×10^{-34} J s). A 6 MeV photon is therefore equivalent to an electromagnetic wave of frequency 1.5×10^{21} Hz. The wavelength, λ, of an electromagnetic wave is related to its frequency through:

$$\lambda = \frac{c}{v}$$

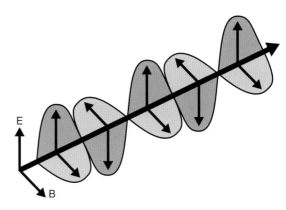

Figure 1.1 Illustration of an electromagnetic wave. Electric (E) and magnetic (B) fields oscillate normal to the direction of travel and to each other.

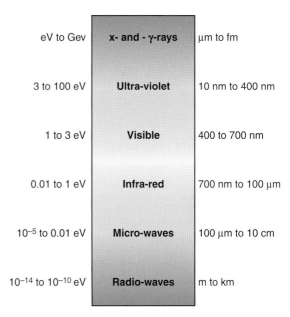

eV to Gev	**x- and - γ-rays**	μm to fm
3 to 100 eV	**Ultra-violet**	10 nm to 400 nm
1 to 3 eV	**Visible**	400 to 700 nm
0.01 to 1 eV	**Infra-red**	700 nm to 100 μm
10^{-5} to 0.01 eV	**Micro-waves**	100 μm to 10 cm
10^{-14} to 10^{-10} eV	**Radio-waves**	m to km

Figure 1.2 The electromagnetic spectrum. Approximate energy ranges are indicated on the left in electron-volts (1 eV = 1.602×10^{-19} J) and wavelengths on the right (adapted from [2]). (1 GeV = 1×10^{9} eV, 1 μm = 1×10^{-6} m, 1 nm = 1×10^{-9} m, 1 fm = 1×10^{-15} m).

Where c is the speed of light. In radiotherapy applications, both discrete energies and energy spectra may be involved. For example, a cobalt-60 source emits two discrete photon energies of 1.17 and 1.33 MeV, while a kV photon spectrum may show a continuous x-ray (bremsstrahlung) spectrum, with discrete (characteristic) energies superimposed on this continuous background. These are illustrated in Figure 1.3.

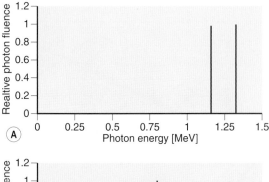

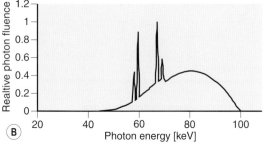

Figure 1.3 Discrete and continuous photon spectra. (A) Discrete photon energies from ^{60}Co [1.173 and 1.332 MeV] and (B) A 100 kV x-ray (bremsstrahlung) spectrum from a tungsten target with superimposed tungsten characteristic lines (from [3]).

Electron shells and binding energy

The term *shell* better describes the allowed, *quantized*, energy levels an electron may occupy around a nucleus, rather than a classical orbit. No energy is lost or gained while an electron occupies a particular shell, and only discrete amounts of energy can be gained or lost by electrons in order to move between shells. The energy associated with a particular electron shell is the sum of the electron's potential energy resulting from the attraction to the nucleus via the nuclear electrotrostatic field and the energy associated with the electron's motion around the nucleus which relates to its angular momentum. For the simplest atom, hydrogen, these quantized energy levels are approximately given by:

$$E_n = \frac{-13.6}{n^2} [eV] \qquad \boxed{1}.\boxed{8}$$

Where n is the principal quantum, or shell, number. Historically, the principal quantum number may also be represented by the letters K (n=1), L (n=2), M (n=3) etc. In order to raise an electron from the first to the second shell, the energy required is therefore E1−E2 =13.6 −13.6/4 = 10.2 eV. In order to remove completely an electron from the nth shell, an amount of energy greater or equal to E_n must be expended. E_n is therefore the binding energy of a particular electron shell. Further quantum numbers relating to angular momentum and spin dictate the maximum number of electrons that can occupy each principal shell. It can be shown that the maximum occupancy of electron

shells is given by $2n^2$, this rule, combined with a further one permitting no more than eight electrons in the outer shell, can be used to determine the electronic structure of atoms, as illustrated for selected elements in Table 1.2. Electrons in an atom will occupy the lowest (most negative) energy states in order to minimize the total energy of the atom. If all the lower electrons shells are occupied, the atom is said to be in its *ground state*. The number of electrons in the outermost shell when the atom is in its ground state is the *valence* and determines the chemical properties of the atom. Atoms which have only one electron (e.g. lithium, sodium, potassium) or one vacancy (e.g. fluorine, chlorine, bromine) in their outer shell are chemically most reactive, while elements with full valence shells (e.g. helium, neon, argon) are chemically unreactive.

Characteristic radiation

The binding energy of each electron shell in an atom is a function both of the principal quantum number, n and of the strength of the electrostatic force, which itself is directly proportional to the atomic number, Z (equation 1.5). The energy differences between electron shells are therefore not only quantized, but are characteristic of the atom's atomic number. An atom may be excited above its ground state by absorbing energy from incoming particles (e.g. photons or electrons) to raise one or more electrons into allowable, but normally empty shells. After a period of time, the atom will return to its ground state as electrons drop from higher shells to lower energy vacancies, releasing a photon of energy, E_γ, to carry away the energy difference between the two shells:

$$E_\gamma = E_i - E_j \qquad \boxed{1}.\boxed{9}$$

The energy of photons produced is therefore dictated by the differences in binding energy between electron shells of the particular atom from which they are emitted and are termed *characteristic radiation*. Figure 1.4. shows the electron shell binding energies and possible electron transitions leading to the production of characteristic photons for tungsten. The higher energy characteristic photons produce discrete lines on the continuous x-ray spectrum produced by an x-ray tube with a tungsten target, as illustrated in Figure 1.3. Distinction is made between electron transitions originating from different shells to the same destination shell by denoting the transition (and characteristic photon) with the final shell letter (K, L, and so on) and adding a Greek letter suffix to indicate the originating shell, as shown in Figure 1.4.

NUCLEAR STRUCTURE

Nucleons (protons and neutrons) are held together within the atomic nucleus by the *strong* (or nuclear) force, which acts only over small distances (10^{-15} m). The collective term

Table 1.2 Filling of atomic electron shells for selected elements.

ELEMENT	SYMBOL	Z	A[1]	DENSITY[2]	PRINCIPAL QUANTUM NUMBER[3]						
					1	2	3	4	5	6	7
Hydrogen	H	1	1	0.09×10^{-3}	1						
Helium	He	2	4	0.18×10^{-3}	2						
Lithium	Li	3	7	0.53	2	1					
Beryllium	Be	4	9	1.85	2	2					
Boron	B	5	11	2.34	2	3					
Carbon	C	6	12	2.26	2	4					
Nitrogen	N	7	14	1.3×10^{-3}	2	5					
Oxygen	O	8	16	1.4×10^{-3}	2	6					
Fluorine	F	9	19	1.7×10^{-3}	2	7					
Sodium	Na	11	23	0.97	2	8	1				
Magnesium	Mg	12	24	1.74	2	8	2				
Aluminium	Al	13	27	2.7	2	8	3				
Silicon	Si	14	28	2.33	2	8	4				
Phosphorus	P	15	31	1.82	2	8	5				
Calcium	Ca	20	40	1.55	2	8	8	2			
Iron	Fe	26	56	7.87	2	8	14	2			
Cobalt	Co	27	59	8.9	2	8	15	2			
Copper	Cu	29	64	8.96	2	8	18	1			
Germanium	Ge	32	73	5.32	2	8	18	4			
Strontium	Sr	38	88	2.54	2	8	18	8	2		
Yttrium	Y	39	89	4.47	2	8	18	9	2		
Molybdenum	Mo	42	96	10.2	2	8	18	13	1		
Technetium	Tc	43	98	11.5	2	8	18	14	1		
Ruthenium	Ru	44	101	12.4	2	8	18	15	1		
Iodine	I	53	127	4.93	2	8	18	18	7		
Caesium	Cs	55	133	1.87	2	8	18	18	8	1	
Barium	Ba	56	137	3.59	2	8	18	18	8	2	
Tungsten	W	74	184	19.4	2	8	18	32	12	2	
Iridium	Ir	77	192	22.4	2	8	18	32	15	2	
Gold	Au	79	197	19.3	2	8	18	32	18	1	

Continued

Table 1.2 Filling of atomic electron shells for selected elements.—cont'd

| | | | | | PRINCIPAL QUANTUM NUMBER[3] | | | | | | |
ELEMENT	SYMBOL	Z	A[1]	DENSITY[2]	1	2	3	4	5	6	7
Lead	Pb	82	207	11.4	2	8	18	32	18	4	
Radon	Rn	86	222	9.7×10^{-3}	2	8	18	32	18	8	
Radium	Ra	88	226	5.5	2	8	18	32	18	8	2
Uranium	U	92	238	19.0	2	8	18	32	18	12	2

[1]Mass number represents the average isotope mass rounded to the nearest integer.
[2]Physical densities are listed in g cm^{-3}.
[3]Historically the principal quantum number, $n = 1, 2, 3...$, may also be expressed as K, L, M ...

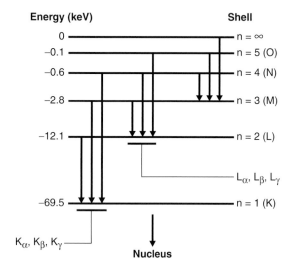

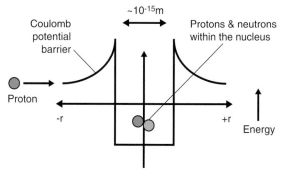

Figure 1.5 Illustration of the electrostatic (Coulomb) and strong force experienced by a charged particle approaching a nucleus. Once within range of the attractive strong force, the repulsive Coulomb force is overcome to hold nucleons together in the nucleus (the binding property of the strong force is represented as negative energy).

Figure 1.4 Electron energy levels and transitions leading to characteristic photons for tungsten. Strictly, each principal shell, *n*, has one or more associated energy levels, only the lowest energy levels for each value of *n* are shown.

for particles that experience the strong force is *hadron* (hence hadron therapy). Figure 1.5 illustrates the forces experienced by a proton being brought toward a nucleus; initially, an electrostatic (Coulomb) force of repulsion between the incoming proton and protons in the nucleus is present, which increases in magnitude (becoming more positive) as the incoming proton is brought closer, according to equation 1.5. Once within range of the strong force, however, the electrostatic force is overcome (the overall force is negative) and the proton is bound within the nucleus.

Plotting the number of protons against the number of neutrons for each stable nucleus results in the *stability line*, shown in Figure 1.6. We see that for low atomic number nuclei, an equal number of protons and neutrons is favoured,

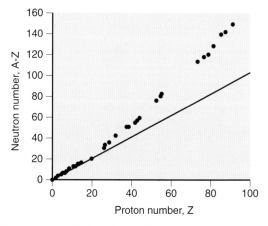

Figure 1.6 Stability line of naturally occurring isotopes (for elements listed in Table 1.2). Filled circles represent stable isotopes while the solid line represents Z=A−Z.

whereas a greater proportion of neutrons provides greater stability for large nuclei. This may be explained by considering the increasing electrostatic force of repulsion between protons in the nucleus as the number of protons is increased.

Evidence suggests that protons and neutrons within a nucleus adopt a shell-like structure analogous to electron orbits and show particular stability when the number of protons or neutrons, or both, corresponds to a *magic number* (2, 8, 20, 28, 50, 82, 126). The strength of the nuclear force is associated with a *nuclear binding energy* which must be overcome to break the nucleus apart. Representing this in terms of mass leads to a *mass-defect*, whereby the mass of a given nucleus is less than the sum of its constituent protons and neutrons. Nuclei with even numbers of protons or neutrons are found to be more stable than those with an odd number of one or both.

RADIOACTIVITY

A nucleus lying off the stability line, shown in Figure 1.6, is unstable and decays by rearranging its nucleon numbers. This is achieved by releasing particles, changing a proton to a neutron or vice versa, or by absorbing nearby particles. The activity of an unstable, or radioactive isotope is the rate at which its nuclei decay, expressed in *Becquerels* (Bq) which correspond to one decay or *disintegration* per second. The *activity* of practical sources is generally represented in MBq (1×10^6 disintegrations per second). The old unit of activity, the *Curie* (Ci) is commonly retained (1 Ci = 37 000 MBq). In the construction of practical radioactive sources, we are also interested in the amount of material that is needed to manufacture a source with a required activity, determined by the *specific activity* (MBq kg^{-1}).

Exponential decay

Suppose we have a radioactive source that decays by an amount, dA (Bq), in a small time, dt (s). If λ is the rate at which the relative activity decreases (s^{-1}), we have:

$$\lambda \, dt = -\frac{dA}{A}$$ **1.10**

Rearranging and integrating over time and activity and applying the condition that the activity at $t = 0$ is A_0, the activity, A, at some time later is given by:

$$A = A_0 \, e^{-\lambda t}$$ **1.11**

λ is the *decay constant* for the nuclide in question. The mathematical form of this expression is identical to that representing the attenuation of photons (see Chapter 2). Figure 1.7 shows the exponential decay in activity for a radioactive source and the linear plot of slope $-\lambda$, that results from a plot of $\ln(A)$ versus time. The nature of the exponential function is that an equal fractional reduction in activity occurs in equal time periods. For example, if a radioactive source of initial activity 160 MBq decays to 80 MBq in 1s, after 2 s

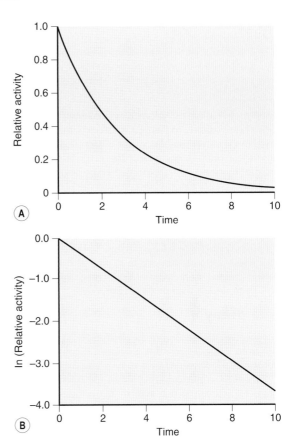

Figure 1.7 Exponential decay of radioactivity. (A) Linear plot showing exponential decrease of relative activity with time, and (B) logarithmic activity axis, giving a straight line of slope $-\lambda$.

the activity will be 40 MBq, after 3 s 20 MBq and so on. The time required for the activity of a radionuclide to fall to half of its initial activity is termed the *half-life* or $t_{1/2}$ (s^{-1}). Substituting $A/A_0 = 0.5$ and $t = t_{1/2}$ into equation 1.11 and rearranging, we obtain ($-\ln[0.5] = \ln[2] = 0.693$):

$$t_{1/2} = \frac{\ln(2)}{\lambda}$$ **1.12**

By definition, after one half-life, the activity of a radioactive source falls to half its initial activity. After two half-lives, the activity will have fallen to one quarter and after n half-lives, the activity, A, is given by:

$$A = A_0 \left(\frac{1}{2}\right)^n$$ **1.13**

Alpha decay

An alpha (α) particle is an alternative name for the nucleus of a helium atom, containing two neutrons and two protons, $^4_2$He. Having both an equal number of protons and neutrons (both of which are *magic numbers*), the helium nucleus is particularly stable and may often be emitted by a heavy unstable nucleus such as radium, uranium or plutonium. In emitting an α particle, the *parent* nucleus decreases its mass number by four and its atomic number by two:

$$^A_Z X \rightarrow ^{A-4}_{Z-2} Y \qquad \boxed{1}.\boxed{1}\boxed{4}$$

For example, radium ($^{226}_{88}$Ra) decays to radon ($^{222}_{86}$Rn) as shown schematically in Figure 1.8A. Energy must be conserved in the transformation, so any difference, Q, between the nuclear binding energies of the *parent* and *daughter* nuclei is shared between the emitted α particle (in the form of kinetic energy) and any photons that are produced:

$$^{226}_{88}Ra \rightarrow ^{226}_{86}Rn + ^4_2He + Q[4.79MeV] \qquad \boxed{1}.\boxed{1}\boxed{5}$$

Being relatively heavy (approximately four times the mass of a proton) and highly charged (containing two protons), α particles are readily stopped in matter. The 4.79 MeV α particle emitted from radium has a range of less than 4 cm in air, or less than 0.004 cm in tissue.

Beta decay

This involves the ejection of an electron (β^-) or positron (β^+) from a nucleus as either a neutron is converted to a proton (in β^- emission) or a proton into a neutron (in β^+ emission). A nucleus lying above the stability line in Figure 1.6 is neutron-rich and, by converting a neutron to a proton, can approach the stability line. Similarly, proton-rich nuclei can undergo the opposite transformation. Observation that the β particles produced display a spectrum of kinetic energies, rather than the discrete energy difference between parent and daughter nuclei, indicates that a further particle must be involved. This particle is the neutrino (v) or its anti-particle ($\bar{v}$). The process for phosphorus 32 ($^{32}_{15}$P) is shown below:

$$^{32}_{15}P \rightarrow ^{32}_{16}S + \beta^- + \bar{v} + Q[1.7MeV]$$
$$n \rightarrow p + e^-; Z \rightarrow Z + 1 \qquad \boxed{1}.\boxed{1}\boxed{6}$$

The Q value of 1.7 MeV is shared between the kinetic energies of the emitted β^- particle (electron) and anti-neutrino, $\bar{v}$ The corresponding energy level diagram is shown in Figure 1.9A, while the general scheme is shown in Figure 1.9B. The spectrum of β particle energies released is indicated in Figure 1.10. The average energy of the emitted β particle is approximately 30% to 40% of the maximum energy, depending on the isotope.

Fluorine 18 ($^{18}_9$F) provides an example of β^+ decay in its transformation to oxygen 18 ($^{18}_8$O):

$$^{18}_9F \rightarrow ^{18}_8O + \beta^+ + v + Q[0.64MeV]$$
$$p \rightarrow n + e^+; Z \rightarrow Z - 1 \qquad \boxed{1}.\boxed{1}\boxed{7}$$

The emitted positron (β^+) travels through matter, rapidly losing kinetic energy through interactions with atomic electrons. It eventually annihilates with an electron (its anti-particle), releasing two photons of 0.511 MeV, traveling in opposite directions to provide momentum conservation. The average energy of the positron, at 0.25 MeV leads to it being stopped within approximately 0.5 mm of the site of emission in tissue. The annihilation photons, on the other hand, at 0.511 MeV each can relatively easily pass

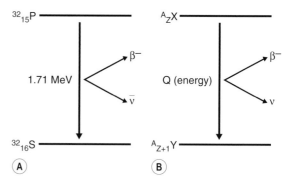

Figure 1.9 Energy level diagram showing (A) the β^- decay of $^{32}_{15}$P to $^{32}_{16}$S and (B) the general process of β^- decay.

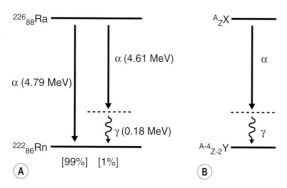

Figure 1.8 (A) α Decay of $^{226}_{88}$Ra. The decay may produce either a 4.79 or 4.61 MeV α particle, the former occurring in 99% of cases. (B) The general decay scheme for α decay.

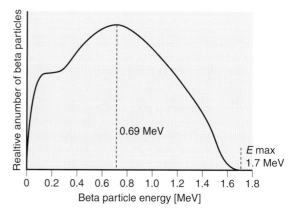

Figure 1.10 β spectrum from ^{32}P.

through tissue. Detection of these coincident photons via positron emission tomography (PET), following administration of a positron-emitting radionuclide to a patient, therefore reveals where the annihilation event occurred and hence where the radionuclide was taken up within the body.

Beta decay frequently occurs by more than one route (or channel) and may be accompanied by photon (γ) emission, as in the case of the β^- decay of $^{137}_{57}$Cs to $^{137}_{58}$Ba, where 95% of the disintegrations are via a meta-stable state (denoted by the letter, m) of barium ($^{137m}_{58}$Ba). $^{137m}_{58}$Ba subsequently decays to stable $^{137}_{58}$Ba, mostly by the emission of a 0.662 MeV photon. This emitted photon is used in brachytherapy with the beta particles being absorbed within the source encapsulation. The energy level diagram for this disintegration is shown in Figure 1.11.

Internal conversion and electron capture

As an alternative to positron emission (β^+ decay), the nucleus of a proton-rich atom may capture one of its own inner shell electrons, via *electron capture* (EC). The captured electron combines with a proton in the nucleus to produce a neutron and neutrino, the latter being emitted from the nucleus carrying kinetic energy equal to the difference in nuclear binding energy between the parent and daughter nuclei.

An excited nucleus may de-excite by emitting a single photon, or by *internal conversion* (IC), in which the excitation energy is transferred to an inner shell electron. The electron is ejected from the atom with kinetic energy equal to the excitation energy minus the electron binding energy; characteristic photons will subsequently be emitted by the atom as the electron shell vacancy is filled.

Decay series and radioactive equilibrium

Large nuclei, such as $^{238}_{92}$U, decay to radioactive daughter nuclei which themselves decay, leading to a decay series, as shown in Figure 1.12. The type of decay occurring at each step can be deduced from the change in A and Z in the figure. The series terminates in a stable isotope of lead.

Where the activity of a parent nucleus decays to a radioactive daughter, the growth of activity of the daughter with time depends on the relative decay constants between parent and daughter. A common example is molybdenum 99 ($^{99}_{42}$Mo) which has an 86% likelihood of decaying to technetium 99m ($^{99m}_{43}$Tc), which subsequently decays by photon emission (140 keV) to stable technetium. In the remaining 14% of cases, molybdenum 99 decays directly by β^- decay to stable technetium. If we assume that there is no daughter product present at time, $t = 0$, and that all parent disintegrations (100%) lead to the daughter product of interest, the activity of the parent, A_p and daughter, A_d, at time, t, are related by [4]:

$$\frac{A_d(t)}{A_p(t)} = \frac{\lambda_d}{\lambda_d - \lambda_p}\left(1 - e^{-(\lambda_d - \lambda_p)t}\right) \qquad \boxed{1}.\boxed{1}\boxed{8}$$

Where λ_p and λ_d are the decay constants of the parent and daughter nucleus respectively and the initial activity of the parent $A_p(0)$ is given by:

$$A_p(0) = A_p(t)e^{\lambda_p t} \qquad \boxed{1}.\boxed{1}\boxed{9}$$

The build up of daughter activity as expressed in equation 1.18 is of relevance to radionuclide generators. If the decay of the parent occurs at a much slower rate than that of the daughter, then $\lambda_d >> \lambda_p$ and equation 1.18 reduces to:

$$\frac{A_d(t)}{A_p(t)} = 1 - e^{-\lambda_d t} \qquad \boxed{1}.\boxed{2}\boxed{0}$$

The right-hand side of equation 1.20 tends to unity for $t >> 1/\lambda_d$, in which case the activity of the daughter and parent radionuclide are the same. This is the situation for ionization chamber consistency check devices containing a strontium-90 source. Strontium-90 undergoes beta decay with a half-life of 28.7 years to yttrium 90, which itself decays via beta decay with a half-life of 64 hours. The activity of the long-lived strontium parent determines and maintains the activity of the short-lived yttrium daughter.

Radionuclides of interest

Table 1.3 lists some common isotopes applied to radiotherapy and nuclear medicine. The choice of isotope for a particular application is based on decay product type (γ, β or α), product energy(ies), half-life, specific activity (activity per unit mass or per unit volume) and availability. β^- particles (electrons) have a relatively short range in tissue, so will deposit energy close to the site at which a radionuclide is taken up in the body. If the site of disease can be preferentially targeted, this leads to significant sparing of surrounding normal tissues in therapeutic applications. If greater penetration is required, of the order of centimetre for brachytherapy, or imaging of radioactivity uptake through external detection of radiation is required, then photons (γ) will be the product of choice.

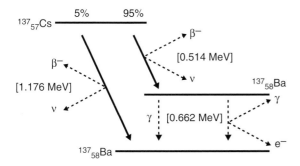

Figure 1.11 Energy level diagram for the β^- decay of caesium-137. Decay from $^{137m}_{58}$Ba is mostly via the emission of a 0.662 MeV photon, but may also occur via internal conversion.

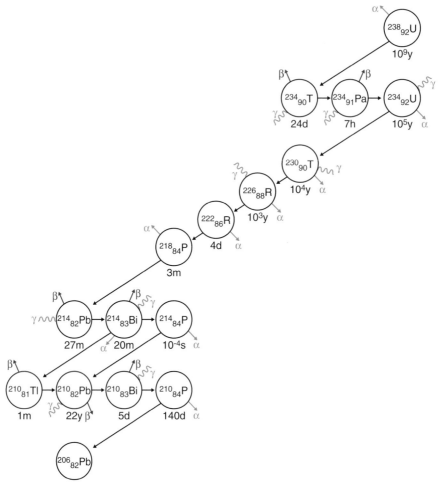

Figure 1.12 Decay series for $^{238}_{92}U$ (redrawn from [5]). Half-lives are indicated in seconds (s), minutes (m), hours (h) and years (y).

Table 1.3 Characteristics of common radionuclides

ISOTOPE	DECAY MECHANISM	APPLICATION(S)	HALF-LIFE
Unsealed sources:			
^{11}C	β+ (2.0 MeV)	PET imaging	20 m
^{13}N	β+ (2.2 MeV)	PET imaging	10 m
^{15}O	β+ (2.8 MeV)	PET imaging	122 s
^{18}F	β+ (1.7 MeV)	PET imaging	109 m
^{32}P	β− (695 keV)	Polycythaemia vera	14.3 d
^{89}Sr	β− (500 keV)	Bone metastases (palliation)	50.5 d
^{99m}Tc	γ (143 keV)	Diagnostic imaging:	6.0 h

Table 1.3 Characteristics of common radionuclides—cont'd

ISOTOPE	DECAY MECHANISM	APPLICATION(S)	HALF-LIFE
^{90}Y	β− (923 keV)	Arthritis	2.7 d
^{131}I	β− (264 keV)	Thyrotoxicosis	
	γ (364 keV)	Thyroid cancer	8.1 d
Sealed sources:			
^{60}Co	β−, γ (1.17, 1.33 MeV)	External beam units	5.26 y
^{103}Pd	EC, γ (21 keV)	Brachytherapy (seeds)	17 d
^{125}I	EC, γ (27-36 keV)	Brachytherapy (seeds)	60 d
^{137}Cs	β−, γ (662 keV)	Brachytherapy (pellets)	30 y
^{192}Ir	β−, γ (300-400 keV)	Brachytherapy (wire)	74 d

REFERENCES

[1] Yao W-M, et al. Review of particle physics. Journal of Physics G: Nuclear and Particle Physics 2006;33:1.

[2] Wilks R. Principles of radiological physics. 2nd ed. Churchill Livingstone; 1987.

[3] Catalogue of diagnostic x-ray spectra and other data. IPEM Report 78. IPEM Publications; 1997.

[4] Attix FH. Introduction to radiological physics and radiation dosimetry. Wiley and Sons Inc; 1986.

[5] Khan FM. The physics of radiation therapy. 3rd ed. Lippincott Williams & Wilkins; 2003.

FURTHER READING

Mayles P, Nahum A, and Rosenwald JC. Handbook of radiotherapy physics: Theory and practice. Taylor and Francis; 2007.

Chapter | 2 |

Radiation interactions with matter

Colin Baker

CHAPTER CONTENTS

INTRODUCTION

Charged and uncharged particles

In this chapter we are mostly concerned with the interactions of electrons and photons with matter, as these are the most commonly used particles in radiotherapy. The dominating feature of any particle is its charge. Electrons carrying a charge of -1.6×10^{-19} C readily interact via the Coulomb force with other charged particles in the matter they traverse, predominantly with atomic electrons and, to a lesser extent, with protons in atomic nuclei. Photons, on the other hand, carrying no charge, interact relatively rarely with matter. The use of clinical proton beams for radiotherapy is increasing as new facilities are constructed worldwide. As charged particles, proton beams passing through matter behave in a similar way to electrons, that is, they readily undergo interactions with atomic electrons. The difference between proton and electron interactions lies in the proton having a mass roughly two thousand times greater than the electron (1.67×10^{-27} kg and 9.11×10^{-31} kg for the proton and electron mass, respectively). The characteristics of proton energy loss in matter makes them highly suitable for radiotherapy, offering distinct advantages over photons and electrons, as will be discussed below. Neutron beams are less often selected as the beam of choice for radiotherapy at the present time, however, they also offer advantages over photon beams for some tumours due to their biological effect on tissue. Being uncharged, neutrons interact in a similar manner to photons and, in fact, produce very similar depth-dose characteristics.

It should be remembered that radiotherapy is not restricted to these particles alone. Ion beams consisting of atomic nuclei stripped of their electrons may also be used (a proton is, after all, a hydrogen atom without its electron). Carbon ions, in particular, have been used to treat a number of cancers in what is, at present, a small number of facilities world-wide and their characteristics are being actively researched. Negative pions (π^-), were also at one time thought to have great potential for radiotherapy due to the nature of their interactions and their energy loss at the end of their range, in particular, which is discussed below. Clinical studies of the use of pions have not demonstrated this advantage to date.

Excitation and ionization

Ionizing radiation, by definition, has sufficient energy to ionize matter. That is, it has sufficient energy to overcome the *binding energy* of atomic electrons. Radiation of energy below the binding energy of a particular electron shell may still interact with an electron by raising it to a higher, vacant shell (see Chapter 1). As a result of this interaction, the atom has gained energy and is left in an *excited state* (Figure 2.1A).

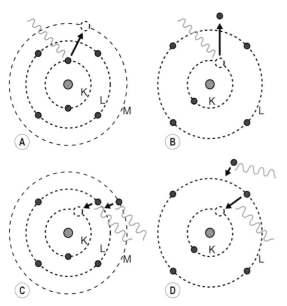

Figure 2.1 Excitation and ionization for a carbon atom. (A) Excitation: an incoming photon raises an inner shell electron to a vacant orbit, the electron has gained energy and, as a result, the atom is left in an excited state. (B) Ionization: an incoming photon ejects a K-shell electron from the atom, the atom is ionized having an overall positive charge. As no scattered photon was produced, the emitted electron has acquired kinetic energy equal to the energy of the incoming photon minus the electron's binding energy. (C) De-excitation: an L-shell electron drops into the vacancy in the K-shell, emitting a characteristic photon, the L-shell vacancy is filled by the electron involved in the original interaction. (D) De-excitation: an L-shell electron fills the K-shell vacancy and a free electron from the medium is captured to the L-shell.

It will eventually lose this excess energy to return to its lowest energy state, or *ground state*. An electron occupying an outer shell relative to the vacancy may achieve a lower energy state by filling the vacancy (Figure 2.1C). The excess energy is released as a *characteristic* photon (of energy equal to the difference in shell binding energies). If this electron is also in an inner shell, it too will leave behind a vacancy which an outer electron can again occupy (Figure 2.1C) losing energy in the form of a characteristic photon. This process results in a *cascade* of electrons moving between shells and a corresponding set of characteristic photons which eventually returns the atom to its ground state.

Even if its own kinetic energy exceeds the atomic electron's binding energy, an incoming particle (electron, photon etc.) may transfer just part of its kinetic energy to an atomic electron to produce excitation. Where the incoming particle transfers more than the binding energy of an atomic electron to the atom, the electron in question is ejected from the atom, with kinetic energy equal to the total energy transferred, minus the binding energy. As a result of losing an electron, the atom has been *ionized* (Figure 2.1B). As well as being chemically reactive as a result of this interaction (the positive ion will seek an electron from its surroundings to return to its uncharged state), any electron ejected from an inner shell will leave a vacancy behind, which represents an excited state. A *cascade* process will then follow as described above as de-excitation takes place (Figure 2.1D).

ELECTRON INTERACTIONS

Range and path-length

Electrons have a negative charge and a relatively small mass. As a result, electron transport through matter is characterized by a large number of interactions through which generally a small amount of energy is lost in each event and a high degree of scattering occurs (Figure 2.2). Because of these frequent interactions, it can often be assumed that electrons lose energy continuously as they traverse matter and to a good approximation the energy loss can be assumed to be at a constant rate. It follows that if electrons (or any other particles) lose energy continuously, then they must have a *finite range*. This is true of all charged particles. Calculated ranges for charged particles can be performed using this *continuous slowing down approximation*, resulting in the *csda range*. If a beam of monoenergetic electrons is incident on a given material and we assume continuous energy loss, then the total distance travelled, or *path length*, must be the same for all electrons in the beam. The depth of penetration, or *range*, will vary due to the different paths traversed by individual electrons as indicated in Figure 2.2. This *range-straggling* leads to a slope in the measured depth-dose curve as illustrated in Figure 2.3A. The steepness of this slope decreases as electron energy is

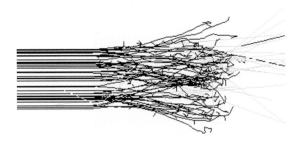

Figure 2.2 Illustration of the frequent interactions, scattering and finite range of electrons traversing matter. A beam of 10 MeV electrons (black) strikes a slab of water from the left. Incident electrons readily scatter, losing energy through collisions with electrons in the medium. Occasionally, energy is lost through x-ray production (bremsstrahlung, indicated by light grey lines). Note that (A) no primary electrons escape the slab as it exceeds the finite range of these electrons, x-ray photons and secondary electrons generated by these photons may leave the slab, and (B) the total distance traveled by an incident electron (path length) is greater than the maximum depth reached (range).

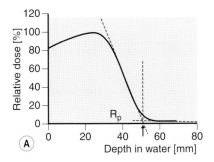

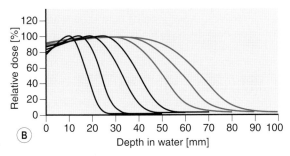

Figure 2.3 Electron depth-dose distribution in water. (A) 10 MeV electron beam, indicating practical range, Rp. (B) Variation of depth-dose with beam energy for (from left to right) 4, 6, 8, 10, 12, 15 and 18 MeV beams.
(Reprinted with the permission of the Clatterbridge Centre for Oncology NHS Foundation Trust: Douglas Cyclotron)

increased, as shown in Figure 2.3B. Note that the dose does not fall to zero immediately beyond the steep region of dose fall-off, due to bremsstrahlung photons being produced (discussed in the next section). The intersection between the slope due to range-straggling and the bremsstrahlung *tail*, gives the *practical range* of the electron beam, R_p. As a guide, for clinical electron beams produced by linear accelerators (approximately 4–20 MeV), the range of electrons in water (or tissue) can be approximated by:

$$\text{Electron range (cm)} \approx \text{Beam energy (MeV)}/2 \qquad \boxed{2}.\boxed{1}$$

An indication of the accuracy of the above expression can be made by comparison with electron csda ranges in water, given in Table 2.1.

Collisional and radiative (bremsstrahlung) energy loss

The last section was concerned with the dominant interaction that a beam of electrons undergoes when traveling through matter, that of collisions with atomic electrons (in the energy range of interest to radiotherapy, at least). These interactions lead to excitation and ionization of the medium traversed, as represented schematically in Figure 2.2. More rarely, electrons from an incident clinical beam will pass near to and interact with the atomic nucleus, again as a result of the Coulomb force of attraction between negatively charged electron and positively charged nucleus. The path (and momentum) of the incident electron is changed under the influence of the nucleus, resulting in a loss of electron energy. This loss of energy appears as a radiated photon, or x-ray photon (radiative energy loss). The term, bremsstrahlung ('braking radiation'), is a helpful descriptive name given to this process, shown

Table 2.1 Electron *csda* (continuous slowing down approximation) ranges in water

ELECTRON BEAM ENERGY (MeV)	*csda* RANGE (cm)
0.1	0.01
0.25	0.06
0.5	0.18
1	0.44
5	2.55
10	4.98
25	11.3
50	19.8
Evaluated using the ESTAR program [1]	

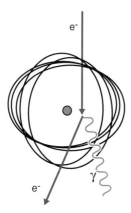

Figure 2.4 Schematic representation of photon production by electrons (bremsstrahlung). An incident electron deflected by the nuclear Coulomb field loses energy, which appears in the form of an emitted photon.

schematically in Figure 2.4. The probability of this interaction occurring is inversely proportional to the square of the incident particle's mass. As a result, bremsstrahlung is only significant for electrons. This important process by which x-ray photons can be produced is described further below.

Stopping power and linear energy transfer (LET)

The rate at which energy from an incident beam of charged particles is lost as it passes through a material is described by the *stopping power*. If an electron of energy, E, loses a small amount of energy, dE, in a small thickness, dx, of material, the stopping power, $S(E)$, is defined by:

$$S(E) = dE/dx \ [\text{MeV cm}^{-1}]$$ **2.2**

If the energy loss is separated into that lost in collisions, S_{coll}, with atomic electrons and that lost through bremsstrahlung (or radiative loss), S_{rad}:

$$S(E) = S_{coll}(E) + S_{rad}(E)$$ **2.3**

If energy is in MeV and distance in centimetres, stopping power has units of MeV cm^{-1}. Alternatively, we may express this in terms of mass stopping power, $S(E)/\rho$, where ρ is the material density (g cm^{-3}). The magnitude of this quantity depends on both the energy of the electron and the material involved. Figure 2.5 shows the variation of electron mass stopping power with energy in water and lead. As stopping power reflects the difference in energy absorption between materials, it is used in radiation dosimetry to convert measured radiation dose between materials. For example, using an air-filled ionization chamber surrounded by water, a direct measurement of energy absorbed, or dose to air, D_{air}, can be made. The dose, D_w, that would be absorbed if the ionization chamber were replaced by water (or a patient) would be given by multiplying by the ratio of mass stopping powers between water and air:

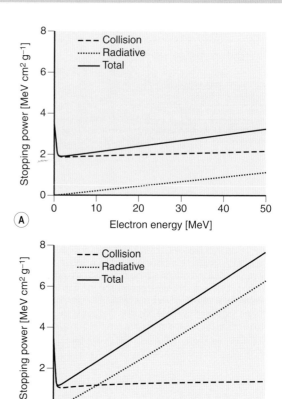

Figure 2.5 Collisional, radiative and total stopping power for electrons. (A) in water and (B) in tungsten. Data calculated using ESTAR [1].

$$D_w = D_{air} \times \frac{S_w(E)/\rho_w}{S_{air}(E)/\rho_{air}}$$ **2.4**

where ρ_w and ρ_{air} are the densities of water and air, respectively. Strictly, the stopping power used in the above expression must be restricted to energy absorbed within the ionization chamber volume and must exclude any energy that is lost from the beam but travels beyond the chamber (site of interaction). For example, energy lost in the form of bremsstrahlung, or collisions in which a large amount of the incident electron's energy is transferred to an atomic electron such that it travels beyond the chamber.

Linear energy transfer (LET) also refers to the amount of energy deposited by ionizing radiation in matter. Units are also energy per unit length, often expressed in keV μm^{-1}. LET is commonly used to distinguish between ionizing radiation in relation to radiobiology; radiation having a higher LET (such as protons, alpha particles) will generally lead to a greater biological effect than low LET radiation (photons, electrons). The smaller length units (μm) for LET reflect its application to energy deposition over subcellular dimensions. A schematic comparison

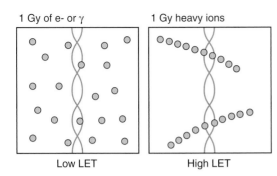

Figure 2.6 Comparison of dose deposition and biological effect for low and high LET beams. Circles refer to ionizing events. The increased track density of ionization events occurring for the higher LET beam leads to greater biological (DNA) damage. This increase in biological damage in comparison to low LET radiation (e.g. photons) can be expressed as a *relative biological effectiveness* (RBE), defined as the ratio of radiation doses required to produce the same degree of biological damage. For example, if an RBE of 1.1 is assumed for protons, then a prescribed proton dose of 70 Gy would achieve the same biological effect as a dose of 77 Gy delivered by photons.

Table 2.2 Percentage of incident electron beam energy appearing as bremsstrahlung for electrons incident on a tungsten target

ELECTRON ENERGY (MeV)	PHOTON YIELD (%)
0.05	0.5
0.25	2
1	6
10	30
50	63
Data calculated using ESTAR [1]	

between energy deposition for high and low LET beams is illustrated in Figure 2.6.

X-ray production

The conversion of electron kinetic energy into photons as a beam of electrons striking a target is decelerated in the nuclear Coulomb field (bremsstrahlung) is the primary method for obtaining clinical photon beams. As suggested earlier, however, for the normal range of energies considered for diagnostic imaging and radiotherapy (20 keV to 25 MeV), electrons are far more likely to interact through collisions with atomic electrons. The efficiency of this process is therefore generally low. The likelihood of bremsstrahlung depends on the atomic number of the material traversed, Z (the total charge of the nucleus) and the energy of the incident electron, E, according to:

$$Probability \sim ZE \qquad \boxed{2}.\boxed{5}$$

The energy of the electron beam is dictated by the maximum photon energy required. The use of high atomic number materials, gives the best yield of photons. Table 2.2 indicates the proportion of electron beam kinetic energy converted to photons for a tungsten target. The remainder of the incident electron's kinetic energy is lost through collisions with atomic electrons in the target, causing excitation and ionization. A large amount of this energy is eventually released in the form of heat, requiring the target to be cooled.

In the bremsstrahlung process, an electron may lose any amount of energy, up to its total kinetic energy. Rather than discrete photon energies, as are observed during de-excitation of atoms, a continuous spectrum of photon energies is produced. An example of the photon spectra produced when electrons are used to generate a 100 kV and 6 MV photon beam is shown in Figure 2.7. Photon spectra are commonly designated by 'kV' or 'MV' to indicate the nominal potential used to accelerate the electrons that created the spectrum. For example, a potential difference of 100 kV between cathode and anode in an x-ray tube will result in 100 keV electrons striking the target, producing a 100 kV photon spectrum. While there is no lower limit on the energy of photons produced, the low energy components of the spectrum are preferentially removed by photon attenuation within the target and other machine components, so that the peak in the spectrum occurs at approximately one-third of the maximum photon energy. Discrete spectral lines can be seen superimposed on the continuous 100 kV spectrum, these are due to characteristic photons being produced during de-excitation of tungsten atoms after inner shell electrons have been excited or ejected through collisions with the incident electron beam. The energies of these characteristic photons correspond to the difference between the binding energies of the inner shell vacancy and the outer shell electron that fills the vacancy. The difference between electron binding energies depends on the atomic number of the target. For tungsten, with a K-shell binding energy of 69 keV and L-shell binding energy of 12 keV, it follows that the minimum energy of a characteristic photon produced by filling an electron vacancy in the K-shell is 57 keV. The same characteristic photons are not observed in the 6 MV spectrum, as they now represent very low energies within this spectrum and are preferentially removed by photon attenuation.

For electrons striking a thin target, photons are produced in all directions. The intensity (or number) in a particular direction depends on the energy of the incident electrons, and the atomic number of the target. For low electron energies (up to 100 keV), the intensity is almost equal in all directions and as

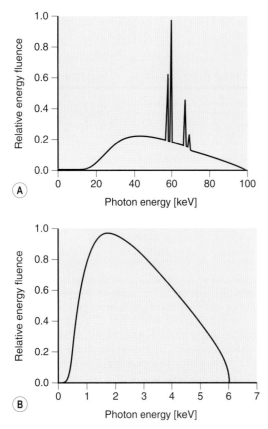

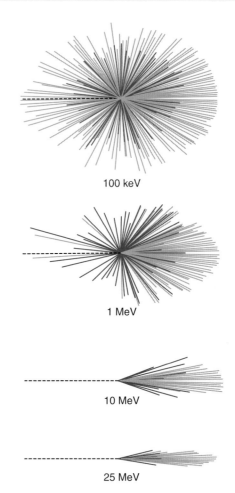

Figure 2.7 X-ray spectra: (A) 100 kV diagnostic spectrum; bremsstrahlung (continuous) spectrum with superimposed discrete characteristic tungsten x-rays [6] and (B) 6 MV photon spectra from an Elekta SL25 linear accelerator [5].

Figure 2.8 Spatial and energy variation of bremsstrahlung produced by electrons incident on a thin target. Electrons are incident from the left (dashed line), bremsstrahlung photons energy is indicated by track length and shade (short/dark = low energy). In each case 2000 bremsstrahlung interactions are simulated from known probabilities.

the electron energy increases, the photons produced become more forward directed. This variation in photon intensity with incident electron energy is illustrated in Figure 2.8, where electrons (indicated by the dashed line) are incident from the left. In this figure, bremsstrahlung production is simulated for a number of incident electrons, with the emitted photon energy and direction sampled from known probabilities (cross-sections). Two thousand photon tracks are represented in each figure, projected from a 3D distribution into a 2D plane. The length and shade of each photon track is representative of the individual photon energy. Note that higher energy photons (lightly shaded, long tracks) appear predominantly in the forward direction. This is one of the reasons for the average photon energy emitted from linear accelerators being lower at angles off the beam central axis.

The observed variation in spatial intensity of bremsstrahlung photons affects the design of x-ray targets. At kilovoltage energies, a reflection target is generally used, where photons produced at right-angles to the direction of incident electrons are extracted for use. At megavoltage energies, a transmission target is required as photons are

mostly travelling approximately parallel to the incident electron beam. This is shown schematically in Figure 2.9.

Beam hardening

In addition to the photon attenuation provided by the target and other machine components (*inherent filtration*), additional filters may be placed in the path of the emerging photon beam, particularly for kV photon beams used for diagnostic imaging (Figure 2.10). The effect of this is to preferentially remove lower energy components from the spectrum, as a result of their higher attenuation. This is a desirable effect as these low energy photons will contribute little to the x-ray image produced, but will be absorbed within the patient, resulting in unnecessary radiation dose. Adding filters in the path of the beam reduces the beam

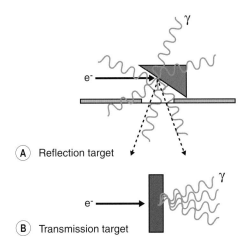

(A) Reflection target

(B) Transmission target

Figure 2.9 Reflection and transmission targets for the production of x-rays: (A) represents the production of a kilovoltage therapy beam and (B) the production of a megavoltage beam.

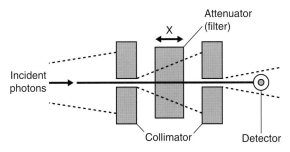

Figure 2.10 Geometry for photon attenuation measurements. Collimators are present to prevent scattered photons from reaching the detector.

intensity (number of photons), but increases the average energy of the beam (or *hardens* the beam) as low energy photons are preferentially removed. Photon attenuation is discussed in more detail below.

PHOTON INTERACTIONS

Exponential attenuation

Figure 2.10 shows an experimental arrangement for measuring the number of photons that reach a detector as a filter, or attenuator, is placed in the beam path. We are interested in measuring how many photons arrive at the detector without undergoing any interaction in the filter, i.e. how many photons are unattenuated. The purpose of the collimators is to prevent any scattered photons, resulting from an interaction in the filter, from reaching the detector and so causing us to overestimate the number of photons that have not interacted. If scattered photons are

excluded, this arrangement is referred to as '*narrow-beam*' geometry. The detector records N photons arriving at the detector for a thickness, x, of filter. If the number of photons reaching the detector changes by an amount, dN, when a thin (infinitely thin) filter of thickness, dx, is placed in the beam and we represent the relative change (dN/N) per unit thickness as μ, we have:

$$\mu\, dx = -\frac{dN}{N}$$ **2**.**6**

By integrating this expression, and applying the condition that for zero filter thickness, N_0 photons are recorded at the detector, it is straight-forward to show that the number of photons, N, transmitted by the filter and reaching the detector when a filter of thickness, x, is placed in the beam is given by:

$$N = N_0 e^{-\mu x}$$ **2**.**7**

Parameter, μ, is the linear attenuation coefficient (units of per unit distance, e.g. cm^{-1}), its value is dependent on the filter material and the energy of the photon beam. In order to compare the effect of varying atomic number on attenuation properties, it is convenient to remove the variation due to material density, ρ. This is achieved by defining the mass attenuation coefficient, μ/ρ. If μ is expressed in units of cm^{-1} and density in $g\,cm^{-3}$, the units of mass attenuation coefficient are $cm^2\,g^{-1}$, the corresponding thickness of filter must then be expressed in terms of mass-thickness (linear thickness × density), $g\,cm^{-2}$.

The mass attenuation coefficient is a macroscopic quantity that, in principle, can be measured relatively simply. It represents the total probability that a photon of a given energy will interact with matter, regardless of the type of interaction. Figure 2.11 shows the variation of mass attenuation coefficient with energy for water and lead. In water,

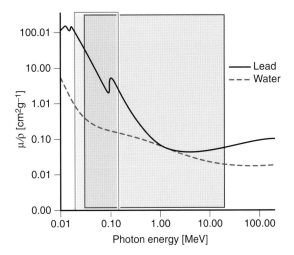

Figure 2.11 Mass attenuation coefficient variation with photon energy in water and lead (data from [2, 3]). The light and dark shaded regions indicate the approximate range of photon energies commonly used for diagnostic imaging and radiotherapy, respectively.

the attenuation coefficient is seen to decrease monotonically as photon energy is increased, up to approximately 50 MeV at which point it begins to increase. For lead, sharp discontinuities are seen around 100 keV (explained below) and the minimum attenuation occurs at a much lower energy of approximately 4 MeV, after which it begins to rise. It follows that the thickness of lead required to provide a chosen degree of attenuation would be greater for 4 MeV photons than it would be for 20 MeV photons. Note that here we are considering monoenergetic photons (MeV), whereas in practice, clinical photon beams contain a spectrum of energies (denoted by MV to indicate this). The effective attenuation coefficients (averaged over all energies in the spectra) in lead for 6 MV and 15 MV beams are roughly equal. The mass attenuation coefficients of water and lead are approximately equal for 1 MeV photons, at 10 MeV the coefficient for lead is a little over twice that of water, whereas at 100 keV, the coefficient for lead is over 30 times that of water. The reason for the particular shape of the attenuation curves for water and lead is explained by the varying probability with energy of the underlying photon interactions that combine to give the total interaction probability and hence attenuation coefficient. These interactions are described in subsequent sections.

The mathematical form of equation 2.7 is identical to that describing radioactive decay. For a chosen material and filter thickness placed in the path of a monoenergetic photon beam, adding additional filters of the same material and thickness will result in the same fraction of beam being transmitted, for example, if 1 cm of a filter results in the beam intensity falling to 70% of its original value, then 2 cm will result in 49% of the original intensity being transmitted. Figure 2.12A shows a plot of relative transmitted photon intensity ($N/N_0 = e^{-\mu x}$) for a monoenergetic beam of photons incident on aluminium filters. Taking natural logarithms of this equation yields a linear function, shown in Figure 2.12B. The slope of the straight line is equal to $-\mu$. For a filter thickness that reduces the intensity to half the original value, we have:

$$\frac{N}{N_0} = 0.5 = e^{-\mu t_{1/2}} \qquad \boxed{2}.\boxed{8}$$

$t_{1/2}$ is denoted the *half-value layer* (*HVL*) or half-value thickness. Rearranging this expression and taking natural logarithms gives:

$$t_{1/2} = HVL = \frac{\ln(2)}{\mu} \qquad \boxed{2}.\boxed{9}$$

For a chosen filter material, the *HVL* of a beam of photons provides a measure of the beam's power of penetration. In the kilovoltage region, *HVL* is therefore used to represent the *quality* of a beam of photons. For a monoenergetic beam of photons, it follows that after one *HVL*, the intensity drops to 50%, after two *HVLs* 25%, after three *HVLs* 12.5% and so on. The presence of inherent filtration for a monoenergetic source of photons would therefore have no effect on the measured beam quality.

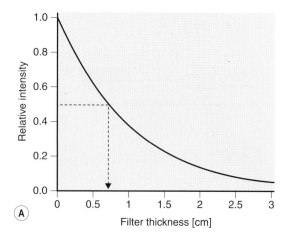

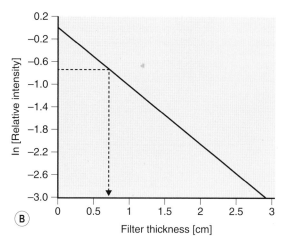

Figure 2.12 Exponential attenuation of monoenergetic photons. (A) Relative transmission versus filter thickness and (B) ln (relative transmission) versus thickness. The HVL of 0.7 cm Al is indicated on each plot.

Attenuation of photon spectra

We have so far considered only monoenergetic beams of photons. In practice, photon beams generated by fast-moving electrons striking a high atomic number target will have a spectrum of energies, as described above. We may expect the attenuation coefficient to decrease as photon energy is increased, i.e. that higher energy photons are more penetrating. In the kilovoltage region, at least, this is indeed the case and is the reason for beam hardening, discussed above. As a photon spectrum (polyenergetic beam) is filtered, lower energy photons will be preferentially removed from the beam due to their larger attenuation coefficients. This results in the average energy of the beam increasing and the average attenuation coefficient decreasing. As a result of this changing attenuation

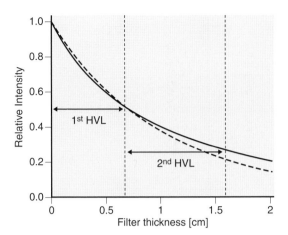

Figure 2.13 Attenuation comparison between a 100 kV photon spectrum (solid line) and a monoenergetic beam (dashed line) of the same first HVL. The first and second HVLs (0.7 and 0.9 cm Al respectively) for the spectrum are indicated. For the monoenergetic beam, the first and second HVLs would be equal, while for a spectrum of energies, the subsequent HVLs increase due to beam hardening, as indicated.

coefficient, the measured transmission curve will no longer be a true exponential. This is represented in Figure 2.13, where successive *HVLs* are no longer constant, but depend on the amount of filtration already present in the beam. Comparison of the first and second *HVL* (HVL_1/HVL_2) gives an indication of the degree of beam hardening occurring and is termed the *homogeneity coefficient*.

Energy absorption

As well as being interested in how many photons are transmitted without interacting in a filter (i.e. remain unattenuated), we may also be interested in the amount of energy that is absorbed in the filter, particularly if we replace the filter with biological tissue. This information is given by the *energy absorption coefficient*, denoted μ_{en}. In a similar approach to that followed for attenuation, we can also define the *mass energy absorption coefficient*, μ_{en}/ρ. These quantities have the same units as their attenuation counterparts. In terms of the geometry shown in Figure 2.10, in order to determine energy absorption, we must detect all unattenuated photons, together with any other energy not absorbed locally. Assuming all charged particles are absorbed (stopped) locally, it is the energy transported away in the form of photons that must be accounted for, i.e. all characteristic photons released from excited atoms following photoelectric interactions, scattered photons resulting from the Compton effect, bremsstrahlung photons produced by charged particles (e.g. Compton electrons) and, finally, photons arising from positron annihilation

following pair-production (if the incident photon energy is high enough). The geometry for this situation then represents *broad-beam* conditions. It follows that the attenuation coefficient for a given monoenergetic photon beam in a given material is larger than the corresponding energy absorption coefficient for the same energy and material as attenuation accounts for both absorption and scatter. Practical measurement geometry will fall between narrow and broad beam conditions. Figure 2.14A compares mass

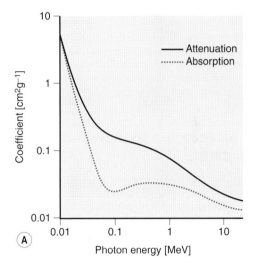

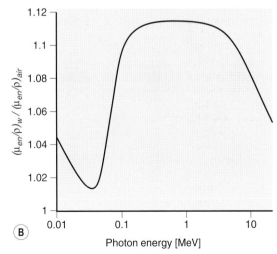

Figure 2.14 (A) Comparison of photon mass attenuation and mass energy absorption coefficients in water. Note that the difference is largest where the Compton effect dominates due to energy being transported away from the site of interaction by Compton-scattered photons. (B) Ratio of water to air mass energy absorption coefficient.
(data taken from [2, 3])

attenuation coefficients and mass energy absorption coefficients in water for the range of photon energies of interest to radiotherapy.

Energy absorption coefficients are used in radiation dosimetry in a similar way to that in which electron stopping powers are used for electron beams described earlier. Taking again the example of an air-filled ionization chamber in water, having determined the dose deposited by photons in the air cavity, D_{air}, the dose to the same region when filled with water, D_w, is given by:

$$D_w = D_{air} \times \frac{(\mu_{en}/\rho)_w}{(\mu_{en}/\rho)_{air}} \qquad \boxed{2.10}$$

(see Figure 2.14B).

The above expression assumes that all electrons set in motion by the incident photons deposit their energy within the chamber. This is a reasonable assumption for kV photon beams. For MV photon beams, however, the ranges of secondary electrons become significant and must be considered.

From attenuation to individual interactions

In the photon energy range of interest for radiotherapy, there are three major interactions that can occur as a beam of photons passes through matter. Figure 2.15 illustrates the interactions occurring in a slab of water when irradiated with a beam of 3 MeV photons. Figure 2.16 shows how the

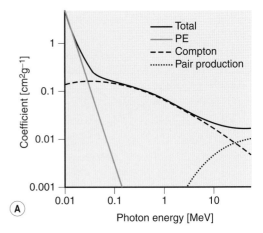

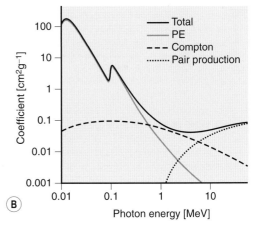

Figure 2.16 Mass attenuation coefficients, showing the relative contributions from the photoelectric effect, Compton effect and pair-production in (A) water (effective Z = 7) and (B) lead (Z = 82). Note the large region of dominance for the Compton effect in water, due to the lower effective atomic number, Z. *(data from [2, 3])*

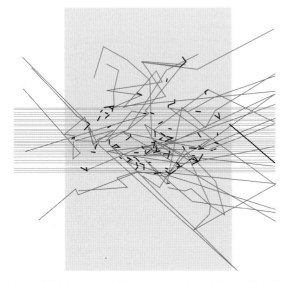

Figure 2.15 Illustration of photon interactions. A beam of 3 MeV photons (light grey) is incident from the left on a 25 cm thick water slab. Photons may escape the slab without interacting, others interact in the water, generating secondary electrons (black) which cause further ionization and may escape the slab if they are generated close to the exit face. Photons may be backscattered from the face of the slab, along with secondary electrons.

individual probabilities of these interactions combine to give the total mass attenuation coefficient, also showing the region of dominance for each interaction type and their variation with atomic between water (Z = 7) and lead (Z = 82). These will be considered in terms of their importance as photon energy increases from the kilovoltage to megavoltage range. The first two of these interactions; the photoelectric effect and Compton effect, are interactions between the incident photon and atomic electrons in the medium traversed. The third, pair-production, occurs between an incident photon and the Coulomb field of the atomic nucleus. At higher energies still, above approximately 8 MeV, photons may undergo interactions directly with the atomic nucleus, releasing neutrons and forming radioactive isotopes. A summary of the energy ranges in which each interaction dominates is shown in Table 2.3.

Table 2.3 Energy regions of domination for photo-electric, Compton and pair-production interactions

INTERACTION	LOW Z (WATER)	HIGH Z (LEAD)
Photoelectric	<30 keV	<500 keV
Compton	30 keV to 25 MeV	0.5 to 5 MeV
Pair production	>25 MeV	>5 MeV

The photoelectric effect

This interaction, shown schematically in Figure 2.17, occurs between an incident photon and atomic electron, generally assumed to be an inner shell electron. If the photon has sufficient energy to overcome the shell binding energy of the electron, it may disappear by transferring all its energy to the electron. The electron is then emitted from the atom, with kinetic energy, *k.e.*, equal to the energy of the incident photon, E_γ, minus the electron binding energy, *b.e.*

$$\text{k.e.} = E_\gamma - \text{b.e.} \qquad \boxed{2}.\boxed{1}\boxed{1}$$

As a consequence of this interaction, the atom is ionized and in an excited state. De-excitation then occurs, releasing characteristic photons, in the same manner as described in Chapter 1 after ionization or excitation by electron interactions. The probability of the photoelectric effect occurring is strongly dependent on the atomic number of the material traversed and on the energy of the incident photon:

$$\text{Probability} \sim Z^3/E^3 \qquad \boxed{2}.\boxed{1}\boxed{2}$$

This strong dependence on atomic number is put to considerable use in diagnostic imaging as it provides clear differentiation between tissues with different atomic number as

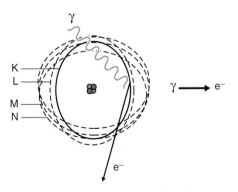

Figure 2.17 Schematic representation of the photoelectric effect. An incoming photon transfers all its energy to an inner shell electron, ejecting the electron with a kinetic energy equal to the photon energy minus the electron binding energy. Electron shells, K to N are indicated.

well as, or in the absence of, differences in physical density. For example, a 70 kV beam of photons passing through a human pelvis is much more likely to interact and be absorbed when passing through bone, with an atomic number of approximately 13, than it is when passing through adjacent soft tissue, with an approximate atomic number of 7. The photon intensity transmitted through the patient therefore clearly distinguishes between bone and soft tissue, providing a high contrast x-ray image.

The large discontinuities observed at approximately 15 and 88 keV for the mass attenuation coefficient in lead, shown in Figure 2.16B are a result of incident photons having sufficient energy to overcome the binding energies of the lead L and K shells, respectively. This large increase in interaction probability around an electron binding energy suggests that a resonance effect is involved, whereby the probability of interaction is highest when the photon energy is close to that of the electron binding energy. This feature in the mass attenuation coefficient curve is referred to as an absorption edge. The photoelectric effect dominates in water, or tissue, for energies up to approximately 30 keV and, in lead, up to approximately 500 keV. The lack of visible absorption edges in water (Figure 2.16A) is due to the lower probability of the photoelectric effect occurring in water, relative to the Compton effect and the low binding energies of the K-shell electrons for oxygen and hydrogen.

The Compton effect

The Compton effect dominates in water between 100 keV and 20 MeV and is therefore the dominant interaction in tissue throughout the radiotherapy energy range of interest for photons. This interaction involves an incident photon interacting with an atomic electron, overcoming the electron binding energy and transferring some of its energy to the electron in the form of kinetic energy and the remainder as a lower energy photon. Unlike the photoelectric effect, no resonance effect is observed and the interaction is likely to occur with outer shell electrons with binding energies far lower than the energy of the incoming photon. As a result, this interaction is often referred to as occurring with 'free' electrons. The interaction is shown schematically in Figure 2.18.

The probability of the Compton interaction depends on the density of electrons in a material, which varies as Z/A. This ratio is almost constant for elements above hydrogen and, as a result, the Compton effect can be considered to be independent of the atomic number of the material the photons pass through and is dependent only on the physical density. It is for this reason that medical imaging with megavoltage photons leads to poorer contrast than imaging with kilovoltage photon beams. This represents a benefit for radiotherapy to soft-tissue tumours, however, as a significant dependence on atomic number would lead to higher absorbed dose being delivered to bone than soft tissue.

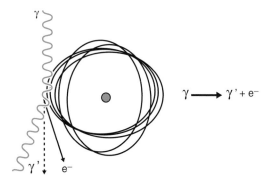

Figure 2.18 Schematic representation of the Compton effect. An incident photon, γ, transfers part of its energy to an electron and a lower energy, scattered photon, γ', is produced.

The average proportion of the incident photon's energy transferred to the electron depends on the incident photon energy. For a 100 keV incident photon, on average approximately 10% of its energy, 10 keV, is passed to the electron, while the scattered photon retains 90 keV. As the incident photon energy increases, however, a higher proportion of its energy is transferred to the electron; a 10 MeV photon transfers an average of approximately 70%, 7 MeV, to the electron and the scattered photon retains 3 MeV. The variation of average energy transferred to the electron via the Compton effect is illustrated in Figure 2.19. These characteristics of the Compton effect have implications for radiotherapy and radiation dosimetry. For kilovoltage photon beams, electrons set in motion through Compton interactions can be assumed to deposit their energy very close to the site of interaction, whereas for megavoltage photons, these interactions produce high energy *secondary* electrons which will travel a significant distance. The latter results in the observed skin-sparing effect of absorbed dose

deposition in tissue by megavoltage photon beams, as electrons set in motion near the skin surface deposit their energy over a significant depth. For example, a 3 MeV photon (approximately the average photon energy in a 10 MV photon spectrum) will provide an electron with an average energy of 1.8 MeV (60%), which will deposit energy over a distance of approximately 1 cm in tissue. The angular distribution of electrons set in motion by the Compton effect is also of interest. For kilovoltage photons, the secondary electrons set in motion are emitted over a wide range of angles from the direction of the incident photon. As the incident photon energy is increased, this distribution of electrons becomes more forward directed.

Pair-production

Above a few MeV, photons may interact with the nuclear Coulomb field to produce an electron-positron pair, shown schematically in Figure 2.20. In this interaction, the photon vanishes and all its energy is transferred to the *rest-mass* and kinetic energy of the electron and position. For an incident photon of energy, E, conservation of energy demands that:

$$E = 1.022 + k.e.\,(e^+) + k.e.\,(e^-)\,[MeV] \qquad \boxed{2}.\boxed{1}\boxed{3}$$

Hence, the incoming photon must have a minimum energy of 1.022 MeV for the interaction to occur. The probability of a photon being attenuated by pair-production is proportional to the atomic number of the material traversed and, for the energy range of interest to radiotherapy, increases gradually with the incoming photon's energy.

$$Probability \sim ZE \quad (E > 1.022\ MeV) \qquad \boxed{2}.\boxed{1}\boxed{4}$$

In water (and soft tissue), pair-production only becomes significant at photon energies above approximately 10 MeV (see Figure 2.16), so accounts for very little of the absorbed dose to a patient undergoing radiotherapy. For higher atomic number materials, pair production becomes significant at lower energies (approximately 3 MeV for lead).

The electron and positron produced will lose energy in the medium traversed, mainly through interactions (collisions) with atomic electrons, as discussed above. The

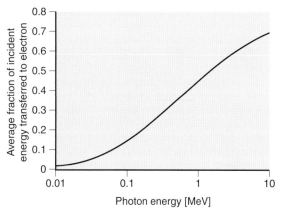

Figure 2.19 Average proportion of photon energy transferred to secondary electrons during the Compton effect. *(derived from [7])*

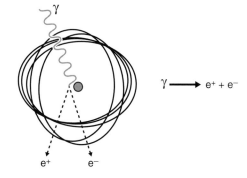

Figure 2.20 Schematic representation of pair production in the nuclear Coulomb field.

positron eventually *annihilates* with a local electron, releasing the remaining positron kinetic energy and rest-mass of the positron and electron in the form of photons. This annihilation event becomes more likely as the positron slows down. If it occurs '*at rest*', i.e. when the positron has lost all of its kinetic energy, the energy of each photon is equal to 0.511 MeV, the electron (and positron) rest-mass. To conserve momentum, these two photons must travel in opposite directions. This feature of positron–electron annihilation is the key to *positron emission tomography* (PET), as coincident detection of the two photons produced reveals information on the position of the annihilation event.

Photons may undergo a similar interaction to the nuclear pair-production interaction described above in the Coulomb field of an electron. However, the probability of this is very low compared to the interaction in the nuclear Coulomb field.

Nuclear interactions

At sufficiently high energies (above approximately 8 MeV, or 15 MV spectra), photons may interact directly with the atomic nucleus, releasing neutrons or protons:

$$\gamma + {}^{A}_{Z}X \rightarrow {}^{A-1}_{Z}X + n$$

$$\gamma + {}^{A}_{Z}X \rightarrow {}^{A-1}_{Z-1}Y + p$$

2.15

These interactions do not lead to a significant patient dose, but the production of neutrons can lead to additional shielding requirements for the treatment room. Activation of linear accelerator components, particularly the photon target, can also occur, which must be allowed to decay to acceptable levels before any intervention, such as machine servicing.

Photon depth-dose and the build-up effect

Figure 2.12 showed how the *transmission* of photons decreases exponentially as the amount of matter traversed is increased. The quantity we are generally more interested in, however, is the absorbed dose received at a depth in tissue and how this varies with depth. This quantity is commonly described as *percentage depth-dose, PDD*:

$$PDD = 100 \times \frac{D(d)}{D(d_{max})}$$

2.16

where $D(d)$ is the measured dose at depth, d, and d_{max} the depth of maximum dose. Example PDD curves for megavoltage photon beams are shown in Figure 2.21. An important feature of these curves is that fact that the maximum dose is not reached at the surface, but at a depth, d_{max}, which is dependent on the energy of the beam. This provides the *skin-sparing* effect of megavoltage photon beams. The dose build-up effect is explained by considering the photon interactions taking place in tissue at the energies involved. Table 2.3 shows us that the Compton effect

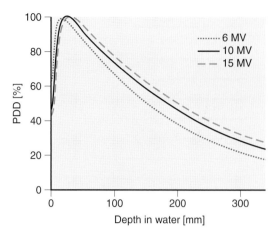

Figure 2.21 Example percentage depth-dose profiles (PDDs) for photon beams in water.
Reprinted with the permission of the Clatterbridge Centre for Oncology NHS Foundation Trust: Douglas Cyclotron

dominates in low atomic number materials, such as tissue, right across the MeV range of photon energies commonly used for radiotherapy. This interaction provides a scattered photon, which generally leaves the site of interaction and a secondary electron which has a finite range over which it deposits its energy. For an incident 1 MeV photon, Figure 2.19 shows us that approximately 0.4 MeV, on average, is passed to the secondary electron, whereas for a 10 MeV incident photon, roughly 6.8 MeV on average would be passed on. This kinetic energy of the secondary electrons is not all deposited at the site of the Compton interaction, but is spread out over the electron's range, which depends on the electron's energy (as shown in Table 2.1). Let's now consider the total absorbed dose from secondary electrons as we move between thin 'layers' from the surface to the depth of d_{max}, in steps of some fraction of d_{max}. As illustrated in Figure 2.22, some energy is deposited in the surface layer by secondary electrons set in motion within this layer and some is transported along with the electrons to underlying layers. Taking a step deeper, we again have a dose from secondary electrons set in motion within this layer, and we have an additional dose contribution from secondary electrons entering from the surface layer (upstream), i.e. we now have contributions from two layers. At the next layer, we have three layers contributing, the one we are in and two upstream. At each successive deeper layer, the number of upstream layers contributing electrons increases, so the total absorbed dose rises, or builds up. This process continues until we are at a depth beyond the range of electrons set in motion in the surface layer, at which point we have reached full build up, at d_{max}. The depth of d_{max}, then, corresponds to the average range of secondary electrons set in motion by the incident photon beam, which increases with photon beam energy, as shown in Figure 2.21 in moving from 6 to 15 MV. In practice, this

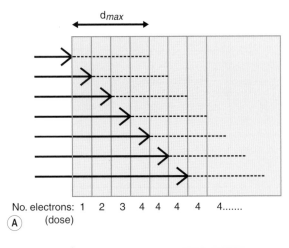

No. electrons: 1   2   3   4   4   4   4   4.......
(A)   (dose)

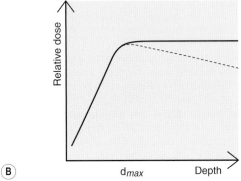

(B)

Figure 2.22 Schematic illustration of dose build-up in MV photon beams. (A) Incident photons (solid lines) interact in each layer, liberating secondary electrons (dashed lines). These electrons deposit their kinetic energy over their (finite) range, here corresponding to four layers. The total dose in each layer is proportional to the number of electrons crossing it (1 to 4). (B) The solid line indicates the build-up of dose in the absence of photon attenuation. The dashed line indicates the exponentially decreasing dose beyond d_{max} due to photon attenuation.

depth will also be influenced by the field size, by contaminant electrons generated in the head of the accelerator and in any beam modifying devices in the path of the beam. If we assume that photon attenuation is negligible over a number of layers, then at d_{max} and beyond, the total number of electrons crossing each layer is constant; the number entering a given layer from upstream equals the number moving downstream (see Figure 2.22). This condition is termed *charged-particle equilibrium* (cpe) and is discussed further in Chapter 3. Note that for kilovoltage photon beams, the energies and ranges of secondary electrons will be very much reduced. For example, a 100 keV photon interacting by the Compton effect will produce, on average, a secondary electron of around 15 keV, which has a range of less than 1/100 mm. Secondary

electrons generated by kV photon beams can therefore be assumed to deposit their energy at the site of interaction in tissue and no dose build up, or skin-sparing occurs.

For a phantom, or patient, irradiated at a fixed *source-to-surface distance* (SSD) with a diverging beam (e.g. that from a small or 'point' source, such as a clinical linear accelerator or x-ray tube), the absorbed dose beyond the depth of d_{max} will decrease with depth due to both increasing attenuation of the incident photons and also due to the increasing distance of the point of interest from the source. This latter effect is known as the *inverse-square law*, as the dose from a point source, in the absence of any attenuating material, will decrease as $1/r^2$, where r is the distance from the source. The derivation of this law is given in Figure 2.23. We can combine the effect of photon attenuation with the inverse-square reduction in photon intensity, to approximate the *PDD* beyond d_{max} as:

$$PDD \approx 100 \times e^{-\mu_{eff}(d-d_{max})} \times \left(\frac{f+d_{max}}{f+d}\right)^2 \quad \boxed{2.17}$$

where μ_{eff} is the effective attenuation coefficient for the beam. The term *effective attenuation coefficient* is used here, as our geometry does not exclude scattered radiation and is likely to represent an average over a photon spectrum. μ_{eff} will therefore vary with field size and depth.

PROTONS AND ION BEAMS

Protons

Carrying the same magnitude, but opposite sign of charge to electrons, protons readily interact with atomic electrons causing ionization and excitation as they continuously lose energy passing through matter. The proton mass, being approximately 2000 times larger than that of an electron, results in protons undergoing far less lateral scattering. As bremsstrahlung losses are inversely proportional to the square of the incoming particle mass, such losses are negligible for protons. Rather than the approximately linear relationship between energy and range, as observed for electrons (where range $\approx$ MeV/2 cm), proton range scales roughly with the square of the proton energy. As protons lose energy far more rapidly than electrons when traversing matter, energies of up to approximately 250 MeV are required to treat deep-seated tumours. Table 2.4 indicates proton ranges for a number of beam energies.

A key difference in the characteristics of energy deposition with depth for protons as opposed to electrons, is the appearance of a Bragg peak, shown in Figure 2.24A. This results from a reduced amount of lateral scattering and a sharp increase in stopping power (dE/dx) as protons slow down in a material (Figure 2.24B). The Bragg peak is ideally suited to radiotherapy as the high dose region is concentrated at depth, protecting both overlying and underlying

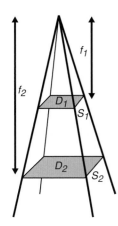

Given a square field of side, s_1 at distance, f_1 the size, s_2, at distance, f_2 is given by:
$s_2 = s_1 \times (f_2 / f_1)$ [1]

Field areas are related by:
$s_2^2 = s_1^2 \times (f_2 / f_1)^2$ [2]

In the absence of photon interactions, the number of photons over each field is constant (=n, say) and the number per unit area (intensity) is therefore:
$I_1 = n/s_1^2$ and $I_2 = n/s_2^2$

The ratio of intensities is therefore:
$I_2/I_1 = s_1^2/s_2^2$ [3]

From [2], we have:
$s_1^2/s_2^2 = (f_1 / f_2)^2$

So, [3] can be written as: $I_2/I_1 = (f_2 / f_1)^2$ [4]
As dose is proportional to intensity, we can replace Is by Ds in [4] to obtain:
$D_2 = D_1 \times (f_1 / f_2)^2$ or $D_2 \propto 1/f_2^2$
This is the inverse-square law; Dose, D_2, is *inversely proportional* to the *square* of the distance, f_2.

Figure 2.23 Illustration of field size scaling and derivation of the inverse-square law.

Table 2.4 Proton range variation with energy (csda range quoted, calculated using PSTAR [1])	
ENERGY (MeV)	**RANGE (cm)**
60	3.1
100	7.7
150	15.8
200	26.0
250	37.9

normal tissue. The Bragg peak is also a characteristic of other heavy charged particle beams, such as carbon ions and pions.

While interactions with atomic electrons is the dominant process by which clinical proton beams (50–250 MeV) lose energy and so deposit dose, an incident proton beam may also interact with the atomic nucleus through *elastic* or *non-elastic* scattering. In elastic scattering events, kinetic energy is passed from the incident proton and the internal structure of the nucleus is unchanged. In non-elastic scattering, the nucleus may be fragmented or left in an excited state, in which case kinetic energy is not conserved. Charged particles (secondary protons, alpha particles etc.) produced during these events will deposit their energy close to the site of interaction, whereas neutrons and photons, being uncharged, may carry energy a significant distance away.

Clinical use of proton beams

In order to deliver a uniform radiation dose over defined target dimensions, at a required depth, the full energy (or pristine) Bragg peak shown in Figure 2.24A must be broadened and range-shifted as in Figure 2.25A. Broadening the Bragg peak can be achieved either by varying beam energy directly or by *passive* scattering of a single energy. The latter is simply achieved by placing different thicknesses of attenuator in front of the patient to vary the depth that protons penetrate. Figure 2.25B shows a Perspex modulator wheel. There are a number of available thicknesses in the wheel, the proportion of each is determined so that the total dose summed over all steps is uniform within the target region.

Carbon ions and pions

In addition to protons, heavier nuclei and other particles may offer potential advantages for radiotherapy due to the physical characteristics of their dose deposition in matter and their relative biological effectiveness (RBE). Beams of carbon ions and pions, in particular, have been applied clinically for radiotherapy. In order to reach deep-seated tumours, the energies of heavy ion beams need to be significantly higher than that of protons. For example, while 150 MeV protons have a range of approximately 16 cm in water, the same penetration depth for carbon ions requires a beam energy of close to 3600 MeV, or 300 MeV for each of the 12 nucleons (6 protons and 6 neutrons) in the ion (often denoted 300 MeV/u).

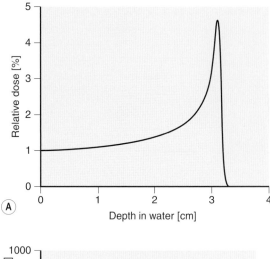

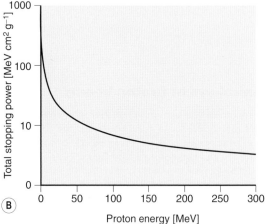

Figure 2.24 (A) Bragg peak for 60 MeV protons in water and (B) proton stopping power in water (data from PSTAR [1]). Notice how the shape of the stopping power curve is reflected in the observed depth-dose curve.

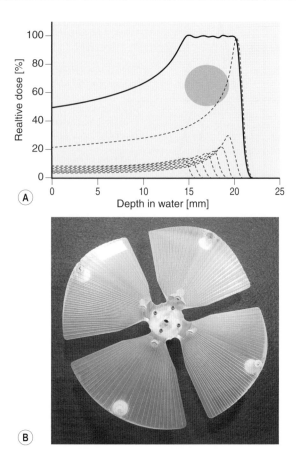

Figure 2.25 Creation of a spread-out Bragg peak (SOBP) for a single proton beam. In (A) the solid line represents the total dose. The uniform dose across the target (circle) is achieved by summing dose contributions from a number of range-shifted Bragg peaks (dotted lines). (B) an example of a perspex modulator wheel, designed to provide the appropriate weighted range-shifting.
(Reprinted with the permission of the Clatterbridge Centre for Oncology NHS Foundation Trust: Douglas Cyclotron)

The LET of carbon ions in the Bragg peak is significantly higher than in the plateau region which leads to an increased RBE across the target region relative to the surrounding low dose region. Hence, in addition to a lower physical dose, normal tissue is spared further due to a lower biological effect. This increased LET in the Bragg peak is a result of nuclear fragments being produced in collisions, which leads to a dose tail following the Bragg peak, illustrated in Figure 2.26A.

Pions, negatively charged particles with a mass approximately 15% of that of a proton and a half-life of 26 ns (2.6×10^{-8} s) can be produced by bombarding carbon or beryllium targets with protons. Pion beams have been used clinically to treat over 500 patients at a small number of centres world-wide. The potential advantage from these particles over alternatives is the '*star effect*' which enhances the dose deposited in their Bragg peak due to their capture by atomic nuclei. This capture process causes the nucleus to become unstable and disintegrate into a number of fragments, each of which has a high LET and very short range in tissue.

NEUTRON INTERACTIONS

Clinical beams of *fast* neutrons, of the order of 60 MV, were the subject of particular interest during the 1970s and 1980s. Being uncharged, they show similar depth-dose

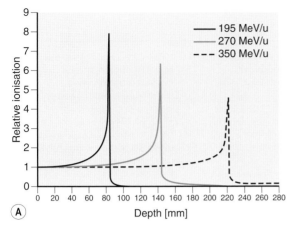

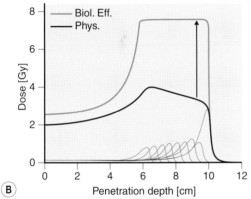

Figure 2.26 (A) Monoenergetic Bragg peaks for carbon ions incident on water. Note the dose tail beyond the peak due to nuclear fragments. (B) Physical dose and biologically effective dose within a clinical target volume for 170 to 220 MeV carbon ions in water. Note the enhanced biological effect across the target region, resulting in preferential damage to tumour.
(Reproduced with permission, M Krämer, GSI, Darmstadt)

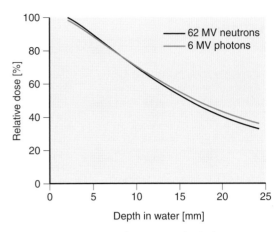

Figure 2.27 Comparison of percentage depth-dose in water at 150 cm source-to-surface distance (SSD) for 62 MeV neutrons. *(Reprinted with the permission of the Clatterbridge Centre for Oncology NHS Foundation Trust: Douglas Cyclotron)*

characteristics to megavoltage photons (Figure 2.27), but offer potential advantages for some tumours in causing a greater degree of irreparable DNA damage which is not dependent on the *oxygen effect*. Low energy (*thermal*) neutron beams are of interest in their application to boron-neutron capture therapy (BNCT). This treatment involves first depositing boron (^{10}B) in the tumour, using tumour-targeting compounds, then applying an external beam of thermal neutrons. These neutrons are captured by boron nuclei within the tumour, creating ^{11}B which subsequently disintegrates releasing helium and lithium nuclei (^{4}He, ^{7}Li), with kinetic energies of 1.47 and 0.84 MeV, respectively. Being highly charged, these particles deposit their energy within a very short distance of the site of their release.

Aside from their therapeutic applications, fast neutrons are also produced in interactions involving high energy photons and protons, as mentioned above. Fast neutrons lose energy primarily through *elastic* collisions with atomic nuclei. In the body, this readily produces *knock-on protons* through collisions with hydrogen, which travel only a short distance in tissue. The proportion of energy that neutrons lose through each collision decreases as the atomic number of the target material increases, with the average energy loss, E, being given by:

$$\frac{E}{E_0} = \frac{2mM}{(m+M)^2} \qquad \boxed{2.18}$$

where E_0 is the incident neutron energy, m the neutron mass (1.67×10^{-27} kg) and M the mass of the target nucleus. Materials with a high hydrogen or other low atomic number (e.g. lithium) content are therefore the most effective in slowing down fast neutrons. Wall cladding with a high proportion of low atomic number material may be used in the maze of bunkers housing high energy photon machines (15 MV and above) in order to rapidly slow fast neutrons produced by photon interactions (*photonuclear interactions*) in the photon target. Once *thermalized*, neutrons are captured by a nucleus (*non-elastic interactions*), for example:

$$n + {}^{1}H \rightarrow {}^{2}H + \gamma [2.2 \text{ MeV}]$$
$$n + {}^{14}N \rightarrow {}^{14}C + p\,[0.6 \text{ MeV}] \qquad \boxed{2.19}$$

In the case of capture by hydrogen (^{1}H), this results in the release of a high energy photon, which itself presents a potential radiation shielding hazard.

REFERENCES

[1] Berger M, Coursey J, Zucker A, Chang J. ESTAR, PSTAR, and ASTAR: Computer programs for calculating stopping-power and range tables for electrons, protons, and helium ions (version 1.2.3), Gaithersburg, MD: National Institute of Standards and Technology; 2005.http://physics.nist.gov/Star.

[2] Hubbell JH, Seltzer SM. Tables of X-ray mass attenuation coefficients and mass energy-absorption coefficients from 1 keV to 20 MeV for elements $Z = 1$ to 92 and 48 additional substances of dosimetric interest. National Institute of Standards and Technlology; 1996. NISTIR 5632.

[3] Berger MJ, Hubbell JH, Seltzer SM, et al. XCOM: Photon cross sections database. National Institute of Standards and Technology; 1998. NBSIR 87-3597.

[4] Mayles P, Nahum A, Rosenwald J-C, editors. Handbook of radiotherapy physics, theory and practice. Taylor and Francis; 2007.

[5] Baker C, Peck K. Reconstruction of 6 MV photon spectra from measured transmission including maximum energy estimation. Phys Med Biol 1997;42:2041–51.

[6] IPEM Report 78 . Catalogue of diagnostic x-ray spectra and other data. Institute of Physics and Engineering in Medicine; 1997.

[7] Attix F. Introduction to radiological physics and radiation dosimetry. John Wiley & Sons Inc; 1996.

FURTHER READING

Central axis depth dose data for use in radiotherapy. A survey of depth doses and related data measured in water or equivalent media. BJR 1996; (Suppl. 25), British Institute of Radiology.

Chapter | 3 |

Radiation detection and measurement

James E. Shaw, Colin Baker

INTRODUCTION

Chapter 2 described the various processes by which photons interact with matter. These interactions produce charged particles (electrons and possibly positrons) which then travel through matter, losing energy by *collision processes* (ionization and excitation of atoms) and through *radiative processes* (production of bremsstrahlung), as illustrated in Figure 3.1.

For photon beams, the transfer of energy from radiation to matter may be seen in two distinct stages:

1. transfer of energy from the radiation to emitted charged particles
2. deposition of energy by the emitted charged particles through collision processes.

The first stage is governed by the interaction coefficients for photons in matter as discussed in Chapter 2. The second stage is dependent upon the energies of the emitted charged particles and their subsequent patterns of energy deposition as determined by their stopping powers. Together, these determine the differences in deposition of energy for differing photon energies and materials. For charged particle beams only the second stage is relevant.

Kerma

The term *kerma*, an acronym for the k*inetic energy released per unit mass,* is used to quantify the first of the above stages. It is defined by ICRU (1) as:

$$K = \Delta E_{tr}/\Delta m$$

where ΔE_{tr} represents the energy transferred from photons to charged particles and is the sum of initial kinetic energies of all the charged particles liberated by uncharged ionizing radiation from an amount of material of mass Δm.

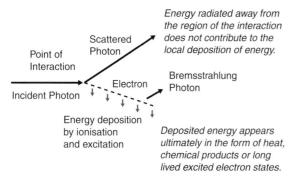

Figure 3.1 Schematic diagram of energy deposition arising from Compton interaction in a matter.

It may be seen from Figure 3.1 that for the Compton interaction illustrated:

1. the energy of an incident photon is shared between a scattered photon and the ejected electron. The scattered photon carries its energy away from the immediate region of the interaction. The term *terma* represents the total energy removed from the beam per unit mass of matter, including that given to the charged particles and that scattered as photons. Terma is therefore always greater than kerma
2. the electron travels through matter losing energy continually until its kinetic energy is exhausted
3. the travelling electron may lose some energy by bremsstrahlung, producing photons which, like the scattered photon, carry energy away from the immediate vicinity. The term *collision kerma* refers to that proportion of kerma that is deposited via collision processes only. Kerma and collision kerma differ only in accounting for the energy that is re-radiated. In body tissues, the energy re-radiated is small, being less than 1%, so these two quantities are almost equal.

Absorbed dose

The travelling electrons deposit energy in matter through which they pass, and so the energy deposited by these electrons is displaced in distance from the site of initial transfer of energy from the photon beam. The amount of energy deposited in a small mass of the material is termed the absorbed dose, which is defined by ICRU [1] as:

$$D = \Delta E_d/\Delta m$$

where ΔE_d is the total energy deposited by these charged particles in a volume element of mass Δm.

The absorbed dose is similar in value to collision kerma, but displaced due to the motion of the secondary charged particles. Absorbed dose equals collision kerma if one of two conditions are met:

1. the distance travelled by secondary charged particles is sufficiently small for it to be neglected, such that energy may be considered to be absorbed by the matter at the point where it is transferred from photons to the charged particles – a condition known as point deposition of dose. This occurs for low energy photons, where the emitted electrons can travel only short distances, as detailed in Chapter 2
2. the energy lost from the region of initial transfer by the movement of charged particles away from that region is exactly compensated for by energy brought into the region by other travelling electrons produced elsewhere – a condition known as energy equilibrium, or more generally as charged particle equilibrium.

Units of kerma and dose

Both kerma and absorbed dose have units of energy per unit mass, the units for which are joules (J) and kilograms (kg), respectively. The gray is used for both absorbed dose and kerma and is defined as:

$$1 \text{ Gy} = 1 \text{ J/kg}$$

Neither absorbed dose nor kerma are material specific and can therefore be related to any matter: a subscript is generally used to indicate the material. Hence K_a and K_w may be used to refer to air kerma and water kerma, respectively. Similarly for absorbed dose.

MEASUREMENT AND STANDARDIZATION OF DOSE

We have seen that when photons interact in matter, an energy pathway is initiated by which energy is transferred to the matter via emission of charged particles which cause ionization and excitation of atoms of the matter. The energy is eventually manifest as heat or as some form of internal potential energy of electrons and atoms within the matter (e.g. chemical bonds, raised electron energy levels).

Systems of detecting radiation utilize specific parts of this energy pathway. Some systems seek to determine energy deposited in matter by measuring the temperature rise (termed calorimetry). Other detection systems look at chemical changes generated by irradiation of the matter (chemical dosimetry), or utilize long-lived excited electron states (e.g. thermoluminescent dosimetry). Still other systems measure the ionization produced by the charged particles in order to calculate the energy transferred to those particles (ionization chamber dosimetry).

This section describes the systems adopted for the measurement and standardization of absorbed dose that underpin clinical practice. Later sections consider other methods of radiation detection and measurement, including other systems for measuring absorbed dose.

Dose standards

It is of particular importance in radiotherapy to ensure that a dose of radiation delivered in any one treatment centre is consistent over time and is consistent also with that delivered in other centre, this being a central part of ongoing quality control. It also allows direct comparison of treatment techniques and results between centre and is essential for multicentre clinical trials to be effective. Consistency of measurements on a national or international basis is achieved through a process of central *standardization*, with all measurements being traceable to an accepted national or international standard. The National Standards Laboratory (i.e. the National Physical Laboratory, NPL in the UK) houses the instruments that are used to determine the *national standard for absorbed dose measurement*. These instruments are purely laboratory instruments that are impractical for routine use within radiotherapy departments.

The UK national standard instruments for the standardization of absorbed dose are of two types:

1. calorimeters for megavoltage photon and electron beams. Calorimeters are used to provide direct determination of absorbed dose [2]
2. free-air ionization chambers for lower energy photon beams from x-ray generators operating at up to 300 kV [3, 4]. These provide direct determination of air kerma from which the absorbed dose to water can be calculated.

Traceability of measurement

In order to ensure consistency of dose measurement between centre, it is necessary for measurements to be traceable back to the appropriate national standard. This is achieved through a hierarchical arrangement shown schematically in Figure 3.2. Dose measuring instruments within individual hospitals (the *field instruments*) are used to measure the radiation beams of radiotherapy treatment units. These are calibrated periodically (i.e. annually in the UK) against a *secondary standard* instrument. The secondary standard instruments are reserved solely for this purpose and are not used to make routine beam measurements. Guidelines on the choice of dosimeter systems for use as secondary standard instruments have been produced by IPEM [5]. Each secondary standard instrument is calibrated periodically (i.e. every 3 years in the UK) by the Standards Laboratory by comparing the response against national reference level instruments that are in turn compared annually with the national standard instrument. The national standards are themselves compared at intervals with equivalent standard instruments developed by standards laboratories in other countries.

Radiotherapy treatment units, such as linear accelerators and kV therapy units, have in-built dose measuring instruments that monitor and determine the amount of dose delivered – these instruments are known as *monitor chambers*. Field instruments are used to calibrate these monitor chambers so that each monitor unit delivers a known amount of radiation. These field instruments may be used to determine not only the amount of radiation delivered, but also the pattern of deposition of energy within matter by measuring dose at different points within the matter. They may be used also to calibrate other dose measuring equipment designed for special purpose measurements, such as *in-vivo dosimeters*.

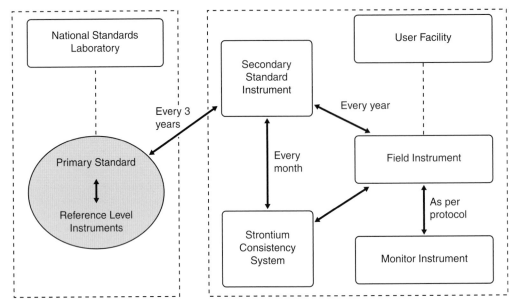

Figure 3.2 Traceability to the National Standard is assured through a chain of intercomparisons, some of which are carried out at the National Standards Laboratory and others are carried out in local radiation beams. Between intercomparisons, calibration is assured using a consistency system.

For the transfer of calibration from instrument to instrument down the chain to be reliable, the method of calibration must be strictly controlled. This is achieved by the adoption of calibration protocols which specify:

- the basis for the standard dose measurement
- the instrumentation and methods for transfer of dose to field instruments by a series of intercomparisons, including specification of any equipment used and any conditions that must exist for the intercomparison to be reliable
- instructions for use of the calibrated dosimeter in routine practice.

Each protocol is specific for an energy range and type of radiation: the protocols for calibration of field instruments are covered in a later section.

Standard calorimeter

In situations where all the absorbed energy is manifest solely as heat, i.e. no energy is 'lost' to form new chemicals or stored in excited electron states, the relationship between radiation dose and change in temperature is given by:

$$\text{Dose (Gy)} = C \times \delta T$$

where C is the specific heat of the irradiated matter (the amount of energy needed to raise the temperature of unit mass of a substance through 1 degree, expressed in units of in $J.kg^{-1}.^{\circ}C^{-1}$) and δT is the change in temperature in degrees Celsius. The equation above assumes no loss of heat to the surrounding environment or structures.

Note that the specific heat may also be expressed in calories rather than joules, in which case an additional numerical multiplier of 4.18 is necessary in the above equation.

The rise in temperature is extremely small – e.g. a beam of x-rays delivering a dose of 5 Gy to soft tissue causes a temperature rise of only $10^{-3}{\circ}$C. Such a small rise in temperature is very difficult to measure accurately and extreme precautions are necessary to prevent heat loss outside the irradiated vessel.

The national standard calorimeter is based on the irradiation of a known mass of graphite (the core of the NPL high energy photon calorimeter measures approximately 20 mm diameter by 3 mm thick) within a graphite phantom. The design of the calorimeter, a photograph and schematic drawing of which are shown in Figure 3.3, has the core shielded by three jackets, each separated by vacuum in order to minimize heat loss. Temperature measurements are carried out using thermistors embedded in the graphite core, the resistances of which change with temperature. In practice, since the amount of heat energy lost from the core to surrounding structures is not negligible and may be difficult to determine, the rise in temperature resulting from irradiation is compared with the rise in temperature produced by heating the core using a known amount of electrical energy, allowing absorbed dose to be determined directly instead of using the above equation.

Graphite has the advantage of having no chemical defect (i.e. all the absorbed energy appears as heat) and a specific heat that is one-fifth that of soft tissue or water, thereby producing greater changes in temperature per unit dose.

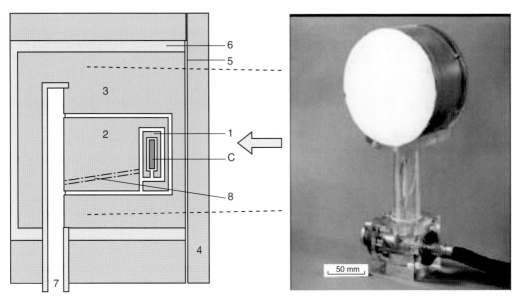

Figure 3.3 Photograph and simplified schematic drawing (redrawn from [2]) of the national standard high energy photon calorimeter, showing the graphite core (C) surrounded by three insulating graphite jackets (1, 2 &. 3). The entire device is housed within a Perspex evacuation vessel (6) which has a thin aluminized mylar front window (5) and which is evacuated via a port (7). A plate (4) suitable for the energy to be measured can be added to the front face. Electrical connections to the core pass through the device (8).

The absorbed dose to water may be calculated from the absorbed dose to graphite using the correction factors determined by Nutbrown [6].

Measurement by calorimetry is largely independent of whether the radiation is delivered continuously or in pulses and of the pulse intensity. It is therefore ideal for measuring radiation from constant-output sources, such as cobalt units, as well as pulsed output from linear accelerators. The pattern of temperature rise (from irradiation) and fall (from leakage of heat away from the core) may be used to determine both the peak and mean dose rates for pulsed radiation sources.

As the standard calorimeter cannot be used in a water tank, a number of specially constructed ionization chambers termed '*reference standard instruments*' are calibrated annually against the graphite calorimeter in a common graphite phantom. These reference instruments are then used to calibrate in turn the secondary standard instruments using a water phantom. The calibration factor provided for each secondary standard instrument is specific to a stated beam quality and depth of measurement, the latter being important as the spectral content of a radiation beam changes with depth. Table 3.1 shows those photon beam qualities at which calibration factors based on absorbed dose to water as determined by the standard graphite calorimeter are provided by the National Physical Laboratory, UK [7, 8]. When used as a basis for calibration in a radiation beam in the user's department, the beam quality

Table 3.1 Photon beam qualities used for therapy level absorbed dose to water calibrations

BEAM QUALITY (TPR$_{20/10}$)	EQUIVALENT BEAM ENERGY	REFERENCE DEPTH (cm)
0.568	60 Co	5
0.621	4 MV	5
0.670	6 MV	5
0.717	8 MV	5
0.746	10 MV	5
0.758	12 MV	7
0.779	16 MV	7
0.790	19 MV	7

The quantity TPR$_{20/10}$ is the ratio of tissue-phantom ratios at depths of 20 cm and 10 cm respectively, used by Standards Laboratories as the specifier of beam quality (see Chapter 2).

A number of Standards Laboratories have developed water calorimeters that directly measure the rise in temperature of a known mass of water. These avoid uncertainties with the national standard instrument in moving from a graphite phantom to a water phantom. Such instruments have been used to confirm doses specified using other systems of dosimetry for photon and charged particle beams and are being increasingly developed as national dosimetry standards [44–48] for that beam must be determined and the appropriate calibration factor obtained by interpolating from the results provided by the standards laboratory. Calibrations in megavoltage photon beams are carried out at the depths shown in Table 3.1 which are beyond the range of contaminating electrons in the radiation beam that have been ejected from the head of the treatment machine [9].

The free air chamber

The free air chamber is the primary standard instrument for kV beams, and is shown schematically in Figure 3.4. The free air chamber effectively determines the energy transferred to secondary electrons as a result of interactions of a photon beam within a defined mass of air, i.e. air kerma (k_a).

A well-defined beam of radiation, confined by external collimators, is incident upon a volume of air located between metal plates that act as electrodes. The radiation causes ionization of the air, resulting in electrons being ejected. These electrons in turn cause further excitation and ionization as they interact with air molecules: the electrons lose kinetic energy with each interaction and will travel an irregular, tortuous path until they come to rest. Each ejected Compton- or photo-electron can produce several hundred ion pairs. An essential requirement of the free air chamber is that the electrons produced by photon interactions lose all their kinetic energy in air and do not reach the metal electrodes. This requirement determines the minimum separation between the metal electrodes, and the overall size of the chamber. For example, measurement of x-rays generated at 200 kV will require a separation of at least 20 cm.

A potential difference, *the polarizing voltage*, is applied between the metal electrodes. This causes positively and negatively charged ions produced in the air to separate, such that positive ions will move towards the negative potential plate while electrons will move towards the other. All ions of one charge sign are collected on one electrode, termed the *collecting electrode*. The charge reaching this electrode is measured and, from this, the number of ions produced may be calculated, since the charge carried by each electron is constant (equal to 1.602×10^{-19} coulomb). The average energy expended by electrons in creating an ion pair, that is allowing for energy lost in exciting atoms as well as energy lost in ionizing them, is well determined from experimental work. Hence, since the number of ions may be determined using the free air chamber and the average energy necessary to produce each one is known, the total energy transferred to secondary electrons by photon interactions can be calculated.

Figure 3.4 shows the physical arrangement. The metal plate that forms the electrode which carries the high tension (HT) polarizing voltage runs the full length of the chamber, whereas the other plate has the collector electrode as the central part only, separated and electrically isolated from adjacent metal plates called *guard rings*, which are held at the same electrical potential as the collector electrode. This arrangement ensures that the electric field within the region of the collector electrode is uniform and perpendicular to that electrode. Any ions produced in air within the region ABCD on the diagram will be collected on the collector electrode, whereas any ions produced outside this region will be collected on the guard rings and will not be included in the measurement.

Charged particle equilibrium

The shaded region in Figure 3.4 indicates the volume of air of interest irradiated by the photon beam, being specified by the cross-sectional area of the photon beam and the length of the collector electrode. The mass of air within this volume depends upon atmospheric conditions (temperature and pressure). Correction for different atmospheric conditions is covered in a later section.

Some electrons (such as trajectory 1) emanating from this region will lose all their kinetic energy within region ABCD and will have the ions collected by the collector electrode. Other electrons (such as trajectory 2) emanating from the air volume will pass beyond the boundaries of region ABCD such that some of their ions will be lost to the collector electrode, thereby reducing the measurement of ionization. However, other electrons emanating from outside the air volume may cause ionization within region ABCD that will be collected and measured as indicated by trajectory 3, thereby increasing the measurement of ionization. *Charged particle equilibrium* is said to exist when the ionization lost from region ABCD is exactly matched by the ionization gained.

Under the conditions of charged particle equilibrium, the total sum of ion pairs generated by the Compton- and photo-electrons ejected from the shaded volume will be equivalent to that determined by measuring the charge collected on the collector electrode.

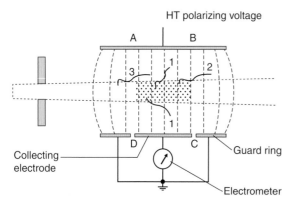

Figure 3.4 The free air ionization chamber. Irradiation of the mass of air shown shaded, defined by the cross-sectional area of the radiation beam and the length of the collecting electrode, results in emission of electrons that lose their kinetic energy by ionization of air. Those ions created within the region ABCD are collected and measured.

For charged particle equilibrium to exist, the path in air before the shaded region is reached must be at least equal to the range in air of the Compton- and photo-electrons. Collimation devices must be sited beyond this range, so that photo-electrons ejected from them cannot reach the measurement region. There must similarly be an equivalent path length of air beyond the distal end of the measurement volume before any exit portal is reached. The whole instrument is therefore very large and unwieldy. Furthermore, it is susceptible to interference from externally generated electric fields and stringent measures have to be adopted to minimizse any such influences.

PRACTICAL IONIZATION CHAMBERS

The Primary Standard instruments described above are complex, sophisticated and sensitive instruments that are unsuitable for routine use within a hospital environment where small, relatively robust, simple instrumentation is needed.

One such instrument is the ionization chamber.

Bragg-Gray cavity theory

The absorbed dose within any medium cannot generally be measured directly and so a surrogate has to be used. Ionization chamber dosimetry is based upon replacing a small volume of the medium by an air cavity within which the ionization of air by the radiation can be measured and from which the dose to the medium can be determined.

When a medium is irradiated uniformly by electrons, then the fluence of electrons (i.e. the energy carried across unit cross-sectional area) will be the same at all points within the medium. If a small air cavity is introduced of size such that it does not perturb the electron fluence (i.e. does not introduce changes to the energy spectrum or numbers of electrons), then the fluence of electrons in the air is the same as in the medium and the cavity is termed a Bragg-Gray cavity. Under these conditions, the energy per unit mass (absorbed dose) imparted to the air (D_a) is given by:

$$D_a = J_a W$$

where Ja is the ionization produced per unit mass of air, W is the average energy lost by the electrons per ion pair formed in the air. If the air is now to be replaced by medium, the energy per unit mass imparted to the medium (D_m) would equal the absorbed dose to air multiplied by the electron mass stopping power for the medium divided by that for air $(S/\rho)^m_a$ (averaged over the energy spectrum of the electrons), i.e.:

$$D_m = J_a W (S/\rho)^m_a$$

This is the basic equation governing the use of ionization chambers in the dosimetry of electron beams. For other charged particle beams, the stopping power ratio for those particles must be used.

Where the medium is irradiated by a photon beam, then photon interactions produce secondary electrons which cause ionization within the air cavity. Provided that interactions of photons with air molecules is negligible, such that all electrons crossing the air cavity arise as secondary electrons from within the medium and that the above conditions relating to constancy of electron fluence are met, then the air volume can be regarded as a Bragg-Gray cavity. The above equation then still holds.

In practice, when using ionization chambers, the air volume is enclosed by a wall of material which differs slightly from both air and the medium. The construction of the chamber may introduce perturbations both to the fluence of electrons crossing the air cavity and to the photon beam itself. A wall of infinitesimally small thickness may be considered as having no impact on either, such that the chamber is effectively an air cavity within the medium. As the wall increases in thickness, then an increasing percentage of secondary electrons crossing the air volume will be from the wall rather than the medium until, in the extreme, all electrons crossing the air volume originate from within the wall. In this situation, the electron fluence across the air volume is the same as the fluence within the wall, and the dose to the wall (D_w) is given by:

$$D_w = J_a W (S/\rho)^w_a$$

Assuming the photon field is not perturbed by the presence of the chamber, then the dose deposited by photons in the medium is related to that deposited in the chamber wall:

$$D_m = D_w (\mu/\rho)^m_w$$

where $(\mu/\rho)^m_w$ is the ratio of mass absorption coefficient for the medium divided by that for the chamber wall.

The conditions for the above to be strictly valid are not met in practice. For measurement of charged particle beams, the fluence of particles may vary with depth and the introduction of the chamber may cause perturbations to this fluence. In measurement of photon beams, the wall of the chamber may be insufficient to stop electrons from outside it reaching the air volume, and the wall of the chamber differs from the medium in its attenuation and scattering of photons. Energy dependent correction factors need to be applied to the above to adjust for these effects.

Dose determination based on calibrated instruments

The above correction factors are not necessary when ionization chambers are used solely as instruments which are calibrated in terms of absorbed dose to water against a suitable primary standard where their effects are taken into account as an intrinsic part of the calibration process. They are required where calibration is in terms of air kerma. Such calibrations are by a series of intercomparisons that are traceable directly to the national standard instruments described above. The absorbed dose is determined using an instrument calibrated in terms of absorbed dose to water (the UK standard for megavoltage photon beams) is given by:

$$D = R.N_D$$

where D is the dose, R is the mean corrected reading and N_D is the absorbed dose calibration factor.

For kV energy photons in the UK, the chamber calibration (N_k) is in terms of air kerma. A factor, $[(\mu_{en}/\rho)w_{air}]$, the ratio of mass energy absorption coefficients for water and air, needs to be included to calculate the dose to water, and a perturbation factor (k) as described above needs to be applied. The equation becomes:

$$D = R.N_k.k. [(\mu_{en}/\rho)w_{air}]$$

The nature and magnitude of the correction factor k depends on whether calibration is carried out in air (for low energy x-rays) or in water. Similar expressions may be derived for other modalities of radiation.

Requirements for practical ionization chambers

Radiation dosimeters based upon ionization chambers have two basic components: the detector chamber which produces electrical charge when irradiated and an associated electrometer, which is an electronic amplifier to which the chamber is connected which is designed specifically for the purpose of measuring charge. The response of the dosimeter represents the response of the chamber to radiation together with the accuracy and consistency of the electrometer in measuring the charge.

Practical instrumentation needs to have a well-determined and predictable, slowly varying response to different energies of radiation, and must be consistent over time.

In addition, other dosimeter requirements are necessary depending upon type of radiation and the nature of the measurement being carried out.

Dosimeter chambers used within Standards Laboratories are specially constructed or selected. Materials used in their construction are fully investigated to determine chemical content and each chamber is meticulously assessed in terms of its assembly and response to radiation. Electronic equipment used to measure the electrical charge is equally carefully designed, constructed and calibrated. The prime requirements here are the elimination of sources of inaccuracy in response and the consistency of that response. The overall accuracy of calibration of these instruments depends upon uncertainties in fundamental parameters being measured and to the extent that systematic uncertainties can be avoided. Overall consistency of calibration is between 0.5 and 1%.

Secondary standard instruments are constructed to less stringent standards, but are required to operate over a range of beam energies and to remain consistent in response between recalibrations by the Standards Laboratories (i.e. 3 years). They must be fully transportable so that they can be used to transfer calibrations to other instruments in beams from different treatment machines, or even across different hospital sites. These chambers maintain an accuracy of calibration around 1%. Guidelines covering secondary standards instruments have been published [5].

Field instruments are used in daily measurements within hospitals. Different types of instrument exist, depending upon the nature of those measurements. Thimble chambers, described in detail in the following section, are generally used for calibration of megavoltage photon beams. Chambers based upon the design of the Farmer chamber [10] feature an air cavity of about 0.6 ml, providing a reasonable balance between the response to radiation and smallness of size, are adequate for measurements in relatively uniform radiation beams with an accuracy of 1–2%. Chambers which have much smaller internal dimensions are used to measure variations in dose distributions, which can be very rapid at beam edges. Here, chambers of 0.1 ml or less may be used, with a trade-off between accuracy of response and spatial resolution. Where there is a rapid variation in dose deposited with depth, such as for measurements in the build-up region of photon beams or in the fall-off region of electron beams, parallel plate chambers are used to ensure good depth resolution for the measurements.

Both thimble ionizations chambers and parallel plate ionization chambers are used widely for routine beam calibration and radiation distribution measurements. Other types of detector systems are useful in particular circumstances and may be used as alternatives to ionization chambers. In particular, in vivo measurements use systems which do not require the application of polarizing voltages, thereby reducing electrical risks to the patient. These various forms of radiation detectors are described within the following sections. Some forms, such as thermoluminescent dosimeters (TLD) have no definitive, maintained calibration and are suitable only for comparative measurements of a radiation dose against a known radiation dose, while other forms (e.g. ionization chambers) do maintain a definitive calibration and can be used as absolute dosimeters.

THIMBLE IONIZATION CHAMBER

A thimble chamber is an ionization chamber that has a central electrode (the collector electrode) in a volume of air that is contained by a thimble-shaped cap which forms the HT electrode which fits closely onto a metallic stem. The central electrode passes through the inside of the stem and is insulated from the metallic stem by a suitable high-quality insulator material such as amber or polythene. This is schematically shown in Figure 3.5. The cap is generally

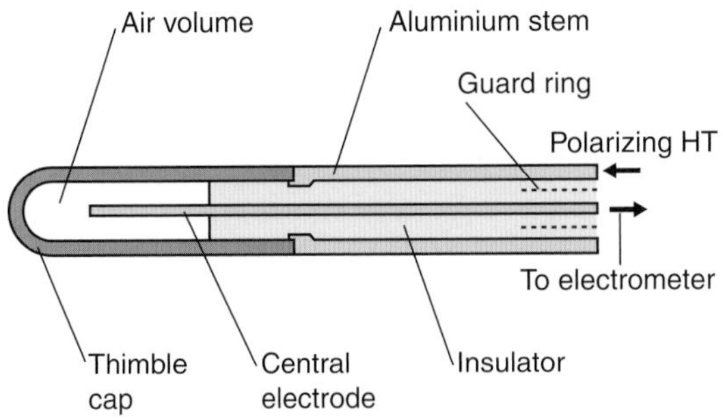

Air volume

Aluminium stem

Guard ring

Polarizing HT

To electrometer

Thimble cap

Central electrode

Insulator

Figure 3.5 Thimble ionization chamber. Ionization produced within the air volume in the thimble cap is collected by the central electrode. The aluminium stem transmits the polarizing voltage to the thimble cap. The guard ring minimizes charge leakage between the outer (HT) and the inner (signal) elements of the interconnecting cable. A thimble chamber of the Farmer type has the chamber linked to the outside via a venting aperture (not shown).

made of a low atomic number low-density material such as graphite, although various plastic materials have been used where the plastic has been manufactured to be conductive (e.g. Shonka plastic: [11]) or has been coated with graphite to be conductive. The central electrode may be made of aluminium or conductive plastic.

A potential difference *(the polarizing voltage)* applied between the outer cap and the inner electrode drives apart any ion pairs produced in the trapped air and prevents ion recombination, but which is insufficiently large to cause ionization of the air itself so that in the absence of ionizing radiation no current flows. A voltage gradient of a few hundred volts per millimetre is generally sufficient for this purpose. In the presence of ionizing radiation, ionization within the air results in the ion pairs being separated, and with the ions of one sign (depending upon the polarity of the polarizing voltage) being collected on the central electrode. The electrometer is generally 'floating', in that the input to it can be at any voltage level with respect to ground without this affecting the reading. In use, the aluminium stem is held at ground potential and the electrometer is floated to the level of the polarizing voltage, so that exposed conductive parts carry no electrical risk to operators. This arrangement allows easy reversal of polarizing voltage as required.

When the chamber is introduced into a photon beam, photo-electric and Compton interactions in the walls of the chamber generate electrons that traverse the air cavity, causing ionization of the air. The wall of the thimble must be sufficiently thick to ensure that all the electrons crossing the air cavity originate in the wall and not in the surrounding material. The wall must therefore be at least as thick as the range of the electrons produced by the photon interactions. However, the wall of the chamber will also attenuate the photon beam and this attenuation will need to be taken into account. If the wall is thick, the attenuation will be large. Practical ionization chambers such as the Farmer

chamber [10] have a wall thickness of about 1 mm. This is sufficient to produce electronic equilibrium for photons generated at kV energies, but is insufficient for megavoltage energies when an additional tight-fitting build-up cap is needed to increase the effective wall thickness. This is particularly important when measurements are made in a phantom constructed from material that differs markedly from the wall material.

The calibration factor of a thimble chamber varies with photon energy. This calibration corrects for wall attenuation, differences in the mass attenuation coefficient between the wall material and water, and perturbations to the photon beam caused when the chamber (and its associated build-up cap, where applicable) are inserted into a water phantom, thereby displacing water. A typical calibration curve for such an instrument in terms of air kerma for photon beams of kV energies is shown in Figure 3.6. The calibration factor rises sharply at low photon energies which limits the lowest energy to which this type of instrument may be used, as small variations in photon energy spectrum for low energy beams can give rise to considerable uncertainties in calibration factor.

The effective point of measurement for the instrument is taken within UK protocols for photon beam calibrations as the chamber centre. The effective point of measurement is forward of the chamber centre for calibration of electron beams. Some international photon calibration protocols are derived for the effective point of measurement being displaced from the chamber centre.

Ionization of the air volume within the cap of a thimble chamber results in a flow of charge onto the collecting electrode. The rate of flow of charge will depend upon the mass of air within the cavity and on the radiation beam intensity. A balance must be made between the physical size of the chamber and on the ability to measure the charge with sufficient accuracy. Chambers with large air volumes (200–2000 ml) must be used to measure the very low dose rates associated with radiation protection measurements. Chambers with volumes of 10–60 ml are

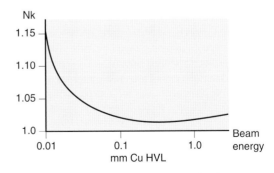

Figure 3.6 Typical variation in air-kerma calibration versus beam energy for a thimble chamber for photon beam energies within the kV range – expressed in terms of their half-value layer (see Chapter 2).

available for measurement of diagnostic radiology beams. For measurement of radiotherapy beams, chambers of about 0.6 ml are used for calibration measurements, while chambers with smaller air volumes may be used for other measurements as described earlier.

Measurement of dose and dose rate

When an ionization chamber is irradiated, a flow of ions is collected by the collecting electrode. The ions may be 'accumulated' and the total charge determined by the electrometer. Such a measurement would be used to determine the radiation dose delivered over the course of the irradiation. The accumulation of charge is effectively achieved by collecting the charge in a capacitor: the voltage across the capacitor plates increases with the charge stored.

The rate at which dose is delivered may be obtained by dividing the measured dose by the irradiation time. This will produce an average value for the dose rate over the irradiation time, although the actual dose rate may vary during the irradiation period. The actual dose rate at any time point within the irradiation period may be determined by measuring the rate of flow of charge. This is achieved by measuring the potential difference produced as the charge flows through a known high-value resistor.

The charge levels referred to above are extremely small for typical radiotherapy doses, typically of the order of nanocoulombs, and dose rate measurements may involve currents of tens of picoamps. The electrometer instrument that measures them must be carefully designed to avoid introducing instrument-induced charges and voltage differences that may interfere with the measurements. Modern instruments are based around purpose-designed high impedence operational amplifiers with low noise levels, able to measure either dose or dose rate, and which can operate over a range of current and charge levels.

THE PARALLEL PLATE IONIZATION CHAMBER

While the thimble chamber described above is suitable for many dosimetry situations, there are circumstances that require alternative chamber designs:

1. for the measurement of low energy photons, the wall of a thimble chamber causes too much attenuation such that the calibration factor is large and varies rapidly with energy. This may lead to considerable uncertainties in measurement of dose
2. the wall of a thimble chamber will also produce too much build up for dose measurements close to the surface for megavoltage radiation
3. in measurement of electron beams, the cylindrical air volume of a thimble chamber causes significant perturbation of the beam that must be corrected for.

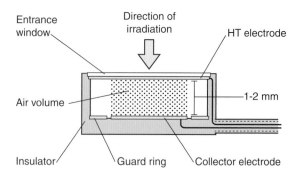

Figure 3.7 Schematic diagram of a parallel plate ionization chamber. Ionization produced within the shaded volume of air is collected by the collector electrode. The guard rings minimize the effects of the chamber walls. The effective point of measurement is the inside surface of the entrance window.

Each of the above may be addressed by use of a different design of ionization chamber. This design has two planar elements: one thin electrode (the HT electrode) forms the entry window for the beam, while a second element consists of the collector electrode surrounded by a guard ring. The air between the electrodes is trapped by insulating walls that form the sides of the chamber and which hold the electrodes apart.

The entry window of such a chamber can be made extremely thin – a few micrometres of plastic material on which a conductive surface (e.g. a graphite layer) has been deposited, but must be sufficiently rigid so as to maintain chamber geometry. For accurate measurement of low energy x-rays, it is important that the materials of the chamber have atomic numbers close to those of water to avoid undue perturbation of the beam. The measuring volume of the chamber (shown as the shaded region in Figure 3.7) is defined by the cross-sectional area of the collecting electrode and the separation between the plates. Interactions with the lateral walls of the chamber generate ions primarily at the edges of the chamber which are collected by the guard ring and not by the collecting electrode.

THE BEAM MONITOR CHAMBER

Linear accelerators and higher energy kV x-ray units have inbuilt ionization chambers to monitor and control the amount of radiation being emitted. For these units, the amount of radiation emitted is specified in terms of *monitor units*, i.e. by the quantity of radiation measured by the inbuilt monitor chamber. The sensitivity of these monitor chambers must be adjusted to give the correct amount of radiation dose per monitor unit – a process known as *calibration*.

Monitor chambers are forms of parallel plate ionization chamber that sample the entire radiation beam emitted from the treatment unit. In linear accelerators, each monitor chamber consists of at least two independent ionization chambers to provide back-up should problems develop with one chamber during patient treatment. One or both chambers may be segmented, having the collector electrode constructed of a number of different and electrically isolated segments, so that assessment of beam uniformity can be made by comparing the current flowing from the various segments. Some monitor chambers are manufactured as sealed units that require no correction for ambient temperature and pressure, but which must be checked to ensure that they remain sealed. Others are manufactured as unsealed chambers that do need correction for temperature and pressure – some modern linear accelerators have in-built pressure and temperature transducers and perform this correction automatically, while others rely on manual adjustment. All monitor chambers must be calibrated regularly (e.g. daily) as specified in the calibration protocol being followed by the treatment centre or in radiation protection guidance.

In linear accelerators, the monitor chamber is situated below the primary collimator and flattening filter/scattering foil carousel, and before the adjustable collimators, as shown in Figure 3.8. In this location, although the chamber is protected as far as practicable from backscatter that arises from the adjustable collimator jaws, it will still be subject to some backscatter. The monitor chamber may also be subject to backscatter from any physical wedges placed in the beam. Variations in backscatter contribute to changes in output with field size and to the apparent effect of the wedge. In kV therapy units, the monitor chamber is located after the exit window of the tube housing and after any added beam filters, so that it samples the final beam. However, the monitor chamber is susceptible to backscatter from the applicator plate and this contributes to differences in output between different treatment applicators.

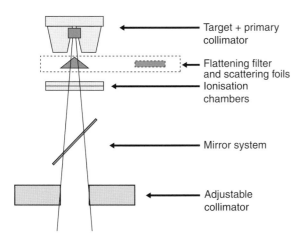

Target + primary collimator

Flattening filter and scattering foils

Ionisation chambers

Mirror system

Adjustable collimator

Figure 3.8 Schematic diagram of a linear accelerator treatment head showing the location of the monitor (ionization) chambers in relation to other components of the head.

INTERCOMPARISONS WITH SECONDARY STANDARD INSTRUMENTS

Transfer of calibration from the primary standard instrument to the field instrument is achieved via a series of intercomparisons. The response of each field instrument is compared with that of a calibrated secondary standard instrument every 12 months (or following repair to the field instrument) at each beam energy and treatment modality at which it is to be used. Where a specific build-up cap was used in determining the relevant calibration factor of the secondary standard instrument, then the same build-up cap should be fitted during intercomparison measurements, even where those measurements are to be carried out in a Perspex phantom.

Intercomparisons are carried out, wherever possible, by placing the field chamber and the secondary standard chamber side by side in the irradiation field and taking simultaneous readings. Several readings should be taken and averaged for each measurement, and the relative positions of the two chambers should be interchanged in order to minimize any effects should the radiation beam produce different dose rates at the positions of the two chambers. The relevant conditions (e.g. type of phantom, depth of measurement, field size) under which these intercomparison measurements and subsequent equipment calibration measurements are made are specified in the appropriate dosimetry protocol. In the UK, separate protocols have been produced by The Institute of Physics and Engineering in Medicine (IPEM) or its forerunner organizations covering:

- x-ray beams below 300 kV generating potential [12, 13]
- high energy (megavoltage) x-ray beams [5, 14]
- electron beams of energy from 4 to 25 MeV [15].

Because of the very different penetration properties of the beams concerned, the first of these is split into three separate sections covering different energy ranges. For very low energy beams (HVL less than 1 mm Al), measurements are specified for the surface of a phantom. For low energy beams (HVL 1–8 mm Al), measurements are specified in air, with no phantom present. For medium energy beams (HVL 0.5–4 mm Cu), which are more penetrating, measurements are specified at depth of 2 cm in a phantom.

STRONTIUM CONSISTENCY CHECK DEVICE

Calibration of instruments is carried out as described earlier. Between calibration sessions, the consistency of each instrument has to be checked using an appropriate consistency checking device.

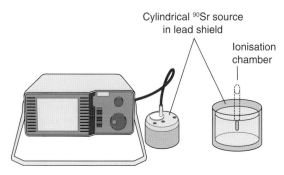

Figure 3.9 Strontium checking device used to check the consistency of a thimble chamber, together with a schematic of the device showing the source wrapped around the chamber.

One such device uses a strontium check source [16] and is illustrated in Figure 3.9. A device of this type for thimble chambers has a ring-shaped source of ^{90}Sr housed within a fully-shielded enclosure, into the centre of which the sensitive volume of the ionization chamber can be accurately placed. ^{90}Sr is a beta emitter and decays at a constant rate with a half-life of 28.7 years. The chamber response within the device is measured at the time at which intercomparison measurements are made. The response to be expected at any subsequent time can then be calculated simply by accounting for radioactive decay, on the proviso that repositioning of the ionization chamber can be carried out with sufficient precision. Different source geometries may be used for different types of ionization chamber, for example planar ^{90}Sr sources may be used to check the consistency of response of parallel plate ionization chambers.

Measurements are carried out periodically (e.g. every month). The chamber response is determined either by measuring the reading achieved for a defined period of measurement or by measuring the time for the chamber to reach a given reading once measurement has been initiated. These measurements ensure the consistency of operation of the measuring device but cannot be used for calibration of the measuring device, since the radiation from ^{90}Sr is not representative of the radiation beams in which the device will be used in clinical practice.

IONIZATION CHAMBER CORRECTIONS

Whenever instruments that are based upon collection of ions produced in air are used to determine absorbed dose, a number of factors in addition to the calibration factor have to be taken into account.

Ion recombination losses

When the air volume of an ionization chamber is irradiated, ion pairs are generated as atoms become ionized. In order to determine the absorbed dose or air kerma accurately, it is necessary to ensure the collection of all the positive or negative ions (depending on polarity) by the collecting electrode. A potential difference is applied across the electrodes to drive the ion pairs apart. If the ion pairs are not driven apart by the applied electric field, they may recombine such that they are 'lost' from collection and the charge is therefore reduced. When ions recombine, the positive and negative ions of an ion pair may recombine with each other (self-recombination), or the negative ion from one ion pair may recombine with the positive ion of a neighbouring ion pair (volume recombination). Both self- and volume recombination result in a reduction in the measured charge. The likelihood of recombination is less where the ions are driven apart rapidly, such as when the polarizing voltage is high.

Recombination is more likely to occur when ions pairs are created close together, both physically and in time. This occurs when measuring high dose rates, or when measuring in beams in which the radiation is delivered in pulses. The radiation from a ^{60}Co gamma beam therapy unit is emitted continuously. The radiation from a modern kilovoltage therapy unit is also virtually continuous, although it does depend somewhat on the type of voltage generator used. For both of these radiation sources, polarizing voltages across a thimble chamber of a few hundred volts is generally sufficient that recombination losses are negligible at dose rates commonly used in radiotherapy. The radiation from a linear accelerator is strongly pulsed: a linear accelerator delivering a dose rate of 4 Gy per minute will deliver the radiation in short pulses, each of a few microseconds duration, the instantaneous dose rate within each pulse being about 40 Gy per second. Under these circumstances, accurate determination of dose requires knowledge of and correction for recombination losses. The amount of recombination may be determined by carrying out measurements using different levels of polarizing voltage across the chamber, applying an empirically-derived equation for the equipment being used or by applying the half-voltage technique [17, 18].

Correction for atmospheric conditions

It has been previously stated that the rate of flow of ions onto the collector electrode will depend on the amount of air enclosed within the thimble of the chamber, and examples have been given of different instrument sizes for measuring in dose rates at typical protection, radiodiagnostic and therapy radiation levels. It is, however, the *mass* of air within the thimble on which the response depends.

For a chamber that is sealed to trap air inside the thimble, variations in atmospheric temperature and pressure will have no impact upon the enclosed mass and will therefore not affect the chamber response. However, the condition of the air within such an instrument may change with time, perhaps due to vapours leaching from the walls of the cap or the surrounding materials. In addition, there is always potential for the seal to fail, allowing some flow of air between the chamber and the environment. If a chamber is unsealed, allowing free passage of air between the inside of the thimble and the general environment, then the mass of air within the thimble will fluctuate with atmospheric temperature and pressure and a correction to any reading will be required to compensate for these changes. As the temperature increases, so the air density falls and the mass of air within the thimble will reduce thereby reducing the chamber sensitivity. As atmospheric pressure rises, so too the density of air increases, increasing the mass of gas within the thimble, thereby increasing the chamber sensitivity. If the assumption is made that air affected by temperature and pressure changes in the same way as an ideal gas, then the ideal gas laws can be applied to determine the magnitude of variation in response. If measurements are made at a temperature of $T°$ Celsius ($°C$) and a pressure of P kilopascal (kPa) using an unsealed instrument, the response may be corrected to what it would have been at a standard temperature of $20°C$ ($293°K$) and pressure of 101.25 kPa by applying the correction factor:

$$Correction = (101.25/P) \times ((T + 273)/293)$$

Most practical field instruments are designed and constructed to be unsealed. The design of such an instrument has to ensure that the thimble does not distort with changes in temperature or pressure so that the volume remains constant. Water vapour can affect the chamber response and the above correction for atmospheric conditions, producing a variation of about 0.7% for change in relative humidity from 10% to 90%. To minimize the impact of relative humidity changes, the secondary standard calibration factor is specified for a humidity value of 50%: variations in chamber response in normal use due to relative humidity changes may generally be ignored.

Chamber stem effect

If the stem of the ionization chamber is within the radiation field, it may perturb the radiation beam and may generate scatter into the air volume of the chamber, thereby affecting the reading (termed the *stem effect*).

During absolute calibration, the chamber is irradiated with a specific field size and a correction is applied for the stem effect with this field size. It is therefore taken into account whenever the calibration factor is applied. There is, however, potential for the effect to increase or decrease for other field sizes.

With well-designed ionization chambers, such as the Farmer chamber, the stem effect is small and variations in it can generally be ignored.

Polarity effect

When an ionization chamber is used to measure charged particles, some of the charged particles may come to rest on the collecting electrode. These will either add to or subtract from the ionization charge being collected, depending upon the charge on the particle and on the direction of the polarizing voltage (whether the collector electrode is collecting positive ions or electrons). The effect is particularly important when using parallel plate chambers to measure proton or electron beams, and can be overcome by averaging measurements taken with both positive and negative polarizing voltage.

A related problem is that, if measurements are carried out in a solid insulating material such as polystyrene, then particles stopped within the material will result in a build up of charge there which will perturb the radiation beam being measured. To avoid this, an insulating phantom should be made of thin sheets of material which allows charge built up in this way to leak away.

ALTERNATIVE DOSE MEASUREMENT SYSTEMS

In the sections above, the primary processes for detection of radiation and measurement of dose centred around calorimetry and ionization of air. National standard and secondary standard instruments are based on these processes, and field instruments of the thimble or parallel-plate chamber design are recommended for routine measurement of radiation output from therapy machines. There are, however, other techniques that are suitable for measurement of dose or dose rate for different circumstances. These are briefly described below and a selection of such devices represented schematically in Figure 3.13.

Film dosimetry

Film has been used as a system for measuring radiation throughout the whole history of radiotherapy. It is particularly useful for measurement of radiation distributions, having applications in phantom measurement of simple and complex radiation beams, in verification of field placements on individual patients, in establishing geometrical accuracy of light beams that delineate radiation beams, and in determination of leakage patterns around the head of a treatment unit.

Film consists essentially of a transparent polyester material (the base) on which is deposited a layer of silver bromide trapped in a gel (the emulsion). The emulsion may be deposited on one side or on both sides of the base. The emulsion is sensitive to light and so must be used in a light-tight packaging or housing. The silver bromine is in the form of small crystals, each crystal being formed as a lattice of negative bromine and positive silver ions. When irradiated, some lattice bonds are broken and electrons are transferred from the bromine to the silver ions, neutralizing those atoms. The presence of neutral silver atoms at key positions of the lattice within a crystal makes the whole crystal 'developable'. In the subsequent development process, the silver ions of developable crystals are converted to atoms of silver. These are fixed in position on the film while the rest of the emulsion, including any non-developable crystals, is removed. The deposited silver absorbs light so these regions of the film appear black while the rest appears transparent. The degree of blackness depends on the relative concentration of deposited crystals which, in turn, depends upon the intensity of radiation at that location on the film. This is measured by shining light through the developed film and measuring the transmitted intensity. A logarithmic scale is used to define the optical density of the film:

$$OD = \log_{10}(I_0/I)$$

where I_0 is the incident light intensity and I is the transmitted intensity. The resultant optical density has to be corrected for the intrinsic density of the developed film base. A graph of optical density against absorbed dose is known as the *dose response curve* and can be produced for any film. Accurate dosimetry requires full knowledge of the dose response curve. The response curve may be effectively linear over a restricted range of doses and simple dose comparisons can be made within this range. Used in this way, film has high spatial resolution unmatched by other measuring systems and can provide a full two-dimensional display of dose distribution (such as variation in dose with depth and position across the beam). However, silver bromide has a high atomic number and therefore the response to low energy photons is greatly increased as a result of increased photoelectric interactions. This makes film unsuitable as an absolute dosimeter and makes accurate comparative measurements difficult in situations where the energy spectrum varies markedly. Although the areas of application of film dosimetry are steadily being reduced as other methods of measurement come to the fore, film dosimetry still has a vital role within radiotherapy. It also has a role in radiation protection dosimetry where the *film badge* has been the historical standard for personal dosimetry, although this is steadily being replaced by other forms of detector.

Radiochromic film

Standard photographic film as described above is sensitive both to ionizing radiation and to visible light. When used for radiation measurements it has to be kept in a light-free container and processed under controlled light conditions. In contrast to this, radiochromic reactions produce direct coloration of a substance by direct absorption of radiation, without the need for chemical processing.

Radiochromic films have been developed that have little or no sensitivity to visible light, but which demonstrate a change in colour when subjected to ionizing radiation.

These may be based upon release of leuco dyes within the material or upon the formation of colored cross-linked polymers from otherwise colourless monomers. The degree of colour change is dependent upon absorbed dose and may be determined by measuring the attenuation of light of specific frequencies that relate to the colour change. Radiochromic films are commercially available which have good response for doses within the range of 0.5–25 Gy and have no high atomic number materials present. Such films therefore have uniform response across a wide range of photon energies. Materials of this type have been used to determine dose distributions for complex radiotherapy treatments and around brachytherapy sources. The most common type is *GAFchromic film* [19]. The principle of polymer cross-linkage is similar to that of polymer gels described in a later section.

Band theory of solids

In individual atoms, outer electrons occupy specific energy levels. When atoms are brought together, as occurs in solid materials, interactions between atoms broaden these specific energy levels into 'energy bands'. Electrons may occupy energy states only within these bands, between which are forbidden zones that normally do not have energy states for electrons to occupy, as illustrated in Figure 3.10.

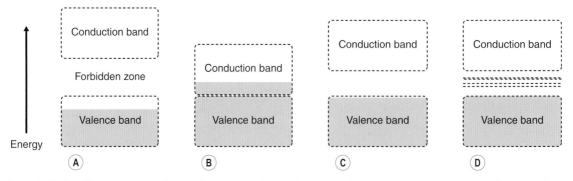

Figure 3.10 Simplified energy level diagram for materials: the shaded regions shows those levels that are normally occupied by electrons for (A) an insulator; (B) a conductor; (C) a semiconductor (undoped); (D) material with impurity levels within the forbidden zone.

The outermost energy bands within the solid material are termed the valence band and the conduction band. Electrons within the valence band are considered as linked to the chemical bonds between individual atoms and are therefore bound in place, although the term 'bound' is used loosely as at normal temperatures such bonds may be continually being broken and reformed. At an energy level slightly above the valence band is the conduction band. Electrons within this band are surplus to any requirements for chemical bonding. At normal temperatures, these electrons are not associated with specific atoms and chemical bonds, but migrate readily through the material. In some materials, there are insufficient electrons to fill the available energy levels of the valence band, such that the conduction band is empty. Where a large forbidden zone exists, these materials are classed as non-conductors or insulators (see Figure 3.10A). Other materials may have more outer electrons than the valence band can accommodate, such that the lower levels of the conduction band are also occupied. In these materials, the conduction band overlaps with the valence band and the forbidden zone disappears, as shown in Figure 3.10B. These materials will generally be good conductors of electricity. There are some materials in which the valence band is just filled, but the conduction band is effectively empty, and a small but significant forbidden zone exists. These materials are classed as semiconductors, illustrated in Figure 3.10C. Any charges injected into a semiconductor will be free to travel through the material. It is to be stressed that this description is overly simplistic but serves as a basis for understanding the principles of solid-state dosimeters.

Impurity bands

The introduction of impurities at low concentrations can alter the structure of the energy bands and may create energy bands that are located between the valence and conduction bands, within the forbidden zone as shown in Figure 3.10D. The properties of the material so formed will depend upon whether these extra bands are normally occupied or empty of electrons, and their actual energy levels. The addition of impurities is critical to the formation of active semiconductor devices (see section below) and to the development and functioning of both scintillator and thermoluminescent materials (see later).

Semiconductor detectors

A number of different types of semiconductor-based radiation detectors have been proposed. This text describes the principles of operation of semiconductor diode detectors and metal oxide field effect transistors (MOS-FET).

These devices use semiconductor material, the most common of which is silicon, to which specific impurities are added at very low concentrations – a process known as *doping*. *n-type* material is doped by an electron donor (e.g. arsenic, selenium) that introduces free electrons into the conduction band. *p-type* material is doped by an electron acceptor (e.g. aluminium, gallium) that effectively introduces additional vacant levels into the valence band. These unfilled levels are termed holes. If electrons are introduced into p-type material, they will fill vacant holes and become 'trapped'.

Diode detectors

When adjacent p-type and n-type doping occurs in a single crystal of silicon, a p–n junction is formed. Conduction electrons in the n-type region will diffuse into the p-type region and become trapped, as shown in Figure 3.11. This results in:

- the region around the interface being devoid of free electrons and unfilled holes. This region is called the depletion layer
- a transfer of electrons (and hence charge) from the n-type to the p-type side of the interface. This transfer of charge generates a small potential difference across the depletion layer.

When this depletion layer is irradiated, electrons are released by ionization creating electron-hole pairs as shown in Figure 3.11C. These drift in opposite directions under the influence of the potential difference across the depletion layer. Electrons will be drawn towards the n-type material while holes will be drawn towards the p-type, causing charge to flow through the circuit in which the

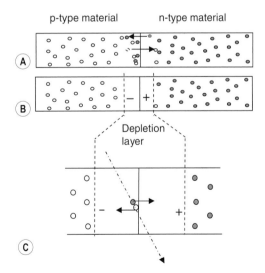

Figure 3.11 Schematic diagram of a p–n junction diode detector. Electrons from the n-type material and holes from the p-type material diffuse across the junction (A), forming a depletion layer across which an internal potential difference forms (B). Electron-hole pairs formed in the depletion layer are pulled apart by the internal electric field (C).

diode is connected. The charge produced is proportional to the dose deposited in the depletion region, and the flow of charge can be measured by an electrometer.

The sensitive region of the diode is very thin, the depletion layer being only a few micrometres in thickness and the cross-sectional area of the silicon crystal being only a few millimetres. However, the sensitivity to radiation is high as the density of the material is over 1000 times that of air in an ionization chamber and the mean energy to produce an electron-hole pair is about one tenth of the energy to create an ion pair in air. Diodes can therefore produce measurable signals from extremely small sensitive volumes that make them particularly suitable for measurements that require high spatial resolution. The absence of any applied polarizing voltage makes diodes particularly useful for in vivo dosimetry.

Diodes have various inherent problems that must be addressed when they are used as radiation detectors. The size of the depletion layer, and hence the sensitivity of the device, strongly depends on temperature [20]. Diodes therefore need to be calibrated at the temperature at which they are to be used. They are constructed from materials with atomic numbers higher than water, making them over-responsive to low energy photon radiation. Their response is therefore sensitive to variations in the energy spectrum of any radiation field such as may be caused by changes in depth, radiation field size and position within the field, or energy setting of equipment being measured. In addition, the construction of the device can influence its angular sensitivity [21, 22]. A further problem is that diodes may suffer radiation damage after receiving high doses of radiation which causes them to change their sensitivity. It has been shown that diodes formed using predominantly heavy p-type doping are less susceptible to sudden change in sensitivity and have longer working lives than predominantly n-doped diodes [23]. The majority of commercial diodes are of this form.

Diodes are used widely in radiotherapy as:

- individual detectors which are used for measuring dose distributions (e.g. depth doses and profiles, particularly where high spatial resolution is required such as in regions of high dose gradient) of radiotherapy beams during initial commissioning and subsequent quality control measurements
- individual or groups of detectors for measurement of radiation doses delivered to patients (in vivo dosimetry)
- arrays of detectors for rapid checking of beam uniformity as part of a quality assurance programme.

MOS-FET detectors

The structure of a MOS-FET is shown schematically in Figure 3.12 which illustrates a device based upon p-doped silicon substrate material onto which layers of heavily n-doped material and SiO_2 are formed. There are three electrical contacts, which are termed the source, gate and drain.

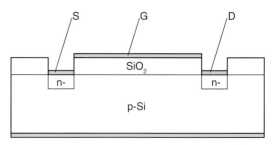

Figure 3.12 Cross-sectional schematic of a MOSFET device. A conducting channel is formed through the oxide layer between the source (S) and the drain (D) when a voltage is applied to the gate (G). The threshold voltage at which this channel is formed is reduced by the effects of radiation.

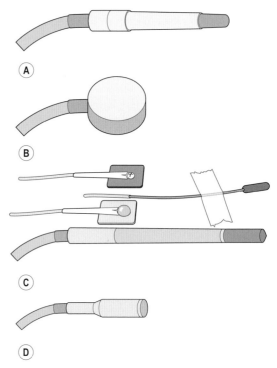

Figure 3.13 Schematic diagram of radiation detectors showing: (A) a Farmer chamber with build-up cap; (B) a parallel plate chamber for electron measurements; (C) a selection of diode detectors for phantom and for in vivo measurements, together with a Farmer type chamber for comparison; (D) a diamond detector.

The source and drain regions may be considered as p–n junctions which are linked by the SiO_2 channel onto which the gate is deposited.

The device operates essentially like a voltage-controlled switch. If a small voltage is generated between the source and the gate with the drain held at the same potential as the gate, then no current flows initially between source and drain until the applied voltage exceeds a specific value (called the threshold voltage), whereupon the device switches and a current starts to flow. The application of the applied voltage causes holes to be drawn to the oxide/silicon surface from both the substrate and from the source and drain regions. A conduction channel between source and drain is formed once the concentration of holes becomes sufficient.

When the device is irradiated, electron-hole pairs are generated within the SiO_2. The mobility of the electrons allows them readily to migrate away, while the holes become trapped at the oxide/silicone surface. These traps, which can survive for a long time, reduce the threshold voltage necessary for the device to switch. The change in threshold voltage is almost linearly related to the radiation dose received by the device.

MOS-FET devices are extremely small (<0.1 mm) and are easily fabricated in various shapes and geometries – such that individual detectors can be used for point doses or planar distributions of detectors to measure complex dose profiles. No electrical connections are necessary during irradiation and the electronic equipment needed for readout is relatively simple, making these devices ideally suited to in vivo dosimetry. They do, however, suffer from the same energy response effects as diode detectors.

Diamond detector

Carbon in the form of diamond is an intrinsic semiconductor with a large energy gap between the conduction and valence bands (5.5 eV). At normal room temperatures, there are very few electrons in the conduction band. If a voltage is placed across a diamond crystal, a tiny current will flow because of these electrons, the magnitude of which is dependent for any given crystal on the applied voltage. The diamond therefore behaves as a resistor.

When irradiated, ion pairs generated within the material increase the number of carriers, and so the resistance falls. The radiation-induced current increases with increasing dose rate. Certain impurities within the diamond can improve the linearity of response between current and dose rate, but the dose–rate response has to be taken into account when using these devices.

A diamond detector consists of a diamond crystal onto which metal contacts have been deposited and to which a voltage of about 100 V is applied. The radiation-induced current is considerably larger than the natural current and so can be measured with precision. Under these conditions, the response is largely independent of temperature. The detector is not readily damaged by radiation so the device has a long operational life. Diamonds may be selected natural diamonds or 'grown' using chemical vapor deposition processes. They are small detectors and so are useful in measuring in high radiation gradients, with good angular response characteristics. Being comprised of carbon, they

are low atomic number devices with electron stopping power values similar to those for water [24].

Summary of direct reading radiation detectors

Various types of radiation detectors have been described in the previous sections. Each type of detector has particular applications for which it is ideally suited. Cylindrical ionisation chambers (Figure 3.13A) are particularly useful as instruments for calibration of megavoltage photon beams. Parallel plate ionisation chambers (Figure 3.13B) are useful when measuring in regions of high dose gradient, such as in the dose fall-off region of an electron beam. Diodes (Figure 3.13C) are useful for in vivo dosimetry. The small size of their detection region makes these devices also useful when measuring in small radiation fields or within beam penumbral regions. Cylindrical forms of these dectectors which include corrections within the design of the device for enhanced low energy photon response are readily available. Diamond detectors (Figure 3.13D) may be used as an alternative to diode detectors and are especially resistant to radiation damage.

Thermoluminescent dosimetry (TLD)

We have seen in the section on the band structure of solids that some materials have a normally empty conduction band. When such a material is irradiated, some electrons within the valence band may be given sufficient energy to excite them into the conduction band, leaving a 'hole' in the valence band. These electrons will eventually lose their extra energy and fall back to the valence band to fill the vacant energy level (hole) there. In doing this, the electron has to lose the energy difference between the two energy levels.

The energy lost in this transition may be a few electron-volts. In some materials, this energy loss is in the form of emission of electromagnetic radiation, akin to the emission of characteristic x-rays from an x-ray target but at much lower energies. This process appears simple, but may actually involve complex energy level changes for both the electron and the hole that are beyond the scope of this book. The result for some types of material is that it is transparent to the electromagnetic radiation released by these transitions, which is then emitted. The energy of the radiation emitted may be within the visible spectrum in which case the irradiated material emits light. Materials of this type are said to be *luminescent* in general. When the electrons excited into the conduction band fall back and emit light immediately, the material is said to be *fluorescent*. Fluorescent screens are used to enhance the response of x-ray film to radiation and are used within some types of portal imaging devices. In luminescent processes, additional energy levels within the forbidden zone as shown in Figure 3.10D, formed either from impurities or as a result of discontinuities in the crystal structure, play a part both in trapping the excited electrons and in the emission of light.

Energy levels immediately below the conduction band form traps for some of the electrons from that band. Electrons falling into these traps may be held there until they gain sufficient energy to move back into the conduction band, from where they can decay back to the valence band. If the trap level is close to the conduction band, then ongoing energy variations from thermal fluctuations will result in traps being emptied rapidly, hence to fluorescence. The further a trap from the conduction band, the longer will be the time for it to empty: traps are therefore characterized by two related features, the distance from the conduction band (the trap depth) and the rate at which it empties (the trap half-life).

In some materials, such as metal-doped lithium fluoride (i.e. doped with magnesium or manganese), the trap levels are well below the conduction band. At normal room temperatures, these traps would empty exceedingly slowly. If, however, the temperature of the crystal is raised, then the additional heat energy imparted may allow electrons rapidly to escape the traps. The light output from the crystal is dependent upon this supply of heat and these materials are termed *thermoluminescent*.

When a thermoluminescent material is irradiated, electrons are transported into the conduction band. A small number of these electrons (perhaps only 1%) fall into the thermoluminescent traps. When the material is later heated to a temperature that allows the traps to empty, light is given off. This process is shown in Figure 3.14. The amount of light is proportional to the number of electrons trapped and hence to the radiation dose delivered to the crystal material. Thermoluminescent dosimetry uses equipment (the TLD reader) that both heats the detector and simultaneously measures the amount of light emitted, as indicated in Figure 3.15.

A material such as lithium fluoride (LiF), which is the most common TLD material in clinical use, will have a number of traps at differing depths. The light output from LiF as a function of temperature of the crystal is known as a glow curve and a typical glow curve is illustrated in Figure 3.16.

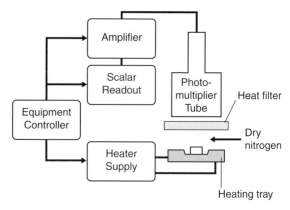

Figure 3.15 Schematic diagram of a thermoluminescent dosimeter readout system. The heat filter protects the photomultiplier tube and reduces thermal counts. The dry nitrogen atmosphere prevents oxidation of the detector surface.

The traps closest to the conduction band empty first, producing the glow peaks labelled I to III. These traps have relatively short half-lives at room temperatures such that the signal falls too rapidly for reliable dose estimates, so the output from these bands is usually ignored. The signal from the higher temperature peaks IV and V are from traps with half-lives measured in years, so that timing between irradiation and readout is not generally relevant – the light from these traps is measured to estimate the dose. After use, the material is thermally annealed, a process which resets the electron energy levels and trap occupancies to their initial values, after which the material may be re-used.

The light output from a specific dosimeter will depend upon a number of factors:

- the amount of intrinsic thermoluminescent material
- the nature and extent of the doping
- the previous thermal history in general and the post-anneal cooling in particular

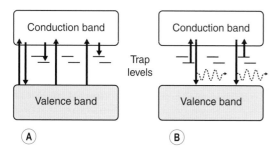

Figure 3.14 Illustration of TLD processes. Irradiation of the material raises electrons into the conduction band. Some of these fall back to the valence band while other become trapped in intervening energy levels, as shown in (A). When heat is applied, the electrons in the traps are raised back into the conduction band and subsequently fall back to the valence band, releasing visible photons as shown in (B).

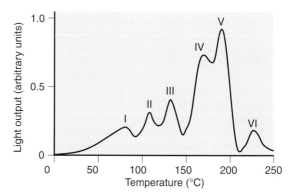

Figure 3.16 Schematic illustration of the glow curve from LiF: Mg,Ti showing the 6 peaks representing different trap depths. *(Redrawn from [25])*

- the radiation history of the material – radiation-induced damage may alter the energy band structure of the material
- the surface condition of the crystalline material – marks and scratches attenuate and scatter the light
- the detailed nature of the readout cycle.

Some of the above cause differences in response between different dosimeters, while others cause differences in response of a single dosimeter from use to use. In addition, the response is not strictly linear with dose but increases with increased dose, a feature known as 'supralinearity'. TLD is not used as an absolute dosimeter (i.e. where the calibration is stable and constant). To address these issues, TLD dosimeters are used in batches, where the dosimeters in each batch have the same handling and general history and where some are selected as measuring dosimeters while others are irradiated to known doses in order to calibrate the batch response in a traceable manner.

Lithium fluoride is the most commonly used TLD material and is available in various forms that include: powder; single crystal chips (size 4 mm×4 mm×1 mm approximately) and rods (size 6 mm long by 1 mm diameter); sintered chips, disks and rods; and Teflon embedded disks and rods. The effective atomic number is slightly greater than that of water leading to over-response of between 1.3 and 1.7 for photon energies of less than 100 KeV, but the response is virtually uniform for megavoltage radiation. The detector response does not vary with dose rate up to dose rates of greater than 10^6 Gy/min. Other materials are available, including lithium borate which has a more uniform energy response at low energies, and calcium sulfate which has a high sensitivity to low energy photons.

TLD materials are currently used as in vivo dosimeters for both surface dose and interstitial measurements. For measurements on the patient surface in order to estimate the dose at the depth of dose maximum, care must be taken to ensure that appropriate build-up is used, both for the patient measurement and also for calibration irradiation. Despite the variations in response described above, TLD is used to provide a traceable postal calibration service both to centres without access to a primary or secondary Standards Laboratory and to check on the accuracy of calibration across various centres as part of clinical trial quality control procedures.

Chemical and biochemical detectors

Energy deposited in matter may be manifest ultimately in various forms, one being altered chemistry, as indicated in Figure 3.1. Radiotherapy relies upon this to a large extent in the process of damaging and destroying tissue cells. In some cells, direct interaction of the radiation with DNA causes irreparable damage leading to death of those cells. In others, radiation-induced chemical changes within the cells produce active free radicals that cause similar damage to DNA.

In some materials, the altered chemical make-up remains and can be detected. Where the effect is stable and proportional to dose, this may be used in chemical and biochemical dosimetry. If the chemical yield is known (number of chemical molecules formed per unit of energy absorbed) then chemical dosimetry could be used as a primary standard. Fricke dosimetry was used for a short period in the past in this way to provide a definitive calibration of electron beams for which the yield was well established.

Fricke dosimetry

Fricke dosimetry is based upon conversion of ferrous sulfate ions (Fe^{2+}) to ferric ions in a weak sulfuric acid solution [26]. The concentration of ferric sulfate is determined by measuring the attenuation of light passing through the solution. Light of a particular wavelength (304 nm) is used as this is attenuated differentially by ferrous and ferric ions. The instrument used for accurate measurement of attenuation at a particular frequency of light is a spectrophotometer. The ferrous sulfate solution has to be carefully prepared and handled to avoid chemical contaminants that can affect the result.

The dose is given by:

$$D = k\Delta A/[\epsilon\ \delta\ \rho\ G\ (Fe^{3+})]$$

where k is a constant, ΔA is the change in absorption (optical density), δ is the optical path length, ρ is the Fricke density, ϵ the difference in molar extinction coefficient, and $G(Fe^{3+})$ is the chemical yield.

This system is not very sensitive such that doses of greater than 10 Gy are required to produce sufficient concentration of ferric ions, but accuracies of better than 2% are readily achievable. The process is effectively insensitive to dose rate and can be used to determine doses up to 400 Gy. The detector is 96% water and is therefore essentially water equivalent. It can be used over a wide range of energies and modalities. Fricke dosimetry has been used in the past by Standards Laboratories to confirm measurements of absorbed dose using other dosimetric techniques.

Ceric dosimetry

Similar to Fricke dosimetry above, ceric dosimetry relies of the reduction by radiation of ceric ions (Ce^{4+}) to cerous ions (Ce^{3+}) in a mixture of ceric and cerous ions in 0.4 M sulfuric acid. The concentration of cerous ions is determined by spectrophotometry using 320 nm light.

Gel dosimetry

The techniques described previously are suitable for producing single point measurements of dose (e.g. ionization chambers) or measurements of two-dimensional distributions (e.g. film). In contrast to these, gel dosimeters allow measurement of three-dimensional distributions. These are ideally suited to determination of distributions arising from complex treatments such as intensity modulated radiotherapy (IMRT). In addition, gel dosimetry is proving useful in situations where other forms of measurement are difficult, such as in dosimetry of very small radiation fields (e.g. stereotactic radiotherapy and proton beams) and measurements around brachytherapy sources where the radiation dose varies rapidly with position relative to the source. Phantoms to hold the gel material can be made to reflect anatomical shapes.

There are currently two forms of gel detectors in use, Fricke gel and polymer gel. For each, various ways of reading out the signal have been developed, the most common of which are magnetic resonance and optical computed tomography (CT). Gel detectors in general are insensitive to dose rates, are effectively water equivalent, and the signal is relatively linear with dose. Overall accuracy is limited (typically around 5%), although spatial resolution is excellent.

Fricke gels and FXG gels

In 1984, Gore proposed the use of magnetic resonance (MR) techniques on Fricke solutions [27] and Fricke-infused gels in which ferrous ions are held within the gel matrix. When reduced by radiation to ferric ions, the spin–spin (T2) relaxation times of linked protein atoms changes. This change in relaxation times in each small volume of the material can be measured using a magnetic resonance scanner. Each measurement is accompanied by a test irradiation that is used to determine the sensitivity of each detector batch to different dose levels.

Although able to produce accurate dose distributions, the process has two main drawbacks. First, measurement is time-consuming and requires ready access to an MR scanner. Secondly, the ferric ions migrate through the gel matrix with time, so that measurements have to be undertaken shortly after irradiation [28].

A development of this technique led to the introduction of Xylenol Orange into the gel mix [29]. This material is photochromic and has the property of changing colour from orange to purple when the mix is irradiated. This change in colour can be determined by measuring optical attenuation of filtered light. A set of two-dimensional slice readouts can be obtained using an optical CT device.

Polymer gels

Polymer gels are based upon the polymerization of monomers embedded in the gel matrix which produces long polymer chains and cross-linkage of polymers [30]. These reduce the T2 relaxation time which can be determined using a magnetic resonance scanner. A common polymer gel in current use is the BANG gel of Maryanski [31] which is based upon polymerization of the monomer acrylamide. This may be produced in forms that allow optical readout using an optical CT device, as radiation induces white opacity in an otherwise transparent material. Because cross-linkage of monomers stabilizes the material, there is no migration away from irradiated areas, such that these devices are stable over time.

BANG gels have to be produced and sealed while under a nitrogen atmosphere to avoid oxygen-induced polymerization affecting the results. This necessity has been removed in newer gel formulations (e.g. MAGIC) in which oxygen in the gel is bound into a chemical matrix which prevents it from causing polymerization, making the production of gels for dosimetry far simpler [32].

Alanine-EPR dosimetry

Alanine is a polycrystalline amino acid (chemical formula $CH_3CH(NH_2)COOH$). When irradiated, stable free radicals are formed within the material. These radicals can exist unchanged for long periods of time, allowing separation of irradiation from the readout process [33]. Some of these free radicals have a single unpaired electron attached to one of the atoms of the radical. The single unpaired electron exists in one of two energy states. When subjected to a magnetic field, these energy states equate to 'spin parallel' and 'spin anti-parallel' states, the difference in energy between them being proportional to the strength of the magnetic field.

The electron normally occupies the lower state, but may be excited into the higher state by absorbing a specific resonant wavelength of electromagnetic radiation of photon energy (hv) equal to the energy separation between the two states, for magnetic field strengths of 300 mT the frequency of about 9 MH, which is within the microwave part of the electromagnetic spectrum. The concentration of free radicals can be assessed by measuring the degree of absorption of this resonant radiation, a process know as electron paramagnetic resonance (EPR – or traditionally electron spin resonance, ESR) [34]. A number of free radicals are involved, the most important one involving the loss of the NH_2 group.

Dosimeters are formed by mixing known quantities of alanine with one or more binding agents to produce a compact, solid detector which has both density and atomic number values that differ only slightly from water and which is suitably sensitive to radiation. The dose response is almost linear from 10 Gy to 10^4 Gy and is largely independent of dose rate. Lower doses down to below 1 Gy can be measured provided that the device is calibrated to account for non-linearity of response at these dose levels. Accuracies of better than 2% are achievable under controlled conditions. The combination of accuracy and stability has led to their being used by a number of Standards Laboratories as a basis for a remote calibration service which rivals the use of thermoluminescent dosimetry. Alanine dosimetry systems are also available commercially. A number of research groups are currently investigating the development of two-dimensional and three-dimensional measurement systems based upon spatially-distributed alanine. Other groups are investigating chemical variations of alanine (e.g. 2-methylalanine) to develop dosimeters more suited to lower dose ranges for in vivo dosimetry [35].

Biological dosimetry

The response of biological systems has been used as an indicator of the dose delivered since the very first applications of radiation to the treatment of human disease. Early dosimetry standards were based upon skin erythema levels, with the absorbed dose determined by the degree of reddening of the skin and on the resultant type of erythema produced. This system was very inaccurate and was abandoned in favour of other physical forms of radiation dosimetry long before the introduction of skin-sparing megavoltage treatments. There are, however, circumstances, such as accidental exposures, where other forms of dosimetry are not applicable and where doses have to be estimated on the basis of the biological responses. There are various possible biological indicators of absorbed dose based upon the response of different biological systems. These include effects on biological molecules and genetic structures, but also include effects on cells and structures.

Biological molecules

The process described earlier in relation to alanine dosimetry in which the concentration of long-lived free radicals can be determined by using electron spin resonance may also be applicable to estimate doses to specific tissues. This process is relatively insensitive, but has been used to estimate doses received around sites of nuclear explosions and accidents [36, 37].

An alternative method to assess absorbed dose is based upon quantifying changes in the chemical composition of body fluids. The concentration of thymidine in blood serum has been shown to be a sensitive indicator of absorbed dose in mice [38], but is unfortunately less applicable to primates.

Genetic structures

The most advanced and established method of biological dosimetry is based upon determining the concentration of chromosome aberrations by counting the number of dicentrics in human peripheral blood lymphocytes [39]. This form of dosimetry is able to estimate doses down to about 0.1 Gy and is used in cases of accidental overexposure.

An alternative method is based upon determining the concentration of micronuclei formed as a result of the radiation exposure. This method may possibly be developed to compete with dicentric concentration analysis [40].

Cells and biological structures

The dose responses for various biological systems are well documented in the literature. Radiation inhibits the production of blood cells and, in males, sperm, and leads to the death of hair follicles – all of which may be used to estimate the absorbed dose shortly after exposure. For high doses of radiation, breakdown of other organs may be used where the absorbed dose exceeds tissue tolerance levels for those organs.

OTHER RADIATION DETECTORS

The ionization chambers previously described may be used to detect and measure both photons and charged particles, provided that the radiation can penetrate the wall or entrance window of the device and also that the ionization current is sufficiently large as to be measurable. Where the radiation intensity is too low for ionization chambers to work satisfactorily, such as in detecting and measuring radiation emitted from a small radioactive source, other more sensitive instruments must be used. The most sensitive devices are 'event counters', able to detect and record individual photon interactions or the passage of individual charged particles. Each interactions results in an electrical pulse which is counted either to give a total number of interactions recorded or the number recorded per unit interval of time to provide a 'count rate'. The decay of a radioactive material may be measured for example by monitoring the fall in count rate with time.

Common types of device that are used in the detection and measurement of low intensity radiation use gas amplification (Geiger-muller counters and proportional counters) and scintillation detectors.

Gas amplification devices

In ionization chambers, the ion pairs produced by particles crossing the air cavity are separated, collected and measured such that the charge collected equates to the number of ion pairs produced. A polarizing voltage is placed across the electrodes of the chamber sufficient to separate the ions and direct them to the electrodes of the device. Any kinetic energy gained by ions as they move towards an electrode is continually removed by collision interactions with other air molecules but the ions do not gain sufficient energy to create additional ionization. If the polarizing voltage is increased, then the charge detected may rise slightly as ion recombination is overcome, but the level will rapidly reach saturation and no further increase in collected charge will occur, as shown in Figure 3.17.

In gas amplification devices, air in the detector chamber is replaced by a gas, the pressure of which is greatly reduced,

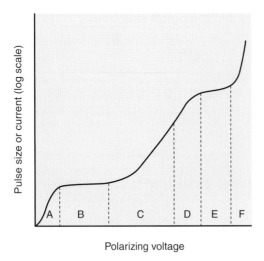

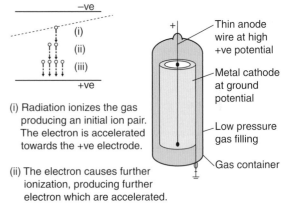

(i) Radiation ionizes the gas producing an initial ion pair. The electron is accelerated towards the +ve electrode.

(ii) The electron causes further ionization, producing further electron which are accelerated.

(iii) The process is repeated, building an electron avalanche.

(A)   (B)

Figure 3.17 Detector pulse size or current as a function of applied polarizing potential. Region A is dominated by recombination of ions. Ionization chambers operate in region B, proportional counters in region C and Geiger counters in region E. Region D represents transition between proportional and Geiger regions, and region F illustrates continuous discharge and electrical breakdown.

Figure 3.18 Schematic diagrams showing (A) the gas amplification process, and (B) a typical Geiger counter.

thereby allowing any ions produced in it to travel much further before interacting with atoms of the gas. If the electric field across the device is sufficiently high, then ions can gain sufficient energy themselves to cause further ionization of the gas, producing additional ion pairs. This leads to an increase in the charge collected. As the polarizing voltage is increased further, these additional ions may also gain sufficient energy to cause further ionization, leading to a cascade effect that produces further increase or amplification of the charge, a process that can be repeated many times, as illustrated in Figure 3.18A. The net result is that the detected pulse of charge is proportional to the amount of ionization produced by the radiation, but is amplified many times. The size of the pulse is determined by both the number of ions initially generated by the radiation and by the amount of amplification that takes place. This is in turn dependent upon the applied voltage across the chamber as shown in Figure 3.17. Gains of many orders of magnitude are possible, and radiation detectors that use this principle are known as *proportional counters*.

If the voltage across the device is further increased, proportionality between initial signal and pulse size starts to break down as the size of the charge avalanche increases. Eventually, the whole chamber volume becomes involved. Ions reaching the electrodes may interact and produce further ions which continue the process. The result is a charge pulse that is determined not by the number of ions initially created, but by the design of the electronics of the detector. Each pulse is the same height and causes

a temporary discharge of the polarizing voltage – this temporary reduction in voltage immediately after a pulse allows the counter to recover and any remaining ions in it to be absorbed. Introduction of special materials known as quenching agents into the gas speed up this residual ion removal. Such detector devices are known as *Geiger counters*.

A typical Geiger counter detector is shown schematically in Figure 3.18B and consists of a small cylindrical metal tube that forms the negative electrode, with a thin wire positive electrode running along the axis of the cylinder. The structure is sealed to enclose the low-pressure gas, typically a mixture of argon and ethanol or neon and chlorine. The structure can be designed as either a side-window device (i.e. where radiation enters through the side of the device) for general radiation detection or as an end-window device (where radiation enters through the end-cap of the device) for beta particle detection, the latter having a thin mica window to allow passage of beta particles. The efficiency of a Geiger counter is high for beta particles, but is very low for x-rays and gamma rays where the reliance is upon interaction with the wall of the device to generate secondary electrons that pass into the chamber cavity.

Each detected event results in an electric pulse, the size of which is independent of the number of ions initially causing the event, but which lasts for a few microseconds. The chamber then has to recover for a period of a few tens of microseconds, a period known as the *dead time* during which it will not respond to any further ionization stimulus. Because the pulse size does not reflect the number of ions initiating the event, the counter cannot distinguish between different types of radiation. Further, the dead time has implications for use in high intensity or pulsed radiation fields. As the radiation intensity increases, so the rate of events increases and the chance of missing pulses because of the extended dead time increases, resulting in under-recording. Similarly, in the pulsed radiation field of a linear accelerator where the pulse lengths are less than the dead time of the detector, the most that a Geiger counter will record will be one count per pulse, regardless of the actual radiation intensity. Hence, Geiger counters cannot be used to measure the intensity of a linear accelerator beam and great care must be exercised when using them to monitor radiation levels around a linear accelerator installation.

The pulse height from a Geiger counter varies only slowly with increasing voltage, as shown in Figure 3.17, making the device relatively insensitive to small changes. At higher voltages, however, the electric field strength can be sufficient in itself to ionize the gas, resulting in continued electrical discharge, or breakdown.

Scintillation devices

Some materials, such as thallium-doped sodium iodide, are known as scintillator materials which are a form of fluorescent material described earlier that emit light when irradiated. Scintillator materials are transparent to the light emitted, and so photon interactions cause short flashes of light in the material. The amount of light emitted is proportional to the energy deposited in the crystal. These short flashes of light can be detected by a photomultiplier tube – a device that converts very low levels of light into measurable electrical pulses. Sodium iodide is hygroscopic and is housed within a container that encompasses the material, prevents ingress of water vapour and reflects light back into the crystal – the inner surface of the container being covered in a reflective coating of titanium dioxide or magnesium oxide. One surface is coupled onto the face of the photomultiplier tube either directly or via a specially constructed light-guide. An optical coupling gel is used whenever two material faces are coupled together to reduce scattering caused by any tiny surface irregularities.

The inner surface of the front face of the photomultiplier tube has deposited on it a material (the photocathode) that causes photo-electrons to be emitted when subjected to visible light. These electrons are accelerated by electric fields within the device onto a series of dynodes. When an electron hits a dynode it causes emission of other electrons which in turn are directed onto other dynodes. Eventually, the avalanche of electrons reaches the anode, from where the electrical pulse is extracted. The electrical pulse from the photomultiplier is proportional to the amount of light hitting the photocathode, which in turn is proportional to the energy deposited by the initial radiation interaction in the scintillator crystal. Thus, a 300 keV gamma ray will, on average, produce a pulse that is twice as large as that produced by a 150 keV gamma ray provided that in both cases the total energy of the gamma ray is absorbed in the crystal.

A *pulse-height analyzer* is a device that has a number of counters each representing one *channel*. Each channel counts the pulses that occur only with a narrow band of pulse heights. Successive channels are set to count increasingly larger pulses. Hence, small pulses will appear in the lower channels and large pulses will be counted in higher channels. When a scintillation detector is connected to a pulse-height analyzer, the spectrum of counts produced represents the spectrum of energies deposited in the scintillator crystal. When measuring monoenergetic radiation (such as gamma rays from a gamma source), those interaction events that result in all the photon energy being absorbed in the crystal will have similar pulse heights and will be counted together in a narrow series of channels that represent this photon energy level. Interactions that result in less energy being deposited in the crystal (such as detection of Compton-scattered photons) will be counted in the wide range of channels below the photopeak channels, as shown in Figure 3.19. Since the positions of peaks in the spectrum represent specific energy levels, scintillation counters are able to differentiate between different energies of incident photons. By matching measured energy levels and their rates of decay against tabulated energies of emissions and half-lives of known radioactive materials, specific radioactive substances can be identified in any given sample. This process is called *gamma spectroscopy*. This process also underlies the principles of operation of the gamma camera used in nuclear medicine.

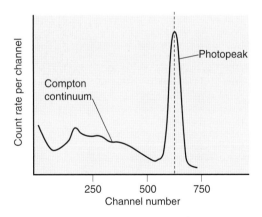

Figure 3.19 Typical pulse-height spectrum from a gamma source that emits a single energy gamma ray. The channel number equates to the energy deposited in the detector and the position of the photopeak is dependent on the energy of the emitted gamma ray. The width of the photopeak is dependent on the energy resolution of the detector system.

The pulse from a sodium iodide/photomultiplier detector has a pulse length of a few microseconds. Additional signals that occur within this time period combine together and appear as an enlarged signal. These will fall outside the main photopeak channels. The chance of two interactions occurring within the short time period will increase as the overall count rate increases, i.e. where the radiation is more intense, resulting in an underestimate of the true radiation intensity. Some plastic scintillators can have much shorter pulse lengths and can be constructed with large surface areas. These can be used to measure higher radiation intensities or to detect and measure radiation distributed over a large area.

Small plastic scintillators connected to distant photomultiplier tubes via long fibre-optic light guides have been used to measure dose distributions in radiotherapy [41]. The high sensitivity of the device allows use of tiny detectors that are of particular use in the measurement of rapidly varying intensities, such as in the penumbra of megavoltage beams or in the measurement of distributions from radioactive eye plaques [42]. More recently, tomographic reconstruction techniques have been applied to the optical signals from liquid scintillators to reconstruct full three-dimensional dose distribution maps around brachytherapy sources and eye plaques [43].

REFERENCES

[1] ICRU. Radiation quantities and units. Report No 33. International Commission on Radiation Units and Measurement; 1980.

[2] DuSautoy AR. The UK primary standard calorimeter for photon beam absorbed dose measurement. Phys Med Biol 1996;41:137–51.

[3] Marsh ARS, Williams TT. 50kV Primary standard of exposure: design of free-air chamber. NPL Report RS(Ext) 54, 182. Teddington: National Physical Laboratory; 1982.

[4] Palmer JA, Duane S, Shipley R, Moretti CJ. The design and construction of a new primary standard free air chamber for medium energy X-rays. Med Biol Eng Comput 1997;35:1086.

[5] Morgan AA, Aird EGA, Aukett RJ, et al. IPEM guidelines on dosimeter systems for use as transfer instruments between UK primary dosimetry standards laboratory (NPL) and radiotherapy centres. Phys Med Biol 2000;45:2445–57.

[6] Nutbrown RF, Duane S, Shipley DR, Thomas RAS. Evaluation of factors to convert absorbed dose calibrations from graphite to water for the NPL high-energy photon calibration service. Phys Med Biol 2002;47:441–54.

[7] Rosser KE, Owen B, DuSautoy AR, Pritchard DH, Stoker I, Brend CJ. The NPL absorbed dose to water calibration service for high-energy photons. IAEA-SM-330/35. In: Proceedings of symposium on measurement assurance in

dosimetry. Vienna: IAEA; 1994. p. 73–81.

[8] NPL. Practical course in reference dosimetry. National Physical Laboratory; 2006.

[9] Lillicrap SC, Owen B, Williams JR, Williams PC. Code of practice for high-energy photon therapy dosimetry based on the NPL absorbed dose calibration service. Phys Med Biol 1990;35:1355–60.

[10] Farmer FT. A substandard x-ray dose-meter. Br J Radiol 1955;28:304.

[11] Shonka RF, Rose JE, Failla G. Conducting plastic equivalent to tissue, air and polystyrene. In: 2nd United Nations Conference on Peaceful uses of Atomic EnergyNew York: UN; 1958. p. 160.

[12] IPEM. The IPEMB code of practice for the determination of absorbed dose for x-rays below 300kV generating potential (0.035mm Al – 4mm Cu HVL, 10–300kV generating potential). Phys Med Biol 1996;41:2605–25.

[13] IPEM. Addendum to the IPEMB code of practice for the determination of absorbed dose for x-rays below 300kV generating potential (0.035mm Al– 4mm Cu HVL, 10–300kV generating potential. Phys Med Biol 2005;50:2739–48.

[14] IPSM. Code of practice for high-energy photon therapy dosimetry based on the NPL absorbed dose calibration service. Phys Med Biol 1990;35:1355–60.

[15] IPEM. The IPEM code of practice for electron dosimetry for radiotherapy beams of initial energy from 4 to 25MeV based on an absorbed dose to water calibration. Phys Med Biol 2003;48:2929–70.

[16] Barish RJ, Lerch IA. Long-term use of an isotope check source for verification of ion chamber calibration. Med Phys 1992;17:203–6.

[17] Burns JE, Rosser KE. Saturation corrections for the NPL 2560/1 dosemeter in photon dosimetry. Phys Med Biol 1991;35:687–693.

[18] Havercroft JM, Klevenhagen SC. Ion chamber corrections for parallel-plate and thimble chambers in electron and photon radiation. Phys Med Biol 1993;38:25–38.

[19] Lewis DF. A processless electronic recording medium. In: Electronic Imaging Proc of SPSE's Symposium. Arlington, Springfield VA: Society for Imaging Science and Technology; 1986. p. 76–9.

[20] Grusell E, Rikner G. Evaluation of temperature effects in p-type silicon detectors. Phys Med Biol 1986;31:527–34.

[21] Rikner G. Silicon diodes as detectors in radiation dosimetry of photon, electron and proton radiation fields. Thesis, Sweden: Uppsala; 1983.

[22] Shi J, Simon WE, Ding L, Saini D. Important issues regarding diode performance in radiation therapy applications. In: Proc 22nd Annual EMBS Int Conference. Chicago; 2000.

[23] Rikner G, Grusell E. Effects of radiation damage on p-type silicon

diodes. Phys Med Biol 1983;28:1261–7.

[24] Khrunov VS, Martynov SS, Vatnitsky SM, et al. Diamond detectors in relative dosimetry of photon, electron and proton radiation fields. Radiat Prot Dosimetry 1990;33:155–7.

[25] Kron T. Thermoluminescence dosimetry and its applications in medicine: Part 1. Physics, materials and equipment. Australas Phys Eng Sci Med 1994;17:175–99.

[26] Fricke H, Morse S. The chemical action of roentgen rays on dilute ferrous sulphate solutions as a measure of radiation dose. Am J Roentgenol Radium Ther Nucl Med 1927;18:430–2.

[27] Gore JC, Kang YS, Schulz RJ. Measurement of radiation dose distributions by nuclear magnetic resonance (NMR) imaging. Phys Med Biol 1984;29: 1189–1197.

[28] Baldock C, Harris PJ, Piercy AR, Healy B. Experimental determination of the diffusion coefficient in two dimensions in ferrous sulphate gels using the finite element method. Australas Phys Eng Sci Med 2001;24: 19–30.

[29] Appleby A, Leghrouz A. Imaging of radiation dose by visible colour development in ferrous-agarose-xylenol orange gels. Med Phys 1991;18:309–12.

[30] Maryanski MJ, Gore JC, Kennan RP, Schulz RJ. NMR relaxation enhancement in gels polymerized and cross-linked by ionizing radiations: a new approach to 3D dosimetry by MRI. Magn Reson Imaging 1993;11:253–8.

[31] Maryanski MJ, Schuklz RJ, Ibbott GS, et al. Magnetic resonance imaging of radiation dose distributions using polymer gel dosimeter. Phys Med Biol 1994;39:1437–55.

[32] Fong PM, Keil DC, Does MD, Gore JC. Polymer gels for magnetic resonance imaging of radiation dose distributions at normal room atmosphere. Phys Med Biol 2001;46:3105–13.

[33] Bradshaw WW, Cadena DG, Crawford GW, Spelzler HAW. The use of alanine as solid dosimeter. Radiat Res 1962;17:11.

[34] Regulla DF, Deffner U. Dosimetry by ESR spectroscopy of alanine. Appl Radiat Isot 1982;33:1101.

[35] Olsson S, Sagstuen E, Bonora M, Lund A. EPR Dosimetric properties of 2-methylalanine: EPR, ENDOR and FT-EPR investigations. Radiat Res 2002;V157:113–21.

[36] Mascarenhas S, Hasegawa A, Takeshita K. EPR dosimetry of bones from the Hiroshima A-bomb site. Bull Am Phys Soc 1973;18:579.

[37] Guskova AK, Barabanova AV, Baranov AY. Acute radiation effects in victims of the Chernobyl nuclear power plant accident. UNSCEAR Report on Sources and Effects of Ionizing Radiation, Appendix 613-631. New York: United Nations; 1988.

[38] Feinendegen LE, Muhlensiepen H, Porchen W, Booz J. Acute non-stochastic effect of very low dose whole body exposure, a thymidine equivalent serum factor. Int J Radiat Biol 1982;41:139–50.

[39] Bender MA, Awa AA, Brooks AL, et al. Current status of cytogenetic procedures to detect and quantify previous exposures to radiation. Mutat Res 1988;196:103–59.

[40] Prosser JS, Lloyd DC, Edwards AA. A comparison of chromosomal and micronuclear methods for radiation accident dosimetry. In: Goldfinch EP, editors. Radiation protection: theory and practice. New York: Institute of Physics; 1989. p. 133–6.

[41] Beddar AS, Mackie TR, Attix FH. Water-equivalent plastic scintillation detectors for high-energy beam dosimetry: 1. Physical characteristics and theoretical considerations. Phys Med Biol 1992;37:1883–900.

[42] Fluhs D, Heintz M, Indenkampen F, Wieczorek C, Kolanoski H, Quast U. Direct reading measurement of absorbed dose with plastic scintillators – the general concept and applications to ophthalmic plaque dosimetry. Med Phys 1996;23:427–34.

[43] Kirov AS, Piao JZ, Mathur NK, et al. The three-dimensional scintillation dosimatery method: test for a ^{106}Ru eye plaque applicator. Phys Med Biol 50:3063–81.

[44] Damen P. Design of a water calorimeter for medium energy x-rays: a status report. CCRI(I)/05-38. Netherlands: NMi Van Swinden Laboratorium; 2005.

[45] Krauss A. The PTB water calorimeter for the absolute determination of absorbed dose to water in 60Co radiation. Metrologia 2006;43:259–72.

[46] Palmans H, Seuntjens JP. Construction, correction factors and relative heat defect of a high purity 4° calorimeter for absorbed dose determinations in high-energy photon beams. NPL Calorimeter Workshop; 1994. p. 1214.

[47] Ross CK, Seuntjens JP, Klassen NV, Shortt KR. The NRC sealed water calorimeter: correction factors and performance. In: Williams AJ, Rosser KE, editors. Proc NPL Workshop on Recent Advances in Calorimetric Absorbed Dose Standards. NPL Teddington; 2000. p. 90–102.

[48] Willaims AJ, Rosser KE, Thomson NJ, DuSautoy AR. Recent advances in water calorimetry at NPL. In: Proc 22nd Annual EMBS International Conference. Chicago; 2000.

Chapter | 4 |

Radiation protection

Mike Dunn

INTRODUCTION

The biological effects of ionizing radiation are described in detail in Chapter 17 of this book, and are summarized in the following section. As there are known risks of radiation exposure, levels of acceptable risk have been specified by international expert groups, principally the International Commission on Radiological Protection (ICRP). Based upon these acceptable risks, dose levels have been recommended and in most cases adopted into national legislative requirements.

In order to understand these dose limits and the associated risks, it is necessary to have an understanding of the dose units that they are measured in and this chapter will explain these dose values. In addition, as there are known risks of radiation, most countries have regulatory requirements that have to be met in order to limit the risk to radiation workers, patients and members of the public arising from the use of radiation. The legislative requirements within the UK will be described and some of the methodology used to comply with these, including personal radiation monitoring, equipment testing, appropriate construction of radiation areas and the administrative arrangements surrounding the application of radiation.

BIOLOGICAL EFFECTS OF RADIATION

The block diagram (Figure 4.1) details the various biological effects that radiation may cause resulting from the absorption of energy associated with the radiation. As will be seen later, different areas of the body have different degrees of radiation sensitivity, which is mirrored in the fact that there are different dose limits for specific areas of the human body.

Almost since the discovery of ionizing radiation, its potential for causing deleterious effects has been known. These effects are caused by the absorption by the human body of the energy associated with the radiation. Such energy absorption can cause ionization (charged particles) and excitation in the body or subsequent chemical changes by the formation of such things as free radicals. The end result, however, is a potential for some form of biological change or damage to occur.

These changes can cause three types of effects, which are summarized below. The first two effects have no known threshold dose below which the effects will not occur and are the origin of the concept of there being no safe dose of radiation.

Stochastic hereditary effects

These effects are expressed not in the exposed individual but in the exposed individual's subsequent offspring or future generations. Effects such as one eye a different colour from the other or, more grossly, one limb shorter or missing, are examples. Genetic defects appear in the population due to many causes, radiation being just one of them, with about one in 200 live births having a genetic defect expressed. As such, the possibility of radiation being the cause of any defect can only be shown statistically, the probability being dose dependent, rising with dose. The current risk estimated by ICRP 60 [1] of severe hereditary effects from radiation is one in 75 000 for a radiation dose of 1 mSv (see below), that is about 375 mSv would double the natural occurrence of genetic defects. That is from one in 200 to two in 200.

Stochastic somatic effects

These effects are expressed in the exposed individual in the form of cancer induction. Again, cancer has a number of causes, radiation being only one. About one in four of the population is likely to have a cancer in their lifetime. The probability of this being caused by radiation increases with dose. The current risk estimated by ICRP 60 [1] of a cancer from radiation is one in 13 000 for a radiation dose of 1 mSv (see below). The extra cancer risk from very low doses is extremely small and, in practice, undetectable in the population. However, the extra cancer risk at higher doses may be detectable using statistical methods. Even after high dose exposure, it is rarely possible to be certain that radiation was directly responsible for a cancer arising in an individual. There are a number of scientific uncertainties in making these estimates of cancer risk at low doses. In 2000, the highly respected United Nations Scientific Committee on the Effects of Atomic Radiation (UNSCEAR) [2]

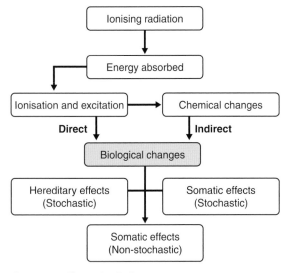

Figure 4.1 Effects of radiation.

suggested that uncertainties in cancer risk estimates may be about twofold higher or lower for acute doses where cancer risk can be directly assessed and a further factor of two (higher or lower) for the projection of these risks to very low doses and low dose rates.

Non-stochastic somatic effects

These effects, sometimes known as deterministic, are expressed in the exposed individual in the form of acute effects of radiation such as radiation burns, hair loss, sterility, vomiting and diarrhoea. These effects will only occur once the level of dose received exceeds the threshold dose for that effect, with the severity of the effect increasing with dose beyond the threshold. Dependent on the area irradiated and the level of dose received, such effects will be displayed by patients undergoing radiotherapy exposures. A picture showing some of these effects is given in (Figure *evolve* 4.2). Details of dose thresholds that need to be exceeded for different effects are given in Table 4.1.

The risk factors quoted above have been assessed from data arising from five main sources of information. These are, the effects noted shortly after the discovery of radiation, evidence from radiation accidents, effects of the atomic bombs exploded in Hiroshima and Nagasaki during World War Two, evidence from radiotherapy treatments and results from animal experiments. These information sources have given data relating to the effects of relatively high doses of radiation, and an assumption is made currently that there is a linear relationship between dose and risk from these high dose data points by extrapolation to the lower dose levels encountered as part of occupational exposure to staff working with radiation. This assumption has not been proven and the relationship may not be linear which would mean that we could be either over- or underestimating the stochastic risks of cancer by using the linear response model.

Table 4.1 Dose thresholds for biological effects

THRESHOLD DOSE (Gy)	AREA IRRADIATED	EFFECT
>0.15	Testes	Temporary sterility
>0.5	Eye	Cataracts
>2.0	Skin	Burns
>2.5	Gonads	Permanent sterility
>20	CNS	Death in hours

DOSE DESCRIPTORS

Two different dose quantities have been quoted in the above text. These are Sieverts (Sv) and Gray (Gy).

The Gray is a measure of absorbed dose or energy in Joules per kilogram as described in Chapter 2. Two other quantities are relevant when discussing radiation protection matters, these are *equivalent dose* and *effective dose* which have the units of Sieverts to indicate a change in dose descriptor.

Equivalent dose

The same absorbed dose delivered by different types of radiation may result in different degrees of biological damage to body tissues. The total energy deposited is not the only factor which determines the extent of the damage. The equivalent dose was introduced to take into account the dependence of the harmful biological effects on the type of radiation being absorbed. The equivalent dose is therefore a measure of the risk associated with an exposure to ionizing radiation. Risks due to exposures to different radiation types can be directly compared when in terms of equivalent dose.

The unit of equivalent dose is the Sievert (Sv) and is defined for a given type of radiation by the relationship:

$$\text{Equivalent dose (Sv) H} = \text{Absorbed dose (Gy)} \times \text{Radiation Weighting Factor } W_R$$

The radiation weighting factor is a dimensionless number which depends on the way in which the energy of the radiation is distributed along its path through the tissue.

The rate of deposition of energy along the track is known as the *linear energy transfer* (LET) of the radiation and has units of keV μm^{-1} measured in water which is considered equivalent to tissue.

Radiation with a high LET (such as protons and alpha particles) is more likely than radiation with a low LET (such as x-rays or beta particles) to damage the small structures in tissue such as DNA molecules. This is because the energy from high LET radiation is absorbed in a small volume surrounding the trail of dense ionization produced by this radiation. The radiation weighting factor is directly related to the LET of the radiation. The radiation weighting factors are used to correct for differences in the biological damage to tissue caused by chronic exposure to different radiations (Table 4.2).

Effective dose

Equivalent dose accounts for the varying biological effects of different types of radiation on a particular tissue type or organ, T. However, it should come as no surprise to find out that the same radiation exposure to different parts of the body can have very different results. If the entire body were irradiated with a uniform beam of a single type of radiation, some parts of the body would react more

Table 4.2 Weighting factors for different types of radiation

RADIATION TYPE AND ENERGY RANGE	RADIATION WEIGHTING FACTOR (W$_R$)
Photons – all energies	1
Electrons – all energies	1
Protons – energy >2 MeV	5
Alpha particles	20
After ICRP60 [1]	

dramatically than others. To take this effect into account, the ICRP have developed a list of tissue weighting factors, denoted W$_T$, for a number of organs and tissues that most significantly contribute to an overall effective biological damage to the body. It should be noted that areas of the body with a high cell turnover are more radiosensitive than areas with a slower cell turnover and thus have a larger weighting factor. Table 4.3 presents values of the tissue-

Table 4.3 W$_T$ values

TISSUE OR BODY PART	W$_T$
Gonads	0.20
Bone marrow	0.12
Colon	0.12
Lung	0.12
Stomach	0.12
Bladder	0.05
Breast	0.05
Liver	0.05
Oesophagus	0.05
Thyroid	0.05
Skin	0.01
Bone surface	0.01
Remainder (adrenals, brain, upper large intestine, small intestine, kidney, muscle, pancreas, spleen, thymus, and uterus)	0.05
Total	1.00
From [1]	

weighting factor W$_T$ based upon standard man which is a 70 kg male. Figures would be different for females, for instance, as they have more radiosensitive breast tissue. As such, the effective dose for a particular examination should not be viewed as a precise figure, but merely a figure giving an indication of relative risk.

To arrive at an effective dose for a particular examination, it is necessary to determine the equivalent dose to the different listed tissues or body parts, multiply these doses by the relevant tissue weighting factor and then sum the constituent parts. The units of effective dose are the Sievert and a worked example is given in Table 4.4.

BACKGROUND RADIATION

We are all exposed to radiation, regardless of our occupation, from 'natural' radiation sources in the environment and from man-made sources. We have no control over the level of exposure to these sources of natural radiation other than by choosing a particular lifestyle. For example, cosmic rays from outer space are attenuated by the Earth's atmosphere and the more atmosphere there is the more the attenuation. This means that people who live at high altitudes or travel in high flying aircraft will get a greater radiation dose from cosmic rays. Other sources of natural radiation and the proportions that they contribute to the overall dose are shown in Figure 4.3.

The major sources of natural radiation are the radioactive gases radon and thoron. Together they contribute over 50% of the average background radiation dose in the UK. These gases are generated in granite rock and, as a consequence, the intensity of the radon exposure varies considerably around the world, being higher in areas were there is more granite rock. In addition, if the rock is cracked the gas can escape into the environment more easily leading to higher levels in the environment. Such a situation exists in Cornwall where the level of radon gas is up to three times the national average. This has consequences in terms of the gas entering the homes of people living in these areas. Since the trend is to insulate homes more rigorously, this can have the effect of trapping the gas in the homes, leading to elevated doses to the inhabitants. Constructing well-ventilated houses and incorporating a special membrane into the foundation of new houses can alleviate this. Installing extraction fans and increasing under floor ventilation may improve older properties. These natural sources contribute an average dose of about 2.3 mSv per annum to a member of the UK population.

Another 0.3 mSv per annum is contributed to by artificial or man-made sources, such as discharges from nuclear power stations, making the average total dose 2.6 mSv. However, the biggest contribution is from the diagnostic uses of radiation where, although the individual doses are small, a large number of x-rays are performed with, on average, every

Table 4.4 Effective dose from a chest x-ray with a skin entrance dose of 500 μGy

ORGAN	% ENTRANCE DOSE	DOSE (μGy)	EQUIVALENT DOSE (μSv)	WEIGHTING FACTOR	TISSUE WEIGHTED DOSE (μSv)
Gonads	0.2	1	1	0.2	0.2
Breast	2	10	10	0.05	0.5
Bone marrow (red)	1	5	5	0.12	0.6
Lung	30	150	150	0.12	18
Thyroid	1	5	5	0.05	0.25
Bone	1	5	5	0.01	0.05
Heart	10	50	50	0.025	1.25
Stomach	5	25	25	0.12	3
Liver	10	50	50	0.05	2.5
			Effective dose (μSv) =		26.35

On the basis of the above ICRP figure of 1 in 13000 cancer incidences per mSv, this implies an additional risk of 1 in 493358

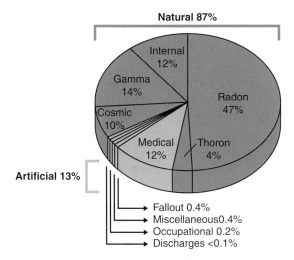

Figure 4.3 The average background radiation levels in the UK is 2.6 mSv per year from the sources detailed in this pie chart. *(Courtesy of the National Radiation Protection Board now the Health Protection Agency).*

member of the UK population undergoing at least one x-ray examination per year. Since this is a controllable exposure to some extent, a great deal of effort has been put into reducing both the individual dose per patient and the number of examinations carried out. This has been brought about by both legislative requirements (see below) and good practice guidelines.

LEGISLATIVE REQUIREMENTS

Until 1985, there were no legislative requirements specifically relating to the use of radiation in place within the UK. The use of radiation in medicine was relatively well self-regulated by compliance with good practice guidelines developed by the professionals involved. The UK's membership of the European Community required the Government to enact a number of legislative requirements, which are common across the Community. These will now be discussed in some detail.

The Ionising Radiations Regulations 1999 [3]

These revised the Ionising Radiations Regulations 1985 and deal with the protection of workers and members of the public from ionizing radiation from any source. The Approved Code of Practice – 'Work with ionising radiation' [4] – supports these. These documents are legally enforceable and breaches of their requirements could lead to prosecution by the regulators, normally the Health and Safety Executive. Good practice guidance is given in the Medical and Dental

Guidance Notes [5]. The Ionising Radiations Regulations require three basic requirements to be met; these are:

1. that no practice involving radiation be adopted unless there is a positive net benefit, either to the exposed individuals or to society, i.e. it can be justified
2. all exposures must be As Low As Reasonably Achievable or Practicable. This is often referred to as the ALARA or ALARP principle. The principle requires that any particular source, the number of people being exposed, and the likelihood of incurring exposures where these are not certain to be received, be optimized to a minimum, taking account of social and economic factors. In practice, there may be a number of options where an assessment would show that costs are not grossly disproportionate. The option, or combination of options, which achieves the lowest level of residual risk, should be implemented, provided grossly disproportionate costs are not incurred. In general, the greater the risk, the more that should be spent in reducing it, and the greater the bias on the side of safety. The judgment as to whether measures are grossly disproportionate should reflect societal risk, that is to say, large numbers of people (employees or the public) being killed at one go. This is because society has a greater aversion to an accident killing 10 people than to 10 accidents killing one person each
3. dose equivalents to individuals do not exceed certain dose limits. The exposure of individuals resulting from the combination of all relevant practices should be subject to dose limits, or to some control of risk in the case of potential exposures. These are aimed at ensuring that no individual is exposed to radiation risks that are judged to be unacceptable from these practices in any normal circumstances.

The revision of these regulations was brought about largely because of a reassessment of the risks of radiation. The new assessment indicated that the risks had previously been underestimated by a factor of about three times. This has meant a reduction in the whole body dose limit by a factor of about three. The reassessment was on the basis of the fact that many of the biological data were based upon the effects observed in the victims of the Hiroshima and Nagasaki bombs. The effects observed were equated to dosimetry data gathered from atomic bombs dropped in the Nevada desert. Unfortunately, the atmospheric conditions in the Nevada desert are very dry in comparison to the humid conditions in Hiroshima and Nagasaki. These humid conditions attenuated the radiation to a greater degree than the atmospheric conditions in the Nevada desert by a difference of about three. As a consequence, the biological effects observed in Hiroshima and Nagasaki were occurring at levels of dose some three times lower than originally thought. This led to a requirement to reduce the previous dose limits by a factor of about three.

Risk assessments

Prior to any work being undertaken with ionizing radiation, the employer is responsible for carrying out a risk assessment. This is in common with the requirement under the Management of Health and Safety at Work Regulations [6] to carry out risk assessments for other work involving hazards. The purpose of this risk assessment is to identify the measures needed to restrict the exposure of employees and other persons to ionizing radiation. The assessment must be suitable and sufficient enough to demonstrate that all hazards with the potential to cause a radiation accident have been identified and the nature and magnitude of the risks arising from those hazards have been evaluated. Where the risk assessment identifies a radiation risk, the employer must take all reasonable steps to prevent any such accident, limit the consequences of any accident that does occur and provide employees with the information, instruction and training to restrict their exposure. These risk assessments should normally be recorded and reviewed regularly to ensure their continued relevance. The factors that should be considered in performing a radiation risk assessment are given in the Approved Code of Practice [4] and include such things as the nature of the sources and the estimated radiation dose rates to which anyone can be exposed.

Dose limits

The annual dose limit has remained largely unchanged for the past 40 years and, despite the new dosimetric evidence, the absolute whole body dose limit per year remains at 50 mSv. However, such a level of dose is only allowable in special circumstances as the dose averaged over a 5-year period must not exceed 20 mSv per year for those occupationally exposed and aged over 18 years old. For those employees under 18 years old, the whole body dose limit is 6 mSv per year. Women of reproductive capacity working with ionizing radiation are subjected to a further dose constraint that the equivalent dose to the abdomen shall not exceed 13 mSv in any consecutive calendar quarter. The current dose limits are summarized in Table 4.5. It should be noted that there are currently no dose limits for patients undergoing examination or treatment with radiation, only that their doses must be as low as reasonably practicable and that any dose given must be justified in terms of the risk to the patient from not carrying out the exposure (see IRMER legislation [7] below).

There are two things to note in Table 4.5. First, there are different dose limits for different areas of the body, as different organs within the body have different radiosensitivities and radiation exposures are very often non-uniform. An area of the body with the quickest cell division and, therefore, the most radiosensitive is the fetus. This, in regulatory terms, is considered to be a member of the public from the point of the dose limit to be applied. A dose limit of 1 mSv to the fetus equates to a dose to the abdomen of the mother

Table 4.5 Current dose limits

	CLASSIFIED WORKERS	UNCLASSIFIED WORKERS	MEMBERS OF THE PUBLIC
Whole body	20	6	1
Individual organ	500	150	50
Lens of eye	150	50	15
Fetus of pregnant worker	1	1	
Dose limits per year in mSv			

of about 2 mSv and is the limit that the employer has to apply for the declared term of the pregnancy. As such, the period of time for the dose limit to be exceeded starts when the worker declares herself to be pregnant to her employer. Secondly, there are three groups of people with different dose limits, classified workers, unclassified workers and members of the public. Classified workers are those workers who, by virtue of the work they undertake, are likely to exceed the dose limits for unclassified workers. Before a worker can be classified, they are required to be declared fit to do so by an appointed doctor. This is a registered medical practitioner who has been appointed in writing by the Health and Safety Executive (HSE). Once a worker has been classified, the employer is legally obliged to issue the worker with an individual radiation dosimeter and keep a cumulative dose record for 50 years of the last entry in it. This must be undertaken by an HSE approved dosimetry and record keeping service. An annual report is sent to a body known as the Central Index for Dose Information (CIDI) of the doses received by all classified persons, with the intention of being able to undertake epidemiological studies in subsequent years and to provide a central record of doses received by a classified worker which, if the worker changes employers, is passed onto their new employer. The reports of any investigation into a real or suspected overexposure of a member of staff or a patient must also be kept for 50 years. The Health and Safety Executive has defined an exposure significantly more than intended as being the reporting criteria to be used in determining if a patient has been overexposed due to equipment failure. This information is given in Appendix 2 of the Guidance Note PM77 [8] – 'Equipment used in connection with medical exposure'. This specifies that notification to the HSE should be made if the dose given to a patient from beam therapy or brachytherapy exceeds 1.1 times the intended dose for a whole course or 1.2 times

the intended dose for any fraction. For unsealed radionuclide therapy, the guideline multiple is 1.2 for any administration.

Although a large number of hospital staff are individually monitored with a radiation dosimeter, very few are classified radiation workers. Possible exceptions are staff such as radiopharmacists, interventional radiologists and radiotherapists handling sealed brachytherapy sources. Radiation monitoring has shown that the vast majority of hospital staff receives less than 0.1 mSv per year from the work they undertake. Nevertheless, employers are obliged to demonstrate that staff working with radiation do not require to become classified and the best way of doing this is to provide them with a radiation monitor.

The whole body effective dose limit for all other persons including anyone below the age of 16 is 1 mSv per year with equivalent dose limits for specific areas in the body as detailed in Table 4.5.

Comforters and carers

A special case is made in the regulations for members of the public who are comforters and carers of patients undergoing or who may have undergone a medical exposure, e.g. a parent who holds a child while being x-rayed or a member of the family of a patient treated with radioactive material who is discharged from hospital with relatively large amounts of radioactive material still in their bodies. To fall into this category, the carer has knowingly and willingly to accept the risks in providing comfort and support to the patient. This means that the carer must be provided with information about the risks by the hospital treating the patient. In this case, there are no specific dose limits for the carer, however, information should be given to them regarding steps to be taken to control as far as reasonably practicable the dose they receive. The National Radiological Protection Board (now part of the Health Protection Agency), a body set up by Government to provide impartial advice on radiation protection matters, has recommended that, in this context, the exposure received by persons acting as comforters and carers should not in general exceed 5 mSv from their involvement in one series or course of treatment. Normally, it should be possible to design procedures that will keep doses received by carers below this level.

There will also be occasions when members of the public who are not comforters and carers and therefore cannot knowingly or willingly be exposed to radiation, come into contact with patients who have undergone a therapeutic administration of a radiopharmaceutical, e.g. sharing public transport or accommodation. In such cases, an effective dose limit of 5 mSv in any period of 5 consecutive years is used. In practice, sufficient action is normally taken by hospitals following accepted practice on release of such patients from hospital for this not to be a problem.

Controlled and supervised radiation areas

If the dose limits are to be adhered to, it is necessary to impose strict controls on how and where radiation generating equipment and radioactive materials are used. Such equipment and material should be housed in areas where sufficient protection is afforded by the surrounding structures so that people in adjacent areas will not get a significant exposure. Where persons are required to enter radiation areas or adjacent locales then engineering controls and design considerations must be used to protect them. For example, concrete walls and door interlocks to terminate an exposure if entry to the treatment room is made, are preferable to mobile lead screens, which may be placed incorrectly or written instruction prohibiting entry, which may not be obeyed.

Radiation areas are defined under UK legislation as being either a controlled or a supervised radiation area. These should have been identified as part of the prior risk assessment (see above).

A controlled area is any area where persons entering are required to follow special procedures to limit the risk of a significant exposure contained within local safety rules, (see below) or where they are likely to receive an effective dose of greater than 6 mSv per year or an equivalent dose greater than three-tenths of any other applicable dose limit. A controlled area must, wherever possible, be defined with reference to physical boundaries, e.g. the whole of an x-ray room must be defined as a controlled area, even though the dose definition of a controlled area would mean that the controlled area perhaps does not extend more than 2 meters from the x-ray tube and patient. Once a controlled area has been defined, access into it must be controlled, wherever practicable radiation warning signs and notices are required to be placed on entrances to the area, explaining the nature of the radiation, e.g. x-rays, gamma rays etc, and the control measures to help avoid the risk, e.g. 'do not enter when red light is on'. An example of such signing is given in (Figure *evolve* 4.4).

Where a source of radiation is mobile, e.g. mobile x-ray unit used on several wards, then such signing would be impracticable and is therefore not used. However, a controlled area is still defined and controlled by the radiographer, e.g. 2 metres around the x-ray set and patient and anywhere in the main beam until it is sufficiently attenuated by a solid object or distance.

In a medical situation, access to a controlled area is limited to four groups of people; these are:

1. the patient undergoing the exposure, for whom there are stringent controls both on the equipment that is used and the process. These are governed by the Ionising Radiation (Medical Exposure) Regulations 2000 (see below)
2. classified workers who are subjected to individual monitoring. Where a classified worker of another employer enters someone else's controlled area, then the owner of the controlled area must make an entry into a passbook carried by the classified worker. This gives an estimate of the dose received by the classified worker while working in the controlled area [9]
3. unclassified radiation workers and others who have been issued with written schemes of work which, if followed, ensure that they do not receive a dose greater than any applicable dose limit
4. regulatory inspectors, who enter to inspect the area for checking compliance with requirements.

A supervised area is any area where a person is likely to receive an effective dose of greater than 1 mSv per year (publics dose limit) or an equivalent dose greater than one-tenth of any relevant dose limit. If a supervised area has been defined, it is necessary to keep the conditions of the area under review to determine if the area needs to be designated a controlled area. Supervised areas should be suitably signed to indicate the nature of the radiation source and warning that a supervised area exists and the risks arising therein.

Local rules, radiation protection advisers and supervisors

Once a controlled or supervised area has been defined, then it is necessary to have written local safety rules, referred to as local rules. These should be drawn up taking into account the findings of the prior risk assessment. These rules must be drawn to the attention of any worker who needs to enter a controlled or supervised area. Among other things, they should contain written schemes of work for safe entry into the controlled areas and contingency plans for any foreseeable accident, e.g. radioactive source spillage. They should also contain the name of the Radiation Protection Adviser (RPA), who needs to be appointed by any employer who has set up a controlled area. Their duty is to advise the employer on compliance with the regulatory requirements, the correct identification of controlled and supervised areas and the prior examination of plans for radiation installations and the acceptance into service of new or modified sources of ionizing radiation. In the Health Service, an RPA is normally an experienced radiation physicist. An RPA is required to have a certificate of competence to act as an RPA, which is issued by an HSE approved certification body every 5 years to candidates who can provide evidence of their suitability to act as an RPA.

In addition, the name of the Radiation Protection Supervisors (RPS) for the area should be included in the local rules. Their responsibility is to supervise that the work with radiation that is being undertaken on a day-to-day basis is in compliance with the local rules. They should also be involved in the preparation of the local rules for the area that they supervise in order to ensure that they are both practical and not prohibitive. To act as an RPS, the person must have received training in a core of knowledge that has been specified by the HSE. They should also be someone in a position of authority and familiar with the work of the area they are supervising. The HSE has also indicated that there should be approximately one RPS for every 20 members of staff working in the radiation areas in order for adequate supervision to be undertaken.

Local rules must contain the following as a minimum:

- identification and description of controlled and supervised areas
- names of RPSs
- arrangements for restricting access to radiation areas
- dose investigation levels. These are levels of dose which, if received, will trigger an
- investigation into the circumstances. They are lower than any applicable dose limit typically 1 mSv to 6 mSv whole body dose
- summary of work instructions, including written arrangements for non-classified persons (schemes of work)
- contingency arrangements for any foreseeable accident or incident.

Radiation safety committee

Ultimate legal responsibility for compliance with the regulations, as with all Health and Safety legislation, lies with the employer. Although not a legal requirement, it is seen as good practice for large establishments, such as hospitals, to set up a radiation safety committee to assist the employer in complying with the regulations and to discuss matters relating to radiation safety including considering reports on any incidents that may have happened. This committee normally has representatives from each area where radiation is used and for each staff group who encounter radiation, together with the RPA and employers' representative. The outcome of the radiation protection committee meetings is very often reported to more general health and safety committees, to ensure as wide as publication of radiation protection matters as possible and to keep employees informed.

The Ionising Radiation (Medical Exposure) Regulations 2000 [7]

These regulations, often abbreviated to IRMER, are designed to protect a patient undergoing treatment or diagnosis with ionizing radiation; they also cover persons exposed to radiation as part of research and medico-legal procedures, such as pre-immigration chest x-rays. These regulations were originally policed by the Department of Health but, following the publication of The Ionising Radiation (Medical Exposure) (Amendment) Regulations 2006 [10], the Health Care Commission now undertake this role. This amendment also required that referrers be registered healthcare professionals.

They define four groups of people with legal responsibility under the regulations.

The employer

The employer is responsible for ensuring there are a number of written procedures in place and that the staff involved adhere to these procedures. The procedures required are as follows:

- procedures to identify correctly the person and the area to be exposed. The majority of errors that occur in procedures involving radiation to patients are due to patient misidentification
- procedures to identify correctly who is entitled to act as referrers, practitioners and operators. It is the responsibility of the employer to decide whom they are willing to let fulfill these roles and to ensure that those undertaking the roles are adequately and appropriately trained. This training has to be role specific and cover those areas relevant to the role being undertaken that are outlined in Schedule 2 of the Regulations. There is also a requirement for staff acting in these roles to demonstrate continuing education in radiation protection of the patient
- procedures to be observed in the case of medico-legal exposures
- procedures to make enquiries of females of childbearing age to establish whether they may be pregnant or breastfeeding. As we have seen, irradiation of the fetus can be detrimental. In addition, radioactive material administered to the mother may be expressed in the breast milk, which would then give a potentially large radiation dose to a breast-fed baby
- procedures to ensure that quality assurance programmes are carried out. These relate to ensuring that these procedures are adhered to and are still relevant and quality assurance programmes performed on radiation equipment as required by the Ionizing Radiations Regulations 1999 [3]
- procedures for the assessment of patient dose and administered activities
- procedures for the use of diagnostic reference levels. These are levels of patient dose which are not expected to be exceeded when good and normal practice regarding diagnostic and technical performance is applied. Levels should be set in terms of easily checked dose parameters such as fluoroscopic screening time or dose area product (DAP) readings. A DAP reading is obtained by the use of a flat bed ion chamber placed upon the collimator of the x-ray unit and it provides a measurement of the dose multiplied by the area of the applied radiation field. As such, the measurement units of a DAP reading are Gy.cm^2. The levels should be set locally with due regard to any national or international data that are available. Such levels have been set by the National Radiation Protection Board, based upon surveys performed across the country and set at the 75th percentile value of the dose distribution found. Over a period, this and changes in technology have had the effect of reducing the doses

given for particular examinations. A local series of diagnostic reference levels should be set for each standard radiological examination, including interventional procedures, nuclear medicine investigations and radiotherapy planning procedures

- procedures for the conduct of medical research involving the exposure to ionizing radiation of the participating individuals where no direct medical benefit is expected from the exposure. This should include the use and setting of dose constraints that are levels of dose associated with the research, which are not allowed to be exceeded
- procedures for giving written information and instruction to patients undergoing treatment or diagnosis with radioactive materials in order for information to be given on how the exposure from the patient can be restricted so as to protect persons in contact with the patient following discharge from the hospital (see comforters and carers above)
- procedures for the carrying out and recording of an evaluation of each medical exposure including factors relating to patient dose. That is a procedure to ensure that no exposure is undertaken without a net benefit to the patient, e.g. if x-ray images were not examined by a radiologist, no benefit would ensue from the exposure
- procedures to ensure that the probability and magnitude of accidental or unintended doses are reduced as far as reasonably practicable. This should include things such as routine servicing and post-servicing quality assurance checks on the equipment.

The employer is also legally obliged to keep training records of those identified as undertaking practitioner or operator roles. They must also draw up and keep up to date an inventory of the radiation equipment at each radiological installation they control. They are also responsible for establishing referral criteria for medical exposures and for making these available to the referrers.

The referrer

The referrer must be a registered medical or dental practitioner or other health professional entitled to act as a referrer under the employer's procedures (see above). The legal responsibility is to provide sufficient detail on the referral request to allow for the correct identification of the patient and, where relevant, their menstrual status. They are also required to provide sufficient details of the clinical problem to allow justification and authorization of the radiation exposure.

The practitioner

The IRMER practitioner is a registered medical or dental practitioner or other health professional who is entitled

by the employer's procedures to undertake this role. Their legal duty is to justify a medical exposure on the basis of the information provided to them by the referrer, taking into account the specific objectives of the exposure, the total potential benefits and risks to the individual undergoing the exposure and the possibility of using alternative techniques which do not employ ionizing radiation but which would attain the same objective.

In radiotherapy applications, there will normally be only one IRMER practitioner, for both the treatment exposures and any concomitant exposures as part of the planning process, e.g. simulation, CT scans and verification images. The number of concomitant exposures is likely to increase as the developing technical capabilities for conformal, image-guided radiotherapy make target and critical organ definition an increasingly important aspect of radiotherapy. Estimation of doses and risks to critical organs in the body from all sources is thus necessary to provide the basis for adequate justification of the exposures as required by IRMER. Although negligible in comparison with the target dose, realistic numbers of concomitant exposures give a small but significant contribution to the total dose to most organs and tissues outside the target volume. Generally, this is in the range of 5–10% of the total organ dose, but can be as high as 20% for bone surfaces [11].

The operator

The operator is any person recognized by the employer's procedures who carries out any practical application of the medical exposure. This covers a range of functions, each of which will have a direct influence on the medical exposure. Some of these will be undertaken in the presence of the patient, e.g. making the exposure, identifying the patient. Other aspects are performed without the patient being present, e.g. machine calibration and radiotherapy planning. Anyone who evaluates a medical image and records the result of this evaluation is also considered to be an operator.

A requirement of the legislation is that practitioners and operators are adequately and appropriately trained and that they undertake continuing education in radiation protection of the patient. Medical and dental practitioners who act as referrers do not require any additional training, although other health professionals performing this role should be trained in the clinical aspects of a patient's presentation that would warrant an exposure.

Medical physics expert (MPE)

An MPE is defined as a state registered clinical scientist with corporate membership of the Institute of Physics and Engineering in Medicine (MIPEM) or equivalent and at least 6 years of experience in the clinical specialty. An MPE is a legal requirement for radiotherapy practices.

They must be full-time contracted to the radiation employer and available at all times for radiotherapy practices. Their roles in radiotherapy are, among other things, to provide consultation on the suitability of treatment techniques, with responsibility for the dosimetry and accuracy of treatment, optimization of treatments by ensuring that equipment meets adequate standards of accuracy and the definitive calibration of radiotherapy equipment and dosimeters.

Legal liability

IRMER requires that any cases of exposures significantly more than intended be reported to the Department of Health in order for them to carry out an investigation. The employer should of course also perform such investigations. In so doing, it should be possible to determine if the IRMER procedures are correct or if they were not adhered to. By failing to adhere to the employers' procedures, individuals take on the legal liability which, in certain circumstances, may lead to a criminal prosecution of that individual.

Radioactive Substance Act 1993 [12]

In order to keep, use and dispose of radioactive materials in the quantities used in a hospital that performs radiotherapy and diagnostic applications of radionuclides, the above Act requires that the premises are registered to keep the material and authorized to dispose of any waste arising from its use. The Department of the Environment pollutions inspectorate regulates this. Registration will detail the maximum activity and number of sources that may be held on the premises of individually named radionuclides. Authorization for keeping and disposal of radioactive waste will be given providing the radiation user has performed an environmental impact assessment, which shows that, in the worse case scenario, doses to members of the public and others who come into contact with the radioactive waste are acceptable and that the disposals follow the best practical means for the environment. Authorizations will indicate the maximum activity of individual radionuclides that may be kept and subsequently disposed of over noted time periods by various routes.

Allowed routes of disposal are:

- in general domestic refuse providing that it is to be disposed of by land filling and that it is below certain very low activity limits and concentrations
- by incineration via a similarly authorized incinerator
- disposal of liquid waste in the sewage system, this is by far the most common route in terms of the activity disposed
- gaseous disposal of radioactive gases normally from a discharge point on the top of a building.

High Activity Sealed Radioactive Sources and Orphan Sources Regulations 2005

These regulations were introduced in an effort to reduce the loss of such sources either through a terrorist act or incorrect disposal. A special registration is required for sources which are designated as High Activity Sealed Sources (HASS). This designation is dependent on the radionuclide involved and its activity and form. If a source falls into an HASS category, additional security arrangements are required to be put in place and the source owner must demonstrate that they have adequate financial provisions in place for its subsequent future disposal. Without this a registration will not be granted.

Administration of Radioactive Substances Advisory Committee (ARSAC)

Regulation 2 of the Medicines (Administration of Radioactive Substances) Regulations 1978 [13] (MARS Regulations 1978) and as amended in 1995 [14], requires that any doctor or dentist who wishes to administer radioactive medicinal products to humans should hold a certificate issued by Health Ministers. The Regulations also established a committee to advise Ministers on applications. This is known as the ARSAC and issues certificates to medical staff (normally of Consultant status) who wish to administer radioactive materials to patients. In order to become certificated, a practitioner is required to demonstrate that they have received IRMER training and an apprenticeship with an ARSAC certificate holder. The certificates issued are hospital location, radionuclide and treatment-type specific.

PROTECTIVE MEASURES

There are a number of protective measures that may be employed, either singularly or, more commonly, in combination to reduce or limit the amount of radiation personnel are exposed to. By minimizing the radiation dose people receive, you will minimize the risk of stochastic effects occurring and eliminate the risk of deterministic effects.

Time

The dose someone receives when exposed to radiation depends on the dose rate of the source and the time spent exposed to it, since high dose rates will give a higher dose in a shorter time. As a consequence, anything that can be done to minimize the time exposed to a radiation source will minimize the exposure. For complex procedures, staff should carry out practice runs with dummy sources until they become proficient in the procedure; for fluoroscopic screening procedures, such as simulation, the use of a last image hold device will minimize the exposure time.

Distance

Radiation arising from a point source reduces in intensity in proportion to the square of the distance from the source. That means doubling your distance would quarter your exposure, quadrupling your distance would reduce the exposure to a sixteenth. As such, this is a relatively easy way of reducing exposure and, importantly from the employer's point of view, does not usually cost anything. The use of long-handled forceps when dealing with radioactive sources will significantly reduce exposure, particularly to the hands. However, in radiotherapy installations, e.g. linear accelerators, as the original source intensity is usually high, the distance required to move to in order to reduce the intensity to an acceptable level makes this method of protection unusable by itself, as the distance required would be in the order of kilometres. Distance is very often employed as a protective measure in linear accelerator installations by the installation of a maze type entrance into the treatment area which requires scattered radiation generated within the treatment area to undergo a number of scattering interactions along the maze corridor before reaching the maze entrance or door, thus increasing the distance the radiation travels and reducing the dose rate. A correctly designed maze can mean no requirement for a radiation protective door to be used at the entrance.

Barriers

By placing an appropriate protective barrier between the radiation source and the area you are trying to protect, the level of the radiation reaching that area will be attenuated and reduced. However, care must be taken in choosing the correct material for the radiation type you are shielding against. If dense materials are used as the initial attenuator for beta particles (electrons), then x-rays will be generated from the attenuating material due to bremsstralung or braking radiation. As a consequence, beta particles should be initially shielded by low-density material, such as Perspex, followed by a denser outer shield, such as lead. The thickness of shielding required is dependent upon the initial dose rate, the dose rate that is required after passing through the attenuator and the energy of the radiation, thickness increasing with any of these. As a consequence, lead aprons, with a thickness of approximately 0.25 mm of lead that are successfully used for shielding personnel using diagnostic x-rays, with a typical energy of 30–60 keV, would be completely inadequate to provide protection from the radiation from a cesium-137 radiation source (energy 662 keV).

Since lead is the most common radiation shielding material, it is normal to quote the amount of protection afforded by different materials in terms of the lead equivalence of that material. The lead equivalence thus forms the basis of comparing one absorber to another at a given radiation energy. At diagnostic x-ray energies, the photoelectric absorption in lead is significant, since attenuation due to photoelectric absorption is proportional to the atomic number of the material cubed and the density. For higher energy radiation where Compton scatter starts to predominate as the attenuation process, the reduction in radiation is proportional to the density of the material. As a consequence, as the energy of the radiation increases, the advantage of lead over other absorbing material diminishes because of the strong interdependence of photo-electric absorption on energy. With radiation above about 1 MeV in energy, where the Compton process predominates, there is no real advantage in using lead since all materials show very similar attenuation properties depending solely on their density.

Contamination

Where unsealed radioactive materials are used, either in the gaseous or liquid state, the possibility of contamination of the surfaces and the environment in which the material is being used needs to be considered. Such contamination may be subsequently internalized within the body either through inhalation, ingestion or absorption through the skin or wounds in the skin. Such absorptions will then counter the protective measures noted above as it will not minimize the exposure time, it will minimize the distance from the source to the tissues and no barriers could be put in place. As a consequence, other controls are essential when unsealed sources are used. These are, source confinement, using trays, fume cupboards, glove boxes etc; ensuring that the environment in which the sources are being used is well ventilated and easily decontaminated and good basic hygiene standards such as wearing gloves and protective clothing and washing hands after dealing with such sources. These simple precautions will help to reduce the risk of internal exposure rather than eliminate it altogether. Adequate contamination monitoring with a radiation detector such as a Geiger counter should also be undertaken.

Building materials

The correct choice of building material is essential for adequate protection of surrounding areas at the least possible cost. Various factors need to be taken into account when specifying the level of protection required and the material with which to protect. The radiation beam itself can consist of three components, primary beam radiation, that is radiation that is in the main beam of the radiation source, this will be the most intense and energetic. Scattered radiation originating from objects such as the patient that the primary beam has struck, this is less intense than the primary beam radiation but is taken to be of the same energy and, finally, for x-ray tubes, linear accelerators and sealed source units, leakage radiation originating from the radiation source housing. This is limited to certain maximum levels by regulatory requirements and typical leakage levels are less than 10% of the maximum allowed. Those factors that need to be taken into account in determining the levels of barrier thickness required are such things as:

- the attenuation properties of the material at the energies of radiation to be used
- the area you are trying to protect, i.e. is it going to contain radiation sensitive material such as film?
- the occupancy of the area to be protected
- the energy of the radiation that is to be used, the higher the energy the greater the penetration
- the possibility of neutron production (see below)
- the beam use factors, i.e. is the area to be subjected to the primary radiation beam at any time and if so for how long, or is it only exposed to scattered and leakage radiation?
- the amount of radiation that is going to be used in a week, more commonly called the workload, e.g. beam on time
- what is above, below and surrounding the area where radiation is being generated
- what is the acceptable exposure level to the areas you are protecting, such areas should be designed to conform to the As Low As Reasonably Practical requirement but, for public areas, should not exceed 1 mSv per year.

Having taken the above factors into consideration, calculations are made to determine the lead equivalence that is needed to protect the areas to the required degree. For diagnostic x-ray and radionuclide uses, the level of protection required varies from about 0.5 mm to 2 mm of lead dependent on whether the barrier is subjected to the primary beam. This is usually achieved either by using sheet lead or concrete. Other material may be used but care must be taken since the design and density of alternative building materials vary. For example, clay bricks come in various densities ranging from 1600 to 2000 kg m^{-3}. In addition, they may be designed to reduce their weight by introducing cavities into the brick. In practice, because of these variables, it is advisable to perform transmission measurements on the intended material before construction with it is undertaken, in order to verify the lead equivalence provided by it. Many lightweight building blocks are available with densities of less than 1000 kg m^{-3} but, by themselves, they are unsuitable for use in a radiation area and need to be used in conjunction with other protective material such as barium (barytes) plaster or lead lining. Conventional plaster is made with calcium sulfate. Replacing the calcium sulfate with barium sulfate to plaster x-ray room walls, significantly increases the attenuation of the wall owing to the relatively high atomic number of barium (56) compared to calcium (20), indeed this is the reason why barium is used in barium meals and enemas. Care needs to be taken with wall and door furniture, such as handles and coat hooks, to ensure that the protection of the barrier

is not compromised. Occasionally, breaches in the protection are essential in order to supply room services such as air conditioning and electrical supply. In such circumstances, thought needs to be given as to how this is achieved. Such breaches should never occur in primary barriers and the use of mazes and careful angulations of the ducting passing through the wall will retain the protective ability. Whenever possible, it is better to take the services through a wall below the level of a solid floor. This is normally tested during room commissioning with the use of a radioactive source and radiation detector. With increasing energy and the photoelectric effect becoming less predominant, lead becomes less favourable as the attenuating medium due to the large amounts that would be required and its tendency to 'creep' or pool under its own weight. As a consequence, for radiotherapy applications, concrete is the usual attenuating medium with occasionally barium concrete being used in areas subjected to the primary beam, particularly where space is at a premium. This type of concrete is relatively expensive and because of its higher density much heavier than normal concrete. The typical wall thickness (primary barrier) for a 10 MeV linear accelerator is of the order of 1.2 meter dense concrete. Lapped steel plate can also be used in conjunction with concrete for an installation where space needs to be conserved, but it is best avoided where neutron production is likely. Such activation is brought about when linear accelerators are operated above 10–15 MV, by photonuclear reactions of the high-energy photons or electrons in the various materials of the target, flattening filter collimator and other shielding materials [19]. Neutron contamination increases rapidly as the energy of the beam increases from 10 to 20 MV and then remains approximately constant above this. Measurements have shown that, in the 16–25 MV x-ray therapy range, the neutron dose equivalent along the central access is about 0.5% of the applied x-ray dose and falls off to about 0.1% outside the field. If concrete has been used to shield from the photons then sufficient protection from the neutrons will be provided by these structures. However, great care needs to be taken if iron or lead is used for part of the shielding as not only is the neutron attenuation poorer but neutron interactions in such material produce gamma radiation. Indeed gamma production can arise in dense concrete which has metal bearing aggregate and care must be taken to avoid this type of aggregate. In such cases, it is necessary to use a combination of shielding materials with a sandwich construction of lead, steel, and polyethylene or concrete. Polyethylene is used as an efficient attenuator of neutrons and the steel or lead is then used as a photon attenuator.

If designing an area where unsealed (e.g. liquid) radionuclides are to be used, then thought needs to be given to ensuring that the floors and walls are constructed and finished in such a way as to make them easy to decontaminate. Decontamination is usually achieved by a washing process, occasionally using caustic solutions. As a consequence, providing the surfaces are easily washable without degradation and are impermeable to the cleaning solutions, then they will be suitable for use. Care should be taken in ensuring that joints between benches, etc. are sealed. Thought also is required in the correct selection of the material used for drains as some radionuclides are absorbed preferentially by plastics.

In conclusion, a number of factors need to be taken into account in designing a radiation room; its walls and barriers must be such that the levels of radiation received by staff, waiting patients and members of the public are kept to a minimum. This can be achieved by the correct use of shielding material. A certified and appropriately experienced Radiation Protection Adviser should always be consulted in any design process involving radiation.

MONITORING OF RADIATION LEVELS

Monitoring of radiation levels can be performed in a number of ways. The Ionising Radiations Regulations only require employers to provide personal radiation dosimeters to their classified radiation workers and to demonstrate that non-classified workers do not need to become classified. One way of avoiding issuing personal radiation monitors to non-classified staff is to perform environmental monitoring and then making a judgment as to the probability of workers requiring to become classified. Environmental monitoring must also be carried out on all new or modified protective structures to ensure that they meet with the radiation protection specification required by the design specification worked out taking into account those matters described in the above section. A number of different instruments can be used to perform this monitoring, each with their own advantages and drawbacks, some of these are now described (see also Chapter 3).

Ion chambers can be used for such measurements; they have the advantage that they have a relatively uniform response over a wide range of energies and can be used to make both dose and dose rate measurements. The lower the level of dose that is to be measured the larger the ionization chamber needs to be in order for there to be sufficient ionization current to make a measurement. Doubling the volume of an ion chamber, will double its sensitivity, all other things being equal. Ion chambers with volumes in excess of 1 litre are available to measure transmission through protective walls. Smaller volume ion chambers are used to measure radiation output in the primary beam of an x-ray unit ranging in volume from about 0.5 to 6 ml. One disadvantage of such devices is that they have a relatively long time constant, which means they do not respond quickly to changes in the incident radiation intensity.

Instruments involving Geiger counters or scintillation detectors are more sensitive than ionization chambers, respond more quickly and use detectors of smaller size. This is because the signals that are initially generated are further amplified. Such instruments are more often used in detecting surface contamination in radionuclide laboratories; their chief disadvantage is that they are energy dependent, their response varying with the energy of radiation being measured. As such, unless the monitor has been calibrated with the energy of radiation being measured the reading will not be correct. Such instruments can be used in diagnostic x-ray installations, together with a radioactive source such as Americium 241 to check the integrity of barriers, at positions such as handles and light switches.

Mains operated radiation detectors are often placed at exits and other strategic places in radiation areas where either the level of radiation may fluctuate or the radiation sources are mobile and a warning is required if the source leaves the area. Detectors with either an audible or visual indication of a high reading are often placed on exit doors of the rooms of patients being treated with radioactive materials such that, if they try to leave the area, an alarm will alert the ward staff. Similar alarms are required in radiotherapy departments, to provide independent confirmation that the source(s) on gamma beam generators or remote after loading units have returned to the safe position.

Personal radiation dosimeters

There are a number of different types of personal radiation dosimeters which can be used to assess the dose individual staff members receive as part of their work activity; these are detailed below, together with their relative advantages and disadvantages. These must be worn when at work and not be exposed to radiation when the person is not at work, as these monitors are used to determine the exposure a person receives as part of their work. This includes those cases where the person undergoes a medical exposure to radiation as part of their care pathway. The dosimeters are usually worn at waist level and changed on a regular basis, normally monthly. If a protective apron is being worn, the dosimeter should be worn underneath, since the whole-body radiation exposure to the trunk is the quantity to be measured. Occasionally, dose is assessed to other areas of the body and providing the dosimeter is small enough can be placed on the fingers, wrists, legs or forehead. These are used to demonstrate that the doses these areas receive are within the dose limits for the individual organs noted in Table 4.5. In order to carry out definitive measurements of dose, which will be accepted by the regulators, the dosimeters used must be of a Health and Safety Executive approved type. To meet this type approval the dosimeters have to meet certain minimum performance and measurement specification.

Direct readout dosimeters

These have a radiation detector associated with an electronic display so that a direct readout of the dose received can be made at any time. More sophisticated devices allow interrogation of the dose time profile via connection to a computer, to help establish when peaks of dose have occurred, and also recording of the dose received. A picture of such a device is shown in (Figure *evolve* 4.5🐭).

The advantage of such dosimeters is that there is no delay in knowing what dose has been received as the equipment provides a direct readout; the disadvantages are that they are relatively expensive (£200–400), susceptible to damage and some are energy dependent so different readings will be obtained on them for the same received dose. Less expensive versions also have the disadvantage that there is no permanent record of the dose received unless logged by the user.

Film badge dosimeters

These consist of an envelope of film placed into a small holder. The holder consists of different thicknesses of different types of material e.g. tin/lead, Dural and different thickness of plastic. The blackening under the different filters is a function of the quality of the radiation to which the whole badge has been exposed. As such, different energies and types of radiation produce different density patterns on the film. For a given radiation quality, the film density is roughly proportional to the exposure, if the exposure is small. The used films are developed with a set of suitable calibration films previously exposed to a range of known doses of gamma rays, together with unexposed films to estimate background and fog effects. A number of empirical methods are adopted by different laboratories to deduce the exposure from the densities measured under the various filters. Film badges are suitable for monitoring doses from photons (15 keV–3 MeV) and beta (E_{max} >500 keV) radiations and with the addition of different filters, they can be used to measure neutron radiation dose. They are ideal for workers who encounter x-ray fields and have a dose range of 0.1 mSv to 10 Sv for $H_p(10)$, that is the penetrating radiation dose at 10 cm depth in tissue. Due to the technique they employ to monitor dose, film monitors provide the ability to detect if radioactive contamination of the dosimeter has occurred. In order to extend the range of exposure covered by the film, one side is coated with a thick sensitive emulsion and the other side has a thinner, less sensitive emulsion. In normal use, the density through both emulsions is measured and the doses of a few percent of the dose limit estimated. High doses make the sensitive emulsion too black for measurement, but it can then be stripped off and a measurement of the density of the thin emulsion alone can be made leading to estimates of up to about 10 Sv.

A typical film badge is shown in (Figure *evolve* 4.6🐭). It will be noticed that there is an open window in the front of the badge which allows the badge identification number to be observed. This is stamped onto the badge with sufficient pressure for the number to be visible on the developed film. Each person monitored will have a number associated with him or her. As a consequence, one should only ever wear the badge issued to you and not one issued to someone else since the dose records will not be correct.

The advantages and disadvantages of film badge dosimeters are as follows:

- use highly sensitivity silver halide film, but not tissue equivalent in its absorption properties, which are energy dependent
- fitted with a range of filters which can fall out of the holder
- distinguishes beta, x-ray, gamma and thermal neutrons
- provides permanent record of an individual's dose which can be reread if there are any doubts about the result
- adverse effects of light and heat can give an indication that a radiation dose has been received
- relatively short shelf-life (months)
- require dark room facilities (development chemicals)
- significant manual handling during assessment
- not washing machine proof, the film emulsion melts making the dosimeter unreadable
- density patterning subject to fading over a period of time and so should be processed within a relative short period after exposure (a month or so)
- doses down to 0.2 mSv accurately readable.

Thermoluminescent dosimeters (TLD)

The TLD consists of a crystal or powder (e.g. calcium sulfate or lithium boride), which is able to record the dose of radiation it is exposed to and store this information. When heated (thermo), the material gives off light (luminescent), the amount of light being given off is proportional to the radiation dose to the material. The material is usually placed in a holder which enables the dosimeter to distinguish between penetrating and non-penetrating radiations; this is done by placing a portion of material underneath a dome of plastic and another portion merely under a thin protective envelope.

- Used as personal and environmental dosimeter
- Use thermoluminescent (TL) materials
- Electrons are raised/trapped at higher energy levels
- The energy is released as light when heated
- Light emitted is converted into an electrical signal
- Light emitted is proportional to incident radiation
- Lithium (LiF:Mn) based TLDs for personal dosimetry: because they are tissue-equivalent
- Calcium (CaF_2:Dy, $CaSO_4$:Dy) based TLDs for environmental monitoring: due to their high sensitivity
- Lithium borate ($Li_2B_4O_7$:Mn) TLDs for high dose range dosimetry
- TL materials are available in many different forms: e.g. powder, hot pressed chips, pellets, impregnated Teflon disks
- Read-out instruments (reader) are required
- Method to heat the TLD material: electrical, hot gas or a radiofrequency heater, heated in an inert gas during read-out
- Device to convert the light output to an electrical pulse
- Light signal is amplified using a photomultiplier

- Small size (only milligram quantities of TL material is needed)
- TLDs can be reused
- Doses down to 0.1 mSv accurately readable

The disadvantages of TLDs are:

- only one reading during heating, cannot be repeated
- subject to fading (due to temperature or light effects)
- requires careful handling to avoid dirt on the dosimeters interfering with light emission.

Optically stimulated luminescent (OSL) dosimeter

These measure radiation through a thin layer of aluminium oxide. During analysis, the aluminium oxide is stimulated with selected frequencies of laser light causing it to become luminescent in proportion to the amount of radiation exposure. This is very similar in principle to the computed radiography imaging plates that are replacing film in diagnostic radiology. The dosimeters give accurate readings down to 0.01 mSv, representing another revolution in dosimetry. This new degree of sensitivity is ideal for employees working in low-radiation environments and for pregnant employees. Another advantage is that they can go through a washing machine cycle without being affected (Figure *evolve* 4.7🖱).

Radiation records

In addition to the personal dose monitoring records mentioned above, a number of other records are also required by the regulators to be kept. These are detailed below.

Contamination checks

In areas using unsealed radioactive materials, regular checks are required to be made on both the personnel working in the area and on the work surfaces of the area to ensure that radioactive contamination is not building up or being spread. Records of these measurements need to be made and are subjected to inspection by both Health and Safety Executive and Department of the Environment inspectors.

Leak tests, disposal and movement logs

All sealed radioactive sources must undergo an annual leak test to verify the integrity of the source housing, in addition, whenever sources are moved from their storage area, a note of where they have gone to needs to be made. Reports of any loss or damage to radioactive sources also need to be kept. The Radioactive Substances Act 1993 requires that records be kept of receipt and disposal of radioactive materials together with the quantities and types of radionuclide (see Radioactive Substance Act above).

Equipment checks and calibration

On an annual basis, contamination monitors, dosimeters and dose rate meters require to be calibrated and the results of this calibration logged. The calibration of such equipment needs to be traceable back to a national calibration standard so that it can be assured that what is measured at one centre will be the same as measured at another. This is often arranged by sending one instrument away for calibration by a national calibration service, such as the National Physical Laboratory, and then cross calibrating other equipment held with the one that was sent away.

Having calibrated the measurement equipment, these can then be used with a degree of confidence for carrying out dose measurements on radiotherapy treatments machines, diagnostic x-ray equipment and for contamination and dose rate measurements. Such measurements in radiotherapy form part of a comprehensive quality assurance programme that is required to be in place in every radiotherapy department to help ensure that the risk of incorrect or inaccurate treatments being given is minimized.

Other requirements

A number of other matters some of which do not directly relate to radiation will now be discussed, all of them are however safety related and are therefore worthy of note.

Transport of radioactive materials

Up until about 10 years ago, it was permissible for professional users of radioactive materials, e.g. a radiotherapist, to transport radioactive materials on the road without any requirements placed upon them for their safe carriage. This professional user's exemption was removed with the introduction of the Radioactive Material Road Transport Regulations. These require that anyone carrying more than certain limited quantities of radioactive material on the road have received adequate and appropriate training, that the material is contained in approved packaging and that the packages and vehicles are labelled and placarded to indicate the risk of ionizing radiation. Anyone involved in the transportation of radioactive materials is also required to appoint a Dangerous Goods Safety Adviser, who needs to be certificated to undertake such a role in the type of dangerous goods they are providing advice on. The advisers' role is to provide guidance to ensure compliance with the regulatory requirements.

Critical examinations, commissioning and quality control

Before new equipment is used clinically, the installer has a legal responsibility to carry out a critical examination of the installation, to ensure that all safety critical parts of the equipment are operating correctly. A report of the examination should be made to the customer who should keep it for reference throughout the life of the equipment. The critical examination should be repeated after any major upgrade or repair to the equipment, which may affect the radiation output or other safety critical factors, e.g. source or x-ray tube change.

Once the installer has performed a critical examination, the user should carry out an adequate number of tests and measurements to establish a quality control baseline and ensure that the equipment is working within the purchasing specification. All safety related features of the equipment should be checked including those associated with the room containing the equipment.

A Medical Physics Expert should be responsible for acceptance testing of the equipment. For radiotherapy equipment, compliance with the Guidance Notes [5], HSG 226 [15], and the appropriate sections of BS EN 60601 [16], relevant to equipment safety should be checked. Further guidance on the acceptance testing and commissioning of radiotherapy equipment can be found in IPEM 54 [17] Commissioning and Quality Assurance of Linear Accelerators and IPEM 81 [18] Physics Aspects of Quality Control in Radiotherapy.

Personal protective equipment (PPE)

A range of PPE (lead aprons, gloves, thyroid shields and eye protectors) should be provided in all diagnostic x-ray rooms and for use with mobile x-ray equipment. When not in use, these should be stored appropriately so as to avoid damaging their protective properties. Lead aprons for instance should never be folded but should be hung on dedicated hangers or rails of sufficiently large diameter to prevent creasing.

All PPE should be visually examined at frequent intervals and any defective items removed from use. Protective clothing must be examined at least annually to ensure that no cracks in the protective material have developed. This has to be done by radiographic or fluoroscopic examination if the protective material is not directly visible. The results of the inspection should be recorded and the protective devices themselves should be individually identifiable, e.g. by a serial number.

Mechanical, electrical and fire hazards

In addition to the hazard from the radiation being generated from radiotherapy and diagnostic x-ray equipment, hazards also arise from the mechanical structure of the equipment in the form of the weight associated with the equipment. Radiotherapy equipment, in particular, normally has a large amount of high-density material (lead or depleted uranium) surrounding the radiation source to ensure that radiation is only directed to the area intended and leakage radiation from the x-ray tube or around the radiation source is minimized. The overall weight of the equipment is also increased by the need for counterbalancing weights in supporting structures. Where megavoltage equipment is concerned, merely rotating the gantry from one position to another involves the acceleration and retardation of several tonnes. Care should be taken in moving such equipment, ensuring that there is nothing in the intended path of travel as a lot of damage can be caused quite easily if such weights crash into something, e.g. a trolley left beside the treatment couch.

Even low voltage electrical equipment has the potential to kill. The voltages that radiotherapy and x-ray equipment work at ranges from a few volts to hundreds of thousands of volts, as a consequence, such equipment should never be operated with wet hands or in wet conditions. All major components of any installation should be visibly connected to 'earth' using either a continuous copper tape or a single core wire covered with a green or green and yellow sheath. These connections should all be brought together at a common earth reference terminal (often labelled as ERT), which is normally a large copper bar placed close to the control console or x-ray generator. All areas of the equipment that is potentially electrically hazardous will be housed in cabinets either behind fixed panels or locked doors. These must always be kept secure and only opened by authorized personnel after they have isolated the electricity supply. In addition, large capacitors may be present and are likely to hold their charge even after the mains supply has been switched off and special precautions need to be taken to discharge them safely before maintenance work is undertaken.

Due to the high voltages employed in radiotherapy and x-ray equipment, there is an increased risk of fire. Due to the requirement for radiotherapy installations to have a minimum number of entrances/exits, such rooms normally only have the one. As such, it is important that any fires starting in such rooms are detected as early as possible and fire detection devices, such as smoke alarms, are essential. In some situations, patients undergoing treatment will be immobilized on the treatment table by securing them to it with treatment moulds. This makes the release of these patients time consuming in an emergency situation such as fire. Rehearsals of removing patients from treatment rooms should be undertaken regularly so staff are aware of problems that they may face. Fire extinguishers should be of a type suitable for tackling electrical fires, the use of water being avoided, as this would present a potential electrocution hazard. Procedures should be in place to provide advice to the fire brigade if a fire occurs in radiation areas and a list of the location of radioactive material should be provided to the fire service on an annual basis. In a fire situation, if the fire brigade see a radiation warning sign they will err on the safe side until the nature of the hazard has been established.

By complying with all the regulatory requirements and guidance, it is possible to remove the risk of acute radiation effects and limit the probability of stochastic effects occurring. As such, anyone working routinely with radiation should be made aware of what is expected of them in terms of protecting both themselves and others from the use of radiation.

REFERENCES

[1] ICRP 60. Ann ICRP 1991;21(1–3). ICRP Publication 60. 1990 Recommendations of the International Commission on Radiological Protection. Pergamon Press.

[2] United Nations. Sources and effects of ionising radiation, vols. 1–2. UNSCEAR 2000 Report to the General Assembly with scientific annexes. United Nations sales publications E.00.IX.3 and E.00. IX.4. United Nations, New York; 2000.

[3] The Ionising Radiations Regulations 1999 – Statutory Instrument 1999 No. 3232. HMSO.

[4] Work with ionising radiation. Approved Code of Practice and Guidance. HSE; 2000.

[5] Medical and Dental Guidance Notes. A good practice guide on all aspects of ionising radiation protection in the clinical environment. Institute of Physic and Engineering in Medicine (IPEM); 2002.

[6] The Management of Health and Safety at Work Regulations 1999 – Statutory Instrument 1999 No. 3242. HMSO.

[7] Ionising Radiation (Medical Exposure) Regulations 2000. Statutory Instrument 2000 No. 1059. HMSO.

[8] Guidance Note PM 77. Equipment used in connection with medical exposure. 3rd ed. Health and Safety Executive; 2006.

[9] HSE. Protection of outside workers against ionising radiation. HSE information sheet Ionising Radiation Protection Series 4. 2000.

[10] The Ionising Radiation (Medical Exposure) (Amendment) Regulations 2006–Statutory Instrument 2006 No. 2523. HMSO.

[11] Harrison RM, Wilkinson M, Shemilt A, Rawlings DJ, Moore M, Lecomber AR. Organ doses from prostate radiotherapy and associated concomitant exposures. Br J Radiol 2006;79:487–96.

[12] Radioactive Substances Act 1993. Chapter 12. HMSO.

[13] The Medicines (Administration of Radioactive Substances) Regulations 1978–Statutory Instrument 1978 No. 1004. HMSO.

[14] The Medicines (Administration of Radioactive Substances) Amendment Regulations 1995–Statutory Instrument 1995 No. 2147. HMSO.

[15] HSG 226. Radiation equipment used for medical exposure. Health and Safety guidance Note 226. Health and Safety Executive.

[16] BS EN 60601. Medical electrical equipment British Standard. From British Standards online at:http://bsonline.techindex.co.uk.

[17] IPEM 54. Commissioning and quality assurance of linear accelerators. IPEM Report No. 54. IPEM; 1988.

[18] IPEM 81. Physics aspects of quality control in radiotherapy. IPEM Report No. 81. IPEM; 1999.

[19] Axton E, Bardell A. Neutron production from electron accelerators used for medical purposes. Phys Med Biol 1972;17:293.

EVOLVE CONTENTS (available online at: http://evolve.elsevier.com/Symonds/radiotherapy/)

Chapter | 5 |

Imaging with x-ray, MRI and ultrasound

Geoffrey P. Lawrence, Carl Tivas, Sarah Wayte

INTRODUCTION

X-ray, magnetic resonance imaging (MRI) and ultrasonic images play a key role in the diagnosis, staging, planning and delivery of treatment and follow up of patients with cancer.

In everyday language, an image is a picture and, more generally, it is a representation of the distribution of some property of an object. It is formed by transferring information from the object to an image domain. In practice, this requires the ordered transfer of energy from some source via the object of interest to a detector system. The detected signal may be processed in some way before being displayed and stored by suitable devices.

Medical imaging modalities covered in this chapter are classified according to the type of energy used to carry information: x-rays, radiofrequency waves and high frequency sound waves.

X-ray imaging enables tumours to be localized with respect to normal anatomical structures and to external markers. Because x-rays travel in straight lines until they are absorbed or scattered, they can produce images which faithfully represent spatial relationships within the body. It is principally for this reason that x-ray images of various kinds are essential to the planning and delivery of radiotherapy. A further reason is that interactions of ionizing radiation with matter are an essential feature of both imaging and therapy, so that information on properties of tissues relevant to treatment planning, such as electron density, may be obtained from suitable images.

Magnetic resonance imaging is an excellent technique for imaging soft tissue, and is often used to diagnose and stage cancer in the head, neck and body. It can also be used to monitor the response to treatment. The extent of the cancer can be seen on anatomical images. Other specialized MRI techniques, such as diffusion weighted imaging and dynamic imaging with a contrast agent can also be used to refine the diagnosis and cancer staging. Magnetic resonance spectroscopy provides information regarding the metabolism of the tumours and can also be used to monitor treatment response.

Diagnostic ultrasound imaging has several advantages over other imaging modalities [1]. It is relatively cheap, safe, gives real time images and has good soft tissue contrast. As well as anatomical detail, ultrasound can exploit the Doppler effect to give information about blood flow and the vascularity in tissues. The distortion of tissue under pressure in ultrasound images can give images related to the elasticity of tissues.

Radionuclide imaging, including PET-CT, which is primarily concerned with the function of organs and tissues is dealt with in Chapter 6.

X-RAY IMAGING

Overview of x-ray imaging process

The energy source in medical x-ray imaging is usually an x-ray tube and electrical generator though, in the case of radiotherapy portal imaging, it is the linear accelerator. As the x-ray beam passes through the patient, some radiation is absorbed or scattered. The intensity of the emerging primary beam varies with position and carries information about the interactions that have occurred in the body. The emerging beam can be detected by a variety of devices, e.g. film/screen cassette, image intensifier, solid state electronic detector. These are typically large area devices and the image is a two-dimensional shadowgraph of the intervening anatomy. Radiographic film is unique in combining all three roles of image detection, recording and display. Image intensifiers are usually coupled to a television camera and display monitors: static images or dynamic (i.e. moving) series may be stored on analogue video media or digitized for storage on DVD or other computer-based media. Digital fluoroscopy and radiography systems use digital computers and their storage and display devices as integral components of the imaging system, as does computed tomography (CT). In CT, the x-ray beam is collimated in the longitudinal direction to a narrow slit and this is aligned with an arc of solid state detectors. The tube and detectors are mounted on a gantry which rotates about the patient. Essentially one-dimensional projection images are acquired from many angles and the data are processed in a digital computer to form images of transverse slices through the patient.

Production of x-rays for imaging

The general topic of x-ray production is covered in Chapter 2. This section highlights some aspects of specific relevance to imaging.

X-rays are generated by causing electrons, which have been accelerated to high energies in a vacuum tube, to collide with a metal target. The electrical supply is normally from a generator, which takes power from the mains three phase alternating current (AC) supply and converts it, using a transformer and associated circuits, to an approximately constant kilovoltage (kV) direct current (DC) output. Older models employed rectification and smoothing circuits which resulted in appreciable ripple on the kV waveform, i.e. the output voltage varied by several per cent over a mains cycle. For this reason, the kilovoltage is specified as the peak value, denoted by the abbreviation kV_p. Modern generators employ converters, operating at a frequency of several kHz, which produce voltage waveforms with very little ripple. Diagnostic imaging work mostly uses accelerating potentials in the range 50 to 150 kV$_p$, though lower values are used in mammography.

At megavoltage energies, as in linear accelerators used for radiotherapy, the x-rays are produced mainly in the forward direction of the electron beam and hence a transmission target is used. At kilovoltage energies, as used in diagnostic x-ray equipment, radiotherapy simulators and CT scanners, x-rays are produced more isotropically and a reflection target is used. This allows the tube to be constructed with a rotating anode (Figure 5.1), which permits the heat generated to be dissipated over a much larger area than with a stationary anode. This is important because more than 99% of the electron beam energy is converted to heat in the anode and less than 1% appears as x-rays. Moreover, to produce images with good spatial resolution, the focal spot must be as small as possible and short exposure times are used to reduce blurring due to patient movement. With a stationary anode, a large quantity of heat would be deposited in a short time over a very small area, resulting in serious damage to the target. In fact, most x-ray tubes offer two sizes of focal spot, the larger being used for higher exposure factors which impose higher heat loading demands on the tube.

The x-rays produced have a spread of energies, i.e. a spectrum as shown in Figure 5.2, and there are two main components. One is the bremsstrahlung produced when electrons experience large accelerations as they pass close to atomic nuclei. This produces the major part of the spectrum, the smooth curve. Superimposed on this is the second component, the line spectrum due to characteristic radiation emitted when orbital electrons move to lower energy levels to fill vacancies which have been caused by ionization. The area under the spectrum represents the total quantity of radiation produced.

The shape of the spectrum determines the quality of the radiation, i.e. its penetrating properties. Increasing the tube current (mA) or the exposure time (s) both increase the quantity of radiation produced but do not affect its quality. Increasing the applied voltage (kV$_p$) increases both the quality and quantity of radiation produced and the output is approximately proportional to kV$_p{}^2$. Other factors, such

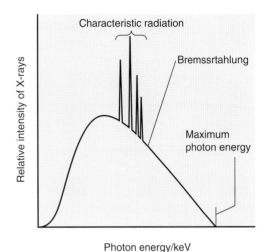

Figure 5.2 X-ray spectrum produced from a tube.

as anode material and filtration of the beam, further affect the quality and quantity of radiation produced. For imaging, the lower energy components are usually selectively reduced by suitable filtration.

Information from absorption/scattering

When x-rays, generated from a suitable source, are incident upon an object, such as the human body, some pass straight through while others interact with the material in the object by processes of absorption and scattering. In biological tissues at kilovoltage energies, the interactions of importance are photoelectric absorption and Compton scattering. The photo-electric effect depends strongly on atomic number Z and the energy E of the x-rays. Calcium, found in bone, has a relatively high atomic number and hence bone strongly absorbs kV x-rays. At megavoltage energies, it is the Compton effect that predominates and this depends primarily on electron density ρ_e.

The beam emerging from the object contains primary radiation together with scattered radiation. It is the varying intensity of the transmitted primary beam which carries useful information to produce an image.

Differential attenuation in the primary beam

Consider the simple situation in Figure 5.3, which shows a slab of some homogeneous material A of thickness x_A and linear attenuation coefficient μ_A, which contains a region of some other material B of thickness x_B and linear attenuation coefficient μ_B. Suppose a parallel x-ray beam of

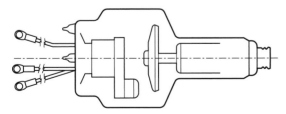

Figure 5.1 X-ray tube construction with rotating anode *(Courtesy of Elekta Ltd).*

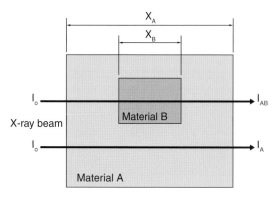

Figure 5.3 Simple inhomogeneous situation to illustrate contrast.

intensity I_O is incident on this slab. Then the intensity of the primary beam transmitted through A is:

$$I_A = I_O \exp(-\mu_A x_A)$$ **5.1**

and that transmitted through both A and B is:

$$
\begin{aligned}
I_{AB} &= I_O \exp(-\mu_A (x_A - x_B)) \exp(-\mu_B x_B) \\
&= I_O \exp(-\mu_A x_A) \exp((\mu_A - \mu_B) x_B) \\
&= I_A \exp((\mu_A - \mu_B) x_B)
\end{aligned}
$$

Hence the ratio of the transmitted intensities is:

$$I_{AB}/I_A = \exp((\mu_A - \mu_B) x_B)$$ **5.2**

By taking the (natural) logarithm of both sides, this may also be expressed as:

$$
\begin{aligned}
\ln(I_{AB}/I_A) &= \ln(I_{AB}) - \ln(I_A) \\
&= (\mu_A - \mu_B) x_B
\end{aligned}
$$ **5.3**

This ratio, which determines the contrast visible in the image, increases with the thickness of B (x_B) and with the difference between the linear attenuation coefficients of A and B ($\mu_A - \mu_B$).

The linear attenuation coefficients for air and bone are very different from those of soft tissue at kV energies, so even quite thin structures containing these materials can be visualized on the x-ray image. The differences between the linear attenuation coefficients for different soft tissues are, however, much smaller and special techniques such as CT are needed to reveal them.

Contrast media

Some structures may be made visible by deliberately introducing contrast agents, such as air or liquids containing iodine or barium, which have a very different value of μ from the surrounding tissues.

Scatter as unwanted background

Scattered radiation generally contributes a more or less uniform background signal to the image, which does not convey useful information but which reduces contrast. The amount of scattered radiation emerging from the patient can be several times greater than the transmitted primary beam, increasing with the energy of the x-ray beam, the size of the area irradiated and the thickness of the body part being imaged. It is possible to reduce the amount of scatter reaching the detector by using anti-scatter grids or by using an air gap technique. The latter relies on an appreciable separation between the patient and the image detector, which is often the case when using a radiotherapy simulator. The principle is illustrated in Figure 5.4, which shows that the amount of scatter reaching the detector falls off much more rapidly than the intensity of the primary beam as this distance is increased.

Anti-scatter grid

The anti-scatter grid consists of an array of long, thin lead strips, separated by some relatively radiolucent spacer material (Figure 5.5). Only radiation travelling perpendicular to the grid can pass through to the detector. Most of the scattered radiation is travelling at other angles and is intercepted and absorbed by the lead strips. Some primary radiation is absorbed too, but the net effect is greatly to increase the ratio of primary to scattered radiation reaching the detector, thus improving image contrast. If the angle between the primary beam and the perpendicular to the grid becomes too great, e.g. towards the edge of large fields, then a significant fraction of primary radiation will be absorbed. This can be overcome by using a focused grid, as shown in Figure 5.6. To avoid shadows from the lead strips producing distracting lines on the image, it is possible to move the grid to and fro laterally during the exposure and thus to blur out those lines.

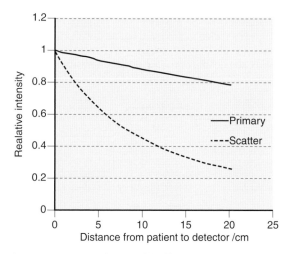

Figure 5.4 Diagram showing fall off in scatter reaching detector with distance.

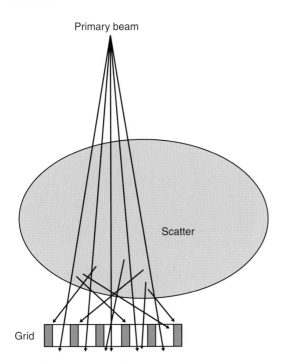

Figure 5.5 Anti-scatter grid principles.

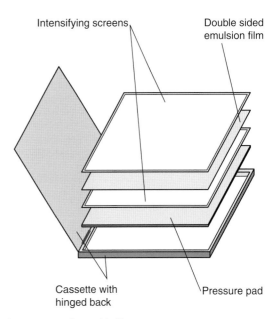

Figure 5.7 Radiographic film cassette.

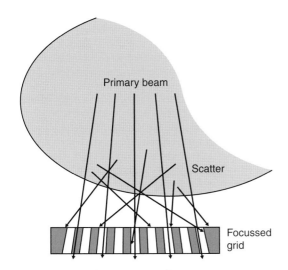

Figure 5.6 Focused anti-scatter grid.

Planar imaging

Film/screen detection

For many years, radiographic film has been used as a combined detector, storage and display device for x-ray images. It is usually used in conjunction with intensifying screens, which have a higher absorption efficiency than film for x-rays and which emit many visible light photons for each x-ray photon absorbed (Figure 5.7).

Radiographic film consists of a transparent polyester base, approximately 0.2 mm thick, usually coated on both sides with an emulsion containing crystals of silver bromide and this, in turn, is coated with a protective layer. When the emulsion is exposed to light or x-rays, some electrons are transferred from bromide ions to silver ions, which are reduced to silver atoms. These form a latent image which is not visible until it is chemically developed, a process in which the remaining silver ions in the affected crystals are also reduced to silver atoms, which cause blackening of the film. The more silver atoms present per unit area in the developed image, the darker the film appears.

Exposed films are normally processed automatically, in several stages:

1. development of the latent image using an organic reducing agent
2. fixing the developed image by dissolving away undeveloped silver bromide from the emulsion
3. hardening the emulsion to protect it from damage; and
4. washing the film and drying it.

Films may be manually loaded into the processor in a darkroom or automatically from suitable cassettes using a so-called daylight processor.

The intensifying screen (Figure 5.8) uses a fluorescent material which emits visible light when irradiated with x-rays and it is this visible light which is then detected by

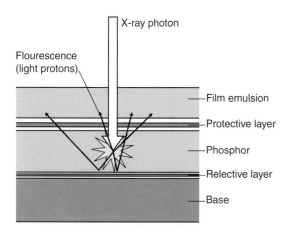

Figure 5.8 Intensifier screen principles.

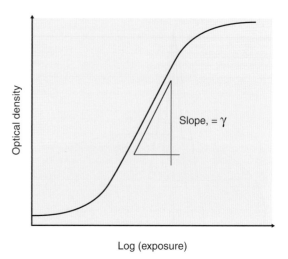

Figure 5.9 Graphical plot of optical density against exposure.

the film. (The same principle is used in image intensifier systems and in some digital imaging devices: see below.) A cassette is used which contains a separate screen for each side of the film and is constructed so as to ensure close contact between screen and film over their whole area. Many visible photons are produced for each x-ray photon absorbed and so the exposure required to produce a given degree of blackening on the film is greatly reduced compared with direct exposure of the film to x-rays. With modern rare earth screens, this reduction may be by a factor of about 1/100.

Characteristic curve

The degree of blackness of the film is measured in terms of optical density (D). If a beam of light of intensity I_o is incident on a piece of film and intensity I_t is transmitted, then:

$$D = \log_{10}(I_o/I_t) \qquad \textbf{5}.\textbf{4}$$

Hence, a region of film which transmits one-tenth of the incident light intensity has optical density 1.0, whereas a region which transmits one hundredth of the incident light intensity has optical density 2.0. A perfectly transparent region would have D = 0.

A graphical plot of D against log(exposure) is called the characteristic curve. A typical example is shown in Figure 5.9. If an unexposed film is developed, its optical density is a little greater than zero because the film base is not perfectly transparent and also because some of the silver bromide crystals are reduced to metallic silver (film fog). Over a range of exposures, the characteristic curve is approximately linear, and the gradient (slope) in this region is known as gamma for that film/screen combination. At very high exposures, all the silver bromide crystals are reduced on development and no increase in D occurs for higher exposures: the film/screen response is said to be saturated.

Contrast is the difference in D between different parts of an image. Under favourable conditions, the human eye can detect density differences as small as 0.02. If the slope of the characteristic curve is steep (i.e. has a high value of gamma), this means that the density increases rapidly over a relatively narrow range of exposure values, so the image has high contrast. On the other hand, only a narrow range of exposures can be represented before the image saturates, i.e. the latitude is low, and careful radiographic technique is needed to ensure that all features of interest are properly imaged. A lower gamma film/screen combination produces lower contrast but can encompass a wider range of exposure levels, i.e. it has greater latitude.

If only a relatively small exposure is required to produce a given density, as in curve A on Figure 5.10, the film/screen combination is said to be fast. Conversely, a slow combination requires a greater exposure to produce the same density (curve B). It might be thought that fast systems would always be desirable, to minimize the patient dose required to produce the image, but this is not necessarily so for two reasons:

1. the image has a more 'grainy' appearance because faster films have larger silver bromide crystals which produce larger individual spots of silver in the developed image
2. fewer x-ray photons (quanta) are used to produce the image and this increases quantum mottle, or noise (see below).

Digital (computed) radiography using photostimulable phosphors

An alternative to imaging on radiographic film is digital radiography using photostimulable phosphor 'plates' as the x-ray detector. These are similar to intensifying screens

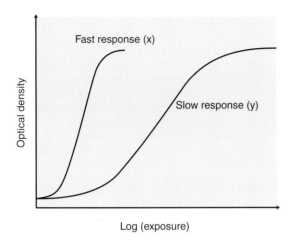

Figure 5.10 Fast and slow film/screen response curves.

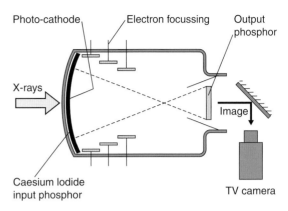

Figure 5.11 TV camera viewing of the intensifier, the II chain.

used with film but, instead of emitting visible light immediately on absorbing x-rays, they store a fraction of the absorbed energy as a latent image by exciting electrons to occupy energy level 'traps' where they remain until stimulated by a suitable light source. This latent image is subsequently read out by scanning the plate with a laser beam, in a light-tight enclosure, and this causes light of a different wavelength from that of the laser to be emitted as the trapped electrons return to a lower energy level in the phosphor. The emitted light is detected by a sensitive photomultiplier tube which produces an electrical signal proportional to the intensity of the light. The electrical signal is digitized and stored in a computer as an image matrix, which might typically contain 2000×2000 pixels (picture elements).

The term computed radiography is sometimes used for these systems to distinguish them from digital radiography using electronic solid state detectors (see below).

Fluoroscopic imaging with image intensifier/TV chain

It is possible to view a time-varying (dynamic) image by using a fluoroscopic system, in which the x-rays are absorbed by a fluorescent material which emits visible light, as in the intensifying screens used with film. Because the brightness of this image is low, an image intensifier is used to increase the brightness and this secondary image is viewed by a TV camera system (Figure 5.11). The TV signal may be recorded in either analogue or digital format.

The image intensifier tube is an evacuated glass envelope with an input phosphor which is typically in the form of a layer of caesium iodide (CsI) crystals. In contact with this is a photocathode, which absorbs the visible light from the phosphor and emits photo-electrons. These are accelerated

through a large potential difference (≈ 25 kV) and focused onto a much smaller output phosphor, which again produces visible light when it absorbs these electrons. As a consequence of the energy gained by the electrons and the fact that they are concentrated onto a smaller area, the brightness of the image at the output phosphor is much higher than at the input. This image is then viewed by a TV camera, usually via a mirror so that the camera is not in the primary x-ray beam.

At each stage in this process there is some loss of fidelity in the image and this can be serious if the electron optics are poorly adjusted or if there is significant interference from external magnetic fields (even the Earth's magnetic field can affect the output image).

Digital fluoroscopy and radiography using solid state detectors

Large area solid state detectors based on amorphous silicon (a-Si) technology are now available as an alternative to the image intensifier. These comprise an array of semiconductor elements, each of which acts as a capacitor storing electric charge and which can be thought of rather like a miniature, solid state ionization chamber. On exposure to radiation, current flows in each element in proportion to the incident intensity, resulting in a spatially varying charge distribution over the array. In fact, the sensitivity of these devices directly to x-rays is rather poor but the signal can be increased by using them in conjunction with a phosphor/photocathode combination (as in the image intensifier), in which case it is the photoelectrons produced in response to irradiation which are actually detected by the a-Si array. The charge pattern can be read out electronically, virtually in real time (unlike computed radiography systems, which require the image plate to be transferred to a reader) and the digital signal stored as an image matrix in a computer. Hence, dynamic imaging can be performed with these systems and pulse mode acquisition is also possible to produce higher quality fluoroscopic and radiographic images.

Assessment of image quality

Magnification/distortion

Because x-rays diverge from a small focal spot and travel in straight lines through the patient before reaching the image detector, the image is magnified as shown in Figure 5.12. Object features which lie in a given plane, parallel to the image detector, are magnified by the same factor. Planes closer to the x-ray source have a higher magnification factor; planes nearer to the image detector have a lower magnification factor. It is often said that a particular image is taken at a certain magnification: strictly this only applies to one specific plane, usually that passing through the isocentre. Any anatomical feature which does not lie in a single plane parallel to the detector will appear distorted in the image, since different parts of it will be magnified to different degrees.

Resolution/unsharpness (geometric/movement)

The resolution of an imaging system is a measure of its ability to represent separate features in the object as separate features in the image. Because no imaging system is perfect, the image of a point in the object is to some degree blurred and sharp edges are rendered unsharp. The image of a point is called the point source response function for the system.

There are several sources which contribute to the unsharpness of an x-ray image: (a) the finite size of the x-ray focal spot, (b) patient movement and (c) resolution of the detector.

(a) X-ray focal spot size

Diagnostic x-ray tubes usually offer a choice of two focal spot sizes: fine (typical diameter 0.4 to 0.8 mm) or broad (typical diameter 0.8 to 1.5 mm). Figure 5.13 shows how such a source gives rise to a penumbra when imaging a sharp edge. The penumbra is wider for a larger focal spot. Because of the bevelled angle of the rotating anode, the apparent size of the focal spot, and hence the degree of blurring, varies across the image in the direction of the axis of rotation of the anode. The blurring is also increased for detail lying in planes with greater magnification. This is especially important for the image of field defining wires in a simulator as these are located relatively close to the x-ray source and are thus greatly magnified (Figure 5.14). Sometimes, especially if the broad focus is used, a double image may be produced: this results from the fact that the focal 'spot' in fact often consists of two relatively intense linear sources of x-rays, separated by a region of lower intensity.

(b) Patient movement

If the patient moves during the exposure, then features will be blurred in the image. This can be minimized by using short exposure times, by asking the patient to keep

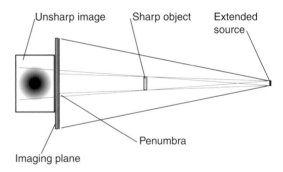

Figure 5.13 How a source gives rise to a penumbra.

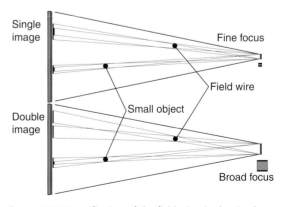

Figure 5.14 Magnification of the field wires in the simulator.

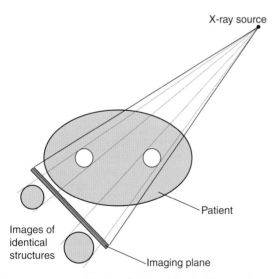

Figure 5.12 Magnification of objects lying in different planes.

still and to hold his/her breath and, if necessary, by using patient immobilization devices.

(c) Detector resolution

The detector resolution is inherently related to the number of distinct and independent samples which are detected within the image. This can be thought of as the spatial sampling rate of the detector. For film, the sampling rate is directly related to the grain size, so for example, if a grain size was 1.0 μm by 1.0 μm, a 1 mm^2 area of film would contain 1 000 000 samples. Hence the sampling rate can be expressed as one million samples per mm^2. With digital systems, the sampling rate is dependent upon the density of sensitive electronic devices which can be manufactured per square mm. This is constantly being increased in order to improve image quality as it is recognized that to ensure adequate detection of a small medical abnormality at an early stage, high resolution is important.

Image signal and noise

An ideal x-ray image would represent the distribution of attenuation coefficient in an object with perfect fidelity. In practice, even the image of a homogeneous object of uniform thickness is not perfectly uniform. The signal exhibits variations about its mean level and these are called noise. Noise can make it difficult to distinguish signal levels which only differ by a small amount, i.e. areas of low contrast in the image.

There are various sources of noise but one which is always present to some degree is quantum noise, or mottle. This results from the fact that any image is made using a finite number of x-ray photons (quanta) and the processes of interaction in the patient and of absorption in the detector are random. This means that there is a statistical variation in the number of photons detected even over an area of uniform attenuation. If the average number of photons per unit area is N, then the statistical uncertainty in the number detected in any particular unit area is $\sqrt{N}$. Expressed as a percentage of the average number this is $100 \times \sqrt{N}/N\%$ or $100/\sqrt{N}\%$. So, relative to the detected signal, the noise decreases as the number of x-ray photons increases, but it is never quite equal to zero.

Other sources of image noise can be the finite size of the fluorescent crystals in intensifying screens, the finite size of silver grains in radiographic film and electrical noise in various components of a TV imaging chain or digital detector system.

Dose

All x-ray imaging procedures, including those discussed below, give some radiation dose to the patient. This is believed to entail a (usually small) risk of harmful effects, such as future cancer induction. It is a requirement of the Ionising Radiation (Medical Exposure) Regulations [2] that the doses from medical imaging exposures should be kept as low as reasonably practicable consistent with the intended purpose. Doses from different procedures can be measured or calculated in various ways. For a given patient, it is often convenient to combine these into an estimate of the total effective dose received, which may be regarded as an index of the total radiation risk from the imaging procedures.

Tomographic imaging

Aims: contrast improvement/ localization in 3D

Planar x-ray imaging is limited in its ability to show low-contrast features, especially in soft tissues, and to allow accurate localization of features in all three spatial dimensions. This results from the fact that it projects a 3-dimensional object onto a 2-dimensional image domain, coupled with limited ability to reject scattered radiation. Tomographic imaging addresses these limitations by imaging selected planes of the patient separately, i.e. 2-dimensional sections of the patient as 2-dimensional images.

Historically, so-called 'conventional' tomography employed linked movements of the x-ray tube with planar detectors to image selected longitudinal planes of the patient in focus, with more distant planes increasingly blurred out into a more or less uniform background. Ingenious methods were devised to optimize the use of these systems and there is continuing interest in digital processing of the component images, e.g. in the technique called tomosynthesis. Although these techniques can improve localization and contrast, they do not reduce the effect of scattered radiation.

CT – Reconstruction from projections

Computed tomography (CT) uses the principle of mathematically reconstructing the internal structure of an object from a set of images of the object taken from different projections. To acquire data from which to reconstruct a single slice, the x-ray beam is collimated to a narrow slit and this is aligned with an arc of solid state detectors. The tube and detectors are mounted on a gantry which rotates about the patient (Figure 5.15). With this set-up it is possible to reject a large proportion of the scatter while detecting the transmitted primary beam with high efficiency. Essentially, one-dimensional projection images are acquired from many angles and the data are processed in a digital computer to form images of transverse slices through the patient. There are several mathematical techniques which can be employed to do this, including Fourier analysis and iterative methods, but most commercial systems use some variant of filtered back projection (FBP). The way in which this works is outlined in Figure 5.16.

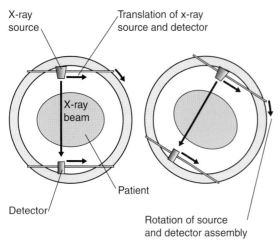

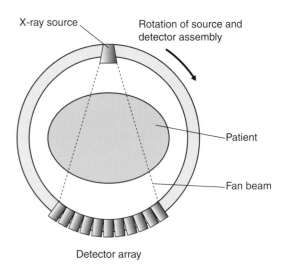

Figure 5.15 General construction of a CT scanner with tube, etc. located.

Figure 5.17 Diagram of a third generation of CT scanner.

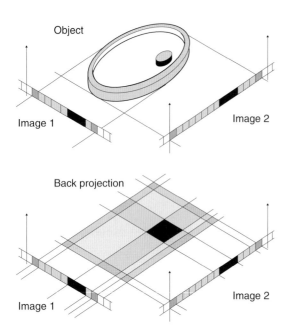

Figure 5.16 The principle of filtered back projection.

Practical configurations

Almost all modern CT scanners are of the so-called third generation design shown in Figure 5.17. (Some fourth generation scanners are in use: these employ a complete, stationary ring of detectors.) Electrical connections with the rotating gantry are made using slip-rings and sliding contactors operating at low voltage, the high voltage generator being mounted on the gantry itself. This allows the gantry

to rotate continuously in the same direction, which is necessary for helical (often known as spiral) acquisitions in which the patient on the table top is slowly advanced through the gantry aperture and data are acquired continuously during several rotations.

Multislice CT

In recent years, multislice CT scanners have become available, in which several arcs of detectors are stacked together longitudinally and the divergence of the x-ray beam can be adjusted so as to irradiate them simultaneously. This permits more rapid collection of projection data from a given length of the patient and makes for efficient use of the x-rays generated by the tube, thus easing the heat loading requirements.

Cone beam CT

It is possible to acquire projection data using devices other than a dedicated CT scanner. Using an electronic planar imaging device and rotating this about the patient during data acquisition, a set of cone beam projections is obtained from which a set of transverse slices can be reconstructed.

Dynamic imaging

Many structures in the body move. Some motion is more or less regularly repetitive or periodic, as in the beating heart or respiratory movement. Some may be quasi-regular, e.g. peristalsis, and others motion intermittent, e.g. swallowing or coughing. A single image will only represent the situation within the time-frame over which it is acquired: if that is short compared with the time over which the movement occurs, then it will be a 'snapshot' of a particular phase of the movement, otherwise it will be a blurred image, averaged over some range of movement.

By taking a time-sequence of images, a so-called dynamic series can be acquired which represents the anatomy of interest at its various positions. This can be useful for diagnosis and staging, e.g. a barium swallow to demonstrate oesophageal or gastric abnormalities, or for planning treatment, e.g. a fluoroscopic study of the chest to demonstrate movement of a lung tumour.

Gated imaging

Where periodic motion is present, gated imaging may be a useful option. This represents data over a typical cycle of the motion as a series of images at different times or phases of the cycle. The image acquisition is linked to some suitable physiological gating signal, e.g. from an electrocardiograph or respiratory monitoring device.

Dedicated radiotherapy systems

Simulator

The radiotherapy simulator is a machine which replicates the movements and geometry of a treatment machine (linac) but uses a diagnostic x-ray tube to produce kV images. It includes beam limiting diaphragms and field-defining wires to allow accurate simulation of the treatment beam and patient geometry. The gantry and couch of the simulator should reproduce all the movements of the treatment machine and to the same accuracy or better (see Chapter 10).

CT virtual simulator

By acquiring a series of CT slices over a suitable longitudinal range, it is possible to generate a digital representation of the body in all three spatial dimensions. This can be used as the basis of virtual simulation, in which digitally reconstructed radiographs (DRR) can be generated to provide beam's eye views (BEV) of the patient from arbitrary directions for various shapes and sizes of field (see Chapter 9).

Treatment verification systems

A check on the accuracy of positioning of treatment fields can be made by acquiring portal images, i.e. images of the transmitted treatment beam emerging from the patient. These may be acquired directly onto film or by an electronic portal imaging device (EPID). Because photoelectric absorption is relatively unimportant with megavoltage x-rays, contrast between bone and soft tissue is much poorer than with kV images so identification of anatomical features depends more on contrast with air.

Manufacturers now offer a range of kilovoltage imaging devices integrated with linear accelerators for image guided radiotherapy (IGRT). These include kV tubes and amorphous silicon imagers mounted on the same gantry at 90° to the megavoltage beam. Such systems can acquire data during a rotation about the patient to produce cone-beam CT images.

Another system employs two fixed x-ray tubes mounted in the floor of the treatment room, used in conjunction with ceiling mounted detectors to acquire oblique views of the patient. The images can be analysed by computer software to compare with reference images to indicate required set-up corrections. It can, however, be difficult for operators to interpret images taken from these angles.

One manufacturer offers a CT scanner in the treatment room so that, by rotating the treatment couch by 90° from the usual treatment position, a CT scan can be obtained with the patient set-up.

MAGNETIC RESONANCE IMAGING

Overview of magnetic resonance imaging process

Magnetic resonance imaging uses a strong magnetic field (typically 0.3 to 3.0 tesla) and radiofrequency (RF) pulses to produce images of the hydrogen distribution within the body. By altering the interval between the RF pulses and the time at which the signals are detected, images with different tissue contrast are produced. Nuclei with odd numbers of protons and neutrons act like tiny magnets. In the presence of a strong magnetic field they have a net alignment with the field. After a pulse of radiofrequency (RF) energy is applied, some of the nuclei will flip and align themselves against the field. After the pulse the nuclei will float back to the original alignment producing an RF signal at the same frequency as the one applied. Images are generated that reflect the distribution of these nuclei within the tissue. So-called T_1 spin lattice relaxation is when the nuclei are aligned in the direction of the magnetic field. The T_2 spin-spin relaxation time is when the nuclei are aligned at 90° to the magnetic field.

Producing a signal

Magnetic resonance occurs when a magnetic field is applied to systems that possess both a magnetic moment and angular momentum. The nuclei of hydrogen atoms are a single proton which has both a magnetic moment and angular momentum. When the hydrogen nuclei or protons in the human body are placed in a strong magnetic field (B_o) they will precess around the direction of the magnetic field at a frequency (f_o) given by the Larmor equation:

$$f_o = \frac{\gamma}{2\pi} B_o \qquad \boxed{5}.\boxed{5}$$

where γ is a constant called the gyromagnetic ratio. $\gamma/2\pi$ is approximately 42.6 $MHzT^{-1}$.

The protons also have a quantum mechanical property called spin. When a magnetic field is applied, the protons

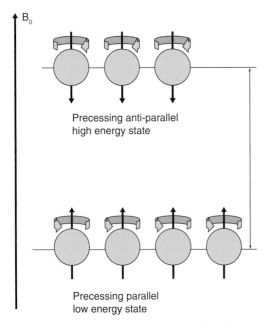

Figure 5.18 Protons precessing parallel or anti-parallel to the applied magnetic field.

can either precess parallel or anti-parallel to the magnetic field, as shown in Figure 5.18. The parallel energy state requires less energy. At a field strength of 1.5 tesla, at body temperature (37°C), the excess of parallel protons is around 4 per million. The excess of parallel protons (or 'spins') in the lower energy state produces a net magnetization vector (M_o) parallel to the magnetic field. By convention, the direction of the applied magnetic field is the z-axis. The net magnetization vector rotates about the z-axis at the Larmor frequency, as shown in Figure 5.19A.

M_o is of the order of microtesla, so in all MR imaging sequences a radiofrequency pulse is applied to detect it. The applied RF pulse needs to be at the Larmor frequency, or it will have no effect. The motion of the net magnetization vector during the radiofrequency pulse in the rotating frame and the lab frame is shown in Figure 5.19. The angle through which M_o is rotated depends on the amplitude and duration of the RF pulse. A 90° pulse will rotate M_o into the x-y or transverse plane.

The rotating magnetization vector induces a voltage in a receiver coil. The detected signal oscillates at Larmor frequency, and decays exponentially, as the individual spin components of M_o rapidly de-phase.

Returning to thermal equilibrium

Once the RF pulse is switched off, the net magnetization vector M_o will return to its thermal equilibrium state parallel to the magnetic field. Felix Bloch described this process, called relaxation, using two different time constants, T_1 and T_2.

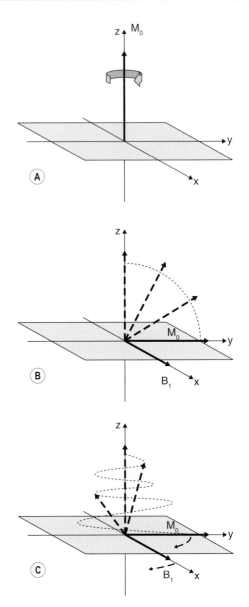

Figure 5.19 (A) The net magnetization vector (Mo) rotating about the z-axis at the Larmor frequency. (B) Motion of Mo in the rotating frame during the application of a 90 RF pulse (B1). (C) Motion of Mo in the lab frame during the application of a 90 RF pulse (B1).

T_1 relaxation is also called longitudinal relaxation, as it governs the rate at which the z-component of M_o recovers. The recovery process occurs when spins which have been excited by the RF pulse give up their energy to their surroundings (or lattice in early experiments). Following a 90° RF pulse, the Bloch equation simplifies to:

$$M_z(t) = M_o\left[1 - e\left(^{-t}/_{T_1}\right)\right]$$ **5.6**

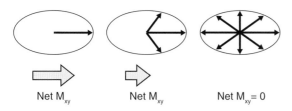

Figure 5.20 De-phasing of transverse magnetization over time shown in the rotating frame.

Table 5.1 T_1 and T_2 relaxation times of common tissues at 1.5 T

TISSUE	T_1 (ms)	T_2 (ms)
White matter	560	82
Grey matter	1100	92
CSF	2060	1000 to 2000
Fat	200	≈ 110

T_2 relaxation occurs because each proton experiences a very slightly different magnetic field strength, as the surrounding protons and molecules move around it on a microscopic scale. As a result, each proton experiences slightly different magnetic fields over time, causing them to rotate at different frequencies (equation 5.5), leading to a de-phasing of the signal in the transverse plane. This de-phasing, viewed in the rotating frame, is shown in Figure 5.20. Following a 90° RF pulse, the Bloch equation simplifies to:

$$M_{xy}(t) = M_{xy}(t = 0)e\left(-t/T_2\right) \qquad \boxed{5}.\boxed{7}$$

As well as the random movement of protons and molecules causing the de-phasing of the protons, de-phasing is also caused by magnetic field inhomogeneities and due to the change in magnetic field at some tissue boundaries. The combined relaxation due to both random spin–spin interactions, and the magnetic field inhomogeneity and changes at some tissue boundaries is called $T_2{}^*$ relaxation.

Imaging sequences

An MR imaging sequence provides spatial information, and also controls the contrast within the image. We will discuss image contrast first using the Bloch equations, and then two-dimensional spatial encoding.

How contrast is altered in an MR image

To produce an MR image, a series of RF pulses must be applied. The reason for this will become clear when spatial encoding of the signal is discussed. The time between the 90° RF pulses is called the repetition time (TR). The echo time (TE) is the time between the 90° RF pulse and the central point of signal detection.

If no transverse magnetization remains when each 90° RF pulse is applied, the signal (S) produced at time TE is:

$$S(TE) \propto M_o\left[1 - e\left(-TR/T_1\right)\right]e\left(-TE/T_2\right) \qquad \boxed{5}.\boxed{8}$$

An image with the contrast dependent on the T_1 times of the tissues is called a T_1 weighted image. From Equation 5.8, to remove any T_2 weighting requires $e(-TE/T_2) \approx 1$ which is achieved by keeping TE«T_2. To make the signal dependent on T_1 requires TR around the minimum T_1 time. Typically, brain imaging at 1.5 T would use a TR of approximately

500 ms and TE of 20 ms. Table 5.1 shows the T_1 and T_2 times of white matter, grey matter, cerebral spinal fluid (CSF) and fat. Equation 5.8, with TR around the minimum T_1 time and TE«T_2, also indicates that tissues with shorter T_1 will produce a higher signal than tissues with a long T_1. So, on a T_1 weighted image, white matter is brighter than grey matter, and CSF is dark. (Fat will also be bright due to its short T_1 time and long T_2 time.)

To produce a T_2 weighted image, with contrast dependent upon T_2 times requires T_1 weighting to be eliminated. Again looking at equation 5.8, this is achieved when $e(-TR/T_1) \approx 0$ which occurs when TR $\approx$ 3 to 5 times T_1. To make the signal dependent on T_2 requires a TE around the T_2 time of tissue. For brain imaging at 1.5 T, the TR is at least 3000 ms and echo times of 80–120 ms would be typical. Equation 5.8, with TR $\geq$ 3000 ms and TE = 80–120 ms, shows that tissues with long T_2 will produce more signal than those with a short T_2. So, from Table 5.1 in a T_2 weighted image, CSF is very bright, and grey matter is brighter than white matter.

A third type of image, called a proton density image, aims to produce weighting dependent only on the density of protons within a given region and independent of the T_1 and T_2 relaxation times. So, again looking at equation 5.8, T_1 weighting is eliminated by using a TR of 3 to 5 times the T_1. T_2 weighting is removed by keeping TE«T_2. The parameters for a brain image at 1.5 T would typically be TR of at least 3000 ms, and TE around 20 ms.

The three image contrasts, and the parameters used to achieve them are shown in Figure *evolve* 5.21 🖱.

How positional information is encoded in the signal

Next, how the signal is spatially encoded to produce an image will be considered. The two-dimensional 'spin warp' [3] imaging method will be described. Other imaging methods are used in MRI, but this method is the most common.

Fundamental to the imaging process are 'gradients' which produce a linear spatial variation of the magnetic field in either the *x*, *y*, or *z* direction. The hardware that produces these gradients will be explained later. When switched on, the gradients produce a linear spatial variation of the magnetic field along their length. This will also produce a linear variation in the rotation frequency of the spins along the gradient (see the Larmor equation 5.5).

The first step of the 2D spin warp imaging process is to select a slice. This is achieved by applying simultaneously an RF pulse and a gradient perpendicular to the slice direction. Figure 5.22 shows a gradient applied along the z-axis (or head–foot direction). At the same time as the gradient is applied, an RF pulse is applied. If the RF pulse is at the Larmor frequency, it will flip the spins which are precessing at the Larmor frequency (in line with the nose on Figure 5.22), and nowhere else. Spins at different slice positions are selected by varying the frequency of the RF pulse, for example, in Figure 5.22, an RF pulse at ($f_o + \Delta f_o$) will flip the spins at eye level. In each case, an axial or transverse slice will be selected. To produce sagittal images, a gradient is applied from left to right across the patient, and for coronal slices from anterior to posterior. Angled slices are produced by applying two gradients at the same time.

Once a slice of spins has been excited, the positions of the spins within that slice need to be determined. Along one dimension/direction of the slice this is achieved using a frequency encoding gradient. In Figure 5.23, the frequency encoding gradient is shown applied horizontally to two different sized test tubes. The signal is collected during the application of the frequency encoding gradient, and Fourier transformed. The Fourier transform of a signal as a function of time, is a signal as a function of frequency. However, by applying the frequency encoding gradient, we have made frequency directly proportional to spatial position. So, the Fourier transform of the time signal is a

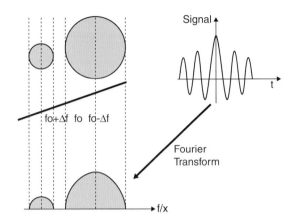

Figure 5.23 The Fourier transformation of the signal as a function of time, produces the amount of signal present at each frequency or spatial position along the x-axis.

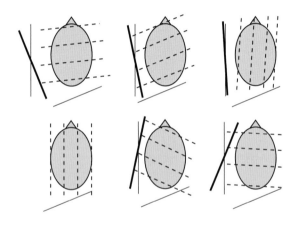

- - - - Lines at the same frequency

Figure 5.24 The phase encoding gradient is shown as a thick black line. As the strength of the phase encoding gradient is varied, the angles of lines of equal frequency change (shown as dotted black lines).

summation of the signal at each position along the gradient. This is shown in Figure *evolve* 5.25 🖰, where the Fourier transform of the signal gives the amount of signal in each column.

How the spatial position in the final dimension of the image is determined is conceptually the most difficult part of the imaging process to understand. For readers who want a much more comprehensive understanding than will be attempted here, I would suggest referring to a good MRI text book, such as 'MRI: From Picture to Proton' [4] or 'Questions and Answers in Magnetic Resonance Imaging' [5]. A gradient, called the phase encoding gradient, is

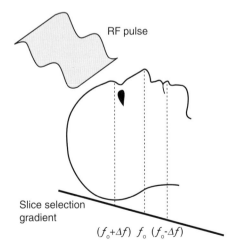

Figure 5.22 Slice selection gradient applied head to foot. An RF pulse at frequency fo will tip all the spins in an axial slice through the nose.

applied along the slice, perpendicular to the frequency encoding gradient. For a 256×256 matrix image, the phase encoding gradient is applied with 256 different amplitudes. In Figure 5.24, some different amplitudes of phase encoding gradient are shown, and it can be seen that these different amplitudes rotate the angle of the lines of equal frequency in the image. The different amplitudes of phase encoding gradient can be thought of as analogous to the different back projections obtained at different tube angles in CT. An RF pulse and slice selection gradient, followed by one of the 256 amplitudes of phase encoding gradient and the frequency encoding gradient, are applied for each signal collected. The signals produced are digitized and stored in turn in a computer. This complete data set (called the k-space data) undergoes a two-dimensional Fourier transform to produce the final MR image of the slice. Figure *evolve* 5.25 🖰 shows the k-space data and corresponding MR image.

MRI scanners

The main components of an MRI scanner are the main magnetic, x, y and z gradient coils, a radiofrequency transmitter coil and a receiver coil. A computer controls the timings of the RF pulses and currents through the gradient coils. Image reconstruction may be performed by the main computer or an additional specialized computer.

The majority of clinical MRI scanners use super-conducting magnets. These currently have field strengths between 0.5 and 3.0 tesla, but there are 7 and 8 T research systems. (The signal to noise ratio increases with field strength, but so does the potential for RF burns and scanner cost.) The super-conductivity (no electrical resistance) is achieved by cooling the wire coils which produce the magnetic field to around $-269°C$ using liquid helium. These magnets have a cylindrical design, with the patients lying inside the bore (or tunnel), and the magnetic field direction aligned with the bore. Figure *evolve* 5.26 🖰 shows a commercial MRI scanner with a super-conducting magnet.

Other types of magnet are available in commercial MRI systems. For example, Figure *evolve* 5.27 🖰 shows an 'open' 0.35 T permanent magnet. Although the magnet is heavy (around 10 tonnes), running costs are low.

The remainder of this section will concentrate on the cylindrical super-conducting magnet system, as it is by far the most common. As the field produced by the magnet is not completely uniform, it must be 'shimmed'. A fixed shim is achieved either passively using small pieces of steel positioned around the magnet, and/or actively using computer determined current magnitudes inside special super-conducting coils called shim coils. As the patient affects the magnetic field homogeneity, additional shimming is also performed each time a patient is imaged. This dynamic shimming uses the gradient coils and sometimes extra (resistive) shim coils.

The RF coils can be used both to transmit the RF pulses and to detect the voltage signal produced. The most common design of coil which both transmits and receives RF pulses is a birdcage coil, Figure 5.28. This coil design produces a uniform RF field with good penetration, and is often used in head and knee coils. Frequently, the RF pulses are transmitted through a 'body' coil which is inside the bore of the magnet, and the signal is picked up by a dedicated receiver coil. At its simplest, this receiver coil is a loop of wire, orientated perpendicular to the main magnetic field. An MRI scanner would typically have five or more different coils dedicated to imaging different body parts, for example head, knee, spine, body, heart and breast coils, and a few general purpose coils for imaging the remaining parts of the body.

Spectroscopy

Single voxel magnetic resonance spectroscopy (MRS) is a technique which produces a spectrum of the metabolites present in a voxel. Most MRS is performed on hydrogen nuclei as they are the most abundant nuclei and MRI systems and coils are already tuned to hydrogen's resonant frequency. MRS can also be performed on ^{23}Na and ^{31}P. In the limited space available here only hydrogen MRS will be discussed.

The voxel which produces the MRS spectrum is normally selected using RF pulses and gradient. For single voxel spectroscopy, two techniques called PRESS [6] and STEAM [6] are commonly used. An Fourier transform of the signal detected from the voxel gives the spectrum (Figure *evolve* 5.29 🖰). A spectrum is produced because each metabolite has a slightly different local magnetic field strength, due to its chemical environment. Therefore, each metabolite resonates at a slightly different frequency. The area under each peak is proportional to the amount of metabolite present. The water peak has to be suppressed, or this would dominate the spectrum.

Chemical shift imaging (CSI) is another spectroscopic technique which produces a matrix of spectra from a matrix of voxels encoded with a phase encoding gradient.

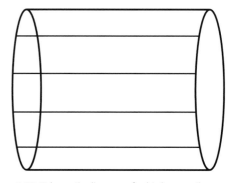

Figure 5.28 Schematic diagram of a birdcage coil.

Clinical applications of MRI in oncology

Anatomical MR imaging is often used in the head, neck, abdomen and pelvis for the detection of cancer, and staging the disease. Contrast agents, which are gadolinium based, and injected intravenously, shorten the T_1 of tissue. Areas of tumour with high vasculature are, therefore, highlighted on T_1 weighted images.

Complete textbooks have been written on the use of MRI in cancer diagnosis, staging, treatment planning and for treatment monitoring. In this section, the application of MRI in brain tumour imaging is briefly outlined. MRI can be used to diagnose and stage cancer in most organs of the body including bladder, pancreas, bowel, and breasts, cervix and ovaries in women, and prostate in men. The use of MRI in bowel cancer will be concentrated on as an example of this vast area.

Brain tumours

MRI scanning is unsurpassed as the ideal imaging medium for the diagnosis of brain tumours. Brain tumours make up around 9% of all adult cancers. Approximately 80% are primary tumours and 20% are secondary.

Figure *evolve* 5.29 🖱 shows images of a large left frontal malignant glioma. Gliomas are the most common type (45–50%) of primary brain tumour. Figure *evolve* 5.30A 🖱 shows the extent of the tumour appears as an area of hyperintense signal on the T_2 weighted image. Pathological processes, such as a tumour or infarction, increase the amount of extracellular water, which can lead to cerebral oedema. T_2 weighted images (Figure *evolve* 5.30A 🖱) are best at showing an increase in the amount of extracellular water, which also appear as hyperintense areas (white). On T_1 weighted images, oedema appears as a hypointense (black) area. A pre-contrast T_1 weighted image of the glioma is shown in Figure *evolve* 5.30B 🖱.

Discrimination between the tumour and surrounding oedema can be helped by the use of gadolinium contrast, which can enhance the tumour in the image. Gadolinium is a rare earth metal with seven unpaired electrons. These unpaired electrons enable nearby protons to align more quickly and shortens the T_1 and T_2 relaxation times. Usually, low grade gliomas do not enhance on T_1 weighted images with gadolinium, however, high grade gliomas enhance avidly, often with a heterogeneous appearance due to haemorrhage or necrosis. Figure *evolve* 5.30C 🖱 shows areas of strong contrast enhancement where the glioma has broken down the blood–brain barrier. However, isolated tumours cells can penetrate beyond the tumour margins visualized using MRI. This is significant with regard to the margins used in planning (see Chapter 9).

The type of brain tumour can usually be determined by its location and appearance. The tumour shown in Figure *evolve* 5.31 🖱 could, from its visual appearance and location, have been a glioma or metastasis.

The single voxel spectrum from the glioma or metastasis is shown in Figure *evolve* 5.32 🖱. For comparison, a spectrum obtained from normal brain tissue was shown in Figure *evolve* 5.29 🖱. The very high level of lactate, and only slightly increased choline level, show that this lesion is likely to be a metastasis.

Body tumours

MRI's role in body cancer diagnosis and staging is vast. As a purely illustrative example, we will look at the role of MRI in staging rectal cancer and the difference that it makes to treatment.

The very close proximity of the rectum to other organs makes the very exact staging of rectal cancer critical. Figure *evolve* 5.33A and B 🖱 shows an early stage of rectal cancer, with the cancer confined within the rectum muscle wall. This patient was managed by surgical resection. Figure *evolve* 5.33C, D and E 🖱 show a patient with the later stage of rectal cancer, the cancer has extended outside the rectal muscle wall along the veins into the surrounding fatty tissue (extra mural venous invasion). This patient required combined radiotherapy and chemotherapy, followed by surgery. MRI was used again at the end of the combined radiotherapy and chemotherapy to monitor the response of the tumour. The patient then had surgery. All patients with rectal cancer will have continued monitoring with CT at 6–12 month intervals, to check for liver and other metastases.

MR images of tumours in the abdomen and pelvis are occasionally fused with CT images for use during treatment planning. The non-rigid nature of the anatomy makes fusion more difficult than in the brain.

ULTRASOUND IMAGING

In this chapter, the emphasis is on the use of ultrasound in imaging. However, above the levels used for diagnosis, it is used in various ways in the treatment of cancer and other conditions. These include lithotripsy, hyperthermia, drug activation and enhancement and high intensity focused ultrasound (HIFU) to ablate soft tissue.

Overview of ultrasound imaging process

Ultrasound is defined as a vibration with a frequency above the upper limit of human hearing at 20 kilohertz (1 hertz = 1 vibration cycle per second). In fact, medical ultrasound most often uses much higher frequencies, usually between 1 and 20 MHz, but sometimes higher frequencies for applications such as acoustic microscopy.

Ultrasound moves as a longitudinal pressure wave through soft tissue with areas of compression and rarefraction travelling through the tissue. Considering a small area of tissue – this will vibrate to and fro along the direction of travel of the ultrasound wave as the pressure wave passes. The amplitude of the ultrasound wave can be defined in various ways, such as the peak pressure, the peak distance displaced or peak velocity of a small area of tissue.

$$C = f \times w$$

where C = speed of sound (m/s), f = frequency (Hz) and w = wavelength (m).

For soft tissues, the average speed of sound is 1540 m/s. So, for medical ultrasound, the wavelength is from about 0.075 to 1.5 mm. The resolution of ultrasound images is related to the wavelength, so higher frequency ultrasound, which has a smaller wavelength, gives better resolution.

The speed of ultrasound in tissue is related to the bulk modulus and the density of the tissue through which the ultrasound travels. The bulk modulus is defined as the change in pressure divided by the fractional change in volume for a material. So, for harder materials, where a given change in pressure will result in a small change in volume, the bulk modulus is large. Higher density results in a lower velocity.

$$C = \sqrt{(B/D)} \qquad \boxed{5}.\boxed{1}\boxed{0}$$

where C = speed of sound (m/s), B = bulk modulus (N/m^2) and D = density (kg/m^3).

$$B = dP/(dV/V) = V \times dP/dV \qquad \boxed{5}.\boxed{1}\boxed{1}$$

where P = pressure (N/m^2) and V = volume (m^3).

The speed of ultrasound in different soft tissues is generally within about ±6% of 1540 m/s. The speed of ultrasound in harder tissues, such as bone, is much higher at about 3200 m/s. Air, which has a low bulk modulus and low density, has a much lower speed of sound at 330 m/s.

For diagnostic purposes, ultrasound gives us information related to the mechanical properties of tissue. Ultrasound is reflected from interfaces between tissues with different mechanical properties. The amount of ultrasound reflected depends on the acoustic impedance of the material.

Considering a small area of tissue, the acoustic impedance is defined as the ratio of the pressure amplitude divided by the velocity amplitude of this small area of tissue as the ultrasound wave passes through it. The acoustic impedance can also be defined relative to the speed of sound and tissue density.

$$Z = \rho \times C \qquad \boxed{5}.\boxed{1}\boxed{2}$$

where Z = acoustic impedance, ρ = density and C = speed of sound in tissue.

The fraction of ultrasound reflected from an interface between tissues of different acoustic impedances can be calculated below.

$$R = (Z_1 - Z_2)^2/(Z_1 + Z_2)^2 \qquad \boxed{5}.\boxed{1}\boxed{3}$$

where R = fraction of ultrasound reflected.

For interfaces between soft tissues, the amount reflected is usually between 0.01 and 1%. For a soft tissue to air interface, 99.9% of the ultrasound is reflected. The practical consequence of this is that ultrasound cannot image beyond gas, so that lung tissue cannot be imaged. Bowel gas can be a problem in the abdomen. Also, the air gap between the ultrasound transducer and the skin must be eliminated using ultrasound gel when scanning. Imaging into and beyond bone is usually difficult as bone both reflects a lot of the ultrasound and highly attenuates the ultrasound beam.

For smooth interfaces between different tissues, reflection will be mirror like, so that the angle of reflection equals the angle of incidence. Also, the transmitted part of the wave may be bent slightly (refracted) due to the difference in sound velocity between the materials. Usually, for soft tissues, the angle of refraction is small and is neglected.

For rough interfaces, the ultrasound will be reflected at a variety of different angles. For small scatterers, which are much smaller than the wavelength, the ultrasound is scattered in all directions. This is called Rayleigh scattering and occurs for instance for red blood cells.

As it travels through tissue, energy will be lost from the ultrasound beam by scattering of ultrasound away from the beam direction and by energy absorption in the tissue. Energy absorption occurs when the coherent vibration of the ultrasound wave is degraded into random motion of the tissue – i.e. heat.

Attenuation of the ultrasound beam is usually proportional to the frequency of the ultrasound, so higher frequency ultrasound is more highly attenuated. This results in a compromise between attenuation and image resolution. For superficial structures, a higher frequency is usually used to give better resolution. For deeper structures, a lower frequency with poorer resolution may be needed to allow sufficient ultrasound to penetrate the tissues.

Ultrasound scanners

Ultrasound machines use piezoelectric materials to generate and detect ultrasound.

The piezoelectric effect was discovered by Pierre and Jacque Curie in 1880 and occurs in some materials where there is a polarized crystal structure. When a piezoelectric material is compressed, it generates a voltage across the crystal structure. An opposite voltage is generated if the crystal is subjected to low pressure. Thus, a piezoelectric crystal will generate an alternating voltage across it as ultrasound passes through it and can be used as a detector. Conversely, if an alternating voltage is applied across a piezoelectric crystal, it will vibrate and hence can be used to generate ultrasound.

The most commonly used piezoelectric material is a ceramic material, lead zirconate titanate (PZT).

Originally, a focused beam of ultrasound was produced by using a flat disk piezoelectric element with an acoustic lens attached to the front. A curved piezoelectric element can also produce a focused beam, but is more difficult to manufacture. Modern ultrasound transducers use an array of many small piezoelectric elements. Focusing can be produced by electronically altering the delay in the pulse applied to each element so that the peak of the ultrasound wave occurs at the focus for all elements. The depth of focus can be altered by electronically altering the amount of delay applied to the elements. Likewise, a stepwise delay across the elements can be used to steer the ultrasound beam.

To produce an ultrasound image, the SONAR (sound navigation and ranging) principle is used. This was originally used to detect submarines. A short pulse is directed along a narrow beam and the depth from which the echoes were generated within the tissue is calculated from the time delay between the transmitted pulse and the echoes return, knowing the speed of ultrasound in tissue. For each pulse transmitted, the amplitude of the echoes can be used to modulate the brightness of the image screen along a line in the image.

By moving the line along which the beam is directed for subsequent pulses, a 2-dimensional image of the amplitude of echoes from the tissue can be built up. This is called a B mode image or brightness mode image (Figure *evolve* 5.34 🖰).

As ultrasound travels very quickly in soft tissue (1540 m/s), each ultrasound image can be acquired very quickly and frame rates of between 5 and 40 images per second can be achieved, allowing real time imaging. This allows following movements of the heart and real time guidance of biopsies from suspicious areas on the ultrasound image.

The movement of blood and tissues can be measured using the Doppler effect. The Doppler effect occurs when a wave is reflected from a moving structure. If the structure is moving towards the sound source, the wavefronts are compressed and this increases the frequency of the ultrasound. Likewise, the frequency is decreased when the structure is moving away from us. The most familiar everyday example of this is a car horn, which sounds higher pitched when the car approaches and lower as the car passes and moves away from us.

Pulsed mode Doppler ultrasound uses repeated sampling of the ultrasound from a sample volume in a blood vessel and gives a detailed real time blood flow velocity spectrum, allowing the changes in flow during the heart cycle to be studied and the blood velocity to be calculated. Figure *evolve* 5.35 🖰 shows a pulsed Doppler mode blood velocity spectrum in the lower half of the image.

It shows the blood flow velocity spectrum (vertical axis) in a small sample volume as it changes with time (horizontal axis). Each peak represents high systolic flow at the start of each heart cycle. The small upper image shows where the sample volume was located.

Colour Doppler ultrasound measures the shift in frequency from moving blood and overlays this on the B mode grey scale image. The colour on the image is coded according to the direction of the flow relative to the beam and the size of the frequency shift, which is related to the blood flow velocity. Colour Doppler images can give an idea of the vascularity of tissue. Figure *evolve* 5.36 🖰 shows a colour flow Doppler image of blood flow in the common carotid artery.

Encapsulated microbubbles can be injected into the blood stream as a contrast agent to increase the reflections from vascular tissue [7].

A newer technique, called elastography, can map out how hard various tissues are [8]. It achieves this by measuring the distortion of the tissues on ultrasound images with and without applying pressure to the tissue. Sometimes, elastography can demonstrate changes in the hardness of tissue surrounding a mass demonstrated on the B mode image. This suggests that infiltration into the surrounding tissue has occurred and that the B mode image alone may underestimate the extent of the tumour local involvement in some cases.

Clinical applications

As previously shown, the dependence of ultrasound imaging on the transmission and reflection at tissue interfaces and the poor transmission through an air–tissue interface limits the clinical applications of ultrasound imaging. It is of no value in examining the lungs or the gastrointestinal tract.

Its use in obstetrics to image the fetus is widely known. The age of the pregnancy, fetal growth and fetal abnormalities can be monitored and detected.

However, ultrasound can identify abnormal structure, size or texture of many different organs in the body. It is used widely in the diagnosis of cancer, assessment of its local extent and staging. Masses can be identified and characterized, helping to differentiate solid masses from benign fluid-filled cysts. Often, the ultrasound appearance of a solid mass is not specific enough to diagnose whether a lesion is cancerous, so needle biopsy of masses is usually performed under ultrasound guidance to define a lesion's histology.

Good images are produced if there is a tissue–fluid interface and, therefore, ultrasound is particularly effective at showing whether lumps are cystic or solid. For this reason, ultrasound is frequently used to examine the breast. Ultrasound can distinguish between solid (often malignant) and cystic (often benign) lumps within the breast. Ultrasound images are influenced by vasculature of the scanned organ and the differences in the blood supply within that organ. This difference may also be used to differentiate between benign and malignant disease within the breast.

Ultrasound is a sensitive technique for detecting metastases within the liver as metastases often reflect the sound wave poorly and produce hypoechogenic areas. The use of gas bubbles as an ultrasound contrast agent can help to characterize the blood supply in liver tumours. Liver tumours often derive their blood supply from the hepatic artery which makes them enhance early on contrast studies. Liver tissue that has a blood supply from the portal vein will enhance later.

Small endoscopic ultrasound probes can be used to assess the invasion of a tumour into the bowel wall and surrounding tissue.

Intracavity probes can be introduced into the body to allow the ultrasound transducer to be as close as possible to the tissue of interest. This allows higher resolution, clearer images to be produced. Trans-rectal and trans-vaginal ultrasound probes can be used in imaging of the prostate, ovary or uterus for instance. Trans-vaginal ultrasound can be used to measure the thickness of the lining of the uterus (the endometrium) and is a sensitive measure for screening for endometrial cancer in patients with post-menopausal bleeding. It also produces good images of ovarian cysts and solid areas within these cysts can be demonstrated which helps decide whether the lesion is likely to be benign or malignant.

REFERENCES

[1] Hoskins P, Thrush A, Martin K, Whittingham T. Diagnostic ultrasound: Physics and equipment. Greenwich Medical Media Ltd; 2002.

[2] Statutory Instrument 2000 No. 1059. The Ionising Radiation (Medical Exposures) Regulations 2000.

[3] Edelstein WA, Hutchison JMS, Johnson G, Redpath TW. Spin warp NMR imaging and application to the human whole-body imaging. Phys Med Biol 1980;25:751–6.

[4] McRobbie DW, Moore EA, Graves MJ, Prince MR. MRI: from picture to proton. Cambridge University Press; 2003.

[5] Elster AD, Burdett JH. Questions and answers in magnetic resonance imaging. Mosby; 2000.

[6] Keevil SF. Spatial localization in nuclear magnetic resonance spectroscopy. Phys Med Biol 2006;51:R579–636.

[7] Rumack CM, Wilson SR, Charboneau JW. Diagnostic ultrasound. 3rd ed. Elsevier Mosby; 2005.

[8] Ophir J, Alam SK, Garra B, et al. Elastography: ultrasonic estimation and imaging of the elastic properties of tissues. Proceedings of the Institute of Mechanical Engineering 1999;213:203–33.

EVOLVE CONTENTS (available online at: http://evolve.elsevier.com/Symonds/radiotherapy/)

Figure evolve 5.21 T_1 weighted image (TR = 554 ms, TE = 13 ms), T_2 weighted image (TR = 5070 ms, TE = 98 ms) and proton density (TR = 370 ms, TE = 15 ms)

Figure evolve 5.25 (A) 'k-space' data stored; (B) the two dimensional Fourier transform of the k-space data

Figure evolve 5.26 An MRI system with a cylindrical super-conducting magnet

Figure evolve 5.27 An open MRI system with a permanent magnet

Figure evolve 5.29 Spectrum from a voxel normal brain tissue showing a high N-acetyl aspartate (NAA) peak, and choline (Cho) levels below those of creatine (Cr). Obtained using a STEAM sequence TE = 30ms

Figure evolve 5.30 (A) T_2 weighted pre-contrast axial image showing a large left frontal lobe malignant glioma. (B) Pre-contrast T_1 weighted axial image. (The same slice position is shown as previous image.) (C) Post-contrast axial T_1 weighted image. The contrast agent clearly defines the area of the glioma where blood/brain barrier has broken down

Figure evolve 5.31 (A) Axial T_2 weighted image of a glioma or brain metastases. (b) Axial T_1 weighted image post contrast

Figure evolve 5.32 Spectrum from the metastasis showing an extremely elevated lactate peak, and slightly elevated choline levels. The spectrum was obtained using STEAM with TE = 30 ms

Figure evolve 5.33 (A) Sagittal image of early stage rectal carcinoma (dark arrow) still contained within the rectal muscle wall (light arrow). (B) Coronal image of early stage rectal carcinoma (dark arrow) still contained within rectal muscle wall (light arrow). (C), (D) and (E) Axial, sagittal and coronal images of a stage 3 rectal cancer, which has extra-mural venous invasion. The dark arrows point to the tumour and the light arrows to areas of extra-mural venous invasion

Figure evolve 5.34 A B-mode transverse image of the neck showing a map of the brightness of reflection of ultrasound from different tissues. Blood vessels are dark on B mode images as blood reflects relatively little ultrasound

Figure evolve 5.35 Pulsed mode Doppler sonogram of flow in the internal carotid artery

Figure evolve 5.36 A colour Doppler image of flow in the common carotid artery. The background B mode information shows the echoes of stationary tissue. Within the colour box flowing blood is colour coded according to the direction of flow and size of the frequency shift, which is related to the blood flow velocity and the angle of the flow relative to the beam direction

Chapter | 6 |

Imaging with radionuclides

Marjorie Rose, Nigel R. Williams

INTRODUCTION

Radionuclide images play a key role in the diagnosis, staging and planning the delivery of treatment to and follow up of patients with cancer.

In everyday language, an image is a picture of something. More generally, it is a representation of the distribution of some property of an object. It is formed by transferring information from the object to an image domain. In practice, this requires the ordered transfer of energy from some source via the object of interest to a detector system.

This medical imaging modality is classified by the radionuclide gamma ray emission which provides the energy for the ordered transfer from the object to the image. Radionuclide imaging is primarily concerned with the function of organs and tissues. The other modalities, x-ray, magnetic resonance imaging (MRI) and ultrasound, primarily convey structural or anatomical information, though the distinction between structural and functional imaging is not absolute. The detected signal is often processed in some way before being displayed. Multimodality combinations of images, as in positron emission tomography and x-ray computed tomography (PET-CT), can provide an especially powerful tool for discriminating between normal and malignant tissues [1].

Nuclear medicine is the science and clinical application of unsealed radiopharmaceuticals for diagnostic and investigative purposes and this includes imaging. A suitable radionuclide or isotope is combined with a pharmaceutical or a molecule which marks a particular biological function or process. The behaviour of this radio-labelled compound is monitored by radiation detectors external to the body, allowing the non-invasive measurement of in-vivo biochemical function, aspects of tissue function, and dynamic biological processes. Localization of functional information is increasingly becoming essential information for cancer diagnosis and radiotherapy treatment.

OVERVIEW OF THE RADIONUCLIDE IMAGING PROCESS

Nuclear medicine departments routinely perform diagnostic imaging and non-imaging procedures and, in many hospitals, undertake radionuclide radiotherapy treatments. However, in this chapter, only radionuclide imaging will be described and therapeutic applications are dealt with in Chapter 7. A radionuclide is an unstable isotope of an element that will spontaneously 'decay' by the emission of particles and/or electromagnetic radiation. The three most common emissions from radionuclides are alpha and beta particles and gamma rays. There are two types of beta particle, beta minus (β^-) and beta plus (β^+), they are both electrons with a negative and positive charge, respectively. A beta plus is referred to as a positron. A gamma ray is a form of electromagnetic radiation and is the only one with sufficient penetrating characteristics to enable it to be detected externally if originating from within the body. Most use is made of a relatively limited number of radionuclides that emit only gamma rays. However, there is a growing use of radionuclides that decay by emitting a positron; this particle is not penetrating but interacts with an electron, both annihilating to form two photons travelling in opposite directions. These photons are penetrating and can be detected as they leave the body. A radionuclide is attached, or labelled, to a pharmaceutical, forming a radiopharmaceutical. This is introduced into the body, most commonly by intravenous injection but also by ingestion and inhalation, and has a known biodistribution

in the body. The distribution of the radiopharmaceutical is related to the physiology or function of an organ, tissue or tissue type; this is in contrast to x-ray, MR or ultrasound imaging which, to a large extent, images structure.

Gamma rays are imaged by a device known as a gamma camera. The device used to detect annihilation photons resulting from the decay of a radionuclide emitting positrons is referred to as a PET camera. Gamma cameras are a large area detection device capable of forming an image of the distribution of a radionuclide within the body. The majority of devices have two detector heads, although it is possible to purchase single or triple head equipment. Imaging with a gamma camera can take place with the detector heads in a stationary position, planar mode, or with the detector heads moving around the body through, typically, 180° or 360°. This mode of acquisition is known as single photon emission computerized tomography (SPECT) or, dropping the reference to computerization (SPET). PET cameras work on the basis of a series of rings of stationary detectors, identifying the location of a nucleus decaying via positron emission, by detection of both annihilation photons within a predefined time (nanoseconds). This is sometimes referred to as coincidence imaging.

The most up-to-date gamma cameras and all PET cameras are now manufactured with an x-ray CT imaging device incorporated into the gantry. In both cases, the primary purpose of this ancillary facility is to allow the use of the structural CT (transmission) images to be converted into an attenuation map [2]. This map is used to correct the functional nuclear medicine (emission) images for variation in body tissue thickness and density. Having the CT imaging incorporated into the cameras allows the emission and transmission images to be acquired sequentially in the same patient imaging session. Assuming there is no patient movement, the data derived from the transmission image can be accurately applied to the emission images. This process is applicable to SPECT images acquired on gamma cameras and all images acquired on PET cameras. Consequently, imaging techniques associated with these devices are known as SPECT/CT and PET/CT. Initially, the CT units were not of a standard comparable to the most up-to-date helical multi-slice devices and the structural images obtained were not of a diagnostic quality. However, gamma cameras and PET scanners can now be purchased with high specification CT units attached and the registration or fusion of high spatial resolution structural images with the sensitive but poor resolution function images results in an imaging device that is extremely effective at identifying and localizing pathology.

GAMMA CAMERAS

Gamma cameras (Figure 6.1) are imaging devices used to detect and record the distribution of a radiopharmaceutical within the body. Gamma rays are detected by a large area crystal of sodium iodide doped with trace quantities of thallium (NaI(Tl)), the crystal structure has the

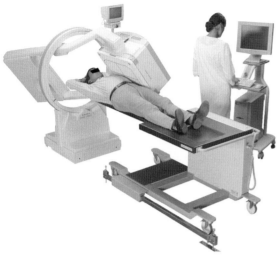

Figure 6.1 Gamma camera.
(Bartec Technologies Ltd)

property of absorbing the gamma radiation and re-emitting photons of visible light; the crystal is referred to as a scintillator. The crystal dimensions vary but are typically 50 cm × 40 cm with a thickness of about 1 cm. Smaller detector systems are available for specialized purposes, such as cardiac or brain imaging. A schematic of a gamma camera detector head is shown in Figure 6.2. Further information

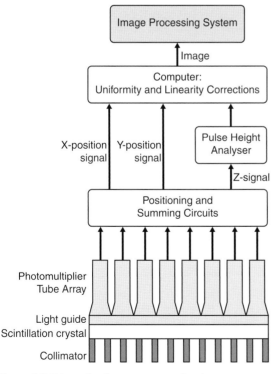

Figure 6.2 Schematic of gamma camera head.

regarding the design of gamma cameras may be found in Cherry et al [3].

The process of recording a single gamma ray event by the camera is as follows:

- a γ-ray emitted from the body and travelling towards the detector, in a direction approximately parallel to collimator holes (parallel hole collimator), will be able to pass through and interact with the NaI(Tl) scintillator crystal
- the γ-ray will be absorbed by the crystal and the energy will be re-emitted as a plume of photons with a wavelength associated with visible light
- the light photons travel through a waveguide to the photomultiplier tube (PMT) array where they are converted into photo-electrons
- the photo-electrons are multiplied between the dynodes of the PMT, amplifying the signal
- circuitry between the PMTs produces information about the position of the detected event
- the total output from the PMT array gives information about the energy of the detected event. Energy discriminators allow photons of a specific energy, usually only unscattered photons, to contribute to the image.

An image of the distribution of radiopharmaceutical within the body is made up of hundreds of thousands to millions of detected events. Each event is individually detected. The crystal, collimator and photomultiplier array are mounted inside a lead shield. Most gamma cameras will have two detector heads and the orientation of these heads is variable. Two important performance characteristics of a gamma camera, spatial resolution and sensitivity, are, to a large degree, influenced by the choice of collimator.

The function of a gamma camera collimator is to permit gamma rays travelling in a predefined direction reaching the scintillation crystal. This is achieved by absorbing all other gamma rays in septa between the holes of the collimator. A number of different types of collimators are available but, by far the most widely used, are parallel-hole collimators.

Parallel-hole collimators consist of a thick lead plate with several thousand small parallel-sided holes perpendicular to the plane of the plate. For this type of collimator, there is a 1:1 relationship between the size of the distribution of imaged activity and its projection on to the crystal. Thus, the size of the image is independent of the distance from the subject to the detector face. The characteristics of a parallel-hole collimator depend on the hole diameter, hole length and septal thickness (lead between the holes). Sensitivity and spatial resolution are inversely related; the higher the sensitivity the poorer the spatial resolution and vice versa. Parallel-hole collimators are designed to image gamma rays of a specific energy range, usually denoted as low, medium and high energy. Imaging Tc-99m requires a low energy collimator. The size of hole, length of septa and number of holes influence the characteristic of a collimator designed for a specific energy. Low energy collimators are available with descriptions such as high sensitivity, general purpose, high resolution and very high resolution. The exact characteristics of each collimator can vary immensely between manufacturers.

IMAGING TECHNIQUES

Planar imaging

Reference has been made to planar and tomographic imaging. Planar imaging can take a number of forms. The simplest is with the camera directed at the part of the body containing the organ or organs of interest and an acquisition of a predefined number of events or period of time takes place. These are sometimes referred to as spot views. Keeping the camera heads in a fixed position but causing the patient to move slowly between the detectors is commonly referred to as whole body imaging. The bone scans shown in the section on Clinical applications utilize this form of imaging. A dynamic acquisition is when a series of images, often sequential and of the same duration, is obtained. With these data, temporal changes in distribution guide the diagnostic results. An example of dynamic imaging is utilized in the section on kidney imaging. A final form of planar imaging is when the acquisition is synchronized to a physiological signal obtained from the patient. A gated blood pool study shown in the section on cardiac imaging is the most widely used form of this mode of imaging. The cardiac cycle is divided into a fixed number of frames, in the example shown 24 frames each of 41 milliseconds. The dynamic acquisition is triggered by the R-wave on the patient's ECG. Images from multiple heart beats are obtained and corresponding frames (first, second, etc.) are summed together to produce a dynamic series representing a composite beat. Without this technique, the quantity of data in each frame would be insufficient to achieve the accuracy of the ejection fraction calculation required.

Tomographic imaging

Tomographic imaging is performed with a gamma camera, by rotating the detector system around the patient while acquiring images. The image data may be obtained with the camera heads stationary at a number of fixed positions around the body known as 'step and shoot' mode, or acquired continuously as the camera rotates. Two-dimensional (2D) cross-sectional images are reconstructed using mathematical algorithms, in a similar way to x-ray CT. The 2D cross-sectional images can be stacked to form a volume of data which gives the appearance of having acquired a 3D dataset.

Knowledge of the 3D distribution of the radiopharmaceutical within the body allows correction for the attenuation of the emitting gamma radiation if the size and density of surrounding structures can be determined. This is achieved with the aid of a CT attenuation map. A CT acquisition represents the variation of x-ray absorption throughout the image volume, a direct relationship can be made between this and the attenuation of the emitted gamma radiation. An example of nuclear medicine images that have been attenuation corrected and fused with the CT structural images is shown in Figure *evolve* 6.6 🖱. Note that the CT device in this example is a low dose unit, not in the diagnostic category.

GAMMA CAMERA PERFORMANCE CHARACTERISTICS

It is essential that gamma camera performance is maintained to achieve the highest possible sensitivity and specificity of each investigation undertaken on it. The performance of gamma camera detectors is characterized by a number of parameters:

- spatial resolution
- sensitivity
- uniformity
- linearity and energy response
- energy resolution
- multiple window registration.

Detailed descriptions of the precise definitions of these parameters, factors influencing their stability, measurement methodologies and how they may be specified during equipment procurement are covered in two publications; IPEM 2003 [4] and NEMA 2007 [5]. Brief outlines are given here.

Spatial resolution. This is the ability to distinguish an object from its surroundings and is a measure of the sharpness of the image. It is defined by a full width half maximum distance and this is about 3 mm for the intrinsic (no collimator) resolution of a current gamma camera.

Sensitivity. This term relates to the number of gamma events per MBq detected by the gamma camera. Described above is the influence the collimator has on the spatial resolution and sensitivity of a gamma camera.

Uniformity. This refers to the variations in count rate across the field of view when the detector is exposed to a uniform source of a gamma ray emitting radionuclide.

Linearity and energy response. These refer to the gamma camera's ability to determine the true location and energy of a gamma ray detected anywhere in the field of view. These are the fundamental parameters that influence detector uniformity.

Energy resolution. Statistical variations in the detection of gamma rays by the crystal and photomultiplier assembly result in a characteristic broadening of the total absorption peak of the energy spectrum. Energy resolution is defined by an energy Full Width Half Maximum.

Multiple window registration. This refers to the ability of the gamma camera to determine the location of a detected gamma event as a function of its energy.

Corrections can be made during data acquisition to overcome some of the non-random defects in camera performance. These include corrections for non-uniformity of sensitivity, non-uniformity of energy resolution, and non-linearity.

There are additional performance characteristics to take into account when performing SPECT imaging and still further with SPECT/CT. SPECT imaging requires the centre of rotation (COR) of the rotating camera heads to be within predefined limits. Failure to do so will result in artifacts on the reconstructed SPECT images. It is also important that the parameters defining the detector heads remain stable at every angle of rotation. SPECT/CT relies on the accurate registration of the SPECT and CT images. The performance of the CT is assessed as for all CT equipment, as covered by IPEM Report 91 [6]. A crucial additional assessment is the alignment of the SPECT and CT data together. Phantoms are routinely used to assess the gamma camera SPECT capability and SPECT/CT alignment.

POSITRON EMISSION TOMOGRAPHY SCANNERS

Dedicated positron emission tomography cameras (Figure 6.3) are designed specifically for radionuclides that decay by positron emission. Scintillator crystals with high stopping power are utilized, examples are bismuth germanate (BGO) and lutetium orthosilicate (LSO). These crystals, coupled to photomultiplier tubes, are positioned in rings around a gantry. Electronic circuitry, designed to register if two crystals detect a photon within a 'coincidence time', usually a few nanoseconds, allow 'true' events to be detected. Many 'single' events will be detected. The size of the crystal elements depends on the make and model, but is generally 3 to 6 mm. The elements are arranged in 360° rings, with typically 15 to 30 rings consisting of the order of 10 000 individual crystal elements. The crystal size is one of the main factors in limiting the spatial resolution, commonly 4 mm (FWHM) [7]. Although systems designed for special purposes, such as brain scanning, can achieve 2 mm. The computer system is able to reconstruct the line connecting two detected events in opposite crystals as a line of response (LOR). Millions of LORs are acquired over a period of time and reconstructed to form cross-sectional images using appropriate image reconstruction software.

Attenuation of the annihilation photons within the body is an issue in the same manner as it is for SPECT imaging. Ironically, although the 511 keV photon energy is much higher and therefore much more penetrating than the Tc-99m 140 keV emission most widely used in SPECT, attenuation effects are more pronounced on the reconstructed images. This is because the majority of detected photons will have had to pass through the equivalent of the total body thickness, the exception being activity located close to the body surface. Correction for the qualitative and quantitative impairment of PET images due to attenuation is achieved by the acquisition of CT attenuation correction maps. CT was introduced for this purpose in the early 2000s and all PET equipment now has diagnostic quality CT units attached. As for SPECT, the primary purpose of the CT is for its correction function, but the quality of the CT greatly enhances the diagnostic capability of the modality as functional and structural information is fused on a single set of images.

RADIOPHARMACEUTICALS

A wide range of radiopharmaceuticals is available [8]. The most common route of administration is intravenous, but radiopharmaceuticals may be administered orally or by inhalation. The intramuscular, intracavity and intrathecal routes are possible, but rare.

When deciding upon the efficacy of a given radiopharmaceutical, the physical and chemical properties of the radionuclide, together with biochemical, physiological and pharmacological properties of the pharmaceutical, must be considered.

The radionuclide

The best possible radionuclide to use for any given procedure will depend upon its properties, which include:

- type of radiation emitted, its energy and abundance
- half-life
- specific activity
- radionuclidic purity
- chemical properties of the element.

Each of these properties is considered below.

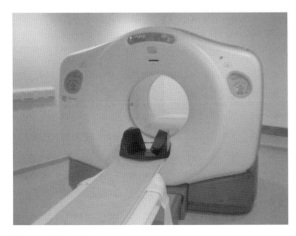

Figure 6.3 Dedicated PET camera.

Type of radiation

Diagnostic imaging involves external detection of the isotope. Therefore, the required physical characteristics include the emission of gamma or x-radiation.

The photon energy should be high enough to avoid serious attenuation in tissue, but low enough to allow the photon to be stopped by and interact with the detector. The design characteristics of a gamma camera favour photons with energies between 75 keV and 300 keV. Selecting radionuclides that have a monoenergetic emission is an advantage as a single energy window will minimize the quantity of scattered radiation contributing to the image. Absorbed radiation dose to the patient will be kept as low as reasonably practicable (ALARP) if the radionuclide has no particulate emission and decays with a high abundance of gamma photons. Technetium-99m does not emit any particles and provides 89 photons of 140 keV for every 100 disintegrations.

Physical half-life

The half-life of the radionuclide must be sufficiently long to allow for production, administration, localization and imaging of the radiopharmaceutical within the organ of interest. At the same time, it should be remembered that the radiation dose to the patient is proportional to the half-life of the radionuclide (see Chapter 1) and therefore the half-life should be as short as possible.

As a rule of thumb, radionuclides are used that have half-lives of similar duration to that of the study. However, there are exceptions and some of these are described and explained with regard to biological half-life (see Chapter 7).

Specific activity

Specific activity should not be confused with radioactive concentration which has units of activity per volume. Specific activity is activity per unit mass and therefore it has units of Becquerel per gram or mole. There is a maximum specific activity for each radionuclide, which depends upon its physical half-life. Specific activity gives an indication of the ratio of radioactive to non-radioactive atoms of the element in the sample.

Generally, it is best to use as high a specific activity as possible. This allows very small quantities to be used which will help to ensure that the radiolabel does not significantly alter the chemical or biological properties of the pharmaceutical to which it is attached. However, carrier-free samples can be difficult to work with because there is so little mass of the element present, for example 500 MBq of carrier-free technetium-99m has a mass of 2 ng.

Radionuclidic purity

Radionuclidic purity is the fraction of the total radioactivity in the sample that is in the form of the desired radionuclide. Radionuclidic contaminants may increase the radiation dose to the patient or degrade the image. Therefore, it is important to have the highest possible radionuclidic purity. Impurities can arise from the manufacturing process, from daughter radionuclides or from parent radionuclides.

Chemical properties

Even if the radionuclide has ideal physical properties, it is of little value if it has no useful chemical properties that it can trace, or if it cannot be efficiently and securely attached to a suitable pharmaceutical. The success of technetium-99m as the radionuclide of choice in diagnostic imaging is due in no small part to the way in which its chemistry has been exploited.

Chemical toxicity is normally not a matter of concern as radiopharmaceuticals are administered in such extremely small quantities, of the order of nanograms. This amount is so small that it is uncommon for the administration of a radioactive material to a patient to cause any interference at all with the physiological effects being investigated.

The ideal radionuclide for imaging

Technetium-99m comes close to meeting the requirements of a near ideal radionuclide for imaging. It has a monoenergetic gamma emission of 140 keV, high abundance, no accompanying particulate emissions, a half-life of 6 hours and decays to an effectively stable daughter product. It is readily available from a molybdenum-99 generator in a chemical form that can be attached to a range of pharmaceuticals.

Mechanisms of localization

Radiopharmaceuticals can be divided into two major categories depending upon whether or not their localization within the body involves their participation in a specific chemical reaction. Many traditional radiopharmaceuticals, such as technetium-99m macroaggregated albumin (MAA) for lung perfusion imaging, are not incorporated into specific biochemical pathways but rely for their utility on the correct molecular size and route of administration. The most exciting developments in recent years have involved radiopharmaceuticals whose precise chemical nature has allowed specific biochemical pathways to be investigated, for example, technetium-99m depreotide (NeoSpect) [9], a synthetic peptide designed to assist in the investigation of a solitary pulmonary nodule.

A more detailed breakdown of mechanisms that determine the localization and behaviour of radiopharmaceuticals is given below.

Diffusion and isotope dilution

Tracers may be used that distribute themselves throughout the space in the body into which they were introduced. Imaging of their distribution can identify the extent of these areas or demonstrate where their natural boundaries have broken down. For example, ventilation imaging, which depends upon the inhalation of a suitable tracer, such as krypton-81m gas, into the lungs where it diffuses throughout the functioning air spaces, allowing them to be visualized.

Isotope dilution is a quantitative method which depends on complete mixing of a radiopharmaceutical throughout a body space. Knowledge of the administered activity and the radioactive concentration of a sample of the fluid within the space once mixing is complete, will allow the volume of the space to be calculated. An example is the determination of red cell mass.

Capillary blockade and cell sequestration

If radioactive particles in the size range 20–50 μm are injected into the vascular system, they will partially occlude the first capillary bed they encounter (the size of capillaries is 8–10 μm). An intravenous injection of half a million technetium-99m labelled particles of MAA will block approximately 0.05% of the capillaries of a normal lung, thus permitting the visualization of the vascular bed of the lungs. A protein such as albumin is chosen for production of the particles, as it will be broken down naturally and removed from the lungs.

Phagocytosis

The reticuloendothelial[1] cells in the body have the capacity to ingest bacteria and small particles in the range 0.01–10 μm. This is known as phagocytosis. If a radio-labelled colloid is injected intravenously, the phagocytic action of the reticuloendothelial cells, in particular the Kupffer cells in the liver, will remove the colloid from the circulation, enabling the organ to be visualized. Areas of non-functioning liver tissue will not remove colloid material.

Metabolic pathway

The metabolic pathway of a huge number of substances can be investigated using radioactive techniques. They may be designed specifically to trace a particular body function, such as technetium-99m-labelled mercapto acetyl triglycine (MAG3) for the investigation of kidney function.

Iodine is incorporated into the hormones produced by the thyroid gland, and a study of the metabolic behaviour of iodine in the body gives valuable diagnostic information

on thyroid function. Radioactive iodine introduced into the body therefore enables iodine metabolism to be studied easily. Iodine-131 and iodine-123 are two radionuclides commonly used for imaging thyroid tissue (see below).

Metabolic trapping

Some radiopharmaceuticals become trapped within the tissue into which they have been transported by metabolic processes. Certain radiopharmaceuticals have been developed specifically to exhibit this behaviour. For example, technetium-99m tetrofosmin and methoxy isobutyl isonitrile (MIBI) were developed to mimic the distribution of uptake of thallium-201 used in myocardial perfusion. Thallium-201 washes out of the tissues quickly but the technetium-99m-labelled analogues are trapped, allowing plenty of time for the distribution of tracer to be imaged.

F-18 fluorodeoxyglucose (F-18 FDG) is the most widely used radiopharmaceutical in PET imaging. It is commonly described as a metabolic marker. Its chemistry is modified by the label so that it becomes trapped with cells and its method of localization comes under the heading of metabolic trapping rather than metabolic pathway (see below).

Antibodies and antibody fragments

Antibodies are large Y-shaped molecules consisting of proteins. They form part of the body's immune response. The body manufactures them as needed to neutralize the threat posed to the body by foreign or harmful material. The material that triggers the antibody response is called the antigen. Antibodies are produced in the body at the site of need. They are not designed to be carried in the blood seeking out suitable receptors but that is what nuclear medicine requires of them as diagnostic or therapeutic agents. One possible solution to this dilemma is to split them into fragments which retain the functionality but are more mobile than the whole antibody.

Antibodies can be raised against substances which are not foreign to the body. For example, there are anti-leukocyte antibodies. These, or fragments of them, can be radiolabeled and used to investigate the distribution of circulating leukocytes and sites of accumulation of them in the body (see below).

Potentially there are an enormous number of antibodies that could be used in nuclear medicine but only a handful is available commercially.

Receptor binding

The experience gained in attempting to label antibodies has paid dividends in the area of receptor labelling. Receptors are found in all areas of the body and their specificity has been exploited in various commercially available products. One example is Octreotide, a somatostatin receptor imaging agent, formulated to be labelled with indium-111. It can be used to investigate and treat neuroendocrine and other tumours (see below).

---

[1]Reticuloendothelial cells are concerned with defense against microbial infection and with the removal of worn-out blood cells from the blood stream (taken from the Oxford Medical Dictionary, 4th edn, (2007), Oxford University Press).

Production and quality control of radiopharmaceuticals

For the vast majority of studies, radiopharmaceuticals are bought from a supplier; either as the labelled compound ready for administration or as a sterile kit containing the chemicals to label the desired radionuclide on site. The chemicals are supplied freeze dried in a vial ready to be reconstituted when needed. The most common type is the technetium-99m 'cold' kit. There are many examples of these. They all contain the pharmaceutical itself, some form of reducing agent to pull the technetium away from its pertechnetate environment and additional material required to bulk out the contents so that they freeze-dry successfully. There may be additional chemicals to buffer the solution to ensure that it maintains the correct pH and other substances required to ensure optimum chemical binding between the radionuclide and the pharmaceutical. The pertechnetate itself is obtained from a molybdenum-99 generator, obtained from a manufacturer once or twice a week, and eluted once or twice a day.

The bulk of the quality control of a radiopharmaceutical or its components is the responsibility of the manufacturer. However, each nuclear medicine department is required to ensure the quality of the radiopharmaceuticals it uses. For the majority of diagnostic tests, intravenous injection is necessary so great care must be taken to produce a radiopharmaceutical in a sterile solution of the correct pH value and free from foreign proteins arising from previous bacteriological activity (pyrogens). To ensure this, they are obtained from an on-site or off-site radiopharmacy which is either licensed by the Medicines and Healthcare Products Regulatory Agency (MHRA) or can claim an exemption under the Medicines Act 1968 [10].

Specialized cabinets are used to provide an environment that caters for the conflicting requirements of the radiation safety of the operator and the need for aseptic production. For radiation safety, it is customary to provide an environment at a lower pressure than its surroundings to contain any airborne contaminants. However, the preparation area must be bathed in pure sterile air at a pressure higher than that of the surroundings so as to avoid inward leakage of non-sterile air and micro-organisms. The labelling of a patient's own cells is classed as a medical procedure and is undertaken in specialized facilities with more stringent requirements for protection of the operator and the product.

Prior to administration, the label on the vial, syringe or capsule, if oral administration, is checked against that prescribed for the procedure. The activity given to the patient is checked independently on a radionuclide calibrator which measures the activity in MBq for the radionuclide specified. The consistency of the radionuclide calibrator is checked daily and its calibration is traceable to national standards. The activity is noted in the patient record. These checks are required under the Medicines Act and the Ionising Radiation (Medical Exposures) Regulations 2000 [11].

If the binding of the radionuclide to the pharmaceutical is poor, the distribution of radioactivity in the body may appear unusual or abnormal. Poor binding can be due to the radiopharmaceutical or one of its components or it may be due to a fault in reconstitution. Radiopharmacies measure the radiochemical purity, usually by chromatography, to check the binding. Unusual distributions in images should be reported to the radiopharmacy for investigation, although other situations can arise that will modify the distribution. For example, a woman who is breastfeeding may exhibit increased uptake of radioactivity due to uptake into milk. Also, prescribed and over-the-counter drugs may affect the distribution of a radiopharmaceutical.

CLINICAL APPLICATIONS

Imaging of the distribution of a radiopharmaceutical within an organ and, in some cases, how it changes with time, enables deductions to be made about the function of the organ. An abnormal distribution may appear as an increase in radioactive concentration above the surroundings or the expected margins, revealing lesions as 'hot spots'; or as reduced activity in the visualized pattern. The appearance of 'hot spots' does not necessarily mean that a lesion is larger than the minimum resolvable power of the gamma camera; if the amount of activity accumulated in the lesion is large enough compared to its surroundings, the lesion will be detected in the image. 'Cold spots' are sometimes referred to as photopenic areas; they are more difficult to detect than 'hot spots' because the margins are blurred with respect to the surroundings.

The purpose of imaging is to investigate organ function rather than anatomical definition. The following provides a brief description of some of the more important clinical applications of radionuclide imaging, directly or closely applicable to imaging cancer.

Table 6.1 is a list of commonly used radiopharmaceuticals with notes on their more important uses, details of the diagnostic reference level, the absorbed dose to the critical organ and the effective dose to the whole body from ICRP 80 [12].

Table 6.2 gives comparative examples of the effective dose from some common radiopharmaceutical investigations and common radiology investigations.

Bone imaging

Bone imaging is the most widely used investigation in nuclear medicine and the majority of referrals relate to patients with known primary tumours and suspected bone secondaries. Bone is made up of collagen and minerals, mainly calcium, phosphates and hydroxides. The minerals

Table 6.1 Examples of some radionuclides in common diagnostic use with critical organ (CO), effective dose (ED) and diagnostic reference level (DRL) activity

RADIONUCLIDE	CHEMICAL FORM	CLINICAL USE	DRL ACTIVITY (MBq)	PHYSICAL HALF-LIFE	ROUTE	CO	DOSE TO CO FROM ACTIVITY (mSv)	ED FROM ACTIVITY (mSv)
Chromium-51	Sodium chromate	Red blood cell volume	4	27.8 days	Red cell labelling and IV	Spleen	6.4	0.7
Cobalt-57	Cyanacobalamin vitamin B12	GI absorption	0.04	270 days	Oral	Pancreas	0.2	0.2
Fluorine-18	Fluoro-deoxy glucose (FDG)	Tumour imaging	400	110 min	IV	Bladder	64	8
Gallium-67	Gallium citrate	Tumour and inflamation imaging	150	78.3 h	IV	Gonads	10	15
Krypton-81m	Gas	Lung ventilation imaging	6000	13 s	Inhalation	Lungs	1	0.2
Indium-111	Indium oxide labelled leukocytes	Infection and abscess imaging	20	2.8 days	Leukocyte labelling and IV	Spleen	110	7
Iodine-123	Sodium iodide	Thyroid imaging	20	13.2 h	Oral or IV	Thyroid	90	4 for 35% uptake
Iodine-125	Human serum albumin (HSA)	Plasma volume measurement	0.2	60 days	IV	Heart	0.1	0.04
Iodine-131	Sodium iodide	Thyroid metastases imaging	400	8.1 days	Oral or IV	Bladder	244	24 for 0% uptake
Technecium-99m	Sodium pertechnetate	Thyroid imaging	80	6 h	IV	Colon	3	1

Continued

Table 6.1 Examples of some radionuclides in common diagnostic use with critical organ (CO), effective dose (ED) and diagnostic reference level (DRL) activity—cont'd

RADIONUCLIDE	CHEMICAL FORM	CLINICAL USE	DRL ACTIVITY (MBq)	PHYSICAL HALF-LIFE	ROUTE	CO	DOSE TO CO FROM ACTIVITY (mSv)	ED FROM ACTIVITY (mSv)
Technecium-99m	Sodium pertechnetate	Meckels diverticulum imaging	400	6 h	IV	Colon	17	5
Technecium-99m	Macro aggregated albumin (MAA)	Lung perfusion imaging	100	6 h	IV	Lungs	7	1
Technecium-99m	Exametazine HMPAO	Regional cerebral bloodflow imaging	500	6 h	IV	Kidney	17	5
Technecium-99m	HM PAO attached to leukocytes	Infection imaging	200	6 h	Leukocyte labelling and IV	Spleen	30	2
Technecium-99m	Pentetate (DTPA)	Kidney renogram imaging	300	6 h	IV	Bladder wall	19	2
Technecium-99m	Pentetate (DTPA) as aerosol	Lung ventilation imaging	80	6 h	Inhalation	Lungs	1	0.5
Technecium-99m	MAG3	Renal imaging	100	6 h	IV	Bladder	11	0.7
Technecium-99m	Phosphonate (MDP, HDP)	Bone imaging	600	6 h	IV	Bladder	29	3
Technecium-99m	Succimer (DMSA)	Kidney imaging	80	6 h	IV	Kidneys	14	0.7
Technecium-99m	MIBI or tetrofosmin	Myocardial perfusion at rest or exercise	400	6 h	IV	Colon	7–10	3–4
Thallium-201	Thallous chloride	Myocardial perfusion imaging	80	73.1 h	IV	Gonads	47	18
Xenon-133	Gas	Lung ventilation imaging	400	5.25 days	Inhalation	Gonads	0.5	0.4

Table 6.2 Effective dose from some common radiopharmaceutical and radiological examinations

RADIOPHARMACEUTICAL EXAMINATION	ACTIVITY (MBq)	EFFECTIVE DOSE (mSv)	RADIOLOGICAL EXAMINATION	EFFECTIVE DOSE (mSv)
[^{18}F] FDG	400	7.8	Chest	0.05
[^{57}Co] Vitamin B$_{12}$	0.04	0.1	Abdomen	1.4
[^{67}Ga] Gallium citrate	150	17	Pelvis	1.2
[^{99m}Tc] Technetium pertechnetate	80	1	Barium meal	3.8
[^{99m}Tc] Technecium phosphonate	600	3	Barium aenema	7.7
[^{201}Tl] Thallous ion	80	18		

form a crystalline lattice known as hydroxyapatite. Following intravenous injection, a bone-seeking agent will be transported to the bone and become adsorbed on to the newly forming hydroxyapatite crystals, thus reflecting the bone-forming (or osteoblastic) activity at a given skeletal site. Hence, areas where there is an abnormally high increase in bone turnover will show increased uptake and will appear as 'hot spots' on the image. Since localization on bone depends on transportation in blood, avascular areas will appear 'cold'. Conversely, areas of locally-increased blood flow may appear as areas of increased uptake on the scan.

All current commercially-available bone-seeking radiopharmaceuticals are based on phosphate-containing compounds which can be labelled with technetium-99m. A variety of analogues is available but the most widely used is methylene diphosphonate (medronate or MDP). Typically, 400–600 MBq of technetium-99m medronate is administered intravenously and, after a period of 3–4 hours (to enable circulating activity to clear), approximately 40% of the injected activity will be localized in the bone, with the major part of the remainder being excreted via the kidneys. Multiple static views or a combination of a whole body image and selected static views are acquired. Tomography may also be helpful. A normal bone scan is shown in Figure *evolve* 6.4 🖱 and a bone scan showing secondary deposits is shown in Figure *evolve* 6.5 🖱.

The bone scan is a very sensitive technique for demonstrating bone lesions and shows changes earlier than conventional x-ray. However, the findings are non-specific and additional cross-sectional imaging (CT or MR) may be required for further evaluation.

Tumour imaging

Nuclear medicine can employ many agents to aid in tumour localization, to follow the progress of treatment. This section describes non-specific tumour agents, such as gallium, thallium and MIBI, as well as several specific tumour agents and studies.

Gallium

Gallium-67 citrate has a long history of use in radionuclide imaging. It was the first agent used for the investigation of infection and has also been used in many different tumour types and in suspected osteomyelitis. Its use has gradually decreased over the years as more specific agents have been developed but it still has a place in the investigation of sarcoidosis of the lung and, in oncology, for the investigation of inflammation or neoplastic disorders, where other modalities have been unhelpful, and in fever of unknown origin.

It is injected intravenously and binds immediately to transferrin which localizes in normal spleen, liver, gastrointestinal tract, kidneys and, to a certain extent, in bone. It also localizes in inflammation, infection and many tumour types. Uptake is therefore widespread and diffuse.

Thallium

Thallium-201 as thallous chloride is handled by the body in a similar way to potassium which is why it has been employed to investigate the parathyroid and myocardial perfusion. Incidental findings on such studies indicated that it could also be taken up by some tumours. The mechanism is uncertain but it has found a role in some centres in the localization of viable tissue, particularly in brain tumour and osteosarcoma.

MIBI

Technetium-99m MIBI was developed to replace thallium-201, and was also noted to localize in tumours while it was under clinical evaluation as a myocardial perfusion agent. It has found an application in the localization of breast tumours.

mIBG

Meta iodobenzyl guanidine (mIBG) is an analogue of norepinephrine (noradrenaline) and guanethidine. It is available radiolabelled with iodine-123 for diagnostic imaging and with iodine-131 for pretreatment dosimetry and therapy. Normal adrenal medulla tissue will concentrate the agent as will neuroendocrine tumours or tumours of neural crest origin, such as phaeochromocytoma, neuroblastoma, carcinoid tumours and medullary carcinoma of the thyroid. Uptake into tumour can be inhibited by many drugs, including tricyclic antidepressants; therefore care must be taken to withdraw any potentially interfering medication well in advance.

Octreotide – somatostatin receptor imaging

Somatostatin is a 14-amino acid peptide found in brain, where it acts as a neurotransmitter, in the gastrointestinal tract, as well as the pancreas, where it is manufactured. It inhibits the release of neuroendocrine hormones, such as growth hormone and insulin.

Somatostatin receptors are found in normal pituitary, pancreas and upper gastrointestinal tract from stomach to jejunum. They are also expressed by a variety of endocrine tumours, such as carcinoid, small cell lung cancer, in tumours of ovary, cervix, endometrium, breast, kidney, larynx, paranasal sinus, salivary gland and some skin tumours, and tumours arising from glial cells in the central nervous system. It can be surmised that somatostatin receptor imaging could therefore be clinically useful in a variety of tumours. However, somatostatin has a half-life of only 2 to 3 minutes in the body so such imaging was not feasible until the availability of Octreotide [8], a somatostatin analogue with a much longer clearance time than the natural peptide.

Octreoscan is a kit which enables the attachment of indium-111 via pentetate to Octreotide to form pentetreotide. Sufficient pentetreotide uptake for visualization can occur with many carcinoid tumours, pituitary tumours, gastrointestinal tract endocrine tumours (although disappointing in insulinoma), small cell lung cancer, medullary carcinoma of thyroid, neuroblastoma, pheochromocytoma, meningioma, Hodgkin's and non-Hodgkin's lymphoma. Many of these tumours may be better visualized with CT and MRI, but pentetreotide imaging may be used to demonstrate small symptomatic tumours and metastatic spread, although hepatic metastases are difficult to visualize because of uptake in normal liver. Evidence of pentetreotide uptake is a guide for therapy with octreotide, especially for carcinoid tumours. Figure *evolve* 6.6 🎯 shows an indium-111 Octreotide SPECT/CT image of a patient with multiple neuroendocrine tumour metastases in the liver.

Oncoscint

Oncoscint [8] was the first monoclonal antibody to be approved by the Food and Drugs Agency (FDA) for use in the USA. It is indium-111 labelled B72.3 or satumomab, a murine monoclonal antibody which targets Tag-72 which is a cell-surface antigen expressed by colorectal carcinoma cells. It may be used for the detection of local recurrence and extra-hepatic metastases in colorectal and ovarian cancer but its role is controversial.

Imaging thyroid cancer

Nuclear medicine imaging of the thyroid plays a minor role in the initial diagnosis of thyroid cancer. Ultrasound and fine needle aspiration (FNA) is the first line imaging technique [13].

The normal function of the thyroid gland includes the concentration of iodine from the circulation, and the synthesis and storage of thyroid hormones. Iodine may also be trapped in the salivary glands and the gastric mucosa. Iodine-131 was once the radionuclide of choice for all thyroid imaging. However, because it delivers a relatively high radiation dose to the patient and it has poorer imaging properties, it has been almost completely superseded by iodine-123 and technetium-99m pertechnetate for routine diagnostic thyroid imaging. Iodine-131 continues to be used for therapy (see Chapter 7) and, in some centres, for whole body imaging in patients who have previously undergone treatment for thyroid cancer and where further disease is suspected.

Figure *evolve* 6.7 🎯 shows a whole body I-131 scan on a patient previously treated for thyroid cancer but with widespread metastases. Sometimes suspected thyroid metastases do not appear 'hot' on the I-131 scan. In such circumstances, they may be designated to be 'not iodine avid' and an F-18 FDG study may be considered for further evaluation.

Cardiac imaging

The commonest cardiac investigation performed in the nuclear medicine department on oncology patients is gated blood pool imaging. It is correctly called equilibrium radionuclide ventriculography but more often termed a MUGA (multiple gated acquisition) scan. It is used to evaluate cardiac function, in terms of left ventricular ejection fraction, prior to and in response to the administration of potentially cardiotoxic chemotherapeutic drugs.

The heart is a muscular organ divided internally by a muscular septum into right and left sides, each side having two chambers. The right and left atria receive blood returning from the pulmonary and systemic circulations. The right and left ventricles are pumping chambers and are more muscular, particularly the left ventricle (LV), which pumps the blood to the systemic circulation.

Left ventricular ejection fraction (LVEF) is one of the major indicators of cardiac function. It can be investigated by means of a MUGA scan which is taken 20–30 minutes following a two-stage injection procedure. A non-radioactive or 'cold' injection of pyrophosphate is followed by 400–800 MBq of technetium-99m pertechnetate, both administered intravenously. Due to the 'cold' pre-injection, labeling of the patient's red cells takes place in vivo. By using the R-wave of the patient's ECG to gate (i.e. control) image acquisition, a series of 16 to 24 images is recorded during each cardiac cycle and stored in time order on computer. Data collection continues for 10 to 15 minutes. Images of adequate spatial resolution for the purpose are obtained by summing images of identical time segments in several hundred cardiac cycles. The MUGA images can be processed to produce amplitude and phase images that aid the delineation of the left ventricle and the demonstration of paradoxical motion. Amplitude refers to the magnitude of the change of the LV image intensity, while phase refers to the timing of the intensity change within the cycle. The LVEF is derived from the maximum counts (C_{max}) and minimum counts (C_{min}) in the left ventricle over the cardiac cycle, Equation 6.1, and is usually expressed as a percentage. All counts are corrected for background.

$$LVEF = (C_{max} - C_{min})/C_{max}$$ **6.1**

The technique is recognized as the 'gold standard' [14] for LVEF estimation among competing modalities as it does not rely on geometrical approximations to the shape of the heart chamber but derives its values from the entire ventricle, including any effect due to paradoxical motion. Figure *evolve* 6.8 shows images from a patient with a normal LVEF.

MUGA scans image radioactive labeled blood within the heart. Blood flow to the heart muscle itself (myocardial perfusion) can be imaged using technetium-99m methoxy isobutyl isonitrile (MIBI) or tetrofosmin. Thallium-201 was once the most common agent but, due to its higher radiation dose, more limited availability and less favorable imaging characteristics, has been superseded in popularity. All of these radiopharmaceuticals distribute themselves within the heart muscle according to blood flow through the coronary arteries. Tomographic images are taken under stress and at rest and the results used in the differential diagnosis of normal myocardial perfusion, ischemia and infarction. These studies have an important role in diagnosis of heart disease in patients with low to medium probability and in prognosis. The LVEF can be derived from gated myocardial perfusion tomography but the results are not as reliable as those from the MUGA, particularly where the position of a substantial part of the myocardial wall must be inferred because there is no blood flow within it. MUGA scanning is used extensively in patients being treated for breast cancer, particularly those receiving Herceptin and the anthracycline group of cytotoxic agents that can be cardiotoxic.

Kidney imaging

The kidney produces urine and disposes of metabolic waste products. It is divided into an outer cortical and an inner medullary region. Urine drains from the medullary region via the renal pelvis into the ureter and thence into the bladder. Several radiopharmaceuticals are available for imaging the kidney and investigating renal function. The choice of pharmaceutical depends on the specific renal function measurements required and the clinical condition being studied.

The commonest reason for renal isotope investigation in oncology patients is to investigate suspected obstruction to urine drainage down the ureters caused by primary tumour masses, such as gynecological pelvic malignancy or bladder and prostate carcinomas, or by secondary metastatic disease spread to lymph nodes in the para-aortic or iliac chains, which lie adjacent to the ureters. The non-imaging test, glomerular filtration rate (GFR) is also common in oncology patients; as part of the algorithm for the prescription of carboplatin or to investigate kidney function prior to and in response to any potentially nephrotoxic drug.

The most widely used radiopharmaceuticals for kidney function imaging are technetium-99m tiatide (MAG3) and pentetate (DTPA). They are suitable for the assessment of individual kidney function, and investigation of drainage. With the kidneys and bladder in the field of view of the gamma camera, up to 80 MBq of technetium-99m MAG3 is injected intravenously. For the following 20 minutes a series of images (generally 20 s frames) is acquired. Regions of interest are defined around the kidneys and bladder and, after suitable background correction, time–activity curves can be generated for each region. This set of curves is termed a renogram. Often, the term is also used to denote the entire investigation.

Figure *evolve* 6.9 shows the renogram results from a patient with one normally functioning kidney and one obstructed kidney.

Other renal agents include technetium-99m dimercapto succinic acid (DMSA), used primarily in the investigation of renal scarring, often in children.

Infection imaging

A patient's own leukocytes (white cells) will accumulate at the site of infection, so one method of localizing infection is to label autologous white cells with a suitable radionuclide. Two are available: indium-111 and technetium-99m. Both labelling processes involve taking up to 200 ml blood from the patient and leaving it to settle under gravity for about an hour. This enables reasonable separation of white cells from the rest of the blood. The cells are incubated with either indium-111 as oxine or tropolonate or technetium-99m as HM-PAO marketed as Ceretec, which was originally developed for cerebral perfusion studies. The labelling technique is not available in many centres as it is labour-intensive, requiring skilled experienced staff and specialized aseptic facilities. An alternative is technetium-99m labelled Leukoscan, or sulesomab, an anti-leukocyte antibody fragment.

The use of gallium-67 citrate in the localization of infection is discussed under its general entry above.

Sentinel node mapping

Lymphatic vessels receive cellular waste and discharge it from the body. The waste is filtered through nodes within the vessels. Metastatic spread from some tumours is carried by the lymphatics and sites of disease are found within the lymph nodes.

Breast cancer is known to spread in this way and almost all of the associated lymph nodes are located in the axilla. A widely used approach by breast surgeons was to perform a full axillary clearance of lymph nodes along with surgical removal of the breast in patients with breast carcinoma. Should histology have subsequently failed to find any evidence of metastatic spread in the nodes, this signalled a good prognosis for the patient. Unfortunately, some of these patients went on to suffer the morbidity associated with the removal of the nodes, including severe oedema of the arm.

A technique has been developed to locate the node(s) nearest to the tumour site; this is referred to as the sentinel node(s). In a subgroup of breast tumour patients a Tc-99m labeled nanacolliod is injected sub- or intra-dermally in the peripheral areola region of the breast quadrant containing the tumour. Many centres will image the breast on a gamma camera post-injection and identify the number and general location of the sentinel nodes. Figure *evolve* 6.10 🖱 shows the sentinel lymph node images of a patient immediately prior to surgery. Injection and imaging, if performed, take place either on the morning of the surgery or the previous afternoon. Patients will have the sentinel nodes located in theatre with the aid of an intra-operative probe system (Figure *evolve* 6.11 🖱). Histological evaluation of the sentinel nodes will influence the patients' subsequent treatment pathway. The technique is now also used for melanoma and vulva tumours and other tumour sites are being investigated.

PET/CT imaging

The increased glucose metabolism of malignant cells compared to healthy tissue makes the positron emitting tracer, fluorine-18 fluorodeoxyglucose (FDG) particularly useful in oncology. Detailed descriptions of clinical PET and PET/CT can be found in Barrington et al [15] and Lin et al [16]. The increased metabolism of glucose in malignant cells is due to upregulation of the enzyme hexokinase and increased levels of the membrane transport proteins GLUT1 and GLUT3. Overexpression of GLUT1 and GLUT3 is primarily seen in the rim of hypoxic tumour tissue. The production of ATP is maintained by upregulation of glucose transport and glycolysis even in the presence of hypoxia. The metabolism of glucose is partly regulated by the transcription factor hypoxia-inducible factor 1 (HIF-1). HIF-1 stimulates the expression of more than 40 genes, including vascular endothelial growth factor (VEGF), insulin-like growth factor 2 (IGF-II), GLUT 1, and 3, and several glycolytic enzymes, e.g. hexokinase 1 and 3. It has been demonstrated that the activity of tumour cell hexokinase, which can be indirectly measured by FDG-PET, is correlated to the growth rate of tumours.

Therefore, determination by PET of the uptake of FDG during and after antineoplastic treatment may be used as an early indicator of response to treatment. The reaction to radiotherapy or chemotherapy treatment may be an initial rise in FDG-uptake, followed by a decrease, the magnitude of which can serve as a marker of treatment response. However, FDG is also taken up in inflammatory lesions giving rise to a non-specificity which presents limitations, and requires caution, in the interpretation of the PET/CT scan. The optimal timing of post-treatment evaluation by PET/CT is not established and is the subject of current research, probably depending on tumour type and treatment modality.

A growing body of literature has now led to FDG-PET being used routinely in the clinic for the detection and staging of malignant tumours, determining the extent of spread of disease (including assessment of the suitability of patients for radical surgery), differentiation of mass lesions, establishing response to therapy, and long-term follow up for detection of recurrent disease.

A great number of other compounds have also been labelled with fluorine-18, such as fluorofatty acids, fluoroamino acids, spiperone derivatives, fluoromisonidazole (FMISO), and fluoroaltanserin. More recently, a fluorine-18 labeled pyrimidine analogue, 3'-deoxy-3'-fluorothymidine (FLT) has shown promise as a marker of tumour cell proliferation. This has the potential to provide more specific and effective PET/CT measurements for monitoring response to therapy. Previously, work on cell proliferation using the equivalent carbon-11 labelled compound, carbon-11 thymidine, has been published by a number of research groups, but it is anticipated that FLT will be superior due to its longer half-life (110 min for fluorine-18, 20 min for carbon-11), allowing simpler metabolite corrections, and longer, more practicable, image acquisition times.

A number of other medium half-life, inorganic positron emitting radionuclides are becoming available. Their half-lives of several hours offer considerable advantages for supply from regional distribution centres. Iodine-124 ($t_{1/2} = 100$ h) or iodine-120 ($t_{1/2} = 1.4$ h) may be used to label tracers and ligands that have been labelled with iodine-123 or iodine-131. 5-Iododeoxyuridine (IUdR), offers potential as a radiotracer for functional imaging of cell proliferation. Bromine-176 ($t_{1/2} = 16$ h) has also been used as a PET label for a variety of compounds, including deoxyuridine deriviatives as proliferation markers and antibodies. Macromolecules, such as peptides (e.g. octreotide) and proteins (e.g. monoclonal antibodies), are also amenable to radiolabelling with such radionuclides. Perfusion and permeability clinical studies have been demonstrated using copper-64 ($t_{1/2} = 12.7$ h) as a label for the perfusion/flow marker copper-64 PTSM (Cu(II)-pyruvaldehyde-bis(N^4-methylthiosemicarbazone)).

Further opportunities are possible using positron emitter generator systems, where the parent radionuclide has a much longer half-life than the daughter. A germanium-

68/gallium-68 generator is already available with parent/daughter having half-lives of 268 days and 68 minutes, respectively. Apart from the demonstrated use of gallium-68 for labelling a variety of tracers and ligands, this generator system may be used as a ready supply of radioisotope for phantom and calibration studies.

Figure *evolve* 6.12 🖰 shows an F-18 FDG PET/CT image of a patient with a lung tumour.

REFERENCES

[1] Lowe VJ, et al. Prospective investigation of positron emission tomography in lung nodules. J Clin Oncol 1998;16:1075–84.

[2] Dendy PP, Heaton B. Physics for diagnostic radiology. 2nd ed. Institute of Physics; 2003.

[3] Cherry SR, Sorenson JA, Phelps ME. Physics in nuclear medicine. 3rd ed. Saunders; 2003.

[4] Institute of Physics and Engineering in Medicine (IPEM). Quality control of gamma camera systems. In: Bolster A, editor. Institute of Physics and Engineering in Medicine. 2003.

[5] National Electrical Manufacturers Association (NEMA). Performance measurements of gamma cameras, NU-1. 2007.

[6] Institute of Physics and Engineering in Medicine (IPEM). Recommended standards for the routine performance testing of diagnostic x-ray imaging systems. IPEM Report 91. IPEM. 2005.

[7] Bailey DL, Townsend DW, Valk PE, Maisey MN, editors. Positron emission tomography. Springer-Verlag; 2005.

[8] Welch MJ, Redvanly CS, editors. Handbook of radiopharmaceuticals, radiochemistry and applications. Wiley; 2003.

[9] Bååth M, Kolbeck K, et al. Somatostatin receptor scintigraphy with ^{99m}Tc-depreotide (NeoSpect) in discriminating between malignant and benign lesions in the diagnosis of lung cancer: a pilot study. Acta Radiol 2004;45:833–9.

[10] The Medicines Act 1968. HMSO; 1968.

[11] SI 1059, The Ionising Radiation (Medical Exposure) Regulations 2000. HMSO; 2000.

[12] ICRP Publication 80. Radiation dose to patients from radiopharmaceuticals. Ann ICRP 1998;28(3).

[13] Schoedel KE, Tublin ME, et al. Ultrasound-guided biopsy of the thyroid: a comparison of technique with respect to diagnostic accuracy. Diagn Cytopathol 2008;36:787–9.

[14] Bartlett ML, Srinivasan G, et al. Left ventricular ejection fraction: comparison of results from planar and SPECT gated blood-pool studies. J Nucl Med 1996;37:1795–9.

[15] Barrington SF, Maisey MN, et al. Atlas of clinical positron emission tomography. 2nd ed. Hodder Arnold; 2006.

[16] Lin EC, Alavi A. PET and PET/CT. Thieme; 2005.

EVOLVE CONTENTS (available online at: http://evolve.elsevier.com/Symonds/radiotherapy/)

Chapter | 7 |

Therapy with unsealed radionuclides

Marjorie Rose, Sue Owens, David Hastings

INTRODUCTION

Internal radiation therapy, radionuclide therapy, targeted radiotherapy and unsealed source therapy are some of the terms used for treatments requiring the systemic administration of unsealed or dispersible sources to patients.

In nuclear medicine, radiopharmaceuticals are chosen for their properties of selective uptake. In diagnostic imaging, this is to distinguish the abnormal from the normal. The abnormal tissue or function may have an increased uptake, decreased or absent uptake, or an abnormal pattern or rate of uptake and clearance of the radioactive tracer. The aim is to obtain the information required with the minimum radiation dose. In therapy, the aim is to convey radiation to target tissues, in order to deliver a sufficient radiation dose to the target with a sparing of normal tissue.

The pharmaceutical is chosen to maximize the ratio between the amount deposited in the abnormal or target tissue and the amount deposited in normal or non-target tissue. The other very important characteristic of the pharmaceutical is the biological half-life, which determines how quickly it is cleared from the body. The radioactive label must be chosen to be suitable for the particular application. The radiobiological effects of the emitted ionizing radiations produce the local therapeutic effect in the target tissue. The important properties of the radionuclide are the type and energy of the radiations emitted and the physical half-life.

Again, choosing a radionuclide for therapy may be contrasted with the ideal for diagnosis. In diagnostic imaging, a radionuclide emitting gamma radiation may be desirable, whereas for treatment, non-penetrating radiations, having a short range in tissue, are required. Gamma photons, when present in therapeutic agents, may contribute a radiation dose to non-target tissues and deliver an external radiation dose to other people. All current routine clinical treatments use beta emitters, although alpha-emitting radionuclides have been used in clinical trials. One of the most commonly used beta emitters is iodine-131, which also emits gamma photons. This enables the distribution in the body to be imaged with a gamma camera and can provide data for dosimetry assessments.

The utility of a radiopharmaceutical depends on the effective half-life. The effective half-life is a combination of the physical and biological half-lives and is given by the formula:

$$\frac{1}{T_{eff}} = \frac{1}{T_{biol}} + \frac{1}{T_{phys}}$$

where T_{eff}, T_{biol} and T_{phys} are the effective, biological and physical half-lives. The effective half-life is the important parameter when estimating radiation dose as it determines the duration and rate of delivery of radiation dose.

Radionuclide therapy has been in use since the 1940s and some treatments have been relatively unchanged for several decades. However, more recently, there has been much research effort dedicated to improving strategies for treatment, developing new radiopharmaceuticals and looking at alternative radionuclides to take advantage of different properties. This is ongoing, but has resulted in introductions such as iodine-131 labelled m-IBG in the 1980s, samarium-153 EDTMP in the 1990s, and now radiolabelled monoclonal antibodies for non-Hodgkin's lymphoma (NHL).

The subject is growing and this text has been limited to products with licences or marketing authorizations, but it should be noted that there are many interesting areas of development, such as the use of yttrium-90-labelled somatostatin analogues for neuroendocrine tumours [1–3].

Please note that where a product is unique to a particular company, the trade name has been given.

IODINE-131 IN THE TREATMENT OF THYROID DISEASE

Iodine-131 (^{131}I) is the radionuclide most widely used therapeutically. Iodine is readily concentrated in the thyroid gland and using ^{131}I, emitting beta particles with a maximum range of 3 mm in tissue, allows a high radiation dose to be delivered to the thyroid and a low dose to the rest of the body. It is most commonly used in the form of sodium iodide[^{131}I] for treatment of benign thyroid disease (thyrotoxicosis and non-toxic goiter) and in thyroid carcinoma. It has no role in medullary thyroid cancer. There are specific guidelines [4–6] from the Royal College of Physicians (RCP) in the UK, as well as from Europe and the USA for using radioiodine in the management of hyperthyroidism and of thyroid cancer. The characteristics of ^{131}I are shown in Table 7.1. As specified by the European Association of Nuclear Medicine (EANM) and the Society of Nuclear Medicine (SNM) [5,6], it is essential that, before any treatment, all thyroid hormones, iodine-containing preparations and supplements and any other medications that could suppress thyroid uptake are discontinued for a sufficient length of time. Almost all thyroid treatments are given orally, as a capsule or as a liquid.

Thyrotoxicosis

In thyrotoxicosis, or hyperthyroidism, the thyroid gland is over-producing thyroid hormones. The possible approaches to radionuclide therapy have included giving sufficient radioiodine to render the patient hypothyroid and giving low activities of ^{131}I in combination with anti-thyroid drugs. However, the RCP recommend that the aim of treatment should be to render the patient euthyroid, while accepting that there will be a moderate rate of hypothyroidism [4]. For a standard case of hyperthyroidism, the RCP suggest a guide activity of 400 to 550 MBq at first presentation. An alternative is to use pretreatment thyroid uptake measurements, with tracer activities of ^{131}I, to calculate the activity to be administered to deliver a prescribed radiation dose. Such calculations require knowledge of the thyroid mass, the percentage uptake and the rate of clearance from the gland, requiring repeated measurements over a period of several days. Some centres may use measured uptake and thyroid mass but assume a

Table 7.1 Properties of the radionuclides used in therapy

RADIONUCLIDE	PHYSICAL HALF-LIFE (DAYS)	BETA MEAN ENERGY (MeV)	BETA MEAN RANGE IN SOFT TISSUE (mm)	GAMMA ENERGY (MeV)	GAMMA % ABUNDANCE
^{32}P	14.3	0.70	3.0	–	–
^{89}Sr	50.5	0.58	2.4	0.909	0.01
^{90}Y	2.7	0.935	3.6	–	–
^{131}I	8.02	0.182	0.6	0.364	81.7
^{153}Sm	1.9	0.22	0.6	0.103	28
^{169}Er	9.4	0.099	0.3	–	–
^{186}Re	3.8	0.33	1.1	0.137	9

standard turnover rate. There have been studies looking at the effectiveness of different treatment schedules and corresponding rates of hypothyroidism [7, 8]. Most treatments in the UK are administered to outpatients, although this will depend on the amount of activity prescribed, the patient's home circumstances and national regulations.

Thyroid tumours

There is also a role for ^{131}I in the treatment of well-differentiated thyroid cancer, when it is administered both for the ablation of thyroid remnant after surgery and for the treatment of metastases. Following total thyroidectomy, the aim of remnant ablation is to destroy any remaining normal thyroid tissue and any microscopic deposits of thyroid carcinoma [9]. The RCP guidelines [4] state that the usual activity administered for ablation is 3.7 GBq but that some centres may use a lower activity (1.1 GBq) and, as for thyrotoxicosis, some use a dosimetric assessment of uptake and clearance in order to prescribe an activity. By destroying any remaining thyroid tissue, the theory is that the only remaining source of thyroglobulin production is any remaining malignant cells, thus making the measurements of thyroglobulin level a sensitive test of any local recurrence or metastatic disease. Metastatic lesions have a lower avidity for iodine than normal thyroid tissue and it is customary to administer higher activities, for instance 7 GBq or more. Treatments for thyroid cancer require an in-patient stay, until the level of radioactivity has fallen sufficiently for safe discharge as outlined in the Medical and Dental Guidance Notes (MDGN) [10]. Gamma camera images, using the 364 keV photons of ^{131}I, may be obtained after treatment to confirm uptake in residual thyroid, recurrence or metastases. Scanning protocols may also be used after surgery and before ablation. It may also be used for instance, to determine the completeness of ablation as part of a patient's treatment. Iodine-123 may provide a suitable alternative, with better characteristics for imaging with a gamma camera. The first report of the use of ^{131}I in treating metastatic thyroid cancer was in 1946 [11]. Even 50 years after that first report, much is being discussed and written about optimization of these treatments.

PHOSPHORUS-32 IN THE TREATMENT OF REFRACTORY MYELOPROLIFERATIVE DISEASE

Phosphorus-32 (^{32}P) is a pure beta emitting radionuclide, with a mean particle range in tissue of 3 mm and a maximum of 8 mm. It is available as a sterile solution of ^{32}P orthophosphate in aqueous solution (sodium phosphate [^{32}P]) which is administered either orally or as normally occurs, by intravenous injection. There is no requirement for an in-patient stay. The most common indication is the treatment of polycythaemia rubra vera (PRV), although the treatment may also be used in essential thrombocythaemia, a rare disorder. In the opinion of the EANM, the use of ^{32}P for this indication is declining. However, there seems to be some agreement that it has a role in patients over 70 who are resistant to other treatments such as venesection and conventional chemotherapy [12].

Treatment regimens vary and are a matter for clinical judgment, with typical activities in the range 150–250 MBq. The EANM Guideline suggests two regimens in current use, based on using either an activity per surface area or a fixed starting activity which is incremented. The use of ^{32}P to treat PRV was first reported in 1955 [13], but Parmentier [12], in a review in 2005 stated: 'Few data are available regarding precise dosimetry in man'. An effective dose (ED) of 2.4 mSv/MBq is given by the International Commission for Radiation Protection (ICRP) in ICRP80 [14], with 11 mGy/MBq for both the bone surfaces and red marrow in ICRP53 [15]. Values of the same order of magnitude may be found in the literature.

INTRA-ARTICULAR AND INTRACAVITARY TREATMENTS

Intra-articular treatment of arthritis and other intracavitary treatments are performed using colloids of beta-emitting radioisotopes. Yttrium-90 (^{90}Y) colloids may be administered intrapleurally or intraperitoneally to treat recurring malignant effusions. In such cases, the amount of activity administered is an order of magnitude higher than for the treatment of arthritis.

For arthritis, radiation synovectomy (or radiosynoviorthesis) means radionuclide therapy of joint synovitis or synovial processes by the intra-articular injection of a colloidal radiopharmaceutical. As a general rule, yttrium-90 silicate/citrate is used for large joints like the knee, rhenium-186 sulfide for medium-sized joints such as the hip, shoulder or ankle and erbium-169 citrate for small joints as in the fingers. A major difference between this treatment and the others discussed in the current chapter is the route of administration, which is intra-articular, rather than oral or IV. The radiopharmaceuticals are colloidal and the particles must be small enough to be taken up in the connective tissue lining of the joint cavity called the synovium. This is achieved through the process of phagocytosis by macrophages in the synovium.

The colloidal particles must also be large enough not to leak from the joint before phagocytosis and the appropriate size range is around 2–10 μm. After treatment, absolute immobilization of the treated joint(s) for 48 hours using splints or bed rest is recommended as this will reduce transport of particles through the lymphatics to the regional lymph nodes.

Yttrium-90 (^{90}Y) is a pure beta emitter (see Table 7.1), and the usual activity per knee joint is 185 MBq. Rhenium-186 (^{186}Re) and erbium-169 (^{169}Er) are mentioned for completeness, as they are used outside the UK and discussed in the literature. The rationale for using each radionuclide in different sized joints may be seen by looking at the average penetration of the beta particles in tissue; 3.6 mm for ^{90}Y in large joints, 1.1 mm for ^{186}Re in medium joints and 0.3 mm for ^{169}Er in small joints. The high energy beta particles emitted by ^{90}Y result in the production of bremsstralung radiation (see Chapter 2), which can be detected externally.

PALLIATION OF BONE PAIN

Radionuclide therapy gives an additional possibility for the palliation of bone pain arising from osteoblastic metastases, which are seen in some cancers with a high prevalence, such as breast and prostate carcinoma. This systemic approach may be used for patients with multifocal osteoblastic metastases, as an alternative to external beam radiotherapy, or for those whose pain is refractory to conventional analgesia or antitumour therapy [16, 17]. Before administration of the treatment, it is essential to verify that there is evidence of focal increased uptake on bone scintigraphy. Such increased uptake is due to an osseous reaction to the development of metastases and, if it is not present on a gamma camera bone scan using a ^{99}Tc^{m} imaging agent (e.g. MDP or HDP, see Chapter 6), there will be no selective uptake of the therapeutic radionuclide and, therefore, no benefit.

The most widely used radiopharmaceuticals for this treatment are ^{89}Sr strontium chloride (Metastron®) and ^{153}Sm lexindonam (ethylene diamine tetramethylene phosphonate or EDTMP: Quadramet®) [18]. The characteristics of ^{89}Sr and ^{153}Sm are given in Table 7.1 with further details in Table 7.2. Two further materials are mentioned in the SNM and EANM guidelines [5, 6], ^{186}Re etidronate (hydroxyl ethylidine diphosphonate or

HEDP) [19] and ^{32}P sodium phosphate [20]. Considering the two more commonly used radionuclides, it should be noted that the physical half-lives are very different, 1.9 days for ^{153}Sm and 50.5 days for ^{89}Sr and there is also a variation in the beta particle energies and hence the mean range in tissue, 0.6 mm for ^{153}Sm and 2.4 mm for ^{89}Sr.

Srontium-89 does not have significant gamma emission (see Table 7.1) and it is not possible to image the in vivo distribution readily. However, studies performed with the surrogate gamma emitter ^{85}Sr have demonstrated uptake at sites of metastases. In contrast, ^{153}Sm emits gamma photons at 103 keV, suitable for imaging with a gamma camera and scans may be performed following treatment to confirm uptake in metastases (Figure 7.1).

IODINE-131 m-IBG THERAPY IN NEUROENDOCRINE DISEASE

Iodine-131 labelled meta-iodobenzylguanidine (m-IBG) is used in the treatment of neurectodermal tumours. Such tumours derive from the primitive neural crest, which develops to form the sympathetic nervous system (SNS): malignant neurectodermal tumours include phaeochromocytoma, neuroblastoma, carcinoid tumours, paraganglioma and medullary thyroid cancer. M-IBG is structurally similar to the catecholamine noradrenaline and has been found to concentrate within secretory granules of cells which produce catecholamines in, for instance, the adrenal medulla. The first report that ^{131}I m-IBG localizes in phaeochromocytoma was in 1981 [21] and in neuroblastoma in 1984 [22].

Before treatment, any drugs known to interfere with the uptake and/or retention of ^{131}I m-IBG must be withdrawn (EANM). A thyroid blocking agent must be prescribed, starting before and continuing for an extended period after treatment, to protect the gland from taking up any free ^{131}I with the subsequent risk of developing hypothyroidism. The dose limiting toxicity is hematological and monitoring of blood counts is essential after treatment.

Table 7.2 Radiation absorbed dose, mGy/MBq for some radionuclides			
RADIOPHARMACEUTICAL	**EFFECTIVE DOSE (mSv/MBq)**	**TYPICAL ADMINISTERED ACTIVITY, A (MBq)**	**EFFECTIVE DOSE FROM A MBq (mSv)**
^{32}P sodium phosphate	2.4	200	480
^{89}Sr strontium chloride	3.1	150	465
^{131}I sodium iodide: carcinoma	0.061	3500	214
^{131}I sodium iodide: thyrotoxicosis	24	400	9600

Figure 7.1 Whole body bone scans on the same patient showing uptake of ^{153}Sm in metastases identifiable on the ^{99m}Tc MDP scans.

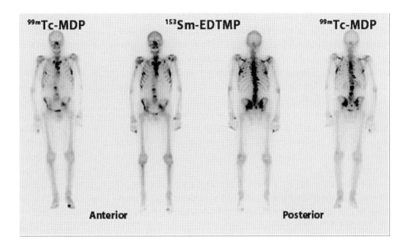

Iodine-123 m-IBG is available for imaging such tumours using a gamma camera and, as part of the preparation for treatment, patients should undergo m-IBG scintigraphy (either ^{123}I or ^{131}I) to confirm uptake in all known tumour sites. Treatment may be prescribed either using a set activity, using an activity per kilogram or by using the results of pretreatment dosimetric measurements with a tracer dose. In this last case, an activity may be prescribed for treatment using a predetermined criterion. For instance, a limit of 2 Gy to the total body has been used in the treatment of children with neuroblastoma [23].

Typical administered activities are between 3.5 GBq and 7 G Bq and patients require admission to an isolation unit for a period of time determined by national regulations. Very careful arrangements must be made for the treatment and nursing of children, who are often under 3 years of age.

The effective dose to a 70 kg adult is 0.013 mSv/MBq, or 46 mSv for 3.5 GBq. The radiation dose to the tumour varies widely.

RADIOLABELED MONOCLONAL ANTIBODIES IN NON-HODGKIN'S LYMPHOMA

In contrast to most of the treatments already discussed, radioimmunotherapy (RIT) using radiolabelled monoclonal antibodies [24] is a relatively recent introduction. RIT has been proven to be effective in follicular non-Hodgkin's lymphoma (NHL) and clinical trials are continuing in this and other forms of NHL, as well as other haematological malignancies. It remains a challenge to deliver sufficient radiation dose with RIT to treat solid tumours, but there has been some progress in clinical trials of locally administered RIT, for instance studies using intra-peritoneal administration to treat malignant ascites [25].

It seems apparent that any text dealing with RIT will be superseded rapidly. In 2005, just two therapeutic radiolabelled antibodies were approved by the FDA for use in the USA, ^{90}Y ibritumomab tiuxetan (Zevalin®) and ^{131}I. tositumomab (Bexxar®).

In both cases:

- the antibody is targeted to CD20, an antigen produced by both malignant and normal B-cells
- the approval is for the treatment of relapsed follicular NHL which is refractory to chemotherapy
- the dose limiting toxicity is haematological.

Yttrium-90 ibritumomab tiuxetan also has EU approval and both materials are being used in on-going clinical trials.

For ^{131}I tositumomab, pretreatment dosimetry is essential, to calculate the therapeutic activity required to deliver a total body dose of 0.75 Gy during treatment. This was established as the maximum tolerated dose in clinical trials. The dosimetry protocol requires measuring the effective half-life in the individual patient following administration of a tracer activity of ^{131}I (185 MBq). The range of treatment activities administered ranges from around 3 to 5 GBq and an inpatient stay in a dedicated facility is required.

With yttrium-90 ibritumomab tiuxetan, there is less individual variation in effective half-life and the treatment is prescribed as 15 MBq/kg, with a maximum of 1.2 GBq.

RADIATION PROTECTION, WASTE AND REGULATIONS

The regulations and the principles behind the radiation protection for the therapeutic use of radionuclides are encompassed within the principles and regulations which apply to all uses of ionizing radiation. These are described in Chapter 4 where the reader will find in particular sections dealing with ARSAC for the administration of radioactive substances, the transport of substances, the statutory instruments governing the general use of radiation and specifically its use for medical applications. In particular, the risk assessment of situations involving the administration of radioisotopes on an individual basis can be required frequently due to particular circumstances. The need for adequate staff monitoring and decontamination provision is also essential for the safe provision of radionuclide treatment.

Consideration of the patients' circumstances in relation to the radionuclide being used is important. Treatments with pure beta emitters, such as yttrium-90, present very little hazard to other people unless the radioactivity is excreted in urine or other body fluids. However, simple hygeine precautions with wound dressings for a short period can also reduce any likely loss of activity and maintain the therapeutic benefit to the patient. By contrast, the administration of ^{131}I with its half-life of 8 days, gamma ray emission at 364 keV as well as the beta particle emission and avidity for the thyroid gland if ingested in the form of iodide presents a more complex problem. Requirements and guidance are drawn from several sources including the IRMER regulations [26] and the MDGN [10]. Patients receiving more than 30 MBq ^{131}I must be assessed individually to ensure that they do not pose a hazard to others. In general, patients receiving less than 800 MBq may go home directly after treatment. A journey time of less than one hour is considered reasonable for ambulance and public transport. Advice should be given about seating position in the vehicle to minimize irradiation of fellow passengers. If conveyed by private car, the driver and patient should be advised regarding journey time and seating position in the car. In addition, certain conditions concerning public transport journey times, places of entertainment, use of cutlery and crockery and contact with young children and pregnant women will be required for the following few weeks.

In circumstances when the activity exceeds 800 MBq, the patient will have to be admitted and cared for in specialized accommodation as follows:

- confinement to a single room with impervious wall finishes and flooring and with coved skirtings to ease decontamination
- the room be designated as a controlled area
- exclusive use of a toilet and shower facility connected directly to a main drain
- suitable warning signage to drainage for maintenance workers
- bed linen, towels and clothing must be monitored for contamination before patient discharge
- visiting by adults should be discouraged for the first 24 hours and restricted thereafter

- visiting by children and pregnant women is forbidden
- emergency decontamination kit and radiation monitor readily accessible
- staff must wear at least gowns and gloves to protect their skin and clothing from contamination
- overshoes should be worn if there is any chance of the floor being contaminated
- if possible, utensils such as cutlery and crockery should be disposable and all waste disposal should be dealt with by authorized personnel
- nursing procedures should be carried out in the minimum time compatible with good nursing care
- a clearly documented procedure must be provided to allow artificial resuscitation of a patient but minimize the risk of radioactive contamination.

Patients who have received radioiodine therapy may not be discharged until the radiation dose which they can potentially give to people they come into contact with is significantly reduced. This is achieved by adherence to simple precautions within specified levels of activity. The limit for discharge is generally held to be when the residual level of activity in the body has fallen below 800 MBq. This limit has no legal standing however, so a careful risk assessment is required before discharge, at whatever level.

The 800 MBq limit for iodine-131 was arrived at by carefully modelling likely patient behaviour and compliance. It corresponds to approximately 300 MBq.MeV, so this figure was initially taken as a suitable limit for discharge of patients who had received other therapeutic radionuclides, such as ^{153}samarium or ^{90}yttrium. Unfortunately, due to differences in half-life and radiation emitted, the extrapolation is not valid [27].

The MDGN [10] contains a table of restrictions which are suitable when discharging patients who have undergone radioiodine therapy for thyrotoxicosis. This includes restrictions on contact with children and any restrictions on the mode of transport used. Self-discharge must be firmly discouraged on the grounds of the hazards to others.

Where risk assessment has shown it necessary, all patients should be given written instructions on leaving hospital about precautions to be taken to minimize the dose to others. This may take the form of a card. Even many weeks after precautions have elapsed, patients may retain enough radioactivity in their bodies to set off radiation alarms at airports. It is wise to question patients on their travel plans prior to discharge and warn them of the possibility of delay.

Following discharge from inpatient accommodation, the room may not be re-used until it has been monitored and declared free from contamination.

In the case of the death of a patient following the administration of a therapeutic dose of radioactivity, due regard must be given to the safety of the relatives, pathologists and undertakers, etc. The MDGN [10] contains a section giving advice on this but a local policy should be written for each treatment offered in that centre.

Staff who prepare, administer or care for patients who have received therapeutic doses should minimize the risk of receiving doses by adherence to good radiation protection principles. They must wear protective clothing when handling the radioisotope, the patient or any articles which may be contaminated. Contaminated goods and clothing must be carefully stored for assay and approved disposal by the medical physics staff. Contamination monitoring should be undertaken by experienced staff and all results recorded. In addition to film or thermoluminescent dosimeters (TLD) badge monitoring, there may be a requirement for periodic monitoring of the staff for inhaled or ingested contamination, e.g. of the thyroid when nursing iodine therapy patients.

Although waste disposal is permitted in gaseous, solid and liquid form and gaseous waste may be encountered from fume cabinets, the majority of waste is liquid and solid. Syringes, swabs, paper tissues and all contaminated material constitute solid waste. Liquid waste arises from radioactive solutions from isotope administration, decontamination procedures and body fluids from patients. The disposal of radioactive waste from a hospital must be organized, carefully controlled and documented in compliance with the UK regulations to avoid hazard to staff patients and the general public. The Environment Agency will have set limits of activity for gaseous, liquid and solid waste for each site in its authorization. The site must show that it disposes of all waste by the *best practicable means* before authorization is granted.

In most cases, the disposal of radioactive excreta from patients is dealt with by discharging to the sewage system. In this way, the hazard to staff involved in collection and disposal is avoided. This is permitted where there is an adequate inactive effluent flow from the hospital to dilute the waste to a low concentration level, and when the toilets reserved for radioactive waste are connected directly to the main drainage system. Similar conditions must also be applied to the disposal of radioactive liquid waste from the laboratories. The waste pipes between the ward/laboratory and the main sewer should be labelled as potentially radioactive.

Some storage facilities are always required for contaminated belongings or storing high activity waste storage until it can be disposed of. An example would be the tubing and bags from peritoneal dialysis. Such storage facilities must be adequately shielded, designed to prevent risk of escape of material and labelled.

Once the activity has decayed to extremely low levels, it can be disposed of with the rest of the clinical waste. Larger concentrations of activity in solid waste or long-lived radionuclides will require special arrangements for disposal through authorized routes but, once again, strict activity limits are imposed.

Detailed records must be kept of all disposals of radioactive materials irrespective of which route has been used. These records should include the type of radionuclide, its activity at disposal, the route of disposal and the date of disposal.

The limits authorized for disposal as liquid waste under RSA93 [28] may be one of the limiting factors in the ability of a hospital to offer radionuclide therapy. Some countries favour the use of delay tanks to store radioactive excreta before release into the environment, however, the ensuing difficulty in ensuring that the control mechanisms on the tanks are functioning correctly without exposing maintenance workers to unacceptable risk has precluded its widespread use in the UK.

REFERENCES

[1] Otte A, Mueller-Brand J, Dellas S, Nitzsche EU, Herrmann R, Maecke HR. Yttrium-90-labelled somatostatin-analogue for cancer treatment. Lancet 1998;351:417–8.

[2] de Jong M, Bakker WH, Krenning EP, et al. Yttrium-90 and indium-111 labelling, receptor binding and biodistribution of [DOTA0,d-Phe1, Tyr3] octreotide, a promising somatostatin analogue for radionuclide therapy. Eur J Nucl Med 1997;24:368–71.

[3] Lewington VJ. Targeted radionuclide therapy for neuroendocrine tumours. Endocr Relat Cancer 2003;10:497–501.

[4] Royal College of Physicians. Radio-iodine in the management of benign thyroid disease. Clinical guidelines: report of a Working Party. Royal College of Physicians; 2007.

[5] Society of Nuclear Medicine. Procedure guidelines for therapy of thyroid disease with iodine-131 (sodium iodide) version 2. Society of Nuclear Medicine; 2005.

[6] Luster M, Clarke SE, Deitler M, et al. European Association of Nuclear Medicine (EANM).Guidelines for radio-iodine therapy of differentiated thyroid cancer. European Journal of Nuclear Medicine and Molecular Immunology 2008;35:1941–59.

[7] Sagel J, Epstein S, Kalk J, Van Mieghem W. Radioactive iodine therapy for thyrotoxicosis at Groote Schur Hospital over a 6 year period. Postgrad Med J 1972;48:308–13.

[8] Pauwels EK, Smit JW, Slats A, Bourquiqnon M, Overbeek F. Health effects of therapeutic use of ^{131}I in hyperthyroidism. Q J Nucl Med 2000;44:333–9.

[9] Robbins RJ, Schlumberger MJ. The evolving role of ^{131}I for the treatment of differentiated thyroid carcinoma. Journal of Nuclear Medicine 2005;46:28S–37S.

[10] Medical and Dental Guidance Notes. A good practice guide on all aspects of ionising radiation

protection in the clinical environment. Institute of Physics and Engineering in Medicine; 2002.

[11] Seidlin SM, Marinelli LD, Oshry E. Radioactive iodine therapy: effect on functioning metastases of adenocarcinoma of the thyroid. J Am Med Assoc 1946;132:838–47.

[12] Parmentier C. Use and risks of phosphorous-32 in the treatment of polycythaemia vera. J Nucl Med 2005;46 (Suppl.):115S–127S.

[13] Lawrence JH. Polycythaemia physiology, diagnosis and treatment. Grune and Stratton; 1955.

[14] ICRP Publication 80. Radiation dose to patients from radiopharmaceuticals, Addendum 2 to ICRP 53 and Addendum 1 to ICRP 72. Elsevier; 1999.

[15] ICRP Publication 53. Radiation dose to patients from radiopharmaceuticals. Elsevier; 1988.

[16] Firusian N, Schmidt CG. Radioactive strontium for treating incurable pain in skeletal neoplasms. Dtsch Med Wochenschr 1973;98:2347–51.

[17] Lewington VJ. Cancer therapy using bone-seeking isotopes. Phys Med Biol 1996;41:2027–42.

[18] Baczyk M, Czepczynski R, Milecki P, Pisarek M, Oleksa R, Sowinski J. ^{89}Sr versus ^{153}Sm-EDTMP : comparison of treatment efficacy of painful bone metastases in prostate and breast carcinoma. Nucl Med Commun 2007;28:245–50.

[19] De klerk JM, Zonnenberg BA, Blijham GH, et al. Treatment of metastatic bone pain using bone seeking radiopharmaceutical Re-186-HEDP. Anticancer Res 1997;17:1773–7.

[20] Roberts Jr DJ. ^{32}P-Sodium phosphate treatment of metastatic malignant disease. Clin Nucl Med 1979;4:92–3.

[21] Sisson JC, Frager MS, Valk TW, et al. Scintigraphic localization of pheochromocytoma. N Engl J Med 1981;305:12–7.

[22] Hattner R, Huberty JP, Engelstad BL, et al. Localization of M-iodi (I-131) benzylguanidine in neuroblastoma. Am J Roentgenol 1984;43:373–4.

[23] Fielding SL, Flower MA, Ackery D, Kemshead JT, Lashford LS, Lewis I. Dosimetry of iodine-131 metaiodobenzylguanidine for treatment of resistant neuroblastoma: results of a UK study. Eur J Nucl Med 1991;18:308–16.

[24] Britton KE, Mather SJ, Granowska M. Radiolabelled monoclonal antibodies in oncology. III. Radioimmunotherapy. Nucl Med Commun 1991;12:333–347.

[25] Sharkey RM, Goldenberg DM. Perspectives on cancer therapy with radiolabeled monoclonal antibodies. J Nucl Med 2005;46 (Suppl. 1), 115S–127S.

[26] Department of Health. The Ionising Radiation (Medical Exposure) Regulations 2000. Statutory Instrument 2000 No 1059. The Stationary Office; 2000.

[27] Waller ML. Estimating periods of non-close-contact for relatives of radioactive patients. Br J Radiol 2001;74:100–102.

[28] Radioactive Substances Act. 1993, The Stationary Office.

Chapter 8

Radiotherapy beam production

John A. Mills, Hamish Porter and David Gill

GENERAL

There is a variety of ionizing radiation beams used in radiotherapy. They range from low energy x-rays involving accelerating voltages as low as 10 kV to megavoltage x-ray beams with equivalent accelerating potentials of up to 25 MV. Electron particle beams in the 4 to 20 MeV energy range are also used. Electron beams and gamma ray beams have also been derived from radioactive sources. The most notable source still being used for a gamma ray beam is cobalt-60.

Neutron beams, proton beams and light ion beams have also been used. At present, neutron beams are no longer widely used, although advantages now recognized with proton and light ion beams have led to an escalation in the number of facilities being set up throughout the world for their clinical use. In addition, there are also development programs to improve our understanding of the absolute dose and of the radiobiological effect of these beams.

Radiotherapy treatment is dominated by the use of x-ray beams, in particular, megavoltage beams between 4 MV and 25 MV, although many of the linear accelerators which produce the megavoltage x-ray beams can also deliver electron beams. Today, the most commonly used treatment delivery system is the linear accelerator which can produce both photon and electron beams. This chapter deals with x-ray and electron beams and their production and also contains a small section on gamma ray beams.

KILOVOLTAGE X-RAY BEAM MACHINES

Deep x-ray and superficial units provide x-ray beams in the keV energy range. The term orthovoltage is also used and this term reflects the arrangement whereby the x-rays are produced in a direction at right angles to that of the accelerating voltage. The units typically take the form of a tube

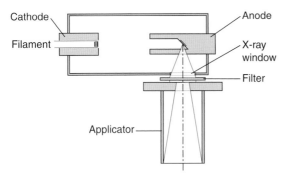

Figure 8.1 Example of an orthovoltage machine.

assembly which can be manually manipulated to direct the beam onto the patient. The source to surface distance is typically in the range of 20 to 50 cm and the field is defined at the surface by a mechanical applicator. An example of such a machine is shown in Figure 8.1.

Tube stand

The tube is mounted on a mechanism commonly referred to as the tube stand (Figure 8.2). The design of the tube stand enables manipulation of the beam direction by the machine operator in order to direct it at the patient's lesion. There are both floor mounted and ceiling mounted stands. The design allows translational and rotational movement of the beam and there may be scales of distance and angle which enable the set-up position or changes to it to be recorded and monitored. Electrical or mechanical brakes are fitted to the rotational axes and translational runners in order that the position can be reliably fixed in position prior to treatment and monitored during treatment.

High voltage circuits

On early machines, step up transformers were used to provide high voltages to excite the x-ray tube. The transformers operated at mains frequency and were very bulky due to the large iron core required.

Modern units employ switched mode power supply techniques, to improve voltage stability and make savings in size and efficiency. The power supply comprises of an input rectifier to convert mains AC to a DC voltage. A switching

Figure 8.2 Orthovoltage machine on a stand.

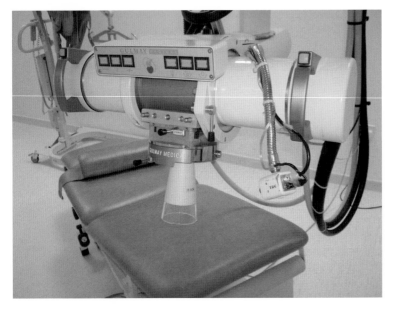

inverter converts the DC to a high frequency (25 kHz) pulsed waveform that is stepped up to 10 kV via a high frequency transformer. Finally, the waveform is rectified and passed through a number of cascaded multiplying stages (Cockcroft-Walton) to produce a DC voltage in the 100 to 300 kV range.

The extra high tension (EHT) voltage is monitored and a control signal fed back to alter the pulse width of the waveform leaving the inverter stage. In this way, a stable voltage is maintained across the x-ray tube.

The intensity of the x-ray beam produced at a particular kilovoltage depends upon the number of electrons emitted from the filament, this tube current is a function of the filament temperature and hence the filament current. The filament drive voltage is controlled electronically to respond to changes in the AC supply and stabilize the beam current. A schematic is shown in Figure 8.3. Typically, for voltages in excess of 200 kV, two high voltage power supplies are used in series.

The HT generator is controlled externally so that safe operating parameters can be set for the particular tube in use. The generator status can also be fed to the operating system to indicate faults, to link into the interlock system to ensure safe treatment and to assist in fault diagnosis.

The high voltage and filament power supply is connected to the x-ray tube by means of a high voltage cable. In order to prevent voltage flash over in the connectors, care must be taken to keep all parts clean and use high voltage insulating grease during assembly and reassembly following maintenance inspection.

Collimation

The anode construction provides the initial collimation of the beam as the x-rays come off the target almost omnidirectionally (Figure 8.4). This is referred to as a hooded anode and the aperture defines the maximum size of conical x-ray beam that could be provided. The collimation is completed by use of an applicator which is fixed directly below the tube aperture and provides the following:

- the base of the applicator consists of a collimator which defines the shape and size of the radiation field at the end of the applicator

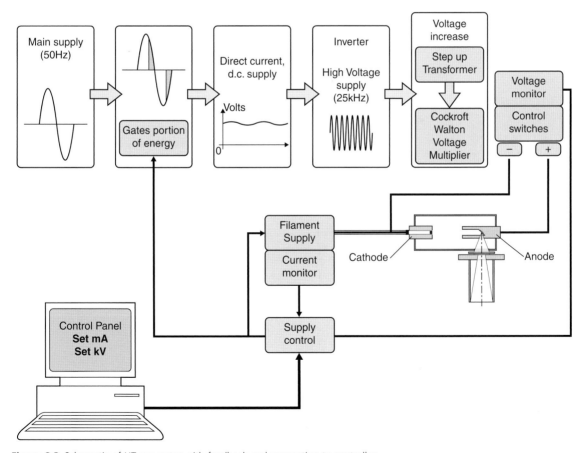

Figure 8.3 Schematic of HT generator with feedback and connection to controller.

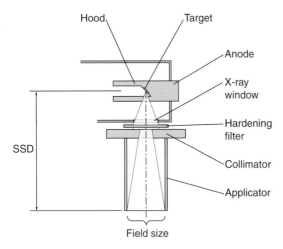

Figure 8.4 Anode construction, hood and omnidirectional emission with applicator to collimate beam and set SSD and define field size.

- the end of the applicator is the shape and size of the radiation beam
- the end of the applicator determines a fixed distance from the source
- the axis of the applicator is mechanically aligned to the axis of the radiation beam.

Beam energy

The x-ray beam from any bremmstrahlung target consists of a range of energies up to the maximum accelerating potential produced by the machine. Hence, for a 120 kV machine, 120 keV will be the accelerated electron energy and, in turn, the maximum x-ray photon energy will be 120 keV. This spectrum of energies is modified using a filter to remove lower energy x-rays and so reduce the dose to the skin. The beam that emerges from the tube through the x-ray window has undergone what is called inherent filtration. However, additional filtration is chosen to provide a beam with the desired depth dose penetration. The energy characteristics of the beam are often referred to as its quality and are dependent upon both the accelerating potential and filtration. The beam quality is normally measured using thicknesses of aluminum or copper and specified in terms of the half-value layer (HVL) which is the thickness of the layer of metal required to reduce the intensity of the beam by half. Typically, when this is measured it is done in a narrow beam, obtained by additional collimation to a broad clinical beam. The measuring ionization chamber is also placed at sufficient distance from the machine, floor and walls to ensure there is no additional scattered radiation. In practical terms, the penetration of the beam is also due to the source to surface distance and the field

size. Depth dose data indicating the penetration of different HVL beams can be compared in the *British Journal of Radiology*, Supplement 25.

Control of output

The stability of the output from the unit is directly related to the electrical stability of the tube voltage and current. Stabilized electrical supplies as described above ensure that this is achieved consistently. Typically, a timer is used to control the amount of dose that is delivered. The timer is normally a countdown device and starts to operate when the treatment is initiated and the voltage and current are supplied to the tube. After the set time has elapsed, the voltage and current are switched off and treatment terminates. A timed exposure requires that the output dose rate is stable and that is dependent upon the electrical control stability mentioned above. There is always an inherent increase in the dose rate as the voltage and the current ramp up to their operating value and this effect is normally taken into account using a transit time to accommodate the underdose which this would otherwise lead to. The transit time is added to the calculated time based upon a nominal dose rate to produce a total set time.

Most modern deep x-ray (DXR) and SXR units utilize a full field ionization monitor chamber through which the beam passes. By measuring the charge released against the absolute dose under particular set-up conditions, it is possible to control the output from the machine by a system which terminates the beam when the accumulated charge equals the required dose. The units of charge from the ionization chamber are referred to as monitor units and the specific dose delivered to any individual patient is achieved by calculating the required number of monitor units to be set.

Skin and eye shielding

Beam collimation is provided on orthovoltage machines with a range applicators which have regular field sizes. These applicators are usually chosen by the user when the unit is purchased. The choice is made to provide a nominal range of sizes for coverage of typical lesions. Often, it is necessary to treat lesions of non-standard size and irregular shape. It is common practice to manufacture a lead cut-out to define the treatment field exactly to the area specified by the radiotherapist. The cut-out is used in conjunction with one of the regular sized applicators to irradiate the treatment area and shield the surrounding normal skin from the rest of the beam. For lesions on the face and in close proximity to the eyes, a lead mask is manufactured based upon a plaster cast of the patient. As well as defining the treatment field and shielding the normal skin and the eyes, the lead mask can also be used to provide direction and localization of the beam (Figure 8.5).

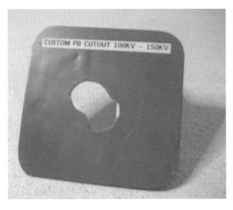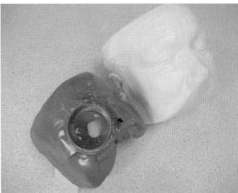

Figure 8.5 Irregular lead cut-out and mask.

To provide effective shielding, the thickness of lead for the cut-out has to be chosen taking into account the energy of the beam. This can be done from tabulated data of attenuation in lead against field size and HVL (beam energy). It is always prudent, however, for the Radiotherapy Physicists to undertake measurements and verify the shielding that is being obtained with the chosen thickness of lead.

When the treatment area impinges onto the eye, it is possible to insert eye shields to provide some protection to the lens. There are commercial lead and tungsten shields available. The problem encountered with eye shields is the contribution from scatter which reaches into the region under the shield from the surrounding field.

Calibration of dose output

As described above, there are two types of exposure control utilized on orthovoltage equipment. For a great many years, it has been done utilizing a timer. However, in more recent years, exposure is controlled by a full field ionization monitor chamber mounted in the radiation beam.

For timer control, the machine operator requires to know the dose rate of the machine and, for ionization chamber control, the response of the chamber must be directly related to an absolute dose. The ionization chamber response is normally quantified in monitor units and calibrated to be dose per monitor unit. Hence, for both systems of control, it is necessary to measure the absolute dose delivered by the beam under a very specific set-up, often referred to as the calibration conditions. The time to be set or the monitor units to be set are then determined using relative factors from the calibration set-up. For example, the specific dose rate may be measured for a 5 cm diameter applicator at 30 cm source to surface distance (SSD). In order to calculate a time to set, relative factors for other applicators, difference in SSD and changes in the irradiated area are used.

The absolute dose is measured in accordance with a protocol or Code of Practice. This ensures uniformity of practice between institutions. It will utilize the absolute dose calibration of the ionization chamber being used for the measurement and this will be traceable to a Standards Laboratory. The calibration can be done in air with the use of mass absorption coefficient ratios to determine the dose to water or tissue. Alternatively, the measurement can be done directly at depth in water. For superficial kV units with HVL values up to 8 mm Al, it is typical to determine the surface dose rate as this is where the dose is to be applied. However, for deep x-ray units with HVL values higher than 8 mm Al, it can be preferable to quote the dose deeper than the surface and closer to the target. In the latter case, it is preferable to calibrate at depth in water.

MEGAVOLTAGE LINEAR ACCELERATOR MACHINES

The workhorse of modern radiotherapy is the linear accelerator which owes its development to the pioneers who worked to produce higher energy beams than the kilovoltage beams upon which teletherapy started. The modern medical linear accelerator was born out of the development of megavoltage treatment machines in the 1950s. At this time, betatrons, auto-transformers and Van de Graff generator designs were utilized to accelerate electron beams to high energy. However, the elegance of acceleration based upon radiofrequency electromagnetic waves became universally adopted to provide high dose-rate megavoltage treatment beams. The fundamental components remain unchanged, although the performance, construction and control systems have been developed considerably to take advantage of modern engineering, technology, electronics and computers. Today, such medical linear accelerators are prolific and provide the vast majority of radiotherapy treatments.

General layout and components

The major core sections of a linear accelerator serve the purpose of producing a high energy electron beam. These components consist of an electron source, a source of radiofrequency (RF) electromagnetic waves and an accelerating waveguide. These core sections can now be found in some custom machines, such as Tomotherapy, and the principles of operation are identical. In this section, however, the description will be with regard to the isocentric gantry mounted machines which are now in widespread use throughout the world.

Besides the major core components, a modern medical linear accelerator consists of a gantry assembly in order to direct the beam into the patient and a radiation head which enables beam shaping. For x-ray beams, the target, which is bombarded by the electron beam to produce the x-rays, is contained in the radiation head. Steering

and stability of the electron beam requires focusing, bending and steering coils. High voltage and high current sources are also needed along with vacuum pumping systems and cooling systems in order to create a stable machine environment for production of the beam.

Figure 8.6 illustrates the typical layout of the major components of a linear accelerator.

The gun filament assembly produces electrons by raising tungsten to a sufficiently high temperature through electrical heating. There are two types of waveguide: standing waves and traveling waves. Although this affects the waveguide structure, both types use electromagnetic waves at a radiofrequency of approximately 3 GHz. In the traveling type, the electrons are carried along on an accelerating wave while the standing type utilizes the electric component of the wave to exert an accelerating force on the electrons.

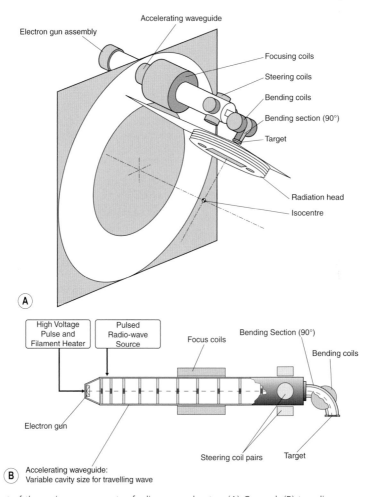

Figure 8.6 Typical layout of the major components of a linear accelerator. (A) General; (B) traveling wave guide;

High Voltage Pulse and Filament Heater

Pulsed Radio-wave Source

Focus coils

Bending Section (90°)

Bending coils

Electron gun

Steering coil pairs

Target

(C) Accelerating waveguide: Fixed cavity size and side cavities for standing wave

Figure 8.6, cont'd (C) standing waveguide.

The source of the radiowaves is either a klystron or a magnetron. The klystron utilizes a low power RF signal from a small cavity oscillator. This is applied to a high power electron stream in the klystron and results in a high power RF wave. By contrast, the magnetron is a multiple cavity device which produces a high power RF wave directly. Waveguide sections transport the RF from the magnetron or klystron to the accelerating waveguide section.

Because electrons are charged particles, there is a tendency for an electron beam to disperse as it travels along the accelerating waveguide. Fortunately, this can be countered by using the interactive force which is applied to any charged particle as it passes through a magnetic field. The magnetic fields that are used to counter this dispersion are produced by focusing coils. These coils are wound around the accelerating waveguide and produce a magnetic field flux parallel to the direction of the electron beam.

This interactive force between a magnetic field and the traveling electrons is further utilized with magnetic fields at right angles to the direction of the electron beam. One of these fields is generated by the bending magnet which bends the electron beam round into a trajectory appropriate for the radiation head. This magnet also plays a crucial role in the selection of the beam energy. By altering the strength of the magnetic field, which can be controlled by the electrical current flowing in the bending magnet coil, the appropriate energy selection can be made.

The other use of magnetic fields at right angles to the electron trajectory is to steer the beam into and out of the accelerating waveguide. It is important to maximize the number of electrons that are accelerated and therefore ensuring the most efficient trajectory of the beam along the guide minimizes the losses experienced. These magnetic fields are produced by the steering coils and control of the electric current within them can be used to adjust the trajectory for efficiency and correct beam alignment through the radiation head.

Beam production is not an energy efficient process and there is a lot of energy dissipated within the machine as heat. The stability of beam production relies on the stability of component dimensions, such as, for example, the RF cavities in the waveguide. These can be subject to expansion and contraction with heating. Hence, there is a need for a great deal of water cooling on the machine; the target, all the magnetic coils, the accelerating waveguide, the RF source and large electrical devices such as transformers. Adequate and stable cooling is essential for effective beam production.

The other essential ancillary aspect of the linear accelerator is the need for the accelerating waveguide to be under high vacuum. For some machine designs, the waveguide is factory sealed while for others vacuum pumps work continuously in order to maintain the high vacuum required.

The gantry construction of the standard medical linear accelerator is referred to as being isocentric. In effect, this means that all the main axes of rotation concerning the gantry, the radiation head and the patient couch intersect approximately though the same point in space referred to as the isocentre This is illustrated in Figure 8.7. The benefit of this isocentric system is that placement of the patient such that the tumour is centred on the machine isocentre simplifies treatment with the superposition of multiple beams.

The x-ray beam

The x-ray beam is produced through bremmstrahlung or 'braking radiation' by bombardment of a tungsten transmission target by the electron beam. The tungsten target is placed directly in the path of the electron beam immediately after it exits from the accelerating waveguide and the bending section. As shown in Figure 8.8, this raw x-ray beam is collimated into the useful beam by the primary collimator. The raw beam has a peak intensity in the

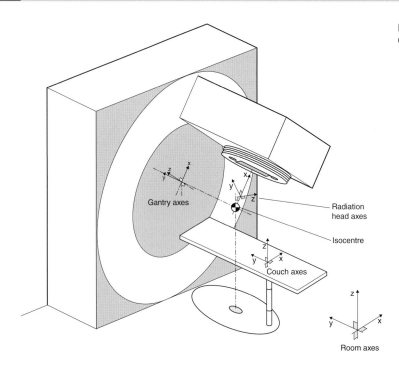

Figure 8.7 LA axes; gantry, collimator and Couch- IEC1217 style.

Gantry axes

Radiation head axes

Isocentre

Couch axes

Room axes

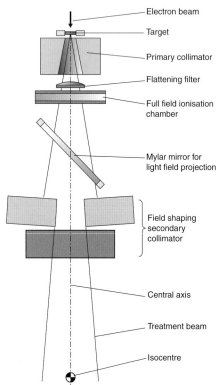

Electron beam

Target

Primary collimator

Flattening filter

Full field ionisation chamber

Mylar mirror for light field projection

Field shaping secondary collimator

Central axis

Treatment beam

Isocentre

Figure 8.8 LA radiation head.

forward direction (Figure 8.9). Conventionally, the aim in radiotherapy has been to deliver as uniform a dose as possible to the tumour. In order to achieve this simply from a direct beam, the raw beam is made uniform or flattened using a flattening filter made from steel. The profile of the flattening filter provides the maximum attenuation in the centre and the detailed shape of the filter is specific to the energy of the x-ray beam.

Following flattening of the beam, the x-rays pass through an ionization chamber before going on to field shaping with the secondary collimators. The ionization chamber consists of three sections and each section covers the full area of the useful beam. The first two sections are the dosimetry channels one and two (Ch-1 and Ch-2). Ch-1 is the primary channel which provides a signal to terminate the beam after a required dose has been delivered. Ch-2 is identical to channel one and acts as a safety back up to guard against excessive overexposure should a fault occur with Ch-1. The third section is a segmented chamber which is used to monitor characteristics of the beam such as uniformity and symmetry. The uniformity refers to the variation of dose across the beam and will be characteristic of the beam energy. The symmetry refers to a tilt in the beam between positions equidistant from the central axis of the beam and is dependent upon the alignment of the electron beam onto the target (Figure 8.10). These signals can be used to control the operation of the machine. For example, the uniformity signal can be used to control the gun filament electron emission and the symmetry signal can be used to control the steering coil currents.

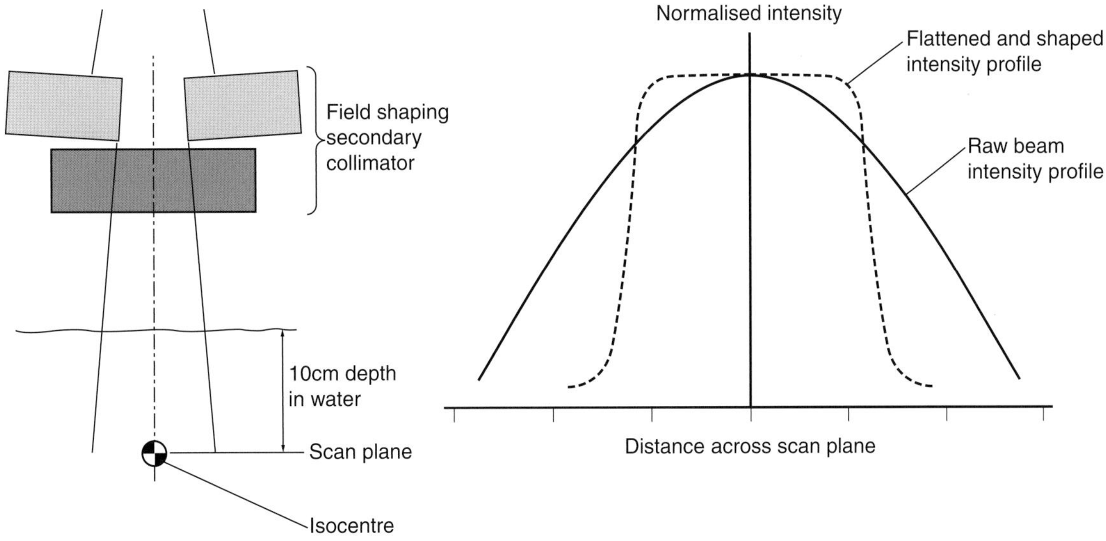

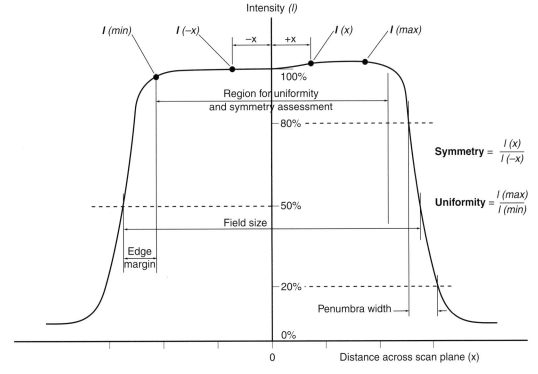

Figure 8.9 Raw beam profile after target and uniform beam under IEC conditions.

Figure 8.10 Uniformity and symmetry profiles.

Final beam shaping is done utilizing the substantial secondary collimation system. In early machines, these consisted of two sets of jaws which could set rectangular field shapes by movement in orthogonal directions. In virtually all modern machines now, these jaws have been replaced entirely or replaced in part or supplemented by multileaf collimation (MLC) with leaf widths at the isocentre ranging from 4 mm to 10 mm. This has provided the opportunity for simplified conformal shaping of the beam to the target volume as well as the

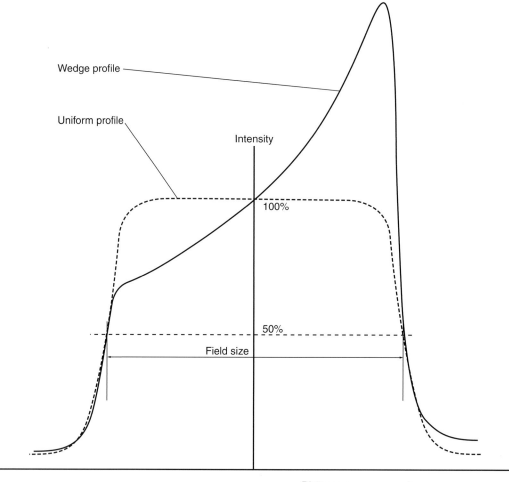

Figure 8.11 A solid wedge photograph and uniform and wedge beam profile.

varying of the beam intensity by rapidly changing the beam shape within the overall field and, in some cases, by dynamic control of the MLC while the machine is radiating.

A standard conventional method of varying the intensity of the beam has been the use of metal wedges placed within the beam to modify the uniformity of the beam profile in a controlled manner. This modification of the beam intensity has been found to be extremely useful in obtaining uniform dose distribution within the target. Figure 8.11 shows the effect which a typical metallic wedge has on the uniform profile. While in the past these wedges were fitted manually by the operator, they can now be provided in two ways. First, by having a metallic wedge mounted on a motorized platform in the radiation head. The wedge can then be automatically moved into and out of the radiation beam. The other way is to have one of the secondary collimator jaws move across the field during radiation. For example, at the start of the radiation, the jaws would be entirely closed with both jaws on the same side of the central axis. As radiation continued, one jaw would open and traverse across to the opposite side of the central axis. The three methods are referred to as fixed wedges, motorized wedges and dynamic wedges.

The electron beam

As well as the x-ray mode of operation, high energy linear accelerators are also used to deliver electron treatment beams. In this mode of operation, the transmission target is automatically moved out of the beam so x-rays are deliberately no longer produced. The electron beam has a very narrow width compared with the required treatment field size and scanning and scattering systems have been

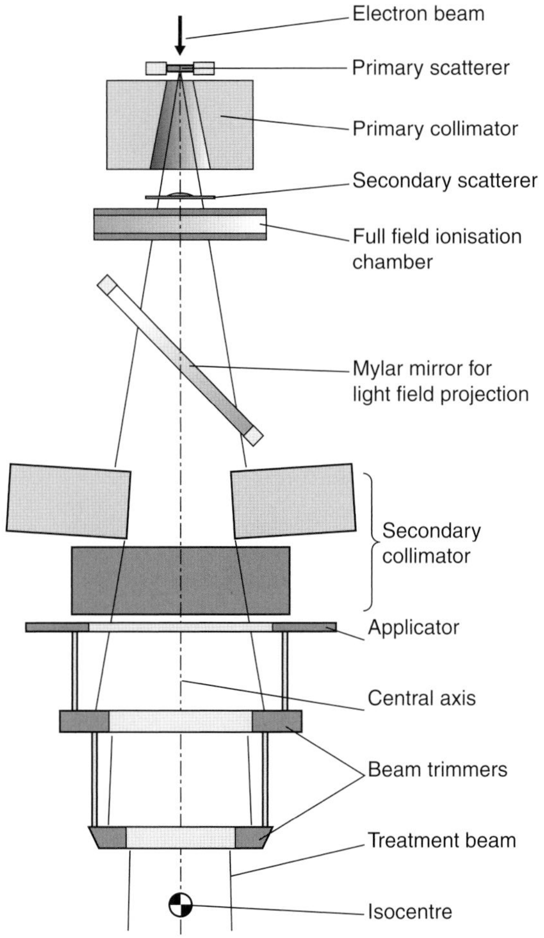
Electron beam
Primary scatterer
Primary collimator
Secondary scatterer
Full field ionisation chamber
Mylar mirror for light field projection
Secondary collimator
Applicator
Central axis
Beam trimmers
Treatment beam
Isocentre

Figure 8.12 Double scattering foil system with applicator for electron beam production.

developed in order to provide adequate field coverage. Scanning techniques employ magnetic fields which enable the electron beam to be steered across the field. However, by far the most predominant technique employs a dual scattering system along with an applicator attachment to the radiation head (Figure 8.12). In the dual scattering system, a primary scatterer is introduced to the electron beam prior to the primary collimator. A secondary scatterer is substituted for the flattening filter and this may be profiled for the specific electron beam. These scatterers and the flattening filter are moved automatically with the energy selection. Typically, a treatment machine would have two photon beams and five or six electron beams, each with a different energy. Both the primary and secondary scatterers are specific to the energy selected. The secondary collimators used for the photon fields set an initial field size as the electron beam leaves the radiation head. The electrons are scattered in air and so an applicator is used to produce a sharp edge to the treatment field at the patient. The applicators have open sides and consist of a set of field trimmers which reduce the field down to the required size. Treatment is done either with the applicator in contact with the patient or with a small stand-off of typically 5 cm. The practice at any centre depends upon local preference. The electron beam passes through the same ionization chamber with multiple sections and segments as the x-ray beam and this controls the delivery of the correct dose and monitoring of the beam as with the x-ray beam.

Control systems

Effective and safe performance of a linear accelerator depends upon two types of control system. The first concerns operation of the systems within the accelerator, for example, the control and tuning of the magnetron. The second relates to the stability controls on voltage and current supplies. The importance of this second type of control is apparent in the use of the bending magnet for energy selection. The supply system for the current is controlled to ensure that a stable current is supplied to the coils of the magnet within appropriate limits. An incorrect current could result in the wrong beam energy being delivered to the patient. While the second type of control is essential, it is not directly controlled by the changes in the radiation beam. One example of a system that is controlled by the beam concerns detection of field symmetry using the ionization chamber in the radiation head. Using the symmetry information, the electron beam is steered using the steering coils in order to maintain a symmetric field (Figure 8.13). In this example, an asymmetry in the field is detected by the segments of the ionization chamber in the radiation head. These signals are electronically or computationally processed in order to alter the current supplied to the steering magnet coils and restore the symmetry of the field.

Satisfactory beam delivery by a linear accelerator relies on the dynamic operation of many control systems. All operate automatically and result in an interplay between the electron emission from the gun, the tuning of the RF source and the steering of the beam along with the stabilization of all the currents and voltages which ensure the correct focusing and bending of the beam.

Alignment of patient to the beam

Both in the x-ray and the electron mode of operation, the radiation beams are set up so that they are aligned with the axis of the mechanical rotation of the radiation head (Figure 8.14). The system for patient–beam alignment can be considered to consist of two parts. The first is indicators which are aligned with the axes of the radiation head rotation and hence the radiation beam. The second is

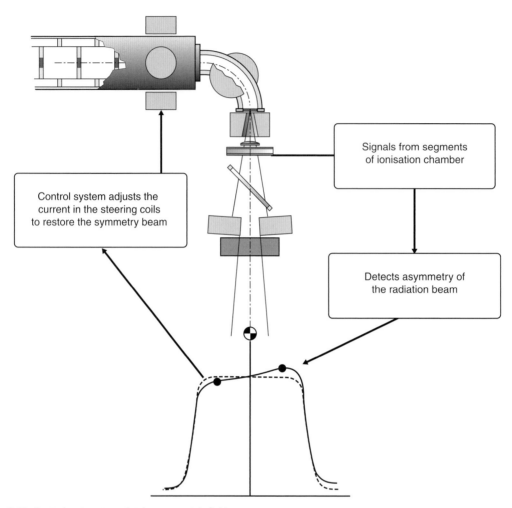

Control system adjusts the current in the steering coils to restore the symmetry beam

Signals from segments of ionisation chamber

Detects asymmetry of the radiation beam

Figure 8.13 Control system to maintain a symmetric field.

indicators which locate the isocentre of the machine in space. In combination, the beam alignment to the patient can be achieved and verified.

There are three main indicators of the radiation beam axis: treatment front pointer, treatment back pointer and light field x-wires. These are illustrated in Figure 8.15 and the pointers are attached to the radiation head during the patient set-up. The light field cross-wire projection is achieved through an optical system in the radiation head. Essentially, this generates a light source which, by using mirrors, is effectively positioned at the x-ray target. Cross-wires are introduced into the light field using a thin transparent film and with the bulb and the cross-wire centre exactly on the radiation head rotation axis, an optical projection of the axis is obtained.

The isocentre is indicated by three optical and mechanical systems. The first uses the treatment front pointer and the tip

of the pointer is set to the isocentre (Figure 8.16). The other indicator is referred to as a distance meter and, effectively, this uses the coincidence between the cross-wire projection and the distance meter projection in order to determine distances from the x-ray source to the surface of the patient (Figure 8.17). The last indicator is independent of the machine and consists of room mounted lasers which, through cylindrical lenses, project sheets through the isocentre providing a set of Cartesian coordinate planes with the isocentre at the origin (Figure 8.18). With the use of surface marks from the planning stages of the patient's treatment preparation, the laser sheets enable the patient to be set up with the isocentre at the appropriate place within the patient.

It is possible to mount a laser on the treatment machine which projects a sheet from the base of the gantry through the isocentre and the axis of gantry rotation. It is possible to

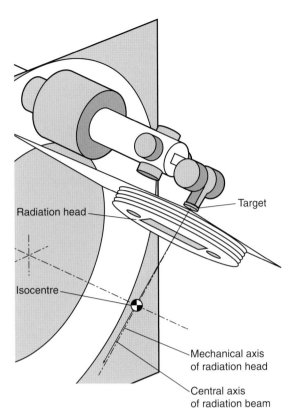

Figure 8.14 Alignment of mechanical and radiation beam axes.

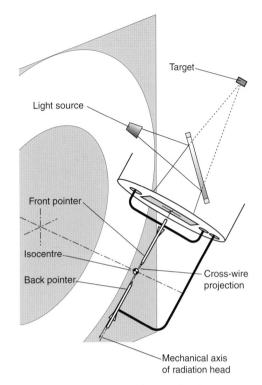

Figure 8.15 X-wires, treatment front and back pointers.

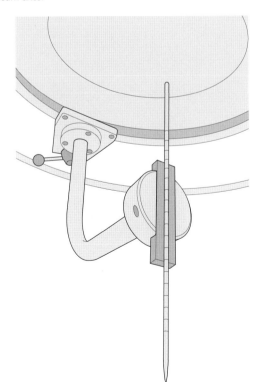

Figure 8.16 Treatment front pointer for isocentre indication.

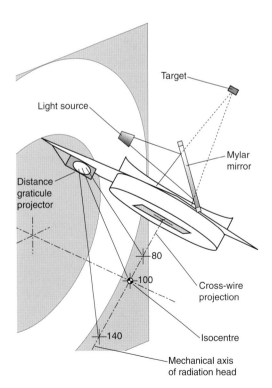

Figure 8.17 Distance meter for isocentre indication.

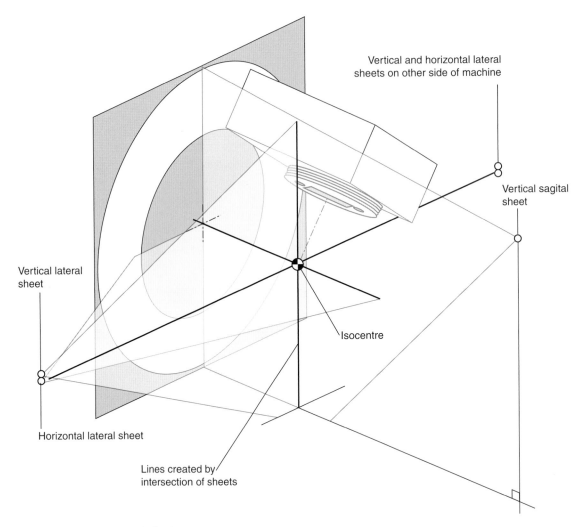

Vertical and horizontal lateral
sheets on other side of machine

Vertical sagital
sheet

Vertical lateral
sheet

Isocentre

Horizontal lateral sheet

Lines created by
intersection of sheets

Figure 8.18 Lasers isocentre indication.

use this sheet in combination with the room sheets instead of a mechanical backpointer (Figure 8.19).

Record and verify systems

The task for the machine operators who deliver the treatment has always involved setting up the patient and the machine and, in some way, having this checked and recorded as independently as possible prior to treatment. The increasing complexity of treatments and the implementation of quality systems with a requirement to demonstrate traceability of the process have made an automatic system essential. With the increasing availability of fast computing systems, record and verify (R+V) systems were developed to fulfill this role. Essentially, the R+V system consists of three distinct components: storage, check and record. The patient prescription is stored, a check is

made that machine parameters at treatment match the prescription and a record is built up of the treatment delivered. The structure of a system is illustrated in Figure 8.20.

For each patient, a treatment parameters file is held and the parameters are downloaded from the R+V system to a treatment machine at each occasion of treatment. The machine is then set up for treatment of the patient by the operators and the R+V system compares the settings on the machine with the values stored in the system file. Any differences must be resolved by the operators before treatment can commence. This will normally be done by adjustment of the patient and machine set-up to bring it in line with the treatment parameters but, in exceptional circumstances, parameters can be over-ridden subject to appropriate checking and supervision. The patient's file is also used to record the dose delivered to the patient on each treatment in order to

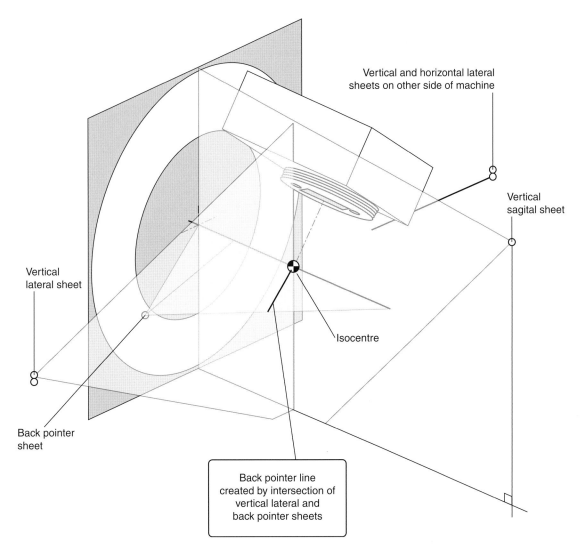

Vertical and horizontal lateral
sheets on other side of machine

Vertical
sagital sheet

Vertical
lateral sheet

Isocentre

Back pointer
sheet

Back pointer line
created by intersection of
vertical lateral and
back pointer sheets

Figure 8.19 Laser backpointer.

maintain an accumulated record of the treatment dose given to the patient.

While these systems provide an invaluable aid to the treatment delivery, it should be borne in mind that such systems can also fail. As with any computerized data transfer process, routine checks are required to check that the system assigns the correct data to a patient's treatment.

Special techniques

Although linear accelerators have been designed to deliver beams which will superimpose on each other within the patient in an effective manner, they have also been adapted to fulfill some other treatment requirements.

One of the major adaptations has been to provide total body irradiation (TBI) treatment with x-rays and total skin electron (TSE) treatment. For both these types of treatment, the limitation of the accelerator is its field size. However, by treating patients at greatly extended distance of up to 4 m, full body coverage has been achieved for megavoltage TBI (Figure 8.21). Likewise, techniques to provide electron fields large enough to cover the entire patient have been devised for TSE. Figure 8.22 shows the well acknowledged Stanford technique, however, there are also techniques which move the patient couch through the beam and techniques which obtain an enlarged field by rotation of the gantry during radiation. For these extended source to patient TSE treatment distances, high dose rates are specially generated on the accelerator in order to reduce the treatment time.

Another adaptation of the linear accelerator has been to supplement the standard field sizes which can be defined

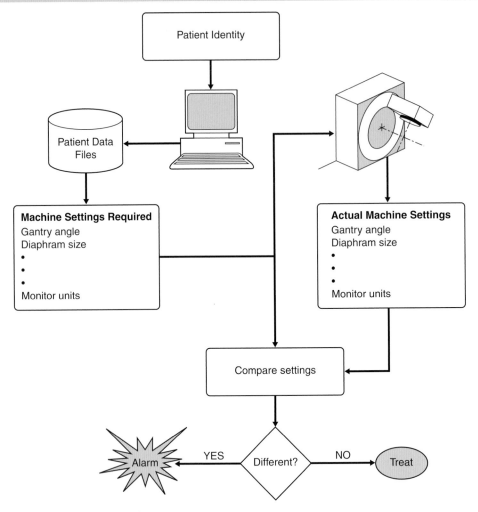

Figure 8.20 Structure of record and verify system.

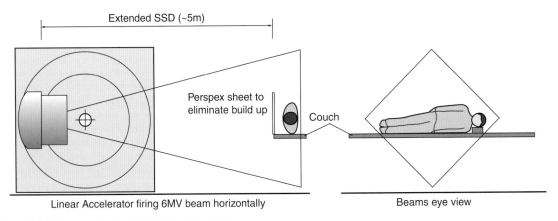

Figure 8.21 Linear accelerator for total body irradiation.

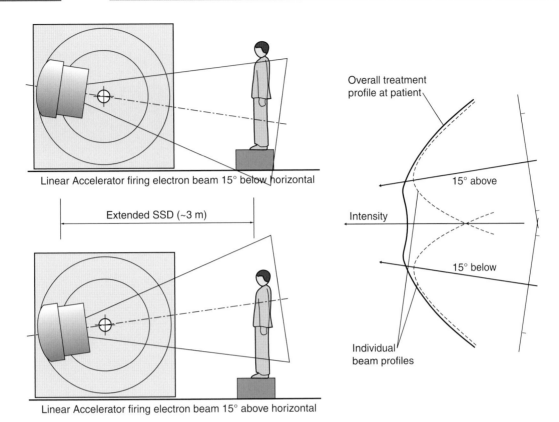

Figure 8.22 Linear accelerator for total skin electron treatment.

with the collimators in the radiation head with fixed narrow beam collimators or a micro multileaf collimator which can define small fields with dimensions of less than 5 cm. These small fields have been used in either static or arcing treatment techniques for accurate stereotactic radiosurgery and stereotactic radiotherapy. These stereotactic techniques are used for cranial tumours, such as brain metastases, and non-malignant arteriovenous malformations (AVM). An early form of dynamic treatment is achieved by rotation of the gantry during irradiation and this can be applied with both megavoltage x-ray and electron beams. Often it is referred to as arc-therapy. In the case of electrons, the technique can be used to treat a large curved surface, such as the side of the chest wall.

GAMMA RAY BEAM MACHINES

The penetrative limitations and high skin dose of even 300 kV x-rays drove the desire for higher energy x-rays. The radioisotope cobalt-60 (^{60}Co) was discovered at the University of California by Seaborg and Livingwood in the 1930s and, in Canada in 1951, it was used for teletherapy. The isotope is produced by neutron bombardment through the following process:

$$59Co + n \rightarrow 60Co + \gamma$$

Nuclear reactors provided an ideal production platform for the substance. The attraction of cobalt-60 was the high energy gamma emission produced in the radioactive decay process (Figure 8.23) and also the relatively long half-life of the isotope of just over 5 years. The energy of the gamma rays are almost four times that of the highest deep x-ray unit.

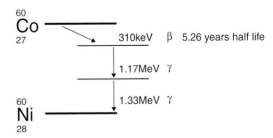

Cobalt-60 decay

Figure 8.23 Cobalt gamma ray decay process.

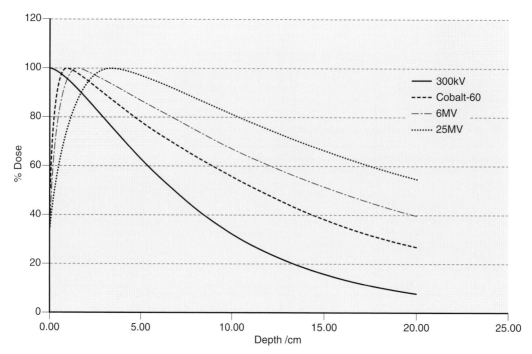

Figure 8.24 300 kV, cobalt, 6 MV and 25 MV DD curves.

The depth dose characteristics of a nominal 10×10 cm cobalt-60 beam at 80SSD is compared in Figure 8.24 to that for a 10 cm diameter, 0.4Cu HVL kilovoltage beam. The latter would typically be produced from acceleration with about 300 kV and appropriate filtration. The depth dose characteristics for a 10×10 cm field size 6 MV and 25 MV beam at 100SSD from a linear accelerator are also shown for comparison.

The advantages are immediately obvious. First, the dose at depth, say 7 cm is increased by almost a factor of 1.5. Secondly, however, the forward scattering of the electrons produced from the photon interactions produces the skin sparing effect with a maximum dose at 0.5 cm depth rather than the surface. Cobalt units provided the clinician with an enormous technical advantage for teletherapy.

The cobalt unit represents an extremely simple method to generate a megavoltage treatment beam. There is no requirement for the highly skilled maintenance and costs associated with linear accelerators and this enables teletherapy to be provided at low cost in situations where technical support is not readily available. This is the enormous potential for these machines: simplicity and economy.

Radioisotope source

The radioactive cobalt-60 source consists of a small container which encapsulates pellets or disks of cobalt with an activity of typically 200 TBq. Typical dimensions of such a source is a 2 cm diameter by 2 cm long cylinder.

Herein lies one of the deficiencies of the cobalt treatment unit as this large source in turn produces a large penumbra in its radiation fields. The source is housed within a large shielded safe which has a shutter mechanism to transport the source into an exposed position. Typical mechanisms are spring-loaded wheels, jaws and sliding mechanism and there were electrical, mechanical, hydraulic and pneumatically driven systems developed. Periodic testing is required to ensure that there is no leakage of radioactive material from the source encapsulation. Swabs are taken of the aperture to the safe in order to detect contamination. Emergency personnel procedures are also required to be in place to ensure that, in the event of a failure of the transport mechanism, the patient can be safely removed from the room and the source returned to the safe by manual means. One noticeable feature of a cobalt head is that it is continually warm. This arises from the radioactive decay and absorption in the shielded housing and, in particular, all the β-decay indicated in Figure 8.23. It is testament to the reality of the energy release from the cobalt source.

Beam collimation

The collimation of the beam is achieved using a system of primary collimator, secondary collimator and penumbra trimmers as shown in Figure 8.25. The primary collimator is adjacent to the source and can form part of the drum assembly within which the source is stored.

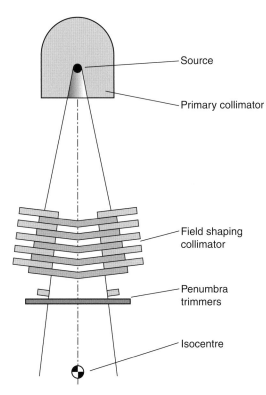

Figure 8.25 Collimation system for cobalt machine.

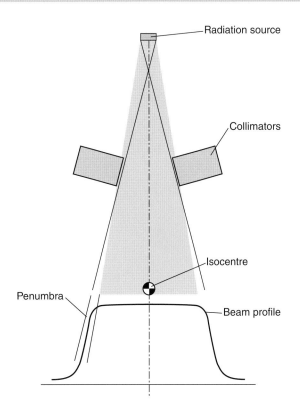

Figure 8.26 Penumbra diagram.

It forms the initial beam which will set the maximum size possible for the final treatment field. The penumbra of a radiation field is dependent upon three aspects: the size of the source, the distance of the secondary collimator jaw from the source and electron scatter at the edge of the beam (Figure 8.26). Scatter really only becomes a problem at very high energies above 15 MV photon beams. However, the radiation source at 2 cm is very large. If then the secondary collimator jaws were placed one above the other, the penumbra across the inner jaws would be larger than across the outer jaws. So, in order to provide a more equitable size in both directions, the jaws are interlaced as shown in Figure 8.25. The distance from the source is extended even further by the use of penumbra trimmers which can be fitted to the ends of the main secondary collimators. Although this technique is effective, it is not always practical because of patient positioning.

Design of gamma-ray teletherapy machines

Initially, there were fixed head cobalt treatment machines followed by rotating gantry mounted machines (Figure 8.27). The rotating gantry machines were arranged

so that the axes of the radiation head rotation and the gantry rotation intersected. This enabled isocentric treatment of the patient with multiple beams intersecting within the target and enhancing the dose there simply by rotation of the gantry. Due to the massive shielding for the radioactive source, the radiation head presented a considerably heavy load for the gantry assembly to accommodate. This led to relatively large displacements between beams at the isocentre and could well be of the order of 10 mm with gantry rotation.

One additional set of movements which was available on several machines was pitch and roll (see Figure 8.27). The advantage of these two movements was that, for some poorly non-ambulant patients, the beam could be directed for treatment with them upright in a chair or even remaining in their bed. Such treatments would be single field and often single shot treatments for palliation. Nevertheless, it provided a valuable treatment technique for the clinician and operator.

In compact rooms, the radiation head was balanced on the gantry by a shield in order to reduce the radiation protection requirements in the room. Wedges were also available for these machines and consisted of metal filters placed on trays directly below the secondary collimators. No dosimetry monitoring was installed to control the radiation delivery. The delivery was controlled by a

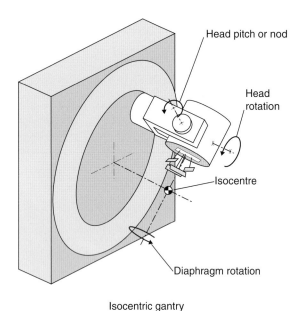

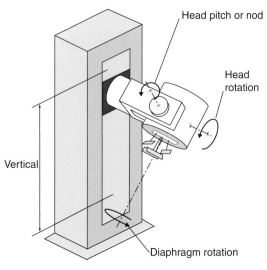

Isocentric gantry   Static gantry

Figure 8.27 Rotational and static gantry cobalt machines.

timer which controlled the period during which the source was exposed to the patient from its safe. Because there was a finite time during which the source would be transported to the fully exposed position, this was accommodated by modifying the exposure time with a transit time. The dose rate of the source was checked periodically by absolute measurement under reference calibration conditions. This would typically be monthly and, in addition, a comparison would be made against the known physical decay prediction in order to insure the purity of the isotope.

CUSTOM TELETHERAPY MACHINES

Although the gantry mounted medical linear accelerator has found extensive use, there have been treatment techniques which have required the adaptation of the linear accelerator and also development of highly specialized treatment machines.

Intraoperative electron beam machines

A treatment technique that has found limited acceptance is to irradiate the tumour bed following resection of the tumour surgically. It is known as intraoperative radiotherapy (IORT). This treatment is done with a single dose during the surgical procedure and with the target exposed to the machine. Because of the localization of the target and relatively shallow depth, electron beams are ideal. There

have been three approaches involving linear accelerators and other more compact electron accelerators. The first approach was to provide a standard gantry mounted linear accelerator in a surgical theater with suitable modifications to eliminate any explosion hazards. This assigns one particular theater for intraoperative treatment. Another approach has been to use a very compact linear accelerator mounted on a mobile assembly which can self propel between theaters. Both approaches, however, utilize the techniques to produce an electron beam from a linear accelerator. Other approaches have utilized compact accelerators, such as a betatron, which are mounted within a chosen theater or on a mobile assembly.

One aspect of note is the alignment of the electron applicator to the target area. Attempts have been made to ensure that there is no direct contact between machine and patient and sophisticated arrangements have been devised for this.

Robotic machines

The isocentric gantry mounting of teletherapy machines provides an efficient method to direct multiple beams at the target with relatively simple movements of the gantry and patient couch. Modern robotic control systems coupled with stereotactic radiographic localization of the patient's position has offered the prospect of delivering multiple beams from virtually any direction in space. Such a highly accurate system has been developed with a compact linear accelerator mounted upon a robotic arm. The location of the patient is determined from two kilovoltage images which, with use of image processing, uses bony anatomy or implanted markers in order to track the position of the patient during treatment and align the machine to ensure the required delivery trajectory of the beam is correctly obtained. This flexibility in the multiplicity of beam delivery directions coupled with high accuracy has enabled complex tumour volumes in close proximity to critical organs to be irradiated. In some cases, the radiation delivery can be achieved when conventional surgery would have so high a risk of complication that it is rendered impossible.

Stereotactic machines

Stereotactic radiotherapy and radiosurgery deliver a high radiation dose to small volumes localized using stereotactic frames in order to ensure a high positional accuracy of the treatment. Although, as mentioned above, a standard linear accelerator can be utilized to deliver such a treatment, machines have also been developed which are dedicated to this purpose. One well known machine is the Leksell gammaknife which consists of a treatment cavity for the head within which there is housed a large array of cobalt sources. The sources array focuses all the beams into a small volume, the dimensions of which are determined by collimators. The positioning of the patient's skull within the treatment cavity is located using a stereotactic frame bolted to the skull and ensures that extremely accurate localization of the compact treatment volume is achieved.

Besides this specialized machine, a standard linear accelerator has been adapted by one stereotactic facility supplier. The machine has been fitted with a high resolution multileaf collimator which is only applicable for very small stereotactic volumes. It is installed within a dedicated room designed with stereotactic kilovoltage imaging facilities to ensure highly accurate tracking of the patient and the target. Adjustment of the patient set-up and movement of the machine is executed to provide accurate dose delivery.

Dedicated intensity modulated machines

Intensity modulation to produce conformal radiation dose distributions based upon inverse treatment planning was promoted by Brahme in the late 1980s. Intensity modulation was not novel having been implemented with mechanical devices including the use of compensators to account for inhomogeneity such as lung within the body. The Scanditronix microtron and racetrack microtron designs attempted to address all aspects of beam modulation, covering energy, beam intensity and beam shaping with multileaf collimation. This machine design provided complete modulation of the beam. However, the basis of the machine was a standard linear accelerator gantry and, in a default condition, the machine reverted to deliver a standard beam identical to that of a standard linear accelerator.

In contrast, the Tomotherapy machine is completely dedicated to intensity modulation delivery. It has been designed to deliver narrow intensity modulated beams which alter in profile as they are rotated around the patient and, in effect, combine to produce a required dose distribution within that slice of the patient. The patient moves through the machine and adjacent slices are stacked together producing a continuous dose distribution throughout the patient tailored to the requirements of the clinician. In fact, the Tomotherapy machine is based upon the gantry design of a CT scanner and it is also able to generate megavoltage CT images for patient realignment prior to treatment. What is notable about this machine is that the original basis of its design was the production of intensity modulated beams for full conformal treatment.

Manufacturers of standard linear accelerators have produced systems which can deliver intensity modulated beams as the machine rotates around the patient. However, while this provides very effective conformal dose distributions efficiently, some of the benefits of a dedicated system like Tomotherapy of simultaneously treatment of multiple targets and also treating the entire length of the patient are lost.

IMAGE GUIDANCE

Megavoltage imaging to verify patient set-up and the location of critical tissue in relation to the radiation field has been carried out for many years with slow film. Because of the poor contrast between soft tissue and bony anatomy at megavoltage energies, attempts were often made to add filtration to the film cassettes to enhance the image contrast. Custom film holders, which could be treated as an accessory, were also made available to facilitate such imaging at any angle of the gantry. Over the past 20 years, electronic systems for both planar and CT imaging of the patient have become available. This development, along with the move to reduce treatment margins on fields, to reduce the dose to critical tissue and increase the dose to the tumour, has, in the interest of accuracy, expanded the role of imaging in radiotherapy. Indeed, it has become such an essential part of the treatment process that linear accelerators are now always supplied with an on-board imaging device.

Planar x-ray imaging

Planar imaging of the field being delivered represents the simplest verification of the location of the field in relation to bony landmarks. Such systems are a logical extension of the slow film used in the past but, with electronic planar devices, there exists an opportunity for image enhancement and automatic comparison between images to quantify patient movement. There are basically two planar imaging systems: a camera viewed fluorescent screen system and a solid state amorphous silicon system. Both types of system can produce high resolution, high contrast images. Therapy imaging techniques involve using the treatment field alone as well as using the treatment field superimposed on a larger field in order to assess better the treatment field's relationship to patient anatomy. Imaging protocols are now widely used to monitor and correct patient position during treatment. These imaging devices are being utilized to make significant decisions about patient position and, as such, their accuracy is of great importance. The devices are mounted on retractable arms attached to the gantry drum and positional corrections for gantry displacement can be required routinely as well as routine image correction parameter determination to account for the deterioration in the imaging devices.

Cone-beam imaging

A logical extension to planar imaging has been to utilize the sequence of images from a complete gantry rotation to generate CT image slices. This has been done for both megavoltage images and kilovoltage images. Of course, for the kilovoltage images, there needs to be a separate kilovoltage radiation source fitted onto the treatment machine. The great benefit from CT imaging is to provide positional information about soft tissue within the patient as opposed to relying on bony anatomy. As opposed to standard diagnostic CT scanners which pass the patient through a slice of radiation, it is more efficient to utilize the entire cone of the radiation beam from the machine or from the kilovoltage source. In effect, the reconstruction process which produces the CT image slices uses the overlap of the divergent beam as the machine rotates around the patient. This gives rise to the term cone-beam CT imaging and the reconstruction is calculated on the entire common volume as opposed to a slice-by-slice basis. The megavoltage CT images can also be used for dose prediction. The imaging devices are again fitted to the gantry using retractable mechanisms which suffer mechanical distortion during gantry rotation. Two aspects are critical here for accurate cone-beam imaging. The first is that suitable corrections are determined in order to reduce imaging artifacts and the second is that the positional registration between the kilovoltage image centre and the megavoltage treatment centre accurately agree.

RADIATION SAFETY

Radiation safety is of paramount importance with regard to radiotherapy treatment machines and relates to several aspects of the machine construction and its operation. The legislative requirements and practical means to achieve effective radiation protection are described in Chapter 4. Another significant aspect with regard to radiation protection is the room design described below.

However, besides these aspects, there is a need for protection of the staff and patients by the provision of machine interlocks and shielding. The radiation head itself is constructed with shielding to minimize the radiation leakage outside the treatment beam. For electron treatment, this is also addressed within the applicator design and the diaphragm settings.

Room door and maze barrier interlocks are installed to try to ensure that no accidental irradiation of staff can occur. Besides these, the treatment machines have many interlocked circuits. These interlocks are of two types. The first type is to ensure that the beam is operating within chosen performance limits. An example of such would be the monitor on a linear accelerator which ensures that the beam is uniform and symmetric about the central axis. Another would be the monitor of the bending current which ensures that the energy of the beam remains stable and would detect any fault in the circuit which could affect it and the energy of the beam. The second type ensures that fitments on the machine are correctly set. An example of this on a kilovoltage machine would be that the filter that had been fitted agreed with that selected at the treatment console. This would typically also be applied to the applicator. On a linear accelerator, a typical example would be to indicate that the target was in position.

One well-established safety system on linear accelerators is the provision of the two monitoring ionization chambers which are completely independent and monitor the entire field. The primary chamber, often referred to as Channel 1 is calibrated to deliver a known dose to a reference point from which doses can be calculated and predicted. The other chamber, referred to as Channel 2, the backup channel is set so that in the event of a Channel 1 failure the difference between the two channels will be detected and the irradiation terminated. Should Channel 1 fail completely, Channel 2 is set so that it will terminate the treatment having delivered a very small additional dose than that intended by the clinician. On linear accelerators there is also a tertiary termination system provided by a timer which should be set so that it would terminate the treatment in the event of both Channel 1 and 2 failures with only a small additional dose being given to the patient.

COMMISSIONING NEW EQUIPMENT

Following the supply of a treatment machine, it is essential that the characteristics of the machine's beams and the performance of the machine is established by measurement. Although this period of commissioning has become an established practice, it is now recognized in legislation such as IRMER 2000. The commissioning period sets out to provide the data upon which all calculations and dose predictions will be made for a patient's treatment. In addition, it provides the baseline set of performance data against which subsequent check or quality control measurements will be made. Besides measuring standard data, such as output factors, depth dose and tissue phantom ratios for example, specific data for beam dose algorithms in computer treatment planning systems along with verification data for the dose predictions are gathered and used for validation. In the case of imaging and any other ancillary equipment relevant commissioning measurements should also be devised.

Quality control

Quality control of the equipment is required to ensure satisfactory operation. It is required routinely and on a periodic basis in order to demonstrate the continued satisfactory operation of the machine. It is required following machine breakdown and repairs to ensure that the operation has been returned to a satisfactory level and, lastly, it is required following adjustments to the running of the machine to ensure again that the satisfactory operation of the machine has been maintained.

As with the commissioning of equipment, the good practice of quality control has grown over the years and is now established in statutory legislation, such as IRMER 2000.

TREATMENT ROOM DESIGN

The details of the treatment room design are very dependent upon the treatment machine, be it megavoltage or kilovoltage. There are two main aspects of room design to consider. The first concerns radiation safety and the protection of personnel while the second relates to the ergonomics of the room. The layout of the room is important to ensure efficient treatment, patient access, as well as machine maintenance.

For radiation protection, many of the features employed and the materials used can also be related to the actual location of the room, either its adjacencies to public areas or whether it is a new room or a re-used and modified room. Although there can be many aspects to detailed room design, there are general features which all room designs utilize to exploit very fundamental characteristics of radiation.

The purpose of the shielding is the protection of members of the public and workers associated with the treatment centre, particularly those who will spend a considerable portion of their working day in the vicinity of the room and involved with patient treatment.

These general features concern first, the direction of the primary beam and providing sufficient shielding to attenuate the direct beam. Also with regard to beam direction, the position of room access and the access of penetrations into the room for services such as electrical supply,

water, cabling for the machine and ventilation should also be placed to avoid primary beam irradiation. Away from the primary shielding, the room walls should be adequate for scattered radiation. While for megavoltage there will be cost savings associated with differentiation between primary shielding and scattered radiation shielding, for kilovoltage the entire room can be shielded for the primary beam.

The next feature concerns room access which may be direct or using a maze. Here, there are considerations such as staff access and also patient considerations about apprehension of being left alone in a room. Direct access requires a substantial shielding door to be fitted in the case of megavoltage and, at kilovoltage energies, the door shielding can also be substantial enough to require a motorized door. For a maze entrance, three aspects are of significance: cross-sectional area, distance along the maze and bends. The area concerns the cross-section of the maze at the room exit and the smaller this can be made consistent with patient access including a bed, the less radiation will enter the maze. Reduction of the cross-section of the maze at the treatment room end by fitting a lintel can make a worthwhile contribution to protection. Secondly, the length of the maze will increase the distance between the entrance and exit and provide a dose reduction. Lastly and significantly, the scatter from a right-angled bend within a maze can make a very significant contribution to reducing the dose.

In Figure 8.28, a typical megavoltage treatment room layout is shown with the features described above indicated for clarity.

For high energy megavoltage beams, one particular aspect of concern is neutron production due to a photon–neutron interaction in the nucleus. This interaction occurs at megavoltage energies and is nominally considered a problem for photon beam energies above 10 MV. Here the aspects described above are not readily applicable and expert advice needs to be sought. Nevertheless, despite the problems which neutrons bring, there are readily available solutions which enable safe room design with direct and maze access, even up to 25 MV. Several aspects concerning neutrons are worthwhile mentioning. The first is that sharp corners in the rooms aid the reduction of the neutron flux. Secondly, care should be taken to avoid metal content in the construction materials including the concrete aggregate as gamma activation can occur trading a neutron problem for a photon problem. This is also the case for wood lining which was considered appropriate in the past. Lastly, specialized lining, including commercial lining substances for the maze and other penetrations can be used to reduce significantly the problem to well below protection limits.

For more details on protection requirements, legislation and the choice of materials see Chapter 4.

Besides safety, the layout within a room for equipment and storage should be given consideration. Adequate

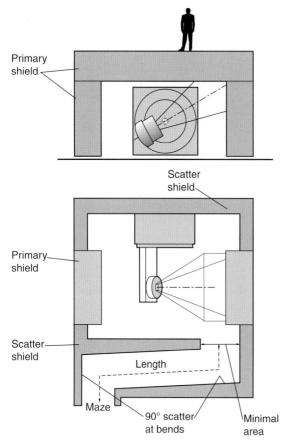

Primary shield

Scatter shield

Primary shield

Scatter shield

Length

Maze

90° scatter at bends

Minimal area

Figure 8.28 Major features of radiation protection for a linear accelerator treatment room.

to the machine and the controls around it, visibility of information screens, and the position of lasers in order to avoid accidental damage are worth consideration. The distance and access from the treatment control area into the room is important to maximize throughput and ease workload. In addition to patient and treatment staff considerations, it is also important to facilitate speedy access to the machine for repairs. This will reduce down time by enabling effective equipment, such as hoists to be used and ensuring that adequate clearance is available for the removal and fitting of components. Lastly, adequate lighting and dimming controls will ease patient set-up and again assist with increasing patient throughput. Similarly, clear and controllable CCTV for both megavoltage and kilovoltage are essential. For kilovoltage in particular, a camera mounted on the treatment head will provide close monitoring of a treatment site, enhancing the safe and effective delivery of the treatment.

CONCLUSION

Linear accelerators have undoubtedly become the mainstay of radiotherapy delivery in the developed world with cobalt teletherapy machines providing simplicity and economic benefits in the less affluent parts of the world. The linear accelerator and its beam shaping, intensity modulation and imaging facilities have provided clinical practice with enormous technical advantages which are now being evaluated in clinical trials. Specialized techniques, such as stereotactic radiotherapy and radiosurgery, have become widely recognized for their clinical benefits and dedicated machines are gradually establishing a niche in treating inoperable sites and providing new treatment opportunities for tackling cancer in patients. With all this technological advance, it remains important to bear in mind not only what is cost effective for treatment but also what can provide the best treatment process for the patient yet gives them the maximum benefit. Hence, there still remains a preference and a role for direct field treatments and even kilovoltage treatment to provide a simple process for say an aged patient or simply to expedite a treatment when intention is palliation and the maximum benefit to the patient is the time they spend away from the treatment centre rather than in it.

storage will ensure that treatment machine accessories, such as applicators and specific patient devices, such as immobilization shells, can be stored properly. This will help to avoid damage which might compromise the treatment because of the incorrect operation of equipment, for example a treatment distance pointer. Also it will avoid the treatment delays that repair would involve to damaged equipment. Similarly, the layout in the room and the access

FURTHER READING

[1] Thwaites DI, Tuohy JB. Back to the future: the history and development of the clinical linear accelerator. Phys Med Biol 2006;51:R343–62.

[2] Karzmark CJ, Morton RJ. A primer on theory and operation of linear accelerators in radiation therapy. 2nd ed. Medical Physics Publishing; 1997.

[3] Stedeford B, Morgan HM, Mayles WPM. The design of radiotherapy treatment room facilities. IPEM; 1997.

Chapter | 9 |

Radiation treatment planning: immobilization, localization and verification techniques

John Conway, Janet Johnson

INTRODUCTION

The treatment planning process consists of a series of patient-related work tasks that eventually result in a custom plan of the external beam treatment and will enable the radiation dose prescription to be applied. The *Radiation Treatment Planning* (RTP) system provides a 3D dose distribution of the beams arranged around the body using a mathematical model of the megavoltage x-ray field. The composite dose map is displayed in relation to the target volume and the critical anatomical structures within the body.

Integral to the planning process are devices that ensure the treatment is reproducible on a daily basis; the most important of these is a method of reducing movement of the patient during treatment, and this is called 'immobilization'. The specification of such a device is dependent on the area of the body for which it is required. For treatments of the head and neck, some form of immobilization device is essential to ensure reproducible set-up and to avoid displacement of the plan isocentre from its intended position. The relatively small field sizes used in the head and neck, compared with pelvic or thorax plans, requires a high degree of beam positional accuracy, because of the proximity to critical organs (e.g. eye, spinal cord), which depends on effective immobilization of the head. Other devices that facilitate reducing movement of the patient are site specific. For example, external beam radiation treatment of the breast utilizes a board that supports the patient at an inclined angle and provides hand grips that raises their arms above their head to meet the requirements for glancing beams arranged to the breast. Other devices stop the patient from moving their legs to reduce lower body movement or can make the treatment more sustainable over the few minutes of the beam exposure time.

Complete eradication of patient movement is impossible to achieve, although reducing this to within acceptable tolerance (e.g. 3 mm for head and neck, 5 mm for thorax and pelvis) is commonly achieved. Another technique to improve beam positional accuracy is to track the movement of the patient or movement of anatomical landmarks using an external device that is integral with the treatment accelerator – this method is called 'Image Guided Radiotherapy' (IGRT)'. IGRT requires monitoring of the patient using a real-time imaging device (e.g. video, ultrasound, x-ray) and the information is compared with the patient plan to correct for any positional inaccuracy. This technique enables a precise level of beam positioning control that can allow for any inadequacies in immobilization or effects of organ movement (e.g. lung displacement during respiration).

Anatomical information of the patient in the treatment position is required in order to undertake 3D treatment planning. The process of 'localization' includes the acquisition of either radiological images from a *simulator* and/or tomographic scanner (e.g. x-ray computer tomography, CT). The localization process provides external contour information and anatomical data that enable definition of planning target volume (PTV) contours and organs at risk (OAR); methods of providing this information range from x-ray CT, magnetic resonance imaging (MRI) through to positron emission tomography (PET). However, the basic requirement, to define the external contour and internal structures for treatment planning, are provided by a CT data set of the patient that can be transferred to the 'Treatment Planning System' (TPS) where attenuation data are converted to 'electron density' values for heterogeneity correction of the megavoltage beam data. Non-x-ray CT imaging modalities cannot provide this attenuation correction.

The production of an optimized treatment plan for external beam megavoltage treatment is highly dependent on the following:

- the size and shape of the PTVs
- the limiting (tolerance) dose to the critical structures (OAR)
- the positional reproducibility of the linear accelerator and couch support system
- limitation dictated by the patient's position within the immobilization device
- selection of optimum beam parameters (e.g. field size collimator rotation).

A customized treatment plan for the patient must be checked prior to first treatment to ensure the accuracy and validity of the plan, this process is called 'verification'.

Verification of the plan can be undertaken on a simulator where radiographic images of each beam portal can ensure the accuracy of the isocentre position and verify the beam size and shape against the treatment plan. Alternatively, a process called 'Virtual Simulation' allows the use of the original CT information to produce a 'Digitally Reconstructed Radiograph' (DRR) of the beam portal that provides a 'virtual film' that is comparable to the simulator image.

PATIENT IMMOBILIZATION

Patient head shells

The majority of patients receiving radiotherapy to the head and neck region are immobilized using a custom made shell that accurately fits to provide effective and reproducible positioning of the head at all stages of planning and treatment. Typically, the process used to fabricate a clear plastic shell, Figure 9.1A requires a plaster cast of the patient's head to be first produced. The transparency of the plastic enables the accuracy of fit to be checked with minor adjustments being made to ensure the shell must be a good fit, achieving the optimal position for treatment, while maintaining patient comfort.

Typically, the following steps are required to produce a full head shell:

1. the patient should assume the position to be adopted in the treatment room; this usually involves a headrest that supports the neck and inclines the head at the required angle for treatment. Separate impressions are taken of the front and back halves of the head
2. an impression of the back half of the patient's head is made using, for example, plaster of Paris bandage or dental alginate, which covers an area up to a coronal plane at the level of the ears
3. before taking a similar impression of the front half of the head a few precautions are necessary to ensure patient comfort. The patient should breathe normally through the nose and 'separating cream' should be used on the skin to enable easy removal of the plaster cast. In some circumstances, a tissue-equivalent mouth insert will be required to depress and fix the tongue
4. the plaster bandage should be shaped carefully round the bony protuberances of the head in order to facilitate good fitting of the shell and to provide effective immobilization. The two plaster impressions front and back must fit uniquely together once they are removed from the patient. Further layers of plaster bandage are applied to the two halves to provide rigidity and, once hardened, are removed from the patient
5. the two halves are fixed together with further plaster bandage over the joints and the impression is filled with a thin mix of plaster and allowed to set overnight
6. the final solid cast is trimmed and sawn in half along a suitable coronal plane. The cast is now ready for vacuum forming
7. the flat surface of each half cast is placed on the vacuum forming machine. A large plastic sheet is heated and stretched into a bubble before the casts are raised and the vacuum applied to form a tight skin around the surface of the molds

8. the excess plastic is trimmed from each shell to provide a flange that enables the two halves to be held together with plastic press-studs. Side supports are molded and attached to the shell to enable it to be fixed to the treatment head support.

Thermoplastic shells

Commercial systems are now widely available that do not require vacuum forming techniques; these perforated thermoplastic materials may be softened in a hot-water bath or warm oven and shaped directly onto the patient, Figure 9.1B. This system utilizes a U-frame in which the attached thermoplastic, when heated and softened, stretches from the tip of the nose to the baseplate, where the U-frame is indexed and locked down. While this system is very easy to use and provides a snug fit for excellent fixation, it also can, in some cases, exhibit shrinkage, leading to patient discomfort due to the stretching of the thermoplastic required with this type of system. Stretching resulting from prolonged use during the course of treatment can lead to inaccuracies in set-up and, although here is a cost benefit from repeated use, sterilization requirements can limit this.

A reinforced thermoplastic is also available that improves rigidity, comfort, and immobilization. Solid thermoplastic reinforcement strips, melted into the perforated sheet, provide rigid fixation and rotational stability necessary for treatments requiring more precise immobilization such as intensity modulated radiotherapy (IMRT) and conformal radiotherapy treatments.

These thermoplastic shells are a particularly attractive alternative to the vacuum formed shells to those sites which do not have extensive pretreatment preparation facilities. The material is easily molded, transparent and the perforations allow visual assessment of the final fit.

Non-shell fixation systems

These systems of head restraint are based on a custom impression of the patient's maxillary teeth and hard palate fixed to a plastic dental bite block (tray). Some designs incorporate a vacuum applied through the bite block that secures it to the maxillary structures; a vacuum pump is placed on the treatment couch and attaches to the mouth tray via a suction tube. Any decrease in pressure indicated by the vacuum gauge is indicative of a misplacement of the bite block. The mouthpiece is attached to two hollow carbon-fiber composite columns mounted on a baseplate by a patient-specific fixation set consisting of a transverse plate and an angle plate. Moving the plates against each other gives enough degrees of freedom to provide exact positioning. Once adjusted, the fixation set stays assembled throughout the entire treatment ensuring precise repositioning for the next fraction. A laser localizer box, consisting of side Perspex plates and top plate, are attached to the baseplate for daily set-up. Etched lines on the plate aid in visualizing the laser lines projected on the plates. This localizer box is removed prior to treatment.

This type of non-shell fixation can be as accurate as head shell methods provided that no displacement of the mouth bite occurs that could compromise the rigidity of the system. Patients that may be unsuitable for shell type immobilization, such as children and phobic patients, will often prefer this technique; however, because of limitations imposed by the system design, it is unsuitable for use with tumours of the lower oral cavity and neck.

Stereotactic frames

Stereotactic frames were originally designed for stereotactic intracranial surgery, biopsy and electrode placement but have since been extensively adopted for radiosurgery head immobilization, Figure 9.1C. The high level of precision required for *radiosurgery*, such as Gamma Knife® and X-knife® systems, necessitates a means of relating three-dimensional patient image coordinates to 3D locations in frame coordinates to submillimeter accuracy. The most common system in use is the Leksell Stereotactic System® Frame which is rigidly attached to the patient's head using four small screws placed with local anesthetic. The frame is shown in figure 9.1C. The frame provides the basis for target coordinate determination and is used to immobilize and position the patient's head within the radiosurgery collimator helmet. The centre coordinates of the target volume are positioned at the intersection of the beams (from 200 cobalt sources for the Gamma Knife®) so that 'target-centering' is always achieved within this geometrically rigid system. Relocatable versions of the stereotactic frame are also available that are closer in design to the 'head-arc fixation' method.

Body immobilization

Numerous techniques are available for immobilization of areas other than the head and neck. The major devices used are best discussed in relation to their site-specific needs:

Breast. Treatment of the breast commonly requires the use of three fields – two coplanar glancing beams to the breast and a supraclavicular field. All fields will often make use of the asymmetric collimators to bring one edge of each field to the beam central axis, thereby removing the effect of beam divergence from that one edge. This does not remove the penumbra, and the alignment of the superior edges of the breast fields with the inferior edges of the supraclavicular fields is critical. To achieve accuracy in this set-up requires careful positioning of the patient so that all fields can be treated without moving the patient. The use of a specially designed breast board is preferred. The device may consist of a support which inclines the patient's upper body and provides an elbow support and/or a hand-grip for the patient to grasp while holding the arm/s above the head;

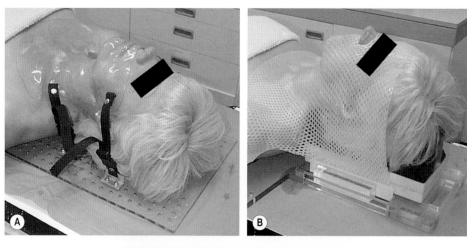

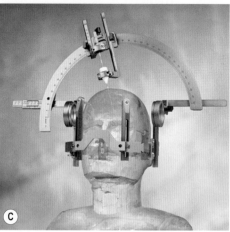

Figure 9.1 (A) Vacuum formed perspex shell, (B) Thermoplastic shell (Orfit), (C) Stereotactic frame (Leksell). *(With kind permission from Elekta).*

all these positions can be varied to meet the individual requirements of the patient's treatment and locked into position, linear and angular measurement scales allow the set-up to be recorded and reproduced at each fraction.

Pelvic region. This is one of the most difficult areas of the body to provide effective immobilization. Some systems utilize a single sheet of thermoplastic over the entire abdomen or pelvis that fixes to a baseplate, this is a larger version of that described for the head. An alternative to this is to use a large sealed plastic bag loosely filled with small expanded polystyrene spheres, Vac-Fix™. The bag is manually formed round the patient while the air pressure in the bag is gradually reduced using a vacuum pump. At approximately half atmospheric pressure, the bag becomes rigid and 'fits' firmly round the patient, preventing any significant movement. The rigidity can be maintained throughout a course of treatment and until the vacuum is released, when the bag and contents may be re-used for another patient. A variety

of shapes and sizes of bag are available to immobilize any part of the anatomy or the whole of the patient, for total body irradiation (TBI), for example. The attenuation in the polystyrene is minimal, but being opaque, consideration must be given to the beam entry ports during the initial evacuation. Radiation damage to the plastic will eventually cause vacuum failure and necessitate the replacement of the bag. Other devices, such as 'ankle stocks' and 'foot rests', can minimize movement by impeding body rotation or slippage on the treatment couch. The use of a 'belly-board' for prone patients, providing a cut-out in the patient support which allows the abdomen to fall anteriorly, ensures that much of the radiosensitive small intestine falls out of the high dose region.

Thorax. For modern radiotherapy, the problems imposed by respiratory movement can be considerable. Normal breathing causes movement of the chest wall and introduces uncertainties with regard to target volume position during treatment. These uncertainties are usually allowed for by introducing appropriate margins to the volume definition at the planning phase. However, these increased margins may have a significant effect on normal tissue doses and therefore have a limiting effect on the target dose. Effective compensation for these movements may involve either tracking of markers on the skin surface or identification of internal lung movement. Tracking the movement of the chest can be achieved using markers that can be followed using video cameras and calculating coordinate shifts that trigger a treatment pause if tolerances are exceeded. The tracking of internal organ movement is called 'Image Guided Radiotherapy'; these systems utilize either ultrasound or x-ray tomographic imaging methods to monitor and compare organ positions with the original CT planning images. This topic will be discussed further later in this chapter.

VOLUME DEFINITIONS

Accurate treatment depends on voluming. The parameters used in defining treatment volumes are described in detail in two documents published by the International Commission on Radiation Units and Measurements (ICRU), Reports 50 and 62 'Prescribing, Recording and Reporting Photon Beam Therapy' [1, 2].

The following are a transcript of the definitions:

Gross tumour volume (GTV) – is the gross palpable or visible/demonstrable extent and location of the malignant growth.
Clinical target volume (CTV) – is a tissue volume that contains a GTV and/or subclinical microscopic malignant disease, which has to be eliminated. This volume thus has to be treated adequately in order to achieve the aim of therapy: cure or palliation.
Planning target volume (PTV) – is a geometrical concept, and it is defined to select appropriate beam size and beam arrangement, taking into consideration the net effect of all the possible geometrical variations and inaccuracies in order to ensure that the prescribed dose is actually absorbed in the CTV.
Treatment volume – is the volume enclosed by an isodose surface, selected and specified by the radiation oncologist as being appropriate to achieve the purpose of treatment.
Organs at risk (OAR) — are normal tissues whose radiation sensitivity may significantly influence treatment planning and/or prescribed dose.

ICRU62 is the supplementary report to ICRU 50 and discusses in more detail the complex factors that account for delineation of the PTV. An *Internal Margin* (IM) is defined to accommodate for the variations in size, shape and position of the CTV as a result of anatomical variations caused by organ movement. An additional *Set-up Margin* (SM) must be then added to allow for the uncertainties of patient–beam position. Whereas the IM is required

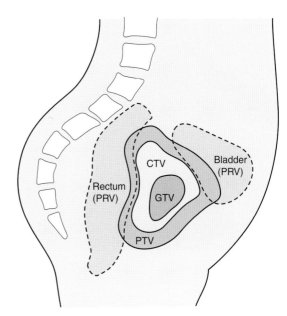

Figure 9.2 Prostate showing GTV, CTV, PTV, Bladder and Rectum.

to allow for a physiological process, the SM is required to allow for the technical factors that cause uncertainties. The SM may be reduced by improved immobilization of the patient and improved set-up accuracy. The IM can only be reduced through techniques such as 'respiratory gating' or 'image guided radiotherapy'. The organs at risk (OAR) volumes will also exhibit the same uncertainties in position and these will also require a margin to be added – the concept of *Planning Organs at Risk Volume (PRV)* is analogous to the PTV (See figure 9.2).

NON-CT CONTOURING DEVICES

Contours are all important in producing dose distributions. The value of radiation treatment planning depends on the reproducibility of the shape of the patient on a day-to-day basis throughout the course of treatment. The couch where the patient contour will be taken therefore should be identical in every respect to the couch on which that patient will be treated. It is imperative that the patient is correctly positioned before the contour is taken for planning purposes. Since the advent of radiotherapy treatment planning, a variety of physical devices has been available for taking patient contours. The simplest of these consists of a material (lead strip, flex curve) that can be bent around the patient and retains the shape while being transferred to paper in order to trace the contour.

Adjustable templates have been used that allow for more complex shapes to be transposed. A large number of

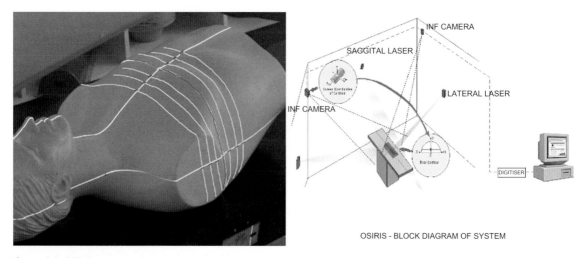

OSIRIS - BLOCK DIAGRAM OF SYSTEM

Figure 9.3 OSIRIS system.
(With kind permission from Qados Ltd)

adjustable pins or rods (3 mm diameter) held in a frame can accurately reproduce the surface shape in an axial plane. The frame is transferred to a drawing board and the contour traced onto paper.

Another simple method of obtaining a contour(s) from an immobilization shell is by fixing the shell within a frame so that a movable pin that can rotate around the plane to be contoured provides radial distance measurements; this system relies on radial coordinate measurements to transpose the contour shape of the required plane to paper. Many of these physical devices involving the use of contact techniques have been superseded by non-contact devices such as laser imaging/optical devices or through the use of computerized axial tomography; the latter will be described in detail in the following sections.

Recently, the use of optical systems, which have the benefit of no direct patient contact, have been introduced to provide both single and multiple contours of the patient in the treatment position. These systems are commonly installed within the simulator room and utilize the in-room alignment lasers (two laterals and one sagittal) that project both an axial and a vertical line on the patient's skin. Multiple views of these laser projections can be imaged by using four CCD cameras, mounted at ceiling height in each corner of the room, focused on the laser lines. Software manipulation of these four images enables a reconstruction of an axial contour and a sagittal contour. Multiple contours of the patient can be acquired by moving the couch either longitudinally (axials) or laterally (sagittals) and capturing images at each position.

This remote method of contour acquisition has many advantages over the physical methods described above; the key benefits are its inherent non-contact with the patient and the technique requires no manual handling of a device. Optical systems provide digital images of the patient's external contour that can quickly and easily be transferred to the

TPS and are generally compatible with the planning software. The ability of these systems to provide 3D skin contours are particularly useful in breast planning where CT planning may be less practical because of limitations of the CT scanner to accommodate patients in the position required for treatment to the breast (see figure 9.3).

PHYSICAL SIMULATION

The treatment simulator is essentially a diagnostic x-ray unit that emulates an isocentric linear accelerator's geometrical movement. The simulator has been an aid to radiotherapy for nearly half a century, and enables highly accurate localization of the target volume, the verification of the proposed treatment plan and, in some cases, even precise visualization of the organs at risk.

The unit allows real-time imaging of the beam portal and a facility to produce x-ray films of each treatment field.

The movements of a radiotherapy simulator are defined in the publication IEC 1217- 'Radiotherapy Equipment – coordinates, movement and scales' [3]. A physical simulator should have at least as good, or better, accuracy in positioning as the treatment unit and its mechanical tolerance must be excellent (e.g. an isocentre accuracy of 1 mm diameter sphere should be possible). The simulator geometry should permit all the required beam directions and field definitions that are achievable on a linear accelerator. Modern physical simulators (e.g. Varian Acuity™) do not have the limitations of the image intensifier systems that have been used for decades. The availability of an amorphous silicon panel to provide a digital imaging device has resulted in simulators that are almost identical to the therapy unit and have few movement constraints.

The simulator couch again needs to be identical to that used on the therapy unit and should have the same range of lateral, longitudinal, vertical and rotational movements. Coordinate scales between the simulator and linear accelerator must be identical. The ability to accommodate all treatment accessories and ensure precise emulation of the patient's position is essential.

The size of image that can be obtained during physical simulation is limited by a number of factors: the physical size of the image detector, the focus–axis distance, the focus–detector distance and the ability to stitch images together using a merge function. Dual and Quad merge techniques allow the acquisition of an image larger than the size of the imager (which is typically 30×40 cm^2). The enlarged image is created by moving the detector plate and acquiring multiple images all of which contain the beam central axis. Software enables these images to be referenced to this common central axis point and aligned accurately to provide extended images in both the horizontal and vertical directions. This facility is particularly useful for large pelvic fields or extended spine fields. Automatic merging of multiple images is less successful when there are significant differences in absorption within the images, e.g. a pelvis where large air gaps cause high contrast gradients.

During the localization procedure, the simulator is used much like a diagnostic x-ray unit where the patient is positioned on the couch in the treatment position and moved while imaging the anatomy. The desired location for field placement requires x-ray visualization in real-time until the required position is reached. In order to minimize radiation exposure to the patient during this procedure, a utility called 'motion control' is available. This function allows the control of field placement, e.g. x/y blades, collimator or field centre by adjusting these parameters on the captured (frozen/stored) image. Subsequent live activation of the imaging system initiated an automatic change to the parameter values and patient position on the physical simulator. The advantage of this function is that clinical decision and minor adjustments can be made on the captured image with a final check made with an x-ray exposure.

A typical head and neck physical simulation procedure is described below (although where a CT based facility is available, this offers a superior method of anatomical localization and contouring).

Localization

The patient is required to adopt the position on the simulator that is optimal for treatment delivery. The immobilization shell is then applied and final checks should be made to ensure that the patient is comfortable, that the head position is appropriate for the treatment being planned and that the contour of the shell fits accurately to the patient. Magnification markers of a known size may be applied to the shell for use during the planning stages.

The couch position is then moved so that the isocentre is approximately incident upon the centre of the proposed

target volume using surface anatomical landmarks. This can then be adjusted using fluoroscopy. Two orthogonal films/images should be taken (typically an AP and a lateral view, although any orthogonal arrangement may be used). It is usually prudent to record positioning details at this stage along with the film exposure factors.

Prior to moving the couch, a contour is taken using an appropriate contouring method which ensures that the film data and the contour data are coincident. This may be taken while the patient is on the couch or, alternatively, the lasers may be used to mark the plane on the shell surface so that a contour can be taken from the shell at a later time.

The size and position of the volume is marked on each film and the data transferred to the TPS for calculation and plan optimization. The plan should be accepted by the oncologist prior to verification.

Verification

Once the optimal treatment plan has been produced based upon the contour and geometric data from the images, the plan must be verified prior to commencement of treatment.

The patient re-attends the simulator and adopts the treatment position using the immobilization shell and positioning details recorded from the localization procedure. Using the parameters from the treatment plan, each field is set up in turn, applying the correct size, shape and direction of the beam. Using fluoroscopy, a comparison can be made between the volume marked at localization and that achieved during verification. Local protocols will specify tolerances for positional accuracy.

Using the light projected field display, the entry points and field borders can be transferred to the shell to ease treatment set-up on the linear accelerator. A verification film/image may be taken as confirmation of the final field portal to be delivered and gantry couch and field data may be transferred via a network to the linear accelerator.

If the beam arrangement is particularly oblique, it may be difficult to interpret the anatomy seen during fluoroscopy and it may be necessary to supplement the beam portal information with an AP and lateral view as a means of accurately confirming the position of the isocentre.

It is difficult to verify intricate beam shaping and multileaf collimator (MLC) configuration using conventional simulation, but this may be achieved either by using a physical device, attached to the accessory mount, which has radiopaque markers to define the leaf positions or by using a digital shape projection device (Figure 9.4).

CT SIMULATION

The term 'CT Virtual Simulation' was first introduced in a publication by George Sherouse in 1987 [4] who recognized that a suitable software package in conjunction with a

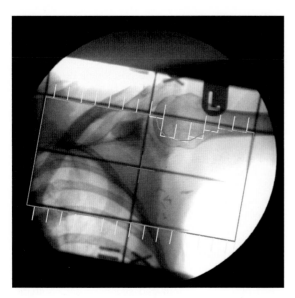

Figure 9.4 MLC fit on image.

diagnostic CT scanner could be developed that would emulate a conventional radiotherapy simulator. In the early 1980s, the use of CT scanners in treatment planning amounted to providing axial images that could be transferred to the TPS. The process of plan optimization and verifying the set-up before treatment was purely a role for the TPS and the physical simulator with no significant manipulation of the 3D CT data to augment this process. At this time, the use of the *Beam's Eye View* (BEV) allowed the visualization of a beam shape relative to the target contour, bony anatomy and other contoured organs. The BEV gave the planner the ability to optimize beam positions, shapes and orientation in the same manner as could be achieved radiographically on the simulator.

In 1983, Goitein et al [5] introduced the use of the *Digitally Reconstructed Radiograph* (DRR), a virtual radiograph or film of the patient. The calculation of DRRs is computationally intensive consisting of ray-line projection, interpolation, line integration and gray scale mapping of the CT data. For many years, the inability for computers to provide fast array processing slowed the introduction of virtual simulation into the treatment planning process.

The automatic registration of the BEV and DRR have provided powerful tools to enable the planner to achieve on the TPS what was available on the simulator but with the added benefits of CT visualization (see figure 9.5A). However, for practical use, the speed of DRR calculation would have to be sub-second to give the planner 'the feel of a simulator'.

In the early 1990s, specialized graphics workstations were introduced that allowed fast 3D array processing for ray-tracing, volume rendering and image reconstruction. Commercial systems became available at this time and,

with the rapid improvement in PC processor speeds over the past 10 years, have resulted in CT Virtual Simulation becoming more available and widely used in radiotherapy (see figure 9.5B).

CT Virtual Simulation is a combination of the physical process of using a CT scanner as an alternative to the physical simulator described above and the virtual process of simulator emulation using software programs.

$$\text{CT Virtual Simulation (CT} - \text{VSIM)}$$
$$= \text{CT localization} + \text{Virtual Simulation (VSIM)}$$

CT localization requires the patient to be supported and immobilized in the same position as for radiotherapy treatment. This can be more difficult compared with the conventional simulator which is designed specifically to mimic the linear accelerator patient support systems. The CT scanner must have a flat-top couch that can accept all these patient support accessories.

The process of marking the patient is facilitated by a laser system consisting of two fixed lateral lasers, the plane of these lasers being offset from the CT aperture plane by typically 500 mm, and a sagittal laser that can be moved laterally to overcome the fixed nature of the CT couch. The laser system can define the origin of a coordinate system that relates to the treatment machine coordinate system by shift distances or, in some cases, define the precise plan isocentre coordinates.

CT scanners used for simulation are invariably diagnostic scanners that have been adapted with flat table-top and external (to the gantry) laser systems. However, the advent of 'large bore scanners' specifically for radiotherapy planning have enabled these systems to be not only complementary but adopted as an alternative to the physical simulator. These new scanners have apertures of 80–85 cm compared with the conventional 70 cm and have scan field of view (SFOV) that are 10–15 cm larger than the diagnostic SFOV. For breast treatments, where the ipsilateral arm is raised above the head and subtends an angle close to 90°, then the large aperture scanners provide increased functionality (see figure 9.6).

The CT simulation process requires a scout (pilot) view to be taken in order to identify the required scan volume and suitable scan parameters. Axial image acquisition can be performed in either axial or spiral mode; the latter enables a continuous movement of the tube/couch rather than stepped movement in the axial mode. The patient CT study is passed to the virtual simulation workstation.

VIRTUAL SIMULATION

The physical simulator provides a real-time image using either a fluoroscopic screen with image intensifier or an amorphous silicon panel; this may be followed by exposure of a radiographic film to provide localization of the

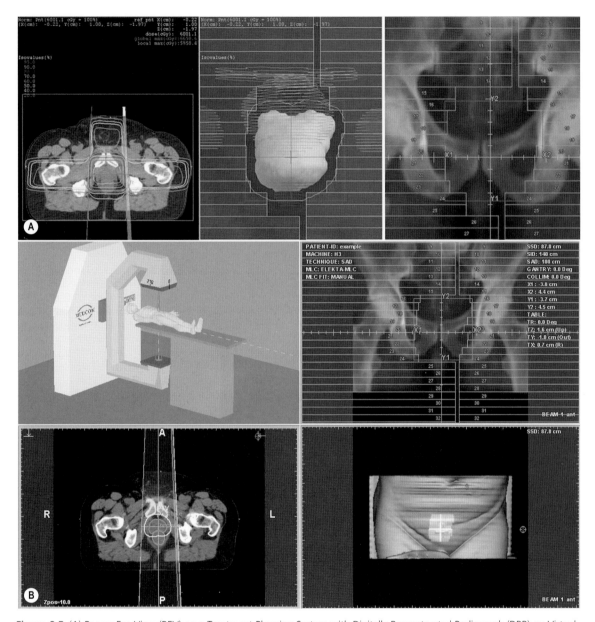

Figure 9.5 (A) Beams Eye View (BEV) on a Treatment Planning System with Digitally Reconstructed Radiograph (DRR) on Virtual Simulator; (B) Screen shot of Virtual Simulator with surface rendering and transverse slice.

treatment volume, visualization of the treatment field and verification of the plan design. Successful implementation of the virtual form of this simulator depends on software manipulation of the CT data.

The CT simulator equivalence to the physical simulator includes software capabilities to contour target volumes and critical structures, placement of treatment isocentre, beam design and generation of digital reconstructed radiographs (DRR). Many of the software control features are also incorporated into 3D planning systems but do not include the ability to provide coordinate information that relates to the patient position on the scanner couch and the provision to mark the isocentre and reference points.

The treatment planning portion of the CT simulation process starts with the definition of a *treatment reference point* that can either coincide exactly with the position of the isocentre or alternatively can be an estimate of its

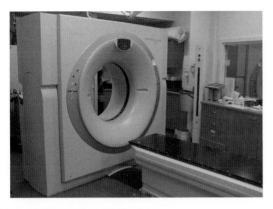

Figure 9.6 Large Bore CT Simulator.

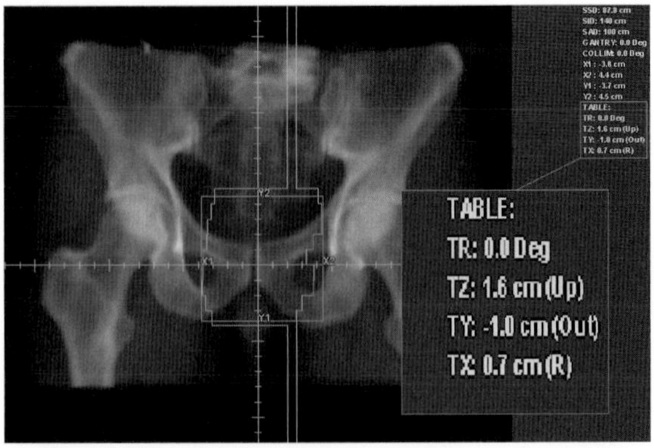

Figure 9.7 BEV/DRR with shift information.

position. The former method will require the definition of the target volume to define precisely the treatment isocentre and will require the oncologist to be present; whereas the latter method does not require the target volume to be defined and the final isocentre position can be found using '*shift coordinates*'. These shift distances, Figure 9.7 are relative to the reference point and can be applied at the first treatment in order to align precisely the isocentre to the target. The shift coordinate method is commonly used in a busy department where there is limited time to wait until targets are contoured or where the oncologist is not available during the scanning session.

A TYPICAL HEAD AND NECK CT SIMULATION PROCEDURE

Localization requires the immobilization shell to be attached to the flat CT couch in order to emulate exactly the patient positioning on the treatment machine. Careful consideration should be given to the design of the head fixation device to enable compatibility between the CT and accelerator table supports.

The scanning parameters are usually a trade-off between maximizing DRR resolution and keeping the number of slices to a manageable size (typically 3 mm slice thickness and 1.5 spiral pitch). The scanning extent is determined from the pilot (scout) view and the external contours are often produced at a remote virtual simulation workstation while previewing the scanned slices.

A reference slice plane is selected and the 'patient reference origin' coordinates created and transferred to the CT couch and/or lasers. The CT longitudinal couch, vertical couch and sagittal laser positions are set to define the 'patient reference origin' and the patient is marked. The patient session is now finished. An alternative

approach is to mark the patient before scanning and to set this position as the 'patient reference origin'.

Virtual simulation requires marking of the GTV, CTV, PTV and OARs; the isocentre and field parameters can then be defined using the TPS. The plan is sent for calculation and optimization to the TPS and exported back to the virtual simulator workstation for verification. The DRRs for all beams are printed (laser imager) and approved by the oncologist.

'*Shift coordinates*' are printed from the relationship between the isocentre to 'patient reference origin' coordinates. These are transferred to the treatment machine with the plan details. Worksheets and DRRs are printed (see figure 9.7).

The advantages of CT virtual simulation can be summarized as follows:

- full 3D simulation allowing unique verification of beam coverage and avoidance in 3D
- beams can be simulated and verified that are not possible with conventional simulation, e.g. vertex fields
- the verification image – the DRR – can contain more information than conventional simulation and can be manipulated to enhance tumour visualization
- there is a much closer connection to diagnostic information with CT simulation allowing integration of multimodality images.

During the early use of CT simulation, it was evident that the inability to image organ movement (e.g. lung) was a significant disadvantage over physical simulation's fluoroscopy. However, the improvement in image acquisition and reconstruction speeds has provided the ability to follow respiratory movement. The technique is often called '*respiratory gated acquisition and 4D viewing*', this method enables images to be acquired at a rate of more than 16 frames per second that enables the full movement of the patient's diaphragm to be visualized within a movie loop. The definition of lung tumour margins can now be assessed in 3D.

MULTIMODALITY IMAGES FOR PLANNING

CT imaging plays a crucial role in radiotherapy planning as it provides the electron density information that is required to correct the absorbed dose for the different tissues through which the beams will pass.

CT imaging also provides excellent definition between tissues having marked differences in x-ray attenuation values (e.g. air/bone/soft tissue), however, the contrast of these images is poor for structures with similar electron densities (e.g. tumour/soft tissue).

Magnetic resonance imaging (MRI) is based on the measurement of radiofrequency radiation resulting from transitions induced between nuclear spin states of hydrogen atoms (protons) in the presence of strong external magnetic fields. Unlike CT, where the signal intensity is dependent on x-ray attenuation and its contrast on the electron density of tissues, MRI depends on the intrinsic tissue properties associated with proton densities and spin relaxation times. Therefore, MRI has the ability to differentiate between tissue of similar density thus providing better delineation, not only of tumour extent, but also of the adjacent critical soft tissue organs.

MRI also provides unrestricted multiplanar, volumetric, vascular and functional information.

Some of the problems associated with using MRI for treatment planning are:

1. inherent *image distortion*, particularly at the periphery of the image (typically 3 mm for heads and up to 15 mm for pelvic images)
2. pixel intensities are not related to electron density values and therefore cannot be used for heterogeneity correction (i.e. density/dose) when calculating treatment plan dose distributions
3. the physical restrictions of the MRI scanner mean that a patient cannot be easily positioned in the treatment position. A quantitative method called *image registration* is used that provides fusion of CT and MRI image studies.

MRI data are transferred to a TPS where the therapy CT images and the MRI images are registered. Manual and automatic methods of registration are now available as part of sophisticated software systems provided with CT simulators. The manual methods involve matching fiducials that are visualized on both CT and MRI; these fiducials are opaque markers or bony structures so that image translation in the three coordinates directions achieve a match between the two studies. The accuracy of image registration can be assessed by the accuracy to which the fiducial markers match.

Once the two image data sets are matched then volume contouring on the MRI images is automatically translated to the CT study. This technique provides the advantages of the MRI images for tumour delineation while maintaining the CT study for accurate calculation of the treatment dose distribution.

Automatic registration methods such as *'mutual information'* use rigid and non-rigid matrix transformations that are able to compensate for rotational as well as translational differences between the two image sets.

New imaging modalities that provide 'functional' or 'tumour kinetic' information for radiotherapy treatment planning are becoming widely accepted. Positron emission tomography (PET) and single photon emission CT (SPECT) produce nuclear medicine images that enable improved staging of malignant disease and improved treatment planning by ensuring that gross tumour volumes are more accurately defined. Information from these functional imaging modalities can be used to design more conformal radiation dose distributions and to prescribe additional dose to specific tumour microregions.

The specific activity of the radiopharmaceutical fluoro-2-deoxyglucose (^{18}F-FDG) produces uptake in malignant tissue that enables highly accurate determination of the extent of solid tumour spread. FDG is taken up by glucose transporters and its concentration can be measured (images) by the retained activity within various tissues. FDG uptake correlates strongly with the presence of cancer.

The introduction of combined PET/CT scanners has improved the availability of this new modality. The PET images are superimposed upon the CT images, both of which are simultaneously acquired during a single scan session. Planning can be performed either in treatment position, requiring modifications to the scanning protocols, or in diagnostic position with image registration being used to accommodate the change in patient position between functional image and treatment planning patient position.

Specialized software can register the PET/CT study with the therapy planning CT study to enable contours on the PET images to be transposed to the planning images.

There is increasing evidence that, in many clinical situations, radiotherapy treatment may be planned more accurately if supplementary functional images of the patient are available. In practice though, the lack of access to PET and the problem of image registration have restricted the use of combined anatomical and functional information:

- PET is prohibitively expensive, which has limited its routine clinical use to only larger oncology facilities
- multimodality image registration is a difficult problem, which is further complicated by the significant anatomical changes that may occur between the different imaging sessions due to surgery, chemotherapy, patient weight change or fluid collection.

PORTAL VERIFICATION AND IMAGE GUIDED TREATMENTS

Portal imaging

Confirmation of the accuracy of the delivered beam is an essential part of quality assurance. This is achieved primarily by imaging the beam portal using the linear accelerator before, during or after a treatment exposure.

This can be achieved using a choice of film. Therapy verification film, a slow film housed in a light proof packet, can be left in place for the full treatment exposure. Alternatively, a faster film housed in a cassette with stainless steel intensifying screens requiring a smaller incident dose can be used, the advantage of this is that it is possible (though perhaps not practical) to develop the image and analyze the outcome prior to delivering the full treatment dose.

The disadvantages of film are the need for on-site processing facilities, the time delay in processing, inability to manipulate the image quality without re-exposure and the resultant long-term storage considerations.

Hardcopy films are now being superseded by electronic or digital forms of imaging. Solid state devices or *electronic portal imaging devices* (EPID) are now becoming integral components of the linear accelerator. These devices may consist of an amorphous silicon detector panel housed on a retractable arm which is an integral component of the linear accelerator gantry. In this way, the panel is always perpendicular to the beam central axis thus avoiding image distortion. Detector panels have a physical size of 30×40 cm and this allows practical imaging of fields, typically 20×25 cm. Image quality from amorphous silicon devices is considerably superior to that which can be achieved with film or optical camera-based systems.

Protocols for the frequency of imaging are determined locally, though typically, these consist of imaging the fields for the first three to five fractions to establish accuracy and reproducibility and then periodically throughout the rest of the course to ensure consistency.

Analysis of the images produced may be qualitative, i.e. an 'eyeball' assessment in conjunction with the software measuring tools or, increasingly, may utilize the assistance of an automatic image registration tool to provide quantitative displacements. The image registration or matching process requires user defined anatomy to be outlined on a reference image (typically the DRR or the conventional simulation image). The same anatomical features are then outlined on the portal image and the software will overlay these contours thus providing a field edge displacement value for the lateral, longitudinal and rotational positions. As a result, it is possible to determine whether the isocentre position is within predetermined tolerances or whether adjustment is required.

There are many advantages to digital imaging systems; physical storage problems are removed – though consideration must be given to the need for future data retrieval. Software tools can be used to manipulate the image to aid viewing and analysis, multiple users can view the image and remote access facilities can be implemented. From a treatment delivery aspect, however, the biggest advantage is the ability for on-line assessment of images and immediate adjustment of patient position to achieve greater accuracy.

Image guided radiotherapy

Conformal radiotherapy depends on geometrical and dose shaping to optimize the dose distribution to the known planning target volume. Techniques to achieve this involve the use of multileaf collimation to shape each field to a beam's eye projection of the PTV (geometric conformality) and intensity modulation of the beam (IMRT) to achieve dose shaping of the beam (dose conformality). These methods do not take into account the fourth dimension to radiotherapy, 'time', which can extend from seconds to days.

A number of time-related factors introduce significant uncertainties in radiotherapy:

1. the movement of target and critical tissues during treatment (seconds – minutes).
2. the movement of organs between treatment fractions (days)
3. the dynamic movement of the beam delivery method (seconds – minutes).

The interplay between the dynamic beam delivery motion and tissue motion during treatment can result in both over- and underdosage of the target volume.

Two questions that have involved considerable debate are: What are the effects of organ motion on treatment planning images? And how can we acquire information on organ motion? The advent of ultra-fast CT acquisition from multislice scanners has enabled time dependent organ position data to be captured This large quantity of data can be used during the treatment planning process but the contouring of the hundreds of image slices is not possible using conventional manual methods. Automatic organ tools (segmentation methods) are being developed that enable tracking of organ movement (*4D imaging*).

During treatment, these organ movements must be also monitored in order to correlate with planning (verification) data.

Four methods of image guided techniques are available:

- radiopaque markers that can be tracked using video cameras
- ultrasound systems that determine organ positions prior to treatment

- diagnostic x-ray systems mounted on the linear accelerator that can provide orthogonal images or CT *(cone beam reconstructed)* images

- treatment-room CT scanners that are adjacent to the linear accelerator and can provide pretreatment or post-treatment CT images.

REFERENCES

[1] ICRU Report 50. Prescribing, recording and reporting photon beam therapy. International Commission on Radiation Units and Measurements; 1993.

[2] ICRU Report 62. Prescribing, recording and reporting photon beam therapy (supplement to ICRU Report 50). International Commission on Radiation Units and Measurements; 1999.

[3] IEC 1217. Radiotherapy equipment – coordinates, movement and scales. IEC; 1996.

[4] Sherouse GW, Mosher CE, Rosenman J, Chaney EL. Virtial Simulation: Concept and Implementation. The Use of Computers in Radiation Therapy. Bruinvis et al, editors. Elsevier, North-Holland; 1987.

[5] Goitein M, Abrams M. Multi-dimensional Treatment Planning: Beam's Eye View, Back Projection, and projection through CT sections. Int J Radiat Oncol Biol Phys 1983;9:789–797.

Chapter | **10** |

Principles and practice of radiation treatment planning

Peter J. Childs, Margaret Bidmead

INTRODUCTION

The goal of treatment planning of external beam radiotherapy is to produce a dose distribution within the patient that will destroy the tumour while sparing as much healthy tissue as possible. The planning role is usually carried out by radiographers, physicists, or technologists with expertise in producing either an optimum plan, or a selection of compromise plans for the clinician to approve. The planner must have sufficient clinical knowledge to understand where compromises may have to be made, either in sparing some of the target volume dose or in accepting higher than desirable doses to radiosensitive healthy tissue.

Most treatment sites will have locally agreed standard treatment protocols and the planner will normally have a limited range of variables with which to optimize the plan.

The planner must take the clinical requirements stated in a prescription and planning request and translate them into the best plan for the individual patient. This must then be presented to the clinician in a clear format so that what in many cases is a complex three-dimensional plan can be readily appraised. Over the years, tools and techniques have evolved to enhance this critical communication between staff groups. The ICRU reports 50 and 62 [1, 2] referred to in Chapter 9 provide an effective methodology of prescribing the volume to be treated and the means of displaying the dose distribution produced by the treatment plan.

The intention of the treatment can drive the complexity of the plan, given that most radiotherapy centres now possess therapy machines capable of delivering highly sophisticated treatments. The cost (i.e. complexity) of the treatment must be balanced against the benefit and, in many instances, the simplest plan is the best plan. The cost may be measured in increased treatment time, which could lead to increased waiting times for other patients. Complex and non-standard plans can also increase the risk of errors.

Where the treatment intent is palliation, for example relief from pain arising from metastatic disease, then a single treatment beam will usually fulfill the purpose. This can be justified as the most important consideration is to give the treatment as soon as possible, with minimal distress to the patient, and the consequences arising from irradiating excess normal tissue do not apply to a patient with a short life expectancy.

Where the treatment intent is curative 'radical' treatment, consideration must be given to short- and long-term side effects arising from the irradiation of healthy tissue. The complexity of a treatment plan is likely to increase, especially when an organ at risk (OAR), also referred to as a critical structure, lies adjacent to the planning target volume (PTV), and the prescribed dose greatly exceeds the tolerance dose of the OARs.

It is important that the planner appreciates the radiosensitivity of normal tissue. OARs can be considered as serial (e.g. spinal cord), parallel (e.g. lungs), or a combination of serial and parallel (e.g. the heart). In a serial organ, if any part of the organ receives a dose above its threshold then there will be total loss of function, e.g. paralysis in the case of the spinal cord. In a parallel organ, part of the organ may be severely damaged but the rest continues to function. Therefore, it is important to consider the volume of the parallel organ that is receiving the damaging dose. For example, the severity of lung pneumonitis significantly increases if the dose exceeds 20 Gy so the plan would be evaluated by considering the volume of lung exceeding this dose – 'V20'. For a patient with two healthy lungs, it would be normal practice to consider both lungs as a single organ.

Table 10.1 gives typical tolerance doses for organs. However, these values should not be taken as absolute, as fractionation affects the ability of normal tissue to repair damage. The quoted dose may represent an increased risk rather than a stochastic threshold above which all patients will be affected. The patient's clinical condition and drugs may affect radiosensitivity of some organs. The complete clinical picture is also important, for example in the abdomen region, the planner must know whether one of the kidneys is already non-functioning as this will enable them to design a plan that may reduce the dose to the healthy kidney at the expense of dose to the already damaged one.

Treatment planning computers offer a variety of tools used to localize treatment volumes, 'virtually simulate' the field arrangement, and to calculate the dose distribution. This chapter covers the production of desired dose distributions to treat a specified PTV and the tools relevant to this process. The majority of radiotherapy treatments are delivered using megavoltage x-rays or electrons from linear accelerators. However, there are some specialized treatment techniques appropriate to a limited range of diseases. These techniques may be delivered with a conventional linear accelerator, or may require specialized equipment such as

Table 10.1 Typical normal tissue tolerance doses for generally accepted risks. Note that these may vary for individual situations due to clinical condition and other therapies increasing radiosensitivity and that correction must be made for different fractionation

ORGAN	TYPICAL DOSE LIMITS	COMMENTS
Spinal cord	45 Gy	Although a serial organ, the length of the cord receiving the dose may be taken into account
Lung	V20 (e.g. <32%) mean lung dose <18 Gy	Normally consider total volume of both lungs (if the GTV or PTV lies within the lung then its volume should be subtracted from the total lung volume and higher V20 volumes may need to be accepted)
Heart	<40 Gy to entire heart No more than 1/3 of heart volume to receive 60 Gy	Normally the heart volume outlined will include blood
Kidney	Whole kidney 12 Gy 1/3 kidney 16 Gy	Essential to ensure unirradiated kidney is functioning or a non-functioning kidney is preferentially sacrificed
Liver	Whole liver <21 Gy 1/3 liver 30 Gy	
Lens	6 Gy	If cataract formation is the concern then consider the consequence of any treatment compromise against future cataract removal
Rectum	% of 2 Gy/fraction dose for 74 Gy prescribed dose Dose (%) Max. vol. 68 60 81 50 88 30 95 15 100 3	An example of a DVH based dose constraint rather than a single volume or dose threshold

the Tomotherapy® device or Gamma knife®. The use of modern treatment delivery equipment with dynamic control of multiple simultaneous movements, such as couch, gantry, and multileaf collimators, may be restricted by the treatment planning process as complex software is required to simulate and calculate dose distributions. Specialist software is required to plan treatments for devices such as Tomotherapy and Gamma knife.

The reasoning behind the prescribed dose required to kill a specific tumour type is discussed in Chapter 17. The treatment planner is given this in the plan request and is solely concerned with delivering this dose at the specified fractionation. However, it is important to have the dose and dose per fraction available at the time of planning as the dose limits to critical structures will depend on the dose rate.

Much of radiotherapy dose and fractionation is based largely on clinical results evaluated over decades. However, better knowledge of how specific tumours and normal tissues respond to radiation, in individuals, or groups of patients, could lead to more effective treatments. If reliable radiobiological data relating to both the tumour and normal tissues are available then it may be possible to prepare a plan based on the effectiveness of the dose delivered rather than the physical dose alone. Inverse planning may be performed by optimizing the dose distribution through the use of normal tissue complication probability (NTCP) and tumour control probability (TCP).

Modern treatment planning is a complex process. As well as striving to meet the optimum clinical objectives, it is also important to comply with local practice for the patient set-up instructions, and local protocols established for reliable and safe treatment delivery. For the beginner, this can be frustrating as, even for basic plans, to some extent the process can only be learnt from one's own mistakes.

PATIENT DATA

The patient contours may be acquired in the form of multiple computed tomography (CT) slices or, in some cases, derived from external contours alone, possibly with some estimation of the dimensions and density of significant internal heterogeneities, such as the lung. The detailed anatomy derived from CT images is the optimum means of obtaining accurate dose distributions as the CT numbers can be converted to electron density maps, which the treatment planning computer (TPS) will use to calculate how the beams are attenuated and scattered. However, CT- density tables can also be manipulated to obtain enhanced digitally reconstructed radiographs (DRRs), so it is important to use a table that is specifically intended for dosimetry rather than imaging (see Chapter 9).

CT is the best imaging modality for radiotherapy in terms of dosimetry and spatial accuracy, but does not always provide the best images for tumour or critical structure localization. Normal practice is to register the diagnostically superior magnetic resonance (MR) or positron emission tomography (PET) images onto the CT images (see Chapter 9). However, it is possible to use the MR images directly for some sites, by applying distortion correction to the MR images and assigning 'bulk heterogeneity' corrections to visible structures such as bone.

When using a TPS with 3D scatter correction, it is important that the CT scan extends beyond the PTV, ideally by at least 2 cm, so that the adjacent anatomy is accounted for in the calculation and not assumed to be air by the TPS.

The contours used for planning must represent the patient contour during treatment delivery – bearing in mind that treatment will take several minutes, whereas CT scans are acquired in seconds. Most contouring techniques, whether CT or external outlines only, are very rapid 'snapshots' compared to treatment delivery times. Therefore, either the planning procedure, or the treatment delivery, must account for patient movement. For the vast majority of treatments, the treatment plan must be designed to account for this patient movement by the addition of margins around the clinical target volume. However, modern technology now offers practical methods of 'gated' treatments that only deliver the dose to the patient while they are in the same position as during the therapy CT scan, or 'tracking' treatments, that can follow the PTV movement. These are discussed in the final section of this chapter.

Figure *evolve* 10.1 shows the effect of patient breathing on a thoracic CT image acquired in spiral mode. The appearance of the liver clearly indicates the breathing motion that otherwise might not be apparent.

Radiotherapy patients may have prostheses, dental fillings, breast implants, and other artifacts present externally or internally. Sometimes these will be present during imaging but may be removed by the time treatment commences (for example, drainage tubes). Where the artifact is made of material similar to tissue density such as breast implants (although some breast implants contain high-density magnets), the CT-density table will correctly allocate the density required. However, for metal implants, the CT scan must be acquired with an extended CT scale and the TPS CT-density table must be extended typically to give Hounsfield numbers of up to 32 000 if metal implants are to be identified and the correct density assigned. Even with artifact

correction tools on CT scanners, there are usually significant artifacts present surrounding metal objects – especially for bilateral hip implants, and a manual overlay of the density may be required (Figure *evolve* 10.2). The use of MR imaging in the presence of non-ferrous implants may provide useful information that may be transferred to the distorted CT dataset.

Cardiac pacemakers present a problem, not only in perturbing the treatment beam, but also in their sensitivity to radiation and electromagnetic interference from linear accelerators. Ideally, pacemakers should not lie in the path of a treatment field and should only receive scattered radiation dose of less than 2 Gy. The cardiologist should be consulted to ascertain the required level of monitoring during and after the treatment.

Contrast may be present in a CT scan, for example, to visualize nodes in head and neck images (Figure *evolve* 10.3), or may be present in the bladder as a result of contrast used elsewhere.

This contrast will not usually be present during the actual treatment, but its presence during planning does not usually have a significant impact on the dosimetric accuracy. However, this should be verified whenever a new contrast-based localization technique is introduced.

Care should be taken to ensure that the CT image represents the treatment set-up. Sometimes, the patient cannot be scanned in the same position as for treatment due to restrictions of the CT scanner aperture, particularly when immobilization devices are employed. For some sites, the scan may be performed feet first into the scanner while the patient may be treated in the head first orientation. In this case, the TPS or scanner software may be utilized to mirror and restack the scans into the treatment position. When such techniques are employed, there must be clearly visible quality assurance (QA) tools to verify that the software has processed the images correctly, such as couch markers identifying the couch superior-inferior and lateral orientations.

The CT couch, immobilization supports, bolus, or non-treatment-related devices may be present in the CT scan. The user should be aware of how the TPS will handle, or ignore, structures that lie outside the patient's external contour and how to compensate for TPS calculations that do not account for beams passing through these structures. High density couch bars on the treatment unit couch may need to be accounted for in plans with beams passing through the couch and, ideally, the positions of these bars should be overlaid on the CT image so that the plan is designed to avoid them.

The planner should also be aware of any anatomical abnormalities in the CT scan that may affect the treatment plan. It may be preferable to avoid regions where surgery has taken place, or to avoid abnormalities unrelated to the disease being treated, such as a hernia.

It is important to appreciate the shortcomings of the TPS algorithms, especially in the presence of heterogeneities.

The build-up effect at internal density boundaries may not be accurate and the 3D scatter distribution may not be accurately modelled. These effects typically lead to the TPS overestimating doses in soft tissue regions (e.g. tumours) surrounded by low density tissue (e.g. lung).

For simple point dose calculations, a water phantom can be used to approximate the patient anatomy. This may be performed manually using tabulated data direct from plotting tank measurements, or by a TPS assuming the patient to be an infinite water phantom. In either case, the actual patient contour may differ significantly from the phantom and where the point dose lies near the patient surface or internal heterogeneities, discrepancies of several percent may exist if comparing against calculations performed with full CT data.

MEGAVOLTAGE PHOTON THERAPY

Treatment beams

The characteristics of a megavoltage beam must be employed to produce an optimum plan for the variety of clinical requirements.

Beam energy

The first parameter the planner selects is the beam energy, by considering the depth of dmax and the penetration properties of the beam (Table 10.2 shows typical values for commonly used energies). Low energy beams, e.g. 4–6 MV are suited to more superficial volumes, e.g. head and neck PTVs, while deep pelvic PTVs will require 10–20 MV. Beam energies above 15 MV do not give a great benefit to the planner, but their frequent use on a Linac can introduce radiation protection problems from neutrons.

The build-up region is a significant feature of the MV beam in that it gives 'skin sparing', allowing doses that would severely damage the skin to be delivered deep into the patient, even from a single beam. However, a PTV that extends from near the surface to a depth requiring MV photons may require bolus to be added to the skin of the patient. By placing this tissue equivalent material on the skin, the build-up region is shifted into the bolus and the maximum dose of the beam is delivered to on or near the skin. Unless the PTV is superficial, the planner should consider the impact of patient immobilization devices on the build-up region.

Asymmetric fields

A standard field set on a treatment machine will be symmetric, i.e. the centre of the field defined by the collimators will be centred on the machine isocentre. Asymmetric fields (i.e. where one or both of the X and Y collimator settings are not equal) have two benefits to the planner. First, they

Table 10.2 Typical depth dose characteristics for 10×10 cm radiotherapy beams

X-RAY ENERGY	SSD (cm)	DMAX DEPTH (cm)	$D_{80\%}$ (cm)	DOSE @ 10 cm (% OF DMAX)
60 kV	30	0	0.5	2
100 kV	30	0	1.0	10
220 kV	50	0	2.5	29
4 MV	100	1.0	5.9	63.0
6 MV	100	1.5	6.7	67.5
10 MV	100	2.3	8.0	73.0
15 MV	100	2.9	9.1	77.0
25 MV	100	3.8	10.9	83.0
Electron energy (MeV)				
4	95	0.9	1.4	1
6	95	1.3	1.9	1
10	95	2.2	3.2	1
15	95	2.6	4.9	3
20	95	2.6	6.7	10

enable a treatment plan isocentre to be located on a convenient anatomical set-up point rather than being restricted to the centre of the PTV. Secondly, they enable the beam divergence of adjacent fields to be matched to one another (see below).

Although un-wedged treatment fields can be considered as delivering a uniform dose across their area, this is not strictly true, especially at points several centimetres away from the central axis. Due to the varying beam energy across the field, this non-uniform dose will also vary with depth. Therefore, manual calculations for asymmetric fields will require the addition of an asymmetric factor to account for the beam profile.

Isocentric plans

For a single field treatment, the machine isocentre may be set to the surface beam entry point (fixed source-to-surface distance (SSD) beam), or at depth. Although the beam characteristics will be slightly different in these two set-ups, there is no significant dosimetric advantage either way, and the treatment method is determined by consistent local practice.

For efficient treatment delivery of multiple beam plans, it is preferable to produce 'isocentric plans'. In this arrangement, the machine isocentre is positioned inside the patient, and typically inside the PTV. Thus, once the patient has been positioned for the first beam, it is only necessary to rotate the gantry and/or couch and collimator angles, to deliver the subsequent beams.

Extended focus skin distance (FSD) plans

Most treatment machines have a maximum field size of 40 × 40 cm so to treat longer volumes with a single field an 'extended FSD' beam is required. Here, the isocentre is positioned outside the patient to take advantage of the beam divergence. Although the daily set up of these plans will be more complex, they have the distinct advantage of avoiding beam matching for PTV dimensions up to 50–55 cm.

Wedges

Megavoltage treatment machines have integral beam modifying techniques which are referred to as wedges (see Chapter 8). They alter the uniform dose distribution of the radiation beam in a simple and controlled manner to produce a dose gradient across the field.

Wedges are essential for most multifield plans to produce a uniform PTV dose and serve two purposes.

First, they allow one field to compensate for the depth dose fall off of another field in the plan (Figure *evolve* 10.4A🖱). Secondly, they compensate for a 'density gradient' in the path of the beam (Figure *evolve* 10.4B, C🖱). The simplest application of this is 'missing tissue' when a beam enters an oblique patient contour, but heterogeneities within the patient may also require correction especially the lungs and large pelvic bones.

There are several techniques used in treatment machines for generating wedge-shaped isodoses (see Chapter 8) and the technology used can influence the plan. Fixed wedges may be positioned in the beam for the entire delivery of the beam. This is less commonly used as it requires each field to be manually set up inside the treatment room but, in some machines, may be the only method of permitting a wedge to be orientated in all four directions in the field. These are described in terms of wedge angle of the isodose distribution that they produce (not the physical shape of the wedge itself).

A 'motorized wedge' is a physical wedge-shaped filter positioned inside the treatment head and is designed to be in the beam for part of the treatment time. This gives the planner a continuous range of wedge angles from zero (wedge out of the field) to typically 55° (when the wedge is in the beam for the entire delivery of that field). These will typically be described by the TPS as the open/wedge segments of the beam.

A 'dynamic wedge' uses no physical wedge in the path of the beam, but generates the wedged isodose effect by moving in one of the collimators across the field during the beam on time. The machine is programmed to deliver either a continuously variable wedge angle or a set of discrete wedge angle values typically 15°, 30°, 45°, 60° and described by the isodose wedge angle that is generated.

For the planner, there are a number of consequences arising from these different technologies.

'Dynamic wedges' tend to produce more penetrating isodoses at the 'thin end' of the wedge with higher doses in the superficial region of the thin end than physical wedges. Physical wedges (fixed or motorized) tend to have more rounded, blunt, profiles.

The wedge direction may be limited, i.e. not both sets of jaws can generate dynamic wedges, or physical wedges cannot be rotated into both collimator planes. When planning with multileaf collimators, this may limit the effectiveness of the multileaf collimator (MLC) shielding if the wedge orientation restricts the planner to a suboptimal collimator rotation (Figure *evolve* 10.5🖱).

Physical wedges (fixed or motorized) significantly attenuate the beam at the central axis and a 60° wedge may typically transmit 25% of the open field dose. Therefore, the treatment time is increased 3–4 fold and this factor can often justify the use of segmented treatments which, although more time consuming to plan, do offer improved PTV dose homogeneity at no additional cost during the treatment delivery.

Compensators

Prior to the advent of asymmetric collimators and modern treatment planning computers, physical compensators offered the only means of varying the dose intensity across the beam area. Although their use is now restricted to a limited range of applications, the concepts of physical compensator design are useful in producing treatment plans.

Compensators can be designed to correct for 'missing tissue' in the beam path so that a uniform dose is delivered at a specified depth plane or a varying depth PTV (e.g. spinal cord). They may be placed on the patient's surface and designed simply to replace the missing tissue with a tissue equivalent material. This is not good practice as there is a complete loss of the build-up effect and rarely has clinical value in megavoltage treatments. A compensator located in the accessory tray of the treatment machine will reduce the loss of build-up and will normally be constructed from high density material such as aluminium or lead sheets, or steel granulate in a moulded polystyrene mold.

Compensators may be used to produce a uniform dose to the spinal cord from an open posterior field or as an approximate missing tissue compensation in TBI treatments, but their widespread use is limited by the labour intensive construction and the need to set them up manually for each field in multiple field plans.

Beam shaping devices

A PTV rarely presents a rectangular contour and beam shaping devices are usually employed to spare the surrounding healthy tissue. Treatment planning should always aim to avoid normal tissue unless this irradiation can be justified, for example, to start an urgent treatment while custom blocks are manufactured or where the treatment intent is palliation.

Blocks

Standard straight-sided lead blocks may be useful in simple and urgent therapy but have some disadvantages:

1. the penumbra is spread, more so the further the block is from the central axis
2. the limited range of block sizes may result in compromised shielding
3. lifting heavy blocks poses a risk to staff and patients.

Blocks are supported on an 'accessory tray' which is mounted at a fixed distance from the radiation source and the tray is usually constructed of Perspex several millimetres thick. This will attenuate the non-blocked part of the beam (this attenuation varying with beam energy) and manual and computer calculations must account for this 'tray factor'.

Customized blocks may be fabricated from low melting point alloy and, in the absence of small leaf width MLCs, can provide high conformity in small fields or where the MLC orientation limits their ability to shield. These can be produced with diverging edges to match the divergence of the beam at all points in the field and thus produce a sharp penumbra.

Multileaf collimators (MLCs)

MLCs provide an easy to use solution to field conformal shaping and also make segmented fields practical in which multiple small beams are treated at the same field position. They do have limitations that must be considered during planning:

- the leaf width (defined at the isocentre) may be too coarse for effective collimation especially of small fields
- the orientation with respect to the wedge may not always provide the optimum shielding (see Figure *evolve* 10.5 🖱)
- there may be unavoidable dose to normal tissue due to interleaf leakage, especially where a backup collimator is relied upon to minimize this effect (Figure *evolve* 10.6 🖱) but cannot be brought up to the field edge due to the shape of the PTV
- where MLCs replace both collimator pairs, one field dimension is limited to increments of the leaf width.

Therefore, the treatment planner must be aware of the limitations of the MLC device and also the abilities of the TPS to calculate accurate distributions.

Segmented fields

MLCs in conjunction with asymmetric collimators make it feasible to generate multiple 'beamlets' within a treatment field. The simplest application can be used to produce a uniform PTV dose by adding small 'top up' beams delivering a few monitoring units (MU) to an area of low dose in an otherwise reasonable plan. These are 'forward planned' in that the planner produces a plan without the top up beams and manually adds this on by effectively shielding out the high dose region on the 'top up' field segment.

Segmented fields can be employed to replace a wedge (physical or dynamic). This is useful where the optimum MLC orientation conflicts with the required wedge orientation. Three segments can typically replace a wedge of 45–60°. Segmented fields can also effectively produce a varying wedge angle across the wedge length.

Intensity modulated radiotherapy

Intensity modulated radiotherapy (IMRT) is a further refinement of this technique in which each of the treatment fields is made up of many segments. The objective is to produce a higher conformity than is achievable with conformal blocked fields. By delivering typically five to seven beams with an individualized intensity profile, the dose is conformed to the volume and normal tissue and critical organs spared. The individual treatment beams for IMRT can be delivered using MLCs in either dynamic or multiple-segment ('step-and-shoot') mode. There are advantages and disadvantages of each method. The design of IMRT plans is impractical by conventional manual techniques and is normally done by 'inverse planning'. The planner specifies the requirements of the plan and the intensity profile is determined by computation to achieve the required dose distribution. The specification must include the relative importance of each requirement as many parameters will be conflicting. For example, if a critical structure lies very close to the PTV and the request is for 10% of the prescription dose to the critical structure but a uniform full dose to the PTV, then this will be impossible to achieve.

Multisegment IMRT is clearly the simpler form of MLC-based IMRT, particularly when a relatively small number of segments are used. As such, the dosimetry is more easily handled, techniques can be implemented using standard 3D planning systems, no complex dynamic collimation control is required so that current MLCs can readily be used. Also, conventional field verification using portal imaging is standard. For complex field modulation, however, many static field segments may be required. There may then be a significant time penalty arising from leaf motion between segments and beam start-up time at the beginning of segments. In particular, the use of small monitor unit increments could result in significant deviations in total dose due to inaccuracies in the dose per monitor unit at small MU settings. Additionally, beam flatness and

165

symmetry should be assessed for small MU increments before such fields are used.

In contrast, while dynamic collimation is potentially more efficient, this advantage may be outweighed by the complexity of the delivery method and beam dosimetry, reproducibility of delivery, maximum leaf speed, the lack of conventional image verification and the need for additional QA dose and fluence measurements.

Dynamic treatment techniques

The IMRT delivery can be more efficient if the segmented treatment is replaced by a continuous exposure with the MLC leaves moving while the beam is on. In this 'sliding window' method each leaf pair sweeps across the beam with the leading and trailing leaf travelling at varying speeds so that the beam aperture varies with time and thus the dose deposited is modulated.

Arc therapy

Most treatment units are capable of continuously irradiating as the gantry is rotated and this was once a popular technique for avoiding high doses to healthy tissues. However, with the introduction of MLC-based conformal treatments, the benefits of static fixed fields became far more advantageous for all but small volume spherical 'radiosurgical' treatments. Improved control of linac motion and dose delivery has made a further refinement of IMRT possible, intensity modulated arc therapy (IMAT). Here, the set of fixed beams is replaced by arcing beams, in which the MLC leaves move as the gantry is arced. This technique has the potential to deliver the best conformality to the PTV in short treatment times.

PLANNING TOOLS, CALCULATION AND DISPLAY

Algorithms for dose calculation in treatment planning systems

There are several algorithms in use in different treatment planning systems in order to calculate dose to a patient. They have varying degrees of accuracy and, in some treatment planning systems, present a choice between a fast calculation and a more accurate dose calculation. For example, a simple fan-line model may be selected to determine field size, gantry angle, wedge etc. and then a more accurate calculation can be used for the final patient treatment plan.

Algorithms can be represented as follows.

Stored beam data models

Stored beam data models are based on the use of measured data which, typically, are stored as fan-line matrices divergent from the source. Generally, this requires a large number of beam measurements to be taken in order to build up a library of radiation beams of different open and wedged field sizes. The Milan-Bentley algorithm was one of the first models of this type and is still in use today in some planning systems.

This algorithm is also frequently used as the method of point dose checking on an independent system. Measurements required are percentage depth doses (PDD's) along the Central Axis (CAX) of the beam and off-axis ratios (OAR's) in the form profiles across the beam (as shown in Figure 10.7A and B), output factors as a function of field size, wedge factors for each wedge, cGy/MU for reference situation with a 10×10 cm field and a knowledge of dmax depth. The planning computer can then interpolate these basic data and apply corrections to produce isodose curves in a tissue equivalent phantom. In order to calculate the dose to a patient, a heterogeneity correction is often applied. This can be done by various different methods, such as bulk density equivalent path length, pixel-by-pixel equivalent path length, power law method (Batho) or the ETAR method. Irregular fields are calculated using scatter integration techniques, such as the Clarkson method.

Pencil beam models

Pencil beam models have been introduced to provide a more accurate method of calculating irregular fields and are therefore more suitable for use in dosimetry of conformal radiotherapy and IMRT inverse planning algorithms. They are, however, still prone to some inaccuracy in very inhomogeneous situations. Figure 10.8 illustrates an example of a pencil beam kernel generated by a Monte Carlo calculation to represent the elemental dose distribution from a single infinitesimal beam element at a specific energy. Multiple elements are then summed to represent the total fluence across the radiation field as shown in Figure 10.9.

There are several limitations of this method in a clinical situation, such as in the calculation of dose to lung, as the side-scatter produced in a real situation is not correctly modelled as illustrated in Figure 10.10.

Three-dimensional techniques

Three-dimensional techniques aim to model fully, radiation transport in three dimensions to provide accurate calculations, taking full account of perturbations to dose-distributions from inhomogeneities of arbitrary shape, position and density. These calculations can give accurate results for beams of irregular cross-section, under and near the edges of beam modifiers and at density interfaces. Convolution techniques are best at this, and the collapsed cone method is the most frequently used of these techniques. These convolve the 3D distribution of primary energy with a point-spread function which describes the transport of energy away from a primary photon interaction site. These convolution algorithms provide very high accuracy with the

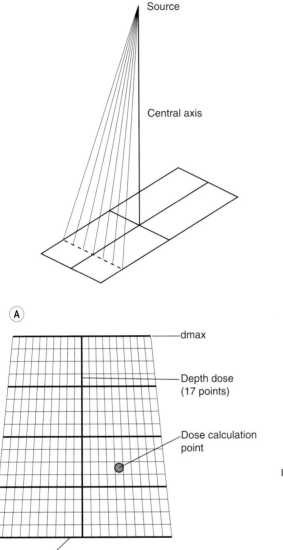

(A)

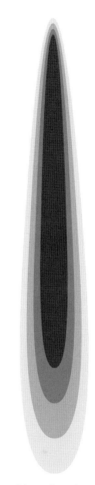

Figure 10.8 The pencil beam kernel.

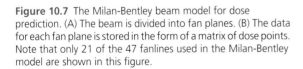

(B)

Figure 10.7 The Milan-Bentley beam model for dose prediction. (A) The beam is divided into fan planes. (B) The data for each fan plane is stored in the form of a matrix of dose points. Note that only 21 of the 47 fanlines used in the Milan-Bentley model are shown in this figure.

inhomogeneities in a patient. Ultimately, Monte Carlo modeling of the interactions from x-ray generation to absorbed dose to patient are the most accurate solution, and are gradually being introduced into TPS with fast, powerful computational ability.

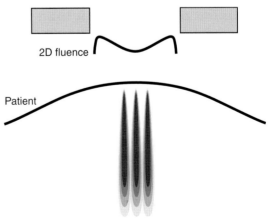

Figure 10.9 The pencil beam model.

Actual situation

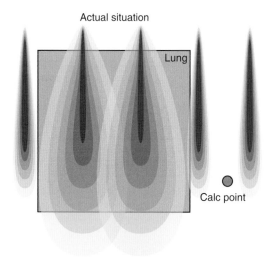

Pencil beam model

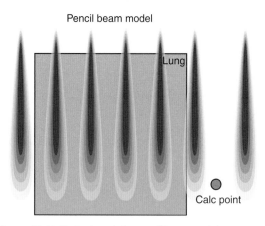

Figure 10.10 Limitation of the pencil beam model to account for changes to lateral scatter affecting a calculation point.

Treatment plan evaluation tools

The ideal radiotherapy treatment plan produces a uniform coverage of the target volume without giving significant dose to surrounding normal tissue. 3D planning is a realistic option for many cases, due to the increased availability of radiotherapy CT scans, virtual simulation, MR, fast computer hardware and improved algorithms. Treatment plans are therefore more difficult to compare and evaluate, hence the need for plan evaluation tools.

Several such tools are in use as discussed.

Isodose distributions

Isodose information is presented as lines or surfaces of equal dose. They show either relative or normalized dose, if the dose is expressed as a percentage of a reference dose or

they give absolute dose, if the dose prescription has been included in the treatment plan. It is a matter of local protocol as to which method is used, although prescriptions specifying different doses to different volumes within the same plan are best displayed in absolute dose.

In order to calculate dose to a surface or volume, a matrix of reference points spread over the volume of interest is required. The number of points and their spatial resolution is always a trade-off between speed and accuracy.

The x and y coordinates of these points are in the transverse plane and the z coordinate is in the superior-inferior plane. The z coordinate is frequently interpolated as the slice thickness of the planning CT scan can vary. The isodose contours are produced by linear interpolation between points, therefore, the separation of these points needs to be small enough to allow sufficient dose detail at organ and PTV boundaries.

Generally, isodose curves are normalized to give 100% to a reference point (such as the ICRU 62 reference point). This makes both the assessment of PTV coverage and the dose uniformity across the volume easier. The aim is usually to cover the PTV with the 95% isodose curve while ensuring the maximum dose within the volume does not exceed 107% [1, 2].

The dose distribution can be displayed on multiple views of reconstructed sections (e.g. transverse, sagittal and coronal sections on a single screen), and also on a 3D reconstruction of anatomy with isodose surfaces displayed.

Useful features are:

- opaque and translucent colour wash displays give a good overall impression of the dose distribution, but can obscure target volumes, so should be interchangeable with conventional isodose lines (Figure *evolve* 10.11🖱)
- zoom and pan facilities
- isodose surfaces displayed as wire frames superimposed on rendered surfaces, with real time manipulation
- a 'volume of regret' is a dose reduction technique applied to the dose distribution. A window of acceptability of dose level is chosen and portions of organs outside this window can be highlighted. For critical organs, this is a one-sided test, where regions where the dose is above the acceptable level are displayed. For target volumes, regions of either too high or too low dose can be shown. This display feature is particularly useful when checking the coverage of arcing beams, e.g. for stereotactic radiotherapy.

Beam's eye view

A useful 3D tool for field placement is the beam's eye view (BEV) which shows the patient's anatomy from the source position of the therapy machine, looking out along the axis of the radiation beam. The BEV approach is useful for identifying the optimal beam angles at which to irradiate the target and avoid irradiating adjacent normal structures, by interactively moving the patient and the treatment beam. Using BEVs, it is possible to set up non-coplanar radiation beams.

- As there can be a great deal of information displayed via the BEV, it is important to show different structures in colour and be able to highlight, include, exclude, shade them interactively while adjusting beam parameters.
- A visual and quantitative representation of machine and treatment couch parameters is also necessary, together with customizable limits and restrictions of beam, collimator and couch angles for specific treatment machines.
- The limitation of BEVs is that it is a one-field presentation, so that field overlap is not immediately observed until the dose calculation is done.
- Another view available on some planning systems is the physician's eye view (PEV) or observer's eye view (OEV) which enables the viewer to look at the patient from all angles to obtain an overview, while multiple fields are being displayed.

An extension of the concept of a BEV is to use a DRR, a digitally reconstructed radiograph. The DRR is reconstructed by various methods from the CT scan data set which has been used for patient voluming and planning. This has the advantage of being the same data set, so that any possible transfer errors which may occur between simulator and CT scanner are eliminated. The accuracy of the reconstruction of the DRR depends on the slice thickness of CT data and the computing tools available to reconstruct the radiographs. CT information can be enhanced to extract more bony structure from the CT data and suppress the soft tissue to obtain an image with well-differentiated bony landmarks. Using such tools, one can also produce an image which is closer in appearance to either a megavoltage portal image or a diagnostic image.

Dose volume histograms

Volume calculations on a 3D treatment planning system provide a large amount of data which can be difficult to interpret and evaluate when displayed as isodose curves on several transverse, sagittal and coronal planes. It is much easier to condense the 3D dose distribution data to a graph which displays the radiation distribution within a specifically defined volume of interest, so that summarizing and analyzing the data are possible. Such a graphical representation is called a dose volume histogram (DVH).

The DVH can be expressed as:

*The summed volume of elements receiving dose in a specified dose interval, against a set of equally spaced dose intervals. This is a **differential** dose volume histogram and shows the absolute or relative volume in each dose interval (bin) directly.*

An example is shown in Figure 10.12 of the evaluation of a breast dose distribution using selected dose bins as the

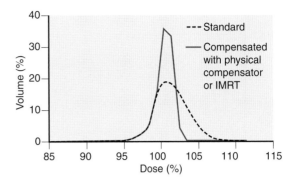

Figure 10.12 Differential DVH comparing a standard and a compensated breast plan.

measure of homogeneity over the treatment volume for two differently compensated plans.

The standard plan gives a wider spread of dose over the volume of interest compared with the compensated plan which shows a large volume receiving much less variation in dose.

More often used are **cumulative** dose volume frequency distributions, which are plots of the volume receiving a dose greater than, or equal to, a given dose, against dose. The volume accumulates starting at the highest dose bin continuing towards zero dose, eventually reaching 100% of the total volume. In most cases, the volume is specified as the percentage of the total volume of a particular structure receiving dose within each interval, however, it may be expressed as absolute volume in some cases.

DVHs can be used during the planning process to check whether the dose is adequate and uniform throughout the target volume. They show that hot and cold spots exist, but do not indicate where they occur, nor whether there are several of them. However, as they do not display spatial information, they should not be the only method of plan evaluation used.

The main use of DVHs is as a plan evaluation tool. They can be used as a graphical way of comparing different treatment plans on a single graph, for specifically identified organs at risk and PTVs. DVH PTV comparisons should show a uniformly high dose throughout the volume, the shape approximates to a step function and a steep slope shows that a large percentage of the volume has a similar dose (Figure 10.13A).

For OARs, the DVH should have a concave appearance (Figure 10.13B) but, for different critical organs, it may be acceptable either to deliver a relatively high dose to a small volume or a small dose to a large volume.

An example of plan comparison for three different dose distributions is shown in Figure 10.14A and B.

DVHs for OARs have a concave appearance. Figure 10.14B shows comparative DVHs for a rectal volume where 50% of the volume is receiving 60, 63 or 66.5 Gy

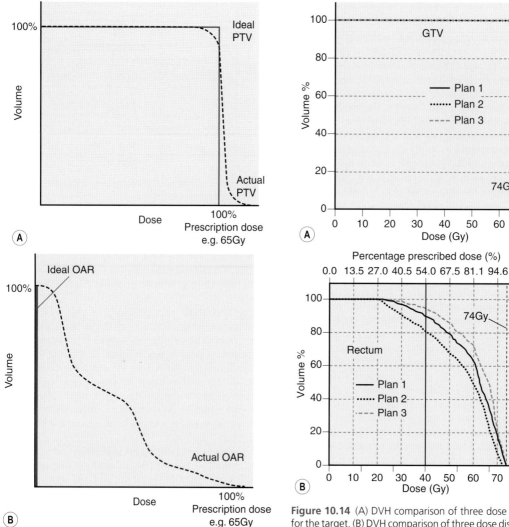

Figure 10.13 (A) Ideal and typical DVHs for a PTV. (B) Ideal and typical DVH for an organ at risk.

Figure 10.14 (A) DVH comparison of three dose distributions for the target. (B) DVH comparison of three dose distributions for the rectum.

depending on the different treatment plan. It is also useful to display both absolute dose and absolute volume, together with normalized values, on the same graph.

DVH calculation requirements and methods

The 3D image is made up of a sequence of CT scans. This can be represented as a 3D grid with cubic volume elements, equally spaced in the x and y directions, but not necessarily in the z direction. The volume of the voxel can then be defined by the product of the x and y grid spacing and the slice thickness. A reasonable resolution for sampling the volume of typical anatomical structures is about 2–3 mm.

Structures with irregular boundaries can give calculation errors when calculating with a regular rectangular grid. Also, structures that are long and thin require a finer resolution in one direction than the other. The ideal solution is to be able to adjust the voxel size dynamically to the dimensions of the structure in x, y and z independently.

The dose for each voxel can be determined at the same time for the outlined volume of interest, by linearly interpolating the dose to the centre of the voxel from the dose matrix. All contributing voxels are collected into the appropriate dose bins of the histogram, for each structure. The user can specify the number and dose interval of the bins to customize the resolution of the DVH plots. These bin values can then be expressed in graphical form. It is important that the dose and volume calculation windows are large enough to include totally all the voxels in any specific structure.

Grid spacing for dose calculation is a compromise. The finer the grid, the greater the calculation accuracy in regions of steep dose gradients, for example close to the beam edges. The disadvantages of a fine grid are the increased computation time and the creation of large data files. In general, two criteria are specified:

1. the desired dose accuracy
2. the maximum acceptable distance between the estimated and actual isodose contours.

For example, 2% dose accuracy or 2 mm isodose positional accuracy will be achieved with a grid spacing of 5 mm.

The range of expected dose values is divided into equal intervals when constructing a histogram. For each interval, the volumes of the voxels receiving dose within that interval are accumulated in the appropriated element of an array, or bin. Cumulative DVHs are obtained by adding volumes accumulated in each bin with the volumes in all bins corresponding to higher dose intervals. For cumulative DVHs, the appropriate dose interval for the bins depends on the dose–response curve for the structure of interest. A dose of 0.5 Gy has been shown to be reasonable, whereas 2 Gy is too wide an interval. Differential DVHs treat the volume in each bin as a separate quantity, and a bin interval of between 2 and 5 Gy is reasonable.

Clinical use and limitations of DVHs

It is not strictly correct to compare plans with different dose computational parameters because different dose calculation algorithms may not handle heterogeneities, or penumbra etc. in the same way. The dose matrix resolution can affect the results of the DVH, especially in regions of steep dose gradient.

Interpretation of the DVH plot is fairly subjective and implications of small differences between DVHs are not well understood. This indicates the usefulness of an objective numeric score, such as TCP or NTCP to provide a 'ranking' when comparing plans. (Small changes in DVH often result in significant differences in the computed TCP and NTCP values.)

DVHs do not indicate the complexity of the field arrangements and will not show any use of 'illegal' couch, collimator angles etc.

In summary, the DVH is a very useful tool for 3D plan comparisons and as an input parameter for TCP and NTCP calculations. TCP and NTCP are quantitative methods of predicting the likelihood of local control. DVHs and the predicted behaviour of the cell population in question are used as input data. There is, however, large uncertainty in the clinical data, so absolute probabilities are not attainable, but relative probabilities can be used to assess different treatment plans. DVHs should, however, be used in conjunction with other plan evaluation tools, especially those which will give spatial information. They can also be used to compare different treatment modalities such as protons and photons when performing treatment planning studies, before doing clinical trials.

Dose surface histograms and dose wall histograms

There are some clinical organs where it could be more relevant to consider the wall of the organ rather than the whole volume, such as the rectum. Dose to rectal wall is more likely to represent patterns of morbidity than dose to volume and 'rectal dose maps' can be extracted from dose surface histograms to give an estimate of areas of high dose which may relate to patterns of morbidity. An example of such a map is shown in Figure 10.15.

Dose statistics

Dose statistics as outlined in Table 10.3 give a simplified view of the dose in a specified structure for evaluation purposes.

Other tools

A publication by Willoughby et al [3] describes a system of evaluating and scoring radiotherapy treatment plans using an artificial neural network. Treatment plans were assigned a figure of merit by a radiation oncologist using a five-point rating scale. DVH data extracted from a large training set were correlated to the physician-generated figure of merit using an artificial neural network, and the net was tested on another set of plans. The accuracy of the neural net in scoring plans compared well with the reproducibility of the clinical scoring and the system is promising for the reliable generation of a clinically relevant figure of merit.

Also useful are:

- side-by-side transverse/sagittal/coronal plans
- video loop stepping through two plans displayed side by side, particularly with colour wash displaying isodoses
- zoom facility over the relevant area to be compared can be useful
- dose at a point interactively integrated and displayed simultaneously on both plans
- dose difference displays
- surface dose display, e.g. on the surface of the spinal cord.

The other aspect of plan evaluation which has not been addressed is the accuracy of the actual dose delivery, which is dependent on complexity of plan, size of margins, reproducibility of set-up etc. Some sort of uncertainty analysis should be developed to include these other aspects of treatment plan evaluation.

Forward and inverse planning

The individual treatment beams for IMRT can be delivered using MLCs in either dynamic or multiple-segment

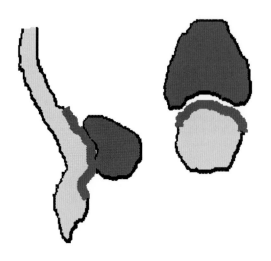

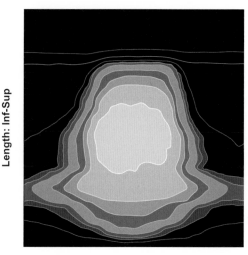

Width: Rt-Lt

Figure 10.15 Dose surface map.

Table 10.3 Definitions of the dose statistics

STATISTIC	DEFINITION
Total volume	The sum of all DVH voxels found within a set of boundary contours
ICRU 50 dose	The specification dose as defined in the ICRU Report 50 [1]
Mean dose	The sum of the doses assigned to each voxel divided by the total number of voxels
Min dose	The dose minimum in the volume
Max dose	The maximum dose in the volume
Volume greater than or equal to the prescribed dose	The sum of all voxels within DVH bins corresponding to a dose greater than or equal to the prescription dose
Volume greater than or equal to the reference dose	The total volume within DVH bins corresponding to a dose greater than or equal to the user supplied reference dose

('step-and-shoot') mode. There are advantages and disadvantages of each method, however, both methods require the intensity of each beam profile to be determined in order to deliver the intended dose to the target, normal tissue and critical structures. Two techniques have been utilized to determine these intensity profiles and these are referred to as forward planning and inverse planning. Forward planning involves the conventional planning technique where an operator applies and modifies beams, assessing the effect on the dose distribution continuously until a satisfactory solution is reached. With inverse planning, this optimization is undertaken by automatic computational manipulation of the intensity profiles based upon constraints specified by the operator or clinician.

Forward-planned IMRT

The step and shoot technique is particularly useful for forward planning, where just segments are used to produce improvements in homogeneity, delivery of integrated boosts, and/or improved sparing of organs at risk.

A simple example is a forward planned breast technique, which retains the preferred tangential beam arrangement, but allows shaping of dose to areas within the breast that would be under- or overdosed without such customized compensation. This is illustrated in Figure *evolve* 10.16B🖱 where the dose uniformity has been improved compared to that in Figure *evolve* 10.16A🖱 by the addition of four segments within the standard field.

Patients with prostate cancer can also be treated using a forward-planned technique. This is done where the aim is simultaneously to boost the dose to the prostate, while delivering a lower dose to prostate + seminal vesicles PTV, within the same treatment fraction. This can be achieved using a three-field technique, with two to three segments per beam. Segment shapes can be determined according to rules based on the patient anatomy and the weights adjusted to give the required dose distribution. Adjustment of segment weights may be manual or automatic.

172

Forward planning can also be used to generate more complex plans, such as the generation of concave dose distributions in the pelvis [4] or head and neck [5]. While the dose distribution of such plans may not be quite as conformal as those produced by inverse planning, they may be an improvement on a standard treatment plan.

These planning methods use optimization, so it is necessary to define dose-volume constraints, as for inverse planning. However, unlike inverse planning, the resultant plan is directly deliverable, to include user-defined restrictions, such as number of segments and minimum segment size, and also incorporates any MLC limitations.

Inverse-planned IMRT

Inverse planning means devising a set of dose constraints which are entered into an optimization routine to generate a solution with usually five or more beams. Essential to this is a fully outlined set of 3-dimensional volumes of interest and defined values as to the acceptable dose levels to be delivered to or avoided by those volumes.

Typical dose constraints for all IMRT plans on the PTV are 99% of the volume needs to receive at least 90% of the prescribed dose, and 95% of the volume should receive at least 95% of the prescribed dose. Simultaneously, there is a constraint that only 5% of the volume receives no more than 105% of the prescribed dose, and 2% of the volume receives no more than 107% of prescribed dose. In addition, there are dose constraints on the organs at risk similar to the dose constraints that would be used for conformal radiotherapy. There may also be the need for constraints to avoid high dose regions throughout the irradiated volume by adding false structures with appropriate dose constraints to force the calculation.

There is a lot of published work on finding class solutions for IMRT plans, in order to define numbers, angles and energies of beams. A number of authors have found that, for some sites, a small number of appropriately selected beam orientations can provide dose distributions as satisfactory as those produced by a large number of unselected equispaced orientations [6, 7]. The general increase in numbers of incident gantry angles means that lower energies are suitable for deep-seated tumours [8], although some groups [9] have preferred to continue using higher energies.

During the inverse planning process, the optimization algorithm will only attempt to cover or spare those volumes that have been completely outlined. It may therefore be necessary to outline volumes where strict dose sparing is not required, however, the planner would prefer to avoid hot spots and ideally reduce the dose within these volumes. A volume that does not strictly relate to anatomy may be drawn in order to apply a dose constraint with a relative low priority that will help to avoid dose 'overspill' in this area. Expanded volumes (i.e. extra margins) can be used to ensure coverage of targets. Depending on the leaf widths and motions this may require differing margins in different directions.

Optimal fluences converted to deliverable leaf motion sequences must take into account the MLC limitations of the machine. This should be considered when choosing beam orientations, selecting gantry and collimator angles to ensure, for example, that the width of the target volumes in BEV is not larger than the maximum beam width that can be delivered at one time.

Each planning system has its own characteristics, therefore, practice with the system when developing class solutions to achieve local planning techniques is important, as is the establishment and participation in clinical trials.

The calculation process is in two stages. First, the TPS calculates the optimum dose fluence for each beam. Then this ideal dose is converted to a deliverable set of segments that the treatment unit is physically capable of. There may be significant differences between the ideal and achievable fluences, so the planning process will be more efficient with access to the final distribution being available during the planning stage. The planner must still ensure that the calculated plan is sensible and deliverable and skilled manual intervention to an inverse plan is usually required. For example, removing very small segments, or those with low MUs. The planner must also be aware of the limitations of the TPS algorithm as there may be significant errors in calculations of small or elongated fields, or fields with small MLC apertures compared with the secondary collimator settings.

BEAM ARRANGEMENTS

This section does not attempt to provide a comprehensive atlas of treatment plans or an in depth planning guidance for each site, but uses a few clinical examples to demonstrate planning techniques.

The first step in preparing a plan is to decide on the position of the isocentre. Although the centre of the PTV might appear to be the best location, in practice, it may be preferable to set the isocentre to predefined skin marks which have been set at the time of CT scanning. The skin marks will have been chosen to lie on a stable skin location, perhaps at a standard anatomical point or height above the couch, and avoiding steep body contour gradients. This results in a simpler and safer set-up and the fields will then be aligned to the PTV by asymmetric collimator settings.

Another strategy is to select the isocentre position based on the internal anatomy of either the PTV or adjacent critical structures. This can minimize the dose to critical structures by eliminating beam divergence without complicating the field arrangement. Examples are breast treatments without the beams diverging into the lung or abutting nodal fields, or brain treatments avoiding beam edges diverging into critical structures, such as the lens. Another aspect regarding choice of internal anatomy relates to the dose computation algorithm and placement of the isocentre in solid material and not in an air cavity in order to improve the dose prediction accuracy at that point for checking.

The beam energy is chosen by considering the depth of dmax and the penetration properties of the beam (Table 10.2 shows typical values for commonly used energies). Low energy beams, e.g. 4–6 MV are suited to more superficial volumes, e.g. head and neck PTVs, while deep pelvic PTVs will require 10–20 MV. Beam energies above 15 MV do not give a great benefit to the planner, but their frequent use on a linac can introduce radiation protection problems due to neutron production.

The build-up region is a significant feature of the MV beam in that it gives 'skin sparing' allowing doses that would severely damage the skin to be delivered deep into the patient. However, a PTV which extends from near the surface to a depth requiring MV photons may require bolus to be added to the skin. By placing this tissue equivalent material on the skin, the build-up region is shifted into the bolus and the maximum dose of the beam is delivered to on or near the skin. Unless the PTV is superficial, the planner should consider the impact of patient immobilization devices acting as build up and increasing the surface dose.

Standard field arrangements may be modified for specific patient situations such as metal hip implants. Here, it is preferable to avoid beams entering through the implant so a three-field arrangement must be modified such as shown in Figure *evolve* 10.17🖱.

Single fields

Most plans are based on the intersecting of multiple field paths to create a high dose region, but single fields may sometimes be the ideal choice especially for superficial PTVs. The spine can be treated with a single posterior field, although this will usually be done as part of a multifield arrangement to treat the whole central nervous system. To cover a PTV length of greater than 40 cm, the field may need to be treated at extended SSD, i.e. the isocentre will be positioned off the skin surface (see Figure *evolve* 10.20🖱). To produce a uniform dose to the cord lying at varying depths, a compensator may be employed, but the most efficient technique is to use top up fields all centred on a single isocentre, delivering a few MU to otherwise underdosed sections of the PTV.

Turned wedges

Wedges are usually most beneficial with the wedge in the plane of the plan (usually the transverse patient plane). However, if the patient contour varies out of this plane, a turned, or longitudinal wedge may be required to produce an even dose in the superior-inferior direction. This may be accomplished by overlying two fields with identical dimensions, but with the collimator rotated 90°. For multibeam plans, it may be possible to achieve uniform dose with a single turned wedge on one field only.

Parallel-opposed fields

The typical isodose distribution arising from a parallel-opposed field is shown in Figure *evolve* 10.18🖱. If the separation is not too great for the available beam energy, then a dose range of +7 to −5% is perhaps just achievable. The high dose regions may present a problem at wide separations and also the hour-glass shaped contour at about the 90–95% level may result in unacceptably low doses at the midplane of the volume. Wedges may be employed where the contour slopes or internal heterogeneities are present and the use of shielding can produce irregular dose distributions conforming to complex PTV shapes. Clinical applications include large pelvis volumes and whole brain treatments.

Beams weighted in 2:1 ratio

The standard parallel-opposed distribution can be modified to deliver a higher dose to one side of the PTV without resorting to a more complex plan. It must be clear what the plan request means by 2:1 weighting. For simple manually calculated plans, it would usually mean that the ratio of MU set is 2:1. However, with computerized plans, a dose reference point may be positioned somewhere other than at the midplane depth so it must be clear to which point the 2:1 ratio applies. The presence of heterogeneities further complicates the issue as the TPS may adjust the set MUs to deliver equal dose from each field to a point by compensating for the different densities each beam has traversed. This demonstrates the potential hazards arising from changing from basic manual calculations to CT-based dosimetry where a seemingly simple request for 2:1 weightings can take on several different interpretations (see Figure *evolve* 10.18🖱).

Breast treatments

The breast can be treated with a parallel-opposed pair, but the technique is generally refined to minimize lung dose by creating a non-diverging edge, either by fully asymmetric fields with the central axis along the field edge, or by slightly angling the fields so that the central axes are not parallel to one another but the back edges are (Figure *evolve* 10.19🖱).

Wedges will usually be required to produce a uniform PTV dose by compensating for the 'missing tissue' and the presence of lung. Due to time constraints, the PTV is not outlined if treating the entire breast and the PTV is normally defined during simulation or virtual simulation and will not be specifically contoured and the gantry angles determined by the accepted amount of lung in the field.

For post-mastectomy 'chest wall' treatments, the contour shape combined with the significant presence of lung may result in open fields or even a wedge orientated with the thin end at the apex of the breast.

A beam of typically 5 MV is adequate for most breast treatments but, as the separation between the medial and lateral field edges increases beyond about 22 cm, a higher energy beam is required. The increased energy results in reduced breast tissue coverage superficially due to the increased build-up depth so should be avoided unless essential.

Segmented fields can produce a more uniform dose especially in larger or irregular outlines (see Figure *evolve* 10.19A–C). Usually, a single segment on one field is sufficient to bring the dose range within ICRU [1, 2] requirements. For left sided breast treatments it may be necessary to shield the heart.

Limb sarcomas

These are usually treated with two opposed fields slightly angled to produce a sharper dose gradient to maximize the drainage channel along the limb. The PTV is often greater than 40 cm long and, for a standard Linac, extended SSD fields are necessary. These require carefully described set up instructions (Figure *evolve* 10.20).

Wedged pairs

For superficial PTVs that extend quite deeply, the wedged pair can produce the optimum dose distribution (Figure *evolve* 10.21). Highly wedged beams are required to maintain a uniform dose across the depth of the PTV. A greater hinge angle tends to produce a more uniform dose gradient and may be necessary for deeper PTVs but is likely to increase normal tissue dose adjacent to the PTV. The exit doses from a two-field plan can be significant for critical structures such as the mouth or cord in parotid treatments and sometimes a lightly weighted third field can be beneficial if the relative weighting of the two fields cannot be adjusted.

Multiple field plans

For PTVs lying deeper in the patient, three or more fields with paths intersecting at the PTV usually offer the best dose distribution for the PTV while avoiding excessive dose to normal tissue. The clinically useful dose will normally only be delivered where all the beam paths overlap, unless complex inverse planning is employed or an intentional dose gradient is required inside the PTV. The field arrangement is designed to ensure that the 'treated volume' conforms as closely as possible to the PTV while complying with critical structure constraints and minimizing the volume of normal tissue irradiated, the 'irradiated volume' as defined in ICRU 50 [1].

Pelvis plans

Three fields will often be sufficient to deliver the required dose to the PTV while maintaining acceptably low normal tissue doses. Unless the PTV extends close to the surface (e.g. some rectum PTVs), a high energy (10 MV or more) is desirable. A posterior plus two lateral fields (as shown in Figure *evolve* 10.22) represent a good starting point for a plan. The wedges on the lateral fields compensate for the fall off in dose from the posterior field and also the 'missing tissue' due to the patient contour. The weightings are adjusted to obtain an acceptable PTV dose while also considering the normal tissue doses in the beam entry path and, in this case, the beam exit path from the posterior field. The lateral maximum doses for typical pelvis patients may be around 80% of the PTV dose, or more for patients with a wide separation. The maximum dose that the posterior field contributes to normal tissue will usually be lower – typically 60% of the prescribed dose due to the presence of more radiosensitive structures within its entry and exit paths. Four fields may be required, especially for large volumes in large patients, a four-field box arrangement being the standard technique.

The lateral fields in the three-field plan may be angled by either a few degrees or perhaps 20° or more. Angling a few degrees posteriorly in a supine patient will produce a sharper dose gradient on the posterior PTV edge which can reduce the dose to the adjacent critical structure, the rectum, in the case of a prostate PTV for example. Angling the fields more posteriorly will reduce the normal tissue doses as the exit dose from one lateral will not contribute so much to the contralateral entrance dose. For some PTV shapes, a better conformality may be achieved with oblique angles but, in many cases, the rectum dose will be increased by the use of posterior oblique fields.

Thorax plans

The optimum field arrangement will significantly depend on the location of the PTV in the chest. Three fields are usually required (but see combined two phase example in the next section) although occasionally, a parallel-opposed pair is the best arrangement. Examples of bronchus PTV field arrangements are shown in Figure *evolve* 10.23. The cord dose tolerance must not be exceeded and the heart dose minimized where relevant. The total left and right lung volume must be outlined so that the total volume is displayed in the DVH. A field arrangement that minimizes the lung volume irradiated should then be found usually by analysing the V20 from the DVH.

The choice of beam energy needs careful consideration as at high energy, the increased path length of the electrons released can be detrimental to the target coverage if the target is adjacent to low density tissue and air. Dose algorithms do not provide accurate dose predictions for these situations and generally the choice of a low energy beam is considered preferable.

Phased treatments

For many sites, the treatment plan will comprise two or occasionally more stages. For example, phase one will deliver dose to a known primary lesion and to surrounding nodal involvement or other disease spread. Phase two will then be a reduced PTV covering the primary lesion only.

Another reason for phased treatment would be to spread the dose to critical structures by employing a different field arrangement in phase two but still targeting the same PTV.

Another form of phased treatments is the use of 'feathered junctions' when treating large PTVs to minimize the risk of over- or underdose occurring at matched field edges and, typically, three phases are employed in this technique. An example is the treatment of the entire central nervous system with a spine field matched to brain fields with collimators angled to follow the divergence of the spine field (Figure *evolve* 10.24🖱).

There may be radiobiological and/or practical advantages in delivering the phases concurrently in each daily fraction rather than consecutively, when a new plan must be produced and checked for each phase.

Oesophagus

Traditionally, the oesophagus has been treated with two phases with the intention of minimizing the cord and lung critical structure doses. Phase one is an anterior-posterior parallel-opposed pair which also irradiates the cord usually to a dose slightly higher than the dose the PTV receives during this phase. As cord tolerance is approached, a phase two plan is introduced, usually an anterior and two posterior oblique fields. The oblique fields avoid the cord completely but it continues to receive an exit dose from the anterior field. Therefore, it is essential to plan the phase two before much of the phase one treatment has been delivered as if the phase two is not started in time, the total cord dose may exceed the tolerance over both phases. This arrangement is intended to minimize lung dose by using the A-P beam arrangement up to cord tolerance. More recently, cardiac toxicity has become a concern, especially where chemotherapy is also administered, and the heart is outlined as a critical structure. The treatment is delivered using a single four-field plan and the lateral fields are angled and conformally shaped to cover the PTV while shielding the heart from as much high dose as possible. Thus, the cord maximum dose, and the lung and heart volume doses are all optimized in a single plan.

Non-coplanar planning

The majority of plans have the central axes of all the fields in one plane – usually the axial patient plane, although a sagittal, coronal, or oblique plane may be preferable in some circumstances, e.g. a wedged pair to treat the orbit (Figure *evolve* 10.25🖱).

Coplanar planning simplifies the planning process as if all beams project the same out of plane dimension then they will each cover the out of plane PTV dimension equally. Beam path lengths through normal tissue are minimized and collimator rotations on opposing fields can be easily matched. For most of the body, coplanar fields are preferable with a few exceptions when small angulations from the treatment plane are used. Examples of such angulations are some breast treatments where floor and collimator rotations are introduced to establish a vertical junction between the breast and nodal fields (Figure *evolve* 10.26🖱) and avoiding the shoulders in lateral neck beams.

One disadvantage of coplanar fields is that the exit path of one field will often overlap the entrance path of another with potentially significant cumulative doses. Non-coplanar plans can be most beneficial in the skull where the beam paths can avoid each other except at the PTV, without increased path lengths due to the approximately spherical body contour. However, greater care is needed to avoid critical structures in three dimensions as beams can deliver significant dose well beyond the PTV area. For example the thyroid irradiated by beams in the sagittal plane treating a brain (Figure *evolve* 10.27🖱).

Field matching

Matching two fields may be essential in order to treat large volumes as described in the section above, with 'feathering' used to spread the uncertainty of the set-up, especially when a single isocentre technique cannot be utilized. Figure 10.28A and B shows how asymmetric fields can simplify field matching and are commonly used, especially in head and neck treatments to match two distinct but abutting PTV shapes into a single treatment.

However, matching may also be necessary when a previous treatment is adjacent to a PTV currently being treated. Matching diverging fields can be complex and a compromise is usually a pragmatic approach, especially in palliative, low-dose treatments. If the planner has confidence in the location of the previous set-up then an attempt to match the beam divergence may be practical. Alternatively the match may be made at a critical structure such as the spinal cord, and the overdose and underdose regions adjacent to the cord is accepted (Figure 10.29).

KILOVOLTAGE PHOTON THERAPY

Kilovoltage beams have very limited penetration so are generally used as a single field to treat very superficial lesions, although opposed fields may be suitable if the separation is small. Depth doses are highly dependent on the filtration as well as the accelerated electron energy and, although the beam energy is commonly described by the accelerating potential in kilovolts (kV), a more accurate description of the beam penetration is the half value

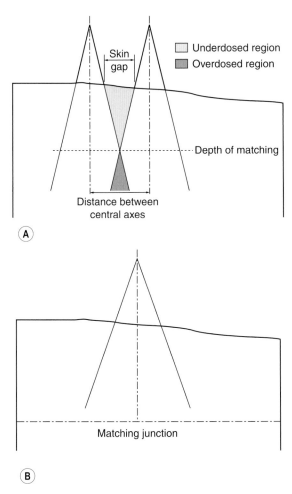

Figure 10.28 Field matching: (A) divergent beams and (B) asymmetric fields.

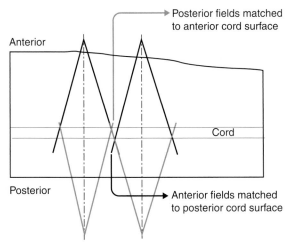

Figure 10.29 Field matching at different depths.

layer (HVL) in terms of mm in Al or Cu (see Chapter 8). Maximum dose is deposited at the surface and the 90% dose level will be approximately 2 mm deep for a 60 kV beam up to 10 mm deep at 220 kV.

The field size may be defined by an applicator attached to the machine, but often a lead cut-out placed on the skin surface defines the field (this need only be 2 mm thick for beam energies up to 160 kV). The sharp penumbra in the high-dose isodoses means that the field can be matched to the PTV edge, although at depth there is some bowing out of the low value isodose contours. The dose deposited is significantly dependent upon the field size due to the contribution of scattered electrons within the patient. Although there is some variation of depth dose with field size, this tends to be pronounced beyond the clinically useful depths so will usually only be relevant if considering the dose to underlying structures. If a lead cut-out on the skin is used, the MU calculation must be based on the cut-out size as well as the applicator output. In this energy range, the electrons are more back and laterally scattered than for MV beams so the factors are referred to as back scatter factors (BSFs), which are the ratio of the dose in air in the absence of the patient to the dose in water at the patient surface (at the same location in the beam). The applicator output may be described by the 'in air output' or with the BSF included. To calculate the dose in a cut-out, the applicator output must be corrected by the ratio of the BSFs for the applicator and cut-out dimensions. This ratio is greater than unity, so that the MU required for the applicator are increased if a cut-out is used.

The 'equivalent square' of the cut-out needs to be calculated or, if tabulating the outputs of circular fields and back scatter factors, then the 'equivalent diameter' may be more appropriate as these areas tend to be more circular than rectangular. For irregular cut-outs and cut-outs on irregular contours, this area measurement is difficult and realistically the output may not be calculated to better than ±2–3% (and probably less accurate for the smallest fields) and may vary by more than this across the area of the cut-out due to the field shape, beam profile, and varying standoff.

Kilovoltage units have short source to skin distances of typically 20–50 cm SSD. Therefore, the inverse square law dependence of output is far more significant than for linac beams. For example, a 1 cm 'standoff' for a 25 cm SSD field results in a drop in output of 8%. It is therefore important to ensure optimum skin apposition to minimize the dose gradient across the PTV.

The limited applicator size means that fields may have to be abutted to treat long PTVs or for high curvature surfaces. The sharp penumbra means that fields can be abutted and give a uniform dose. The most practical method of achieving this is to use lead on the skin to define the junction rather than an applicator. Care should be taken to ensure the beams are as parallel to each other as possible to minimize overdosing at depth.

ELECTRON THERAPY

Electron beams provide an ideal treatment for superficial PTVs extending from the skin surface to typically up to 5 cm deep. The major advantage over photon beams is the sharp fall off in the dose at depth. However, it should be noted that at higher electron energies (>15 MeV), the slope is not so steep and underlying tissue may receive a significant dose. The radiobiological effect is the same as that for x-rays.

The electron field is defined by an applicator which, depending on design, may be placed in contact with the skin, or with a small standard standoff. The beam may be further conformed by the addition of standard 'end-frames' (a range of circles or rectangles) placed at the end of the applicator, or custom cut-outs may be constructed for individual patient PTV shapes.

The majority of electron treatments are not computer planned as the set up is fairly straightforward and the patient can be considered as a uniform water medium. In these cases, standard depth doses and output factor charts may be employed to select beam energy and calculate the MU required. However, there are many commonly encountered sites where a computer calculated dose distribution would be of benefit, such as in the presence of heterogeneities, e.g. bone, lung, or air cavities, or where there is oblique incidence of the electron beam to the patient surface which can cause significant changes in dose deposition.

Manual calculations are usually based on the central axis depth dose of a standard 10 cm × 10 cm field but it is important to understand the limitations of applying these standard data to real clinical conditions. Electron beams interact with patient contours in unexpected ways and these interactions vary significantly over the clinical range of electron energies (typically 4–20 MeV) so computer planning, or experimental verification can be essential in some treatments.

The widely used computer pencil beam algorithms provide a reasonable estimate of dose in heterogeneous media but should be used as an indication of dose distributions rather than determining absolute dose. Most treatment planning systems require extensive data input in order to generate MU calculations for the wide range of field sizes clinically required, and the full commissioning of electron planning is often considered impractical.

A recent innovation is the use of Monte Carlo algorithms for electron beam calculation. This offers the potential for more accurate dose distributions and equally usefully, MU calculation for irregular cut-outs.

Energy and depth dose characteristics

Figure 10.30 shows how an electron beam energy is selected for a specific PTV depth. At low energies, the surface dose may be less than 95% of the prescribed PTV dose and bolus may be needed to shift the isodoses deeper within the patient (Figure 10.30). Bolus may also be used to modify the treatment depth if a limited range of electron energies is available. The bolus may be applied to the patient skin (in the form of wax or other flexible tissue equivalent material), or it may be more convenient and comfortable for the patient if the bolus is attached to the end of the applicator, when a solid material such as Perspex may be used. In the latter situation, standoff of up to about 5 cm between the bolus and the patient surface will produce the same penetration of the beam in the patient as if the bolus had been applied directly to the skin surface.

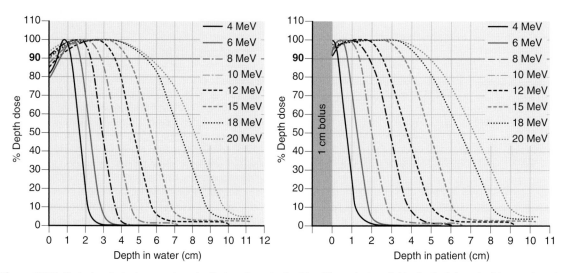

Figure 10.30 Typical central axis percentage depth doses in water for 10 × 10 cm electron fields. On the left, no build-up and, on the right, with build-up.

If the 90% isodose is selected to cover the PTV and the dose prescribed to this isodose, then this will result in a 111% maximum dose at dmax. However, this will always be within the PTV. The 90% or 95% isodose is selected as they provide a useful range to cover the PTV, while the 100% peak would, at most beam energies, be of insufficient range to deliver the prescribed dose to more than a few millimeters in depth.

Penumbra

The penumbral region of any treatment beam determines the field margin that must be applied around the PTV. In electron fields, this is not so easy to define as in photon fields, as the penumbra varies significantly with depth (Figure 10.31). The clinician must appreciate the dose profile and whether adequate coverage at the field edges will be achieved. If coverage of the 95% isodose at the dmax depth is the only point of interest then the margin can be taken as 'A' in Figure 10.31A. However, for small fields in particular, the rounded profile of the 95% contour becomes significant and the field could be described as being entirely formed of penumbra as shown in Figure 10.31B.

Standoff and stand in

It may be impossible to position the applicator at the standard treatment position. For example, neck treatments may be obstructed by the shoulders, or the patient surface may present a variable SSD across the field area. The inverse square law cannot usually be applied in the same way as for photon beams produced by the same treatment machine as each electron energy has a 'virtual source distance' due to the multiple sources of electrons ranging from the scattering foils through to the photon collimators and the electron applicator. Therefore, either standard standoff

correction tables should be used, or an inverse square calculation made, based on the virtual source distance. Where the patient contour varies within the field, it is a matter for clinical judgment as to where the prescribed dose is delivered and where an over- or underdose is acceptable.

Patient contour effects

If an electron beam is incident on a steep gradient in the patient contour, then the uniform scattering that produces the standard isodose and depth dose characteristics no longer exists, and the light field projected onto the skin gives a misleading indication of good coverage. Electrons are cascaded along the edge of the gradient to greater depths before depositing their dose. For shallow gradients, this effect may only result in a small modification to the depth dose but, for steep gradients, the cascaded electrons deposit a significant dose, often beyond the targeted volume. All these effects are highly energy dependent and therefore require a reliable planning algorithm or careful experiment to confirm the actual dose distribution. Whenever practicable, this situation should be avoided. The beam angle of incidence should be carefully set up by gantry, collimator, and couch rotations to minimize non-orthogonal incidence. If the electron beam is incident on a cavity such as the ear, then the ear should be filled with a wax plug or wet gauze. Bolus should always extend beyond the field edge so as to avoid a sharp gradient and variations in bolus thickness should be gradual. It may be necessary to employ bolus to block up some target volumes, e.g. around the ear pinna or nose, to provide lateral scatter into the PTV and to generate the uniform dose distribution predicted by the standard isodose distributions. Note that field defining collimation will not produce a significant scatter contribution due to self-absorption. However, shielding within the field must be coated with wax or similar materials to prevent backscattered electrons from enhancing the dose to adjacent tissue. Examples of internal shielding are nasal and mouth shields to prevent the beam from penetrating beyond the PTV.

Heterogeneities

Bone will attenuate an electron beam due to its higher density and this can be advantageous where the PTV lies above bone as this reduces the dose to underlying tissue. Lung and other air cavities can be a significant hazard in electron beams as their transmission is minimal compared to water and the electron beam entering lung will not be significantly attenuated until it reaches the lung tissue interface. Therefore, great care should be taken when using higher energy beams (greater than 12 MeV) to ensure that the dose limits of critical structures underlying the air cavity are not exceeded. The commonest example of this is in electron breast boosts where the heart may receive a significant dose.

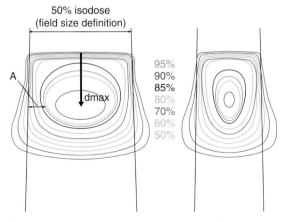

Figure 10.31 Electron isodose distributions for fields (A) 8 × 8 cm and (B) 3 × 3 cm.

The use of CT planning can demonstrate the effects of heterogeneities, but unless the calculation algorithm has been verified under all conditions, the isodose distributions should be considered 'for indication only'. CT planning can be useful for identifying the depth of critical structures, e.g. the spinal cord in neck node treatments even if the TPS dose calculation is not used.

Field matching

A perfect match between electron–electron or electron–photon fields is not possible and a compromise is always needed – either to underdose at the junction and risk recurrence or overdose and accept potential tissue damage. The underdose or overdose regions are not in the same location and are dependent on the electron beam energy. Typically, a gap at the skin surface between the 50% isodose edges of an electron and photon beam of 2 mm will give an acceptable compromise. No gap will produce doses of typically 120% or more, while a 5 mm gap will result in a significant low dose region of 70%. Angling the photon beam a few degrees away from the electron beam will give a very small reduction in the overdose region. The use of 'spoilers', e.g. Perspex build-up in the electron beam can broaden its penumbra and make the set-up less critical [10].

Matching two electron beams is similarly very difficult and will often be complicated by the fact that the beams are not parallel to one another as the reason for matching is to cover a large or highly curved contour (e.g. the skull). The match border on a curved surface may be created by a lead strip which shields the surface from one field and is then positioned on the other side of the junction to shield the surface from the abutting field. Even with careful immobilization, such junctions are prone to significant over- or underdosing, especially with oblique fields and where the lead cannot be perfectly positioned in direct skin contact. Therefore, junctions should generally be 'feathered' by moving the junction two or three times during the treatment course to reduce severe over- and underdosing. However, many electron treatments are 'boost fields' so a high-dose region of 120% of the boost dose may only be present for say 25% of the overall treatment and thus represents a total dose of 105%.

Verification measurements should be performed with thermoluminescent dosimetry or film to estimate the dose distribution in unusual electron treatment set-ups.

Special electron techniques

The majority of electron treatments are undertaken with direct single fields using the standard beams on the linear accelerator. However, there are two established special techniques which, although not used widely, are worthy of description.

Arcing electron treatment

Initially, many treatment sites appear good candidates for arcing electron therapy – where multiple fixed fields are replaced by a single beam arcing over the patient and thus eliminating problems of matching junctions. However, in practice, arcing therapy is of no practical value in all but a small number of cases. Figure 10.32 shows the cross-sectional view of an arc with a narrow slit beam (typically 2–5 cm wide), centred on a deep isocentre, sweeping over the patient. The arc commences and terminates with the slit irradiating shielding so that each part of the patient receives the same exposure to the slit beam.

Figure 10.32 shows why this treatment is rarely applicable to widespread surface lesions. The dose to each point depends on the dose rate of the treatment machine, the slit width, and the time that each point of the patient is in the beam. This in turn depends on the arcing speed but, more crucially, it also depends on the distance from the isocentre. If Points A and B in the diagram are at the same depth and the SSD at Point B is 3 cm greater than at Point A then the dose at Point B will be approximately 6% less than that at Point A due to the inverse square law. However, Point B is closer to the isocentre so the sweeping beam will spend much longer irradiating this point than Point A resulting in a much higher dose at this point. Therefore, contours with any significant variation in curvature will introduce large dose ranges across the arc. There are few sites where this can be achieved for more than 30° of arc and the back is probably the best location for this treatment. The head is unlikely to be a site where arcing therapy offers any advantage over fixed fields even when matching of abutting fixed fields is the alternative.

In principle, varying the slit width during the arc could adjust the output, but this requires specialized technology to perform and is not available as a standard treatment option. A specialized treatment planning computer is also

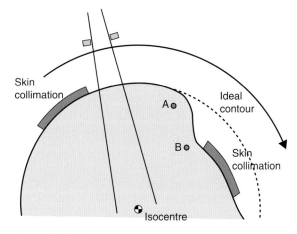

Figure 10.32 Electron arc treatment.

required to design this complex treatment as the contour will vary along the slit as well as around the arc. As arcing beams have entirely different characteristics to fixed fields of the same energy, and the inevitable variation of contour through the arc, many hours of pretreatment phantom measurements and in vivo verification during the treatment are required to design the treatment.

Total skin electron irradiation (TSEI) or (TSET, total skin electron therapy)

The treatment of mycosis fungoides and similar malignancies requires irradiation of the entire skin surface and, given the rarity of the disease, this complex treatment delivery is performed at only a few specialized centres. An even dose distribution is required to a depth of only typically 6 mm for the 90% isodose level, but often encompassing the entire skin surface of the body. It is extremely difficult to come close to achieving 95 to 107% uniformity however complex the treatment technique may be.

A wide variety of techniques has been developed to attempt to achieve this dose coverage. A small single field at an SSD of 1–2 m which scans, or arcs, over the patient is one option, but the commonest technique is to use an extended SSD of between 3 and 7 m so that the patient is covered in one or two beams. The dose rate of a standard linac is increased to reduce treatment times and the dose delivered in daily fractions over several weeks, for example 36 Gy in 1 Gy daily fractions, as not all treatment positions are delivered in each fraction. The x-ray component of the electron beam is in the range of 1–4% of the maximum electron dose for these techniques, so the whole body dose is not normally of concern.

Beam energies of between 4 and 10 MeV are usually employed, although the energy at the patient is reduced by scattering in air, and energy degraders and scattering screens placed in the beam to improve dose uniformity and appropriate beam penetration. The standard depth doses will not be applicable under these conditions and extensive commissioning work is required to determine depth dose and dose rates under these unique treatment conditions. The patient is usually standing and will adopt a different pose at each fraction to be treated effectively at different beam angles to deliver an even dose and to minimize self-shielding. Additional static fields may be required to boost regions that have not received sufficient dose due to self-shielding or extreme obliquity of the incident beam, e.g. the soles of the feet and top of the head.

Evaluation of the dose delivered is difficult as the dose from different beams with a wide range of angle of incidence must be measured at very shallow depths. Thermoluminescent dosimetry is ideal in this area. There is limited scope for precise treatment planning for individual patients prior to treatment delivery and in vivo dosimetry is important in verifying the delivered dose to the individual patient and potentially leading to small adjustments in treatment position in subsequent fractions.

DIFFERENCES BETWEEN KILOVOLTAGE AND ELECTRON THERAPY

While both modalities are suited for superficial treatments, the mechanism of dose deposition is different, resulting in clinically significant differences in the features of the dose distribution.

Depth dose characteristics will usually favour electron beams due to the sharp fall off in dose beyond the PTV, although if the prescribed dose is to be delivered to the patient, surface bolus material may be required for lower energy (typically <10 MeV) electron beams. This is due to the build-up effect present in electron beams, but which is negligible in kV x-ray beams where the maximum dose is at the surface.

The predominant interaction of a low energy kV photon beam is photoelectric absorption with a probability of interaction in tissue approximately depending on Z^4 (Z being the atomic number). Therefore, there is an enhanced dose absorption in bone, which can be significant if high doses are prescribed to superficial regions with underlying bone, such as the scalp. At 100 kV (3 mm Al HVL), the dose absorption in bone will be 4.5 times greater than in water. By 300 kV (3 mm Cu HVL), this is reduced to 1.05 times the water dose as Compton interactions predominate and the atomic number of the absorbing material is no longer significant.

The relatively high energy of electrons in an electron beam compared with those generated in a kV beam results in a large range and they can therefore penetrate into tissue well beyond the field edge. The consequence of this is a much broader penumbral region than is present in a kV x-ray beam, and this penumbra varies with depth. Therefore, the use of electron beams to treat PTVs very close to critical structures, such as the lens, should be avoided if possible. The sharp penumbra of a kV beam makes it the ideal modality where critical structures are adjacent.

The SSD of a kV machine will typically be far shorter than a linear accelerator usually ranging from 25 to 50 cm. Therefore, the inverse square law dependence of dose will be far more significant in kilovoltage than electron treatments, e.g. a 2 cm air gap results in a dose reduction of approximately 12% at 30 cm SSD compared with a reduction of approximately 4% for an electron beam at a standard linear accelerator SSD.

There is usually less demand on a kV treatment machine than on a linear accelerator, so where the physical differences in the beam are of no clinical significance, then the use of kV may reduce departmental waiting times and facilitate a treatment starting sooner than on a linear accelerator. For a few patients, the increased treatment time arising from the lower dose rates of a kilovoltage unit compared to those from a linear accelerator may be a disadvantage.

SPECIAL TECHNIQUES

Over the past 20 years, highly specialist treatment techniques have been developed often with dedicated treatment machines. Although often some form of the treatment can be delivered on a standard linear accelerator with specialized accessories or modification, there are also examples of highly specialized treatment facilities being developed in order to exploit and explore the potential of the special technique.

Total body irradiation

TBI is employed in the treatment of leukaemia in order to kill leukaemic cells and to suppress the immune system prior to a bone marrow transplant. The target site is therefore all malignant stem cells, immunocytes (cells of the immune system), and bone marrow stem cells, while the most important critical structure is the lung, as radiation induced pneumonitis is a common side effect and can limit the total dose administered. TBI is administered in conjunction with chemotherapy prior to bone marrow transplant so a reliable treatment delivery is essential as once the chemotherapy commences, the bone marrow transplant cannot be delayed.

The only practical radiotherapy technique is to give a uniform dose to the entire body (including the skin). There are wide variations in the delivery technique, the dose administered, the dose specification point, and the dose rate [11]. However, most techniques employ a standard linear accelerator beam with the patient at an extended SSD of approximately 4 to 5 m treated with lateral fields. A Perspex sheet is placed in the beam to reduce the depth of the build-up region and bolus may be placed close to the patient to even out the body contour and provide a more uniform dose. The low density of lung means that the thorax will receive a higher dose than the rest of the trunk so it is important to provide some form of lung compensator, which can range from positioning the patient's arms over the chest to MLC compensation.

The beam characteristics will differ considerably from those at the standard treatment distance so extensive measurements are required to establish a TBI technique. The effect of scatter from the wall behind the patient, the floor, and the air, all create a unique beam condition, and these affect not only the patient dosimetry, but also the measuring devices such as TLD and diodes which must also be calibrated in these conditions.

Treatment planning may be based on CT data if the treatment planning computer can accurately account for extended SSD fields. However, all techniques rely on in vivo dosimetry to confirm or establish the MU required.

These surface dose measurements must be carefully related to the dose at depth – usually the midplane dose at the abdomen, or dose to lung, and may be significantly influenced by electron contamination and the unpredictable scattered radiation doses in this set-up.

Stereotactic radiotherapy and radiosurgery

The term 'stereotactic' means the 3D localization of a point in space by a unique set of coordinates that relate to a fixed external reference frame (Figure *evolve* 10.33). The first radiotherapeutic use of stereotactic radiotherapy (SRT) was in the treatment of brain tumours, following the principles that had evolved with its neurosurgical use. Although mainly used in the brain, stereotactic principles can be used to treat any tumour site in the body, provided that a good, reproducible fixation system is used, whether the treatment is given in single or multiple fractions.

Stereotactic radiosurgery (SRS) is the technique by which narrow, well-defined beams of radiation are focused precisely onto a small target. This single fraction treatment can be given using cobalt-60 (gamma-knife), linear accelerators, protons, heavy ions or tomotherapy.

It is particularly used in brain radiotherapy because of its highly focused nature and the importance of reducing dose to sensitive structures, such as brain stem and optic nerves. As the patient fixation, target localization, treatment delivery and verification is so precise, the PTV margins around the GTV are generally smaller than for conventional treatment.

Gamma units

These machines use a helmet containing 201 cobalt-60 sources arranged in a $160°$ sectored array. These are focused to a target with the aid of tungsten secondary collimating shells that define treatment spheres of 4, 8, 14, or 18 mm in diameter. This is extremely precise and can give a dose delivery to within $±0.4$ mm. It is simple to operate and mechanically robust. The disadvantages are that it is expensive, limited to the treatment of brain tumours and requires the 201 cobalt sources to be replaced about every 8 years.

Linacs

Much more universally available is the use of conventional linear accelerators to deliver precise small field radiotherapy. The beams are usually defined either with customized tertiary collimators or more usually microleaf collimators (leaf-size between 2 and 5 mm at the isocentre). The other requirements for precise delivery are an adjustable stereotactic frame and bracket, fiducial markers, stable and precise lasers and customized quality assurance tools, dosimetric phantoms and procedures. Access to MRI, CT and angiographic imaging and a method of treatment verification are also essential.

Stereotactic treatment planning

There are specific stereo planning systems available but, increasingly, conventional treatment planning systems have a separate package for stereotactic radiotherapy. For treatment planning, however, the user is required to characterize and measure small field radiation beams. Measurements include beam profiles (OAR) plus either a central axis depth dose curve (PDD) or Tissue Maximum Ratio (TMR) curve for each field size measured. A lack of lateral electronic equilibrium with narrow photon beams means small detectors with high spatial resolution should be used. OAR's are often measured with film such as Kodak XV2, EDR or Gafchromic EBT, all corrected for dose/density non-linearity. PDD and TMR data are usually measured using small volume (0.1 cc) ion chambers or p-type diodes. Attention to the effects of collimator scatter, MLC leaf shape and transmission need consideration, so beam data measurement is best done in 'typical' treatment conditions. This is true whether demountable collimators or MLC are used. Generally, a separate 'treatment machine' for stereotactic procedures can be stored within the beam data of the treatment planning system.

Imaging of the patient in the treatment frame is an important part of the precision of the procedure. MR is an essential imaging tool for the brain and therefore high precision therapy distortion correction image registration software is an important part of the planning system. CT data provide the basic data set against which other imaging modalities are registered.

Treatment planning requires the facility to plan multiple non-coplanar arcs focused to one or more isocentres, or to use multiple, fixed, non-coplanar conformal beams (conformed with either custom blocks or MLCs). Planning systems will generally allow planning with dynamic non-coplanar conformal arcs linked to a microleaf delivery system. This directly replaces the original multiple arcs of pencil beams produced with tertiary collimators. IMAT (intensity modulated arc therapy) is also available.

DVH analysis of brain treatment plans has shown that three to five arcs provide sufficient normal tissue sparing (while giving good dose uniformity to the PTV). However, if stereotactic treatment is being used for young patients or for benign conditions, it is relevant to consider increasing the number of arcs to reduce the exit dose to the whole body from any sagittally orientated arcs.

For larger, irregular target volumes (35–70 cc), four to six fixed, non-coplanar fields are probably a better technique, with either conformal blocking or MLC defined shielding based on the BEV of each portal.

Figure 10.34 shows DVHs comparing three different beam configurations used in a stereotactically planned, elliptically shaped brain lesion. The sparing effect of conformal beam shaping for four and six fixed fields compared to a spherical treatment volume produced by single isocentre, multiple arcing with a circular collimation is clearly shown.

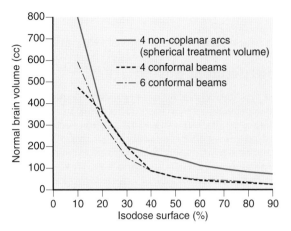

Figure 10.34 A simple comparison for an ellipsoid volume.

Although multileaf collimators make it very efficient to produce conformality, conventional 1 cm leaf systems are often unacceptably coarse for SRT and SRS. The added efficiency of the MLC device always has to be balanced against the 'gold standard' of target conformation given by customized lead alloy blocks.

TREATMENT PLAN CHECKING

A treatment planning system will be tested during commissioning and this will include evaluating correct data transfer to the record and verify network and treatment unit, and comparing the dose delivered to a phantom with that calculated by the treatment planning system. However, there is an ongoing requirement to check individual treatment plans as each plan is unique and may be susceptible to both operator and inherent software errors. The checking process should be a thorough review before releasing the plan for treatment and is to some extent dependent upon local equipment and practice but should include the following:

- the appropriateness of the plan (does it follow protocol), is any complexity, or a non standard plan justified
- no collision of patient, immobilization devices etc., with the treatment head
- beams passing through the couch or immobilization devices are not significantly attenuated or the transmission has been corrected for
- correct patient data used and identified, correct image registration if applicable
- correct prescription, including dose per fraction
- PTV coverage and dose homogeneity in all planes and organ at risk doses evaluated by DVH and inspection of each slice

- isocentre position set up instructions are correct and unambiguous
- imaging data such as orthogonal DRRs, are correct.

Independent dose check

The TPS dose calculation must be independently checked, either manually, or most likely, using a separate dose calculating computer, which should use a different beam data set and perform a different calculation to that of the main planning system. Usually, the dose check will use a simpler calculation method, so differences between the plan and the check calculation will be expected in certain patient situations, such as the presence of heterogeneities, small, and/or highly wedged or asymmetric fields, but these differences should be predictable. Once the limitations of the checking algorithm are established, a dose check tolerance can be set with $\pm 2\%$ tolerance and an action level of $\pm 3\%$ being typical values.

Plan checking at treatment

Although record and verify systems make set-up errors less likely than when daily manual input of field parameters are used, the plan data should include enough information, such as a scaled patient outline or SSDs for each beam, to confirm that the plan is being delivered correctly. Portal imaging is highly effective in checking beam positions but it is critical that the image data sent to the treatment unit are correct and clearly represent the isocentre positioning.

In vivo beam entrance and/or exit dose measurements may be performed and these require appropriate data from the planning computer for example applying the correct build up depth for the measurement device.

Even with a perfect set-up, the patient anatomy (both external or internal) may change from when the planning data were acquired, and the plan may need to be adapted, either with a simple adjustment of monitor units or, in some cases, a complete replan is required.

REFERENCES

[1] ICRU Report 50. Prescribing, recording and reporting photon beam therapy. International Commission on Radiation Units and Measurements; 1993.

[2] ICRU Report 62. Prescribing, recording and reporting photon beam therapy. (supplement to ICRU Report 50). International Commission on Radiation Units and Measurements; 1999.

[3] Willoughby TR, Starkschall G, Janjan NA, Rosen II. Evaluation and scoring of radiotherapy treatment plans using an artificial neural network. Int J Radiat Oncol Biol Phys 1996;34:923–30.

[4] Vaarkamp J, Adams EJ, Warrington AP, Dearnaley DP. A comparison of forward and inverse planned conformal, multi segment and intensity modulated radiotherapy for the treatment of prostate and pelvic nodes. Radiother Oncol 2004;73:65–72.

[5] Tomsej M, Gregoire V, Vynckier S, Scalliet P. Sparing parotids and increasing conformity in laryngopharyngeal treatments: development of a new conformal technique, description of a complete quality assurance program and first results. Radiother Oncol 2001; 61(S1):S45.

[6] Bragg CM, Conway J, Robinson MH. The role of intensity-modulated radiotherapy in the treatment of parotid tumors. Int J Radiat Oncol Biol Phys 2002;52:729–38.

[7] Das IJ, Kase KR, Tello VM. Dosimetric accuracy at low monitor unit settings. Br J Radiol 1991;64:808–11.

[8] Clark CH, Mubata CD, Meehan CA, et al. IMRT clinical implementation: prostate and pelvic node irradiation using Helios and a 120-leaf multileaf collimator. J Appl Clin Med Phys 2002;3:273–84.

[9] Pirzkall A, Carol MP, Pickett B, et al. The effect of beam energy and number of fields on photon-based IMRT for deep seated targets. Int J Radiat Oncol Biol Phys 2002;53: 434–42.

[10] McKenzie A. A simple method for matching electron beams in radiotherapy. Phys Med Biol 1998;3465–78.

[11] Plowman PN. A review of total body irradiation. Br J Radiol Suppl 1988;22:135–44.

FURTHER READING

Drzymala R, Holman MD, Yan D, et al. Integrated software tools for the evaluation of radiotherapy treatment plans. Int J Radiat Oncol Biol Phys 1994;30:909–19.

Austin-Seymour MM, Chen GTY, Castro JR, et al. Dose volume histogram analysis of liver radiation tolerance. Int J Radiat Oncol Biol Phys 1986;12:31–5.

Brown AP, Urie MM, Barest G, et al. Three-dimensional treatment planning for Hodgkin's disease 1991;21:205–15.

Chen GTY, Austin-Seymour MM, Castro JR, et al. Dose volume histograms in treatment planning evaluation of carcinoma of the pancreas. In: Proceedings, Eighth International Conference on Uses of Computers in Radiation Therapy. IEEE; 1984.

Coia LR, Galvin J, Sontag M, et al. Three-dimensional photon treatment planning in carcinoma of the larynx. Int J Radiat Oncol Biol Phys 1991;21:183–92.

Emami B, Purdy JA, Manolis J, et al. Three-dimensional treatment planning for lung cancer. Int J Radiat Oncol Biol Phys 1991;21:217–27.

Kutcher GJ, Fuks Z, Brenner H, et al. Three-dimensional photon treatment planning for carcinoma of the nasopharynx. Int J Radiat Oncol Biol Phys 1991;21:164–82.

Munzenrider JE, Doppke KP, Brown AP, et al. Three-dimensional treatment planning for para-aortic node irradiation in patients with cervical cancer. Int J Radiat Oncol Biol Phys 1991;21:229–42.

Shank B, LoSasso T, Brewster L, et al. Three-dimensional treatment planning for post-operative treatment of rectal carcinoma. Int J Radiat Oncol Biol Phys 1991;21:253–65.

Shipley WU, Tepper JE, Prout GR, et al. Proton radiation as boost therapy for localized prostatic carcinoma. J Am Med Assoc 1979;241:1912–5.

Simpson JR, Purdy JA, Manolis JM, et al. Three-dimensional treatment planning considerations for prostate cancer. Int J Radiat Oncol Biol Phys 1991;21:243–52.

Solin LJ, Chu JCH, Sontag MR, et al. Three-dimensional treatment planning of the intact breast. Int J Radiat Oncol Biol Phys 1991;21:193–203.

Drzymala RE, Mohan R, Brewster MS, et al. Dose volume histograms. Int J Radiat Oncol Biol Phys 1991;21:71–8.

Wambersie A, Landberg T, Chavaudra J, et al. ICRU Report 50: Prescribing, recording, and reporting photon beam therapy. International Commission on Radiation Units and Measurements; 1991.

Jain NL, Kahn MG, Drzymala RE, Emami B, Purdy JA. Objective evaluation of 3D radiation treatment plans: a decision-analytic tool incorporating treatment preferences of radiation oncologists. Int J Radiat Oncol Biol Phys 1993;26:321–33.

Niemierko A, Goitein M. Dose-volume distributions: A new approach to dose-volume histograms in three-dimensional treatment planning. Med Phys 1994;21:3–11.

Bohsung J, Gillis S, Arrans R, et al. IMRT treatment planning – A comparative inter-system and inter-centre planning exercise of the QUASIMODO group. Radiother Oncol 2005 Sep 8.

Weber DC, Bogner J, Verwey J, et al. Proton beam radiotherapy versus fractionated stereotactic radiotherapy for uveal melanomas: A comparative study. Int J Radiat Oncol Biol Phys 2005;63:373–84.

Lu Y, Li S, Spelbring D, et al. Dose-surface histograms as treatment planning tool for prostate conformal therapy. Med Phys 1995;22:279–84.

Garcia-Vicente F, Zapatero A, Floriano A, et al. Statistical analysis of dose-volume and dose-wall histograms for rectal toxicity following 3D-CRT in prostate cancer. Med Phys 2005;32: 2503–2509.

Nioutsikou E, Webb S. Reconsidering the definition of a dose-volume histogram. Phys Med Biol 2005;50:17–9.

Niemierko A. Reporting and analyzing dose distributions: a concept of equivalent uniform dose. Med Phys 1997;24:103–10.

Deasy JO, Niemierko A, Herbert D, et al. Methodological issues in radiation dose-volume outcome analyses: summary of a joint AAPM/NIH workshop. Med Phys 2002;29:2109–27.

Bortfeld TR, Kahler DL, Waldron TL, Boyer AL. X-ray field compensation with multileaf compensators. Int J Radiat Oncol Biol Phys 1994;28:723–30.

Convery DJ, Rosenbloom ME. The generation of intensity-modulated fields for conformal radiotherapy by dynamic collimation. Phys Med Biol 1992;37:1359–74.

Convery DJ, Webb S. Generation of discrete beam-intensity modulation by dynamic multileaf collimation under minimum leaf separation constraints. Phys Med Biol 1998;43:2521–38.

Damen EMF, Brugmans MJP, van der Horst A, et al. Planning, computer optimization, and dosimetric verification of a segmented irradiation technique for prostate cancer. Int J Radiat Oncol Biol Phys 2001;49:1183–95.

De Gersem W, Claus F, De Wagter C, et al. Leaf position optimisation for step-and-shoot IMRT. Int J Radiat Oncol Biol Phys 2001;51:1371–88.

Eisbruch A, Marsh LH, Martel MK, et al. Comprehensive irradiation of head and neck cancer using conformal multisegmental fields: assessment of target coverage and noninvolved tissue sparing. Int J Radiat Oncol Biol Phys 1998;41:559–68.

Evans PM, Donovan EM, Partridge M, et al. The delivery of intensity modulated radiotherapy to the breast using multiple static fields. Radiother Oncol 2000;57:79–89.

Galvin JM, Chen X-G, Smith RM. Combining multileaf fields to modulate fluence distributions. Int J Radiat Oncol Biol Phys 1993;27:697–705.

Henrys A, Taylor H, Bedford J, Tait D. Optimizing the use of multileaf collimators in the treatment of colo-rectal cancer. Clin Oncol 2003;15 (Suppl. 2):S18.

Kestin LL, Sharpe MB, Frazier RC, et al. Intensity modulation to improve dose uniformity with tangential breast radiotherapy: initial clinical experience. Int J Radiat Oncol Biol Phys 2000;48:1559–68.

Shepard , et al. Med Phys 2002;29:1007–18.

Spirou SV, Chui CS. Generation of arbitrary intensity profiles by dynamic jaws or multileaf collimators. Med Phys 1994;21:1031–41.

Stein J, Bortfeld T, Dörschel B, Schlegel W. Dynamic x-ray compensation for conformal radiotherapy by means of multi-leaf collimation. Radiother Oncol 1994;32:163–73.

Sternick ES, Bleier AR, Carol MP, et al. Intensity modulated radiation therapy: what photon energy is best? In: Leavitt , Sharkschall , editors. Proceedings 12th International Conference on the use of computers in radiation therapy. Salt Lake City; May, 1997. p. 418–9.

Svensson R, Källman P, Brahme A. An analytical solution for the dynamic control of multileaf collimators. Phys Med Biol 1994;39:37–61.

Intensity-Modulated Radiation Therapy Collaborative Working Group. Int J Radiat Oncol Biol Phys 2001;51:880–914.

Adams EJ, Cosgrove VP, Shepherd SF, et al. Comparison of a multileaf collimator with conformal blocks for the delivery of stereotactically guided conformal radiotherapy. Radiother Oncol 1999;51:205–209.

Belec J, Patrocinio H, Verhaegen F. Development of a Monte Carlo model for the Brainlab microMLC. Phys Med Biol 2005;50:787–99.

Brada M. Radiosurgery for brain tumours. Eur J Cancer 1991;27:1545–8.

Blomgren H, Lax I, Naslund I, Svanstrom R. Stereotactic high dose fraction radiation therapy of extracranial tumors using an accelerator; clinical experience of the first thirty-one patients. Acta Oncol 1995;34:861–70.

Cosgrove VP, Jahn U, Pfaender M, Bauer S, Budach V, Wurm RE. Commissioning of a micro multi-leaf collimator and planning system for stereotactic radiosurgery. Radiother Oncol 1999;50:325–36.

Gill SS, Thomas GT, Warrington AP, Brada M. Relocatable frame for stereotactic external beam radiotherapy. Int J Radiat Oncol Biol Phys 1991;20:599–603.

Graham JD, et al. A comparison of techniques for stereotactic radiotherapy by linear accelerator based on 3-dimensional dose distributions. Radiother Oncol 1991;22:29–35.

Gross MW, Engenhart-Cabillic R. Normal tissue reactions after linac-based radiosurgery and stereotactic radiotherapy. Front Radiat Ther Oncol 2002;37:140–50.

Hartmann GH, et al. Precision and accuracy of stereotactic convergent beam irradiations from a linear accelerator. Int J Radiat Oncol Biol Phys 1993;28:481–92.

Kooy HM, et al. Image fusion for stereotactic radiotherapy and radiosurgery treatment planning. Int J Radiat Oncol Biol Phys 1994;28:1229–234.

Kooy HM, Dunbar SF, Tarbell NJ, et al. Adaptation and verification of the relocatable Gill-Thomas-Cosman frame in stereotactic radiotherapy. Int J Radiat Oncol Biol Phys 1994;30:685–91.

Laing RW, et al. Stereotactic radiotherapy of irregular targets: a comparison between static conformal beams and non-coplanar arcs. Radiother Oncol 1993;28:241–6.

Leksell LT. The stereotactic method and radiosurgery of the brain. Acta Chir Scand 1951;102:316.

Lutz W, Winston KR, Maleki N. A system for stereotactic radiosurgery with a linear accelerator. Int J Radiat Oncol Biol 1988;14:373–81.

McKerracher C, Thwaites DI. Assessment of new small-field detectors against standard field detectors for practical stereotactic beam data acquisition. Phys Med Biol 1999;44:2143–60.

Serago CF, Houdek PV, Hartmann GH, Saini DS, Serago ME, Kaydee A. Tissue maximum ratios (and other parameters) of small circular 4, 6, 10, 15 and 24 MV x-ray beams for

radiosurgery. Phys Med Biol 1992;37:1943–56.

Siddon RL, Barth NH. Stereotactic localization of intercranial targets. Int J Radiat Oncol Biol Phys 1987;13:1241–6.

Sweeney RA, Bale RJ, Vogele M, Foerster S, Auberger T, Lukas P. A simple and noninvasive vacuum-mouthpiece based head-fixation system for high-precision radiotherapy. Strahlenther Onkol 2001;177:43–7.

Tepper JE, editor. Stereotactic radiosurgery. Semin Radiat Oncol 1995;5.

Tepper JE, Webb S, Evans P, editors. Innovative technologies in radiation therapy. Semin Radiat Oncol 2006;16.

Thomson ES, Gill SS, Doughty D. Stereotactic multiple arc radiotherapy. Br J Radiol 1990;63:745–51.

Tsai J, Buck BA, Svensson GK, et al. Quality assurance in stereotactic radiosurgery using a standard linear accelerator. Int J Radiat Oncol Biol Phys 1991;21:737.

Verhaegen F, Seuntjens J. Monte Carlo modelling of external radiotherapy photon beams. Phys Med Biol 2003;48:R107–64.

Walton L, et al. The Sheffield stereotactic radiosurgery unit: physical characteristics and principles of operation. Br J Radiol 1987;60:897–906.

Warrington AP, Laing RW, Brada M. Quality assurance in fractionated stereotactic radiotherapy. Radiother Oncol 1994;30:239–46.

EVOLVE CONTENTS (available online at: http://evolve.elsevier.com/Symonds/radiotherapy/)

collimators. Also, the Y1 collimator has not been brought in optimally to cover the MLCs to minimize interleaf leakage. In the right image, the isocentre has been shifted in the X leaf direction by half the width of the MLC leaves, thus optimizing the margin around the PTV

Figure *evolve* 10.11 Tumour and nodal volume in the left image with the right image showing an IMRT plan delivering different doses to the tumour and nodal volumes

Figure *evolve* 10.16 The use of additional segmented fields within the two wedged fields which alone produced the dose distribution on the left (A) improves the dose uniformity to that shown in the right image (B)

Figure *evolve* 10.17 Modified three-field beam arrangement to avoid prosthesis

Figure *evolve* 10.18 Isodose distributions produced by parallel-opposed beams. Left image beams are equally weighted, central image weighting is 2:1 at mid-plane and right image weighting is 2:1 at point A

Figure *evolve* 10.19 (A) Varying the wedge angle and relative beam weightings may not produce a satisfactory dose distribution especially when considering all the slices in a CT contour set. (B) By adding a segmented field, the high-dose regions (shown in green) can be shielded and the lower dose regions thus boosted. A longitudinal wedge may also assist in this process. (C) The result of using a segment field on the plan in (A)

Figure *evolve* 10.20 Sarcoma with parallel-opposed fields, isocentres outside target

Figure *evolve* 10.21 Left image shows transverse view of wedged pair with low weighted 'segment' field used to boost the dose to part of the PTV(shown in blue). On the right, the BEV of boost field showing partial shielding of the cord

Figure *evolve* 10.22 Three-field rectum treatment

Figure *evolve* 10.23 (A–D) Bronchus treatment. (E) Segments used in the left anterior oblique field in (C) instead of a wedge

Figure *evolve* 10.24 CNS junction

Figure *evolve* 10.25 Planning in the sagittal plane to avoid adjacent critical structures, in this case the contralateral eye

Figure *evolve* 10.26 Breast junction

Figure *evolve* 10.27 Non-coplanar skull

Figure *evolve* 10.33 Fiducial marker system with isocentres shown

Chapter | 11 |

Brachytherapy

Paul Symonds, Charles Deehan

INTRODUCTION

The use of discrete gamma ray sources to irradiate tissues is usually referred to as *brachytherapy* and falls into three distinct applications. *Interstitial therapy* is where the sources are implanted directly into the diseased tissues. *Intracavitary therapy* is where the sources are arranged in a suitable applicator to irradiate the walls of a body cavity from inside, in effect the sources are placed in the heart of the tumour in both of these cases. The use of *surface applicators* is where an external surface of the patient is treated by locally applied sources arranged on an appropriately shaped applicator. While the use of gamma-emitting surface applicators has been largely replaced by the use of electron beams and will not be covered in this chapter, limited use is made of *beta plaques* and these will be briefly described.

Treatment times vary from:

- A short period of time which may be measured in minutes as in the case of temporary implants
- A long period, over the effective life-time of the radionuclide during the decay phase, in the case of permanent implants.

In brachytherapy, most radionuclides are photons emitters, however, beta or even neutron-emitting sources are used for some applications. The present chapter describes the physical aspects of sealed sources and how they are used in brachytherapy.

INDICATIONS FOR BRACHYTHERAPY

The extent of the neoplasm must be known precisely as treatment is often given to a relatively small volume and 'geographic miss' is otherwise likely.

The site should be accessible for both inserting and, where appropriate, removing sources and allowing satisfactory geometric positioning of those sources.

ADVANTAGES OF BRACHYTHERAPY

The probability of local tumour control increases with increasing radiation dose, however, so does the probability of normal tissue damage. Brachytherapy allows the delivery of a highly localized radiation dose to a small tumour volume, increasing the chance of local control. There is a sharp fall off of radiation dose in the surrounding normal tissue, therefore, the risks of complication are reduced.

The overall duration of brachytherapy is relatively short, and can vary from a minute or two to several days depending on dose rate, prescribed dose and treatment distance from the radiation source. Constant low dose rate irradiation (below 1.0 Gy/hr) takes advantage of the different rates of repair and repopulation of normal and malignant tissue to produce differential cell killing. Hypoxic cells are relatively resistant to radiation treatment. Reoxygenation may occur during low dose rate radiotherapy with initially resistant hypoxic cells becoming well aerated and sensitive. Often in brachytherapy treatments, the dose distribution within tumour volume is not homogeneous. Treatment is often prescribed to the minimum dose received around the periphery of the treated volume. Areas close to the radiation sources in the centre of the tumour volume often receive up to twice this dose. Hypoxic cells are situated in avascular, sometimes necrotic, areas in the centre of tumours and the higher doses received here help to compensate for the relative radioresistance of these hypoxic cells. Irregular shaped tumours can be treated by judicious positioning of radiation sources and critical surrounding normal tissues can be avoided. At higher dose rate (above 12.0 Gy/hr) the radiobiological issues considerations are similar to those of external beam treatments.

DISADVANTAGES OF BRACHYTHERAPY

Many of the sources used in brachytherapy emit gamma rays and nursing and medical staff may be exposed inadvertently to low doses of radiation from the patient. Staff exposure can be minimized by afterloading techniques or the use of low energy radionuclides (see below).

Large tumours are usually unsuitable for brachytherapy. However, brachytherapy may be employed as a boost treatment following reduction in size by external beam radiotherapy and/or chemotherapy.

The radiation dose falls off rapidly from the sources, therefore, in order to treat the required tissue volume adequately, accurate geometric positioning is critically important. The spatial arrangement of sources used varies depending on the type of source applicator, the anatomical position of the tumour and the surrounding dose limiting normal tissue. Accurate positioning of sources or applicators requires special skill and training and this is not universally available.

Surrounding structures, such as lymph nodes that may contain overt or microscopic cancer, will not be irradiated by the implant or intracavitary treatment.

RADIONUCLIDES IN BRACHYTHERAPY

Gamma emitters

Radium, which has a half-life of 1600 years, and its alpha emitting gaseous daughter product radon, were used for many years as the major source of gamma rays for brachytherapy. The major source of gamma rays is the gaseous daughter product radon. When they were used, radium tubes and needles had to be gas tight and frequently checked for leaks (for radium the mean photon energy is 0.78 MeV). The gamma rays used are highly penetrating and very thick lead shields are required to provide adequate radiation protection. Other radionuclides with more suitable properties are now available and as a result this material is no longer in use.

The ideal radionuclide should have the following properties:

Radioactivity

At low gamma ray energies photoelectric effect can cause the absorbed dose in bone to be higher than that of soft tissue. Emission energy should therefore be high enough to minimize this but be low enough to reduce the level of scattered radiation and satisfy radiation safety requirements and sheilding cost constraints. A useful working range lies between 0.2 and 0.4 MeV. Where present unwanted charged particle emissions should be easily screened, radionuclides should also have no gaseous disintegration products and have a high specific activity.

Half-life

For temporary implants the half-life should be long enough so that radioactive decay does not need to be taken into account when calculating treatment times. Although most centres do not now keep a permanent stock of radionu-clides, where these are kept a very long half-life is desirable to avoid frequent replacement of stock.

Material properties

Sources should be small to enable easy delivery to (and retrival from) afterloading carriers which may have tightly curved loops. Some material can still be obtained in the form of flexible radioactive wire, e.g. Iridium-192, which can be cut into appropriate lengths with minimal risk of contamination. It is also highly desirable that the radionu-clide should be non-toxic, insoluble, not prone to break up or easy dispersal if the source container is broken and should be able to undergo frequent sterilization without suffering damage.

Although none of the currently available radionuclides satisfies all of the above criteria, those in common use satisfy several. Radionuclides are therefore chosen for dif-ferent uses where they are suitable. Developments in the production of radionuclides in nuclear reactors, which began following World War II, account for one source of these materials, the other being naturally occurring materi-als. All sources have a *recommended working life* beyond which the manufacturer will not guarantee the integrity of the source.

Half-life and specification of source strength

Radioactive decay is characterized by a period called the half-life of decay, $T_{1/2}$. In simple terms, this is the time taken for the activity of a source A_0 at time t = 0 to decay to half of its value or $0.5A_0$. During the next period, $T_{1/2}$, the activity will decay to half of that again or $0.25A_0$ and so on. The process is an exponential one and can be modelled using the equation:

$$A = A_0 Exp^{(-\lambda t)} \qquad \boxed{11.1}$$

where A_0 is the activity at time $t = 0$ and A the activity at time t. The factor λ is the decay constant and $\lambda = \ln2/ T_{1/2}$

Absorbed dose

The absorbed radiation dose rate, D_r, in tissue can be calcu-lated from the reference air kerma rate. Kerma rate (K_r) is an acronym for kinetic energy, (dE_r), released per unit mass (dm) and is defined as:

$$K_r = \frac{dE_r}{dm} \qquad \boxed{11.2}$$

The special unit for kerma is the gray (Gy) and the relation-ship between kerma and dose rate, D_r is:

$$D_r = K_r(1 - g) \qquad \boxed{11.3}$$

The dose rate D_r is less than kerma rate K_r by a factor $(1-g)$, this takes account of the energy lost by processes like bremsstrahlung and the production of delta rays (high energy electrons) produced by the electrons as they interact with matter and which are not absorbed in the

volume dm. The factor g (<1) is the fraction of the energy lost in the bremsstrahlung process and the production of delta rays.

Gamma emitters

Caesium-137

As a fission product derived from spent uranium fuel rods used in nuclear reactors, Caesium-137 has no gaseous daughter products and largely replaced radium as the nuclide of choice in the 1960s. It has a very useful half-life of 30 years and a somewhat less penetrating 0.662 MeV (mean) gamma ray than radium which was used some dec-ades ago, which emitted gamma rays of 0.780 MeV (mean). It was favoured for gynaecological insertions and was exten-sively used in low dose rate (LDR) and medium dose rate (MDR) afterloading systems from the late seventies but has now been largely replaced by high dose rate (HDR) after-loading systems using iridium-192.

It is an alkaline metal but, as a compound of chloride or sulfate, it is chemically stable, however, these salts are sol-uble and, therefore, for clinical sources it is mixed with other materials to reduce the risk of being absorbed by tis-sue should the source capsule break. When used with LDR afterloading systems, it was most commonly in the form of spherical pellets. This was achieved by mixing the caesium with glass to form beads which could be encapsulated by spherical stainless steel shells. These pellets could then be used in the form of a source train. Caesium was also incorporated into zirconium phosphate for needles and tubes used for manual interstitial and intracavitary brachy-therapy. Sources are doubly encapsulated and have a recommended working life of 10 years, during which their activity falls by approximately 20%.

Iridium-192

Iridium-192 with a mean gamma energy of 0.370 MeV and half-life of 74 days is now being widely used, taking advantage of its high specific activity and the properties of a flexible wire, in which form it has many advantages over traditional radium or caesium needles. It has been in use since the late 1950s, first in the form of seeds, by Henschke, and then a few years later in the form of wire and hair-pins at the Institute Gustave Roussy in Paris. Coils of thin wire (0.3 mm diameter) can be cut to conve-nient lengths and inserted into flexible nylon tubes or rigid hollow afterloading needles similar to hypodermic needles, which have been previously implanted into tumours (see Figure 11.1A and B). The active iridium–platinum core is 0.1 mm in diameter and contained within a sheath of platinum 0.1 mm thick. This sheath is adequate to filter out most of the beta-rays produced as a result of the decay process. Beta emmissions are pre-dominantly at energies of 0.530 MeV and 0.670 MeV. Thicker wires, 0.6 mm in diameter, in the form of hairpins (see Figure 11.1C and D) can also be inserted directly

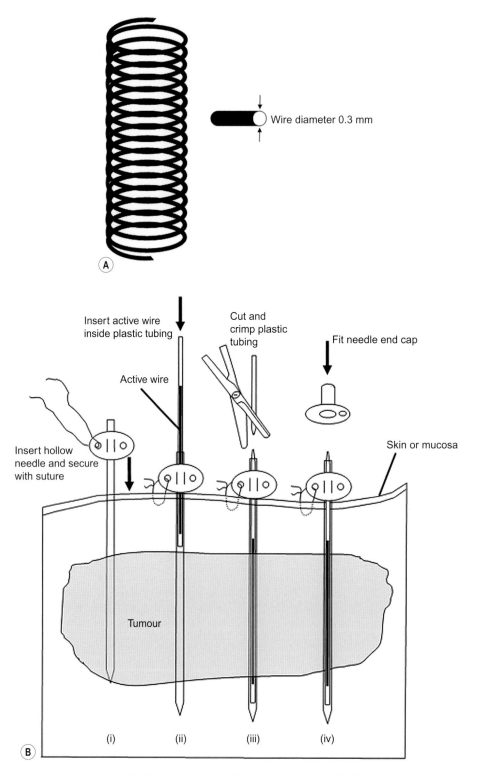

Wire diameter 0.3 mm

Figure 11.1 Iridium-192 wire implants. (A) Wire is supplied in 500 mm length, coiled. (B) Wire is inserted using needle guides. (i)- Hollow needle is inserted and sutured in place. (ii)- Active sheathed wire is inserted down the needle. (iii)- Non-active part of sheath is cut and crimped. (iv)- Wire is secured by a screw-on end cap.

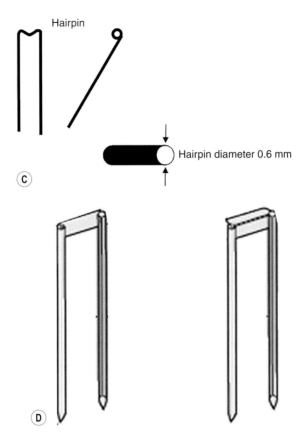

Figure 11.1, Cont'd (C) Thicker wires in the form of Single and Double Hairpins may be used. (D) Gutter guides are inserted into the treatment volume and hairpins are pushed into the guides, sutured in place and the guides removed.

into tumours through suitable introducers. In the USA, iridium is available in the form of seeds sealed in thin nylon coated ribbon. Although iridium in the form mentioned here is generally used for low dose rate treatments, it can also be used as a high activity source for HDR systems (see Figure 11.2A and B).

As iridium produces gamma rays of mean energy 0.370 MeV, lead shields of only 2 cm in thickness provide very good protection. The only major disadvantage of iridium is the relatively short half-life, therefore, fresh material should be used for each implant, at low dose rate and HDR sources are normally renewed every 3 months.

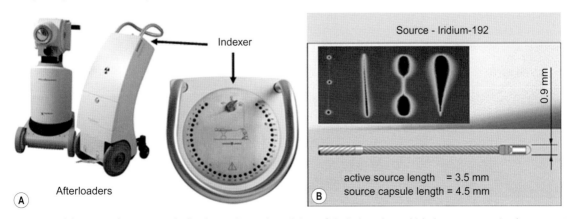

Figure 11.2 (A) Two Nucletron HDR afterloaders and an enlarged view of the indexer into which the source transit tubes connect. (B) ^{192}Iridium HDR source and dose distributions.
(By kind permission of Nucletron UK Ltd).

Iodine-125

Iodine[125] with a half-life of 60 days is used for permanent implants of the prostate. It has been used clinically since the early 1960s and is the daughter product of xenon-125 which is produced by an (n-gamma) reaction.

The low photon energy of iodine-125 means that the half-value layer (HVL) thickness of lead required for protection is only 0.02 mm and, in tissue, this HVL is in the region of 1.7 cm. As well as having a relatively short half-life, the gamma rays produced by this radionuclide (27–35 KeV) are of very low energy and very little radiation is emitted from the patient following the implant.

Cobalt-60

Treatments of retinoblastoma have been effected using cobalt-60 ophthalmic applicators of similar construction to the ruthenium applicator (see beta emitters below). Their longer half-life was an advantage, but the high-energy gamma radiation gave higher doses to other vital structures, e.g. the lens, macula and optic nerve, than with the ruthenium beta particle radiations. The cobalt-60 applicators had a useful dose rate of typically 0.06 Gy min^{-1} at the surface, reducing to 50% at $\approx$2 mm.

Beta emitters

The major use of plaques emitting beta ray radiation is in the treatment of eye tumours. Plaques can be made of strontium-90 or ruthenium-106/rhodium-106.

Strontium-90

The strontium-90 ($T_{1/2} = 28.7$ years) compound is incorporated in a rolled silver foil bonded into the silver applicator and formed so that it presents an active concave surface of 15 mm radius to the cornea, with a surface filtration of 0.1 mm silver. Strontium-90 is only useful when in radioactive equilibrium with its daughter product, yttrium-90 ($T_{1/2} = 2.7$ days). The silver filter is designed to absorb low-energy beta particles from the strontium decay (0.546 MeV max, range in water 1.2 mm) while transmitting the higher-energy beta particles from the yttrium-90 (2.27 MeV max., range in water $\approx$11 mm). The back of the applicator is finished with a much thicker (0.9 mm) layer of silver to reduce the transmitted dose rate to a relatively safe level. A variety of plaques is available, each designed to give a useful dose rate of approximately 1 Gy min^{-1} at the surface reducing to 50% at $\approx$2 mm (Figure 11.3).

Ruthenium-106

Ruthenium-106 ($T_{1/2} = 369$ days) is a fission product of uranium and decays with a low-energy beta emission to rhodium-106 ($T_{1/2} = 30s$) which has a higher-energy beta emission, namely 3.54 MeV max. The ruthenium applicator is made of silver with a window thickness of 0.1 mm

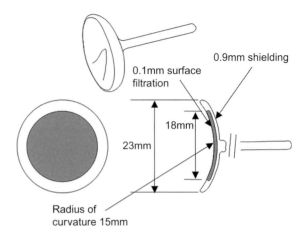

Figure 11.3 The strontium eye plaque is fabricated so that low energy beta radiation is filtered out allowing therapy to be given with higher energy beta radiation.

of silver and a thicker protective layer of 0.9 mm of silver on the back. The spherical radius of the window is 12 mm. The applicator is designed for suturing to the sclera for 7–10 days. The useful dose rate is typically 0.1 Gy min^{-1} at the surface reducing to 50% at $\approx$2.7 mm. A 15 mm acrylic visor is recommended to protect the eyes of the operator when using the ruthenium applicators.

Neutron emitters

Californium-252 has been used in the past to treat gynaecological tumours in particular. It is made by bombarding plutonium-239 with neutrons in a high flux reactor. Californium decays by alpha emission with a half-life of 2.64 years a process which effectively determines the overall practical half life of this source. However the most desirable property of this radionuclide is that it emits neutrons as a result of a process known as spontaneous fission with a half life of 85 years. Neutrons produced have an average energy in the range 2.1–2.3 MeV, also produced x-rays with an energy in the range 0.5 to 1 MeV. In theory, these sources should be more effective against hypoxic tumours. However, these theoretical advantages have never been convincingly demonstrated clinically and the radiation hazards involved have markedly restricted the use of these substances. The specific activity of ^{252}Ca is high and therefore can be made up into small sources which are suitable for brachytherapy applications.

RADIOBIOLOGY OF BRACHYTHERAPY

As with any radiation treatment, brachytherapy exploits differences between intrinsic radiosensitivity, repair and repopulation of normal and malignant cells. The major difference between brachytherapy and external beam treatments is seen in the marked variation in dose and dose rate distributions seen around the arrangement of radioactive sources. Close to radiation sources in any implant where the dose rate is high enough both normal and malignant cells will be killed regardless of their radiosensitivity. Further out from the sources in regions of low dose rate the killing effect will be much smaller and most radiosensitive cells will survive. Between these extremes is a region where differential cell killing will occur. The effects of cell proliferation during a low dose rate treatment lasting several days are complex. Normal tissue may undergo cell cycle arrest at the G1/S boundary and P^{53} mediated repair of radiation damage. By contrast, tumour cells may contiue to proliferate and enter the G2 and M phases of the cell cycle. Then, the accumulated radiation damage may lead to the death of malignant cells. Radioresistant hypoxic cells are often found in the centre of tumours, however, as sources are normaly implanted within the mass of the tumour even relatively resistant cells will be killed because of the presence of the high dose levels. The death of hypoxic cells may allow for reoxygenation of hypoxic tumour cells elsewhere within the treatment volume. The effects on hypoxic cells situated some distance from the sources are more complex. Ling measured oxygen enhancement ratios (OER) as a function of dose rate over the range 276 Gy/h to 0.89 Gy/h. The OER initialy increased from 3.0 to 4.0 (dose rate 20–60 Gy/h), then fell to 2.4 at the lower dose rates.

This finding implies that hypoxic cell killing is increased at dose rates in the range frequently used in practice.

The linear quadratic formula can be used to calculate biological equivalent doses (BED) for both brachytherapy and external beam treatments [1]. The proposed threshold BED for rectal complications is 90 Gy_3 (i.e. calculated with an α/β of 3 Gy), and for 50% morbidity rate is 190 Gy_3. The dose tolerance of the bladder is not so clearly known. The threshold for late morbidity in the bladder ranges from 100 to 125 Gy_3.

DOSIMETRY

Radioactive material is implanted into tissues according to distribution rules which vary according to the system used. In Europe, the classical Parker-Paterson and Quimby systems have largely been superseded by the Paris system, which is particularly suitable for iridium wire implants.

Dosimetry for iridium wire

Wire of the same linear activity is used and sources are arranged in parallel, straight, equidistant lines 18–20 mm apart and are 20–30% longer than the length of the treated

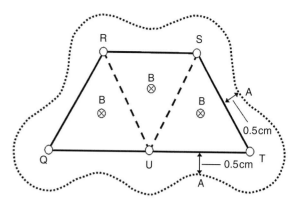

Figure 11.4 Volume implanted wires Q, R, S, T and U running perpendicular to the plane shown. Basal doserate points B and the dose contour A, representing 85% of the mean Basal Doserate.

volume. In a volume implant, sources in cross-section should be arranged in either equilateral triangles or squares (Figure 11.4).

The dose to the tumour can be calculated by hand using suitable graphs, such as Oxford cross line curves or by computer. The average basal dose rate (the arithmetic mean of minimum values between sources) is first calculated. The treatment dose (such as 65 Gy in 7 days, classically 10 Gy per day) is prescribed to the reference dose line (85% of the average basal dose). A similar method of calculation is used for hairpins. The prescription point for surface applicators, such as moulds, and some intracavity treatment is usually 0.5–1 cm from the applicator.

Dosimetry for gynaecological treatments

The dose that can be given during gynaecological brachytherapy is limited by the tolerance of the surrounding normal tissues including the cervix, uterus, upper vagina, bladder and rectum [2]. The uterus and cervix are highly tolerant of radiation. Excessive dose can cause serious late - damage to the upper vagina, bladder or rectum. A survey of British patients treated in 1993 for carcinoma of cervix by radical radiotherapy found 6% of patients developed serious late affects within 5 years of treatment [3].

In the treatment of carcinoma of cervix, the most frequently used prescribing point is the Manchester A point, defined as a point 2 cm lateral to the uterine canal and 2 cm above the cervical os. Anatomically, this point is said to be where the uterine artery crosses the ureter (see Figure 11.5).

The dose received at this point was found to be of predictive value for late radiation damage to ureter, bladder, rectum and other pelvic organs.

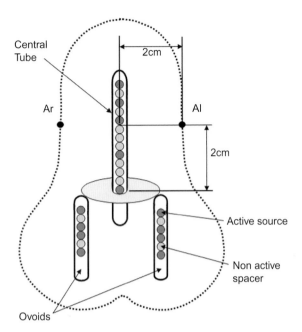

Figure 11.5 MDR source positions and the Manchester A points.

An alternative method of prescribing is to treat to tolerance the surrounding normal tissues. The maximum rectal dose can be either measured directly or more commonly calculated using orthogonal radiographs. This dose is often expressed as percentage of the A point dose and, in most centres, is between 60 and 70% of the A point dose given by brachytherapy.

A growing number of centres are prescribing by making use of CT and MR imaging. This image guided brachytherapy makes use of many of the planning tools and features developed for external beam treatment planning. Data sets acquired using different imaging modalities can be co-registered to allow accurate delineation of tumour and organs at risk and different treatment options can be compared using dose volume histograms.

Types of implants

Implants can be classified as manually (see below) inserted, afterloaded or remote afterloaded. Manual insertion of radiation sources should be avoided if possible owing to the radiation hazards to operating staff and nurses. Afterloading is when radioactive material is loaded into hollow needles, catheters or applicators which have been inserted into the tumour area previously. Manipulation of these "cold" applicators carries no radiation hazard for medical and nursing staff so that time can safely be taken to ensure optimal source geometry.

Most implants are of the removable type. The radiation sources are removed after delivery of the prescribed treatment dose. However, permanent implants can be performed using relatively short half life isotopes such as Iodine-125 which are implanted into tumours (particularly early prostate cancer) in the form of seeds which remain after the radiation has decayed completely.

GYNAECOLOGICAL CANCER

Manual loading and afterloading

From when brachytherapy was first introduced up until the mid-1970s, brachytherapy sources were loaded into rubber applicators and positioned by hand. Sources remained in place during the treatment and then were manually retrieved. This, of course, had the consequence that staff involved in the process from beginning to end were exposed to ionizing radiation.

In the late 1970s, sources with a high specific activity were readily available, for example cesium-137. In addition, developments in computer controlled delivery (microprocessors) and new flexible carriers made it possible to produce devices that could automatically deliver and retrieve treatment sources.

Manually inserted low dose rate (LDR) cesium with or without supplementary x-ray treatment can produced excellent tumour control rates unsurpassed by more modern methods of brachytherapy. The serious complication rate was also low, at 5% or less. Such results remain the gold standard against which modern techniques must be judged. The most widely used technique was the Manchester system in which preloaded sources were placed in the uterus and against the cervix (see Figure 11.5).

The dose rate at point A was approximately 0.5 Gy/h, which proved to be biologically very advantageous. A typical regimen used to treat an early stage 1_b carcinoma of cervix was two insertions of approximately 72 hours given 1 week apart to give a total dose of 75 Gy to point A.

The International Commission of Radiation Units and Measurement (ICRU) Report 38 [4] has proposed that volume (defined as height, thickness and width) enclosed by the 60 Gy isodose line from combined brachytherapy and external beam treatment should be used for reporting (but not prescribing) absorbed dose following gynaecological treatments. This concept has been accepted in parts of Europe but not in the USA or the UK [5].

Although most centres have discarded manually inserted sources, a few centres still treat carefully selected patients, such as those who are frail and elderly or are bleeding heavily from a cervical tumour. Frail patients tolerate manually inserted sources better than the more rigid (and uncomfortable) afterloading applicators. Manually inserted sources along with appropriate gauze packing are an excellent haemostat.

Afterloading machines

For gynaecological cancer high dose rate (HDR) is currently the most widely used method of brachytherapy treatment delivery in the UK although a few Medium/Low Dose Rate (MDR or LDR) and Pulsed Dose Rate (PDR) units are still in use. Applicators, dwell times and in some cases source trains have been configured to produce similar isodose patterns as manually inserted Manchester type caesium sources.

During insertions, the cervical os is dilated sufficiently to allow a rigid central tube to be placed in the uterus. Usually the central tube is 5 cm or less in length than the uterine canal to prevent 'tenting' of the uterus. As comparative studies have shown, after loading applicators tend to be more anterior in the pelvis than manual sources some operators use a shallow angle uterine tube to reduce the dose to the bladder.

Ovoid applicators are then placed against the cervix in line with the flange on the central tube. Gauze packing is placed beneath and above the ovoids to reduce the dose, particularly to the rectum and to the bladder.

The position of the applicators can be checked in theatre using an imagine intensifier. The dose rate to the rectum, base of bladder and prescription point is calculated from orthogonal radiographs and a treatment time is prescribed taking into account tolerance of normal tissues.

Then radioactive material can delivered under computer control to the intrauterine and vaginal applicators. In the case of HDR treatments a single source is most commonly used which tracks its way along the applicators halting at predetermined postions for specific periods called dwell times. In this way the overall average dose distribution is achieved when the tracking process is complete. Figure 11.2A shows a typical treatment unit, autoradiographs are also shown in figure 11.2B which illustrate how the dose distribution can be shaped by selection of different dwell postions and times. The HDR source can be seen in Figure 11.2B fitted to the tip of its transport cable which is used to deliver and retrieve the source. Alternatively MDR treatments use programmable arrangments of radioactive and non-active dummy pellets which are moved backwards and forward pneumatically into the applicators (see Figure 11.5.). Although much less common a second alternative involves the use of PDR techniques where a source of intermediate activity between HDR and MDR is used. The source delivery system is the same as with HDR but the dwell times are arranged in such a way that the resulting average dose rate distribution is similar to that seen with manually inserted LDR.

After loading applicators tend to be more uncomfortable than manually inserted sources carriers, however, with higher dose rates the treatment time is considerabley shorter. Dependant on source strength HDR dose rate is commonly around 53.5 Gy per hour to the Manchester point A compared with 1.8 Gy per hour with MDR. The dose rate from manually inserted LDR sources is 0.5 Gy per hour. Increased dose rate has a greater biological effect which needs to be accounted for and this is done by reducing the overall dose and delivering the treatment in a number of separate fractions.

MDR systems are steadily being replaced by HDR afterloading devices using high activity iridium sources. Treatment is completed in a matter of minutes. Rather like external beam irradiation, HDR treatments are fractionated. The ideal fraction scheme for HDR treatments is unknown. The linear quadratic formula is often used as a guideline to formulate HDR fractionation regimens. An analysis by Colin Orton and colleagues has provided useful experience based data [6]. Orton recommends that the dose to point A should be no greater than 7 Gy per fraction. Overall doses need to be reduced because of the increased dose rate. Overall HDR doses should be reduced by 50–60% compared to LDR treatments.

PERMANENT PROSTATE IMPLANTS

This technique is usually restricted to patients with early stage disease with favourable prognostic features [7]. These are patients with stage T1 and T2 tumours with pre-treatment PSA levels less than 10 mg/ml, and Gleeson scores of 6 or less. Patients with significant outflow obstruction symptoms are unsuitable for this technique owing to high instances of acute urinary obstruction following the implant process. Implantation is performed with the patient in the lithotomy position [8]. Prior to implantation, the transrectal ultrasound (TRUS) volume is determined using an ultrasound probe and this volume has been reported in the range 14.2–84.4 cc [3]. A needle guidance template attached to ultrasound apparatus is placed against the perineum. Hollow needles are inserted through the template under TRUS guidance with supplementary fluoroscopic screening if necessary. Iridium-125 seeds are introduced through these hollow needles in a prearranged pattern. Approximately 80 to 100 may be used in each implant (see Figure 11.6) and the dose delivered to the prostate before the seeds decay completely is about 160 Gy.

In general, this technique is tolerated well and patients can be rapidly discharged from hospital. The results of this technique depend partially on patient selection and partially on the experience of the team treating the patient. Typical relapse-free 5-year survival figures quoted are between 79 and 94%.

BRONCHIAL CANCERS

The possible major indication for intraluminal brachytherapy in carcinoma of bronchus is obstruction of a major airway. A fine catheter can be introduced through the tumour

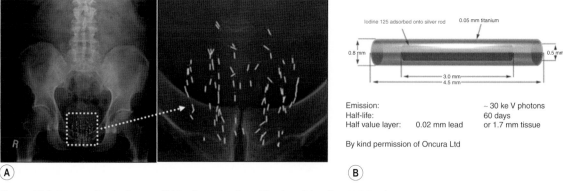

Figure 11.6 Prostate Brachytherapy. (A) Radiograph of seed implant (B) Iodine-125 Seed. *(By kind permission of Oncura Ltd).*

using a bronchoscope. This allows a high dose iridium source to be introduced into the bronchus. The typical dose is 15 Gy 1 cm from the iridium source given in a single fraction.

There has been only one randomized control trial that compared single exposure of bronchial brachytherapy with external beam radiotherapy (30 Gy in eight fractions). External beam radiotherapy reduced symptoms better than endobronchial treatment and there was modest but significant survival gain for those treated with external beam treatment.

OESOPHAGUS

An endoscope is used to place a suitable catheter through the oesophageal tumour. A high dose iridium source or, less frequently, caesium pellets in the medium dose rate Selectron are introduced into the catheter to treat the tumour. One limitation of brachytherapy is that the tumour can only be treated up to a distance of 1 cm from the source. A major use of intraluminal brachytherapy is as a palliative treatment to relieve either bleeding or dysphagia. Typical results following a single fraction of 15 Gy are improvement in dysphagia in 67% of patients 4–6 weeks after therapy and 47% of patients had complete relief of symptoms.

Intraluminal brachytherapy allows the escalation of dose to the tumour while protecting the surrounding dose limiting structures such as lung, heart and spinal cord. However, the results of clinical trials so far have shown that the addition of brachytherapy as a boost treatment does not appear to have improved results compared with external beam radiotherapy alone or concomitant chemotherapy with radiotherapy.

BILE DUCT CANCER

Primary biliary cancer is a rare condition. For this reason, studies in the use of intraluminal brachytherapy have tended to be small, non-randomized trials. Iridium wire or, preferably, a high dose rate iridium source from an after-loading machine, can be introduced into the bile duct via an external biliary drain leading to tumour shrinkage and relief of jaundice. Infection in the form of ascended cholangitis is the major complication of this technique. It is doubtful whether brachytherapy offers any significant advantage over biliary stenting or other forms of biliary decompression in this disease.

BREAST CANCER

The purpose of interstitial implantation in the treatment of breast cancer is usually to boost the radiation dose at the site of excision. If possible, flexible polythene tubes are inserted at the time of surgical excision of the breast lump (see Figure 11.7). However, it is more common to insert the tubing postoperatively. An advantage of peri-operative installation of tubing is that the radiotherapist knows the exact site of the excised tumour. Iridium wires can be inserted later.

Many centres have abandoned the use of postoperative iridium implantation to the tumour bed as the cosmetic results, particularly postoperative fibrosis, seem inferior to those seen following electron boosts. A major current use for interstitial implantation is as part of a treatment programme for inoperable breast cancer. Often, chemotherapy will be used to reduce the size of the tumour. If the tumour is then operable, the patient will proceed to surgery, if not, external beam radiotherapy can be

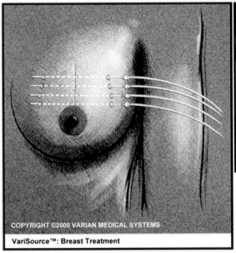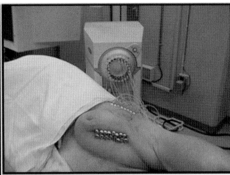

COPYRIGHT ©2000 VARIAN MEDICAL SYSTEMS

VariSource™: Breast Treatment

Figure 11.7 HDR afterloader for breast treatment using Iridium-192 stepping source. The source travels along flexible polythene tubes which have been inserted in theater.
(By kind permission of VARIAN UK Ltd).

administered followed by an interstitial boost treatment. Depending on the size of the residual breast tumour this can be given using either a single or double plane of iridium sources. Sometimes to ensure precise geometry, rigid needles are used secured in a template rather than flexible plastic tubes.

TONGUE AND FLOOR OF MOUTH

A T1 or T2 tumour on the lateral edge of the anterior two thirds of tongue can be very satisfactorily treated by iridium hairpins. Larger tumours are usually treated first by external beam radiotherapy (with or without chemotherapy) and the implant is used merely as a boost treatment. In French centres, sometimes brachytherapy of the tongue is accompanied by a functional neck dissection to treat the lymph nodes in the suprahyoid region of the upper neck.

Under general anaesthetic the tongue is both inspected and palpated to find out the full extent of the tumour. Gutter guides (see Figure 11.1B) are inserted to the tumour-bearing structure at 12 mm intervals under fluoroscopic control. The most posterior gutter guide is inserted first and attempts are made to keep all subsequent gutter guides parallel with this. Three gutter guides (occasionally four) are inserted to treat the tumour with a 1 cm margin of normal tissue. Once the operator is satisfied about the geometry of the implant, iridium hairpins are then inserted into the gutter guides. The hairpin is pressed down using a surgical hook and then the gutter guides are removed. The iridium is secured to the dorsum of the tongue by a stitch around the crossbar of the hairpin. The length of hairpins depends on the size of the tumour but usually 4 cm long

hairpins are inserted. A typical dose for a low dose rate implant is 65 Gy given over 6–7 days.

ANAL CANCER

Implantation is rarely used as the sole treatment of anal cancer. Patients are initially treated with external beam radiotherapy to doses of 40–45 Gy over 4–5 weeks. Patients with tumours greater than 5 cm also should receive chemotherapy, either mitomycin-C and 5-fluorouracil or cisplatin-based combinations.

After 1–2 months to allow the tumour to regress and the reaction to settle, the patient undergoes an implant which is carried out under general anaesthesia. A horseshoe-shaped jig is placed against the anal skin and up to eight hollow needles are inserted 1 cm apart through the jig to cover the area of the tumour plus a safety margin. The needles extend beyond the tumour for two reasons. The first is to include occult disease and a margin of 1 cm is usual. The second is to compensate for gradual reduction of radiation dose at the end of the implant. Fifteen percent is added to length of the iridium at each end to ensure the clinical volume receives the full dose. A hollow syringe barrel is inserted into the anus to allow the escape of flatus or faeces. The jig is stitched against the patient's skin and the needles are secured by a locking bar. The iridium is later inserted to give a dose of 15–25 Gy in 2–2½ days to the reference isodose line using the Paris system. This technique has yielded an impressive 93% three-year survival in a series of 48 patients with tumours under 5 cm. Six out of a total of 79 patients (7.6%) developed severe late complications.

199

FUTURE TRENDS

There is an increasing trend to treat early prostate cancer with brachytherapy. This modality seems very attractive to patients as the treatment can be completed in as little as 24 hours and theoretically avoids some of the complications of both external beam radiotherapy and radical surgery. However, there have been no randomized trials comparing the three modalities. The Sloan Kettering Memorial Institute in New York has a huge experience of both external beam and brachytherapy in the treatment of early prostate cancer. A retrospective analysis of patients treated at the Memorial showed 5-year disease-free survival was slightly better after external beam compared with brachytherapy.

In the treatment of gynaecological HDR systems have largely replaced LDR or MDR afterloading systems. HDR has the advantage that treatment can be carried out in a few minutes during a short general anaesthetic. Theoretically, HDR is more likely to cause normal tissue damage than LDR. However, this has not been seen in practice and is thought to be largely due to the effects of fractionation. HDR brachytherapy treatment is usually divided into two or three fractions, given over weekly intervals, of less than 7 Gy to point A.

Image guided brachytherapy has been a feature of prostate Iodine-125 implant treatment for the last three decades where ultrasound has been use to locate the protate and organs at risk as well as guide the placement of seeds. In the coming years with easier access to imaging other areas of brachytherapy work are likely to benefit more an more from image guided techniques. There also is growning interest in the development of combined brachytherapy and chemotherapy schedules which may lead to significant advances in the treatment of cervical cancer [9].

Within the last few years is has become more difficult to obtain iridium-192 wire in the UK. The future trend is to carry out implants using remote afterloading machines. Although HDR machines are mainly used for gynaecological insertions they can also be used to deliver interstitial or even surface of skin treatments. They can be used as the sole method of treatment or to deliver a boost doses after external beam radiotherapy.

A typical example of this is the treatment of prostate cancer. Plastic catheters can be inserted under general anaesthetic using needles inserted through a template under ultrasound control. A high intensity iridium source can then move into each of the catheters to occupy pre-determined dwell positions for specific times. HDR treatments given in 2 to 4 single fractions for early prostate cancer are an alternative to permanent iodine-125 seed implants.

Patients with locally advanced prostate cancer were treated in a randomised control trial either by external beam radiotherapy only or by external beam plus an HDR brachytherapy boost. The patients receiving a brachytherapy boost had a 15% improvement in local control (assessed by PSA measurements) compared to those treated by external beam only.

Pulsed dose rate machines typically delivering a dose rate of 1 Gy per hour try to reproduce the therapeutic results seen following iridium-192 wire implants. A series of catheters are inserted into the treatment volume. The iridium-192 source enters the catheters once an hour to deliver a dose of 1 Gy to the treatment volume over a few minutes. As radioactive material is only present for a few minutes during each hour the patient may have visitors or receive nursing support between each pulse of radiation.

Except for prostate and gynaelogical cancers, brachytherapy will probably be a 'niche' area suitable for patients being referred to only a few centres where resources and experience can be concentrated.

REFERENCES AND FURTHER READING

[1] Dale RG, Jones B. The clinical radiobiology of brachytherapy. Brit J Radiol 1998;71:465–83.

[2] Sundar S, Symonds P, Deehan C. Tolerance of pelvic organs to treatment for carcinoma of cervix. Clin Oncol 2003;15:240–7.

[3] Denton AS, Bond J, Mathews S, et al. National audit of the management and outcome of carcinoma of the cervix treated by radiotherapy in 1993. Clin Oncol 2000;12:347–53.

[4] International Commission on Radiation Units and Measurement. Dose and volume specification for reporting intracavitary brachytherapy in gyneacology. ICRU report 38. Maryland: Bethesda; 1985.

[5] Aird EGA, Jones CH, Joslin CAF, et al. Recommendations for brachytherapy dosimetry. British Institute of Radiology; 1993.

[6] Orton CG, Seyedsadr M, Somnay A. Comparison of high and low dose-rate remote afterloading for cervix and the inportance of fractionation. Int J Radiat Oncol Biol Phys 1991;21:1425–34.

[7] Moule RN, Hoskins PJ. Non-surgical treatment of localised prostate cancer. Surgical Oncology 2009;18:255–67.

[8] Acher P, et al. Prostate brachytherapy: dosimetric results and analysis of a learning curve with a dynamic dose-feedback technique. Int J Radiat Oncol Biol Phys 2006;65:694–8.

[9] Vale CL, Tierney JF, Davidson SE, Drinkwater KJ, Symonds P. Substantial improvement in UK cervical cancer survival with chemoradiotherapy: results of a Royal College of Radiologists' Audit. Clin Oncol 2010;22:590–601.

Chapter | 12 |

Networking, data and image handling and computing in radiotherapy

John Sage

CHAPTER CONTENTS

INTRODUCTION

Technology is so much fun but we can drown in our technology. The fog of information can drive out knowledge. Daniel Boorstin

Computers permeate every aspect of modern radiotherapy. With their application, we can deliver ever more intricate treatments. However, every technological innovation comes at a cost – in equipment, maintenance and added complexity. With care, these costs can be kept in balance and benefits to the patient achieved.

Computing in radiotherapy has developed as computers have grown more powerful. In 1965, Gordon Moore, co-founder of the computing giant Intel, predicted that microchip complexity would increase exponentially for at least 10 years [1]. In fact, Moore's law still holds today, with processors doubling in complexity approximately every 2 years. Moore's law typifies the growth in all aspects of computing. Hard disk drive capacity nearly doubles each year while the cost per gigabyte nearly halves [2].

This growth has consequences for radiotherapy. The useful lifetime of any item of computer software or hardware is going to be fairly short. In the NHS, a lifetime of 5 years is used for IT equipment, compared to 10 years for a linear accelerator [3]. This growth also needs to be considered when planning for long-term needs. It will be more costly to purchase 5 years' data storage immediately than it will be to buy half now and half in 2 years' time, at a quarter of the cost.

History

For many decades, radiotherapy was developed without computers. Isodose planning and linear accelerators both pre-date the use of computers. In the 1960s, the first investigations were made into using computers for radiotherapy. Such use required access to one of the small number of large 'mainframe' computers, probably at a university, since personal computers were not invented until the 1970s. The first widespread use of computers was for calculating isodose distributions, replacing laborious manual calculations. In the late 1970s, the first use was made of computed tomography (CT) data for radiotherapy planning. This required a magnetic tape reader connected to the planning system to read the CT scanner tapes.

As networking technology became available, it was possible to connect computers directly together. However, CT scanners still used different file formats. In 1985, the American College of Radiology and the National Electrical Manufacturers Association created a standard for medical images called ACR-NEMA. In the third version, in 1991, the standard was developed to specify how systems should communicate directly. To mark this change a new name for the standard was used: 'Digital Imaging and Communication in Medicine', or DICOM 3.0.

In the 1980s, the first record and verify systems appeared. Later, it became possible to transmit plans from the planning computer to the record and verify system, driven by the use of multileaf collimators in the 1990s. It was also in the 1990s that electronic portal imaging devices were developed. Accompanying them was a need to obtain reference images in electronic form, whether digital simulator images or digitally reconstructed radiographs.

At the turn of the millennium, radiotherapy centres were filled with computer systems transferring data. Managing these could be difficult and expectations frequently exceeded the realities of what could be achieved. These frustrations led to the recent development of radiotherapy, or oncology, information systems. These act as a central hub of the network: receiving and organizing data from various sources. This coordination of data is going to be vital for the era of image guided radiotherapy.

Benefits and hazards of computerization

The more advanced techniques that we practise would not be possible at all without the assistance of computers.

Intensity modulated radiotherapy would be totally unfeasible without computers or data communication. Even simple techniques are enhanced by the use of computers. If data are transferred directly between computers there is less chance of human error. The use of record and verify systems has certainly reduced the number of random human errors at the point of treatment delivery [4].

Ultimately, the hazards of computerization relate to our increased dependence on computer systems and the faulty assumption that they are reliable. Computers and networks do fail. A radiotherapy department that is reliant on a system can be crippled if that system is the victim of component failure, a virus, or even theft.

As systems become more complicated, they are harder to check for errors. It should never be assumed that the computer is correct. Furthermore, computers do not remove the risk of human error altogether. Proper use of a system relies on operators performing tasks correctly. If they do not then incorrect information can be passed down the line and used at a later stage. Where errors do occur in computerized systems they may affect a series of patients or a single patient for every fraction of their treatment [5].

In order to reduce these risks, we need to reverse the assumption that the computer is reliable. Key checks should be made, during system testing and for individual treatments. Is the isocentre correct? Is the patient reference position correct? Where there are multiple data sets, has the correct one been used for the treatment? When every plan had to be calculated and delivered manually, each person involved had to understand fully the technique and the treatment. Now that the treatment can be delivered at the touch of a button, that level of understanding is critical to detect errors.

NETWORKING

Networks are commonly described as having a number of layers. In one of the simpler descriptions, the TCP/IP model, four layers are described [6]. In order to understand these layers, we draw a comparison with the postal system (Table 12.1).

Because the network is layered in this way, any changes that occur in one layer do not affect the others, so you do not need to write a new application because you have bought a new modem.

Link layer: physical infrastructure

Two computers can be connected by a single cable. But what if four computers need to be connected? It is possible to connect them via a network loop so that a packet of data sent by A is visible to B, C and D, but will only be picked up by the computer it is intended for. The problem with this is

Table 12.1 The four network layers of the TCP/IP model

LAYER	NETWORK	POSTAL
Link	The infrastructure of cables, switches, modems and so on which allow information to be moved from one place to another	The infrastructure of vehicles and sorting offices which allow post to be moved around
Network	The addressing system which allows a single computer to be identified and for data to be routed to it	The addressing system which allows post to be directed to the correct destination
Transport	The process of packing the data and sending it into the network. Also the process of receiving data from the network	Taking letters to the post office to send and picking up received letters
Application	Defining the data to be sent and interpreting any data received	Writing and reading your post

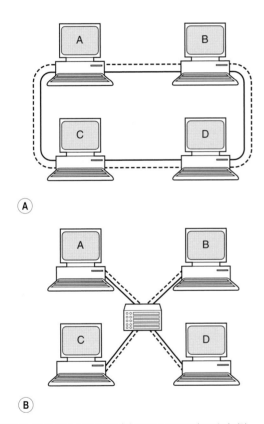

Figure 12.1 Network loop (A) versus network switch (B).

that it would be impossible for A and B to communicate at exactly the same time as C and D. The solution is to have each computer connected to a central network switch or hub. The switch only makes connections that are in use and prevents network traffic on one part of a network affecting another part (Figure 12.1).

In a very large network, such as a hospital, there will be a large number of such switches, controlling and routing the flow of data in the hospital. In such a large network, the computers may be organized into subnetworks, or subnets. Access between subnets is controlled by 'gateways' which can prevent unauthorized access between areas (Figure 12.2).

Network layer: addressing

When you type 'www.estro.be' into a web browser, how does your computer connect to the computer that contains the homepage of the European Society for Therapeutic Radiotherapy and Oncology? Each domain name is registered to a computer address called an IP address which consists of four numbers. Your computer initially sends a request to a directory to find out the correct IP address. Then it sends a request to that IP address to retrieve the correct web page.

Inside a private network, such as a hospital, computers are still referenced using an IP address. Special ranges of numbers are reserved for use in private networks to avoid confusion with Internet traffic. On many windows computers, it is possible to see the network configuration by typing the command 'ipconfig' at a command prompt[1]. If you do this, and your computer is attached to a network, you will see something like that shown in Figure 12.3.

This tells us that our computer is in the network domain hospital.nhs.uk. The first two numbers of the IP address are among those reserved for private networks. That tells us that this computer cannot be seen by the Internet. The second two numbers in the IP address will be unique for this computer within the hospital. The subnet mask describes the range of IP addresses that are in our local subnet; in this case the IP addresses 192.168.123.1 through to 192.168.123.255. The default gateway is the IP address of the computer or switch that our computer must go though in order to access the network outside the local subnet, such as the Internet.

---

[1]To get a command prompt: click on the start button, select 'run' and type cmd in the box and select OK.

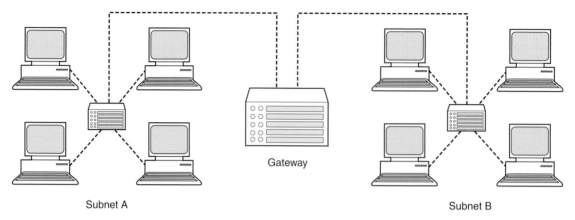

Figure 12.2 Two subnets separated by a gateway.

```
Windows IP Configuration
Ethernet adapter Local Area Connection:
  Connection-specific DNS suffix  . : hospital.nhs.uk
  IP Address . . . . . . . . . . : 192.168.123.45
  Subnet mask. . . . . . . . . . : 255.255.255.0
  Default Gateway  . . . . . . . : 192.168.123.1
```

Figure 12.3 Sample output of ipconfig.

```
Pinging 192.168.123.1 with 32 bytes of data:

Reply from 192.168.123.1: bytes=32 time<1ms TTL=255
Reply from 192.168.123.1: bytes=32 time<1ms TTL=255
Reply from 192.168.123.1: bytes=32 time<1ms TTL=255
Reply from 192.168.123.1: bytes=32 time<1ms TTL=255

Ping statistics for 192.168.123.1:
  Packets: sent = 4, Recieved = 4, Lost = 0 (0% loss)
Approximate round trip times in milli-seconds:
  Minimum = 0ms, Maximum = 0ms, Average = 0ms
```

Figure 12.4 Sample output from ping.

Transport layer: send and receive

The simplest form of data transport is the 'ping', which is used for the testing of data connections. If you still have a command prompt open on your computer type 'ping 192.168.123.1', replacing the IP address here with the IP address of your gateway (Figure 12.4).

Your computer has just packaged a data packet and sent it into the network addressed to the gateway. On receipt, the gateway sends a return package back to your computer. The ping command is often one of the first tools used when testing a network connection. A successful ping proves that both the link layer and the network layer are working correctly.

There are a lot of different potential connections that a computer can make. In the example above, how did the

gateway know that this single data packet came from a ping request and that it should send a return message? Also, how can a computer make multiple connections of different types without them getting confused? Each computer has a whole series of network 'ports'. When a computer receives a data packet addressed to port number 7, it knows that this is a ping request and responds accordingly, whereas requests for web pages are normally addressed to port 80. Imagine having a whole series of slots outside your house and the postman sorting them out for you into bills, junk mail and so on.

Application layer: the program

The final layer is the program itself, which is often the hardest part. Just because you can send a letter to anywhere in the world, it does not mean that they will be able to understand what you have written.

Network security

Because the modern radiotherapy department is so reliant on the network, it is important to protect it against various hazards. There is also a legal requirement to protect patient data and often a minimum security level which must be reached to connect to the hospital network. These are summarized in Figure 12.5.

Dicom

As described previously, dicom stands for 'Digital imaging and communication in medicine' and is produced by the National Electrical Manufacturers Association in the USA. Dicom is a constantly evolving standard with a number of working parties and regular releases [7].

Dicom is often mistakenly considered as a data file format. While there is a file format within dicom, it is primarily a data transfer protocol, a means to move medical

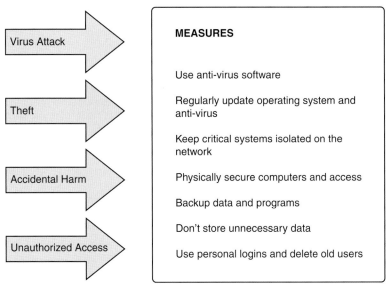

Figure 12.5 Potential impact of network hazards and measures to mitigate them.

images between systems. Dicom aims to be a complete specification for such transfer and specifies requirements over all the network layers.

The second common misconception about dicom is that two dicom compliant devices will communicate correctly. This mistake is the root cause of a great deal of anxiety. Given the huge variety of medical imaging equipment, dicom is not prescriptive. There is a great deal of variation possible within the standard. Where there is variation, dicom provides us with a common language to describe the functionality of a system and check whether two systems are compatible.

Dicom services

Dicom connections are not always about the transfer of images from one computer to another. A connection may be in order to print an image, send a worklist to a scanner, or find patient images. Each of these possibilities is called a *service class*. Furthermore, in any transaction there will be a *service class provider* (SCP), and a *service class user* (SCU). So, a server may offer the storage class as SCP and a number of systems may send images to it as SCU.

Dicom communication

To establish a dicom connection we need two critical pieces of information. First, we need to know the IP address of the computer we wish to connect to. Secondly, we need to know which network port the dicom program is monitoring. Port 104 is reserved for use by dicom programs and is normally the correct port. However, this is not always the case, a single computer may even run several dicom servers on different ports. With these two pieces of information, we

are able to establish communication with the dicom server, but this does not necessarily mean that the connection will be successful.

The security of dicom servers varies widely. Some will communicate with any system that has the correct address and port. This makes setting the system up easy but security will be poor. Others will make further checks. Each dicom program has a name, called an *application entity title* (AET). Most servers will refuse a connection to a system that does not call it by the correct name. Furthermore, many servers will check the AET of the requesting system against a list of known AETs.

Upon connection, the two systems perform what is known as a 'handshake'. They swap credentials. They determine whether the action that is being requested is supported and whether to continue with the action. Then information is exchanged and the association is closed.

Dicom data objects

One key problem in sending data between imaging systems is defining the exact meaning of the information sent. Dicom solves this through the use of a data dictionary. Each possible piece of information about the image, called a *data element*, is catalogued and given a code. The exact definition of the information for each code is contained in the standard.

Any *data object*, such as a radiotherapy plan or a CT image, will consist of a collection of data elements relevant to that object. The dicom standard details which data elements are mandatory for a given object and which are optional. Another new term, the service-object pair (SOP), is used to describe the application of a particular service class to a data object. We may talk about a general *SOP class*, such as CT image storage, or even a particular *SOP instance*, one specific stored CT image.

Figure 12.6 shows an example minimal CT object. Each row of the diagram shows the entry for each of the separate data elements. For each data element there is a two number code which relates that element to the dicom data dictionary. The data elements are grouped by the first number. In this example, group 0008 is the identity group and contains all the elements which help uniquely identify this object. Group 0010 is the patient demographics group, group 0018 the CT parameters group, and so on. The last of all of the data elements contains the actual image data itself.

One special class of data element, the *unique identifier* (UID), consists of a long numeric code. This code must be truly unique and may not be reused. In the sample below, there are three kinds of UID. The values for the SOP class UID are defined in the standard and each code describes the object. In this case, this is the code for a stored CT image. The SOP instance UID is the unique code for this object. No other dicom object in the world may have the same UID. In this way, a dicom server can tell if it is sent the same image twice and can disregard one of them. The study instance UID is the unique code for this study for this patient. All images in this study will contain the same study instance UID and a dicom server can use this correctly to group images together.

Dicom conformance

Whereas the CT object in the example above is a valid CT object according to the standard, it contains very little information and would probably be rejected by many dicom servers. This is the problem. By allowing manufacturers to choose which data elements are contained in the data object, the standard creates room for incompatibility. It becomes very important for manufacturers to describe exactly how their system behaves, which data elements are important and which are ignored.

The dicom standard specifies a common format for such descriptions, the *dicom conformance statement*. It should be possible to determine whether two systems will be able to communicate successfully by comparing their dicom conformance statements. In practice, these documents are quite long and an incompatibility might be difficult to spot.

RADIOTHERAPY DATA

Data storage

Data storage essentially comprises a number of switches, which are on or off. The smallest size of data storage is one switch, called a bit, which can store a one or a zero. More bits are used to store larger numbers. If eight bits

```
0008 0008  Image Type                      ORIGINAL\PRIMARY\AXIAL
0008 0016  SOP ClassVID                    1.2.840.10008.5.1.4.1.1.2
0008 0018  SOP Instance VID                1.2.345.6.789.8.76.5.4321.0.10
0008 0020  Study Date                      20021011
0008 0060  Modality                        CT
0008 0090  Referring Physician             DR
0008 1030  Study Description               SAMPLE CT SCAN

0010 0010  Patient Name                    Walter/Miller
0010 0020  Patient ID                      01234

0018 0050  Slice Thickness                 5
0018 0060  KVP                             130
0018 5100  Patient Posistion               HFS

0020 000d  Study Instance VID              1.2.345.6.789.8.76.4.4321.0
0020 0010  Study ID                        123
0020 0013  Image Number                    10
0200 0020  Patient Orientation             L\P
0020 0032  Image Position Patient          -200\-500\-40
0020 0037  Image Orientation               1\1\0\0\1\0

0028 0004  Photometric Interpretation      MONOCHROME2
0028 0010  Rows                            512
0028 0011  Columns                         512
0028 0030  Pixel Spacing                   0.9\0.9

7fe0 0010  Pixel Data                      _
```

Figure 12.6 A minimal stored CT dicom object.

are used then a number from 0 to 255 can be stored, called a byte. A kilobyte (kB) is equal to 1024 bytes. A megabyte (MB) is equal to 1024 kB, a gigabyte (GB) is equal to 1024 MB and a terabyte (TB) is equal to 1024 GB.

Image quality

There is a trade-off between the quality of the image and the space it takes up. For reference, a standard CT slice uses 512 kB. To illustrate this section, a test image is used which also requires approximately 512 kB, Figure 12.7A.

Dimensions and scale

Many images are two dimensional. We frequently also use three-dimensional data sets consisting of two-dimensional images. A CT series might comprise 50 slices at 5 mm spacing, requiring 25 MB. Time sequences can also be considered as a series of 2D frames. As the number of points increases in any dimension, so does the image size. In Figure 12.7B the image only requires 8 kB of storage, 64 times less. However much of the detail is lost at this resolution.

Bit depth

The bit depth describes the number of shades of grey between the maximum and minimum possible values. In medical imaging, most images are either 8 bit, with 256 levels of grey, or 16 bit, with 65 536 levels of gray. It is widely accepted that a person cannot discriminate between more than 256 shades of grey. However, a user may interrogate 16 bit images by changing the contrast window to examine different grey levels more clearly.

Compression

There are two kinds of compression. Lossless compression reduces the size of the data, generally to about half, without any alteration of the data, Figure 12.8A. Lossy compression has greater ability to reduce the size of the data but at the expense of some degradation of the data, Figure 12.8B. Lossy schemes can achieve much greater compression with almost undetectable reduction in image quality. However, they are often considered inappropriate for medical applications where any subtle change might affect patient treatment.

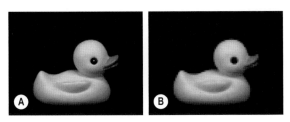

Figure 12.7 (A) Test image (B) at reduced resolution.

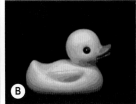

Figure 12.8 (A) 4 bit image showing significant degradation for only 50% space saving (B) Compressed image taking up just 2% of the original space, but differences are visible.

Colour

Colour images can be considered as separate grey-scale images for the red, green and blue components. These are combined to form a final image, Figure 12.9. Colour images are most often stored as 24 bit images. That is three frames of 8 bits each.

Radiotherapy data types

Given the huge range of definitions found between different manufacturers, it will be easiest to consider these in the context of the range of data objects defined within dicom. These fall into two groups: general image data types and those data types specific to radiotherapy, commonly referred to as dicom RT.

Tomographic images

In radiotherapy, CT images are used extensively with magnetic resonance imaging (MRI) and positron emission tomography (PET) becoming more widespread. All of these are well defined in dicom. However, at present, most radiotherapy systems will only accept images with a simple transverse imaging geometry. As the use of 3D images increases, it is anticipated that manufacturers will increase the range of acceptable imaging geometries.

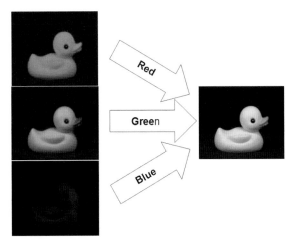

Figure 12.9 Three 8 bit images combine to form a 24 bit colour image.

Planar images

Ideally, all planar images in radiotherapy should be presented as true RT images, described below. However, many manufacturers have not implemented this and still use one of several dicom data objects appropriate for simple planar images.

Curves, annotations and overlays

There is scope in dicom to store and send any annotation that has been made on an image. Some manufacturers use these to attach additional information to an image, such as anatomical outlines. Any use of these which is more than just the simple display of annotation tends not to be transferable across manufacturers.

RT structure set

The RT structure set describes anatomical outlines that have been defined on tomographic data. It is used for the transfer of target volumes and organs at risk between planning systems. The structure set object specifically references the UID of each of the images on which it was defined. In this way, a system can check that it does not load a structure set onto the wrong set of images.

RT plan

The RT plan contains all the required information to deliver a radiotherapy treatment. It is possible for an RT plan to describe an external beam or a brachytherapy treatment. If the RT plan was created using target volumes from a CT dataset, it will reference the UID of the RT structure set from which it was defined.

RT dose

The RT dose object contains the result of the dose calculation. There may be a single dose object for each calculated slice or a full 3D calculation in a single object. Dose objects may also contain dose volume histograms.

RT image

The RT image data type is used for all radiotherapy planar images. There are several differences between an RT image and a standard planar image. RT images contain much more precise details about the imaging geometry and explicitly specify the type of RT image, digitally reconstructed radiograph (DRR), portal image or so on. RT images also allow the aspects of the RT plan which are relevant to that beam to be attached to the image, such as gantry angle, jaw positions and beam shaping.

RT treatment summary

The RT treatment summary is less widely used and is often overlooked. It contains a record of the treatment that was delivered.

Data burden

The build-up of patient data can represent a serious problem for the radiotherapy department. Without care, it is possible for a system, such as the planning system, to fill up completely, with a risk of system failure, loss of data and disruption to the service. The additional build-up of data is often an unforeseen side effect of service development. For example, a breast patient planned with virtual simulation may require fifty times the data storage of a patient planned with a conventional simulator and a digitized outline.

Measures can be taken to manage the radiotherapy data burden:

- avoid increases in patient data for which there is no clinical benefit, such as inappropriate dose grid size or unnecessary imaging
- good housekeeping. Delete any patient plans or images which are not used clinically
- consider whether data are being stored multiple times. Identical CT data may be being stored on the CT scanner, the virtual simulator, the planning system and on a central disk
- assess data requirements for any new technique and ensure facilities are in place
- monitor the rate of data build-up and the capacity of clinical systems. Investigate any unforeseen increase in data and any system regularly greater than 80% full
- plan future data requirements.

With fewer datasets being stored there is also a reduced risk of patient mistreatment as a result of an incorrect data set being used.

The example shown in Table 12.2 demonstrates the total data storage commitment for an example lung patient. In this example, the greatest storage commitment is for the dose distributions on the planning system. There are three reasons for this. Dose values are often stored as high precision numbers which require 32 bits. Secondly, they are often stored as 3D cubes, so there are a lot of data points to be stored. Thirdly, as in this example, a separate dose grid may be stored for each field to allow beam weighting to be altered without a full recalculation. Not all planning systems are the same in this regard.

Data security

Backup

It is critical that the data are not lost in the event of a failure of the system on which it is stored. In order to achieve this, the data need to be copied to a second location. There are many ways in which this can be achieved. In Figure 12.10A, the data are written by the computer to a hard disk. Overnight an automatic program copies the data to a digital tape. The scheme shown in

Table 12.2 Data for an example lung patient

ITEM	NO.	FORMAT	MEMORY
Planning CT	80	512×512×16bit	40 MB
CT outlines	1		5 kB
Treatment plan	1		5 kB
DRRs	3	512×512×16bit	1.5 MB
Dose distribution	3	200×200×200×32bit	91.5 MB
Simulator verification	3	1024×1024×8bit	3 MB
Portal verification	24	1024×1024×16bit	48 MB
		Total	184 MB

DRRs: digitally reconstructed radiographs

Archive

As patient data are acquired, computer systems may become full and old data need to be transferred to an archive to release storage capacity. Archive is very similar to backup and the two are often confused, but they fulfil very different roles. Backup is very short term in scope. Today's data are stored in case of a catastrophe tomorrow. Archival is long term in scope. Archived data will need to be kept for years. It is important that sufficient records are kept to enable the data to be located in the future. Furthermore, one must have the means to read the data. It is pointless storing patient data if it can only be read by a planning system that is no longer available.

If data are archived to a physical medium such as tape or CD, then the long-term life of the medium will need to be considered. As the archive grows the number of media being stored will grow and may take up a significant amount of space. Because disk storage is so cheap, it is feasible to create a hard disk archive, and simply purchase new disk storage when it fills up. Some systems are now being written with this in mind and have no archive facility. All of the data are available all of the time.

SOFTWARE DEVELOPMENT

Frequently, there comes a time when available products do not meet the immediate need and a centre must consider in-house developed software. Even the simplest spreadsheet can be considered as software and should be developed with care. One of the worst series of radiation therapy incidents, the Therac 25 incidents, had poor software design and testing as the root cause [8].

Detailed advice on the management and validation of software projects is available. One excellent example is 'General Principles of Software Validation; Final Guidance for Industry and FDA Staff', which is available online [9]. In particular, I recommend the section entitled 'Software is different from hardware' which details a series of reasons why care must be applied to software development.

A software development project can be considered as having five main areas of effort, which are shown in Figure 12.11. Frequently, the only area of effort which has allocated resources is the actual computer programming itself, with all other effort taking place on an ad-hoc basis. This approach is inefficient as the software will need constant reworking as the specification changes during the project. This approach is also unsafe as it often leads to software coming into use without proper documentation and with only superficial testing and training. In the more safe approach shown, only 20% of the effort is actually spent on computer programming.

In the specification and design work area, it is important clearly to describe the requirements for the project. This will include the functionality and any technical

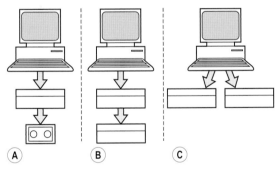

Figure 12.10 Backup schemes: (A) backup to tape, (B) backup to disk, (C) mirrored disks.

Figure 12.10B is similar except the data are copied overnight to a second hard disk drive. This has the advantage that the copies can be retrieved without any time delay. In Figure 12.10C, the data are written immediately to two separate independent disk drives. This scheme is known as drive mirroring.

It is important to ensure that backups performed by any method can actually be read. It is known for systems to be backed up every night but when they are actually required the tapes are useless. As the number of computer systems and the amount of data in a department grows, then backup can be a significant technical problem.

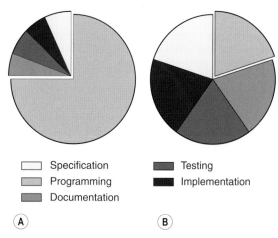

	Specification		Testing
	Programming		Implementation
	Documentation		

(A)   (B)

Figure 12.11 Division of effort in software development projects. (A) What is often perceived as required. (B) A much more realistic and safe approach.

requirements. Important decisions, such as the programming language to be used, should not be left solely to the programmer as this will affect the ability of a centre to support the software in the future. This phase should also include a risk assessment of the impact of software failure and consequently any safety requirements.

Documentation is vital to maintaining a safe software system. Not just user manuals but clear technical documentation and description of the operation of the computer code itself. It is not sufficient for all documentation to be written retrospectively as important details can be forgotten.

Testing can also be undertaken throughout software development and should be undertaken by both the programmer and a second party. The testing program should relate closely to the system specification and especially the risk assessment.

Finally, the implementation of the system needs to be planned with various 'what if' scenarios considered and all training, technical and user, undertaken in a timely manner. Ideally, the whole project will be managed by an individual or small team who will be able to sign off the project when all aspects are complete. Various software quality assurance systems exist [10,11] and should be considered for critical software projects, however, the principles outlined here can be applied to all software projects large or small.

CONCLUDING REMARKS

This simple introduction to the use of computers in radiotherapy will, regrettably, by the very nature of the subject be out of date almost instantly. It is important to obtain up-to-date guidance on specific aspects. One guide worthy of specific mention is IPEM report 93, 'Guidance for Commissioning and QA of a Networked Radiotherapy Department' [12]. The field of radiotherapy computing overlaps traditional work boundaries and there are frequently problems with IT professionals who do not fully understand the requirements of radiotherapy as much as radiotherapy professionals who do not fully understand the technicalities of IT. Out of this situation a new breed is rising, the radiotherapy IT specialist. Such people will be extremely important to ensure that we continue to reap the benefits of computerized radiotherapy.

REFERENCES

[1] Moore G. Cramming more components onto integrated circuits. Electronics Magazine 19 April 1965.

[2] Walter C. Kryder's law. Sci Am 2005;07–25.

[3] NHS Finance Manual. http://www.info.doh.gov.uk/doh/finman.nsf.

[4] Muller-Runkel R, Watkins S. Introducing a computerized record and verify system: its impact on the reduction of treatment errors. Med Dosim 1991;16:19–22.

[5] Patton G, et al. Facilitation of radiotherapeutic error by computerized record and verify systems. Int J Radiat Oncol Biol Phys 2003;56:50–7.

[6] Cerf V, Kahn R. A protocol for packet network intercommunication. IEEE Trans Commun 1974;COM-22:637–48.

[7] http://medical.nema.org.

[8] Leveson N. Safeware: system safety and computers. Addison-Wesley; 1995. Available at:

http://sunnyday.mit.edu/papers/therac.pdf.

[9] http://www.fda.gov/cdrh/comp/guidance/938.pdf.

[10] ISO/IEC 9126. Software product evaluation—Quality characteristics and guidelines for their use. ISO; 2001.

[11] http://www.tickit.org.

[12] Kirby M, et al. IPEM report 93: Guidance for Commissioning and QA of a Networked Radiotherapy Department. IPEM; 2006.

Chapter | **13** |

Quality control

John A. Mills

GENERAL

The process of measurement, testing or inspection devised to ensure that the function and the performance of a device is achieving a required level is referred to as *quality control* (QC). The requirement for routine quality control is recognized in the statutory Ionising Regulations (IRMER) [1]. The level required may be set out in Standards agreed by a national or international agency. For example IEC60601 [2], the general standard for medical devices was set by the International Electrotechnical Commission (IEC) which is part of the International Standards Organisation (ISO). IEC60601 was adopted by the European Union and thus became a Standard for the UK. Many parts of this standard concern the safety of radiotherapy treatment machines and simulators and one part particularly relates to the performance requirements and quality control of megavoltage treatment machines [3, 4]. Standards may also be set with respect to what is considered to be good practice or they may be set upon locally based experience. For example, radiotherapy physicists in the UK have identified good practice in many aspects of radiotherapy and published this in a document [5] referred to as

IPEM81. An example of a locally set tolerance may be that the field size on a megavoltage treatment machine can be made to lie within ±1.5 mm when another type of machine can achieve ±1 mm for the same amount of work.

Effective quality control needs to fulfill two roles. One is to demonstrate the correct performance of a system and the other is to detect deterioration of the system in order to take corrective action. Demonstration and detection are, in fact, two sides of the same coin. The boundary between each side is set in accordance with appropriate limits chosen with regard to the distribution of a measured parameter as shown in Figure 13.1 for the example of a 10 × 10 field.

Quality control immediately following a repair of equipment demonstrates that performance has been restored or detects problems with the repair.

In radiotherapy, quality control has become increasingly significant over the past 20 years. It has been recognized that, in order to achieve and maintain high standards of safe and effective dose delivery, there is a need for not only quality assurance systems which ensure safe, effective and traceable processes, but also for effective quality control checks to demonstrate and ensure satisfactory operation of equipment. In 1985, the ICRP [6] recognized the role that quality control played in the protection of the patient in radiotherapy. The hazards of radiation to normal tissue were well known and the risk of oncogenesis [7–9] further complicates the use of radiation in cancer treatment. These concerns were reinforced by accidents [10], some of which were due to safety failures, others due to performance failures and, of course, some due to human error. It has been clear that the absence or deficiencies of quality control had

an adverse affect in some of these accidents. Many accidents highlighted the need for standards to be established in both safety and performance.

The acceptable variation in dose delivery has been identified from clinical experience and radiobiological studies to be ±5% [11, 12]. This gives some perspective on the seriousness of, for example, the Exeter accident in 1988 [13] when a 25% overdose was delivered to many patients between February and July of that year. Systems of quality control checks endeavour to ensure that treatment equipment operates both safely and effectively.

A COMMITMENT TO QUALITY CONTROL

For quality control to be effective, there must be a commitment to examine aspects of a machine's operation. It is self-evident that provided an aspect does not show itself up in clinical practice and is never measured, it is never a problem. The saying 'leave well alone' comes to mind.

The Exeter overdose was apparent in skin reactions and raised concerns. However, that in itself did not prompt a measurement check, yet this was an overdose of 25%.

> ... it is seen that even a person whose treatment had started as early as mid February would not necessarily have shown any abnormal signs until about mid May [13].

An underdose may well go on for a much longer period of time and the incident at Stoke [14], when an underdose of approximately 20% continued for several years, serves as a demonstration of this.

At Exeter, there were clinical concerns by the end of May and the beginning of June 1988. On July 4, the calibration of February 12 was still thought to be correct by the Physics Department and it was not re-measured. No further measurement would have taken place until August. The IPEM dosimetry survey [15] measurement, which revealed the error, was done on July 12.

This indicates that it is essential that the staff group responsible for the equipment's performance must look, measure and check. Measurements can reveal problems much quicker than clinical outcome will reveal them. The difficult decision that needs to be made is what to look at, how to look at it, how often to look at it and how to judge what we find and what to do about it.

SAFETY, POSITION AND DOSE

There are two aspects to dose delivery. First, the physical amount of dose and, secondly, is it in the correct position. Both aspects are significant and, in addition to safety systems, are the key to satisfactory radiotherapy performance.

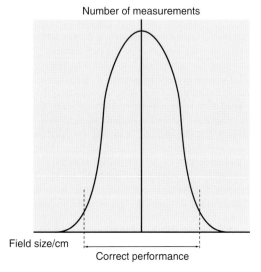

Figure 13.1 Illustration of limits chosen to encompass what is considered to be satisfactory performance within the distribution of measurements of a parameter. For example, one side of a field size dimension, such as the X jaw of a 10 × 10 field.

When we consider the many and various components within the radiotherapy process, these two aspects are identifiable as where uncertainty in the treatment delivery can occur. For example, the calibration of CT number for dose prediction is a dose aspect while the movement accuracy of the scanner and processing of the image matrix will be a positional aspect.

FREQUENCY, TOLERANCES AND FAILURE TRENDS

The classical assumption for performance deterioration is a linear change with time. Consider a tolerance of ±3% in dose delivered with action being taken at that level to restore the performance to the required value. Figure 13.2 illustrates such a change in performance with time.

Considering the effect of the length of the time period t:

t = 1 day

If t was one day then, depending upon when a patient was treated and assuming they attended at the same time each day, then their dose for the entire treatment will be different by between 0% and −3% over the full course of treatment.

t = 5 days

For all treatments of duration greater than or equal to 5 days, the variation from the required dose will be approximately −1.5%. For treatments of 4 days or less, the variation will be between 0% and −3% depending upon the day and the number of days treated. For example, a 3-day treatment on days 2, 3 and 4 will have a mean difference of −(0.6% + 1.2% +1.8%)/3 = −1.2%. However, an 8-day treatment on days 1 to 8 will have a mean difference of −1.575%

t = 20 days

For treatments of duration greater than or equal to 20 days, the variation from the required dose will be about −1.5%. For treatments of 19 days or less, the variation will be between 0% and −3% depending upon the day and the number of days treated.

Hence the length of t can have a variable effect on the dose delivered to the patient.

t = Total treatment time (T) or greater

If t is long, say several times as long as a total course treatment time, T, where typically that can be between 3 to 6 weeks, the following occurs compared to having t equal to T. The variation in the dose is shown in Figure 13.3.

This shows that the final batch of patients could be receiving a dose difference up to almost double that for a period of t which is about as long as a fractionation regimen. The deterioration may not be controllable. There is, therefore, a need to choose a tighter tolerance for this parameter.

Indeed, the performance deterioration is likely to be far from linear and more likely to be non-linear as in Figure 13.4.

This has significance for the interval between checks, although that needs to be balanced against resources. For example, frequent recording of parameters on a machine will perhaps pick up the deterioration in a parameter as it begins. However, in order to do this effectively without any automated recording and analysis system requires sufficient staff to run-up a machine, taking note of parameters

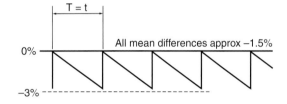

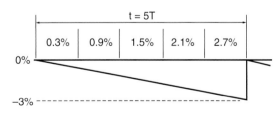

Figure 13.3 Change in performance represented by a linear change of a parameter over a time period when t=T, (upper) and t=5T, (lower).

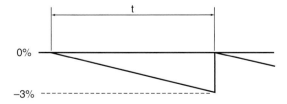

Figure 13.2 Change in performance represented by a linear change of a parameter over a time period t after which corrective action is taken to restore the performance.

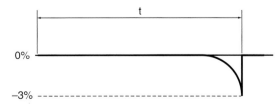

Figure 13.4 Change in performance represented by a non-linear change of a parameter over a time period t after which corrective action is taken to restore the performance.

213

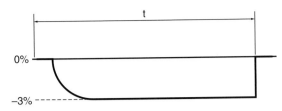

Figure 13.5 A worse case non-linear change of a parameter over a time period t after which corrective action is taken to restore the performance.

and using the machine in different modes and energies in order to vary many settings on the machine.

When a parameter is satisfactorily checked and it lies within tolerance it demonstrates compliance. If at the next check the parameter is found to be outside of tolerance then the assumption will be made that it has deteriorated linearly since the previous check. However, the worst case of deterioration will be as in Figure 13.5.

By identifying parameters with such a trend in deterioration, increased sampling or adaptive sampling can be justified.

MEASUREMENT AND UNCERTAINTY

When a measurement is made, the 'best estimate' of the parameter is determined and not its exact value.

The best estimate of a parameter is normally the mean of a number of measurements and the spread in the measurements gives an indication of the variation in the best estimate due to measurement conditions, measurement equipment, experimental set-up and other factors which contribute to the variation of the measurements upon which the best estimate is based.

Typically, the best estimate is thought of in terms of a Gaussian distribution with a mean, M and standard deviation, σ representing the best estimate and the variation respectively (Figure 13.6).

The question that follows is how certain can we be that the best estimate is close to the true value of the parameter? This can be quantified in terms of the distribution. For example, 95% of the area under the Gaussian distribution lies within plus and minus two standard deviations of the mean, $\pm 2\sigma$. Hence, there is a 5% uncertainty that the true value does not lie within $\pm 2\sigma$ of the best estimate, M.

NULL HYPOTHESIS

This is an essential aspect of all statistical analysis. The null hypothesis (H_0) is the hypothesis that the measurement M is not different from the reference value R. Consider a measurement with a best estimate mean M and standard

deviation σ_M. If the null hypothesis applies with 95% confidence then R lies within the boundaries of M $\pm 2\sigma_M$.

Put another way, the null hypothesis asks: is the best estimate M which has been measured *really different* from a reference value R? If the reference value lies within $\pm 2\sigma$ of the best estimate then this is unlikely because we are 95% confident that the real value lies within this region. The answer to the question is therefore no, they are not different and the null hypothesis applies.

Hence, we start off on the basis that within the variation of our measurement the best estimate is not any different from the required reference value, R unless R lies outside the $\pm 2\sigma$ region of the best estimate (Figure 13.7).

It is on the basis of the null hypothesis, the best estimate, M and the uncertainty, σ_M in the best estimate that a decision can be reached as to whether a parameter is in tolerance or not.

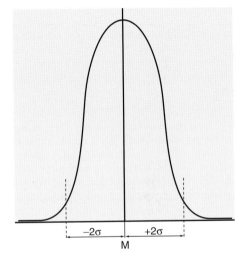

Figure 13.6 Best estimate of a parameter indicated by the mean M and standard deviation σ.

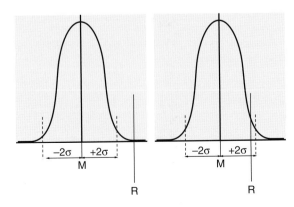

Figure 13.7 A mean of a measurement M with respect to a reference value, R.

The $\pm 2\sigma$ region also indicates what a significant tolerance level would be. On the basis that 95% of measurements will lie within this region, a tolerance equal to $\pm 2\sigma$ provides a realistic limit outside of which the performance should be evaluated.

COMBINING VARIANCES AND TOLERANCES

The variation in a parameter due to several factors is a compound of the individual variation of each factor. The generalized method to determine an overall variance is to combine all the variances as follows. Since the variance equals the square of the standard deviation:

$$\text{Total variance} = (\sigma_{Total})^2 = (\sigma_1)^2 + (\sigma_2)^2 + \ldots + (\sigma_n)^2$$

13.1

This is known as combining the variations in quadrature.

This can be applied not only to measurements but also to the tolerances. It assumes that the variations in each factor occur at random.

As an example, let the measurement technique have a standard deviation of $\pm 0.5\%$ and the intrinsic standard deviation of the machine's performance for the measured parameter also be $\pm 0.5\%$. These values can be combined as in equation 1 to give

$$(\sigma_{Total})^2 = (0.5)^2 + (0.5)^2 = 2 \times 0.25 = 0.5 \quad \textbf{13.2}$$

This results in $\sigma_{Total} = \pm 0.707\%$ and this gives 2σ to be approximately $\pm 1.4\%$.

SETTING A TOLERANCE TO ACCOUNT FOR THE STANDARD DEVIATION IN A MEASUREMENT

Consider that we have a reference value R for a parameter which we do not want to have vary by more than $\pm 3\%$. Then the lowest value which R should have will be $0.97 \times R$ and the greatest will be $1.03 \times R$. Let a measurement be made and the mean is $M = 0.97 \times R$. Since there will be a standard deviation σ associated with this measurement, the 95% boundaries of $\pm 2\sigma$ will lie either side of $0.97 \times R$. This indicates that there is as much chance of the parameter lying below $0.97 \times R$ as above $0.97 \times R$. We are only 50% confident that the parameter has not gone below $0.97 \times R$.

If we want to have a greater confidence from the measurement M that the parameter has not dropped below $0.97 \times R$, then a greater amount of the distribution associated with M and σ needs to lie above $0.97 \times R$.

For example, since 95% of the distribution associated with a mean M lies between $\pm 2\sigma$ of the mean, then 2.5% of the distribution lies below $M - 2\sigma$ and 2.5% lies

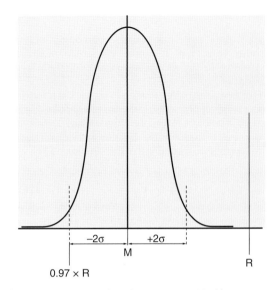

Figure 13.8 A mean value of measurement M with respect to a 3% difference from a reference value, R.

above $M + 2\sigma$. Hence, if $0.97 \times R$ were equal to $M - 2\sigma$, 97.5% of the distribution would lie above $0.97 \times R$ (Figure 13.8). Therefore, we could be 97.5% confident that the parameter was greater than $0.97 \times R$.

This indicates that, in order to ensure with 97.5% confidence from measurement that a minimum variation of $0.97 \times R$ is not exceeded, a limit measurement M_L, where $(M_L - 2\sigma) = 0.97 \times R$ would be required. This limit, M_L is the tolerance that would be used for monitoring the parameter, where $M_L = 0.97 \times R + 2\sigma$. The same analysis can be applied to the upper value, $1.03 \times R$ which the parameter should not exceed. This results in an upper tolerance value of $M_U = 1.03 \times R - 2\sigma$.

In essence, to take into account the uncertainty in a measurement, represented by σ, the tolerance limits need to be tighter than the variation which is to be allowed in a parameter.

Continuing with the example above, where the measurement technique had a standard deviation of $\pm 0.5\%$ and the intrinsic standard deviation of the machine for the measured parameter was also $\pm 0.5\%$. The combination results in 2σ being 1.4%. This means that to ensure with 97.5% confidence that the variation in the parameter does not exceed $\pm 3\%$ from its reference value R, a tolerance of $\pm 1.6\%$ is required.

COMBINED TOLERANCES

A very relevant aspect of combined differences relates to setting tolerances for the individual parameter which contributes to an overall effect. This can be illustrated with the factors used to determine the dose delivered:

$$D = M.O.W.T.S.C \qquad \boxed{13.3}$$

where D is the dose, M the number of monitor units and the other terms, O, W, T, S and C represent output, wedge, tray, source to surface and machine calibration factors respectively.

If we assume that the variation in the factors is independent, it is appropriate to apply the same method of combining the tolerances as was applied for standard deviations in equation 13.1. Therefore, the variation in the dose D can be written as follows, assuming that the variation on M is zero:

$$(\sigma_D)^2 = (\sigma_O)^2 + (\sigma_W)^2 + (\sigma_T)^2 + (\sigma_S)^2 + (\sigma_C)^2 \qquad \boxed{13.4}$$

If we choose D to be within $\pm 2\%$, then the tolerance on C needs to be less than $\pm 2\%$ if all the other factors are not required to have zero tolerance, which of course is impossible. If we allow D to lie within $\pm 3\%$, take the tolerance on C to be $\pm 1\%$ and let all the other tolerances be equal then a value for the tolerance on each of the other factors would be $\pm 1.4\%$. If they are all equal then the tolerance on all factors are $\pm 1.3\%$.

MAINTENANCE AND CATASTROPHES

It is important to bear in mind that not all aspects of equipment performance can be maintained. Catastrophes are inevitable and these are usually exhibited by component failure. They can also occur due to human error. Although some devices and components can be replaced, or action taken to monitor performance and replace components before failure, not everything can be maintained. Provision needs to be made as best as possible for catastrophes. Such provision is to enable routine treatment provision to be maintained while equipment repair is completed.

SHORT-TERM, LONG-TERM AND IMMEDIATE MONITORING

Constantly monitoring a parameter demonstrates performance up until the point at which it is considered that unacceptable performance has been detected. Hence, the data collected through QC measurements can be used not simply in a pass or fail fashion but to examine trends in performance and, if possible, use these as predictors for maintaining the performance of equipment.

One routinely used but simple trend technique is when a double tolerance level is set to monitor a parameter. Let these levels be $\pm a\%$ and $\pm b\%$ where b>a. Results outside $\pm b\%$ are considered to require immediate attention while results outside $\pm a\%$ and also within $\pm b\%$ must occur on a number of subsequent occasions in order for action to be taken.

There are three major categories of quality control. Each involves drawing conclusions from measurement data obtained from different methods of monitoring: immediate monitoring, short-term and long-term monitoring. For treatment machines, each method provides different but appropriate means by which to evaluate and maintain performance as follows.

Immediate monitoring. In this category, the immediate effect on the performance of the machine is determined from the response to changing a control parameter. Using this approach, the optimum tuning of a circuit or system can be determined. The monitoring of the machine can involve both external and internal output signals. Internal parameters which alter as a consequence of the changed parameter can provide system response information and externally monitored characteristics of the beam, such as beam symmetry and energy, can also provide response information.

Long-term monitoring. Many parameters on a machine alter slowly as components age or their performance deteriorates. In order to correct and compensate for the deterioration, including replacement of a component, long-term data trends provide an indication as to when action is required. For example, this may be used to indicate the need to adjust a parameter which requires adjustment continuously over time in order to maintain the performance within an adequate value. Or it might indicate when the end of life of the device can be expected in order to schedule replacement and avoid treatment delays and interruption due to machine breakdown or lack of component availability. The data might again come from internal parameters of the machine or from measurements made independent of the machine. Inevitably, data are difficult to record, log and process. In particular, for measurements on the radiation beam, the results cannot be gathered in an entirely automatic manner and any system which can assist with the recording and processing of these data is invaluable.

Short-term monitoring. In contrast to immediate and long term, short term endeavours to determine the performance of the machine during a treatment day. Only internal parameters of the machine are recorded during the day for subsequent processing. By analysis of such recorded data, it is possible to identify deteriorating overall performance of the machine and schedule periods for attending to the machine. Although only internal parameters are monitored, it can be useful to compare the processed results with appropriate daily measurements of external beam characteristics.

THE RADIOTHERAPY PROCESS

Quality control has a role throughout the entire radiotherapy process due to the significant technology that each aspect relies upon. The purpose of quality control in each aspect can be identified in terms of dose, position or safety and it contributes to ensuring effective overall treatment delivery.

Overview

The radiotherapy process can be considered to consist of three major aspects. *Acquisition* is the first major aspect, when information is gathered about the target for the radiotherapy and the regions which surround the target. *Analysis* of this information permits determination of the most appropriate way to deliver the treatment. *Delivery* of the treatment is the third and final aspect. Hence, we can identify three distinct aspects of the process: acquisition, analysis and delivery.

It can be seen that one piece of radiotherapy equipment can be involved in different aspects. For example, the simulator can contribute first to acquiring information about the patient and then can be used to verify the treatment delivery as part of the analysis prior to treatment delivery.

Acquisition

Patient information that is not determined from clinical examination and physiological and biochemical testing is almost entirely obtained through imaging. The focus of the information is the computed tomography (CT) scan which forms the basis for dose prediction. This is supplemented with magnetic resonance imaging (MRI) and positron emission tomography (PET) imaging, the use of which relies upon accurate image registration in order to ensure in turn accurate target localization.

The radiotherapy simulator still continues to contribute significantly to gathering data about the patient in many clinical situations. However, the manipulation of large CT data sets with virtual simulation has proved to be increasingly useful. In brachytherapy, localization of the radioactive sources or the applicators is readily obtained radiographically with a simulator or with a C-arm radiographic device and it is also done with CT imaging supplemented by MRI.

Analysis

Treatment simulation is now accomplished predominantly with virtual simulation using a CT data set. With a simulator, the analysis is often performed during the acquisition of the data. However, with virtual simulation, more extensive analysis can be undertaken without clinical pressure. Dose prediction remains a significant part of the analysis in order to determine an adequate dose distribution in the target while sparing critical tissue. The simulator can again be used to validate a treatment delivery and confirm the localization of the tumour, based upon the intended treatment delivery.

Delivery

The final stage is the treatment delivery based upon the data acquisition and the data analysis. The uncertainty in both these preliminary aspects will have an impact upon the overall uncertainty in the final treatment delivery.

The majority of radiotherapy treatment delivery takes place with teletherapy machines, such as linear accelerators, orthovoltage and cobalt machines, However, low dose rate (LDR), high dose rate (HDR) and manual brachytherapy insertions must be considered along with the administration of radioactive substances.

THE RADIOTHERAPY TECHNOLOGY

The previous section demonstrates the need for quality control across the radiotherapy process. The purpose and extent of the quality control for each technological device utilized throughout these aspects can now be considered in context.

CT scanner

The quality control for the CT scanner relates to ensuring the alignment of the patient with respect to the scanner is appropriate and accurate and also that any patient density information is appropriate for dosimetry calculations. Table 13.1 lists areas of consideration which are typical but not comprehensive.

MRI, PET and image registration with CT

The CT image data set forms the basis for dose prediction and the MRI and PET images aid target volume localization. Hence, the MRI and PET registration with the CT image data needs quality control checks which will ensure that the geometric alignment between these images and the CT images is accurate and that volume sizes and dimensions are not transferred incorrectly from one to the other.

Radiotherapy simulator

There are two aspects to simulator quality control. One aspect concerns the image quality, including contrast and resolution, as well as the dose delivered to the patient from

Table 13.1 Six aspects of a CT scanner that require quality control

1	Patient alignment lasers
2	Couch movement
3	Slice thickness
4	Image size
5	Image geometry
6	Hounsfield numbers for range of materials

fluoroscopy. The other aspect is very close to the checks required to ensure the satisfactory performance of a treatment machine from a mechanical, optical and radiation alignment perspective. Since the simulator can form the basis for treatment or verification, ideally, its performance should be better than the treatment machine which it is simulating.

Virtual simulator

The basis for performance of the virtual simulator lies with the performance of the CT scanner. However, quality control checks can be used to ensure that the manipulation of the CT data sets does not introduce any geometrical distortions which could compromise the perception of the alignment of the machine to the patient. While it can be argued that once software is initially verified there will be no change in its performance, there is a need for adequate quality control checks to be done after any software upgrades. Also, since the data set originates from the CT scanner, periodic checks may well identify problems which are due to some changes in the scanner or in the process of handling the data.

C-arm radiographic imaging system

C-arm radiographic devices often provide the imaging facilities essential for dose prediction in brachytherapy treatment as well as source position verification. For dose prediction, the geometric accuracy of the system needs to be subject to quality control. To ensure safe levels of radiation exposure and satisfactory imaging performance, quality control is also required.

Isocentric linear accelerators and cobalt machines

Besides ensuring the satisfactory operation of safety interlocks, there are many aspects concerning the performance of these machines that require routine quality control. These aspects concern mechanical and optical alignment as well as the performance of the radiation beam in terms of its alignment to the optics and mechanics of the machine and the relative dose distribution within the beam, normally referred to as symmetry and uniformity. Both the mechanical and radiation performance are prerequisites for the correct delivery of absolute dose and the final quality control checks are to ensure that an accurate dose is delivered. With linear accelerators, there may well be multiple energies for both photon and electron modes. Quality control needs to be performed for all energies and radiation modes. Table 13.2 lists checks that are typical but not comprehensive.

Orthovoltage teletherapy machines

Orthovoltage treatment machines require mechanical, radiation field and dosimetry checks in a similar fashion

Table 13.2 Twelve aspects of linear accelerators that require quality control

1	isocentre determined by the radiation beam
2	isocentre indicators, e.g. distance meter
3	Light field size, symmetry and x-wires
4	Patient alignment lasers
5	Radiation beam symmetry with gantry angle
6	Radiation field size
7	Radiation field alignment to optical field
8	Couch isocentric and vertical movement
9	Beam energy
10	Dose variation with gantry angle
11	Dose linearity and reproducibility
12	Absolute dose

Table 13.3 Seven aspects of orthovoltage machines that require quality control

1	Focal spot to applicator alignment
2	Applicator dimensions and orthogonality
3	Large field uniformity
4	Beam energy
5	Dose variation with tube angle
6	Dose linearity and reproducibility
7	Absolute dose

to the megavoltage machines. One fundamental aspect is the alignment of the focal spot to the mechanical assembly of the applicators and tube attachment. Once this is accurately established then accurate mechanical alignment of the applicators will ensure adequate performance. Table 13.3 lists checks that are typical but not comprehensive.

Afterloading brachytherapy machines

High, medium and low dose-rate machines all require quality control checks for safety and performance. With this equipment, the mechanical aspects concern the positional accuracy of the radiation source and then ensuring that the dummy source indicators, which are used for

Table 13.4 Five aspects of brachytherapy machines that require quality control

1	Source position autoradiograph
2	Dummy source agreement with autoradiograph
3	Timer
4	Air kerma rate measurement
5	Absorbed dose of simulated treatment

planning radiographs, accurately reflect the source positions. Finally, of course, measurement of the absolute dose checks source activity, timer and positional accuracy. Table 13.4 lists checks that are typical but not comprehensive.

Patient positioning

Besides patient laser alignment systems, there are active systems which often use stereotactic cameras to monitor the position of the patient. For these systems, quality control is required to ensure that detected displacements are accurate and also that the relationship of the displacements to the isocentre are accurate if the system is calibrated to that point.

Treatment verification

Treatment verification systems have become routinely used to monitor treatment machine settings prior to treatment and to record the machine settings when the radiation exposure was delivered to the patient. Some amount of quality control is required to make sure that both aspects of the system are taking place correctly. In particular, the machine operators now rely on the automatic detection of inappropriate settings before irradiation, especially with conformal and intensity modulated techniques which make this unavoidable. The high complexity of treatment delivery now also requires an automated record of the treatment to be acquired.

Computer systems and networking

Computer systems and networks have become an established and essential part of radiotherapy treatment. Such systems handle critical data across the entire radiotherapy process. Quality control of the computer systems and networks aims to ensure that data are transferred between the various stages of the process accurately. It can also serve to identify the limitations within the system and to monitor these. For example, resolution changes which may occur within image sets as they are processed after acquisition. The integrity of the treatment requires that the data intended for treatment can be stored, accessed and transferred correctly.

Measurement equipment

One of the most important requirements for quality control is the use of the correct measurement equipment. It is essential to ensure the accurate operation of the measurement devices that are used to undertake the quality control measurements. From a ruler and spirit level used in mechanical checks to film densitometers used for radiation field size measurements and calibrated ionization chambers and electrometers used for absolute dose measurements, all equipment requires quality control.

GETTING THINGS IN BALANCE

There are three aspects which need to be balanced when dealing with a problem:

- clinical effect of performance
- resource of manpower and equipment required to correct
- component availability for repair or correction.

All problems can be considered as a balance between the three and this can assist in determining how to deal with a problem (Figure 13.9). The clinical effect really relates to the performance of the machine and making a judgment about how significant treating the patient with the performance compromised to a known extent will be. The resource required is the man-hours required and the skill and expertise available and required to restore the machine's performance. The component availability relates to whether a component is affordable, whether it is available in stores, or was it too expensive to keep on the shelf at the hospital and therefore needs to be ordered.

The balance can be illustrated by considering two extremes: high clinical impact and minimal component cost and very high component cost but insignificant clinical impact (Figure 13.10).

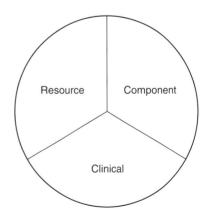

Figure 13.9 The three aspects to be considered in equipment problems and restoring performance.

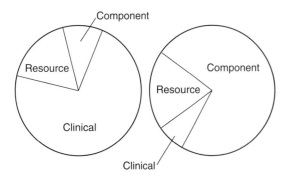

Figure 13.10 Illustration of the split between the three aspects to be considered in equipment problems and restoring performance for two extreme situations.

On the one hand, if the clinical significance is small and the resource and/or part availability is large, then the work can be scheduled for planned maintenance (PPM). However, on the other hand, if the clinical significance is great, then an immediate repair will be appropriate.

There is no easy answer to the numerous situations between the two extremes. This has to rely on the skill, knowledge and insight of the scientists and technicians involved in the work.

Quality control coupled with planned maintenance forms an essential component in ensuring that safe and effective radiotherapy is achieved.

QUALITY CONTROL CHECKS AND SCHEDULING FOR MEGAVOLTAGE MACHINES

The scheduling of routine quality control should be chosen to suit the local circumstances. For many types of equipment, this can be accommodated within normal working hours. However, in the case of treatment machines, this may not be possible due to the lack of treatment capacity and patient demand. Suitable guidance as to the frequency of checks and the types of tests can be found in both IEC60601:9076 [6] and IPEM81 [5]. Both documents provide guidance for checks to be conducted on a monthly to 12-monthly frequency. The IEC document does not specify weekly checks. An estimate of the total time for the checks suggested is approximately the same based upon experience of nominal times. This amounts to between 117 and 128 hours per year which compares favorably with 1 to 2 hours per week and one half day per month which requires 120 hours. If this time is taken from the normal working day then it amounts to only about 5% of the total normal time.

With an increasing number of treatment machines in a single centre, the time and resource for QC increases and scheduling techniques are required to accommodate it.

CONCLUSION

Quality control and planned maintenance are a requirement of IRMER [1]. They are both often seen as an unnecessary intrusion into the routine treatment of patients. It can become very frustrating for treatment personnel when the performance of a treatment machine needs to be checked and confirmed following the repair after a breakdown. It is, however, apparent from previous incidents that measurement of a physical parameter could have averted incorrect treatment over a lengthy period before clinical indicators indicated a problem.

It is important to be able to put the checks on performance into context. This can be done in relation to the treatment planning and dose prediction undertaken for the treatment of a patient. For example, considerable effort is used on occasions to achieve a dose distribution satisfying the ICRU 50 [16] criteria of −5% to +7% across the target. The performance of the machine can compromise this due to several factors. A non-uniform beam due to energy change or tilted beam due to poor steering could change this by ±6%. The variation in the factors used for calculation of the monitor units in combination with the dose calibration of the machine could also change this by up to ±6%. Geometric misalignment between the radiation beam and the beam indicators can result in dose differences, particularly in regions of high dose gradient such as wedged or modulated fields. It is worth bearing in mind that, typically, within 5 mm of a radiation field's geometrical edge, a dose variation of up to ±10% can result from the order of a 1 mm discrepancy.

A random combination of these many factors throughout the treatment cannot be guaranteed and the performance variation that might result without adequate quality control and planned maintenance could well negate or even swamp the variation expected from the planned dose prediction.

A comprehensive system of quality control for all the equipment used in radiotherapy will ensure that accurate and reproducible treatment is being delivered.

REFERENCES

[1] Statutory Instrument 2000 No. 1059. The Ionising Radiation (Medical Exposures) Regulations. 2000.

[2] British Standards Institute. BSEN 6061-1-1:2002. Medical electrical equipment. General requirements for safety. Collateral standard. Safety requirements for medical electrical systems.

[3] British Standards Institute. BSEN 60976:2001. Medical electrical

equipment – Medical electron accelerators – Functional performance characteristics.

[4] British Standards Institute. BS 5724-3.1: Supplement 1: 1990: Medical electrical equipment – Part 3: Particular requirements for performance – Section 3.1 Methods of declaring functional performance characteristics of medical electron accelerators in the range 1 MeV to 50 MeV – Supplement 1. Guide to functional performance values.

[5] Institute of Physics and Engineering in Medicine. IPEM Report 81. Physics Aspects of Quality Control in Radiotherapy.

[6] ICRP Publication 44. Protection of the patient in radiation therapy. Pergamon Press.

[7] Travis LB, et al. Cumulative absolute breast cancer risk for young women treated for Hodgkin lymphoma. J Natl Cancer Inst 2005;97:1394–5.

[8] Lorigan P, Radford J, Howell A, Thatcher N. Lung cancer after treatment for Hodgkin's lymphoma: a systematic review. Lancet Oncol 2005;6:773–9.

[9] Amemiya K, Shibuya H, Yoshimura R, Okada N. The risk of radiation-induced cancer in patients with squamous cell carcinoma of the head and neck and its results of treatment. Br J Radiol 2005;78:1028–33.

[10] IAEA Safety Report Series No 17 Lessons learned from accidental exposures in radiotherapy. 2000.

[11] Dutreix A. When and how can we improve precision in radiotherapy? Radiother Oncol 1984;2:275–92.

[12] Herring DF, Compton DMJ. The degree of precision required in the radiation dose delivered in cancer radiotherapy. Br J Radiol 1971; (Suppl. 5):51–8.

[13] The Exeter District Health Authority. The Report of the Committee of Enquiry into the overdoses administered in the Department of Radiotherapy in the period February to July 1988. 28 November, 1988.

[14] West Midlands Health Authority. Second Report of the Independent Enquiry into the conduct of isocentric radiotherapy at the North Staffordshire Royal Infirmary, 1994.

[15] Thwaites DI, et al. A dosimetric intercomparison of megavoltage photon beams in UK radiotherapy centres. Phys Med Biol 1992;37:445–661.

[16] ICRU Report 50 Prescribing, recording, and reporting photon beam therapy. International Commission on Radiation Units and Measurements. 1993.

Chapter | 14 |

Quality management in radiotherapy

Jill Emmerson, Julie Clark, Caroline Mansell

INTRODUCTION – WHAT IS QUALITY?

There are many different, well-documented theories and approaches to quality and quality management [1]. Approaches to quality have seen a shifting emphasis and have evolved through the following stages:

1. inspection and remedial action
2. identifying improvements and taking steps to prevent mistakes occurring
3. doing things differently, i.e. modernization.

This is reflected in the history of quality in radiotherapy [2], such that the interpretation of quality has widened and can now be applied to every aspect of the service, incorporating many local, professional and national standards. It is not possible to cover every aspect of quality in detail in a single chapter. This chapter aims to provide an overview of quality and quality management and their significance to radiotherapy, outline the requirements of the international quality standard BS EN ISO 9001, signpost readers to further information on a number of quality initiatives and promote an integrated approach to quality management in UK Oncology Centres.

There are many different definitions and perceptions of quality and several terms associated with quality that are important to describe from the outset. Quality may be defined as fitness for purpose or conformance to requirements, but it is more than this.

Quality is the totality of features and characteristics of a product or service that bear on its ability to satisfy stated or implied needs [3].

In other words, it is the degree to which a product or service satisfies the requirements of the user. Some definitions do not take costs into account. However, quality is about meeting customer requirements, stated or implied, while also keeping costs to a minimum.

Another often used term is quality control (QC): 'the part of quality management focused on fulfilling quality requirements, [4].

In radiotherapy, quality control does not only apply to controlling the performance of the equipment, but also to controlling the performance of radiotherapy processes.

Quality assurance (QA) refers to 'the part of quality management focused on providing confidence that quality requirements will be fulfilled' [4] or: 'a systematic process of verifying that a product or service is meeting specified requirements' [5].

Quality assurance incorporates risk assessment, determining what might go wrong, or what is critical to get right, then planning the process and putting procedures in place to ensure that a reliable service is provided. Aspects to be included should be operational, including legislative and educational requirements; physical and technical checks to verify correct functioning of equipment; and clinical aspects, including patient care and management. This can be achieved through activities such as documentation, training and ongoing review of existing processes.

Quality management (QM) is 'the coordinated activities to direct and control an organization with regard to quality' [4]. The underpinning philosophy, to get the process and the service right first time, applies to all parts of the organization, involving managing all functions and activities to achieve quality.

A quality system (QS) is the organizational structure, responsibilities, procedures, processes and resources which must be in place to implement quality management.

A quality management system (QMS) is a management system to direct and control an organization with regard to quality [4].

There are a number of documented approaches to quality, including total quality management (TQM), continuous quality improvement (CQI) and business process re-engineering. From these different approaches, it is possible to identify a number of recurring key themes:

- management commitment
- staff involvement
- identification of clear requirements or standards
- identification of clear processes, broken down into identifiable steps

- a focus on the prevention of problems
- recognition that quality is a continual process.

The steps to achieving any quality initiative must include the following stages:

- analysis of current service
- identification of recommendations for change
- implementation of change
- evaluation of the impact of change.

The main aim of quality in radiotherapy is safe and effective treatment. In addition to ensuring that all treatments are optimized, a quality system should ensure that all possible measures are taken to prevent inappropriate exposures from occurring [6].

HISTORY OF QUALITY IN RADIOTHERAPY

There are a number of well-documented radiotherapy incidents [7–12], which have occurred both in the UK and internationally (Table 14.1). These have led to hundreds of patients receiving incorrect doses of radiation which, in turn, may have led to the possibility of the treatment intent being compromised or causing unnecessary and distressing acute and late side effects of treatment. Subsequent outcomes in the UK have included key reports which have contributed to the development of quality management systems in radiotherapy.

It is notable that, throughout numerous reported incidents, a number of recurring themes can be identified as contributing factors. These include:

- lack of communication, especially at staff group interfaces
- training, competency and supervision issues
- lack of up-to-date procedures, protocols and documentation
- no independent check/calibration
- inadequate identification of clear responsibilities.

It is of the utmost importance that the radiotherapy community shares information and learns from past mistakes [6,20]. Departments should also search for, correct, monitor and learn from their own incidents. Departments open themselves up to risk if there are workload or time pressures or if there is an insufficiency in:

- attention to detail, alertness or awareness
- procedures or checks
- resources, e.g. qualified and well-trained staff
- coordination, communication and clear responsibilities [6].

All of these factors are encompassed by ISO 9001 and should be incorporated into a department's quality management system. They are areas that should be kept under regular review with a view to continual improvement.

Table 14.1 Chronology of quality development in radiotherapy in the UK

YEAR	EVENT	REFERENCE
1988	Exeter. Overdose, 207 patients affected	
1988	Thwaites Report: detailed root cause of Exeter incident.	[13]
	DoH working party, chaired by Professor Bleehen, to investigate the application of quality assurance to radiotherapy to reduce the probability of incidents occurring in other centres.	
1982–1991	Stoke. Underdose, 1045 patients affected	
1991	Bleehen Report: Quality assurance in radiotherapy (QART). Took the form of a quality standard and provided a formal system for managing quality in radiotherapy. It was based on the Quality Standard BS 5750, Part 2, 1987 (the predecessor of ISO 9001), a quality standard which was generic to a range of industries and services and thus, open to a degree of interpretation and translation. DoH funded two pilot sites, Bristol and Manchester: • To implement a quality system to see if it was feasible. • To prepare manuals that would serve as examples to other radiotherapy departments	[14]
1994	Stoke: report from investigation.	[15]
1994	Sample documents from two pilot sites published and DoH recommendation for all departments to develop their own quality management system (QMS)	[16]
1994	BS EN ISO 9001:1994 replaced BS5750	
2000	BS EN ISO 9001:2000 replaced BS EN ISO 9001:1994	[17]
2006	Incident at Beatson Oncology Centre	[18]
2006	Report into overexposure at Beatson	[19]
2008	Redacted Independent review of the circumstances surrounding a serious adverse incident	[12]

QUALITY MANAGEMENT SYSTEMS

A quality management system (QMS) is a set of interrelated or interacting processes which provide a framework for an organization to manage its activities in order to achieve its quality policy and quality objectives. Management system standards, such as ISO 9000 (see below), provide a model to follow in setting up and operating a quality management system. The ISO 9001 requirements are based on eight quality management principles (QMP), the key elements of which are illustrated in Figure 14.1.

QMP 1 Customer focus

A service should understand and strive to meet the needs and expectations of its customers. In radiotherapy, this would include not only external customers, such as patients and carers, the Commissioning Health Authority and the Primary Care Trust, whose respective requirements and expectations may well be different from each other, but also internal customers, such as sections within oncology, e.g. mould room, radiotherapy physics and treatment machines.

QMP 2 Leadership

Management is responsible for creating an environment in which quality can flourish. The department's management team must establish a clear quality policy with related objectives which are achievable, realistic, incorporate other initiatives and are communicated to all staff.

QMP 3 Involvement of people

All staff should be fully involved in the service and should be able to use all of their abilities to the benefit of the organization.

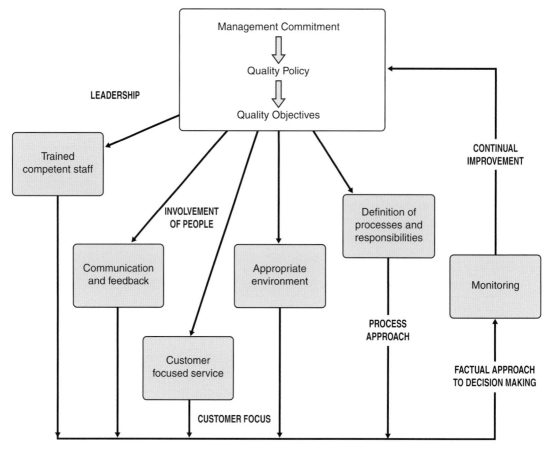

Figure 14.1 Key quality management principles underpinning ISO 9001:2008.

QMP 4 Process approach

Quality should be process driven, i.e. all resources and activities should be managed as a process, giving consideration to both inputs and outputs.

QMP 5 System approach to management

A clear understanding of the organization's aims and all the interrelated processes involved in achieving objectives will maximize efficiency. Processes should be integrated to ensure improved efficiency, especially where there are interfaces between different key areas or staff groups, such as the planning department and pretreatment.

QMP 6 Continual improvement

Systems, such as audit, should be in place for continual measurement, review and improvement of a department's processes and service.

QMP 7 Factual approach to decision making

All decisions should be evidence based, supported by appropriate data and information. For example, there should be appropriate data collated to support future service planning and developments.

QMP 8 Mutually beneficial supplier relationships

Any supplier has an effect on quality and a healthy relationship between an organization and its suppliers, both internal and external, enhances the ability of both to ensure a high level of quality is maintained.

ISO 9000

ISO 9000 is a family of documents that provides an international standard code of practice for quality management systems. It is designed to be generic so that it is independent of any specific industry and therefore applicable to both manufacturing and service industries, including healthcare. It consists of:

- ISO 9000 Quality management systems – Fundamentals and vocabulary (last published 2005 [21])
- ISO 9001 Quality management systems – Requirements (last published 2008 [22])
- ISO 9004 Quality management systems – Guidelines for performance improvements (last published 2000 [23], due for republication 2009 [24] with a new focus on 'sustained success').

The standards themselves are subject to a review programme to ensure that they remain relevant. There were major changes when ISO 9001:2000 was introduced, whereas the publication of ISO 9001:2008 included only minor amendments.

The scope of a department's QMS defines the activities included within the QMS and is determined by the organization. There are variations between oncology departments: some include just radiotherapy whereas others include planning and dosimetry, medical physics, chemotherapy, clinical trials and clerical areas. ISO 9001 is the standard against which an organization is assessed. It specifies the requirements a QMS must meet but not how the organization should meet them.

The ISO 9001:2008 [22] standard comprises nine clauses, listed in Box 14.1.

Clause 0, Introduction, describes a 'process approach' and compatibility with other management systems. Clause 1, Scope, specifies the type of organization that the standard is applicable to. Clause 2, Normative references, gives reference to the document ISO 9000:2005 [21], which is necessary for the application of the ISO standard. Clause 3, Terms and definitions, defines what particular terms, e.g. product, mean within the concept of ISO 9000. The remaining clauses, 4–8, contain the requirements against which departments are assessed.

These requirements are based on the eight quality management principles outlined above. Table 14.2 illustrates

the quality management principles which underpin the clauses of ISO 9001. The ISO 9001:2008 requirements are very much based on the Plan – Do – Check – Act cycle [22], as illustrated in Figure 14.2. Clauses 4–8 and their requirements are described further below, with the relevant quality management principles (QMP) indicated in brackets.

Clause 4 Quality management system (QMP 2, 4, 5, 6, 7)

This describes the basic requirements for establishing a QMS and does include some duplication of requirements contained in other clauses, but this serves to emphasize the key actions required. Although the 2000 version of ISO 9001 shifted the emphasis from documentation to a process-based approach, implementation of a QMS does require a certain amount of documentation. ISO 9001:2008 stipulates that there must be a quality manual, often referred to as the Level 1 document, containing documented statements of a quality policy and quality objectives. In addition, there should be written procedures for:

1. control of documents (Clause 4)
2. control of records (Clause 4)
3. internal audit (Clause 8)
4. control of non-conforming product (Clause 8), e.g. complaints, clinical incidents
5. corrective action (Clause 8)
6. preventive action (Clause 8).

Box 14.1 **The clauses of ISO 9001:2008**

0 Introduction
1 Scope
2 Normative references
3 Terms and definitions
4 Quality management system
5 Management responsibility
6 Resource management
7 Product realization
8 Measurement, analysis and improvement

Table 14.2 Quality management principles underpinning ISO 9001 clauses

CLAUSES OF ISO 9001:2008	QUALITY MANAGEMENT PRINCIPLE (QMP)							
	1	2	3	4	5	6	7	8
4. Quality management system		√		√	√	√	√	
5. Management responsibility	√	√		√	√	√	√	
6. Resource management	√	√	√	√			√	
7. Product realization	√	√	√	√	√	√	√	√
8. Measurement analysis & improvement	√	√		√		√	√	

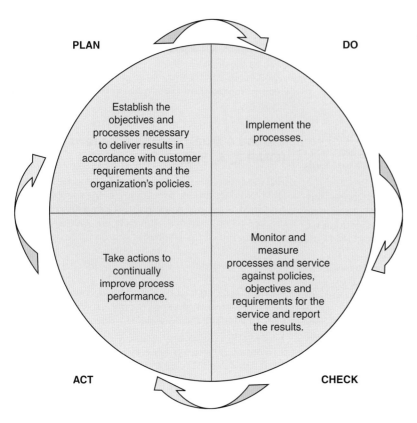

PLAN

DO

Establish the objectives and processes necessary to deliver results in accordance with customer requirements and the organization's policies.

Implement the processes.

Take actions to continually improve process performance.

Monitor and measure processes and service against policies, objectives and requirements for the service and report the results.

ACT

CHECK

Figure 14.2 The plan– do– check– act cycle applied to ISO 9001:2008.

A QMS will also contain all or some of the following:

- department procedures
- process flow charts
- clinical protocols
- work instructions (detailed instruction about how a task should be carried out)
- forms
- data
- reference documents.

Control of all these documents includes regulating their development, approval, issue, identification, amendments, distribution, storage, security, obsolescence, retention and disposal. Similarly, records produced, such as training records, patient treatment records, equipment maintenance records and records of complaints and incidents, must be regulated for the duration of their life cycle. A record may be any document that provides evidence of activities performed. Records must be legible, identifiable and retrievable. A department must define what its quality records are, how they are stored, who has responsibility for them, how long they should be retained and the method of disposal. Departments must ensure they incorporate legislative [25, 26], national [27–29] and local requirements into their control of documents and records policies.

Clause 5 Management responsibility (QMP 1, 2, 4, 5, 6, 7)

Specific areas of management responsibility outlined in this clause include:

- evidence of management commitment
- determining, meeting and enhancing customers' requirements
- an established quality policy which reflects the vision of the organization
- established quality objectives which are based on the quality policy and business objectives, and aim to fulfill the needs of the customers
- management review meetings to review the effectiveness of the QMS and the department's performance against objectives, and to identify further improvements
- ensuring the availability and effective allocation of the resources required to fulfil the department's objectives.

Clause 6 Resources (QMP 1, 2, 3, 4, 7)

The resources required to provide a service and fulfill the department's objectives are categorized by ISO 9001:2008 as listed below. The management team is responsible for determining and then providing the resources to implement and maintain the QMS, continually improve its effectiveness and enhance customer satisfaction.

- Human resources. For example: there should be sufficient numbers of staff who are trained and competent [30]
- Infrastructure. This includes buildings, utilities, IT and support services. It includes not only the purchase of but also the correct maintenance of treatment machines and other equipment
- Work environment. This encompasses physical, social and psychological factors associated with the work environment. For example, health and safety, local rules and radiation protection.

Clause 7 Product realization (QMP 1, 2, 3, 4, 5, 6, 7, 8)

This clause, the largest of ISO 9001:2008, describes and includes the processes and steps involved from identifying the need for a service, to creating and providing it. In planning the provision of a particular service to fulfill requirements, consideration must be given to:

- customer requirements and how they are identified
- resources required, e.g. skill mix of staff, equipment
- documentation requirements, e.g. are detailed work instructions required?
- the activities required to verify, validate and monitor the process at critical stages, e.g. what checks should be in place at each stage?
- records that should be maintained, e.g. patient records, equipment records [27]
- statutory and regulatory requirements, e.g. radiation protection [31]
- customer communication, e.g. obtaining customer feedback and handling complaints
- purchasing, e.g. equipment specifications, and use of reliable suppliers
- service provision, including, for example, the use of work instructions, suitable equipment, monitoring and checking processes, identification and traceability issues. Examples could include the identification of the patient and their accessories throughout the treatment process, traceability of any equipment used and the storage of records such as patient notes
- the control of measuring and monitoring devices. This applies to any method used to monitor whether the service provided meets the determined requirements. It could be applied to satisfaction surveys, but also to the calibration of measuring equipment.

Clause 8 Measurement, analysis and improvement (QMP 1, 2, 4, 6, 7)

One of the key points of emphasis in ISO 9001:2008 is continual improvement. To establish how a department can improve its service, it must be able to identify standards to strive for, measure its performance and monitor outcomes against requirements and expectations, analyze the findings and identify potential improvements. Departments should develop indicators and measures which are meaningful to them and which they can use to measure improvement. Key requirements of this clause include:

- monitoring customer satisfaction to assess whether the service provided has met with customers' expectations, e.g. using information from customer surveys, complaints [32], compliments and user groups
- internal audit. Quality audits are the measurement component of a QMS and, through independent examination, should provide objective evidence of:
  - effective implementation of the organization's processes
  - achieving the organization's objectives
  - conformance to ISO 9001 requirements
- monitoring systems at identified points of a process to detect any problems or faults and prevent errors from occurring, e.g. calculation checks
- measurement systems to verify performance against targets, e.g. waiting time targets
- control of a non-conforming product. If any problems, such as complaints, are detected by the monitoring systems in place, there should be clear systems in place to record and correct them and to prevent them escalating
- analysis of data. Organizations need to identify sources of data, for example, clinical incidents, machine down time and waiting time data, which give an indication of performance. These data should be analyzed to identify whether there are opportunities for improvement
- improvement. The previous requirements lead on to implementing continual improvement. Immediate remedial action is required in response to an error, non-compliance with a procedure or a complaint. Corrective action is necessary to identify the cause of a problem and prevent it recurring. Methods of preventive action should be in place to identify any potential faults or risks in processes in order that action can be taken to reduce the likelihood of occurrence.

Further reading on ISO 9000 should include the standards themselves. In addition, there are many textbooks which interpret how to apply the requirements [33]. Figure 14.3 illustrates the process of implementation of a QMS through to ongoing surveillance visits.

THE RADIOTHERAPY PROCESS

ISO 9000:2000 [4] defines a process as: 'A set of interrelated or interacting activities which transforms inputs into outputs.'

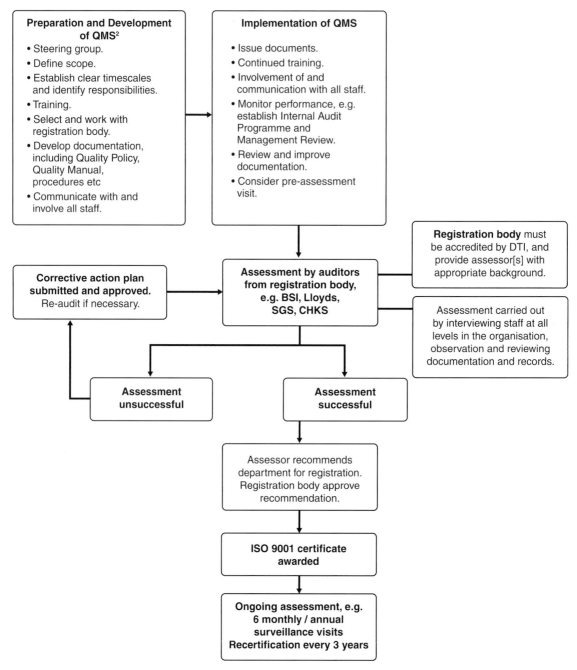

Figure 14.3 The route to ISO 9001 registration.

The ISO 9001:2008 standard adopts a process-based approach and requires systematic identification and management of an organization's processes and the interaction between them. To adopt a process-based approach, a radiotherapy department should consider the following:

- identify each process carried out
- what are the inputs?
- what are the outputs?
- how are they measured?
- what are the critical interfaces with other processes?
- have responsibilities been clearly identified?

Processes are best illustrated with a diagram or flow chart. An example, relating to the treatment process, is shown in Figure 14.4. It is important to remember that a process

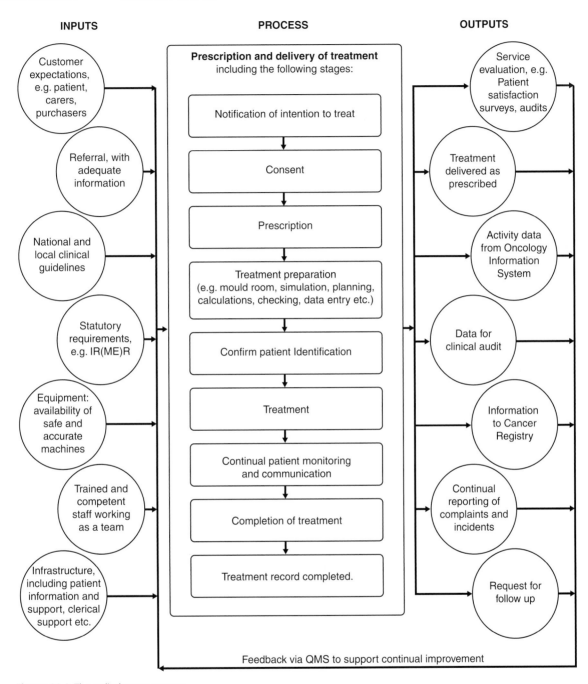

Figure 14.4 The radiotherapy process.

can be defined at many levels. A core process (e.g. treatment) will be made up of a number of subprocesses. Figure 14.5 illustrates an example of the interaction between a department's core processes. For each process, it is important to consider the key elements of the ISO 9001 requirements, for example, in addition to the list above:

- are resources allocated effectively?
- is the work environment suitable for the task?

- are staff trained and competent?
- are training records up to date?
- how do you know if your customers' expectations have been fulfilled?
- how are complaints or other problems resolved?
- how could potential improvements be identified?

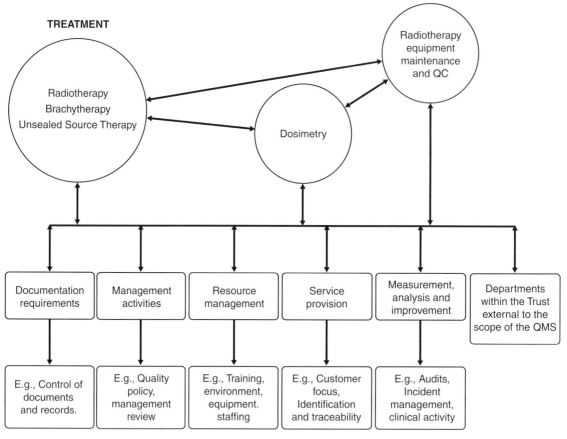

TREATMENT

Radiotherapy
Brachytherapy
Unsealed Source Therapy

Radiotherapy
equipment
maintenance
and QC

Dosimetry

| Documentation requirements | Management activities | Resource management | Service provision | Measurement, analysis and improvement | Departments within the Trust external to the scope of the QMS |

| E.g., Control of documents and records. | E.g., Quality policy, management review | E.g., Training, environment, equipment. staffing | E.g., Customer focus, Identification and traceability | E.g., Audits, Incident management, clinical activity |

Figure 14.5 The interaction of processes in a radiotherapy department.

- what are the arrangements for ensuring calibration equipment remains within specification?
- is identification and traceability, e.g. of equipment and patients, maintained throughout the process.

AN INTEGRATED APPROACH TO QUALITY AND OTHER INITIATIVES

Quality in the NHS

Quality may be measured in a number of ways and there are a number of standards, measures, targets and improvement initiatives within the NHS, both generic and specific to cancer services. Key examples of this include Clinical governance (Box 14.2) and National Cancer Peer Review (Box 14.3). Table 14.3 lists a number of other initiatives and documents that have contributed to the development of quality in UK radiotherapy departments. Many of these

complement each other or have common characteristics, and should not be considered in isolation. They reflect the same principles that underpin quality management systems and are all designed with the same ultimate objective – to improve the patients' experience [34], whether this is by, for example, improving treatment outcome, reducing waiting times, reducing the risk of incidents, improving communication with patients or improving patient facilities. Meeting such standards gives an indication that an acceptable level of quality has been achieved and allows inter comparison. Obviously, getting the right measure of quality is important. For example, waiting times measure the speed of throughput for patients but have no bearing on the standard of treatment delivered. This chapter has discussed the principles of quality management systems but this is only part of developing and maintaining a quality service. An effective QMS should be a tool to help implement, integrate and measure any new initiative introduced into a department. For example, most UK radiotherapy departments who have undergone the peer review process

Box 14.2 **Clinical governance**

The concept of Clinical Governance was first defined in 'A First Class Service: Quality in the New NHS' [35] as 'A framework through which NHS organizations are accountable for continuously improving the quality of their services and safeguarding high standards of care by creating an environment in which excellence in clinical care will flourish.'

To demonstrate accountability an NHS organization must have systems in place which address aspects of the service. These include:

Strategic planning/supply and demand
* Planning a service to meet the needs of a public, managing resources taking into account population served and recommendations or guidelines from professional bodies relating to staffing and equipment

Management structure/leadership
* Clearly defined lines of management and authority
* Staff management and training
* Recruitment
* CPD
* Appraisals
* Mandatory training requirements
* Introduction of new developments or techniques

Risk management
* Incident reporting (including treatment errors and near misses)
* Infection control
* Health and safety

Information management/sharing information/communication
* Confidentiality
* Patient records
* Data Protection Act
* Networks
* Multidisciplinary groups
* Cross-organization groups
* Information to patients, staff, GPs, Trusts, and external bodies

Clinical effectiveness
* Research
* Clinical audit

Public involvement
* Patient groups
* Surveys
* Complaints

Box 14.3 **National Cancer Peer Review (NCPR) [36]**

The NCPR programme is managed by the National Cancer Action Team and is an integral part of the NHS Cancer Reform Strategy [37] and the overall NHS Cancer Programme, led by the National Cancer Director.
* 2000: 'Cancer Standards', applicable to all aspects of cancer treatment, e.g. site-specific standards, including radiotherapy, were introduced as part of the NHS Cancer Plan [34], to introduce national standards of practice for cancer centres.
* 2004: the standards were revised and renamed Cancer Measures [38]. The topics contained in the Cancer Measures are subject to ongoing review and updates.
* 2008: updated Manual for Cancer Services
    – Revision of quality measures – clinically relevant, reduced number
    – New self-assessment process from May 2009
* Since 2008, compliance with the Cancer Measures is assessed by:
    – Annual validated self assessments
    – Externally verified self assessments (sampled)
    – Peer review visits (targeted)
* A peer review team consists of multidisciplinary professionals with knowledge of the area they are assessing, but independent of the network they are reviewing.
* The aims of NCPR include:
    – To ensure services are as safe as possible
    – To improve the quality and effectiveness of care
    – To improve the patient and carer experience
    – To undertake independent, fair reviews of services
    – To provide development and learning for all involved
    – To encourage the dissemination of good practice
* Key principles of NCPR:
    – Clinically led; national consistency in delivery of programme; developmental; peer on peer; focus on coordination within and across organizations; integration with other review systems; user/carer involvement
* NCPR in the future:
    – Greater focus on self-assessment and internal QA; improved value for money; responsiveness to NHS changes; continued emphasis on clinically led peer review; greater emphasis on outcomes

as part of the National Cancer Peer Review programme have found that using documentation describing working practices, which was already present in the QMS, has made the whole experience much easier. The following paragraphs on risk management, clinical incidents, audit and patient focused care give more detail on some of the most important areas where a robust QMS can ensure smooth interfaces between different initiatives.

Table 14.3 Overview of quality initiatives in oncology and the NHS

	YEAR	INITIATIVE, REQUIREMENT OR PUBLICATION	COMMENT	FURTHER INFORMATION AVAILABLE FROM: (LAST ACCESSED JANUARY 2009)
1.	October 1991	Patients Charter	Defined standards of care that patients could expect to receive from the NHS, for example, waiting times. 2001: replaced by 'Your Guide to the NHS: getting the most from your National Health Service' 2008: superseded by 'Best practice guidance for your guide to local health services'	http://www.pfc.org.uk/node/633 http://www.dh.gov.uk/en/Publicationsandstatistics/Lettersandcirculars/Dearcolleagueletters/DH_090451
2.	1992	Chartermark	The government's national standard for customer service excellence. Now closed to new applicants and replaced with the Government's new standard, Customer Service Excellence, March 2008	http://www.cabinetoffice.gov.uk/chartermark/criteria.aspx www.chartermark.gov.uk http://www.cse.cabinetoffice.gov.uk/homeCSE.do
3.	July 1993	'Reducing Delays in Cancer Treatment.' Joint Council for Clinical Oncology (JCCO)	Provided waiting time targets for cancer treatments	http://www.rcr.ac.uk/docs/oncology/pdf/reducingdelaysincancertreatment.pdf
4.	1995	NHS Litigation Authority (NHSLA) established.	Special health authority with responsibility for implementing risk management and handling negligence claims within the NHS	www.nhsla.com
5.	April 1995	Calman-Hine Report 'A Policy Framework for Commissioning Cancer Services'	Major review of cancer services in the UK. Main principles and areas for future development were: • Accessibility to services • Education • Information • Patient centered services • Primary care team involvement • Social care • Data monitoring	http://www.dh.gov.uk/en/Publicationsandstatistics/Publications/PublicationsPolicyAndGuidance/DH_4071083

Table 14.3 Overview of quality initiatives in oncology and the NHS—cont'd

	YEAR	INITIATIVE, REQUIREMENT OR PUBLICATION	COMMENT	FURTHER INFORMATION AVAILABLE FROM: (LAST ACCESSED JANUARY 2009)
6.	December 1997	The New NHS: Modern, Dependable	Government white paper which formed the basis for a 10-year programme to modernize and improve healthcare	http://www.dh.gov.uk/en/Publicationsandstatistics/Publications/PublicationsPolicyAndGuidance/DH_4008869
7.	July 1998	A First Class Service: Quality in the New NHS	Document which set out the government's strategy for reorganizing and modernizing the NHS. Defined the concept of Clinical Governance – see Box 14.2	http://www.dh.gov.uk/en/Publicationsandstatistics/Publications/PublicationsPolicyAndGuidance/DH_4006902 www.cgsupport.nhs.uk
8.	June 2000	Organisation with a Memory	This report was the result of the findings of an expert group set up to examine ways of learning from adverse events in the NHS	http://www.dh.gov.uk/en/Publicationsandstatistics/Publications/PublicationsPolicyAndGuidance/DH_4065083
9.	July 2000	NHS plan	Outlined the vision of a health service designed around the patient. Main areas in need of improvement: • Efficient use of more and better paid staff • Reduced waiting times • Improvements to facilities	http://www.dh.gov.uk/en/Publicationsandstatistics/Publications/PublicationsPolicyAndGuidance/DH_4002960
10.	September 2000	NHS Cancer Plan	Set out a 5- year plan. Main areas identified were: • reducing waiting times in the system • promoting the empowerment and involvement of patients • adoption of national standards of practice • Cancer Research Networks • Cancer Information Strategy • Cancer Services Collborative • Cancer Networks	http://www.dh.gov.uk/en/Publicationsandstatistics/Publications/PublicationsPolicyAndGuidance/DH_4009609

Continued

Table 14.3 Overview of quality initiatives in oncology and the NHS—cont'd

	YEAR	INITIATIVE, REQUIREMENT OR PUBLICATION	COMMENT	FURTHER INFORMATION AVAILABLE FROM: (LAST ACCESSED JANUARY 2009)
11.	2001	National Patient Safety Agency (NPSA)	An agency, linked to the Department of Health (DoH), set up to lead and contribute to improved, safe patient care by informing, supporting and influencing organizations and people working in the health sector. This includes the National Reporting and Learning Service (NRLS)	http://www.npsa.nhs.uk/
12.	April 2001	Building a Safer NHS	Followed on from 'An Organization with a Memory' (June 2000) with emphasis on patient safety	http://www.dh.gov.uk/en/Publicationsandstatistics/Publications/PublicationsPolicyAndGuidance/DH_4006525
13.	April 2001	Modernization Agency/Cancer Services Collaborative Improvement Partnership (CSCIP)	Supported the NHS in modernizing services and improving experiences and outcomes for patients	www.cancerimprovement.nhs.uk
14.	January 2003	Commission for Public and Patient Involvement in Health (CPPIH)	Aimed to ensure public involvement with healthcare services by setting up and supporting patient forums. Abolished March 2008 and replaced with Local Involvement Networks (LINks) to give public and patients a stronger voice in how their health and social care services are delivered	http://www.dh.gov.uk/en/Managingyourorganisation/PatientAndPublicinvolvement/DH_076366
15.	March 2004	Healthcare Commission (formally Commission for Healthcare Improvement, CHI)	The Healthcare Commission took over the functions of several organizations including CHI. Responsibilities include awarding the annual performance ratings for all NHS Trusts, and enforcement of the Ionising Radiation (Medical Exposure) Regulations 2000 (IR(ME)R) in England	www.healthcarecommission.org.uk http://www.healthcarecommission.org.uk/guidanceforhealthcarestaff/nhsstaff/managingrisk/useofionisingradiation.cfm

Table 14.3 Overview of quality initiatives in oncology and the NHS—cont'd

	YEAR	INITIATIVE, REQUIREMENT OR PUBLICATION	COMMENT	FURTHER INFORMATION AVAILABLE FROM: (LAST ACCESSED JANUARY 2009)
16.	June 2004	NHS Improvement Plan	This document built on The NHS Plan (see July 2000) and set out the priorities for the NHS up until 2008.	http://www.dh.gov.uk/en/Publicationsandstatistics/ Publications/PublicationsPolicyAndGuidance/ DH_4084476
17.	July 2004	Standards for Better Health	To establish basic standards for NHS health care. Seven main areas identified are: • Safety • Clinical and cost effectiveness • Governance • Patient focus • Accessible and responsive care • Care environment and amenities • Public health Each year all health organizations are assessed by the Healthcare Commission against the standards within each of these areas ('Annual Health Check') and are awarded a star rating	http://www.dh.gov.uk/en/Publicationsandstatistics/ Publications/PublicationsPolicyAndGuidance/ DH_4086665
18.	April 2005	National Institute for Health and Clinical Excellence (NICE)	An independent organization responsible for providing national guidance on prevention and treatment of ill health	http://www.nice.org.uk/
19.	November 2006	Cancer Waiting Targets	Defines target waiting times (generally 31 or 62 day targets) for cancer referrals to treatment	http://www.dh.gov.uk/en/Publicationsandstatistics/ Publications/PublicationsPolicyAndGuidance/ DH_063067
20.	May 2007	National Radiotherapy Advisory Group report (NRAG) Radiotherapy: developing a world class service for England	Report from a specialist group with the remit to review current radiotherapy services in England, maximizing efficiency and future developments	http://www.dh.gov.uk/en/Publicationsandstatistics/ Publications/PublicationsPolicyAndGuidance/ DH_074575

Continued

Table 14.3 Overview of quality initiatives in oncology and the NHS—cont'd

	YEAR	INITIATIVE, REQUIREMENT OR PUBLICATION	COMMENT	FURTHER INFORMATION AVAILABLE FROM: (LAST ACCESSED JANUARY 2009)
21.	June 2007	Complaints monitoring: Making experiences count	Reviewed and suggested improvements to the NHS Complaints System	http://www.dh.gov.uk/en/Policyandguidance/Organisationpolicy/Complaintspolicy/index.htm
22.	July 2007	Chief Medical Officer Report Radiotherapy, The Hidden Dangers.	Identified the areas of radiotherapy with the maximum risk potential for errors	http://www.dh.gov.uk/en/Publicationsandstatistics/Publications/AnnualReports/DH_076817?IdcService=GET_FILE&dID=144555&Rendition=Web
23.	September 2007	NHS Next Stage Review – Our NHS, Our Future	A review of the way the NHS delivers healthcare, looking at how it can become fairer, more personalized, effective and safe, setting out immediate and longer term priorities. Final report launched June 2008	http://www.ournhs.nhs.uk/
24.	December 2007	Cancer Reform Strategy	Builds on NHS Cancer Plan (September 2000)	http://www.dh.gov.uk/en/Publicationsandstatistics/Publications/PublicationsPolicyAndGuidance/DH_081006
25.	April 2008	Towards Safer Radiotherapy	A joint report published by the British Institute of Radiology, the Institute of Physics and Engineering in Medicine, the National Patient Safety Agency, the Society and College of Radiographers and The Royal College of Radiologists. A multidisciplinary working party reviewed the incidence and causes of incidents in radiotherapy and methods of detection, prevention, reporting and learning from these with the aim of reducing errors in radiotherapy	https://www.rcr.ac.uk/docs/oncology/pdf/Towards_saferRT_final.pdf
26.	2008	WHO Radiotherapy Risk Profile. Technical Manual	Comprises two parts, the first is an international review of patient safety measures in radiotherapy practice and the second sets out WHO's Radiotherapy Risk Profile and analyses the radiotherapy process, from patient assessment to treatment verification and monitoring	http://www.who.int/patientsafety/activities/technical/radiotherapy_risk_profile.pdf

Risk management

Patient and staff safety is foremost in all NHS Trusts and risk management is one element of a quality management system that healthcare organizations must ensure they address, particularly in such high risk specialties as radiotherapy. Risk management includes risk identification, risk assessment and risk minimization [1], thus preventing faults rather than acting after something has gone wrong. It should be integrated into all organizational structures and activities. For example, all radiotherapy equipment is subject to a strict maintenance programme and rigorous QC checks (see Chapter 13) and there is evidence to demonstrate that checks at a number of stages within the treatment process can provide an effective error prevention system [18, 39]. Examples of risk management include:

- existing checking processes should be under review to ensure that they add value. Any redundant checks should then be eliminated
- introducing an additional check or the use of a checklist may not be effective in preventing an error
- can the risk of involuntary automaticity [40], where staff carry out checks automatically and see or hear what they expect to see, rather than what is actually written or said, be reduced or eliminated?
- are the checks in place truly independent? For example, a second calculation should be carried out separately and the result compared with the first calculation, rather than the checker reviewing the original calculation
- if a junior member of staff has carried out a task under supervision, staffing levels should ensure that the supervising member of staff should not then be responsible for checking that task
- is there a risk of latent threats [41] which may lie dormant for months, such that patients are exposed to risk before a mistake actually occurs or the risk is detected?

A key element of risk management is the reporting of incidents and near misses and then learning from them.

Clinical incidents

The National Patient Safety Agency (NPSA) [42] was established in 2001 with a mandate to identify issues relating to patient safety and to find appropriate solutions that would improve safety for patients. It encourages health organizations to be open in reporting incidents and to learn from them. There are a number of tools available for use in managing clinical incidents, such as incident decision trees, root cause analysis and The London Protocol for systems analysis of clinical incidents [43]. There is a long history of incident reporting in radiotherapy [39, 44–46] both in the UK and internationally. However, since there has been:

- no unified approach
- no standard definitions for the terminology in use, such as 'near miss', or
- no defined classifications, such as level of impact, source or root cause,

it has been difficult to compare error rates and to define any standards. A multidisciplinary working party [41,47], including representation from the Royal College of Radiologists (RCR), the Institute of Physics and Engineering in Medicine (IPEM), the Society and College of Radiographers (SCoR), the British Institute of Radiology (BIR) and the NPSA was established in 2006, and has now published a report containing recommendations for a national system to support the reporting, analysis and learning from radiotherapy incidents [48].

Clinical incident records and reporting

As part of their QMS, radiotherapy departments should operate a system for defining and recording radiotherapy incidents (including actual errors and near misses), either via the Trust system, a local system or a combination of both so that data can be monitored for trends, and information can be fed back to staff. Major incidents are reportable under different regulations to various agencies, including:

- National Patient Safety Agency (NPSA). Any incident involving harm to a patient
- Healthcare Commission. Under IR[ME]R [49], any radiation incident where a patient has been exposed to ionizing radiation to an extent much greater than intended, other than those due to a malfunction or defect in equipment
- Health and Safety Executive (HSE). Under the Ionising Radiations Regulations 1999 [31], any incident leading to a dose much greater than intended occurring as a result of malfunction or defect in any radiation equipment. Guidance note PM77 [50],'Equipment used in connection with medical exposure' includes advice on such incidents
- Medicine and Healthcare Products Regulatory Agency (MHRA). Under The Medical Devices Regulations 2002 [51], incidents and faults relating to medical equipment. Medical Device Alert MDA/2007/001 gives further advice
- HSE. Under the Reporting of Injuries, Diseases and Dangerous Occurrences Regulations (RIDDOR) [52], any injuries that have resulted in a member of staff being off sick for 3 or more days.

Action following an incident should be considered carefully by departments, including disclosure to the patient [53] and support for staff involved. Communicating honestly and sympathetically with patients and their families is a vital component in dealing effectively with errors or mistakes [54]. An apology can be an expression of regret and sympathy and not necessarily an admission of guilt [55].

Audit

Audit is a key requirement of a quality management system and has a long history both in the NHS, including medical, clinical and multiprofessional audit, and in oncology [56]. There are many definitions of 'audit' [57]. For example:

A systematic, independent and documented process for obtaining audit evidence and evaluating it objectively to determine the extent to which audit criteria are fulfilled [4]

where, in the above definition, audit criteria are a set of policies, procedures or requirements and audit evidence consists of records, statements of fact or other information relevant to audit criteria which is verifiable. A definition of clinical audit is included in Box 14.4.

It is important to distinguish audit from research. In the most simplistic terms, research tells us the most effective way to do things and how to achieve the best results and audit tells us if we are doing that [1].

All audits are cyclical in nature (Figure 14.6) and have the same key features, such as defining audit criteria to evaluate findings against. Audits are a valuable tool for ensuring continual improvement. Many departments will have a clinical audit programme that is developed independently to the QMS internal audit programme. Whereas clinical audits may focus more on outcomes, for example, the effect on health or on patient experience, QMS audits aim to verify processes, particularly at the interfaces, highlight any areas of concern and identify areas for potential improvement. An integrated approach to both QMS and clinical audits could encompass a range of audit projects and provide a comprehensive audit programme.

Patient focused care

Patient focused care is an approach to quality improvement which is geared specifically to health, rather than derived from industry [1]. It is underpinned by a philosophy which puts patients at the centre of the health service. In today's world, patients' expectations have increased [61], as too has their intolerance of failure or complications. Their final perception of the quality of service received will result from a comparison of their expectations with their actual experience. The most common complaints concern delays, incorrect treatment and morbidity [55], perception of professional competence and efficiency of process. There is a long history of public and patient participation in the UK [62], leading to user involvement being at the centre of the development and evaluation of services, extending from the establishment of Community Health Councils in 1974, and including a number of the initiatives included in Table 14.3. In particular, the development of user

involvement in cancer services was driven by the Calman–Hine report [63] and then re-emphasized in the NHS Cancer Plan [34]. At the heart of the current modernization agenda is the empowerment of the customer or user while the hopes, fears, aspirations and expectations of patients need to be central to decisions about their care. Current national policies make it clear that all NHS cancer services are responsible at a local level for developing user involvement in service evaluation, planning and delivery. In practical terms, the development of patient and carer input can be achieved in various ways including questionnaires, complaint monitoring, focus groups, interviews, websites, newsletters,

---

Box 14.4 Clinical audit

'Clinical audit is a quality improvement process that seeks to improve patient care and outcomes through systematic review of care against explicit criteria and the implementation of change. Aspects of the structures, processes and outcomes of care are selected and systematically evaluated against explicit criteria. Where indicated changes are implemented at an individual, team, or service level and further monitoring is used to confirm improvement in healthcare delivery' [58].

Clinical audit, initially termed 'Medical Audit', was introduced to the NHS by the 1989 White Paper, Working for Patients. It has continued to evolve and is now well established in the NHS, forming a key component of the clinical governance framework. Guidance on audit is available from NICE [58] and the NHS Clinical Governance Support Team [59]. It is monitored by the Healthcare Commission as a requirement of the 'Standards for Better Health' [60].

Clinical audit:

- is a specific form of audit that involves measuring clinical practice against standards
- provides a framework to improve the quality of patient care in a collaborative and systematic way
- should be owned by healthcare professionals. They carry out the audit, discuss the results and then make improvements to practice. Other forms of audit, to a greater or lesser extent, may involve someone coming in to 'audit' you
- should be patient focused, develop a culture of continuous evaluation and improve clinical effectiveness by examining patient outcomes
- is essentially all about checking whether best practice is being followed and making improvements if there are shortfalls in the delivery of care.

A good clinical audit will identify or confirm any problems and then lead to changes that should result in improved patient care.

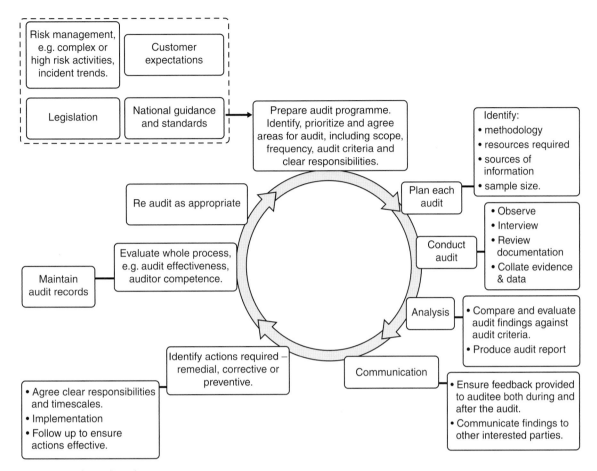

Figure 14.6 The audit cycle.

workshops, user involvement training programs, suggestion boxes, facilitating support groups, patient liaison services and user councils [62]. Service users can be involved in a systematic way and user involvement practices built into the way in which care is organized and delivered.

Obviously, all patients want to receive accurate treatment, with minimal waiting time to start. But what else is important to patients? Often it is the simple things that make the biggest difference [61]:

- a smiling friendly face to greet you rather than an empty reception desk or staff who are too busy to acknowledge your presence
- a pleasant waiting area with comfortable seating and a variety of up-to-date reading material
- easy availability of drinks and maybe snacks
- car parking – minimal waiting and spaces available close by
- effective communication and provision of information
- easy access to the building – no long walks or numerous swing doors or stairs.

IMPLEMENTATION OF NEW TECHNOLOGY AND NEW TECHNIQUES

Technology in radiotherapy has developed at an unprecedented rate over the last decade and so have the treatment techniques that are employed. Introducing any new development, equipment, software [18, 41] or change in procedure, however small, carries with it the risk of error and must be managed carefully [64], with full evaluation of safety issues and final authorization. Satisfactory management can include, for example:

- setting up specialist multidisciplinary groups to evaluate fully all implications and inviting feedback from all staff groups involved
- visiting/liaising with other departments who already utilize the technique/technology
- carrying out a full risk assessment of implementing the new technique/technology

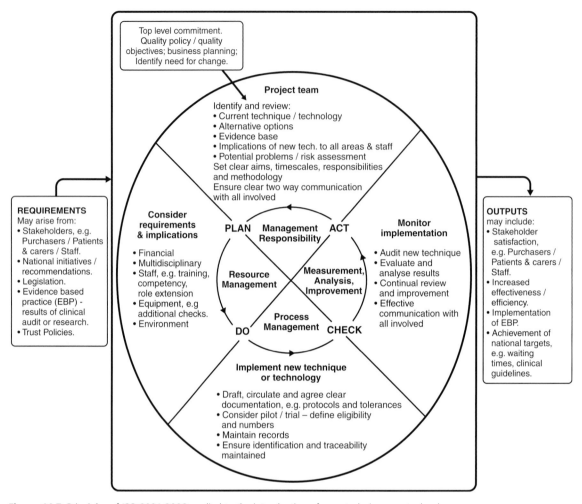

Figure 14.7 Principles of ISO 9001:2008 applied to the introduction of new techniques or technology.

- developing clear guidelines as to when and how new techniques/technology may be used
- identifying and developing clear documentation detailing procedures to be used
- a review of the number of staff and training needs.

Figure 14.7 illustrates how the principles of ISO 9001 can be applied to the safe introduction of new techniques or technology. It is vital that attention is paid to the recurrent themes identified in error reporting as outlined in this chapter. For example, provision of adequate training and assessment of competency.

CONCLUSION

There is a long history of technically focused QA programmes in radiotherapy. However, in response to a number of pressures, the emphasis has shifted towards more comprehensive quality management systems. Departments must build on what they have in place and develop a culture of continuous improvement, encouraging all staff to be involved. A multidisciplinary approach will generate service wide problem identification [2]. It may be argued that a QMS is costly to implement and maintain and that there is a risk of running a system without addressing vital quality issues. However, if a system has management commitment and is run effectively, although it may not prevent disasters or eliminate human error [46], it will:

- reduce an organization's exposure to the common elements behind disasters
- ensure that an organization has systems in place to prevent problems escalating into disaster
- provide the tools to react quickly to put things right
- reduce the risk of major errors and reduce the frequency of minor errors [2].

Historically, ISO 9001 has received criticism for being too generic since it is up to the organization to set a number of its own standards. To implement a system effectively, and gain the most benefit, oncology and radiotherapy departments should implement the ISO 9001 requirements in such a way as to provide a framework which ensures an integrated approach to the numerous quality standards, targets and initiatives that they are required to fulfill. A quality management system is not just about achieving certification, it is to ensure that the best possible treatments are provided within the resources available. Departments with systems in place should continue to improve and develop their QMS, incorporating recommendations from:

- the investigations and reports of publicized errors
- national and international multidisciplinary working parties, such as the group set up to develop incident reporting [41], the NPSA working party developing a safety package for radiotherapy and the World Health Organization [65].

REFERENCES

[1] Parsley K, Corrigan P. Quality improvement in healthcare, putting evidence into practice. Stanley Thornes; 1999.

[2] Kehoe T, Rugg L-J. From technical quality assurance of radiotherapy to a comprehensive quality of service management system. Radiother Oncol 1999;51:281–90.

[3] BS4778 Quality vocabulary. Availability, reliability and maintainability terms. Guide to concepts and related definitions. British Standards Institute; 1991.

[4] BS EN ISO 9000. Quality management systems – Fundamentals and vocabulary. British Standards Institute; 2000.

[5] Department of Health. National standards, local action. Health and social care standards and planning framework. HMSO; 2004.

[6] Radiation safety in external beam radiotherapy: radiological protection of patients. IAEA; November 2008. Online. Available: http://rpop.iaea.org/RPoP/RPoP/Content/InformationFor/HealthProfessionals/2_Radiotherapy/RadSafetyExtBeamRadiotherapy.htm.

[7] IAEA Safety Report Series no 38. Applying radiation safety standards in radiotherapy. International Atomic Energy Agency; 2006.

[8] Borras C. Overexposure of radiation therapy patients in Panama: problem recognition and follow up measures. Pan American Journal of Public Health 2006;20:173–87.

[9] ICRP Publication 86. Prevention of accidental exposures to patients undergoing radiation therapy. Pergamon Press; 2001.

[10] IAEA Safety Report Series No 17. Lessons learned from accidental exposures in radiotherapy. International Atomic Energy Agency; 2000.

[11] Summary of ASN report nn 2006 ENSTR 019 – IGAS no RM 2007-015P on the Epinal radiotherapy accident. November 2008. Online. Available: http://www.asn.fr/sections/main/documents-available-in/documents-available-in-english/downloadFile/attachedFile_ unvisible_3_f0/ASN_report_n_2006_ENSTR_019_-_IGAS.pdf?nocache=1174581960.71.

[12] Toft B. Redacted independent review of the circumstances surrounding a serious adverse incident. November 2008. Online. Available: http://www.who.int/patientsafety/news/Radiotherapy_adverse_event_Toft_ report.pdf.

[13] The Exeter District Health Authority. The Report of the Committee of Enquiry into the overdoses administered in the Department of Radiotherapy in the period February to July 1988. 28th November, 1988.

[14] Department of Health. Quality assurance in radiotherapy; report of a Working Party. Bleehen, et al., editors. HMSO; 1991.

[15] Baldwin Report. Report of an investigation into the conduct of isocentric radiotherapy at the North Staffordshire Royal Infirmary between 1982 and 1991. Second report, March 1994, W Midlands Health Authority; 1994.

[16] Department of Health. Quality assurance in radiotherapy: a quality management system for radiotherapy. HMSO; 1994.

[17] BS EN ISO 9001. Quality management systems – Requirements. British Standards Institute; 2000.

[18] Mayles W. The Glasgow incident – a physicist's reflections. Clin Oncol 2007;19:4–7.

[19] Report into unintended overexposure of Lisa Norris at Beatson, Glasgow. Scottish Executive; October 2006.

[20] Radiation Oncology Safety Information System (ROSIS). 26 January 2009. Online. Available: www.rosis.info.

[21] BS EN ISO 9000. Quality management systems – Fundamentals and vocabulary. British Standards Institute; 2005.

[22] BS EN ISO 9001. Quality management systems – Requirements. British Standards Institute; 2008.

[23] BS EN ISO 9004. Quality management systems – Guidelines for performance improvements. British Standards Institute; 2000.

[24] British Standards Institute (BSI). Updates to ISO 9001 and ISO 9004. 21 November 2008. Online. Available: http://www.bsigroup.com/en/Assessment-and-certification-services/management-systems/Business-areas/Quality-Management/ISO9001-and-ISO9004/.

[25] Freedom of Information Act, HMSO; 2000. Online. Available: http://www.opsi.gov.uk/Acts/acts2000/ukpga_20000036_en_1 26 January 2009.

[26] Data Protection Act, HMSO; 1998. Online. Available: http://www.opsi.gov.uk/ACTS/acts1998/19980029.htm 26 January 2009.

[27] Department of Health. The Records Management: NHS Code of Practice. HMSO; 2006. Online. Available: http://www.dh.gov.uk/en/Policyandguidance/Organisationpolicy/Recordsmanagement/index.htm 26 January 2009.

[28] Report on the review of patient identifiable information (The Caldicott Report). HMSO; 1997. Online. Available: http://www.dh.gov.uk/en/Publicationsandstatistics/Publications/PublicationsPolicyAndGuidance/DH_4068403 26 January 2009.

[29] Department of Health. The NHS Confidentiality Code of Practice, HMSO; 2007. Online. Available: http://www.dh.gov.uk/en/Policyandguidance/Informationpolicy/Patientconfidentiality andcaldicottguardians/DH_4100550 26 January 2009.

[30] Griffiths S, Craig A, Abraham M. Radiographer roles and risk management in radiotherapy, and a UK survey. Journal of Radiotherapy in Practice 2006;5:137–46.

[31] The Ionising Radiation Regulations, HMSO; 1999. Online. Available: http://www.opsi.gov.uk/si/si1999/19993232.htm 26 January 2009.

[32] NHS Complaints Procedure. 12 December 2007. Online. Available: http://www.dh.gov.uk/en/Policyandguidance/Organisationpolicy/Complaintspolicy/NHScomplaintsprocedure/index.htm.

[33] Hoyle D. ISO 9000 quality systems handbook. Butterworth-Heinemann; 2001.

[34] Department of Health. The NHS Cancer Plan: a plan for investment, a plan for reform. HMSO; 2000.

[35] Department of Health. A first class service: quality in the new NHS. 1998. Online. Available: http://www.dh.gov.uk/en/publicationsandstatistics/publications/publicationspolicyandguidance/dh_4006902 26 January 2009.

[36] National Cancer Peer Review Programme. 20 January 2009.

[37] Department of Health. Cancer Reform Strategy. 2007. Online. Available: http://www.dh.gov.uk/en/Publicationsandstatistics/Publications/PublicationsPolicyAndGuidance/dh_081006 20 January 2009.

Online. Available: http://www.cquins.nhs.uk/.

[38] Department of Health. Manual for Cancer Services. 2004. Online. Available: http://www.dh.gov.uk/assetRoot/04/13/55/97/04135597.pdf 20 January 2009.

[39] Holmberg O, McClean B. Preventing treatment errors in radiotherapy by identifying and evaluating near misses and actual incidents. Journal of Radiotherapy in Practice 2002;3:13–25.

[40] Toft B, Mascie-Taylor H. Involuntary automaticity: a work system induced risk to safe healthcare. Health Serv Manage Res 2005;18:211–6.

[41] Williams MV. Radiotherapy near misses, incidents and errors: radiotherapy incident at Glasgow. Clin Oncol 2007;19:1–3.

[42] National Patient Safety Agency (NPSA). Online. Available: www.npsa.nhs.uk/ 26 January 2009.

[43] Taylor-Adams S, Vincent C. Systems analysis of clinical incidents, the London protocol. Clinical Safety Research Unit, Imperial College London; 23 November 2008. Online. Available: http://www.csru.org.uk/downloads/SACI.pdf.

[44] Munro AJ. Hidden danger, obvious opportunity: error and risk in the management of cancer. Br J Radiol 2007;80:955–66.

[45] Verstraete J, Huyskens DP. Use of QA forms to register procedural errors in a radiotherapy department in an attempt to improve the overall process: a pilot study. Journal of Radiotherapy in Practice 2002;3:43–50.

[46] TaiKeung Y, et al. Quality assurance in radiotherapy: evaluation of errors and incidents over a 10 year period. Radiother Oncol 2005;74:283–91.

[47] Williams M, Erridge S. Towards safer radiotherapy. Synergy 2008; April, 18–22.

[48] The Royal College of Radiologists, Society and College of

Radiographers, Institute of Physics and Engineering in Medicine, National Patient Safety Agency, British Institute of Radiology. Towards safer radiotherapy. The Royal College of Radiologists; 2008. Online. Available: www.npsa.nhs.uk/EasySiteWeb/GatewayLink.aspx?alId=11378 23 November 2008.

[49] Department of Health. The Ionising Radiation (Medical Exposure) Regulations. 2000. Online. Available: http://www.dh.gov.uk/en/Publicationsandstatistics/Publications/PublicationsPolicyAndGuidance/DH_4007957 26 January 2009.

[50] Health and Safety Executive. Guidance Note PM77. 3rd ed.

[51] The Medical Devices Regulations. HMSO; 2002.

[52] Health and Safety Executive. The reporting of injuries, diseases and dangerous occurrences regulations (RIDDOR). 1995.

[53] Weselake T, French J. The ethics of disclosure perspectives of radiation therapists and patients regarding disclosure of radiation therapy errors. Can J Med Radiat Technol 2004;35:10–7.

[54] NPSA. Being open policy. 2005. Online. Available: www.npsa.nhs.uk/nrls/improvingpatientsafety/patient-safety-tools-and-guidance/beingopen/ 23 November 2008.

[55] McNee SG. Clinical governance: risks and quality control in radiotherapy, Br J Radiol 2001;74:209–12. Online. Available: http://bjr.birjournals.org/cgi/content/full/74/879/209 23 November 2008.

[56] Tobias, et al. Clinical governance and revalidation: a practical guide from the faculty of clinical oncology. Royal College of Radiologists; 2003.

[57] Henwood S, Knapp K. Research, audit and CPD. Are they compatible? Synergy 2007 March, 24–27 April, 22–25.

[58] NICE. Principles for best practice in clinical audit. Radcliffe Medical Press; 2002.

[59] Clinical Governance Support Team. A practical handbook for clinical audit. CGST; 2005.

[60] Department of Health. Standards for better health. 2004. Online. Available: http://www.dh.gov.uk/en/publicationsandstatistics/publications/publicationspolicyandguidance/dh_4086665 20th January 2009.

[61] Clinical Oncology Patients' Liaison Group. Making your radiotherapy service more patient friendly. 2nd ed. Royal College of Radiologists; 2007. Online. Available: http://www.rcr.ac.uk/

index.asp?PageID=149&PublicationID=256 23 November 2008.

[62] Tritter J, Daykin N, Evans S, et al. Improving cancer services through patient involvement. Radcliffe Medical Press; 2004.

[63] Department of Health. A policy framework for commissioning cancer services – a report by the Expert Advisory Group on Cancer to the Chief Medical Officers of England and Wales: Guidance for purchasers and

providers of cancer services. HMSO; 1995.

[64] Dixon P, O'Sullivan B. Radiotherapy quality assurance: time for everyone to take it seriously. Eur J Cancer 2003;39:423–9.

[65] World Health Organization. Radiotherapy risk profile. Technical manual. WHO Press; 2008. Online. Available: http://www.who.int/patientsafety/activities/technical/radiotherapy_risk_profile.pdf February 2009.

Section | 2 |

Chapter | 15 |

Epidemiology of cancer and screening

David Hole, Paul Symonds

CHAPTER CONTENTS

THE CANCER PROBLEM

In 2000, malignant tumours were responsible for 12% of the nearly 56 million deaths worldwide from all causes. In many countries, more than a quarter of deaths are attributable to cancer. In 2000, 5.3 million men and 4.7 million women developed a malignant tumour and altogether 6.2 million died from the disease. Cancer has now emerged as a major public health problem in developing countries, matching its effect in industrialized nations.

Cancer rates could further increase by 50% from 10 million new cases globally in 2000 to 15 million new cases in the year 2020. This increase will mainly be due to steadily ageing populations in both developed and developing countries and also to current trends in smoking prevalence and the growing adoption of unhealthy lifestyles. However, there is clear evidence that healthy lifestyles and public health action by governments and health practitioners could stem this trend, and prevent as many as one third of cancers worldwide.

Lung cancer is the most common cancer worldwide, accounting for 1.2 million new cases annually; followed by cancer of the breast, just over 1 million cases; colorectal, 940 000; stomach, 870 000; liver, 560 000; cervical, 470 000; oesophageal, 410 000; head and neck, 390 000; bladder, 330 000; malignant non-Hodgkin's lymphomas, 290 000; leukaemia, 250 000; prostate and testicular, 250 000; pancreatic, 216 000; ovarian, 190 000; kidney, 190 000; endometrial, 188 000; nervous system, 175 000; melanoma, 133 000; thyroid, 123 000; pharynx, 65 000; and Hodgkin's disease, 62 000 cases.

In developed countries, the probability of being diagnosed with cancer is more than twice as high as in developing countries. However, in rich countries, some 50% of cancer patients die of the disease while, in developing countries, 80% of cancer victims already have late-stage incurable tumours when they are diagnosed, pointing to the need for much better detection programmes. The main reasons for the greater cancer burden of affluent societies are the earlier onset of the tobacco epidemic, the earlier exposure to occupational carcinogens, and the Western nutrition and lifestyle. However, with increasing wealth and industrialization, many countries undergo rapid lifestyle changes that will greatly increase their future disease burden.

CANCER IN THE USA

Cancer, after heart disease, is the second leading cause of death. One of every four deaths in the USA is due to cancer. It is estimated that, in 2003, 1.33 million Americans would receive a new diagnosis of invasive cancer (excluding basal and squamous cell skin cancers) and over 0.5 million Americans will die of this disease. The most common cancers among men were prostate, lung and colorectal and among women were breast, lung and colorectal. For both sexes, these cancers made up over 50% of the new cases diagnosed in 2000. Age-adjusted incidence rates for all cancer sites combined were essentially stable from 1995 through to 2000 with increases in breast cancer among women and prostate cancer in men being offset by long-term decreases in lung cancer among men.

The four most common cancer killers – lung, breast, prostate and colorectal – all declined in the late 1990s. The steep decline in lung cancer rates in men and the recent slowing of an increase in rates in women are steps in the right direction and further progress will require rigorous application of strategies known to be effective in reducing tobacco use. Death rates from breast cancer are falling despite a gradual, long-term increase in the rate of new diagnoses. This has been attributed to the successful implementation of more effective adjuvant treatment and the increased use of mammography screening. However, higher rates of late-stage disease exist in some population groups such as women who lacked health insurance and recent immigrants.

Prostate cancer death rates have been declining since 1994, while incidence rates have increased dramatically since this time. Much of the increase is due to the wider use of prostate specific antigen (PSA) screening rather than a major increase in symptomatic disease. Colorectal cancer death rates have been declining since the 1970s with steeper declines beginning in the mid-1980s. This is probably due to improving surgical techniques and, more recently, the introduction of adjuvant treatment regimens.

Cancer in Europe

The International Agency for Research on Cancer has recently produced estimates of the number of new cancers developing and the number of deaths due to cancer which are likely to have occurred in 2004. Of an estimated total of 2 886 800 incident cases of cancer (excluding non-melanoma skin), the most common forms were lung (381 500 cases), colorectal (376 400 cases) and breast (370 100 cases). Among men, the top five cancers were lung, prostate, colorectal, bladder and stomach. Among women, the most common cancers were breast, colorectal, lung, endometrium and ovary. In terms of mortality, it is estimated there were 1 711 000 cancer deaths, with the main causes being lung (341 800 deaths), colorectal (203 700 deaths), stomach (137 900 deaths) and breast (129 900 deaths). With nearly 3 million new cancers and 1.75 million deaths each year, cancer remains one of the most important public health problems in Europe. As the European population ages, these numbers will increase even if the age-specific rates remain constant. Lung, colorectal, stomach and breast cancers account for nearly half of all cancer deaths in Europe and point very clearly to the priorities for cancer control action.

While many countries, particularly in the European Union, have seen falls in the age-standardized mortality rates for cancer over the past 20 years, there are a few notable exceptions (Greece, Spain, Portugal). Many of the countries from Central and Eastern Europe exhibit increasing trends with lung cancer a particular problem.

EPIDEMIOLOGY OF CANCER

Terminology

Epidemiology is the study of the occurrence, distribution and causes of disease. It can be divided into three main components – descriptive, analytical and experimental.

Descriptive epidemiology is concerned with the variation in frequency (incidence or mortality) of a disease over space, time and in relation to age, sex and socioeconomic status. *Analytical epidemiology* is the study of the relationship between potentially causal risk factors (e.g. cigarette smoking, asbestos, ionizing radiation) or their proxies and the development of disease. *Experimental epidemiology* involves observing the effects of controlling relevant adverse risk factors (e.g. stopping cigarette smoking) or promoting possible preventative factors (e.g. beta-carotene).

The *incidence rate* of any disease is the total number of new cases occurring over a given period of time (a year) among a given number of people (usually 100 000 for cancer). This is different from the *prevalence rate*, which is the number of cases of a particular disease alive at a given point in time. This should be qualified by a statement as to how far back in time cancer patients are considered to be at risk from their disease – this is often taken as referring to cancers diagnosed within the previous 5 years. The *mortality rate* is the number of deaths attributed to the cancer in a given period of time (a year) among a given number of people (usually 100 000 for cancer).

Crude incidence or death rates are defined as the *total* number of cancers or deaths divided by the *total* population. Crude rates are of limited value since they do not take account of the differing proportions of people in particular age groups between populations. The crude rate in a particular population may exceed that of another country simply because it contains a higher proportion of elderly people. The *age-standardized incidence or death rate* takes account of the effect of age distribution on rates by attributing a weighting system to each of the age-specific rates. A choice of weighting systems exists – the two most common are the *world standardized population* and the *European standardized population*. When comparing cancer incidence rates in countries with very different proportions of elderly people (e.g. those in the developing world versus those in the developed world), the world standard is recommended. This is known as the world standardized rate (WSR). For comparison of countries with more similar proportions of elderly people, the European Standard is preferable. This is known as the European standardized rate (ESR).

An alternative method of expressing relative incidence or mortality is known as the *standardized incidence ratio (SIR) or the standardized mortality ratio (SMR)*. This is an overall measure of incidence (mortality) which compares the observed number of cases (deaths) in a particular population with the expected number of cases (deaths) that would have been anticipated in a standard population (e.g. national) if the age-specific incidence (death) rates were the same. This is usually expressed as a ratio of 100 if the observed and expected rates are the same, and greater than 100 if the rate in the population of interest is higher than that for the standard (national) rate. SIRs are useful in comparing cancer incidence between socioeconomic or particular occupational groups.

SURVIVAL AND CURE IN CANCER

What do we mean by 'cure' for a cancer patient? Technically, it is when the survival for that patient is the same as that for the general population from which they originate – their 'excess' risk of death becomes zero. Thus, it makes sense to talk of 'cure' of, for example, a small basal cell carcinoma treated by surgery or radiotherapy where recurrence or persistent disease is uncommon. However, for other cancers, particularly breast cancer, the possibility of local or distant recurrence remains for many years after the tumour has been 'successfully' removed surgically. This likelihood increases substantially for larger tumours with nodal involvement and adverse histological features. Thus, *survival rates* are quoted as a measure of success but should be qualified by the length of follow up – usually 5 years.

Five-year survival is often interpreted as 'cure'. While this is true of many tumours, it is not true of breast cancer, as suggested above. For breast cancer, 10-, 20- or even 30-year survival figures are more appropriate end-points because of the long-term pattern of relapse and death from the disease. Survival may be with or without evidence of cancer. For this reason, the terms *disease-free survival* or *recurrence-free survival* are commonly used to define the outcome of treatment. These results require an elaborate system of clinic follow up. Yet, it is only from painstaking analysis of this kind that we can derive a sound knowledge of both the natural history of cancer and the effects of treatment. Survival data are commonly presented plotted graphically as curves which allow the comparison of different treatments for different stages of disease over time.

In studies of patients treated for cancer, a variety of ways is used for describing their survival. *Crude survival rate* refers to the percentage of patients alive a given number of years (n) after treatment. This is not valid unless all the patients included have been followed up for at least n years. More often, a sizeable proportion of patients have been followed up for a shorter time than n years, and the *life table or Kaplan-Meier method* is more appropriate. This method uses information from all the patients for the time intervals for which they have been followed. Thus, someone who has been in the study for 1 year will contribute to the first year survival estimate, those in for 2 years will contribute to the first and second year survival estimates, and so on. There is an underlying assumption that all patients are subject to the same time-specific probability of dying from a particular cancer whether or not they have been followed for all or part of the follow-up period of study. This method can be used for calculating survival rates for all causes of death (*overall survival rate*) or for a specific type of cancer (*cancer-specific survival rate*). Patients who die from causes other than cancer of interest (i.e. from intercurrent disease) are considered to have been withdrawn from the study at the point in time that their death occurred.

An alternative method for dealing with the problem of intercurrent deaths or mortality from natural causes of the patients studied is to introduce an age correction (*age-corrected survival rate*), which adjusts for the fact that some deaths would be expected in the cohort normally, and that this will vary with age and sex. Thus, the age-corrected survival rate enables direct comparisons between cohorts of patients with different age and sex distributions.

Outcome of palliative care

Survival figures are essential for estimating the success of treatment aimed at cure but are of limited value in assessing the effects of palliative treatment. The main aim of palliative treatment is the relief of distressing symptoms. Palliative radiotherapy or chemotherapy may sometimes restrain tumour growth sufficiently to prolong the patient's life for a few months or sometimes years. In this case, a better measure of survival would be the *median survival time*. This is calculated by ranking the survival times in ascending order and choosing the middle value. It is subject to the proviso that all survival times for patients still alive, which are less than the middle value, are excluded and the median recalculated.

EPIDEMIOLOGY AND THE PREVENTION OF CANCER

The principal role of epidemiological studies in cancer has been the identification of risk factors, the assessment of their likelihood of being causative agents and, ultimately, whether their avoidance offers a practical solution for reducing the cancer burden. Most of the research effort has been directed at identifying factors associated with an increased risk of cancer but it is equally legitimate to try to identify factors which are associated with a decrease in risk. One, often misunderstood concept, particularly by the general media, is that the findings of epidemiological studies are indicative of causal effects. In fact, epidemiological studies will only ever identify associations.

Criteria for causality

After individual epidemiological studies of cancer have been summarized and the quality assessed, a judgment is made concerning the strength of evidence that the agent or exposure in question is carcinogenic for humans. Several criteria are considered:

- a strong association (a large relative risk) is more likely to indicate causality than a weak one
- associations that are replicated in several studies of the same design or using different epidemiological approaches or under different circumstances of exposure are more likely to represent a causal

relationship than isolated observations from single studies
- if the risk of the disease increases with the amount of exposure, this is considered to be a strong indication of causality
- demonstration of a decline in risk after cessation of or reduction in exposure in individuals or in whole populations also supports a causal interpretation
- although a carcinogen may act upon more than one target organ, the specificity of an association (an increased occurrence of cancer at one anatomical site or of one morphological type) adds plausibility to a causal relationship
- where an increase in exposure in a population and an increase in the incidence of a cancer are apparent, there must be a sensible latency (20+ years for solid tumours, 3+ years for blood-borne cancers) between the timings of the two increases
- there is evidence from animal models of a link between the exposure and the occurrence of the cancer
- there is a biological mechanism in humans for a link between the exposure and the cancer
- bias and confounding can be ruled out as possible explanations for the association.

It is not necessary for all of these criteria to hold for a judgment to be made that causality exists.

One current area of controversy that currently concerns public health is the impact of chronic low levels of exposure of known carcinogens. Two examples would be the impact of ionizing radiation to the general population and leukaemia risk, and the effect of inhaling second-hand tobacco smoke among non-smokers and lung cancer risk. In both cases, the first criterion listed above would not be expected to hold – the relative risks are likely to be low because the level of exposure is (relatively) low. In these circumstances, a more appropriate interpretation would be that the level of risk should be compatible with an acceptable extrapolation from the dose–response relationship observed for higher levels of exposure.

Such studies have played a major role in establishing occupational hazards in several industries (e.g. bladder cancer in aniline dye workers) and the link between lung cancer and smoking.

Epidemiology can assist in the prevention of cancer in a number of ways. First, it can show differences in the incidence of cancer in different populations and correlate them with differences in the prevalence of a potential causal factor. Secondly, it can test a hypothesis about the relationship between the occurrence of the disease to an aspect of the affected individual's constitution or exposure to some environmental factor. Thirdly, it can test the validity of a causal relationship by seeing whether the disease can be prevented or its incidence reduced by changing the prevalence of the suspected agent. A good example of the latter is the reduction in lung cancer observed among doctors since they gave up smoking cigarettes.

AETIOLOGY

Lung cancer

Tobacco

Lung cancer is currently still the largest single cause of death from any cancer in the world as well as being the most common incident cancer (excluding non-melanoma skin cancer). However, it was a rare disease at the start of the 20th century, but exposures to new etiological agents, particularly tobacco, and an increasing lifespan led to enormous increases in numbers of cases. While tobacco had been used throughout the world for many centuries, the 20th century pandemic was a result of the introduction of manufactured cigarettes on a mass scale. Its addictive properties led to sustained exposure of inhaled carcinogens. Scientists in Nazi Germany conducted some of the earliest research on the links between smoking and lung cancer, but their results were generally dismissed as propaganda. In the early 1950s, case-control studies in Britain and the USA suggested a strong association. Three major cohort studies were initiated at that time – UK doctors, US veterans and the American Cancer Society volunteers – and their findings corroborated the earlier observations as well as identifying other cancers and causes of death as also being strongly linked to cigarette smoking. For a smoker, lung cancer risk is related to cigarette smoking in accordance with the basic principles of chemical carcinogenesis. Risk is determined by the number of cigarettes smoked (dose), the number of years of smoking (duration) and the intensity of exposure (inhalation, tar levels). After taking these factors into account, women are at least as susceptible as men. An increase in risk of lung cancer (relative to a non-smoker) is consistently evident at the lowest level of daily consumption, and is at least linearly related to increasing consumption.

Doll et al reported on 50 years' worth of observations of the UK doctors study initiated in 1951. It is only now that the emergence of the full hazards for persistent smokers can be gagged as it requires a study of men whose cigarette consumption as young adults was already substantial when those who are now old were young. Men born in the 1920s in the UK may well have had the most intense early exposure as widespread military conscription of 18-year-old men, which began in 1939 and continued for decades, routinely included provision of low cost cigarettes to the conscripts. The (relative) risks of lung cancer for all levels of smoking range from 7.5 for light smokers (<15/day) to 25.4 for heavy smokers (≥25/day) as compared with lifelong non-smokers. These levels of risk are higher than previously observed, highlighting the fact that earlier analyses have underestimated the full effect of persistent cigarette smoking.

The introduction of lower tar cigarettes was one mechanism by which it was hoped to reduce the risk of lung cancer. In practice, the reduction in risk has been far less than might be have been expected on the basis of reduced exposure and, in a recent analysis of the American Cancer Society cancer prevention study II, there was no difference in risk for men or women who smoked brands rated as very low (≤7 mg tar/cigarette) or low (8–14 mg) compared with those who smoked medium tar (15–21 mg) brands. There was an increase in risk for those who smoked high tar (≥22 mg) brands, these tended to be non-filter brands. The explanation for this phenomenon is described as 'compensatory' smoking. Addicted smokers who switch from a higher to lower tar cigarette can maintain their nicotine intake by blocking ventilation holes, increasing the puff volume or the time during which the smoke is retained in the lungs. As a result, the actual dose of toxicants to the smoker may be higher than is predicted by machine-measured yields. Thus, reducing the use of higher tar cigarettes will provide limited public health benefits.

Smoking cessation is by far the most effective means of reducing the risk of lung cancer among active smokers. There is a steady upward trend in lung cancer risk between lifelong non-smokers, those stopping between the ages of 25 and 34 years, 35–44 years, 45–54 years, 55–64 years and continuing smokers. Thus, there is substantial protection even for those who stop at 55–64 years, and progressively greater protection for those who stop earlier, up to as much as a 90% reduction in those stopping between 25 and 34 years.

On a global scale, the rise in cigarette consumption in developing countries such as China and India is alarming. Going on the current worldwide smoking patterns, whereby about 30% of young adults become smokers, there will be about 7 million lung cancer deaths worldwide unless there is widespread cessation. Convincing the next generation not to start smoking remains a major public health imperative.

Involuntary smoking

The question as to whether involuntary smoking poses a significant risk of lung cancer has received considerable scientific interest since 1980. Involuntary (or passive) smoking is exposure to second-hand tobacco smoke, which is a mixture of exhaled mainstream smoke and side stream smoke released from the smouldering cigarette and diluted with ambient air. Involuntary smoking involves exposure to the same numerous carcinogens and toxic substances that are present in tobacco smoke produced by active smoking, which is the principal cause of lung cancer. This implies that there will be some risk of lung cancer from exposure to second-hand tobacco smoke.

More than 50 studies, based on over 7300 non-smoking lung cancer cases, have examined the association between involuntary smoking and the risk of lung cancer in never-smokers, especially spouses of smokers, from many countries during the last 25 years. Most showed an increased risk, especially for persons with higher exposures. To evaluate the information collectively, in particular from those studies with a limited number of cases, meta-analyses have been conducted. The excess risk of lung cancer has been identified as being of the order of 24% and this excess could not be explained by chance, potential biases or confounding. Moreover, a recent international working group of 29 experts convened by the IARC Monograph Program concluded that second-hand smoke is carcinogenic to humans.

Interestingly, an association has also been shown between exposure to environmental tobacco smoke (ETS) in infancy and risk of lung cancer in adulthood among 60, 182 lifelong non-smokers who participated in the EPIC (European Prospective Investigation into Cancer and Nutrition) study.

With passive smoking now implicated as a cause of lung cancer as well as being a contributing factor in increasing coronary heart disease, the emphasis has now moved to what action public health policy makers should advocate and what legislation government should enact. The whole of the UK and Ireland have imposed bans on smoking in enclosed workspaces to protect the health of workers and a number of other countries are actively considering or recommending legislation. One of the additional benefits of such restrictions has been a reduction in the rate of 'active' smoking among the population at large.

Asbestos

It has been known for many years that exposure to asbestos is a major cause of lung cancer. In 1999, a meta-analysis of 69 cohort studies found a standardized mortality ratio (SMR) of 163 for lung cancer, but a substantial heterogeneity existed largely attributable to the different cumulative exposure to asbestos in various cohorts. These cohorts comprised workers from a variety of industries – mining, textile and manufacturing, insulation, asbestos-cement factories and shipyards – and risk was closely related to level of exposure in the different industries. Type of asbestos was also observed to be relevant, with chrysotile fibres being considered less carcinogenic than amphiboles.

Asbestos dust and cigarette smoke are both causes of lung cancer. What is less clear is the effect of the combination of the two carcinogenic agents. Initially, two hypotheses existed about the way asbestos and cigarette smoking interact. In one, it is assumed that asbestos produces the same additional risk in men who smoke cigarettes as in those who do not (additive hypothesis); in the other, it is assumed that asbestos produces an effect that is proportional to the effect of the other agent (multiplicative hypothesis). The additive hypothesis explains the data less well than the second, but the fit to the latter is not particularly convincing. Until recently, no other hypotheses have been considered even though the multiplicative hypothesis is just one of infinitely many putative forms of synergism.

One often quoted study by Hammond et al estimates relative risks of 1, 5, 11 and 53 for no asbestos exposure

and never smoked, asbestos exposed and never smoked, no asbestos exposure and ever smoked and exposed to both carcinogens. These results clearly favoured the multiplicative model but it has not proven to be generalizable to other studies. Indeed, a recent analysis of the Quebec chrysotile miners and millers cohort concluded that an additive model provided the best fit to their data but cautioned that there seems no good reason to believe that interactions should conform to any simple theory.

The situation with regard to mesothelioma is far simpler in that asbestos exposure is a causal factor but cigarette smoking is not. The disease is rapidly fatal, most of those affected dying within a year of diagnosis. There is a long latent period between first exposure to asbestos and diagnosis of mesothelioma that is seldom less than 15 years and often exceeds 60 years. In all, 85% of deaths are among men, and the risk is highest in occupations with substantial exposure to asbestos. Shipyard workers have been a particularly susceptible group in that considerable exposures were to be found during the 1940s, 1950s and into the 1960s when ships were being repaired and the merchant fleet was being rebuilt after the World War II. Incidence rates of mesothelioma in Clydebank, one of the main centres of shipbuilding in Scotland, reached such a peak in the early 1990s that it registered as the fourth most common male cancer in the local population.

While mesothelioma is almost exclusively due to inhalation of asbestos fibres, it is of note that, in specific areas of Turkey, a high incidence of mesothelioma has been observed in conjunction with environmental exposure to erionite. Erionite occurs as a fibrous component of some zeolite deposits and has been identified as a component of soil and building materials in these areas.

With asbestos clearly established as an occupational carcinogen, more interest surrounds the issue of whether 'domestic' or environmental exposure poses an increased risk. Domestic exposure and increased risk has been observed among the wives of South African Cape miners who brought home contaminated working clothes for cleaning. Air pollution from asbestos mines and factories does represent exposure. Fibre concentrations in the lungs of (non-mining) residents near the chrysotile mines in Quebec are up to 10 times higher than the average Canadian. The critical question is whether this level of exposure represents an increased risk of the disease. The answer to this question is almost certainly yes as there appears to be no evidence that a threshold level exists below which there is no (excess) risk of mesothelioma. There might exist a background level of mesothelioma occurring in the absence of exposure to asbestos, but there is no proof of this and this 'natural level' is probably lower than 1 case/million/year.

Radon

Underground miners exposed to radioactive radon and its decay products have been found to be at an increased risk of lung cancer. Indoor exposure to radon has been associated with a marginal increase in risk of lung cancer.

Chemoprevention

Chemoprevention is defined as the reduction of the risk of cancer development through the use of pharmaceuticals or micronutrients. There has been consistent evidence that high intake of fruit and vegetables is associated with some reduction in risk of lung cancer. Thus, it has been suggested that micronutrients and macronutrients present in our diet may act as cancer inhibiting substances. Epidemiological studies have verified that B-carotene is inversely related to lung cancer risk and a number of randomized controlled intervention trials have been undertaken. The settings have varied but the largest trials have targeted high-risk smokers (ATBC study, Physicians Health Study) or asbestos workers (CARET study). None of these trials showed a reduction in lung cancer incidence or mortality, and two of them even suggested an increased risk, albeit small. Clearly, our understanding of the mechanism by which relatively short-term intake of retinoids and carotenoids affects the development of cancer in large populations is insufficient to use this approach as a specific lung cancer control procedure.

Colon cancer

Incidence rates for cancer of the colon vary greatly across the world. High rates are found in some states in the USA, Australia and Argentina. Incidence rates in northern and western Europe are generally somewhat lower. In developing countries, incidence rates are substantially lower. Studies of migrants suggest that environmental factors rather than ethnic or genetic factors play a major role in its aetiology. Most studies have involved migrants moving from low-risk to high-risk areas, such as Chinese and Japanese to Hawaii or the rest of the USA, or southern Europeans to North America or Australia. In general, the risk in migrants approximates that of the new country with rates increasing with increasing duration of stay, presumably as their lifestyles merge with that of the host country.

Over time, the incidence of colon cancer has been rising, slowly in high-risk areas but more rapidly in areas where the risk was formerly low. These changes have been accompanied by changing ratios between the subsites within the colon at which tumours occur, with left-sided tumours (of the descending and sigmoid colon) becoming more frequent.

Risk of colon cancer is closely related to diet and other lifestyle factors. International comparisons have suggested increased risks with increased intakes of dietary fat and a decreased intake of cereal grains and dietary fibre. Analytical studies within populations have shown a deficiency of vegetables and fruits and a sedentary lifestyle as being associated with an increased risk. However, attempts to identify independent roles for specific macronutrients have proved unsuccessful, with the exception of over-consumption of

energy. Thus, dietary associations with colon cancer are characterized as typical of the 'western' diet, without being able to tie in any specific components. The recurring problem has been to explain the association of colon cancer with a disparate group of dietary and lifestyle factors.

More recently, epidemiological studies have started to demonstrate a close association between colon cancer risk and evidence of insulin resistance. Insulin resistance is a condition in which higher levels of insulin are needed to dispose of plasma glucose, and it is associated with an increased risk of type 2 diabetes. The mechanism begins with the excess dietary energy provided by the high-risk diet. This excess energy elevates the intravascular levels of insulin and energy substrates. The excess hormone exposure and excess energy available to epithelial cells stimulate cell signalling pathways to increase the proliferation, presumably favouring cells with defective cell cycle control.

Also, agents are now being identified that significantly inhibit experimental colon carcinogenesis. The following mechanism has been proposed: focal loss of epithelial barrier function resulting from a failure of terminal differentiation results in the leak of an undefined toxin and a local inflammatory response characterized by evidence of the activation of the COX-2 enzyme and an oxidative stress with the release of reactive oxygen intermediates. The resulting focal proliferation and mutagenesis give rise to aberrant crypt foci and adenomas.

These two mechanisms, insulin resistance acting throughout the body and focal epithelial barrier failure acting locally, can describe most of the known relationships between diet and colon cancer risk.

While the vast majority of colon cancer cases occur 'sporadically' in the general population, a number of specific disease groups – Crohn's disease, ulcerative colitis and familial polyposis – are subject to increased risks. For example, colorectal cancer in ulcerative colitis only accounts for 1% of all colorectal cancer cases, it accounts for one-sixth of all deaths in ulcerative colitis patients. The overall prevalence of colorectal cancer in any ulcerative colitis patient is estimated to be 3.7%. However, there is general agreement that the colorectal cancer risk is highest in those with extensive disease of long duration. Overall, incidence rates build to cumulative probabilities of 2% by 10 years, 8% by 20 years and 18% by 30 years.

Screening

Colorectal cancer is one of the few internal cancers that are amenable to secondary prevention, that is, prevention by detection of preclinical lesions. The precursor of advanced colorectal cancer is either an adenomatous polyp or a flat neoplastic area. In order to prevent premature death, people aged 50–69 years are the main focus of attention.

Screening by the fecal occult blood test (FOBT) is currently considered the optimal screening strategy in terms of cost-effectiveness. FOBT identifies persons at risk, though falling short of being definite for cancer. In general, the test is positive in about 2% of those screened. The sensitivity of the test is around 50% for cancer (i.e. of all screened persons who have cancer, 50% will be detected) and around 10% for polyps. The predictive value of a positive test is around 10% (i.e. out of 10 persons with a positive test, only one will have cancer).

Endoscopy, using either the flexible sigmoidoscope or the colonoscope is the most definitive means of detection but has limitations. The major weakness is the limited reach of the former (somewhere between the sigmoid colon and the splenic flexure). The colonoscope permits exploration of the colon with a low false negative rate for polypoid lesions of at least 10 mm in diameter. However, patient compliance is poor, the cost of the procedure is high and perforation is an acknowledged morbidity which, although uncommon, may be of consequence in large series.

FOBT has been assessed in randomized trials. In two European, population-based, trials conducted in the UK and Denmark with a biennial non-rehydrated FOBT, the compliance was about 60%, about 4% of individuals tested underwent colonoscopy and the reduction in mortality was about 15%. Screening by sigmoidoscopy has been evaluated in case-control studies. Less compliance has been observed but a higher yield of detection with mortality reductions of up to 50% being claimed with good compliance.

Options for population based screening in countries with high rates of colorectal cancer include: annual FOBT, biennial FOBT, annual FOBT + sigmoidoscopy every 5 years, sigmoidoscopy every 5 years, colonoscopy every 10 years, and colonoscopy once in a lifetime. Cost and compliance will be the major determining factors.

Breast

The majority of cancers exhibit a consistently increasing rise in incidence rates with age. Breast cancer is one of a number which do not adhere to this rule, highlighting the fact that the frequency of a disease is a function of duration of exposure rather than age per se. Among pre-menopausal women, incidence rates steeply with age. For those women in their fifties, the incidence rate remains relatively steady (sometimes referred to as Clemmensen's hook) and thereafter starts to rise again but at a much less steep gradient than is observed for pre-menopausal women. The examination of the shape of age-specific incidence curves can give indications as to causal factors, particularly those that change over a person's lifetime, such as hormonal factors. Thus, for breast cancer it would seem to indicate that the factors related to pre-menopausal breast cancer may well be different to those which cause post-menopausal breast cancer. Add to this the observation that the incidence of pre-menopausal breast cancer has remained stable over time while post-menopausal breast cancer rates have been slowly, but steadily increasing over

time and it may well be that pre-menopausal and post-menopausal breast cancer should be considered as two separate diseases in etiological terms.

Reproductive factors have been consistently related to (post-menopausal) breast cancer in that early age at first full-term pregnancy and high parity are associated with lower levels of the disease. Furthermore, risk is increased in women who have early menarche or who have late menopause. Obesity, related to various alterations in plasma levels of total and bioavailable sex steroids, is also a strong risk factor. As circulating levels of sex steroids are regulated by a range of factors, including insulin and insulin-like growth factors, this may provide the link between many observations regarding excessive energy intake and increased risk of cancer.

The 'oestrogen excess' hypothesis stipulates that risk depends directly on breast tissue exposure to oestrogens. Oestrogens increase breast cell proliferation and inhibit apoptosis in vitro and, in experimental animals, cause increased rates of tumour development when oestrogens are administered. This theory is consistent with the epidemiological evidence showing an increase in breast cancer risk in post-menopausal women who have low circulating sex hormone-binding globulin and elevated total and bioavailable oestradiol.

Two developments in the second half of the 20th century, the oral contraceptive pill and hormone replacement therapy (HRT), have impacted on the risk of breast cancer. Oral contraceptives, in the form of oestrogen–progestogen combinations, were introduced in the early 1960s and rapidly found widespread use in most developed countries. Preparations of oral contraceptives have undergone substantial changes over time, reducing the potency of the oestrogens, adding in different progestogens and using biphasic and triphasic pills. A small increase in risk has been observed in current and recent users of combined oral contraceptives (a relative risk of about 1.2), but this association is unrelated to duration of use or type and dose of preparation, and 10 years after cessation of use, the excess risk disappears. Causation has not been clearly established and one suggestion has been that it could be the result of detection bias due to the increased attention to the occurrence of breast abnormalities in women regularly visiting their doctor for contraceptive prescriptions.

HRT is used to treat the symptoms of menopause and, during the 1990s, up to one-third of all menopausal women in the USA and many European countries used HRT for some period. A small increase in breast cancer risk is correlated with longer duration of oestrogen replacement therapy use in current and recent users. The increase seems to cease several years after use has stopped. Initially, there appeared to be no difference in breast cancer risk between long-term users of all hormone replacement therapy and users of oestrogens alone, although two recent studies have suggested that HRT may pose a greater risk than oestrogens alone.

A second 'oestrogen–progestogen' hypothesis postulates that compared to an exposure to oestrogens alone (as in post-menopausal women not using any exogenous hormones), risk of breast cancer is increased further in women who have elevated plasma and tissue levels of oestrogens in combination with progestogens. This theory is supported by observations that post-menopausal women using oestrogen-plus-progestogen preparations for HRT have a greater increase in risk than women using oestrogens alone.

Screening

No practical strategies exist which can be recommended for the prevention of breast cancer and so considerable effort has been aimed at developing methods of early detection. Mammography can detect preclinical cancer, that is, before it is palpable or before it causes symptoms. Tumours detected and treated at an early stage would be expected to be associated with a better survival rate than those detected symptomatically. However, as some breast cancers are characterized by early systemic dissemination, the actual effectiveness of screening is not at all clear. In this context, a number of large randomized trials were undertaken to evaluate its effectiveness on a population basis. The analysis of these trials has shown that in women aged 50 to 69 years, mammography screening can reduce mortality from breast cancer by 25–30%. For women in the age group 40–49 years, screening efficacy is significantly less.

The only true measure of success of a screening programme is an associated reduction in mortality. Survival rates can theoretically improve without extending length of life by the simple expedient of bringing forward the date of diagnosis while the date of death remains the same. This is known as lead-time bias. Analysis of trial data suggests that screening brings forward the date of diagnosis by an average of about 3 years, but this will vary considerably on an individual basis depending on how long the tumour remains in the 'screen-detectable' phase. This raises a second phenomenon known as length-time bias. The argument is based on the well-founded assumption that tumours grow at varying speeds in different women. Slow-growing tumours will therefore remain in the 'screen-detectable' window for longer than fast-growing tumours. Hence, a screening programme will tend to pick up slow-growing tumours disproportionately more than fast-growing tumours. If slow-growing tumours are also more amenable to cure then survival rates will tend to be artificially inflated as they will tend to include a larger proportion of better prognosis tumours.

A sizeable number of developed countries have now established national or subnational screening programmes. Eligible age ranges vary, the repeat interval varies, some use single view mammography, others use two view and independent double reading of mammograms is recommended but not always adhered to. One of the 'side effects' of the introduction of national breast screening programmes has been the necessity to overhaul the referral and management pathway for breast cancer generally. Now, designated surgical units provide specialist expertise to manage breast cancer, particularly those women with impalpable tumours, and pathologists and oncologists with a special interest in breast cancer and clinical nurse specialists combine to form a multidisciplinary team for the management of the disease.

The effectiveness of routine national breast screening programmes has been questioned. There is general agreement that the extent of the reduction in mortality has been lower than that experienced in the trial situation. Under optimal conditions with a high compliance rate, a mortality reduction of 20% appears achievable. In reality, this may be more in the region of 10–15% on current data. One of the major problems in trying to assess the reduction in mortality due to screening now is that other factors have come into play, which were not operating at the time when the trials were being conducted. Before the late 1980s, no decline in mortality had been seen, but then a smooth downturn occurred in Europe, North America and Australia. These changes accelerated in the early 1990s but the fall occurred too soon after the widespread availability of mammography to be a consequence of it. More likely, the success of adjuvant therapy based on tamoxifen and chemotherapy was the major cause of this trend. Thus, the concurrent changes in improved adjuvant therapy, better and more focused surgical services, protocol driven management and a better awareness of breast cancer and its symptoms among the general population make it almost impossible to isolate the contribution that breast screening is now making. However, there is no denying the fact that more women are being diagnosed with smaller tumours and consequently can safely be offered conservation surgery rather than radical mastectomy.

Stomach

On a global scale, mortality from stomach cancer is second only to lung cancer. The areas with the highest incidence rates are in Eastern Asia, the Andean regions of South America and Eastern Europe. There is marked geographical variation in incidence between countries and among different ethnic groups within the same locale. Migration studies show that the risk of cancer changes within two generations when people move from high-incidence to low-incidence areas. For example, Japanese immigrants to the USA retain their original risk, whereas subsequent generations share the incidence of the host country. No matter what level of incidence, there has been a general decline worldwide. In most European countries, it has fallen by more than 60% during the past 50 years.

Dietary risk factors include inadequate intake of fresh fruits and vegetables, high salt intake and consumption of smoked or cured meats or fish. There is good evidence that refrigeration of food also protects against this cancer by facilitating year-round consumption of fruit and vegetables and probably by reducing the need for salt as a preservative. Vitamin C, contained in vegetables and fruits and other foods of plant origin, is probably protective and so too are diets high in whole-grain cereals, carotenoids and allium compounds.

Conditions that cause an excessive rate of cell proliferation in the gastric epithelium, thus increasing the chance of fixation of replication errors induced by dietary and endogenous carcinogens, include *Helicobacter pylori* infection, gastric ulcer, atrophic gastritis and autoimmune gastritis associated with pernicious anaemia. Gastritis is associated with increased production of oxidants and reactive nitrogen intermediates, including nitric oxide. There is increased expression of the inducible isoform of nitric oxide synthase in gastritis. Gastritis and atrophy alter gastric acid secretion, elevating gastric pH, changing the gastric flora and allowing anaerobic bacteria to colonize the stomach.

Screening

About 80% of western patients with stomach cancer present with advanced tumours. Screening for early disease by x-ray (photofluoroscopy), followed by gastroscopy and biopsy of suspicious findings, has been widely used in Japan since the 1960s. It is a costly approach to prevention and the results have been controversial. With the background incidence now falling substantially, screening has not been considered as a national priority in most other countries.

Prostate

Prostate cancer is the third most common cancer in men in the world. In the majority of developed and developing countries, prostate cancer is the most commonly diagnosed neoplasm affecting men beyond middle age. In recent times, incidence rates of prostate cancer have been influenced by the diagnosis of latent cancers whose presence has been suggested by screening of asymptomatic individuals. In the USA, for example, the introduction of screening using prostate-specific antigen (PSA) testing has led to an enormous increase in the diagnosis of prostate cancer, making it by far the most commonly diagnosed cancer in men.

The distribution of mortality rates is less affected than incidence by the effects of early diagnosis of asymptomatic cancers and is thus a more reliable way of comparing rates of the disease. High rates are found in North America, northern and western Europe, Australia/New Zealand and the Caribbean. The difference between China and the USA is 26-fold and, within the USA, black populations have higher rates than white, who in turn have rates considerably higher than populations of Asian origin.

The causes of prostate cancer are not well understood. Development of this malignancy is a multistep process associated with a long natural history. The initiation of preneoplastic lesions and microscopic cancer is probably influenced by environmental factors which implies a case for lifestyle causes and primary prevention. The strong association of race, familial and geographic patterns and the weak link

of many of the risk factors proposed suggests a significant role for genetic–environmental interactions in determining patterns of disease. The role of hormones, particularly androgens, is obviously important given the impact of orchidectomy on progression. Genetic polymorphisms in the androgen receptor may be more important than any imbalance of hormones in the circulation. A diet characteristic of Asian countries, essentially a low fat intake with consequent low body weight and an intake of relatively high levels of phytoestrogens, may provide the means of restraining the growth and progression of prostate cancer. A strategy for prevention would be to increase the intake of phytoestrogens, essentially isoflavonoids, lignans and possibly certain flavonoids.

Screening

Secondary prevention of prostate cancer is feasible, but is subject to controversy, since the capacity to detect early disease must inevitably result in the overtreatment of some individuals with substantial costs to society in exchange for decreased mortality. PSA testing is widely used for the early detection of prostate cancer. Elevated levels of PSA are closely, but not definitely, associated with the presence of a tumour. Using a cut-off level of 4 ng/ml for normality, 25% of patients diagnosed with prostate cancer will have levels below this value. Of men with moderately raised levels (4–10 ng/ml) 25% will have cancer but this rises to 60% when PSA levels are greater than 10 ng/ml.

In order to improve the sensitivity of the PSA analysis, it should be combined with a digital rectal examination. This will provide an assessment of the volume of the gland since PSA is also released into the bloodstream of patients with benign prostate hyperplasia and other prostatic diseases. Additionally, different age-specific reference values for the 'cut-off' threshold are of value – 2.5 ng/ml for age group 40–49 years and 3.5 ng/ml for age group 50–59 years. Any patient who asks for a PSA test should be counselled about the risks and benefits in relation to the procedure and its outcome.

Some national authorities have recommended screening for the detection of prostate cancer, starting at the age of 50 for men with at least a 10-year life expectancy. A slight but definite decrease in mortality has been observed in countries where PSA has been widely used in screening different cohorts of men, although the reason for the decrease in mortality has become a major subject of controversy. The general expectation that the earlier detection of prostate cancer inevitably provides a unique chance for cure has to be balanced against the clear prevalence of overdiagnosing a disease which may never become symptomatic during a man's lifetime.

Ultimately, resolution of the true benefit of screening will only be achieved on the basis of the results of large randomized controlled trials. One such trial in Europe has recruited 180 000 men randomized between diagnosis and treatment in screened men versus controls. In the USA,

74 000 men have been enrolled in a trial of screening for prostate, colorectal and other cancers. Collaboration has led to the development of the International Prostate Screening Trial Evaluation Group which will provide a sound basis for the scientific evidence to decide on the merit of large population-based screening programmes.

Cervix

Cancer of the cervix is the second most common cancer among women worldwide with about 470 000 new cases diagnosed each year. Eighty percent of cases of cervical cancer occur in developing countries where, in many regions, it is the most common cancer of women. The highest incidence rates are in South America and the Caribbean, sub-Saharan Africa, and South and South-Eastern Asia.

Incidence and mortality have declined markedly in the last 40 years in western Europe, USA, Canada, Australia and New Zealand, mainly in relation to extensive screening programmes based on exfoliative cervical cytology, typically by means of the Pap smear. Nevertheless, in several countries, notably the UK, Australia, New Zealand, and in central Europe, there have been increases in risk in younger women, probably the result of changes in exposure to risk factors. These changes are most evident for adenocarcinomas, which share to some extent the same aetiological agents of squamous cell carcinomas, but for which cytological screening is ineffective in countering the increase in risk.

Molecular studies have shown that certain human papillomavirus (HPV) types are the central cause of cervical cancer and cervical intraepithelial neoplasia (CIN), the pre-invasive state. It is now clear that the well-established risk factors associated with sexual behaviour, such as multiple sexual partners and early age of starting sexual activity, simply reflect the probability of being infected with HPV. HPV DNA has been detected in virtually all cervical cancer specimens. The association of HPV with cervical cancer is equally strong for the two main histological types: squamous cell carcinoma and adenocarcinoma. Over 100 HPV types have been identified and about 40 can infect the genital tract. Fifteen of these have been classified as high-risk, three as probably high-risk and twelve as low-risk. However, since only a small fraction of HPV-infected women will eventually develop cervical cancer, there must be other exogenous or endogenous factors which, acting in conjunction with HPV, influence the progression from cervical infection to cervical cancer. In assessing of the role of these co-factors, it should be recognized that HPV is very much the dominant effect. Co-factors which have been identified as being associated with an increased risk include high parity, smoking and long-term use of oral contraceptives.

Screening

By far the best-established screening method for cervical cancer is the Papanicolaou ('Pap') smear. Population-based screening programmes using the Pap smear were initiated in British Columbia in 1949 and in regions of Norway in 1959 and Scotland in 1960. Since then, programmes based on the Pap smear have been introduced in many developed countries.

No randomized trials have ever been performed to assess the efficacy of such a method of cervical screening. The main evidence is indirect, being based on the trends in the incidence of, or mortality due to, cervical cancer in relation to screening intensity and the risk of cervical cancer in individuals in relation to their screening history. Nationwide programmes were established in Finland, Iceland and Sweden; in Denmark, programmes covered about 40% of the female population and in Norway only 5%. In Iceland, cervical cancer mortality fell by 80% between 1965 and 1982, compared with 50% in Finland, 34% in Sweden, 25% in Denmark and 10% in Norway. More recently, the effect of cytologic screening on the incidence of cervical cancer has been examined in 17 populations covered by cancer registries between the early 1960s and late 1980s. Compared with the time before the introduction of screening, the age standardized incidence rates decreased by at least 25% in 11 of the 17 populations, with the largest effect occurring in the 45–55 year age groups.

Oesophagus

Cancer of the oesophagus is the sixth most frequent cancer worldwide. About 412 000 new cases occur each year, of which over 80% are in developing countries. While squamous cell carcinomas occur at high frequency in many developing countries, adenocarcinomas are essentially a tumour of more developed, industrialized countries. Differences between the incidence of oesophageal cancer in distinct geographical areas are more extreme than observed for any other cancer. An 'oesophageal cancer belt' in Asia stretches from northern Iran through the central Asian republics to Henan province in north-central China. Incidence rates are as high as 200 per 100 000 per year and, in some areas, there is a female predominance. In Europe, high rates occur in Normandy and Brittany in France and in the north-east of Italy. In these areas, high rates occur specifically in males.

Consumption of tobacco and alcohol, associated with low intake of fresh fruit, vegetables and meat, is causally associated with squamous cell carcinoma of the oesophagus worldwide. In developed countries, about 90% of the squamous cell cancers are attributable to tobacco and alcohol, with a multiplicative increase in risk when individuals are exposed to both factors. Risk factors for oesophageal cancer in developing countries vary by region, with oral consumption of opium by-products an important factor in the Caspian Sea area, betel chewing in South-East Asia, drinking of scalding hot beverages, such as mate, in South America and environmental factors including nitrosamines, contamination with fungi and deficiency of vitamins A and C in parts of China.

Melanoma

There are about 133 000 new cases of melanoma worldwide each year, of which almost 80% are in North America, Europe, Australia and New Zealand. Incidence is similar in men and in women.

Malignant melanoma of the skin occurs predominantly in white-skinned populations ('Caucasians') living in countries where there is high intensity ultraviolet radiation, but this malignancy afflicts to some degree all ethnic groups. Assessed in relation to skin colour, melanoma incidence falls dramatically as skin pigmentation increases and the disease is very rare in dark-skinned people. The highest incidence of melanoma occurs in Australia where the population is predominantly white, there is an average of six hours of bright sunlight every day of the year and there is an essentially outdoors lifestyle. The lifetime risk of developing melanoma in Australia is 4–5% in men and 3–4% in women.

Dark-skinned people have a low risk of melanoma in Africa and South America, the sole of the foot, where the skin is not pigmented, is the most frequent site affected in the context of a low incidence. Asian peoples have a low risk of melanoma despite their paler skins; naevi in Asian people, though common, are predominantly of the acral-lentiginous type, which have low malignant potential. Marked increases in incidence and mortality are being observed in both sexes in many countries.

It is estimated that 80% of melanoma is caused by ultraviolet damage to sensitive skin, i.e. skin that burns easily, fair or reddish skin, multiple freckles, skin that does not tan and develops nevi in response to early sunlight exposure. Prevention of melanoma is based on limitation of exposure to ultraviolet radiation, particularly in the first 20 years of life.

Ultraviolet radiation is particularly hazardous when it involves sporadic intense exposure and sunburn. Most damage caused by sunlight occurs in childhood and adolescence, making this the most important target group for prevention programmes. Established but rare risk factors include congenital naevi, immunosuppression and excessive use of solaria. While melanoma may occur anywhere on the skin, the majority of melanoma in men is on the back, while in women the majority is on the legs. The difference in site incidence is not completely explained by differential exposure to ultraviolet light.

Head and neck

Cancers of the oral mucosa and oro- and hypopharynx can be considered together, as there are similarities in epidemiology, treatment and prognosis. The geographic patterns and trends in incidence for these cancers vary depending upon the anatomical subsites concerned, a phenomenon that is often explicable by the influence of risk factors, such as tobacco use and alcohol consumption. A high incidence of these cancers is observed in the Indian subcontinent,

Australia, France, South America (Brazil) and Southern Africa.

The highest incidence among males is reported in Bas-Rhin and Calvados in France, whereas among females the highest occurrence is observed in India. Cancers of the mouth and anterior two-thirds of the tongue generally predominate in developing countries, whereas pharyngeal cancers are common in developed countries and in Central and Eastern Europe.

Smoking and drinking are the major risk factors for head and neck cancer in developed countries, in the Caribbean and in South American countries. Smoking is estimated to be responsible for about 41% of laryngeal and oral/pharyngeal cancers in men, and 15% in women worldwide and these proportions vary among different populations. Tobacco smoking has also been found to be an important risk factor for nasopharyngeal cancer in otherwise low-risk populations. These risk factors have been shown, for laryngeal and oropharyngeal cancers, to have a joint 'multiplicative' or synergistic effect. In the Indian subcontinent, chewing tobacco in the form of betel quid (a combination of betel leaf, slaked lime, areca-nut and tobacco with or without other condiments), bide (a locally hand-rolled cigarette of dried temburni leaf containing coarse tobacco), smoking and drinking locally brewed crude alcoholic drinks are the major causative factors.

Reverse smoking (in which the lit end of the cigarette is placed in the mouth so that an intense heat is experienced) is a risk factor for cancer of the hard palate. Oral snuff use is an emerging risk factor for oral cancer, particularly among young males in the USA.

A generally impoverished diet, particularly lacking in vegetables and fruits, is another risk factor for oral cancer. Consistently, studies also indicate a protective effect of a diet rich in vegetables and fruits (20–60% reduction in risk). Oral human papillomavirus (HPV) infection (transmitted sexually or perinatally) is associated with an increased risk of head and neck squamous cell carcinoma development.

Infection with Epstein-Barr virus is important in the ateiology of nasopharyngeal cancer. This virus is not found in normal epithelial cells of the nasopharynx, but is present in all nasopharyngeal tumour cells, and even in dysplastic precursor lesions.

Lymphoma

Lymphoma covers a heterogeneous group of neoplasms of lymphoid tissue. Traditionally, lymphomas have been categorized as either Hodgkin's disease (HD) or non-Hodgkin's lymphoma (NHL), these distinct entities having different patterns of behaviour and response to treatment.

Geographically, NHL is most common in developed countries (52% of the total cases globally, and the seventh most common cancer in more developed countries), although in the developing world, there are areas of moderate to high incidence in some Middle-Eastern countries (Saudi Arabia, Israel) and in parts of sub-Saharan Africa. Much of the latter's high rate is due to the high incidence of Burkitt's lymphoma, an aggressive subtype of NHL.

NHL incidence rates have risen dramatically in the last 20 years, particularly in developed countries, including western Europe, North America and Australia. In part, this reflects better diagnosis and changing classification systems. However, this is by no means the complete explanation. Also, the fact that NHL is a complication of AIDS (occurring in up to 5–10% of AIDS cases in developed countries) does not completely account for the increasing trend. In contrast to incidence, mortality rates have, in general, been declining as a consequence of improvement in therapy.

In developed countries, HD incidence reaches a peak in young adults, whereas in developing countries, HD occurs mainly in children and in the elderly. In developed countries, incidence has fallen over the last 20 years.

Patients with HIV/AIDS or who have received immuno-suppressant therapy have a higher risk of developing NHL. Viral infection such as HIV-1, HTLV-1, and Epstein-Barr virus (EBV) are also associated with NHL. Infection of the stomach with *Helicobacter pylori* is associated with gastric lymphoma. There is also an increased risk of NHL among persons with a family history of lymphoma or haematological cancer.

A subtype of HD cases, the mixed cellularity type, has been linked to the EBV. Overall, around 45% of cases may be attributable to EBV. The presence of EBV in tumours seems also to be related to age and socioeconomic circumstances. EBV is involved in the aetiology of Burkitt's lymphoma, especially in cases in tropical Africa, where over 95% of tumours contain the virus. The proportion of EBV-positive tumours is much less in the sporadic cases of HD occurring in Europe and North America. The singular geographic distribution of Burkitt's lymphoma is not explicable on the basis of EBV alone, however, since infection by the virus is ubiquitous, suspicion has fallen upon intense malarial infection as predisposing to Burkitt's lymphoma in the presence of EBV infection. The risk of HD is also increased in patients with HIV infection.

Leukaemia

Leukaemias comprise about 3% of all incident cancers worldwide, with about 257 000 new cases occurring annually.

A relatively high incidence is evident in the USA, Canada, western Europe, Australia and New Zealand, while rates are generally low in most African and Asian countries with rates less than half those in the former group. The trends in overall incidence of leukaemia have generally been stable or slowly increasing. However, a substantial reduction in death rates from leukaemias, particularly in childhood, has been observed since the 1960s, thanks to advances in treatment and consequent improvement in survival.

Leukaemia has a peak in incidence in the first four years of life, which is predominantly due to acute lymphoblastic leukaemia (ALL), the most common paediatric malignancy, accounting for nearly 25% of all such disease. After infancy, there is a steep decline in rates of leukaemia with age, lowest incidence being at 15 to 25, after which there is an exponential rise up to age 85.

The usual form of the disease in adults is acute myeloid leukaemia (AML), accounting for 70% of all cases. The more differentiated, or chronic forms of leukaemia are predominantly adult diseases, rarely occurring below the age of 30, and then increasing progressively in incidence with age. Chronic myelogenous leukaemia (CML) accounts for 15–20% of all case of leukaemia. For patients over 50, chronic lymphocytic leukaemia (CLL) is the dominant type of leukaemia.

The cause of most leukaemias is not known. A range of risk factors has been predominantly, although not exclusively, associated with particular leukaemia subtypes. Ionizing radiation (nuclear bombs, medical procedures), and occupational exposure to benzene are associated with acute myeloid leukaemia.

Leukaemia (mainly acute myeloid) may occur in a small proportion of cancer patients treated with chlorambucil, cyclophosphamide, melphalan, thiotepa, treosulphan or etoposide, as well as certain combination chemotherapy. Leukaemia has followed induction of aplastic anaemia by the antibiotic, chloramphenicol. Certain risk factors, such as Down's syndrome, have been identified for childhood leukaemia but, generally, the causes of the disease are not known. Some studies have shown a risk of childhood leukaemia with exposure to high-level residential extremely low frequency electromagnetic fields, but causality has not been established.

Infection with the virus HTLV-1 has been established as a cause of leukaemia. This virus is responsible for adult T-cell leukaemia, a disease mainly observed in tropical countries and Japan, and rarely in the USA and Europe. In experimental animals, particularly in mice, there are many retroviruses, which can cause a variety of leukaemias, but such retroviruses have not been identified in humans.

REDUCING THE RISKS OF DEVELOPING CANCER

Based largely on our current knowledge of the aetiology of cancer, it has been estimated that 80% of malignancies are preventable. To put the environmental causes of cancer in perspective, their relative proportions have been summarized in Table 15.1. The striking feature is the high proportion due to dietary factors and to smoking (30% each). Changing dietary habits could potentially reduce the risk of cancer, possibly by a third. The main cancers involved are those of the stomach, colon and rectum, and breast.

Table 15.1 Major causes of cancer

FACTOR	AGENT	TYPE OF CANCER	RELATIVE CONTRIBUTION TO RISK
Tobacco	Polycyclic hydrocarbons e.g. benzopyrene Nitrosamines e.g. N-nitrodimethylamine volatile aldehydes, e.g. formaldehyde Metals, e.g. cadmium	Lung, larynx, oesophagus, pancreas Bladder	30%
Alcohol		Oral, pharynx, larynx, oesophagus and liver	1–4%
Interacting with tobacco smoke			up to 10%
Diet	Rich in animal fat and protein, low in fresh fruit and vegetables Obesity and sedentary lifestyle contributing factors	Colon, breast, prostate and endometrium	30%
Chronic infections			
Epstein-Barr virus (EBV)		Lymphoma and nasopharynx cancer	
Human papilloma virus (HPV)		Cervix and oropharynx	20%
Hepatitis B and C		Liver	
Schistosomiasis		Bladder	
Helicobacter pylori		Stomach	
Food contamination			
Aflatoxins		Liver	Varies up to 20% in hot/humid parts of the world
Pesticides		Pancreas, breast, lymphoma/leukaemia	
Pollution of air, water and soil	Arsenic in water Asbestos, specific Skin	Lung	Varies 1–4 %
Pollutants such as benzopyrene, engine exhaust Tobacco smoke		Bladder	
Medicinal drugs			
Hormones, cytotoxic chemotherapy		Kidney, bladder Leukaemia	
	Phenacetin	Uterus, breast	
Sunlight			
Ultraviolet radiation	Melanoma and non-melanomatory	Skin cancer	Up to 80% of all cases of melanoma
Occupation	See Table 15.2		4–5%
Ionizing radiation		See Table 15.3	

The EC has produced a 10-point code for the general public, summarizing the ways in which certain common cancers can be prevented.

Reducing tobacco smoking

Every country should give high priority to tobacco control in its fight against cancer. Unchecked, smoking will cause more than 10 million deaths from cancer (mostly lung cancer) in the next decade.

The UK Government has made health warnings mandatory on commercial tobacco products and on advertisements for tobacco. To achieve substantial reductions in tobacco consumption, additional measures will be required. These could include banning advertising of tobacco, its consumption in public places and working environments, increasing taxation on tobacco, reducing tar content in cigarettes and setting up clinics for smokers to help them break the habit.

There is a great need for effective and carefully evaluated school education programmes which include tobacco abstinence as a major goal.

Modifying alcohol consumption

After smoking, alcohol is the second most important cause of cancer. It may be responsible in some countries for up to 10% of deaths from cancer. Cancers of the mouth, larynx, pharynx, oesophagus and liver are certainly caused in part by alcohol. It probably has a role in the aetiology of some breast and rectal cancers. For several tumours, the risk rises with the quantity consumed to more than tenfold for lifelong non-drinkers. Alcohol and tobacco smoking act as synergistic carcinogens (i.e. the combined effect is greater than that of either alone). This combination accounts for the very high incidence of these tumours in France, where they are often multifocal. Alcohol probably acts as a co-carcinogen rather than a carcinogen (i.e. it promotes rather than initiates carcinogenesis). Spirits may have a slightly stronger carcinogenic effect than other alcoholic beverages.

Any policy on moderating the consumption of alcohol has to take account of a number of facts. First, many people find it pleasurable. Secondly, moderate amounts (2–3 units per day) protect against coronary thrombosis, though heavy drinking has other undesirable social consequences (e.g. violent behaviour and road accidents). Thirdly, its carcinogenic effects are largely in conjunction with smoking tobacco. Thus, the risk of cancer induction by alcohol in non-smokers is relatively small.

Ultraviolet light

Exposure to ultraviolet light has been increasing with the reduction of the ozone layer, caused by chemical pollution. An increase in the incidence of all forms of skin cancer can be expected. The principal culprits are the *chlorofluorohydrocarbons* (CFCs). These are components in, for example, aerosol sprays, refrigerants, and solvents for cleaning electronic equipment. However, to put the contribution of commercial sources of CFCs into context, one volcano in Antarctica emits 100 tons of chlorine every month, substantially more than the combined output of CFCs from deodorants over the same period. Nitrogen oxides from vehicle exhaust fumes also deplete the ozone layer. International agreements have been reached, aimed at eliminating the use of CFCs.

Occupational exposure

A wide variety of occupations are known to carry the risk of exposure to carcinogens. However, they only represent a relatively small number of cases of cancer deaths (4% in the USA). In 1987, 246 agents were classified by the International Agency for Research on Cancer as definitely (50), probably (37) or possibly (159) carcinogenic to humans. These included industrial processes, industrial chemicals, pesticides, laboratory chemicals, drugs, food ingredients, tobacco smoking and related stimulants. Drugs and industrial chemicals represent the largest risks. There are many other occupations where an agent is thought to be carcinogenic to workers but a causal link has not been established. Some of the known occupational hazards are listed in Table 15.2. Of these, exposure to asbestos dust, aromatic amines and the products of burning fossil fuels are the commonest. Measures to prevent occupational exposure include labelling of products as carcinogenic, and prohibiting the marketing and use of certain substances, e.g. the four aromatic amines (naphthylamine, 4-aminobiphenyl, 4-nitrodiphenyl and benzidine) and blue asbestos (crocidolite).

It is thought that preventive methods are likely to have little impact on the mortality from occupational cancers in the near future. The detection of tumours at an early stage by screening is likely to have a greater effect on mortality. Screening of urine by cytology among workers in the dyestuff and rubber industries has long been practiced.

Diet

Diet influences carcinogenesis in a variety of ways: carcinogens may be eaten; food substances may be converted to carcinogens once ingested; and dietary components may modify the ways in which the body metabolizes and responds to carcinogens. The only component of food that has been found to be strongly linked to the development of cancer is *aflatoxin*. This is a product of the fungus *Aspergillus fumigatus*, which often contaminates damp cereals in tropical countries. It causes primary liver cancer, although the data are unclear since there is a high incidence of hepatitis B, itself associated with liver tumours, in the same group of patients.

Table 15.2 International Agency for Research on Cancer (IARC) Class I, Occupational carcinogenesis (strong evidence of an association with human cancer)

AGENT	CANCER SITE/CANCER	MAIN INDUSTRY INDUSTRY/USE
4 Aminobiphenyl	Bladder	Rubber
Arsenic and arsenic compounds	Lung, skin	Glass, metals, pesticides
Asbestos	Lung, pleura peritoneum	Insulation, filter Material, textiles
Benzene	Leukaemia	Solvent, fuel
Benzidene	Bladder	Dye/pigment manufacture
Beryllium and beryllium compounds	Lung	Aerospace/metals
Bis (chlormethyl) ether	Lung	Chemical intermediate/ether by-product
Cadmium and cadmium compounds	Lung	Dye/pigment manufacture
Chloramethyl Methyl ether	Lung	Chemical intermediate/by-product
Chromium (VI) compounds	Nasal cavity, lung	Metal planting dye/pigment Manufacture
Coal-tar pitches	Skin, lung and bladder	Building materials Electrodes
Coal tars	Skin, lung	Fuel
Ethylene oxide	Leukaemia	Chemical intermediate/Sterilizing agent
Mineral oils, untreated and mildly treated	Skin	Lubricants
2-Naphthylamine	Bladder	Rubber dye manufacturers
Nickel compounds	Nasal cavity, lung	Metallurgy, alloys, catalysts
Shale-oils	Skin	Lubricants, fuels
Silica, crystalline	Lung	Stone cutting, mining foundaries
Soots	Skin, lung	Pigments
Strong-inorganic acid mists containing sulfuric acid	Larynx, lung	Metal batteries
Talc containing asbestiform fibres 2, 3, 7, 8	Lung	Paper, paint
Tetrachloro-dibenzo-para-dioxin (TCDD)	Multiple organs	Contaminant
Vinyl chloride	Liver	Plastics monomer
Wood dust	Nasal cavity	Wood industry

Bracken fern containing nitrates is suspected of causing oesophageal cancer, particularly among the Japanese. Salted fish is implicated in the aetiology of nasopharyngeal cancer, possibly as a co-carcinogen with the Epstein-Barr virus.

Diet may be indirectly related to carcinogenesis. One example is fibre, which seems to have a protective effect against colorectal cancer. A second is obesity, which is associated with an increased incidence of cancer of the endometrium and of the gallbladder in women. Consumption of saturated fat is implicated but not proven as a cause of breast cancer. A third is vitamin A (retinol) and its derivatives, retinoids, which may inhibit the full malignant transformation of cells and prevent tumour formation.

Dietary measures likely to reduce the risk of cancers are:

- high-fibre diet
- reducing saturated fats
- plenty of fresh fruit and vegetables (owing to the presence of antioxidants such as vitamin E).

Ionizing radiation

The whole spectrum of sources of ionizing radiations, both natural and man-made, has been calculated to contribute 1.5% of all fatal cancers. The sources of radiation exposure in the UK are shown in Table 15.3.

It is estimated that exposure to radon gas from domestic buildings may be responsible for 1% of lung cancer in Europe. Concentrations of radon gas in excess of 400 Bq/m^3 (about 1 in 1000 homes) will expose the

occupants to 20 mSv per year. The lifetime risk of fatal cancer from this exposure is about 10%. The carcinogenic risks of ionizing radiation have been revised upwards since 1988. Current estimates of risk are two to five times higher. However, it is unclear whether these revised estimates apply to very low levels of exposure to natural background radioactivity.

The role of ionizing radiation in the causation of cancer is mainly derived from occupational exposure. Early evidence came from the development of lung cancer among miners at Joachimstal in Czechoslovakia and Schneeberg in Germany. Lung disease had been known to occur among these workers since the 16th century. It was subsequently appreciated that the disease was lung cancer due to radioactive radon gas in the mines.

The main source of evidence of the effects of ionizing radiation in man are the survivors of the atomic bombs dropped on Hiroshima and Nagasaki in 1945. The incidence of acute and chronic leukaemia was significantly raised within a radius of 1.5 km from the epicentre. The highest incidence occurred 6–8 years afterwards. For cancers other than leukaemia, the latent period was longer (15–20 years) among victims who received 1 Gy or more; indeed the incidence is still higher over 50 years later.

It is assumed that there is no threshold below which cancers cannot be induced by ionizing radiation. Indeed, children who received only 0.01–0.02 Gy in utero when their mothers were irradiated had an additional 1 in 2000 risk of cancer. At low doses, the risk of developing cancer is probably proportional to dose, although much uncertainty remains.

Reducing the levels of radon gas from domestic buildings requires a number of measures. First, systematic surveys are needed to identify buildings which pose a hazard. Levels of radon gas can be reduced by alterations to the floors and installation of extractor fans.

Table 15.3 Estimated annual dose of ionizing radiation received by a member of the general public (mSv)

External terrestrial radiation	0.4
Cosmic radiation	0.3
Ingestion of naturally occurring radioactive substances	0.3
Inhalation of radon progeny	2.4
Use of ionizing radiation and radioactive substances in medicine (mainly diagnostic x-rays)	1.5
Fall out from nuclear weapons testing	<0.01
Nuclear power plants	<0.01
Reactor accident in Chernobyl	<0.02
Use of radioactive materials and ionizing radiation in industry, research and at home	<0.01
Occupational exposure	<0.01

POLLUTION

Atmospheric pollution has been suspected to be carcinogenic, ever since the incidence of lung cancer was found to be higher in cities than in the country. The combustion products of coal are known to contain carcinogenic hydrocarbons. However, since the atmosphere is polluted by a wide variety of substances, often in small quantities, the assessment of carcinogenic risk is very difficult. The situation is further complicated by the contribution to atmospheric pollution of tobacco smoking. In the past, pollution probably accounted for about 1% of cancers. Atmospheric pollution in the UK is now falling with stricter rules on the burning of fossil fuels. The evidence suggests that the current burning of fossil fuels, arsenic and asbestos will contribute to much less than 1% of future cancers.

Chemoprevention

The oral cavity, lung and colon have been the commonest primary sites subject to attempts at chemoprevention. Beta-carotene, synthetic retinoids, calcium and a variety of vitamins reduce the risk of developing oral cancer. A trial of alpha-tocopherol and beta-carotene showed no protective effect against the development of lung cancer.

Among patients in China at high risk of oesophageal or stomach cancer, treatment with vitamin and mineral supplements reduced the incidence and mortality of these tumours. These populations have a 20% incidence of oesophageal dysplasia.

Trials of adjuvant tamoxifen have showed a reduction in the risk of contralateral breast cancer. Trials are ongoing to determine whether tamoxifen can prevent the disease among women at high risk on the basis of their strong family history of the disease. Antioxidants, e.g. vitamins A and E, are thought to act by reducing DNA damage early in the process of carcinogenesis. It seems most likely that chemoprevention with such agents should occur early in life if they proved to be effective. The cost-effectiveness of chemoprevention needs to be carefully considered. Preventive treatment may have to be continued for several decades, which may prove very expensive when compared to the numbers of lives saved.

CONCLUSION

The negative impact of cancer on individuals and communities can be greatly reduced through cancer control programmes. While the scope of cancer control extends from prevention and screening to management of disease, rehabilitation and palliative care, successful prevention can make a huge contribution to reducing the global cancer load, and compared to the other strategies at a relatively low cost. As this involves changes in lifestyle for many individuals, it is critical that the medical and public health professionals engage with populations in embracing 'healthy' living as a shared goal.

FURTHER READING

Boyle P, Ferlay J. Cancer incidence and mortality in Europe, 2004. Ann Oncol 2005;16:481–8.

Harris JE, Thun MJ, Mondul AM, et al. Cigarette tar yields in relation to mortality from lung cancer in the cancer prevention study II prospective cohort. 1982–8. Br Med J 2004;328:72.

Doll R, Peto R, Boreham, et al. Mortality in relation to smoking: 50 years' observations on male British doctors. Br Med J 2004;22 Jun.

Doll R, Peto R, Wheatley K, et al. Mortality in relation to smoking: 40 years' observations on male British doctors. Br Med J 1994;309:901–11.

Passive smoking

Boffetta P. Involuntary smoking and lung cancer. Scand J Work Environ Health 2002;28(s):30–40.

Hackshaw AK, Law MR, Wald NJ. The accumulated evidence on lung cancer and environmental tobacco smoke. Br Med J 1997;315:980–8.

International Agency for Research on Cancer IARC Monograph 83: Tobacco smoke and involuntary smoking. IARC Lyon 2002.

Asbestos

Goodman M. Cancer in asbestos-exposed occupational cohorts: a meta-analysis. Cancer Causes Control 1999;10:453–65.

Hammond EC, Selikoff IJ, Seidman H. Asbestos exposure, cigarette smoking and death rates. Ann N Y Acad Sci 1979;330:473–90.

Liddell FD, Armstrong BG. The combination of effects on lung cancer of cigarette smoking and exposure in Quebec chrysotile miners and millers. Ann Occup Hyg 2002;46:5–13.

Colon cancer

Potter JD, Slattery ML, Bostick RM, et al. Colon cancer: a review of the epidemiology. Epidemiol Rev 1993;15:499–545.

Bruce WR, Giacca A, Medline A. Possible mechanisms relating diet and risk of colon cancer. Cancer Epidemiol Biomarkers Prev 2000;9:1271–9.

Breast cancer and hormones

International Agency for Research on Cancer IARC Monograph 72. Hormonal contraception and post-menopausal hormone therapy. IARC Lyon 1999.

World Health Organization. Guidelines for controlling and monitoring the tobacco epidemic. WHO; 1998.

Chapter | 16 |

Biological and pathological introduction

John R. Goepel

Radiotherapy is used almost exclusively for the treatment of cancer and related conditions. It is thus very important to have a reasonable understanding of this disease. This chapter contains an outline of the basic characteristics of cancerous cells, and the conditions that can cause cancer. There is consideration of the natural history of untreated cancer, and of the ways that different types of cancer are named and classified.

GROWTH: PROLIFERATION, DIFFERENTIATION AND APOPTOSIS

Growth is the process of increase in size and maturity of tissues from fertilization through to the adult. When normally controlled, the different parts of the body take on their correct size and specialist functions, and relationship to one another. Furthermore, throughout life these attributes continue despite the need for replacement and repair. This is all a reflection of accurate control of the timing and extent of cellular proliferation, cell-to-cell orientation and organization, and *differentiation*. Differentiation is the process of a cell taking on a specialized function; this is usually associated with a change in its microscopic appearance. It is also usually a one-way commitment, with relative or complete loss of the ability to continue proliferating. Also important is the ability to delete cells which are no longer needed, by a process called *apoptosis* or programmed cell death. This is used in the development of the fetus, and in maintaining or adjusting the size of a structure in the adult. Apoptosis is also used to delete defective cells.

Growth disorders

Hypertrophy is an increase in the size of an organ due to an increase in the size of its constituent cells. The left ventricle of the heart becomes hypertrophic if it has to work harder because of hypertension.

Hyperplasia is an increase in size because of an increase in the number of cells. The adrenal cortex will become hyperplastic if there is excessive adrenocorticotrophic hormone to stimulate it. However, it will return to normal if the stimulus is reduced again.

Metaplasia is a change from one type of tissue to another. Smoking induces a change of the bronchial lining from the usual respiratory mucosa to a squamous epithelium, with resultant loss of mucus-producing and ciliated cells. It is also potentially reversible.

Neoplasia (literally a new growth), in contrast, is an irreversible process once initiated: it is the main subject of this chapter. It is also called cancer, or a tumour, though the latter is sometimes used to denote any swelling.

NEOPLASIA

A neoplasm can be defined as a lesion resulting from the autonomous or relatively autonomous abnormal growth of cells which persists after the initiating stimulus has been removed; i.e. cell growth has escaped from normal regulatory mechanisms. The abnormality affects all aspects of cell growth and apoptosis to varying degrees. Proliferation continues unabated, irrespective of the requirements of the organ in which the neoplasm is situated. This, combined with loss of control of the normal relationships between cells, often results in the new tumour cells replacing and insinuating themselves between the adjacent normal tissues, a process called *invasion*. Loss of differentiation accompanies, and often correlates with, failure of proliferation control and invasiveness. Failure of apoptosis may also be a major contribution to the survival of abnormal cells.

Benign and malignant neoplasms

Neoplasia is not a single disease, but rather a common pathological process with a multitude of different varieties and clinical outcomes. One fundamental division is between *benign* and *malignant* tumours. Benign tumours will remain localized, with generally relatively little effect on the patient. In contrast, other tumours are locally destructive, may spread to involve other parts of the body, and ultimately result in the death of the patient. Figure 16.1 and Table 16.1 show some of the differences between benign and malignant neoplasms. Further aspects of the classification of tumours are discussed later in this chapter.

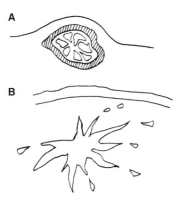

Figure 16.1 The difference between a benign tumour A contained by a definitive capsule and a malignant tumour B actively invading the tumour bed.

Table 16.1 Characteristics of neoplasms		
FEATURE	**BENIGN**	**MALIGNANT**
Growth rate	Slow	Variable, may be rapid
Margin	Encapsulated	Invasive
Local effect	Little	Destructive
Differentiation	Good	Variable, may be poor
Metastases	No	Frequently
Usual outcome	Good	Fatal

The term *cancer* (Latin for 'crab') is very ancient, and there are several explanations for its usage. Some say it reflects the tenacious grip the disease has on its victim, some that it describes the radiating prominent veins that may surround an advanced superficial tumour. Others contend that it describes the irregular infiltrative profile of some tumours, e.g. of breast. Suffice it to say that cancer is a common colloquial term that is generally applied to any malignant neoplasm.

Though the behaviour of tumours, particularly malignant ones, may seem very odd, it can generally be explained by the excessive or inappropriate expression of genes that are present in all cells. The tumour continues to be dependent upon an adequate blood supply (though many acquire the capacity to induce new vessels). Also, many of those which arise from hormone-dependent tissues (e.g. breast, prostate) continue to show a degree of dependence on those hormones. This can be exploited to therapeutic advantage by giving anti-hormone treatment.

CARCINOGENESIS

The causes of cancer are numerous, and mechanisms of its production are complex, but some of the principles will be presented. There are two avenues of thought to follow: one at the molecular and genetic levels, the other concerned with causative associations. It is not always easy to relate these to each other. Underlying the mechanistic approach is the assumption that cell behavior is controlled by the genes expressed (which ones, and how strongly), bearing in mind that these can be influenced by chemical messages relayed from outside the cell. Every cell contains the entire genetic code, but only expresses those genes appropriate to its own situation. In cancer, this has gone wrong, particularly with respect to proliferation, differentiation or apoptosis. We can generalize to say that multiple abnormalities need to have occurred between normality and cancer, and that this reflects a *multistep* process. Only those cells capable of division are at risk of transforming into a neoplasm. This excludes terminally differentiated cells such as circulating red cells, the uppermost keratinized cells of the skin, and adult voluntary muscle and nerve cells.

Initiation

This describes the first step towards neoplasia. It reflects a change at the molecular level of how a cell can function, escaping in some small way from a control mechanism. Nothing can be seen microscopically at this stage. Substances that can initiate neoplasia are called *initiators* or *carcinogens*.

Promotion

No more will come of the initiated cell unless it continues to divide. Further abnormalities of cell function (i.e. gene expression) arise over a period of time. Substances that enhance this process are called *promoters*.

Progression

Neoplasms are *clonal*, i.e. are derived from a single cell. For this to happen, a cell and its progeny must acquire and sustain a growth advantage over other cells throughout succeeding cell divisions. This eventually results in visible alterations at the microscopic level. Not all the daughter cells will be identical, giving rise to differences between individual cells or subclones; this is called *pleomorphism*.

Clinical cancer

Finally, the neoplasm becomes manifest as a clinically significant tumour. Unless removed, it will continue to progress with a general tendency towards further loss of growth restraint, and acquisition of the capacity to spread to other parts of the body (metastasize).

Oncogenes and tumour suppressor genes

The function of a cell is critically dependent on the expression of its genes. In cancer, it has been observed that there may be both inappropriate levels of expression of otherwise normal genes, and abnormalities of genes. Though copying of the genetic code from one cell generation to another is very accurate, it is not perfect. An abnormal copy or *mutation* may give rise to a protein with excessive function or reduced function, or may fail to produce a protein at all, resulting in no function. Alternatively, it may be the control of the gene which is altered, so that there is increased or decreased expression resulting in excess or deficient protein product and hence function. An *oncogene* is an altered gene which contributes to cancer development when its expression is increased. The normally functioning counterparts of these genes are often concerned with control of cell proliferation.

In contrast, *tumour suppressor genes* are those which, when totally absent or non-functioning in a cell, permit the emergence of neoplasia, i.e. their presence prevents neoplasia. Given that all normal cells will have two copies of each gene (one on each chromosome pair), the development of neoplasia by this means requires loss or mutation of both copies.

It must be stressed that clinical cancer does not reflect a solitary abnormality of one of these genes, but rather the final result of a combination of several errors of function. The gradual accumulation of multiple genetic defects is typified by the progression of a benign polyp in the colon to a cancer over about 10 years. How is it that a cell can acquire so many abnormal genes? The explanation in several situations is that there is failure of the screening of the cell's genetic code for abnormalities, or defective repair of incidental genetic damage. The protein p53 is important in assuring the integrity of the genome, and it is frequently defective in cancer cells. Similarly, the failure of DNA repair can result in much more rapid accumulation of mutations – the *mutator phenotype*.

Defective apoptosis has several consequences with regard to cancer. Inappropriately increased expression of *BCL-2*, which inhibits apoptosis, is a major reason for cell accumulation in some tumours, for example follicular lymphoma. Failure of apoptosis may contribute to survival of defective cells and also cell survival in abnormal environments such as occurs during invasion and metastasis. Finally, many cancer treatments rely on induction of apoptosis to kill tumour cells, so these will be less effective if apoptosis is defective.

Blood vessels

The development of cancer cells into a clinically important mass requires establishing a blood supply, a process called *angiogenesis*. New capillaries form under the influence of vascular endothelial growth factors (VEGF); platelets are the main source of VEGF in the blood. VEGF may be secreted directly by tumour cells, particularly when stimulated by hypoxia, but also when tumours abnormally express a range of other oncogenes, for example epidermal growth factor receptor (EGFR) and Her2. Her2 is important in many breast cancers, and is a therapeutic target for trastuzumab (Herceptin). Drugs are also becoming available to target angiogenesis, for example the VEGF antibody bevacizumab (Avastin).

Heredity and cancer

The great majority of common tumours do not seem to have any relationship to hereditary factors. However, some rare tumours do, and have led to an understanding of tumour suppressor genes. The pioneering work of Knudson on families of patients with multiple retinoblastomas (a tumour of the eye) indicated first that there must be two genetic events. In due course, it became clear that one defective gene was inherited by the patient, while its corresponding gene on the opposite chromosome became defective, or was lost, in some cells during the growth of the eye. With both retinoblastoma (Rb) genes now defective, the cells proceeded to neoplasia.

It is apparent that a minority of common tumours run in families because of the same sort of mechanism. For example, breast cancer kindreds may be passing on the *BRCA-1* or *BRCA-2* genes, and also be associated with carcinoma of the ovary or colon, (these genes code for DNA repair). In familial adenomatous polyposis, a defective APC gene results in adenomas and colon cancers, while in hereditary non-polyposis colon cancer (HNPCC), one of a number of mismatch repair genes or abnormal hypermethylation is involved, giving rise to colon cancer by a different molecular biology route. These issues are taken further in the relevant sections about breast cancer or colon cancer. An inherited risk of malignancy does not imply that it is certain that a cancer will arise in a particular individual.

Physical agents

Ionizing radiation

There is no doubt that ionizing radiation can cause cancer. Direct damage to DNA (i.e. the chemical basis of genetic information), and damage mediated via ionization of water can result in mutation of genes. The damage is randomly scattered throughout the genetic code, but can include sites critical to the development of cancer by the usual sequence of initiation, promotion and so on. Traditionally, it has been thought that radiation causes a somatic mutation in a normal cell. The earliest event is probably genomic instability. Subsequently, there is a multistep sequence of genetic events. This typically results in an interval of many years between exposure and clinical cancer. The source of radiation does not matter from the point of view of causing cancer, though it will affect the sites at risk.

Ionizing radiation can lead to loss of tumour suppressor genes and activation of proto-oncogenes. Oncogenes may also be activated as result of point mutations. Gene amplification can lead to activation and overexpression of a proto-oncogene. It had previously been thought that mutagenesis only occurred in normal cells traversed by radiation particles. However, normal cells can undergo change without such damage by virtue of what is termed the 'bystander effect'. The mechanism of this bystander effect is not clear but it could be due to secretion of factors (as yet unidentified) from irradiated cells that influence the survival of adjacent non-irradiated cells.

The dose at which carcinogenesis occurs may be tissue specific. Actively proliferating tissues within or adjacent to the irradiated volume (e.g. in the pelvis), and having a high capacity for proliferation not inhibited by radiation, will carry a risk of radiation-induced malignancy at lower doses than in slowly turning-over tissues such as connective tissue.

Industrial exposure

Early workers with x-rays unknowingly induced tumours, and other radiation damage, in their hands. Today, diagnostic and therapeutic radiation also carry this risk to patients and staff alike, necessitating stringent safety regulations. Some mineworkers are exposed to high levels of radon, which is inhaled and may cause lung cancer (a risk increased by cigarette smoking). Radon- induced lung cancer has been linked to mutations of *p53*, a tumour suppressor gene. This mutation differs from those seen in lung cancer induced by smoking. Another industrial association was with the painters of luminous watch dials. These ladies pointed their brush with their lips, thereby taking in minute quantities of radium. Some of the material remained near the jaw, while some was absorbed and passed to bone marrow, where the alpha emissions resulted in bone necrosis, tumours and marrow failure. In all cases, there was the usual long time delay between exposure and clinical cancer.

Atomic bomb survivors have been followed up very carefully. There has been an excessive number of cases of leukaemia, mainly 7–12 years after exposure, and also a larger number of other cancers from about 20 years later onwards.

Ultraviolet light

The shorter wavelengths of solar ultraviolet light, UVB, are capable of damaging the DNA of various skin cells, resulting in mutations and eventually cancers. Melanin pigment protects against UV penetration to the deeper layers of cells. The common tumours, basal cell and squamous cell carcinomas, seem to result from chronic overexposure; malignant melanoma correlates better with acute and intense exposure.

Chemicals

Coal tars, oils and cigarette smoke

Percival Pott, in 1775, described carcinoma of the scrotal skin in chimney sweeps, and attributed it to the soot. Similarly, mule-spinners in mills developed tumours due to the oil that soaked their clothing and, even today, motor mechanics are at risk from lubricating oils. However, the greatest problem at present from this group of chemicals is cigarette smoke. This contains many known *carcinogenic* substances, including benzo[a]pyrene, a potent carcinogen also present in coal tars. Not only do smokers have a very greatly increased incidence of lung cancer, they also have a higher risk of cancer at several other sites, such as the bladder. Chemicals that are able to cause tumours are called *direct carcinogens*, but most require metabolism to the active chemical so are called *procarcinogens*.

Aniline dyes and the rubber industry

Workers in the chemical industry, particularly those involved in making dyes, were found to develop bladder cancer. A similar risk was noted in the rubber-processing industry. The chemical implicated, β-naphthylamine, needs to be metabolized in the kidney, thus releasing the active ingredient into the urine.

Asbestos

Many particulate minerals are now recognized as carcinogenic, including asbestos. The blue asbestos (crocidolite) particles used for insulation are easily inhaled when very small but are then retained within the lung. Over a period of decades, they may then cause tumours of the pleura (malignant mesothelioma); they also correlate with bronchial cancer, particularly if associated with smoking.

Hormones

Are endogenous chemicals such as hormones carcinogenic? There is no doubt that hormone levels are important in hormonally responsive organs and their cancers. Whether the hormone is actually carcinogenic, or simply contributes to the process of carcinogenesis by promoting cell proliferation is debatable; the latter is more probable. The relationship between oestrogens and endometrial cancer is discussed in Chapter 27. Breast and prostate cancers are also likely to relate to hormonal influences. As mentioned earlier, hormonal manipulation is an important therapeutic tool in cancer treatment.

Viruses and cancer

As viruses contain genetic material, and gain access to the inside of cells, they have long been suspected of having a role in carcinogenesis. This speculation has been fuelled by finding close similarity between some viral genes and oncogenes. Viruses are clearly responsible for a variety of tumours in several species, such as leukaemias in mice and cats and sarcomas in chickens. In humans, common skin warts are self-limiting benign tumours caused by a virus. Over recent years, these human papilloma (wart) viruses (HPV) have been found to be a large family of related organisms, some of which correlate closely with cancer of the uterine cervix and similar tumours. Similarly, Epstein-Barr virus, which is very widespread and causes infectious mononucleosis, is closely associated with tumours such as Hodgkin's Lymphoma, Burkitt's lymphoma (a high-grade non-Hodgkin's lymphoma), and nasopharyngeal carcinoma.

Infectivity and cancer

Some patients, or their relatives, worry that cancer may be infectious. It is possible to allay these fears and assure them that this is not the case. The association with viruses mentioned above is a rare sequel to agents widely present in the community; the cancer cannot be passed on.

Immunity and cancer

The immune system exists to detect and eliminate foreign substances, from isolated molecules to whole organisms. This is effected by antibodies and cells, principally lymphocytes. In the development of a tumour, it is quite possible for new or inappropriate substances to be produced. From this one would predict that tumours would sometimes be antigenic, i.e. provoke an immune response. This does seem to be the case. There are several examples of rare and common tumours with evidence of an immune response, generally the presence of numerous lymphocytes within and around the tumour. Tumours of rectum and breast, and seminoma of the testis all vary in the density of tumour-infiltrating lymphocytes. Studies of patients have correlated the density of lymphocytes with survival, often showing an advantage to those with an immune response. However, the effect is not large, and is easily obscured by better treatment to all patients.

With malignant melanoma of skin, there is slightly more evidence to suggest a significant favorable immune response in some patients. Microscopic examination sometimes shows areas of apparent regression within the primary growth. There are also some patients with advanced melanoma who respond to stimulation of their immune system against the tumour (immunotherapy).

Despite these few encouraging observations, it is obvious that the majority of clinical cancer is beyond the capability of the patient's immune system. In some cases, there is evidence that tumour cells may simply evade it.

Immune surveillance

The normal immune system actively seeks foreign material, apparently screening everything against its memory bank to distinguish self from non-self. This may allow the detection and elimination of some cancers before they are clinically established. For example, renal transplant patients require drugs to suppress their immune response in order for the new kidney to survive. These patients have many more skin tumours than would otherwise be expected, possibly as a result of loss of immune surveillance. Patients with AIDS suffer from a wide range of tumours, but this does not necessarily imply that loss of immune surveillance is the key event. Many patients with defects of the immune system (either as a result of disease or treatment) have an increase in tumours of lymphocytes, but this is probably a different phenomenon.

Injury and cancer

To be acceptable as a cause of cancer, an injury would need to be severe enough to have caused tissue damage, there must be evidence that the site was previously normal, and that the tumour arose at the site of injury. Finally, the time interval must be long enough to be plausible, generally several years. The mechanism is presumably via a non-specific induction of cell division as part of the repair process, rather than anything actually carcinogenic. There are a few instances that fulfil these criteria, but the usual circumstance is simply that the injury draws attention to a pre-existing tumour.

PRECANCEROUS LESIONS

There are a number of conditions in which there is an increased risk of the subsequent development of cancer. Some are disorders that are not of themselves neoplastic, but carry a risk of cancer. Others are more like a halfway house in which the process of development towards cancer is recognizable as neither normal nor cancer. Some are benign tumours that may change to be malignant. In none is the development of cancer inevitable, though the risk and time scale vary greatly. Some examples are given below.

- *Undescended testis* is an abnormality of development: it carries a high risk of neoplasia.
- *Paget's disease of bone*, a condition of middle to late adult life, has a risk of osteosarcoma, a tumour otherwise seen in adolescence.
- *Solar keratosis* is a warty skin lesion due to sun exposure; it may progress to cancer.
- *Leukoplakia*, a whitish patch in the mouth or vulva, is a descriptive term including several conditions. Some run the risk of cancer later.
- *Dysplasia* may be detected at several sites (e.g. stomach), and indicates a microscopic abnormality of cells with some, but not all, features of cancer.
- *Carcinoma-in-situ* may be seen on a surface (e.g. cervix) or within the lumen of a duct (intraduct carcinoma of the breast). This has all the microscopic features of cancer, but the cells are still confined to their normal anatomical limits, i.e. have not invaded.
- *Adenomatous polyp* of the large intestine is a benign tumour. However, it may develop into a malignant tumour. In the condition familial adenomatous polyposis, there are so many polyps (thousands) that malignancy becomes inevitable (Figure *evolve* 16.2) In addition to the malignant potential of adenomas, it is now becoming apparent that large hyperplastic polyps of the right colon, and those with a serrated surface epithelium, can also progress to cancer but by a different molecular pathway.

An important consideration is that the detection of some of these conditions allows surgical intervention before cancer becomes established.

Field change

Although an individual tumour arises from a single cell, within the vicinity of that cell there are often other cells part-way through carcinogenesis. Removal of the tumour, or its precursor lesion, may be followed by the local development of further lesions. This is regarded as a field change across the whole area. An example would be the appearance of cancer on the tongue following removal of one from the buccal mucosa.

NATURAL HISTORY AND SPREAD OF CANCER

As stated earlier, *benign* tumours remain localized, often separated from surrounding tissue by a capsule. The tumour has relatively little effect on the adjacent structures, unless it arises in a particularly critical site, and surgical removal is curative. In contrast, *malignant* tumours show a capacity to invade, frequently recur after surgery, spread to other sites and result in the death of the patient. The initial or *primary* site of tumour growth thus gives rise to separate secondary tumours, or *metastases*. Some tumours, such as *basal cell carcinoma* of skin have an intermediate behavior; they invade locally but do not give rise to metastases.

In summary, spread may occur in several ways (Figure 16.3):

- by local invasion
- by lymphatic vessels
- by blood vessels
- across cavities.

Local invasion

As the tumour invades, adjacent tissues are displaced and destroyed to be replaced by tumour. The tumour margin is ill-defined and irregular. Surgical removal therefore needs to include a generous extent of normal tissue. Failure to do so results in some tumour being left behind, which proliferates and gives rise to *local recurrence*. Radiotherapy is frequently used after surgery in order to prevent this situation. The invasion often follows anatomical tissue planes; it may be temporarily halted by some dense structure such as bone, until this is also eroded.

Functional effects

The effects a tumour produces will depend upon the site involved; a knowledge of anatomy and physiology allows prediction of many symptoms. Thus, a tumour in the head of the pancreas will soon obstruct the bile duct, so that the patient becomes jaundiced (Figure *evolve* 16.4🖱). A tumour of the left lung may obstruct its bronchus, with resulting pneumonia from infection of retained secretions. Further local invasion of this mass will compress the recurrent laryngeal nerve; the patient's voice is altered. Further growth may obstruct the superior vena cava passing through the mediastinum, causing swelling of the face and arms.

A tumour just beneath the skin can so stretch it and impair its nutrition that it breaks down to form an ulcer. This is then liable to infection or bleeding. Pain and weakness will occur when peripheral nerves are affected, e.g. Pancoast tumour at the apex of the lung invading upwards to compress nerves to the arm and hand.

The extent of local invasion dictates the extent of surgery necessary to remove it and, indeed, may render the tumour inoperable if critical structures are involved. However, the usual reason why a tumour is 'inoperable' is because of metastatic disease. Sometimes it is worth debulking the tumour, but surgery alone is insufficient to cure the patient.

Metastasis

By lymphatic vessels

Invasive tumours readily penetrate the thin wall of lymphatics. Then fragments of tumour are carried downstream to lodge in one or more local lymph nodes. If the tumour cells survive this journey and proliferate in the node they form a *metastasis*, or secondary tumour. Further dissemination may proceed to other lymph nodes along the chain, e.g. from pelvic to para-aortic to supraclavicular nodes. Some primary tumours remain tiny, yet have massive nodal deposits. If the node capsule is breached by tumour, the whole mass becomes fixed to surrounding structures.

Figure 16.3 Metastasis or secondary spread. Tumours can spread by a variety of routes including local spread, spread through the lymphatics, via the blood and across cavities. *(Reproduced from Calman, Smyth and Tattersall, Basic Principles of Cancer Chemotherapy, Macmillan, 1980 with permission of Palgrave).*

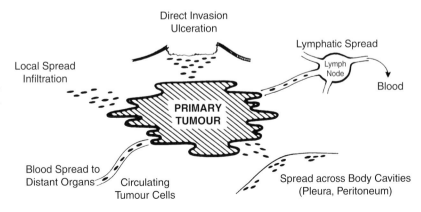

By blood vessels

Thin-walled blood vessels are similarly at risk of tumour invasion, and again fragments of tumour float passively downstream. (Single tumour cells are generally destroyed by non-specific defense mechanisms in the blood.) These then lodge in the next capillary bed, where they may develop into metastases. Though this can happen in any tissue, the liver, lungs and bone are by far the most frequent sites for secondaries (Figure *evolve* 16.5🖱).

Across cavities (transcelomic)

Access to the *pleura* enables tumour cells to seed themselves around the pleural cavity, forming numerous further deposits or seedlings. These may be associated with secretion of fluid into the cavity, with resultant impairment of respiration. An identical process may occur in the peritoneum; the fluid accumulation is called *ascites*. Malignant cells may settle on the ovaries, or all over the omentum. Related to this, some intracranial tumours, such as medulloblastoma of the cerebellum, may disseminate by the cerebrospinal fluid, seeding over the surface of the brain and down the spinal canal (Figure *evolve* 16.6🖱).

Implantation

Occasionally cells may be implanted in the scar by the surgeon's knife while removing a tumour, or through a pleural or abdominal paracentesis drainage site.

Functioning tumours

Many tumour cells continue certain cell functions related to their tissue of origin but, in some, this has a profound effect on the patient. Tumours of endocrine glands typically produce an excess of their hormone. The problem is that the tumour is no longer responsive to the usual control of secretion. Thus, an adrenal cortex tumour will produce steroids despite switching off its pituitary drive, and Cushing's syndrome will result.

In other circumstances, the hormone production is quite inappropriate for the tumour site. Many lung tumours produce substances that mimic the function of parathyroid hormone, antidiuretic hormone, or adrenocorticotrophic hormone. Again, it is not subject to the normal control of secretion, and the clinical consequences may be severe. Some of the other effects that tumours may have, such as profound weight loss, could be due to secretions as yet unidentified.

Cause of death from cancer

As the word 'malignant' implies, death is the natural consequence of untreated cancer. Sometimes the tumour will have grown locally and spread in a predictable manner.

In other cases, the primary site remains undetected despite widespread metastatic deposits. Some tumours show relentless progression, and run their course in a few months; others take many years, with long intervals of apparent dormancy.

Many patients with locally advanced or metastatic cancer become bedridden and die from bronchopneumonia, inanition and/or metabolic disturbance. Sometimes there may be liver failure due to numerous liver secondaries. Often the actual cause of death is unclear. It is important to consider carrying out a post-mortem examination if there is reasonable doubt about the cause of death. Patients with cancer are still at risk of non-neoplastic conditions such as coronary artery disease. This is particularly likely in patients who smoke. Indeed, smoking may have given rise both to the primary tumour (e.g. in the lung, oral cavity or pharynx) and to ischemic heart disease.

It is important to make a judgment as to whether the patient died from cancer or from an unrelated condition, since this influences cancer mortality statistics. Where a patient has remained disease free from cancer for more than 5 years, and the cause of death is said to be cancer, this conclusion should be questioned. However, late relapses can occur after 5 years, in breast cancer, for example. Alternatively, a new primary may develop, especially in head and neck cancer.

STAGING OF CANCERS

It is of the greatest practical importance in many cases to estimate the extent of the spread of a tumour at the time of initial diagnosis. This process is called *staging*. Staging often influences the choice of treatment, and can provide valuable information on prognosis. Staging may include clinical, pathological, radiological, and biochemical information. This enables similar groups of patients to be compared between different oncology centres nationally and internationally. A number of staging classifications are in use. The simplest and oldest classification is as follows:

Stage 1: Tumour confined to the organ of origin
Stage 2: Local lymph nodes invaded
Stage 3: Distant nodes invaded, or local spread beyond the organ of origin
Stage 4: Blood-borne metastasis present.

This is still used with some cancers, though often with slight modification to bring in subcategories, as with the FIGO system for cervix cancer. The UICC (International Union Against Cancer) has worked towards international agreement on the staging of many tumours, coding them on the TNM system.

TNM classification

This includes a description of the primary tumour (T), nodal spread (N), and distant metastases (M). It provides a succinct summary of the extent of malignancy in the patient.

T1–3: Generally based on the size and/or extent of the primary
T4: The most advanced local disease, often with invasion of adjacent structures
N0: No nodes palpable
N1: Mobile nodes on the same side as the primary
N1a: Nodes not considered to contain tumour
N1b: Nodes considered to contain tumour
N2: Mobile nodes on the opposite side (N2a and N2b as above)
N3: Fixed, involved nodes
M0: No evidence of distant metastasis
M1: Distant metastasis present

Thus, a very early cancer would be categorized as T1N0M0, and a very advanced one as T4N3M1. The details of how to categorise a tumour vary between sites; the TNM classification for breast cancer is shown in Table 26.3.

The clinical staging may differ from the pathological staging. For example, a tumour in the breast may be measured clinically as 2 cm in diameter and thus be staged as T1. However, when actually measured directly in the mastectomy specimen it might be 3 cm in maximum diameter, and thus be pathologically T2 (abbreviated as pT2). Most staging classifications are based on the clinical extent of spread.

Radiological information may influence staging. For example, in carcinoma of the cervix, the presence of an obstructed kidney on ultrasound or other investigation (in the absence of a non-neoplastic cause), automatically indicates stage 3b.

The staging of testicular cancer is an example where biochemical information (the presence of serum tumour markers alpha-fetoprotein and human chorionic gonadotrophin) is included. If the tumour is clinically confined to the testis but tumour markers are rising, it is classified as stage 1, marker positive (Mk+).

HISTOLOGICAL GRADING: DIFFERENTIATION

In an effort to predict the future course of a tumour, an estimate is made of how malignant it is for a particular site and type of tumour. Generally speaking, the closer a tumour cell resembles its normal counterpart, i.e. the better it is differentiated, the more orderly and slower its growth. Thus, histological examination allows tumour *grading* on the basis of the extent of differentiation. Attention is given to the nucleus (how abnormal it is and how often mitosis is observed), and the cytoplasm (the extent to which normal structures are seen) (Figures *evolve* 16.7 & 16.8 🖱).

For most of the common tumours, the pathologist divides them into descriptive categories: well differentiated, moderately differentiated and poorly differentiated. Undifferentiated tumours lack sufficient features to allow more than a broad classification, as do anaplastic tumours (see below under Classification of neoplasms) (Figure *evolve* 16.9 🖱).

Limitations of grading

Some tumours show a tight correlation between histological grading and behavior, such that treatment is guided by this information. Cancer of the bladder is one of these. However, the tumour stage is of overriding importance. Some tumours (e.g. pancreatic islet) have a very variable rate of clinical progression, but uniform histology: grading in this circumstance is misleading if attempted. Other tumours vary considerably from one microscopic field to another: in general, the outlook will depend upon the worst areas, but these could be missed without adequate sampling. Finally, the organ of origin is important: a well-differentiated cancer of the skin carries an excellent prognosis, whereas in the lung it may not.

GROWTH RATE OF CANCERS

As indicated in the section on carcinogenesis, there is usually a considerable time between initiation of a tumour and its clinical detection. Part of this time is taken by the process of becoming a cancer cell, and part by growing to sufficient size to be found. The latter can be measured as the time taken for it to double in diameter, its *doubling time*. A mass 1 mm in diameter would represent about one million cells: this could result from one cell, and each of its subsequent daughter cells, dividing 20 times. A word of caution is needed before theorizing further. Once a tumour exceeds about 2 mm it is essential for it to have its own blood supply: this, together with other supporting structures, is the tumour *stroma*. In some tumours, the stroma is very scanty, while in others it constitutes the majority of the mass. (The character of the stroma also influences what the tumour feels like on palpation; most breast cancers are hard because of abundant, dense stroma.) Thus, calculations about how many cancer cells there are in a tumour of a certain size will be incorrect if they ignore the stroma.

Another consideration is that the clinical growth of a tumour will be the result of the balance between cell proliferation and loss. It will be influenced too by the growth fraction or proportion of cancer cells actually proliferating. Many cancer cells in a tumour cease to proliferate as they differentiate, or produce non-viable daughter cells. Furthermore, if the vascularity of the stroma is inadequate there will be necrosis.

Though a cancer produces an expanding mass, this is a reflection of loss of control of growth. The actual rate at which individual cancer cells divide is *slower* than comparable normal tissues. If there is a very sudden increase in the size of a tumour, it will probably reflect internal hemorrhage or fluid accumulation. (On the other hand, a slow-growing mass which begins to grow faster may have changed from benign to malignant.)

Observation of established clinical cancers has shown that doubling times vary widely, but average about 2 months. Leaving aside the question of whether this is true for the first 20 doublings to reach 1 mm size, it would require about a further 10 doublings (i.e. 20 months) to reach 1 cm diameter, at which point it might be detectable. Many tumours are 2 cm or more in diameter before they produce symptoms, so a considerable time has elapsed between the first emergence of a clone of cancer cells and the clinical disease. In comparison with that, the remainder of its course, if unchecked, is liable to be over after five or so more doublings. Metastatic deposits may be disseminated during the preclinical period, only to appear after removal of the primary. If the doubling time is considerably more than 2 months the whole process takes on a much longer time scale.

Bearing these matters in mind, there is no fixed length of disease-free interval that equates with a cure. However, for practical purposes 5 years disease free is tantamount to cure for many of the common tumours, with breast cancer as a notable exception. The earlier detection of a cancer at a minute size increases the possibility of removal before metastases develop. However, the tumour has been around for a long time. Prolonged post-operative survival in these patients may simply reflect 'earlier diagnosis' rather than 'longer survival', a phenomenon called *lead-time bias*.

Spontaneous regression of cancer

Occasionally, a tumour may regress and disappear without treatment, though the original diagnosis could have been erroneous. Most of the reported cases are renal cell carcinoma, malignant melanoma and gestational choriocarcinoma. In all these instances, immunological mechanisms are thought to be responsible. Some cases of lymphoid tumours fluctuate in size, and may temporarily disappear, only to return later. In some cases of neuroblastoma, a primitive tumour of nerve cells, there is subsequent differentiation and growth ceases.

CLASSIFICATION OF NEOPLASMS

Table 16.2 lists examples of tumour nomenclature. In general, the names are built up from one part to describe the tissue type, and another to indicate its behavior. All end in 'oma' to denote a lump, a suffix almost restricted to neoplasms, though a few other terms are in use, such as hematoma for an accumulation of blood. Most malignant tumours fall into the following broad categories:

- carcinoma
- sarcoma
- lymphoma.

Table 16.2 Types of neoplasms

TYPE	BENIGN	MALIGNANT
Epithelial		*Carcinoma*
Squamous	Papilloma	Squamous carcinoma
Transitional	Papilloma	Transitional cell carcinoma
Basal cell	Papilloma	Basal cell carcinoma
Glandular	Adenoma	Adenocarcinoma
Mesenchymal		*Sarcoma*
Smooth muscle	Leiomyoma	Leiomyosarcoma
Striated muscle	Rhabdomyoma	Rhabdomyosarcoma
Fat	Lipoma	Liposarcoma
Blood vessels	Angioma	Angiosarcoma
Bone	Osteoma	Osteosarcoma
Cartilage	Chondroma	Chondrosarcoma
Lymphoid tissue		*Lymphoma*
		Hodgkin's lymphoma
		Non-Hodgkin's lymphoma
Plasma cell		Multiple myeloma
White blood cells		Leukaemia
Intracranial and neural		
Supporting cells		Glioma
Meninges	Meningioma	
Cerebellum		Medulloblastoma
Retina		Retinoblastoma
Sympathetic nerve	Ganglioneuroma	Neuroblastoma
Pigment cells		
Skin or eye	Mole or nevus	Malignant melanoma
Gonad		
Germ cells	Dermoid cyst	Malignant teratoma (Figure *evolve* 16.10 🖱) Seminoma
Placenta		
	Hydatidiform mole	Choriocarcinoma

The majority of tumours arise from epithelium (surface lining cells). Benign ones are called *papilloma* (Figure *evolve* 16.11 🖱) or *adenoma*; malignant ones *carcinoma*, often with a prefix to give the cell type. Carcinoma is Greek for 'crab' but is used in a more restricted sense than cancer and applied only to epithelial malignancy, which makes up 75% of cancer.

Squamous epithelium lines the skin, where it is called epidermis, the upper aerodigestive tract (mouth, pharynx, larynx, oesophagus), anus, vagina and cervix. It is present in the bronchi if there is metaplasia. *Transitional cell epithelium*, (or *urothelium*) lines the renal pelvis, ureters and bladder.

Glandular (secretory) epithelium lines the gut from stomach to rectum, and forms the related secretory glands (salivary, pancreas, biliary tract and liver), endocrine glands (pituitary, thyroid, parathyroids, adrenals), kidneys, ovarian surface, endometrium and breast (Figure *evolve* 16.12).

Sometimes the tumour name is combined with a description of shape or function. If a *cyst* is formed it may be cystadenoma or cystadenocarcinoma, both of which are common in the ovary. Mucin-secreting variants would be mucinous cystadenoma.

Sarcoma denotes any tumour of mesenchymal origin (supporting structures). They are much less frequent than carcinoma. Metastasis from sarcomas is generally blood-borne, and few give rise to lymph node secondaries (Figure *evolve* 16.13).

Lymphomas are malignant tumours of lymphoid cells; many are classified as Hodgkin's lymphoma, leaving the remainder as non-Hodgkin's lymphoma. Some are closely related to leukaemias (tumours of white blood cells).

There are many tumours that do not easily fit the guidelines mentioned such as testicular teratomas: some are in Table 16.2 and others are referred to elsewhere in this book under the relevant organ Refer to Figure *evolve* 16.10 (Teratoma) (Figure *evolve* 16.14).

Undifferentiated tumours

Some tumours lack obvious features to allow their identification or classification. An undifferentiated carcinoma or sarcoma cannot be ascribed to any subcategory. An anaplastic tumour could be carcinoma, lymphoma or sarcoma. As these different categories have major therapeutic consequences, it is important to attempt a more detailed diagnosis. Simple microscopy can now be supplemented by special staining procedures, many of which involve detecting cell components with antibodies. The presence of the leukocyte common antigen (CD45), B-cell (CD20) or T-cell (CD3) markers would indicate a lymphoma, whereas finding cytokeratins would suggest a carcinoma (Figure *evolve* 16.15). As tumours have deranged genetic function there are sometimes unexpected findings. Electron microscopy sometimes helps. There are other approaches such as cytogenetics, which depends upon finding characteristic abnormalities of the chromosomes. These are most often loss or gain of part or the whole of a chromosome, or translocations in which two chromosomes break and are rejoined with the fragments on the wrong chromosome, for example t(11;22).

Most oncology centres arrange for many of their patients' tumours to be reviewed before treatment. Diagnosis and classification of rare or undifferentiated tumours form a considerable part of such work.

EVOLVE CONTENTS (available online at: http://evolve.elsevier.com/Symonds/radiotherapy/)

Chapter | 17 |

Molecular, cellular and tissue effects of radiotherapy

George D.D. Jones, Paul Symonds

INTRODUCTION

One of the most successful and useful modalities in the clinical treatment of cancer is the local eradication of a patient's tumour using external beam radiotherapy (RT). In addition to this, external beam RT is also used in the palliation of cancer-associated symptoms, for example, to treat pain or spinal cord compression, to shrink tumour masses or to relieve bleeding. The local treatment of a patient's tumour via external beam RT is accomplished by (i) the precise and focused delivery of radiation to kill tumour and tumour-associated cancer cells by conforming, and more recently modulating, the delivered radiation dose to the target volume, and (ii), by exploiting the differences in the response of tumour and normal tissue to irradiation. Through largely empirical studies, this has led to curative external beam RT protocols of typically $\approx$2–3 Gy being delivered in daily fractions to the tumour site over 4–7 weeks; the exact dose and fractionation schedule depending on the clinical situation and the tolerance of the normal tissue being co-irradiated. Indeed, in many instances, it is the likelihood of normal tissue damage that limits the total dose that can be delivered to the tumour site. Overall, however, the exact basis for the success of RT in eliminating cancers is still poorly understood, appearing to depend on differences in intrinsic sensitivity, ability to proliferate, and repair capacity between both normal and malignant tissues.

In the last 30 years, radiobiology has gone someway to providing explanations and reasoning for these empirically derived schedules and, while many of the advances in RT have been realized via the optimization of treatment delivery schedules and technologic improvements in the physical targeting of dose, biologic discoveries, particularly those investigating the molecular and cellular response to irradiation, continue to point the way towards new and more effective methods/protocols of treatment. Indeed, there is every hope that this biologic information will aid individualization of RT, both in terms of improved treatments and superior patient selection.

The aim of this chapter is to describe some of the pertinent molecular and cellular principles and phenomena that underpin current radiation treatment practice, to relate this to outcomes observed in the clinic, and to provide insight into possible future developments and potential pitfalls in radiotherapy and radiobiology research. Clearly, this is a vast field, so this chapter will concentrate largely on the molecular, cellular and tissue radiobiology of low LET (linear energy transfer) radiation. Only brief mention of other radiations (i.e. heavy particle) will be made, while other delivery techniques (i.e. brachytherapy) are covered in detail elsewhere in this book.

IONIZING RADIATION, FREE RADICAL GENERATION, SUBCELLULAR RADIOGENIC DAMAGE

Radiations interact with matter by transferring energy to the molecules of the absorbing material. Indeed, radiations of wavelengths $<10^{-6}$ cm have sufficient photon energy to eject orbital electrons from the atoms of the absorber's molecules, leading to their *ionization*. As the most abundant molecule in a cell is water, the main product of this initial process in a cell is an ionized water molecule ($H_2O^{+\bullet}$); these radical cation species then interact with other water molecules to form hydroxyl radicals ($^\bullet OH$) (Figure 17.1A). The initially ejected electrons (e^-) may possess sufficient energy themselves to cause further ionizations until their energy is dissipated and they become solvated to give an aqueous electron (e^-_{aq}) and/or combine with other species to generate reducing species such as hydrogen atoms ($H^\bullet$) or superoxide ($O_2^{\bullet -}$). Ionizing radiation is non-discriminatory in that all molecular species in a cell may be damaged. However, DNA is considered to be a key molecular target for the deleterious effects of ionizing radiation in cells. $^\bullet OH$ radicals are highly reactive and, together with the less reactive reducing

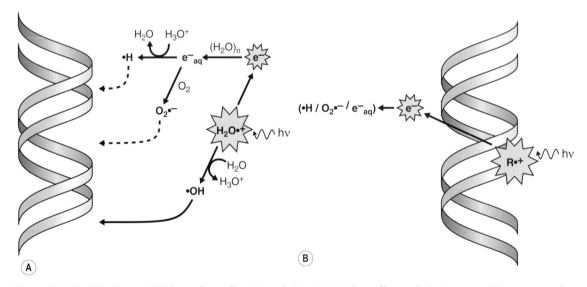

Figure 17.1 The (A) indirect and (B) direct effects of ionizing radiation. In the indirect effect, radiation interacts with water to produce hydroxyl free radicals ($^\bullet OH$) which, in turn, react with the DNA producing damage. In the direct effect, the radiation interacts directly with the DNA to produce damage. While both direct and indirect effects damage DNA, it is suggested that only indirect events happening within 2 nm of the DNA damage the DNA. Indirect effects dominate for low LET ionizing radiations. (The $^\bullet$ 'dot' refers to an unpaired electron of a free radical, and the dashed lines reflect the lower reactivity of the reducing species with DNA, as compared to the high reactivity of $^\bullet OH$).

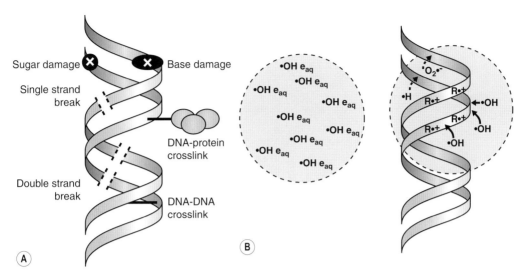

Figure 17.2 (A) The types of damage produced by radiation. (B) The concept of multiply damaged sites being produced by a cluster of ionizations impinging on the DNA and its local environment. Energy deposition for x-rays is not uniformly absorbed, but deposited in discrete events of high energy sufficient to generate a number of ion-pairs. Should this happen in pure water this will generate locally several $^{\bullet}OH + e^-$ pairs, however, should these events overlap the DNA both the direct and indirect effects will contribute to MDS formation.

species, may damage DNA via the so-called *indirect* effect (Figure 17.1A). Radiation can also directly ionize the DNA leading to *direct* damage of the DNA's bases or sugar-phosphate backbone ($R^{+\bullet}$) (Figure 17.1B); although the distinction between *direct* and *indirect* damage is not always clear as electrons and radical cations produced in the DNA and DNA-associated water may lead to further ionizations/oxidations in the DNA macromolecule and its surrounding microenvironment.

Through *direct* and *indirect* effects, radiation causes a wide range of damage in DNA, including strand breaks, base or sugar damage and cross-links between macromolecules (i.e. DNA–DNA or DNA–protein cross-links) (Figure 17.2A); the frequency of these DNA lesions is shown in Table 17.1. In general, it is considered that the DNA double-strand break (DSB) is the most critical for the lethal effects of radiation; evidence for this is a follows:

- under a variety of experimental conditions, it is the relative level of induced or unrepaired DSBs that best correlates with cell killing
- a single DSB is lethal to yeast
- enzymatically produced DSBs (produced by inserting DNA restriction enzymes into cells) gives the same pattern of chromosome damage and lethality as radiation
- microbeam irradiation has shown the cell nucleus to be the most radiation sensitive site in the cell
- the extreme radiosensitivity of some mutant cell lines is due to defects in DSB repair.

Table 17.1 Types and frequency of radiation-induced damage

TYPE OF DAMAGE	APPROXIMATE NUMBER PER Gy PER CELL
DNA double-strand breaks	40
DNA single-strand breaks	1000
DNA–protein cross-links	150
DNA–DNA cross-links	30
Base damage	2000
Sugar damage	1500

However, not all DSBs are the same, as the chemical nature of the strand break ends and the separation between the constituent single strand breaks can vary considerably, as can the proximity of other types of lesions. Indeed, the influence of the proximity of induced lesions has been shown to affect the reparability of damage and this is relevant because low LET radiation (x-rays and γ-rays) can produce multiple ionizations in isolated events (termed *spurs* and *blobs*). When these isolated events occur close to or overlap the DNA molecule (see Figure 17.2B), several lesions may be formed within a region of a few base-pairs

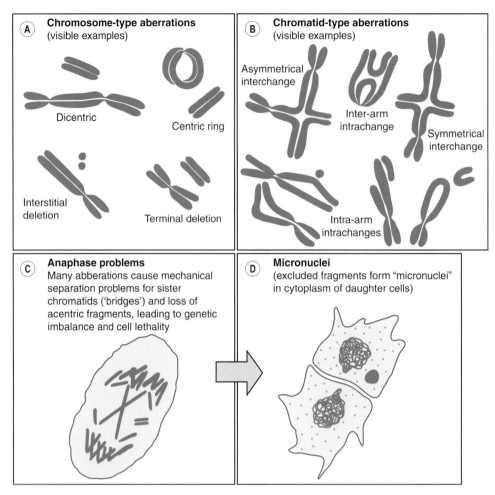

Figure 17.3 Some examples of radiation-induced chromosomal structural changes – solid stained. (A) *Chromosome-type* aberrations – all breaks and rejoins affect *both* sister-chromatids at the same locus. Only forms that produce acentric fragments are visible with solid staining. However, there is much hidden damage present, some of which is transmitted to future cell generations. (B) *Chromatid-type* aberrations – all breaks and rejoins affect *only one* of the sister chromatids at any one locus. Compared with chromosome-type changes, many more forms are visible with solid staining, but hidden damage still occurs. The observed frequencies always vary with post-irradiation sampling time, so there is never a fixed yield to set against a given exposure dose. Ionizing radiation can produce both types; the type recovered at first post-irradiation division depends upon the duplication status of the target chromatin, chromosome-types arising from pre-replicated chromatin. (C) Many forms lead to mechanical separation problems at anaphase ('inter-cell bridges') and acentric fragments are usually excluded from the daughter nuclei, leading to 'micronuclei' in their cytoplasm. (D) The exclusion of any visible fragment means the loss of many megabases of DNA. These bridges and fragments are the primary cause of cell lethality and genetic imbalance.
(Courtesy of Dr John Savage)

producing so-called *multiply damaged sites* (MDS), as described by Ward.

On a larger scale, radiation damage to chromosomes and chromatids leading to aberrations involving breakage and rejoining of chromosome/chromatid fragments (e.g. translocations and ring formations) are observed in many irradiated cells (Figure 17.3). As these events appear to correlate radiation-induced cell killing, such damage is considered an important aspect of the radiation-induced effects in many cells. Furthermore, chromosome damage may be a very sensitive indicator of environmental radiation exposure in an individual.

RECOVERY, DNA DAMAGE REPAIR AND CELL SIGNALLING

Recovery

Much of the DNA damage induced in cells is subject to repair (see below), with initial evidence coming from 'recovery' studies, such as split dose and delayed plating experiments. For the former, the effect of a dose of radiation was observed to be less if it is split into two fractions delivered a few hours apart and this was attributed to the 'sublethal damage recovery' (SLDR) or 'Elkind repair'. For the latter, it was observed that cells irradiated in a non-growing state, and left in this state for increasing periods of time, showed enhanced survival. This has been termed 'potentially lethal damage recovery' (PLDR). Both SLDR and PLDR are practical definitions in that they reflect the decrease in cell kill when RT is prolonged using lower dose rates or fractionated (SLDR) or delivered to a tissue in a non-proliferative state (PLDR). Both are believed to have a basis in DNA repair capacity, although there is some evidence that they do not reflect the same repair processes. It has been suggested that some resistant tumours owe their resistance to substantial PLDR, though this is controversial.

DSB repair and cell signalling

Each of the types of radiation-induced DNA damage is repaired by one of several DNA repair pathways (Table 17.2). Of particular significance to the deleterious biological effects of radiation is the repair of DNA DSBs. Consequently, intricate damage response pathways have evolved to repair DSBs. Two principal recombinational DSB repair pathways, that employ mostly separate protein complexes, have been recognized; *homologous recombination repair* (HRR) and *non-homologous end-joining* (NHEJ) (Figure 17.4A). Briefly, DSB repair by HRR requires an undamaged template molecule that contains a homologous DNA sequence, typically on the sister chromatid in the S and G2 phases of the cell cycle (see later). In contrast, NHEJ of two double-stranded DNA ends, which may occur in all phases of the cell cycle, does not require an undamaged partner and does not rely on extensive homologies between the recombining ends. It is likely that the balance between NHEJ and HRR in the removal of DSBs depends on the type and location of the lesion. Of note, however, is that NHEJ, unlike HRR, is inherently error prone and possibly mutagenic; that is, this process is potentially unable faithfully to restore the original DNA sequence. Still, NHEJ is considered to be the dominant DSB repair pathway in mammalian cells. The study of these pathways has proved to be a rapidly evolving field of research over the past few years and considerable interest has been generated by the realization that defects in HRR and, in some cases, NHEJ can be causally linked to impaired DNA replication, genomic instability, human chromosomal instability syndromes, cancer development, and cellular hypersensitivity to DNA-damaging agents.

Both NHEJ and HR DSB repair are facilitated by the sequential recruitment of a variety of DNA repair proteins and co-factors to the sites of DNA damage. For example, in NHEJ (see Figure 17.4B), Ku autoantigen, a DNA end-binding heterocomplex of two proteins (Ku70 and Ku80) binds to DSB sends, and then recruits and activates the DNA-dependent protein kinase catalytic subunit (DNA-PKcs) to form the active kinase DNA-PK, and possibly the MRE11/RAD50/NBS1 (MRN) complex, whose exonuclease activities may be required for trimming back DNA strands to areas of micro-homology. A DNA polymerase then fills any gaps and the XRCC4/ligase IV heterodimer

Table 17.2 Pathways involved in the repair of DNA damage

REPAIR PATHWAY	TYPE OF LESION	INVOLVED IN RADIOSENSITIVITY?
Base excision repair (BER)	BD, AP site, SSB	Yes
Homologous recombination repair (HRR)	DSB	Yes
Non-homologous end joining (NHEJ)	DSB	Yes
Nucleotide excision repair (NER)	CL, dimers, bulky adducts	?
Transcription coupled repair (TCR)	BD, dimers, bulky adducts	?
Mismatch repair (MMR)	Mismatched bases	?

AP, abasic site; BD, base damage; CL, cross-links; DSB, double strand break; SSB, single strand break.
(From Steel 2002, with permission of Hodder Education.)

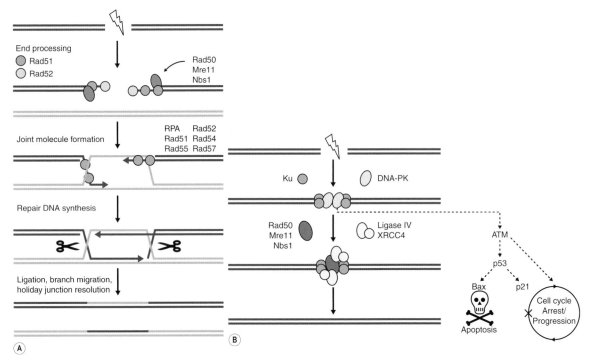

Figure 17.4 DNA double strand break repair; (A) homologous recombination repair (HRR) and (B) non-homologous end-joining (NHEJ). NHEJ is error prone while HRR uses a non-damaged homologous template and is therefore error free.

seals the breaks by forming a phosphodiester bond. Importantly, however, DNA-PK also appears to trigger signal transduction pathways that are involved in stress responses leading to apoptosis (leading to the elimination cells bearing excessive or irreparable damage), cell cycle arrest (allowing cells more time for repair) or cell progression. This is an example of an important concept, developed from studies in molecular radiobiology, that cells possess sensors of induced damage and that these act to link damage to a cell's ultimate response through intricate cell signaling pathways. Patterns are now emerging that allow critical molecules and pathways to be recognized linking DNA damage and DNA damage repair to classical outcomes of radiation exposure.

A major unanswered question, which is now the focus of increasing research, is the extent to which variation in the level of expression/activity of DNA repair enzymes plus enzymes and proteins involved in downstream signalling, influences the outcome of RT. Given the highly ordered nature of the described protein machines, small structural changes introduced by single amino-acid changes in individual proteins may alter the activity of the complex significantly. Indeed, there is increasing evidence that mild reductions in DNA repair capacity, assumed to be the consequence of common genetic variation in the human population (polymorphisms), affect cancer predisposition and, by inference, may possibly modulate the response to radiation treatment as well.

Epigenetic radiation signalling mechanisms

Although, traditionally, nuclear DNA has been considered to be the key target for the biological effects of ionizing radiation, numerous studies have now revealed several non-genomic 'epigenetic' targets that influence a cell's response to ionizing radiation. Radiation-induced damage to cytoplasmic, mitochondrial and membrane structures, changes in redox balance and protease activity have all now been suggested to mediate cellular responses to ionizing radiation. These include ceramide production from plasma membrane-derived sphingomyelin and activation of numerous signalling pathways including inflammatory-type pathways, mediated by proinflammatory cytokines (e.g. tumour necrosis factor α (TNF-α) and cytokine IL-1) and other cytokines and cytokine receptors, plus cell adhesion molecules and proteases/antiproteases. These responses play an important role in tissue recovery and remodelling following irradiation (see later). Another example of the epigenetic radiation-induced signalling includes expression of epidermal growth factor receptor (EGFR), which has a prosurvival effect. Pharmacological inhibition of this pathway leading to cell sensitization can be achieved with EGFR-binding antibodies or small molecule inhibitors of the EGFR tyrosine kinase (e.g. Gefitinib (Iressa) and Tarceva (erlotinib, OSI 774)).

Another factor to consider is the bystander effect, an intercellular signalling pathway now described in several studies. These responses appear to be cell-type dependent, and they consist of broad cellular changes including gene activation, induction of genomic instability, differentiation, and changes in apoptotic potential. This appears to be mediated, at least in part, by diffusible substances, since the effect occurs when 'bystander cells' are physically separated from the irradiated cells. While the diffusible substance remains to be identified, contenders include nitric oxide and/or cytokines being released to mediate membrane dependent signaling events. Consequently, the entire tumour microenvironment may need to be taken into account when considering the consequences of cancer cell irradiation.

RADIATION-INDUCED CELL KILLING

As already mentioned, the objective of RT is to kill cancer cells while limiting damage to the surrounding normal tissue and this is achieved in part by exploiting the differences in the response of tumour and normal tissue to irradiation. One of the best known and most studied differences between tumour and normal tissue is the manifestation of hypoxia in tumours.

Tumour hypoxia, oxygen effect and reoxygenation

In order to grow, solid tumours need to develop their own blood supply through the process of *angiogenesis*. However, the formation of this neovasculature tends to 'shadow' tumour growth, consequently, a growing tumour's nutrient and oxygen demands can exceed the capacity of the host's blood supply. Furthermore, the chaotic nature of tumour vasculature coupled with the limited diffusion of oxygen in a highly proliferating tumour (see below) results in areas of chronic and sustained hypoxia and nutrient deprivation. In addition, areas of acute reversible hypoxia are also found which may be the result of physiological defects in the new vessels (leading to temporary closure of blood vessels), transient flow instability or changes in fluid pressure.

The relevance of hypoxia to the radiation treatment of cancer is that laboratory studies have demonstrated that cells irradiated in the absence of oxygen are considerably more resistant to the lethal effects of radiation than those irradiated in oxygen (Figure 17.5). This is partly due to molecular oxygen reacting with the induced DNA radicals to produce chemically irreparable peroxy radicals (Figure 17.6A). Thus, in effect, oxic cells suffer more DNA damage. The degree of sensitization by oxygen in often quoted as an *oxygen enhancement ratio* (OER), which is the ratio of doses needed to produce a given biological effect in the presence and absence of oxygen (see Figure 17.5). For most cells and tissues, the OER has a value of around 2.0–3 (*ca.* 2 at clinically relevant doses).

Numerous studies have linked hypoxia to poor RT outcome. The number of hypoxic cells has been shown to be

an important factor following the irradiation of human tumours. This has been shown by direct and indirect clinical studies. One of the most important studies was by Tomlinson and Gray in 1955. They examined sections of human bronchogenic carcinoma specimens and showed that there were cords of viable cells close to blood vessels. By contrast, 150–180 µm from blood vessels there were areas of necrosis. The width of the viable tissue (150–180 µm) was equal to the calculated diffusion distance of oxygen from blood vessels beyond which cells were unable to survive. They postulated that radioresistant hypoxic cells were present within the areas of necrosis. It is possible to measure oxygen tensions in accessible tumours, such as carcinoma of cervix, by directly inserting Eppendorf electrodes into the tumour. The degree of hypoxia within tumours has been correlated to clinical outcome; tumours with large areas of hypoxia tend to persist after RT, while those tumours that are better oxygenated are more likely to be controlled.

In addition to its effects on DNA damage, laboratory studies have shown that hypoxia can also trigger genetic mechanisms that may give tumour cells additional survival advantages. Hypoxia induces the expression of a number of genes, in particular genetic programs that are under the control of hypoxia inducible factor 1 (HIF-1). HIF-1 is recognized as a key mediator of gene expression in hypoxic

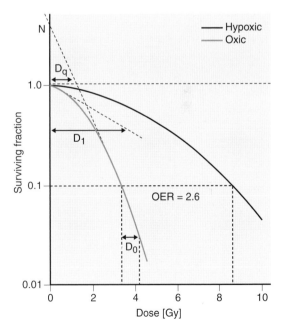

Figure 17.5 Survival curves (and derived measures) for mammalian cells exposed to low LET radiation under oxic or hypoxic conditions. Since the slopes of the initial and final slopes depend on the presence of oxygen, the OER is 2.5–3.0 for high dose-related effects (2.6 for 10% survival in the figure) but is typically less for lower dose-related effects.
(From McBride, Dougherty and Milas 2002, with permission of John Wiley & Sons)

tumours. The range of its downstream target genes is extensive. Some of these (i.e. vascular endothelial growth factor (VEGF), erythropoietin and TNF-α) are clearly aimed at increasing angiogenesis and oxygen delivery, so driving tumour growth. HIF-1 regulated mechanisms also control the acidity of tumour tissue and may further enhance tumour growth and radioresistance. Importantly, hypoxia can induce apoptosis by a mechanism dependent upon a drop in extracellular pH. Although, intuitively, this process would be expected to reduce the tumour cell population, it can in fact provide a selective pressure for the emergence of apoptotic-resistant subclones (see Figure 17.6B). In this way, hypoxia may select for cells with p53 mutations (since cells expressing wild-type p53 tend to undergo apoptosis more readily) and these tumours will have an anti-apoptotic, more malignant phenotype.

Cells that are initially hypoxic may become more oxygenated during a fractionated course of RT. Following a fraction of RT, most of the radiosensitive aerobic cells in a tumour will be killed and the surviving fraction will be predominantly hypoxic. If sufficient time is allowed before the next fraction of radiation, some of the tumour cells will oxygenate through the process of *reoxygenation* and, if this is efficient, the presence of hypoxic cells does not greatly affect the response of the tumour. However, the speed of reoxygenation varies widely, occurring within a few hours in some tumours and several days in others.

In order to reduce the number of hypoxic cells in a tumour, in the past, patients have been irradiated in hyperbaric oxygen chambers breathing oxygen at three atmospheres pressure. Breathing in hyperbaric oxygen has been shown to be advantageous in some tumours (locally advanced head and neck

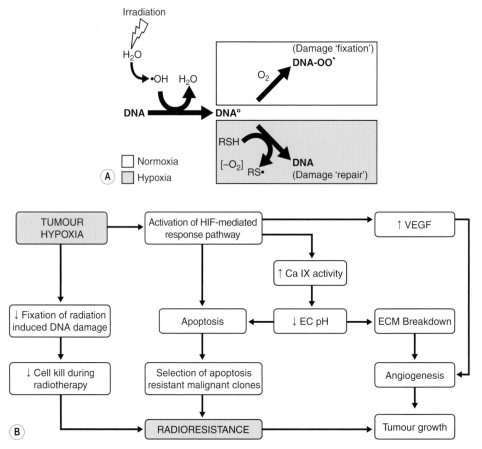

Figure 17.6 (A) The pivotal role of oxygen in the fixation of radiation-induced DNA damage. Ionizing radiation generates hydroxyl free radicals ($^\bullet$OH) that lead to the formation of DNA-centered radicals (DNA$^\bullet$). In the presence of oxygen, this damage becomes fixed. However, under hypoxic conditions, endogenous thiols (RSH) are able chemically to repair this damage (by donating hydrogen), effectively contributing to radioresistance. (B) Schematic diagram showing the role of hypoxia in causing radioresistance. In addition to its physical effects on the 'fixation' of radiogenic DNA damage, hypoxia triggers specific patterns of gene expression, mediated by HIF-1α. CA IX is pivotal in this response, causing acidification of the extracellular space, promoting extracellular matrix breakdown and apoptosis which, in turn, may provide a selective pressure favoring apoptosis-resistant subclones.

cancer) but not in others (cervical cancer). However, because of the dangers of fire, explosion and fits within the hyperbaric oxygen chamber, this treatment has fallen into disrepute. A class of electronaffinic drugs that mimic the damage-fixating radiosensitizing effects of oxygen, the nitroimidazoles, were evaluated as radiosensitizers. It was postulated that such agents would diffuse out of the tumour blood supply and, unlike oxygen, which is rapidly metabolized by tumour cells, would be able to diffuse further and reach the more distant hypoxic cells, and thus sensitize them. The drug misonidazole produced impressive results in the treatment of mouse tumours but neurotoxicity prevented this drug being of clinical value in patients. More recently, nimorazole has been shown to increase the locoregional control in patients with advanced head and neck cancer in a Danish study, but this drug is not in widespread use. However, reduction in the toxicity of the sensitizing compounds and the ability to identify tumours with significant hypoxic fractions has restored faith in the potential for this approach. One potentially fruitful opportunity for further development in this area centres on the recognition that cells can react to hypoxia by switching on specific genes (i.e. glucose transporter 1 (GLUT-1) and carbonic anhydrase 9 (CA 9)). This will not only allow the identification of hypoxic cells but may allow the specific targeting of hypoxic cells in gene therapy approaches. In addition, the use of drugs that are specifically activated in hypoxic areas (i.e. tirapazamine (SR4233) and AQ4N) have also been studied.

The cell cycle and sensitivity to irradiation

The radiosensitivity of cells varies throughout the cell cycle. Most cells are more vulnerable in the G2/M phase of the cell cycle (as the cells have little time to repair radiation-induced damage before the cells divide) and least vulnerable in late S-phase (possibly due to an increased opportunity for homologous recombination). Normally, within the tumour, individual cells are in different phases of the cell cycle. If their cell division could be synchronized in some way so they would be in a sensitive phase of the cell cycle during treatment, this would increase the effectiveness of RT. Although it is possible to synchronize the population of cells in tissue culture, it has not proved possible to do so in clinical practice. A number of drugs have been used to try to produce a cell cycle block leading to increased killing by radiation. A typical example is hydroxyurea, which produces a late G2/M phase block. However, in practice, this drug has not been shown to increase radiosensitivity of tumours.

Low-dose hyper-radiosensitivity

Typically, most cell lines exhibit *hyper-radiosensitivity* (HRS) to very low radiation doses (<10 cGy) that is not predicted by back-extrapolating the cell survival response from higher

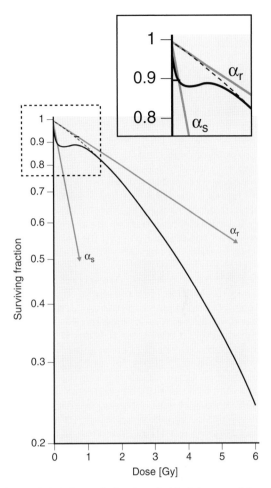

Figure 17.7 At low radiation doses (<10 cGy) many cell lines exhibit hyper-radiosensitivity which is characterized by a slope (α_s) that is considerably steeper than the slope predicted by back-extrapolating the cell survival response from higher doses. The magnified insert shows the low dose region over 0–1.4 Gy. The transition over ≈20–80 cGy from sensitive to resistant response has been termed a region of increased radioresistance (IRR). The dashed line represents the fit of the linear quadratic model. At doses below 1 Gy, the linear quadratic model, using an initial slope of α_r, substantially underestimates the effect of irradiation; this domain is better described by the steeper initial slope α_s.

doses (Figure 17.7). This is typically manifest as an initial steep decline in the cell survival curve. However, as the dose is increased above ≈30 cGy, there is increased radioresistance until, at doses beyond about 1 Gy, radioresistance is maximal. At higher doses, the cell survival follows the usual downward-bending curve with increasing dose. The precise operational and activational mechanism of the process is still unclear but Marples and Joiner, who originally discovered the phenomenon, propose the noted increased radioresistance (IRR) to be caused by an increase in the extent of DNA repair of cells in the IRR region.

Patterns of cell death after irradiation

Historically, radiation has been considered to kill cells largely by means of a 'mitotic cell death' in which proliferating cells undergo a general breakdown (i.e. 'necrosis', see below) when they attempt to divide with radiation-damaged chromosomes. This holds true for many cells but it is clear that some cells, notably those of some normal tissues, die via a morphologically distinct mechanism known as 'apoptosis'. The differences between apoptotic and necrotic cells are listed in Table 17.3. Cells lethally injured by radiation typically execute one or more divisions before dying. The number of divisions depends on the size of the radiation dose but after a dose of 2 Gy, two or three attempts to divide may be made. The progeny of these cells may all die or a proportion may survive to contribute to the reproductive (clonogenic) pool. In the 'interphase death' process, whereby cells die before they divide, cells die 2–6 hours after irradiation. These tend to be radiosensitive cells such as lymphocytes, spermatagonia and hair follicles and only relatively low doses of radiation are required.

Apoptosis is an important mechanism of normal tissue homeostasis and is a form of 'programmed cell death'. It is a mechanism for eliminating cells that have sustained high levels of potentially deleterious, irreversible damage. It is now recognized as being the outcome of a sequence of biochemical signals, usually requiring the involvement of p53 gene products, that ultimately result in the activation of a series of enzymes (caspases) that degrade cellular proteins and DNA endonucleases that cut DNA in regularly repeated regions that are not protected by nucleosomal proteins. The latter results in the fragmentation of DNA into multiples of 80–100 base pairs which produce a characteristic ladder pattern when the DNA is separated in an agarose gel. The significance of this is that apoptosis is under specific genetic control and, therefore, susceptibility to radiation-induced apoptosis may be amenable to manipulation. Apoptotic cells undergo phagocytosis by neighbouring cells and inflammation is not induced.

Within a few hours there is no trace of the dead cell. For this reason, apoptosis was underestimated in the past as a source of cellular loss. The frequency by which cells undergo apoptosis varies in different tumour types. For example, lymphomas have a high incidence of both spontaneous and treatment-induced apoptosis, whereas high-grade gliomas do not.

Necrosis is a pathological process that is not a component of normal tissue haemostasis and may occur in tumours due to prolonged nutrient and oxic deprivation. This involves the loss of membrane integrity, an increase in cell size with the release of lysosomal enzymes with a subsequent inflammatory response. Necrosis can follow vascular injury, changes in pattern of perfusion through the tumour or may be the mode of death of cells that lack an adequate apoptotic pathway.

Models of radiation cell survival

As radiation-induced cell killing is exponential rather than arithmetic in nature, it is traditionally illustrated as the logarithm of survival plotted against linear dose. A typical survival curve produced by low LET radiation (x- or γ rays) is shown in Figure 17.5. There are two components to this curve. First, there is an initial slope (designated D_1) and shoulder, then at higher doses the curve becomes steeper and straighter as survival decreases exponentially with dose. Cell killing is measured in the exponential part of the curve by using the value D_0, which is the dose sufficient to reduce the survival fraction by 37% ($1/e$) and in so doing the radiation induces on average one lethal event per cell. The size of the shoulder is regarded as giving an indication of the repair capacity of the cell and can be quantified by the quasi threshold dose Dq.

There have been several mathematical models developed to describe cell survival curves, including the *multitarget equation*, the *multitarget with single hit equation* and the *linear quadratic equation*. The oldest, the multitarget theory, presumed that the cell contained a number of critical targets all of which have to be inactivated to bring about lethality. However, studies with human tumour cells indicate that the initial shoulder is not absolutely flat, so the simple multitarget equation is not appropriate. The linear quadratic model is a better description of cell killing, particularly at lower dose. This assumes that radiation can produce both non-recoverable and repairable lesions. Non-repairable damage is referred to as the alpha component (represented as αD on a logarithmic scale) and is considered induced linearly by 'single hit' mechanisms, while the beta component (βD^2) describes the quadratic cell inactivation by the accumulation and possible interaction of repairable damage induced by 'multiple hits'. When plotting cell survival, alpha-type damage is represented by a straight line and beta damage by a curve (Figure 17.8). The ratio of alpha-beta (α/β) is the dose at which single and multi-hit mechanisms contribute equally to cell killing; that is $\alpha D = \beta D^2$.

Table 17.3 A comparison of some of the morphological features of apoptosis and necrosis

NECROSIS	APOPTOSIS
Cells swell	Cells shrink
Mitochondria dilate and other organelles dissolve	Organelles retain definition for a long time
Plasma membranes rupture	Cells dissociate from surrounding cells
Nuclear changes 'unremarkable'	Chromatin condensation and 'regular' DNA degradation

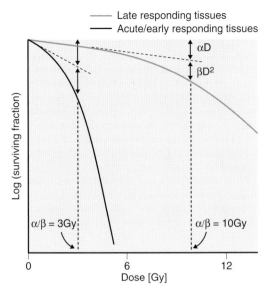

— Late responding tissues
— Acute/early responding tissues

αD

βD²

Log (surviving fraction)

α/β = 3Gy

α/β = 10Gy

0   6   12

Dose [Gy]

Figure 17.8 Dose–response relationships for early- and late-responding tissues. The relationship for late-responding tissues is more curved than for early-responding tissues, which in the linear-quadratic formula translates into a larger α/β ratio for early than for late effects.

The α/β ratio is used to define survival curve characteristics and classify cellular and tissue responses to RT. Acute/early responding tissues, which express radiation damage days or weeks after irradiation, have high α/β values of 7–20 Gy (typically around 10 Gy) (see Figure 17.8). Well-oxygenated tumours have even higher ratios. In contrast, late responding tissues, which express radiation damage months to years after RT have low α/β values of between 0.5 and 6 Gy (typically ≈3 Gy). The survival curves of cells in late responding tissues are significantly more curved than those with high α/β ratios. Late responding tissues, such as the spinal cord, are much more sensitive to changes in fraction size than acute responding tissues, such as skin or the mucosa of the mouth. Generally, tumours have α/β ratios similar to acute responding tissues. One exception may be prostate cancer that has a low α/β ratio.

The importance of these values is that they can be used to calculate isoeffect relationships in RT, and calculations of parameters like the *biologically effective dose* (BED) are important when manipulating fractionation regimens. The BED, in effect, is the dose required to produce a given biological effect when the radiation is given as an infinitely large number of very small fractions or as a single dose at extremely low dose rate. For a given treatment, the BED can be calculated if the α/β ratio of the dose-limiting tissue and the tolerance dose for a given fractionation regimen are known. Using the BED, the relationship between tolerance dose and dose per fraction can be worked out for new fractionation regimens.

Attempts to introduce biological mechanisms into the models has lead to the *lethal, potentially lethal damage* and *repair saturation* models, though the actual mechanisms are rudimentary and poorly defined. Furthermore, the recently discovered phenomenon of low-dose HRS (see above) deems that the older (and indeed some of the more current) models of radiation cell killing cannot be considered as adequate.

RADIATION EFFECTS IN NORMAL AND MALIGNANT TISSUE

As mentioned above, both DNA and epigenetic sites are important initiators of radiation-induced signalling responses following exposure. Indeed, many of the effects seen at the tissue level in the clinic (i.e. recovery and remodelling) are the manifestation of these pathways. Cellular responses to irradiation include induction of early response genes (e.g. v-jun sarcoma virus 17 oncogene homologue (avian) (JUN), v-fos FBJ murine osteosarcoma viral oncogene homologue (FOS), and early growth response 1 (EGR1)), which can bind to specific DNA sequences to modulate the expression of other genes. Also, intermediate and late genes are induced, such as TNF-α, platelet-derived growth factor (PDGF), transforming growth factor (TGF) β, and fibroblast growth factor 2 (basic) (bFGF), which are involved in premature terminal differentiation of fibroblasts by ionizing radiation and therefore mediate fibrosis as a late response to RT. Also, a growing body of evidence appears to support the hypothesis that chronic oxidative stress serves to drive the progression of radiation-induced late effects. Some of the pathways that mediate these effects are now revealed, but their importance is still the subject of current debate and the focus of continued research. What follows is a brief description of the effects of radiation at a tissue level.

Acute responses of normal tissue

Following large single x-ray treatment, such as a single fraction of 10 Gy to treat bone metastasis, cytokines and proteases, products of cell signalling and from cell killing (apoptosis and necrosis), are released from the irradiated tissue and interact with normal macrophages and lymphocytes. This may bring about erythema of treated skin within hours, oedema and may be the source of nausea and vomiting associated with RT. The acute effects of RT are normally seen in tissues with a high cellular turnover rate, such as gastrointestinal mucosa, skin, bone marrow and mucosa of the upper aerodigestive tract. These effects are usually seen after 2–3 weeks during a fractionated course of radical RT lasting 4–7 weeks.

Acute reactions are due to cellular loss. A good model is the acute reaction in skin, especially if the patient is treated with kilovoltage radiation. After about 14 days, hair loss (epilation) occurs. This is followed by erythema. If the dose is high enough this may be followed by dry desquamation. As the skin is shed there is a serous exudate, which is referred to as moist desquamation. Healing depends on initial recovery of the skin stem cells, which usually regenerate most of their number before differentiating to restore function. This process is normally complete within a few weeks. A similar effect is seen within the mucosa of the upper aerodigestive tract. Cells are lost from the mucosa following RT leading to a characteristic radiation reaction. Initially, there is erythema of the mucosa followed by mucosal cell loss. This denuded area is covered by a white membrane containing inflammatory exudate and dead cells and is usually white in colour. In the normal mucosa, only about 15% of stem cells are undergoing cellular division to replace normal cell loss. The majority are in the resting phase (G0) of the cell cycle. After about 10–12 days into a standard course of RT, virtually all surviving stem cells are dividing to replace cell loss from RT. Usually within a few weeks of completing a standard dose of RT the mucosa has healed, but if a very high dose has been given sufficiently to destroy the stem cell pool, the patient may be left with a persisting area of ulceration within the treated area.

Subacute reactions of normal tissue

Some tissues, such as neural tissue, have a much longer normal turnover time than skin or oral mucosa. The effects of radiation may not be seen until several months after treatment. A typical example is Lhermitte's syndrome following irradiation of the spinal cord. A few weeks after treatment the patient complains of electric shocks radiating down to fingers and toes especially if they flex their neck. This is due to partial temporary demyelination of the spinal cord. There is often an interval of 9–18 months before late effects are seen in cell populations with a slow rate of proliferation such as nervous tissue, kidney, blood vessels, subcutaneous tissue and bone or cartilage. Initially, damage to the slowly proliferating vascular endothelium was thought to be the common cellular injury linking most late effects. Undoubtedly, damage to blood vessels is important but, for example, with late demyelination of the brain there is also loss of oligodendrocytes and subsequently neurons as well as damage to small blood vessels. Similarly, in the kidney, there is loss of renal tubular cells as well as vascular injury. In late responding tissues, such as jejunal mucosa, cell loss is rapid and there may be evidence of radiation-induced cell loss within 24 hours of irradiation. By contrast, in the kidney there may be no histological evidence of cell depletion for many months after RT. If a high enough radiation dose has been given to destroy all the clonogenic tubular cells, the tubules will not regenerate. If one or more tubular clonogenic cell per nephron survives, the tubule may well regenerate over several months.

The effect of radiotherapy upon tissues

All tissues have different cellular populations within them and may undergo both acute and late damage. A typical example is the effects on skin and subcutaneous tissue. If the radiation dose is moderate, any acute reaction may settle without any late effects. However, if there has been marked depletion of the epidermal proliferating cell compartment, the skin may be thin (atrophic) and may be white owing to loss of pigment-producing cells. There may be also permanent loss of hair. The tissues of the dermis may be replaced with fibrous tissue leading to thickening of the subcutaneous tissues and loss of elasticity. The thickening of tissues around joints, such as the shoulder, may lead to marked reduction in shoulder movement. The walls of arteries may be replaced by fibrous tissue leading to narrowing of the lumen and thrombosis. This is often followed by compensating dilation of skin capillaries leading to telangiectasia of the skin. These red blood vessels on the skin surface may be very disfiguring.

Ultimately, perhaps following a minor insult such a trauma or infection, the skin may necrose leading to a non-healing ulcer.

The tolerance of normal tissues

The dose that can be given to tumours is limited by the tolerance of normal tissues. The tolerance depends on the overall radiation dose, fraction size and the time between fractions. Overall treatment time and the volume irradiated are lesser factors, but the type of radiation used is also very important. Megavoltage x-rays spare the skin compared to kilovoltage (250–300 kV). Absorption in bone and cartilage is also much less with megavoltage x-rays and there is less risk of necrosis.

By and large, acute reactions settle with simple medical measures. It is the late effects that are most feared as target organ damage can be severe and capacity for recovery is usually small. Such injuries are very difficult to treat surgically as the blood supply to heavily irradiated tissues is very poor. The frequency of late effects depends upon the site and the stage of the tumour. The aim of RT following lumpectomy for breast cancer is local control of the breast cancer plus a cosmetically acceptable breast. The late serious complication rate following breast irradiation should be very small (less than 0.5%). In early larynx cancer, the incidence of serious necrosis is only 1–2%, although the incidence rises with more advanced disease. One of the highest frequencies of late effects is seen in the treatment of cancer of cervix. In a national audit of patients treated in 1993, the incidence of serious late injury was 6%.

The tolerance of organs that have rapidly proliferating cells may be quite low. The tolerance of both lungs to megavoltage RT is 20 Gy given in 15 fractions over 3 weeks. The kidney has a similar tolerance. The tolerance of the whole liver is 25 Gy given again over 3 weeks. The incidence of radiation myelitis of the spinal cord is 1–5% with doses of 50–54 Gy given in 1.8 or 2 Gy fractions.

Retreatment

Conventional wisdom is that heavily irradiated tissue will not tolerate a retreatment. Previous high dose irradiation may limit the tolerance of the tissue to retreatment but, in some cases, further RT is possible. Factors governing the possibility of further therapy include the amount of cell depletion, the time elapsed since the previous treatment and the dose given and fraction size used. Clinical examination is sometime extremely useful to decide whether the patient can be retreated. If the skin has marked late changes with extensive subcutaneous fibrosis, retreatment may well be impossible. Similarly, radiological investigations may show evidence of late radiation damage, such as pulmonary fibrosis, which may preclude further radiation treatment. Primate studies have shown a modest but significant repair of radiation damage of the spinal cord. There seems to be about a 40% recovery in radiation tolerance following a dose of 44 Gy given in 2.2 fractions by 2 years after treatment.

Response of tumours to radiation

Tumours may have numerous mitoses visible on histological examination but they only grow slowly. A classical example is the slow-growing basal cell carcinoma of skin. In this tumour, virtually all cells produced following cell division are lost by apoptosis and necrosis and only a small number of the progeny of the dividing tumour adds to the tumour mass. In most carcinomas, over 90% of cells are lost in this way and are referred to as the cell loss factor. The potential volume doubling time (i.e. the time to go from a volume of $2 cm^3$ to $4 cm^3$) in many tumours is in the order of 60 days. Without cell loss, tumours have the potential to grow much faster than this. Mitotic count, S-phase count and bromodeoxyuridine labelling index would suggest that, in many tumours, they have a potential doubling time of 3–8 days. Although the growth potential of many tumours is extremely rapid, owing to the high cell loss factor, in practice they grow much more slowly.

Cell loss factor may influence the rate of tumour regression during RT. Tumours with a high spontaneous cell loss factor will regress more rapidly during therapy regardless of whether the tumour was growing quickly or slowly before treatment. However, what will govern ultimate outcome is the number of clonogenic tumour cells surviving the radiation treatment. Classically, only one clonogenic cell needs to survive; the tumour will then regrow. Many squamous cancers have high loss fractions and regress quickly. By contrast, the cell loss factor in prostatic cancer is much smaller and these tumours shrink much more slowly after a lethal dose of radiation.

The growth fraction is the number of cells that are in cycle. In solid tumours, these are usually less than 20% of the cells. Tumours with a high growth fraction may shrink more rapidly than those with a smaller growth fraction, however, unless all clonogens are sterilized, these tumours may also rapidly regrow. Tumour growth fraction and repopulation may be increased following radiation treatment. Experiments have shown that there can be rapid regrowth of the clonogenic population of the tumour even while the tumour mass is regressing.

Modification of fractionation patterns

Repopulation during fractionated treatment is one reason why tumours persist after RT. This may be overcome by giving two or three treatments daily. A fraction size less than 2 Gy is normally given to reduce the late effects in tissues, although acute reactions may be enhanced. Interfraction intervals should be as long as possible, but there should be at least 6 hours between treatments. The use of fraction sizes less then 2 Gy is usually referred to as hyperfractionation and treatment schedules shorter than standard treatments are usually called accelerated treatment. Patients with well- or moderately well-differentiated tumours seem to have the greatest capacity for repopulation during RT and seem to be the group most likely to benefit from accelerated treatment.

OTHER RADIATION MODALITIES

Heavy particle radiotherapy

Neutrons were perceived as a solution to the hypoxic cell problem as, in experimental systems, hypoxic cells were more sensitive to neutrons than conventional x- or gamma rays. However, in practice, neutron irradiation was found to be no more effective than conventional fractionated photon RT. Moreover, many trials had to be abandoned because of the severity of severe late effects associated with neutrons. This treatment is no longer used.

By contrast, treatment with protons looks more promising. The relative biological effect of protons is similar to x-rays and the physical characteristics of a proton beam has potential marked depth dose advantage in the treatment of some tumours. The distribution of charged ion beams in tissue is entirely different to those of photons (x- and γ rays). Protons increase their rate of energy deposition as they slow down with increasing penetration finally stopping and releasing an intense burst of ionization called the Bragg peak. By selecting a suitable proton energy, it may be possible to release most of the energy of a proton beam within the tumour if the Bragg peak is superimposed over the tumour-bearing area.

FUTURE TRENDS (AND PITFALLS)

New technologies

With many of the advances in RT having been realized via technologic improvements in the physical targeting of the radiation, work is continuing in this area to delivery superior instruments. *Intensity-modulated radiotherapy* (IMRT) is latest form of three-dimensional conformal RT, designed to address a major limitation of conventionally delivered RT;

namely, the inability to restrict the treatment beam to the tumour-bearing tissue. However, the move from conventional conformal RT to IMRT involves more fields and a larger volume of normal tissue being exposed to lower doses. In addition, the number of monitor units is increased by a factor of two to three, increasing the total body exposure, due to leakage radiation. Both factors will tend to increase the risk of second cancers, with IMRT estimated approximately to double the incidence of second malignancies compared with conventional RT from about 1% to 1.75% for patients surviving 10 years. The numbers may be even larger for longer survival (or for younger patients), but the ratio should remain the same. *Image guided radiation therapy* (IGRT) consists of a linear accelerator with an integrated 3D volume imaging functionality. This allows an image of the tumour site with CT-like quality to be acquired and reconstructed immediately before treatment, with the patient already set up in the treatment position. Consequently, if the patient needs to be moved, the treatment table can be controlled remotely to do so. Alternatively, if the tumour is no longer where it was or has changed shape or size, then the treatment plan or conformal setting can be modified as appropriate. If the tumour is likely to move during treatment (for example a lung tumour during respiration) then appropriate margins can be set using sequential imaging. This allows the radiotherapist to address directly clinical concerns regarding organ motion and deformation and uncertainties in repeating and maintaining the set-up of the patient, thereby inspiring clinical confidence in the practice of advanced radiation therapy techniques.

Molecular studies

An important future aim of molecular/biologic studies in RT is to increase the therapeutic ratio to increase tumour control and/or to decrease late effects by predicting outcome on an individual basis to select the most appropriate treatment for each patient. Also, molecular/biologic studies should enable development of new combined-modality treatments such as RT and concurrent biological therapies or chemotherapy in a scientifically rational manner. The advent of the 'Omic' technologies holds great promise for the future development of molecular studies in RT. *Gene expression arrays* (cDNA and oligonucleotide arrays) allow investigation of large numbers of patients' genes and show variation in gene expression among tumours with similar histological features. In diffuse large B-cell lymphomas, there is a very different overall survival between two such groups using this assay. Genes that would be expected to be good candidates for prediction of radiosensitivity include DNA repair genes and genes related to cell cycle control, growth regulation, and differentiation. *Proteomic* technologies may also have a role in investigation of radiosensitivity as it can provide a more accurate indicator of protein function than gene expression arrays by taking into account post-translational modifications.

In summary, radiobiology has reached a stage where specific molecular and cellular pathways and responses are being related to the various outcomes of RT. Such studies are exposing new potential targets for therapeutic manipulation of radiation responses. The well-established efficacy of RT, together with the accumulated knowledge of many decades of treatment, provides a robust platform from which to launch novel approaches to extend the usefulness and increase the efficacy of RT. Combined with the molecular evaluations of the probability of tumour cure and normal tissue complication, as well as the more precise delivery of dose, the future of radiobiology in RT research looks bright.

FURTHER READING

Books

Hall EJ. Radiobiology for the radiologist. 5th ed. Lippincott Williams and Wilkins; 2000.

King RJB. Cancer biology. 2nd ed. Prentice Hall; 2000.

Steel GG. Basic clinical radiobiology. 3rd ed. Arnold; 2002.

Chapters in books

Kiltie AE. Radiotherapy and molecular radiotherapy. In: Knowles MA, Selby PJ, editors. Introduction to the cellular and molecular biology of cancer. 4th ed. Oxford University Press; 2005. p. 414–27.

McBride WH, Doughert GJ, Milas L. Molecular mechanisms in radiotherapy. In: Alison M, editor. The cancer handbook. John Wiley & Sons; 2002. p. 1359–69.

Journal reviews

Barcellous-Hoff MH, Park C, Wright EG. Radiation and the microenvironment – tumorigenesis and therapy. Nat Rev Cancer 2005;5:867–75.

Connell PP, Kron SJ, Weichselbaum RR. Relevance and irrelevance of DNA damage response to radiotherapy. DNA Repair (Amst) 2004;3:1245–51.

Ward JF. Complexity of damage produced by ionizing radiation. Cold Spring Harb Symp Quant Biol 2000;65:377–82.

Willers H, Dahm-Daphi J, Powell SN. Repair of radiation damage to DNA. Br J Cancer 2004;90:1297–301.

Chapter | **18** |

Principles of management of patients with cancer

Paul Symonds, Cathy Meredith

INTRODUCTION

The diagnosis of a malignancy is only the beginning of a cancer patient's journey and throughout this time decisions about how to best manage and care for patients have to be addressed. Before seeing the oncologist, the majority of cancer patients will have been given their diagnosis, most frequently in the outpatient department rather than a hospital ward. The importance of this event cannot be overemphasized and the manner of communicating this information is pivotally important.

When patients do meet their oncologist for the first time, the presence of a family member or friend can be helpful, as the family member can provide emotional support, help in recall of the conversation and can ask supplementary questions. This can be important at a time when patients will be seeking to try to understand their condition and what the future may hold for them. There is little doubt that the majority of patients with cancer want as much information as possible. This often includes the elderly and the incurable. The first, sometimes initially unspoken, question is 'is it curable?' and after that 'is it treatable?' At some point, most want to know the options there are for treatment and the side effects of possible treatments. Absorbing this information can be traumatic and often patients cannot take in this complex web of information in one consultation. Support nurses, or other healthcare

Table 18.1 10 steps to breaking bad news

1. **Preparation**
   Know all the facts before the meeting, find out who the patient wants present and ensure privacy and chairs to sit on.

2. **What does the patient know?**
   Ask for a narrative of events by the patient (e.g. 'How did it all start?')

3. **Is more information wanted?**
   Test the waters but be aware that it can be very frightening to ask for more information (e.g. 'Would you like me to explain a bit more?')

4. **Give a warning shot**
   e.g. 'I'm afraid it looks rather serious' – then allow for a pause for the patient to respond.

5. **Allow denial**
   Denial is a defence, and a way of coping. Allow the patient to control the amount of information.

6. **Explain (if requested)**
   Narrow the information gap, step by step. Detail will not be remembered but the *way* you explain will be.

7. **Listen to concerns**
   Ask 'What are your main concerns at the moment?' and then allow space for expression of feelings.

8. **Encourage ventilation of feelings**
   This is the *key* phase in terms of patient satisfaction with the interview because it conveys empathy.

9. **Summary and plan**
   Summarize concerns, plan treatment, foster hope.

10. **Offer availability**
    Most patients need further explanation (the details will not have been remembered) and support (adjustment takes weeks or months) and benefit greatly from a family meeting.

professionals, who are present in the clinic, can provide useful reinforcement and clarification of patients' questions. Often the oncologist needs to cover the ground more than twice.

This whole process involves relaying information that can severely alter a patient's view of their future and is challenging for the giver of the information as well as the patient. A useful guide in this process is the ten-step approach to giving bad news (Table 18.1). This model advocates good preparation, finding out what patients want to know, allowing denial and listening to concerns. It also recognizes the importance of encouraging the ventilation of feelings and the important role played by relatives.

The most important decision at this time is whether the patient should be treated radically with cure as the aim of treatment. But radical treatment may be associated with treatment-induced morbidity and, occasionally, mortality and it is therefore vital to ensure that it is the appropriate route to be taking. Unfortunately, a number of patients will be unsuitable for a radical approach to treatment and palliation will be the appropriate option.

The next question is which is the best treatment modality or modalities for that particular patient. Clearly, the patient needs to have been fully investigated before such decisions can be taken and usually these investigations will have been carried out prior to referral to the oncologist. However, supplementary investigations may need to be carried out. These may include examination under anaesthetic, endoscopy and appropriate radiological investigations such as computed tomography (CT), magnetic resonance imaging (MRI) or isotope bone scans. As the diagnosis of cancer has such possible dire implications, all patients should have histological proof of the diagnosis, if this is possible, especially if radical treatment is planned. To make appropriate management decisions the clinician must take into account tumour and patient factors (listed below).

Frequently, the patient's management may have been discussed in a multidisciplinary team meeting (MDT) where the patient's pathology and radiological investigations will have been reviewed. The decision is usually made about whether cure is possible and the appropriate treatment modality. However, only one or two of the treating team may have met the patient at this stage and decisions made at the MDT meeting may not survive the consultation with the patient and oncologist. When discussing treatment options, the patient's wishes are paramount. However, in practice, the majority of patients will accept the careful reasoned advice of their doctors. Very occasionally, patients ask for radical treatment when this is futile. Somewhat more frequently, such requests come from relatives. However, a doctor is not obliged to provide a treatment that they conscientiously feel is not in the patient's best interest.

FACTORS GOVERNING CLINICAL DECISIONS

Tumour factors

Organ of origin

The organ in which the cancer develops is an important factor affecting both outcome and treatment. Complete surgical removal of brain tumours is usually impossible, as a complete excision would normally damage vital parts of the brain, leading to either death or an unacceptable neurological deficit. Similarly, the brain is sensitive to ionizing radiation and this limits the dose of radiotherapy that can be given. However, in other sites, such as the kidney, a complete organ can be removed with impunity.

Histological type

Identification of the precise histological type of a tumour governs both treatment and prognosis. For instance, basal cell and squamous carcinomas arising from the epidermis of the skin have a good prognosis and the treatment is straightforward. By contrast, melanomas arising from pigment-producing cells (melanocytes) have a much more serious outlook.

Degree of differentiation

The pathologist can grade the degree of differentiation. Well-differentiated tumours look like the tissue of origin and poorly-differentiated tumours may look primitive and do not look like the tissue from which they arise. For instance, well-differentiated thyroid cancer has a good prognosis and is relatively easily treated by such measures as surgical excision and radioiodine. Anaplastic thyroid cancers rapidly spread and respond poorly to any treatment.

Tumour staging

Where possible, tumours should be staged using the international T, N and M classifications. T stands for primary tumour stage, which is usually decided by the tumour size. N stands for the presence or absence of lymph node metastases, the usual method of spread in carcinomas and some sarcomas. M represents the presence or absence of distant metastases. In practice, other staging systems have been developed and are referred to in the preceding chapters.

Tumour size

In general, the larger the tumour the lower is the chance of cure either by surgery or radiotherapy. It may not be possible to excise completely a large tumour. Similarly, a large tumour treated by radiotherapy contains more clonogenic tumour cells (cells capable of forming colonies of cells following radiotherapy) and an increased proportion of radioresistant hypoxic cells. Stage Ib carcinoma of cervix is tumour confined to the cervix, but this stage is subdivided into stage Ib1 (less than 4 cm) and Ib2 (greater than 4 cm). By and large, stage Ib1 tumours are treated by radical hysterectomy and stage Ib2 by chemoradiotherapy.

Locoregional spread

Spread to regional lymph nodes usually indicates a poorer prognosis and the need for more aggressive therapy. Patients with squamous carcinoma of head and neck with spread to regional lymph nodes may be treated by a radical neck dissection along with primary radiotherapy or surgical excision of the affected organ. As spread to lymph nodes in breast cancer is often associated with occult distant spread, such patients usually receive adjuvant chemotherapy following surgery.

Distant metastases

The presence of distant metastases may suggest that attempts to remove the primary tumour completely are futile, as is the case in lung cancer. However, such metastases may be chemosensitive and a high probability of cure may be possible. A typical case is testicular teratoma where high cure rates are seen following cisplatin-based chemotherapy.

Tumour site

Tumour site may determine the treatment modality. For instance, the skin on the back of the hand or the shin does not tolerate radiotherapy well. There is an increased risk of skin necrosis at these sites compared to elsewhere in the body. Surgery is often the preferred treatment for basal cell or squamous carcinoma in these areas. However, small basal cell carcinomas on the eyelid are often better treated by radiotherapy than surgery.

Operability

Many factors must be taken into account before deciding to treat the patient by radical surgery. A patient may have other illnesses than cancer that may make the risks of surgery or anaesthesia extremely high (see below). The tumour's size or involvement of adjacent structures may prevent complete removal of the cancer. The site of origin has also got to be taken into account together with the chance of complications following surgery and the functional result.

Removal of inguinal lymph nodes is an important part of the treatment of carcinoma of the vulva. However, groin wounds are slow to heal and may become infected, especially in elderly people. The high risk of complications may be a contraindication for this type of surgery in the very elderly. Functional and cosmetic results are extremely important in head and neck surgery. Before the decision is made to remove a cancer, it must be possible to reconstruct the appropriate part of the upper aerodigestive tract and guarantee reasonable function and cosmesis.

Pathological examination of the excised tissue

At first, surgery may be planned as the sole method of treatment modality. However, pathological examination of the excised tissue may change this decision. If the pathologist finds that tumour extends to surgical margins, the chance of tumour recurrence is very high indeed. Postoperative radiotherapy may then be required. Radiation treatment may also be required depending on the degree of spread within the organ. The chance of microscopic spread to the pelvic lymph nodes is associated with the degree of differentiation of endometrial cancer and the degree of spread into the myometrium. Following simple hysterectomy, patients with poorly-differentiated tumours and/or deep spread into the myometrium are often offered postoperative radiotherapy to reduce the chance of pelvic recurrence.

Patient factors

Age

As a general rule, patients aged up to 75 years tolerate surgery or radical radiotherapy well. However, the biological age of the patient needs to be taken into account as well as the chronological age. A fit patient in their 80s will tolerate radiotherapy well but younger patients with serious general medical conditions may find treatment side effects intolerable. Many elderly patients may have chronic medical problems, such as chronic obstructive airways disease or ischaemic heart disease. These co-morbid conditions may increase the risks of surgery to an unacceptable degree. Similarly, they may affect outcome after radiotherapy. Patients with poor pulmonary function are not suitable for radical treatment for lung cancer. The lung may become fibrosed around the irradiated tumour. This will have no effect in a fit patient but the loss of even a small amount of lung function may cause respiratory failure in someone with chronic obstructive airways disease. Patients with ischaemic heart disease may have poor normal tissue perfusion. This may increase the number of radioresistant hypoxic cells within the tumour and also affect the ability of normal tissue to repair damage following radiation treatment.

Performance status (Tables 18.2 and 18.3) provides a crude but very effective method for judging response to treatment, especially with chemotherapy. Poor performance status is associated with shorter life expectancy. Patients with performance status three (in bed more than 50% of the time) are often not suitable for radical treatment. A paradox is that, although these patients have marked symptoms and the most to gain from chemotherapy, they are the group least likely to respond to this treatment. The highest response rates are seen in those with performance status zero or one.

Patient preference

Patient's preference should be taken into account. For instance, Stage Ib carcinoma of cervix can be treated equally

Table 18.2 Karnofsky performance status scale	
100	Normal, no complaints
90	Normal activity, minimal signs or symptoms
80	Normal activity with effort, some symptoms
70	Caring for self, unable to work
60	Needs occasional assistance but able to cater for most needs
50	Needs considerable assistance and frequent medical care
40	Disabled, needs special care
30	Severely disabled, needs hospital care
20	Very ill, in hospital, needs supportive care
10	Moribund
0	Dead

Table 18.3 UICC performance status scale	
Grade	
0	Able to carry out normal activity
1	Able to live at home with tolerable symptoms
2	Disabling symptoms, but less than 50% of the time in bed
3	Severely disabled, greater than 50% of the time in bed but able to stand
4	Very ill, confined to bed

well by radical surgery or radiotherapy. By and large, younger and fitter patients are offered radical hysterectomy and older or more obese patients tend to be treated by radiotherapy. However, the individual patient may have a preference for one modality or the other.

Chance of cure

Decision making is easy if the chance of cure is high. A typical case is a T1 larynx cancer, which carries a chance of cure better than 90%. The side effects of radiotherapy to the larynx are tolerable even in the very elderly. By and large, patients with a 30% or better chance of cure are offered radical treatment. In more advanced disease with a poorer outlook, a lot depends on the patient's age and fitness. For instance a T4 carcinoma of bladder carries a 10–25% chance of cure. A fit middle-aged man may be offered intensive chemotherapy prior to removal of the bladder and construction of an ileostomy, whereas the right treatment for an unfit, elderly man may be palliative radiotherapy in order to suppress symptoms from his bladder cancer.

Treatment modality

Increasing use of multimodality treatment has rather blurred the once clear-cut rules for treatment by the various modalities.

Surgery

Surgery, traditionally, was important for establishing the diagnosis and finding the extent of spread of the cancer. Increasingly, diagnosis is made without operation using sophisticated imaging techniques such as MRI or CT scanning. Histological proof may be obtained by fine needle or tru-cut biopsy. Radical surgery is still the treatment of choice for many adenocarcinomas, particularly arising in the stomach, colon, thyroid and kidney.

Palliative surgery

Prior to palliative surgery, the risks and benefits to the patient need to be carefully measured and the patient's potential life expectancy needs to be taken into account. Surgery is particularly useful in dealing with obstruction of an organ. A classical case is the relief of large bowel obstruction by a colon cancer by a colostomy. However, palliative surgery may be inappropriate in patients with multiple small bowel obstruction. This is often the case in ovarian cancer where the risks of surgery outweigh the benefits. Advanced fungating breast tumours are much less common than they were 25 years ago, but surgery offers a rapid method of relieving the unpleasant odour and bleeding associated with such tumours. The pinning of the broken bone, which is often followed by palliative radiotherapy, may relieve pain following a pathological fracture.

Radical radiotherapy

The decision to treat the patient by radical radiotherapy depends on the tumour and patient factors previously discussed. The precise regimen will depend on the potential radiosensitivity of the tumour, the size of the treatment volume and the proximity of dose-limiting critical tissues. Seminoma of the testes is among the most radiosensitive tumours. The doses required to control small volume disease in the para-aortic lymph nodes are 25–30 Gy in 15 fractions over 3 weeks. By contrast, large lymph nodes containing metastatic squamous carcinoma may not be controlled by doses as high as 70 Gy given in 35 fractions over 7 weeks.

What governs radiation dose is the tolerance of the surrounding normal tissues. The small bowel is the most sensitive tissue in the pelvis and the chance of serious small bowel damage rises steeply with doses exceeding 50 Gy given in 25 fractions over 5 weeks. Radiation damage to the spinal cord can be catastrophic leading to permanent paralysis. In the treatment of tumours in the head and neck, oesophagus and bronchus, care must be taken to restrict the spinal cord dose to 45–50 Gy in 25 fractions over 5 weeks.

The side effects of radical radiotherapy may be marked. For instance, the mucositis associated with treatment of head and neck cancer may prevent the patient swallowing and they may require nasogastric or PEG (percutaneous endoscopic gastrostomy) feeding. However, acute side effects are normally self-limiting and settle in a few weeks with the help of simple supportive measures. It is a probability of late radiation damage that limits the dose to the tumour. In the treatment of breast cancer, the incidence of serious late effects should be vanishingly small and certainly less than half a percent of those patients treated. As the life-threatening nature of the tumour increases, the patient and the oncologist may be persuaded to take greater chances. Serious damage is seen in the larynx following treatment for a T3 (fixed vocal cord) tumour in 1–3% of patients. In patients with inoperable cervical cancer, the only realistic chance of cure is chemoradiotherapy. Some of the highest complication rates associated with radiotherapy are seen following the treatment of cervical cancer. On average, 6% of patients require surgery to try to correct late damage following treatment.

Palliative radiotherapy

Palliative treatments can make up between one-third and one-half of the workload of any department. The aim of such treatment is to relieve local symptoms in advanced cancer. An important part of the treatment is that there should be minimal upset. Treatment should be simple and a minimum number of fractions should be used. Symptomatic relief should be rapid.

Up to 80% of patients with bone metastases have significant pain relief within 3 weeks of a single radiation treatment of 8–10 Gy. Pain relief will be complete within half of these patients. Other important indications for palliative radiotherapy are the relief of haemoptysis, cough, dyspnoea and mediastinal obstruction in lung cancer. These symptoms can be suppressed in between 50 and 80% of patients by a course of radiotherapy lasting up to a week, with minimal side effects.

However, some symptoms require longer radiotherapy treatments. Tumours involving nerves, such as the brachial plexus (Pancoast tumours from the apex of the lung) or the lumbosacral plexus, produce pain of a very unpleasant quality that is difficult to relieve with opiate analgesia. Relief of such neuropathic pain may require 4–5 weeks' radiotherapy treatment. Typically, neuropathic pain from advanced rectal cancer can be relieved in two-thirds of patients with doses of 45–50 Gy given in 4–5 weeks. Radiotherapy can prolong life in some incurable tumours. Randomized controlled trials have shown that the average survival of patients with glioblastomas of the brain following optimal surgery and radiotherapy is only a year. However, 6 weeks' radiotherapy increases a patient's survival by, on average, 9 months compared to treatment with surgery and best supportive care. When making the decision to offer a patient 6 weeks' radiotherapy, one needs to balance life expectancy that is taken up by the radiotherapy treatment and the associated fatigue with the survival benefit associated with a treatment which is unlikely to cure the patient. Elderly or more infirm patients are probably better treated by a simple scheme of 30 Gy given in six fractions three times a week over 2 weeks rather than 60 Gy given over 30 fractions.

Chemotherapy

Chemotherapy can be given as the sole source of treatment when there is a high chance of cure. Only a small number of tumours are highly chemosensitive and these include the lymphomas, testicular teratoma and choriocarcinoma. Chemotherapy frequently cures children with Wilms' tumours, rhabdomyosarcomas and acute lymphoblastic leukaemia. Chemotherapy may be given prior to radiotherapy or surgery to reduce the tumour in size. This is often referred to as neoadjuvant treatment. Increasingly, radiotherapy and chemotherapy are given together. This is of proven value in the treatment of carcinoma of cervix and squamous carcinoma of anus. Clinical trials are continuing in other tumour sites, particularly in the treatment of carcinoma of oesophagus and squamous carcinoma of the head and neck. Chemotherapy may be of palliative value only in advanced breast cancer or carcinoma of the colon but, in the treatment of small volume disease following surgery, adjuvant chemotherapy may improve cure rates. Chemotherapy improves 10-year survival in node positive breast cancer by about 10%. A similar survival advantage is seen following adjuvant chemotherapy in Duke's stage C colon cancer.

Support services

During and after cancer treatment, a wide range of services to provide the patient with physical, psychological and social support should be available. The most important single individual is the general practitioner. The general practitioner needs to be appraised of the patient's progress, the likely side effects of cancer treatment and what can be done at home to treat these side effects. They also need to be informed of what is the patient's likely prognosis. This is especially true if the treatment is palliative, as the general practitioner has a key role to play in the provision of continuing care. There is a wide range of specialist nursing services. Some have a relatively restricted role, such as stoma care nurses who provide practical advice on the management of bowel (colostomy and ileostomy) and urinary (urostomy) stomas. Increasingly, specialist nurses are attached to multidisciplinary teams in areas such as breast, gynaecological and CNS cancer. They have multiple roles in giving the patient specialist advice and psychological support. Last, but not least, is a range of national and local support services such as Macmillan Cancer Support.

There are important support nurses in the community, such as Macmillan and Marie Curie nurses. As well as providing advice on symptom control and emotional support for both patient and family, they also have a most important liaison role. They can act as a link between the patient, the general practitioner and hospital services. District nurses play an important role of care at home providing basic services such as bathing, dressing of wounds and giving medicines by injection.

Adequate nutrition is important following both radical and palliative radiotherapy and hospital- and community-based dieticians help with the special dietary needs of patients. Patients may also require the help of the prosthetic services. For some patients, one of the most distressing side effects of chemotherapy or radiotherapy to the head is hair loss. A good quality wig may help to maintain the patient's appearance and maintain morale. Other cosmetic prostheses that are important are replacements for eyes and sometimes ears or noses. Prosthetic limb fitters may be required to provide replacement limbs following amputation.

A patient with cancer may be the main breadwinner for the family, therefore, his or her illness may cause acute financial problems. Medical social workers and the Department of Health and Social Security may be able to provide financial support both from the State and from charitable bodies. Last, but not least, is a range of national and local support services such as Cancer BACUP or Macmillan Cancer Support.

Palliative care

In a regional oncology centre, at least 50% of the work is the treatment of advanced disease. Patients may be judged incurable from the outset and the aim of treatment is the relief of physical and psychological distress. Subsequently, patients who were thought initially to be in the curable category (such as carcinoma of breast) may develop advanced disease and may require the same type of care. Oncology centres will have developed their own systems of care to support these patients and this should interface well with their home or hospice care.

Ideally, patients should be cared for at home with the help of the general practitioner and district nurses. Specialist Macmillan nurses make a significant contribution to this process and, increasingly, organizations such as Marie Curie provide 'hospice at home' services.

Patients who have symptoms that cannot be controlled at home or when their nursing care is too complex may need admission to hospital or, ideally, to a specialist hospice. Hospices provide a more homely, less institutional and quieter environment than the noisy, busy hospital ward. The higher staff to patient ratio gives more time for patients to talk about their illnesses. The hospice team has the distinctive knowledge and skills needed to provide spiritual and emotional support for patients at this challenging time. Often, after symptoms have been controlled, patients may be able to return home perhaps to return to the hospice at a later date. Such patients while at home can be helped by attendance at the hospice day centre. As well as checking that the patient's symptoms are controlled, hospice day centres provide a social environment for patients and can allow other family members a respite from care to continue employment.

One of the main aims of a hospice is symptom control. These include pain, anorexia, nausea, vomiting, dysphasia, dyspnoea and lack of energy.

Pain control

Up to three-quarters of patients with advanced cancer may have some degree of pain. Up to 80% of patients may have pain at multiple sites. The three most common sources of cancer pain are bone metastases, compression of nerves and soft tissue disease.

Pain has both physical and psychological dimensions. Anxiety or depression may accentuate the perception of pain and lower the pain threshold. Physical conditions such as hypercalcaemia may also physiologically increase the degree of pain. The treatment of hypercalcaemia may be a pain control measure by itself. The basis of pain control is to establish the causes of pain and, if possible, eradicate the source of pain. The patient may benefit from a single radiotherapy treatment. However, come what may, the pain should be controlled by suitable analgesia if this is possible.

Ideally, all analgesics should be given by mouth. Mild or moderate pain may respond to simple analgesias, such as paracetamol or aspirin. The non-steroidal group of analgesics, such as diclofenac, may be useful, especially for bone pain. They can, however, cause gastric irritation and should be used with caution in even mild degrees of renal failure. Codeine or dihydrocodeine are useful for moderate pain but, unlike morphine, the dose of these drugs cannot be escalated. Increasing the doses above 60 mg four times a day just produces toxicity and not an increase in analgesia.

Morphine is still a standard analgesic for severe pain. In patients with normal renal and hepatic function, the metabolic half-life of morphine is two and a half hours. It therefore needs to be given no less frequently than four hourly. Morphine serum levels are stable after six half-lives, therefore, in practice morphine doses can be escalated every 12 hours. An initial dose of oral morphine should be chosen according to the patient's age, size and the degree of pain. This may vary between 5 and 30 milligrams. This is usually given in the form of either morphine sulfate tablets or an elixir. The dose can be rapidly escalated if necessary. When pain control is achieved, the total morphine dose over 24 hours can then be added up. This is a guide for the prescription of a strong acting analgesic such as MST (morphine sulfate continuous tablets). These tablets contain morphine in a cellulose matrix that is slowly released over a 12-hour period. If the patient has been receiving 30 mg of morphine elixir every four hours, the total morphine dosage in 24 hours

is 180 milligrams. This can be given in the form of 90 mg of MST every 12 hours to provide sustained pain control. If the patient cannot swallow, diamorphine is a useful substitute. This is highly soluble in very small quantities of water and can be given subcutaneously either by intermittent injection or continuously using a syringe driver. Diamorphine has roughly twice the potency of morphine when given by injection and three times the potency of oral morphine. Virtually all opiates cause constipation and patients should be routinely prescribed a laxative. A common side effect is nausea but this usually settles within 5 days.

Respiratory depression is rarely a problem but, if the patient develops significant respiratory oppression, morphine can be temporarily stopped and restarted at a lower dose. Occasionally, very high doses of morphine can cause myoclonic twitching of limbs.

About 10–15% of patients are intolerant to morphine because of either prolonged nausea or a dysphoric reaction. Alternative preparations are fentanyl patches, hydromorphone or oxycodone. In the treatment of neuropathic pain, tricyclic drugs, such as amitriptyline, or anticonvulsants such as gabapentin or sodium valproate often help symptoms. Occasionally, patients with neuropathic pain may require a nerve block. Sites where this can be carried out are in the intercostal nerves in the ribs, the brachial plexus when this is involved by an apical lung tumour, coeliac axis plexus following infiltration by a pancreatic cancer or involvement of the lumbar-sacral nerve plexus by pelvic cancer. These nerve blocks are technically very demanding. Usually a long-acting local anaesthetic is injected to check that nerve block will bring about adequate analgesia. If the pain is relieved this could be followed by a further injection using phenol or alcohol to destroy the nerve.

Dyspnoea

Shortness of breath can be more frightening than pain and sometimes more difficult to treat. Treatment of the underlying cause is often useful, such as aspirating a pleural effusion or abdominal ascites. If there is a strong anxiety component, an anxiolytic, such as diazepam, may be helpful. Morphine depresses the respiratory centre but this side effect is beneficial in reducing tumour-induced dyspnoea. As in the control of pain, the ideal route of morphine administration is by mouth but, if necessary, the patient may require diamorphine by syringe driver. As in other forms of dyspnoea, oxygen can be very helpful along with psychological support from staff.

Nausea and vomiting

There are many causes of nausea and vomiting in advanced cancer patients. Drug-induced vomiting is one of the most common. This may be also a symptom of renal or hepatic failure. Vomiting without a headache can be a feature of raised intracranial pressure.

5HT3 antagonists, such as granisetron or ondansetron, are probably the most effective drugs in the treatment of radiotherapy- or chemotherapy-induced nausea and vomiting. Where nausea and vomiting are associated with a strong anxiety component, antiemetic drugs, such as prochlorperazine or haloperidol, are often useful.

Anorexia

Anorexia is often multifactorial in origin. The most common cause is the underlying malignancy. It is thought that the cancer stimulates the release of cytokines from the immune system, which induce anorexia. Anorexia though may be due to treatment (radiotherapy or chemotherapy) or the physical effects of cancer, such as pain or intestinal obstruction. Dietetic advice may be helpful and a small amount of alcohol before meals may stimulate the appetite. Steroids are the most effective antianorexic agents. It is worth trying prednisolone at 30 milligrams over a 7-day period. If this increases appetite, the dose can be reduced to a maintenance dose of 5–10 milligrams. Progesterones, such as megestrol acetate, do improve appetite, however, they can cause ankle oedema and have been associated with an increased risk of thrombosis.

At least a quarter of patients with advanced cancer have significant depression. Virtually all patients with advanced cancer have a feeling of sadness and a sense of loss. Antidepressant medication should be considered sooner rather than later. The selective serotonin re-uptake inhibitors, such as fluoxetine or sertraline, are better tolerated than the traditional tricyclic antidepressants. They often work faster than the 3 weeks often quoted. Counselling, relaxation therapy and other measures are also useful adjuncts in the treatment of anxiety and depression.

Context of care

It is apparent that there is a multiplicity of professionals essential to the treatment and care of patients. These individuals work across the Health and Social Care sectors where the potential for a breakdown in communications is obvious. It is one of the challenges facing modern provision of cancer services that these groups are able to work together as a team to enable patients to be provided with a seamless service. This is now well recognized and encouraged by a host of Government initiatives designed to improve cancer services across the UK.

FURTHER READING

Department of Health. The NHS cancer plan. HMSO; 2000.

Kaye P. Breaking bad news: a ten step approach. EPL Publications; 1996.

Meredith C, Symonds P, Webster L, et al. Information needs of cancer patients in west Scotland; cross sectional survey of patients' views. Br Med J 1996;313:724–6.

NHS Executive. Improving the quality of cancer services. HSC/021. NHS Executive; 2000.

Chapter | 19 |

Chemotherapy and hormones

Anne L. Thomas

INTRODUCTION

Chemotherapy is the use of cytotoxic (cell poisoning) drugs to control tumour growth. Over the last 30 years, there have been advances in the management of several solid tumours and haematological malignancies, such as testicular teratoma, the leukaemias, childhood cancers and choriocarcinoma. Over 70% of childhood cancers are now curable and the cure rate for teratoma is over 95%. What has been more challenging is the use of cytotoxics in the management of the common tumours, such as non-small lung cancer, breast and bowel cancer. These tumours often present in the metastatic stage and are relatively resistant to chemotherapy. Despite intense research, chemotherapy for these tumours remains palliative in intent rather than curative.

One of the major drawbacks of cytotoxic agents is that they affect all rapidly dividing cells, and do not discriminate between normal tissues and tumours, hence, the toxicity of chemotherapy. We are now entering an exciting era in oncology with new targeted therapies becoming available. These novel agents are designed to exploit our increased understanding of molecular oncology and will hopefully be more successful in overcoming drug resistance and reducing the side effects of treatment.

Hormone therapy is another systemic treatment for cancer. It may involve inhibiting the production of endogenous hormones or introducing synthetic ones. There are now many different hormone preparations available and they play a vital role in the treatment of tumours such as prostate and breast cancer.

General indications for chemotherapy

There are four main ways in which chemotherapy can be used in the treatment of cancer. First, it is used as the primary treatment for patients with advanced cancers for which no alternative treatment exists. This is sometimes called palliative chemotherapy and is essentially used to palliate the symptoms of cancer. Adjuvant chemotherapy is the use of cytotoxic drugs after the primary tumour has been controlled by either surgery or radiotherapy. Here, the rationale is to eradicate subclinical micrometastatic disease and reduce the risk of recurrence. Examples of this would be in the treatment of bowel and breast cancer. Neoadjuvant (or primary) chemotherapy is used to debulk the primary tumour in an attempt to make the definitive treatment, for example surgery, successful. An example of this is neoadjuvant therapy of large breast primary tumours so that conservative local surgery rather than mastectomy is made possible. The fourth setting is to use chemotherapy directly into the tumour site, for example, into the blood supply of liver metastases from colorectal cancer.

Development and testing of anti-cancer agents

Cytotoxic therapies have been discovered in a variety of ways. First, some drugs have been developed de novo based on distinct properties that should confer anti-tumour effect. Alternatively, a range of compounds are produced and then screened against a selection of resistant tumour cell lines. Those with significant activity are then taken forward. Once this first generation drug is discovered then analogues with superior pharmacological properties (for example less toxicity, more convenient administration), are synthesized. Of course, one should not forget the past serendipitous discovery of drugs, such as cisplatin. Once an agent has been shown in its preclinical assessment to have sufficient activity against animal tumours, with acceptable toxicity, it can be considered for clinical evaluation. There are three phases of clinical assessment.

Phase I studies

In *phase I* studies, the main aim is to establish the maximum tolerated dose and the safety of the agent under investigation. Such studies are often performed with the informed consent of patients for whom standard therapy has no role. The starting dose is determined by preclinical data and is usually a tenth of the lethal dose (LD_{10}) in rodents. In phase I studies, pharmacokinetic studies (how the body handles the drug, for example by metabolism) and pharmacodynamic studies (assessing the impact of the drug on the physiology of the body) are conducted.

Phase II studies

Once a drug is found to have acceptable side effects it is taken forward into phase II studies to study its efficacy in a specific tumour type. The type selected is usually ascertained from the responses to therapy seen in the cell lines and sometimes from activity demonstrated in the phase I setting. The main outcome is to achieve a response rate which is at least comparable with the standard agent in that setting. Now there is a vogue actually to randomize some phase II studies so that either the drug can be compared with the standard or two different dose schedules could be studied. Gaining these data as early as possible in a drug's development obviously enables the pharmaceutical company to withdraw a drug as soon as possible if activity is disappointing or, alternatively, fast track drugs with impressive potential.

Phase III studies

In phase III studies, the new drug is compared against the gold standard in a randomized fashion. The main endpoint is survival but toxicity data are collected and also quality of life and health economic data. The cost effectiveness of the drug has to be assessed and deemed to be acceptable before the drug can be licensed and marketed.

Assessing tumour responses

It is essential that there is standardization of how tumours are measured and responses defined so that studies can be interpreted accurately. A number of different response criteria are available, but the system used most commonly now is RECIST (Response Criteria in Solid Tumours). In this system, the lesions are measured in one dimension, longest diameter (LD). A *complete response* is defined as eradication of all known disease based on two assessments at least 4 weeks apart. A *partial response* (PR) represents a reduction of at least 30% in the sum of the LD of target lesions maintained for at least 4 weeks. *Progressive disease* (PD) represents an increase of 20% or more in the sum of LD of lesions or the development of new lesions. *Stable disease* (SD) occurs when the measurements are either not good enough for a PR but also not bad enough for PD.

The evaluation of targeted therapies

With the advent of targeted therapies, such as anti-angiogenic treatment, and epidermal growth factor inhibition, it has become apparent that there are difficulties in assessing these agents using conventional study design endpoints. This is because the classic endpoint of the maximum tolerated dose may not actually be the biologically active dose. Moreover, these agents may be cytostatic rather than cytotoxic. This means that stabilization of disease is the best response that can be expected and the classical endpoint of reduction in tumour volume is not reached. It is therefore imperative that the actual target of these drugs is known and assays are incorporated into the study design as some 'surrogate' endpoints. An example of this would be the studies that investigated the activity of trastuzumab, the HER-2/erbB2 growth factor inhibitor, in breast cancer. Here, assays were carried out in tumour biopsies to ensure that the HER-2 receptor was indeed being targeted. It is envisaged that over the next few years there is going to be a change in study design with novel validated endpoints.

PRINCIPLES OF CYTOTOXIC THERAPY

To understand the rationale of cytotoxic chemotherapy it is important to recognize the features of tumour growth. The asymmetric sigmoidal growth curve, the 'Gompertzian growth curve' (Figure 19.1) describes the natural history of tumour growth. By the time that a tumour is clinically detectable, the majority of its growth has already occurred. In the early exponential phase of growth, the rates of tumour cell growth and tumour cell loss are proportional to the tumour cell burden at any point. Since most anticancer agents are more toxic to proliferating cells and most tumours are in a relatively slow phase of growth when diagnosed (i.e. they lie high and towards the plateau of the Gompertzian growth curve), it explains the limited effectiveness of chemotherapy for many cancers. The reason for tumour cytoreduction (e.g. by surgery) before chemotherapy is to bring the tumour to a lower point on the growth curve when the growth fraction of the tumour rises. The concept of moving the tumour down the Gompertzian curve underpins the rationale of adjuvant chemotherapy.

Unfortunately, it is not only the proliferating cells that must be eradicated by chemotherapy but also the small population of clonogenic cells mainly in G_0 phase. This explains some of the inherent problems of tumour chemoresistance. Cytotoxic drugs prevent cell division by inhibiting DNA replication. Unfortunately, these agents are not specifically acting against malignant cells, and damage both normal and malignant proliferating cells. A careful balance has to be kept between toxicity to the tumour and to the patient's normal tissues. What distinguishes normal and malignant cells is the failure of the malignant cell, unlike normal cells, to recover from cytotoxic damage. It is exploitation of these differences that underpins the role of targeted therapies.

Drug resistance

A variety of host factors influence the response to chemotherapy, these include the growth fraction of the tumour, the availability of the drug to the tumour and drug resistance. Resistance to chemotherapy may be intrinsic or acquired. Some tumours are intrinsically chemoresistant and show no response to treatment de novo. In other tumours, there is an initial response followed by relapse due to acquired resistance. Acquired resistance may have a variety of mechanisms. These include:

1. changes in the cell membrane impeding drug transport (e.g. of methotrexate)
2. DNA repair of drug-induced lesions (e.g. caused by cisplatin)
3. utilization of alternative metabolic pathways (e.g. 5-fluorouracil)
4. increased production of a target enzyme (e.g. dihydrofolate reductase binding to methotrexate)
5. modification of the target enzyme, enabling it to recognize the difference between true and false metabolites (e.g. 6-mercaptopurine).

The multiple drug resistance gene (*MDR1*) encodes P-glycoprotein. The latter is a membrane-associated efflux pump that is widely found in normal cells and serves to protect them from drug-induced damage. Normally, P-glycoprotein is found in very low levels, however, cancer cells can overexpress *MDR1* so conferring resistance to a variety of chemotherapeutic agents. In addition, *p53*, the 'guardian' of the genome and an important mediator of apoptosis (programmed cell death) may be mutated and give rise to chemoresistance in a number of solid tumours.

The reasons for drug resistance are not fully understood. It is common to find that a tumour responds to a particular

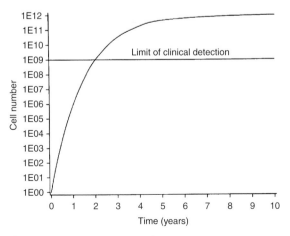

Figure 19.1 Gompertzian growth curve.

drug or combination of drugs for a period of time and then ceases to do so. It is thought that within many tumour populations there are genetically determined drug-resistant cells. When the chemosensitive cells have been killed, the resistant population may proliferate. Drug resistance to repeated exposure to a single agent will usually result in cross-resistance to other compounds of the same class of drugs. This is probably due to common transport mechanisms and pathways of metabolism and intracellular cytotoxic targets. However, cancer cells that have become resistant to one class of drugs may retain sensitivity to another class of drugs. Most drugs have a variety of mechanisms of drug resistance.

Some drugs which show excellent cell kill in vitro fail to do so in vivo. There may be multiple reasons for this. For example, if the tumour is in a sanctuary site, such as the central nervous system (CNS), the drug does not cross the blood–brain barrier and is therefore ineffective. There is also evidence that some tumours exhibit drug resistance that is partly due to host factors which modify the pharmacokinetics of the anticancer agent in vivo. Chemotherapy is most effective in killing proliferating cells. While the growth fraction is high in many chemosensitive tumours, such as the lymphomas and testicular teratomas, it is relatively low in many common tumours, e.g. colorectal cancer. Finally, in parts of the tumour the blood supply tends to be poor. This not only results in an inadequate concentration of drug reaching the tumour, but also the hypoxia reduces the growth fraction.

Selection and scheduling of chemotherapy agents

In an attempt to improve the curative potential of chemotherapy, agents with proven anticancer properties against a particular tumour but with different mechanisms of action and, as far as possible, non-overlapping toxicities are combined. This is known as *combination chemotherapy*. For example, in treating breast cancer, three agents – cyclophosphamide, methotrexate and 5-fluorouracil (known as CMF) – all have activity against breast cancer as single agents. However, their response rate as a combination (around 40%) is two- to three-fold that of their response rates as single agents. Thus, the overall response is at least additive if not synergistic.

Most schedules of chemotherapy administer the drugs on an intermittent basis to take advantage of the growth kinetics of malignant cells and normal tissues. After each pulse, the normal and malignant cell populations decline due to killing of cells in mitosis. The lowest level of the blood count is known as the *nadir*. However, whereas the bone marrow recovers to its previous level, the malignant cell population does not. With each subsequent course, this difference is accentuated. If the interval between pulses is too short, toxicity may prevent the delivery of further pulses on schedule, conversely, if the interval is too long, the tumour may regrow between courses. The total dose that can be administered is limited by the tolerance of normal tissue. Toxicity is often cumulative and may be irreversible. For example, the major dose-limiting toxicity of the anthracycline, doxorubicin is cardiotoxicity.

High-dose chemotherapy

Higher than conventional doses of chemotherapy can be delivered if the primary organ toxicity is to the bone marrow and there is minimal toxicity to other organs. Dose intensity is recognized to be important, particularly in chemosensitive tumours. Bone marrow toxicity can be overcome by autologous bone marrow transplantation. Normal bone marrow is harvested from the patient before high-dose chemotherapy. It is then returned to the patient at the time of chemotherapy to support the bone marrow through the period of neutropenia and thrombocytopenia. While high-dose strategies have been extremely useful in haematological malignancies, the results from similar approaches in solid tumours have been disappointing.

ROUTE OF ADMINISTRATION

The route of administration is governed by the solubility, chemical stability and local irritant properties of the agent. The simplest route, and the one that patients prefer, is the oral route. Patients can take their tablets at home with intermittent outpatient visits to monitor treatment. Unfortunately, many cytotoxic drugs are unstable and inactivated in the stomach, rendering them ineffective. Intravenous injection is the commonest route of administration of cytotoxic agents since it gives direct access to the systemic circulation. It can be done by delivery of a bolus dose or by infusion. Continuous infusions can be given (e.g. 5-fluorouracil) linked to a battery-operated pump worn around the patient's waist. The risks of intravenous administration are the introduction of infection and damage to the tissues around the site of administration if extravasation occurs.

It is possible to administer intraperitoneal chemotherapy, for example, in ovarian cancer. However, the drug absorption is variable and there are concerns about adverse effects, such as the development of adhesions. Intra-arterial administration has the advantage of delivering the drug in high concentration to the tissue supplied by the artery. Its limitations are the complexity of administration and the difficulty in correctly identifying the arterial supply of the tumour. Its main use is in the infusion of chemotherapeutic agents into the hepatic artery of patients with liver metastases from colorectal cancer. Intrathecal injection is used to deliver drugs in high dose into the CNS. Many cytotoxic drugs do not cross the blood–brain barrier and are therefore unable to kill tumour cells within the CNS. Methotrexate is the agent most commonly given by this route, for example, when the meninges are involved in lymphoma.

SIDE EFFECTS OF CHEMOTHERAPY

The main normal tissues damaged by cytotoxic therapy are those with rapidly dividing cell populations: the bone marrow, the gastrointestinal epithelium, the hair and the germ cells of the testis. By contrast, there is little effect on non-proliferating tissues, such as skeletal muscle and nervous tissue. The most common side effects of individual cytotoxic drugs are shown in Table 19.1. The most dramatic improvement in the management of side effects was with the development of the 5-hydroxytryptamine antagonist antiemetics. More recently the Neurokinin-1 antagonist aprepitant has improved the emesis of patients undergoing cisplatin based chemotherapy. Typical antiemetic regimens are shown in Table 19.2. Other drugs that have improved drug delivery have been the recombinant growth factors for red (erythropoietin) and white cells (human granulocyte colony-stimulating factor (G-CSF)). These agents stimulate the release of progenitor cells from the bone marrow and are useful in the treatment and prevention of anaemia and neutropenia.

CLASSIFICATION OF CYTOTOXIC DRUGS

The available agents may be divided into a few broad groups on the basis of their mechanism of action:

- alkylating agents
- antimetabolites
- mitotic inhibitors
- topoisomerase inhibitors
- miscellaneous
- hormones.

Some cytotoxic drugs act only on particular phases of the cell cycle (cell-cycle specific), while others act throughout the cycle (cell-cycle non-specific).

Alkylating agents

The main antitumour action of alkylating agents is the binding of an alkyl chemical group (R-CH2) to DNA, so inhibiting its synthesis. They also bind to RNA and other cell proteins, but these reactions are much less cytotoxic. The majority of alkylating agents have two available alkyl groups with which they can bind with DNA. Cross-linking may occur between a single strand of DNA or between two separate strands. Alkylating agents with this capacity to cross-link are called *bifunctional* and are more cytotoxic than alkylating agents with only one available alkyl group for binding to DNA.

The intravenous alkylating agents are nearly all vesicants and are irritant to the skin and other tissues if they extravasate out of the vein. In general, they do cause nausea and vomiting but this is usually controlled with antiemetics. They all cause myelosuppression, alopecia and temporary amenorrhoea. Nitrosoureas are a group of similar drugs whose main mode of action is alkylation. Specific examples of alkylating agents and nitrosoureas with specific side effects and main uses are shown in Table 19.3.

Antimetabolites

Antimetabolites are structurally similar to normal metabolites involved in nucleic acid synthesis. They are divided into three groups: folate, purine and pyrimidine antagonists. They substitute for their normal purine and pyrimidine counterparts in metabolic pathways, resulting in abnormal nuclear material that fails to function normally, or bind to enzymes, so inhibiting protein synthesis.

Folate antagonists

Methotrexate is the classical example. A number of co-factors are necessary for the synthesis of purines and pyrimidines. The reduction of folic acid is essential for the production of these co-factors. A key reaction in this process is the reduction of dihydrofolic acid to tetrahydrofolic acid by means of an enzyme, *dihydrofolate reductase*. Methotrexate is structurally similar to folic acid and has a much greater affinity for dihydrofolate reductase than does folic acid. Methotrexate therefore binds preferentially to dihydrofolate reductase and inactivates it. As a result, tetrahydrofolates cannot be made and purine and pyrimidine synthesis is inhibited. Methotrexate can be given orally, intravenously or at low dose intrathecally (Figure 19.2).

The metabolic block on the activity of dihydrofolate reductase can be bypassed by administering an intermediate metabolite, folinic acid (also known as leucovorin). Folinic acid is a tetrahydrofolate which provides an alternative source for continuing nucleic acid synthesis. The cytotoxic action of methotrexate and its toxicity can be diminished by administrating folinic acid. This is termed 'folinic acid rescue' and is particularly useful after high dose methotrexate therapy has been used. The main side effects of methotrexate are on the bone marrow and on the gastrointestinal tract. The nadir of the white count is at 10 days. Anorexia, nausea and vomiting are the first symptoms, followed 4–6 days later by oral and pharyngeal mucositis and diarrhoea. Conjunctivitis may occur as a result of accumulation of the drug in tears. Renal failure may complicate high-dose therapy. Liver damage (ranging from elevated liver enzymes to cirrhosis), lung injury (mainly fibrosis) may complicate prolonged therapy. Alopecia is uncommon. Methotrexate is used most commonly in non-Hodgkin's lymphoma, acute lymphoblastic leukaemia, breast cancer, and choriocarcinoma. Over the last ten years, new antifolates have been developed including pemetrexed. This is a multi targeted pyrroloprimidine based antifolate. When polyglutamated, it targets a number of folate dependent enzymes, for example, DHFR and TS. It has activity in a number of tumour types including non-small cell lung cancer and mesothelioma.

Table 19.1 Side effects of treatment

	ALOPECIA	GI TOXICITY	NEUROTOXICITY	CARDIOTOXICITY	UROLOGICAL TOXICITY	MYELOTOXICITY	SKIN CHANGES	LUNG TOXICITY	ALLERGIC REACTIONS
Cyclophosphamide	+	+			+	+			
Ifosfamide	+	+	++		++	+	+		
Chlorambucil		+				+	+		
Thiotepa		+				+	+		
Busulphan		+			+	+	+	+	+
Procarbazine		+	+			+	+	+	+
CCNU		+				+		+	
BCNU		+				+	+	+	
Dacarbazine		++				+	+		+
Mitoxantrone		+		+		+			
Temozoamide	+	+				+	+	+	
Mitomycin C		+				+			
Melphalan		+				+	+	+	+
Methotrexate		+	+		+	+	+		
6-Mercaptopurine		+				+	+		
Fludarabine		+			+	++		+	
5-Fluorouracil		+		+		+	+		
Cytosine arabinoside		+				+	+	+	

Drug								
Gemcitabine	+				++	+	+	+
Vincristine	+	++			+	+	+	
Vinblastine	+	+			+		+	
Vinorelbine	+	+			+	+	+	
Paclitaxel	+	++			+	+	+	+
Docetaxel	++	+			+	+	+	+
Doxorubicin	++	+	++		++	+	+	
Epirubicin	+	+	+		+	+	+	
Actinomycin D	+	+			+	+	+	+
Bleomycin	+					+	+	++
Cisplatin	+	+		++	+		+	
Carboplatin	+	+		+	+		+	
Oxaliplatin	+	++			+		+	+
Etoposide	+	+			++	+	+	+
Topotecan	+	+			+			
Irinotecan	+	++		+	+			
Asparaginase	+	+			+		+	+
Hyroxyurea	+	+			+	+	+	

+: minor toxicity; ++: moderate to high toxicity

Table 19.2 Typical antiemetic regimens

GRADE OF EMESIS	ANTIEMETIC PROTOCOL
Low	Metoclopramide 20 mg IV if required Metoclopramide 10–20 mg orally (PO) tds PRN
Moderate	5HT$_3$ antagonist PO and dexamethasone 8 mg PO then Metoclopramide 20 mg tds Dexamethasone 4 mg bd Both for 3 days
High	5HT$_3$ antagonist PO and dexamethasone 8 mg PO then 5HT$_3$ antagonist PO for 1 day Dexamethasone 4 mg bd for 3 days Metoclopramide 20 mg tds PRN
Second-line antiemetics	
Acute emesis	Give the antiemetic protocol for next grade of emesis
If already at 'high' give metoclopramide regularly, consider alternative antiemetics	Add in aprepitant 125 mg PO pre chemotherapy and 80 mg PO for 2 days post chemotherapy
Delayed emesis (>24 hours post chemotherapy)	Consider lengthening course of steroids, add in aprepitant and consider alternative antiemetics
Anxiety component	Add Lorazepam 1 mg PO or sublingually tds PRN. This can be started 1–2 days prior to chemotherapy
Alternative antiemetics	Domperidone rectally 30–60 mg 4–8 hourly PRN Haloperidol 1.5 mg tds PRN Cyclizine 50 mg tds PRN or regularly or levomepromazine 6 mg qds PRN

Purine antagonists

6-Mercaptopurine is a purine antagonist and inhibits a number of enzymes involved in the synthesis of the purine bases, adenine and guanine, which thus inhibits the synthesis of DNA. It is normally given orally and used in the treatment of leukaemia. The main toxicity is on the bone marrow (leukopoenia and thrombocytopoenia) and the liver. The nadir for white count and platelets is at 15 days.

Raised serum bilirubin is the most common feature of liver toxicity. This usually returns to normal on withdrawing the drug.

6-Thioguanine is also a purine antagonist and is an analogue of guanine. It may be given orally or intravenously but is now very rarely used in practice.

Fludarabine is a more recently developed antipurine. It is an adenosine analogue and is currently the most active single agent in the treatment of chronic lymphatic leukaemia. It is also active in the treatment of lymphomas. Its main limiting side effect is myelosuppression which can be very severe.

Pyrimidine antagonists

5-Fluorouracil (5-FU) is a fluoropyrimidine that inhibits DNA synthesis by inhibiting the main enzyme in pyrimidine synthesis and thus the formation of cytosine and thymine. In addition, it is erroneously incorporated into RNA instead of uracil and inhibits RNA synthesis. 5-FU is metabolized intracellularly in a number of steps to the active fluorodeoxyuridine monophosphate (FdUMP), this then forms covalent bonds with thymidylate synthase and its cofactor 5,10-methylene tetrahydrofolate, creating a complex which inhibits the formation of thymidine from deoxyuridine monophosphate (dUMP), so inhibiting DNA synthesis (see Figure 19.2). One problem with 5-FU is that elevated dUMP levels may overcome the inhibition of thymidylate synthase, thereby causing chemoresistance. Specific thymidylate synthase inhibitors, e.g. raltitrexed, have therefore been developed. Unfortunately, despite initially encouraging results, raltitrexed has not been as useful against colorectal cancer as predicted. In reality, it appears only to have a role in treating patients with cardiac problems as it is has a safer cardiac profile than 5-FU.

Historically, it was only possible to give 5-FU intravenously as the oral bioavailability of 5-FU was too unpredictable. The development of the oral fluoropyrimidines tegafur-uracil (UFT) and capecitabine have overcome this. In particular, capecitabine, is an interesting compound as it was formulated to be preferentially activated in the tumour. Capecitabine is metabolized to 5-FU in a three-step enzymatic reaction with tumour-selective generation of 5-FU through exploitation of the higher level of thymidine phosphorylase in tumour compared with normal tissue. The pharmacokinetics of orally administered capecitabine essentially mimics a continuous infusion rather than bolus 5-FU. To be able to prescribe an oral formulation of 5-FU is an enormous advantage as, understandably, patients prefer to take tablets and the potential risk of central line complications is avoided.

The main toxicities of 5-FU are to the gastrointestinal tract (diarrhoea, nausea and vomiting) and myelosuppression. The severity of the toxicity depends on the scheduling of 5-FU. For example, it is well recognized that giving 5-FU as a continuous infusion over 48 hours (De Gramont schedule) produces fewer side effects than giving the drug once every day for 5 days every month (Mayo schedule). Rarely, if a

Table 19.3 Summary of alkylating agents and nitrosoureas

NAME	ROUTE OF ADMINISTRATION	MAIN USE	NADIR	SPECIFIC SIDE EFFECTS
Cyclophosphamide	PO or IV	Non-Hodgkin's lymphomas, breast, ovary, sarcomas	9–15 days	Hemorrhagic cystitis due to the urinary metabolites of the drug, Treated with Mesna
Ifosfamide	IV	Sarcomas	5–10 days	As above Encephalopathy Nephrotoxicity
Chlorambucil	PO	Low grade lymphoma	8–15 days	GI upset
Melphalan	PO or IV	Myeloma	14–21 days	Mucositis
Thiotepa	IV	High dose therapy	28 days	Myelosuppression
Busulfan	PO	Chronic myeloid leukaemia	28 days	Lung fibrosis Prolonged myelosuppression
Procarbazine	PO	Brain tumours Hodgkin's	28+ days	CNS toxicity
CCNU (Lomustine)	PO	Brain tumours, lymphomas	28+ days	Delayed myelosuppression
BCNU (Carmustine)	IV	High dose, lymphomas	28+ days	Pulmonary fibrosis Delayed myelosuppression
DTIC	IV	Melanoma	21 days	Myalgia
Temozolamide	PO	Brain tumours	10–14 days	Myelosuppression
Mitomycin C	IV	Gastric, breast	14–28 days	Prolonged neutropenia

patient has genetic deficiency of the dihydropyrimidine dehydrogenase, very severe toxicity can result including neurological effects. 5-FU is widely used in a number of tumours, especially those of the gastrointestinal tract.

Cytosine arabinoside is an analogue of deoxycytidine. It is a competitive inhibitor of the enzyme DNA polymerase. Its principal action is as a false nucleotide competing for the enzymes which are responsible for converting cytidine to deoxycytidine and for incorporating deoxycytidine in to DNA. It can be given by intravenous or subcutaneous routes and is used mainly in acute leukaemias. The main side effects are bone marrow suppression, nausea, vomiting and diarrhoea.

Gemcitabine is a second-generation pyrimidine analogue. It is metabolized by nucleotide kinases intracellularly to the active diphosphate and triphosphate and inhibits DNA synthesis. Side effects include nausea and vomiting, myelosuppression, flu-like symptoms, rashes and oedema.

Gemcitabine is the standard therapy for pancreatic tumours and also is used in non-small cell lung cancer.

Mitotic inhibitors

There are two major classes of mitotic inhibitors, the vinca alkaloids and the taxanes. The vinca alkaloids are naturally occurring or semisynthetic compounds found in the periwinkle plant (*Vinca rosea*): vincristine, vinblastine and vinorelbine. They inhibit formation of the microtubule spindle on which the chromatids line up during metaphase in mitosis and therefore prevent cell division. They are all given intravenously and, despite being similar in structure, have differing side effects. Vincristine is used in lymphomas, leukaemias and breast cancer. It is vesicant locally and neurotoxicity is the main dose-limiting toxicity. This presents in the form of a sensorimotor peripheral neuropathy (paresthaesiae in fingers, muscle cramps, paralytic ileus,

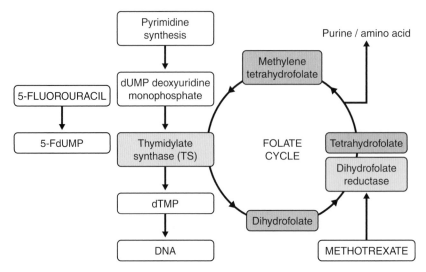

Figure 19.2 Enzymatic pathway for 5-FU and methotrexate.

constipation). Vinblastine is also a sclerosant, but myelo-suppression, especially thrombocytopenia, is the main dose-limiting toxicity. Neurotoxicity is less severe than with vincristine. It is used mainly in lymphoma, testicular teratoma and non-small cell lung cancer. Vinorelbine is the most recently discovered vinca alkaloid and causes less alopecia and neuropathy than the older agents. It can however cause significant constipation. It also has the advantage of being available for intravenous and oral administration.

The taxanes are an important class of anticancer drugs in the field of oncology. Although they also have an effect on the formation of the microtubule spindle, they differ from the vinca alkaloids since they promote the assembly of the microtubules spindle and inhibit its disassembly. Paclitaxel is an extract from the bark of the Pacific yew. Initially, its development was hampered by the limited supply of the primary source and also its poor solubility in water. With the development of docetaxel, the semisynthetic analogue from the needles of the tree, the supply was no longer threatened.

The most important antitumour activity of these drugs has been seen in breast and ovarian cancer. Both drugs are given intravenously and there has been a great deal of work involved in optimizing the scheduling. Despite being closely related, there are some differences in their toxicity profiles. Both have myelosuppression as one of the major limiting side effects with the nadir occurring at days 8–10 post-infusion. A relatively rare but important side effect of paclitaxel is a hypersensitivity reaction with dyspnoea, urticaria and hypotension. Patients therefore receive prophylactic steroids and H2 inhibitors as premedication. Paclitaxel also produces a peripheral neuropathy characterized by sensory symptoms in a glove and stocking distribution. This can be permanent. A newcomer to the field is abraxane, a novel nanoparticle

albumin bound paclitaxel. It has fewer hypersensitivity reactions and is licensed for use in metastatic breast cancer.

Docetaxel is characterized by a unique fluid retention syndrome with the development of oedema and weight gain. As with paclitaxel, a premedication is used. Skin toxicity may occur and this produces a widespread itchy erythematous rash and nail changes characterized by discolouration, ridging and onycholysis – the nails lift up from the nail bed. Liver toxicity can occur if patients with impaired liver function are not given a dose reduction. Stomatitis and diarrhoea are more common with docetaxel. All taxanes cause alopecia.

Currently, a new group of mitotic inhibitors, the tubulin polymerizing agents, are in development. These agents show promise as early studies suggest they have a wider tumour activity profile, for example in tumours that are taxane resistant. To date significant toxicity has been associated with these agents and Ixabepilone is the only agent to date approved for use in breast cancer.

Topoisomerase inhibitors

Topoisomerases are enzymes involved in the coiling and uncoiling of DNA. There are two types. Topoisomerase I inhibitors bind to double-stranded DNA and cause a single strand break in DNA. The camptothecin analogues topotecan and irinotecan are topoisomerase I inhibitors. Topoisomerase II exists as alpha and beta isoenzymes. They undergo covalent bonding to complementary strands of DNA and cleave both strands. Topoisomerase II inhibitors prevent the relegation of DNA cleaved by topoisomerase II and produce protein-linked breaks in DNA. Epipodophyllotoxins are examples of topoisomerase II inhibitors. The anthracyclines inhibit both type I and type II topoisomerases and therefore will be discussed in this section too.

Camptothecin was the first topoisomerase I inhibitor to be discovered. Its further development was hindered by toxicity and it was not until its analogues topotecan and irinotecan were developed that the usefulness of this group of drugs became apparent. Topotecan was the first camptothecin analogue approved for clinical use and is now used in ovarian cancer and small cell lung cancer. It can be given intravenously or orally with the latter being far more convenient. The major side effects are neutropenia and nausea and vomiting. Interestingly, although the neutropenia can be profound, the nadir is very short lived and therefore is seldom complicated by sepsis.

Irinotecan is a semisynthetic derivative of camptothecin. Its active metabolite SN-38 binds to the topoisomerase I enzyme-DNA cleaved complex and prevents religation thus causing double strand breaks. SN-38 is mainly cleared by the liver and the drug can only be used with caution in patients with abnormal liver function. Irinotecan has a role in the treatment of colorectal cancer and is active in patients with 5-FU resistant disease. The major side effects are diarrhoea and myelosuppression. These can occur concurrently with fatal outcome if the diarrhoea is not controlled correctly. Irinotecan is also used in the management of upper gastrointestinal malignancies.

Etoposide (VP16) is the most widely used epipodophyllotoxin. Like 5-FU, it is a good example of a schedule-dependent drug as it is more effective given over 5 days than on 1 day. It can be given orally or intravenously and the dose-limiting toxicity is bone marrow suppression. The nadir is at about 16 days. Nausea, vomiting and anorexia are relatively minor but more marked if etoposide is given orally. Alopecia is also common as is mucositis. Etoposide is used mainly in Hodgkin's disease, non-Hodgkin's lymphoma, small cell lung cancer, and testicular teratoma.

Daunorubicin, doxorubicin (Adriamycin) and epirubicin are the principal anthracycline antibiotics. They are produced from different strains of fungi (*Streptomyces*). The mechanisms of their cytotoxic action are not fully understood. They induce formation of topoisomerase-DNA complexes and prevent the enzyme from completing the religation of the ligation–religation reaction. In addition, they insert part of their planar structure between two adjacent base pairs (intercalation), causing single and double strand breaks. They also can undergo chemical reduction to form free radicals.

Doxorubicin and epirubicin are given intravenously and the main toxicity is to the bone marrow, gastrointestinal tract and the heart. The nadir of the white count is at 10 days. Epirubicin causes slightly less vomiting than the other two anthracyclines. Daunorubicin and doxorubicin and, to a much lesser extent, epirubicin, cause cumulative cardiotoxicity and there is a maximum recommended total dose. Acute cardiac toxicity is manifest by arrhythmias and abnormalities of electrical conduction. The chronic effect is a cardiomyopathy (pericarditis and congestive cardiac failure) and, thus, anthracyclines should be avoided if there is previous history of cardiac failure or ischaemic heart disease. Their use is widespread in lymphoma, breast cancer,

sarcomas, lung cancer, Wilms' tumour, and acute myelogenous leukaemia (daunorubicin).

In an attempt to improve the antitumour effect of doxorubicin, a liposomal preparation called doxil (Caelyx® in the UK) has been developed. Essentially, the doxorubicin molecule has been formulated in a fat 'bubble'. The body's reticuloendothelial system fails to recognize the molecule as being foreign, hence the term 'stealth liposome', and therefore the drug has a longer half-life. The side effects of doxil are generally less than for doxorubicin except for the development of a hand foot syndrome called palmar plantar erythrodysaesthesia. It is used in breast cancer and ovarian cancer.

Miscellaneous

Platinum analogues

The platinum drugs are widely used in a variety of tumours such as testicular teratoma and seminoma, ovarian, cervical, non-small cell lung cancer and osteosarcoma. Cisplatin and carboplatin inhibit DNA synthesis in a similar way to alkylating agents. They form cross-linkages (adducts) between a pair of their chlorine atoms and the guanine molecules of opposing DNA strands (interstrand linkages), but differ in that they also bind to bases on the same DNA strand (intrastrand linkages). Both drugs are administered intravenously and are predominantly excreted in the urine. Cisplatin causes severe nausea and vomiting which can be prevented with $5-HT_3$ antagonists and aprepitant the NK-1 antagonist. In addition, cisplatin causes renal impairment and therefore it is essential that pre- and post-treatment hydration be used. The peripheral nerves and auditory nerves are sensitive to cisplatin and patients may develop high frequency hearing loss and peripheral neuropathy. Carboplatin has the advantage of much less emesis, ototoxicity, nephrotoxicity and neurotoxicity. The dose-limiting toxicity is to the bone marrow, particularly to platelets. Unlike the other chemotherapy agents, carboplatin is dosed depending on the renal function of the patient rather than the patient's body surface area.

Oxaliplatin is the most recent platinum analogue to be licensed. It is a third generation platinum compound and differs from the other platinum drugs by having a large 1,2 diaminocyclohexane (DACH) ligand in its structure. It is thought that the presence of the DACH group renders the molecule non-recognizable by the mismatch repair process. This means that the DNA repair mechanisms that are responsible for platinum resistance are not so effective. Oxaliplatin therefore is useful in tumours where cisplatin has failed and also in colorectal cancer, a tumour type not classically treated by platinum agents. Oxaliplatin does not have the nephrotoxicity associated with carboplatin, although it does have a striking neurotoxicity. Patients develop a peripheral neuropathy with cumulative drug exposure. They also develop an acute neuropathy that is characterized by cold-induced tingling (paraesthesia) in the fingertips and toes after infusion. This can also affect the throat on drinking cold drinks and the patient develops a feeling of choking. Oxaliplatin is usually administered with 5-FU chemotherapy, as in combination, they are synergistic.

Non-anthracycline antibiotics

Actinomycin D is a highly toxic drug, which is only given intravenously. It is used in the treatment of some sarcomas and causes significant myelosuppression, oral ulceration, nausea, vomiting, diarrhoea, alopecia and skin rashes.

Bleomycin intercalates with DNA strands causing single and double strand breaks. It inhibits DNA synthesis and, to a lesser degree, RNA synthesis. It is usually given intravenously, although can be given intramuscularly, subcutaneously, or intrapleurally (for pleural effusions). The main toxicity is to the lung and progressive fibrosis occurs causing non-productive cough and dyspnoea. Respiratory complications of general anaesthesia are increased. Occasionally, patients have an immediate life-threatening anaphylactic reaction, although fever and chills are more common. Skin changes are common with pigmentation, erythema, and thickening of the nail bed. There is little myelosuppression and so it is often used in combination with other agents. The main use of bleomycin is in the treatment of testicular teratoma, although it is also used in lymphoma.

Enzymes

Asparaginase is used mainly in the treatment of leukaemia. It is an enzyme that degrades asparagine, an essential amino acid for protein and nucleic acid synthesis. Tumour cells, unlike their normal counterparts, have no or little asparagine synthetase, the enzyme necessary for making asparagine. When asparagine levels fall, both protein and nucleic acid synthesis are inhibited. It is used in the treatment of acute leukaemias and the most common side effect is a hypersensitivity reaction.

Hormones

There is a group of cancers where the mainstay of treatment is hormone therapy. These include breast, prostate, and endometrial tumours. In recent years, an increase in the understanding of the molecular biology of hormone receptors has greatly improved the treatment of these cancers, in particular breast cancer. Remissions may last for years and symptomatic benefit may be substantial, and even dramatic, during this period. While the administration of hormones avoids the morbidities particular to surgery, radiotherapy and cytotoxic chemotherapy, side effects are seen, some of which are unacceptable (e.g. masculinizing effects of androgens in women with breast cancer) and

can be dangerous (e.g. cardiovascular morbidity from diethylstilbestrol for prostate cancer). A careful balance has to be struck between toxicity and benefit in tumour control. There are five main areas that will be discussed:

- antioestrogens
- aromatase inhibitors
- gonadotrophin-releasing hormone analogues
- antiandrogens
- female hormones.

Antioestrogens

Tamoxifen is the most important synthetic antioestrogen preparation. First, it blocks the oestrogen stimulation of breast cancer cells by competitive binding to oestrogen receptors (ER). It also has weak oestrogenic action, raising levels of sex hormone binding globulin, which binds to freely circulating oestrogen and so reduces the amount of free oestrogen available to bind to oestrogen receptors. The binding of oestrogen to the ER reduces the synthesis of growth factors and stimulates the production of progesterone receptors. Tamoxifen is used in women whose breast tumour cells are found on immunohistological staining to express oestrogen or progesterone receptors. It is indicated as adjuvant therapy in early breast cancer in pre- and post-menopausal women and also in recurrent and advanced breast cancer.

The oestrogenic properties of tamoxifen are responsible for both its activity and toxicity. In general, tamoxifen is tolerated well, however, women do experience significant hot flushes and also an increase in incidence of endometrial cancer. On a more positive note, tamoxifen can prevent cardiovascular events and also osteoporosis in post-menopausal women. In an attempt to overcome the negative aspects of tamoxifen, other selective oestrogen receptor modulators (SERMS), have been developed. These include those that are tamoxifen-like including toremifene, fixed ring compounds such as raloxifene and selective oestrogen receptor down-regulators (SERDs) such as fulvestrant. There has been a significant amount of work carried out to understand the mode of action of these compounds further and this information will inform the use of these compounds both as chemoprevention agents, and as therapy for early and advanced breast cancer.

Aromatase inhibitors

Aromatase inhibitors play an important role in the endocrine management of adjuvant, advanced and recurrent ER-positive breast cancer. The earliest of these aromatase inhibitors was aminoglutethimide, a drug now considered to be outdated due to the development of selective aromatase inhibitors with superior side-effect profiles. In post-menopausal women, oestrogen synthesis occurs peripherally (e.g. adrenals and fat) as the enzyme aromatase converts androstenedione to estrone. Aromatase inhibitors block this conversion

Table 19.4 Summary of aromatase inhibitors

GENERATION	NON-STEROIDAL	STEROIDAL
First	Aminogluthemide	Testolactone
Second	Fadrozole	
Third	Anastrazole	Exemestane
	Letrozole	

and are therefore extremely valuable drugs for post-menopausal women with breast cancer. In premenopausal women, oestrogen synthesis is governed by gonadotrophin-releasing hormone stimulating the ovary. Aromatase inhibitors are therefore only useful in premenopausal women who have been oophorectomized. There are a number of first, second and third generation aromatase inhibitors available as shown in Table 19.4. Common toxicities of these drugs include nausea, headache, hot flushes and weight gain. Unlike tamoxifen, aromatase inhibitors may decrease bone density and predispose to osteoporosis. Although clear molecular differences exist between these two types of aromatase inhibitors, significant clinical differences have not been forthcoming from the studies to date. There may be some non cross resistance between the groups as switching from one to another can confer a modest improvement in outcome. A Cochrane analysis has found that in metastatic breast cancer, aromatase inhibitors show a survival benefit compared to other endocrine therapy although there is limited data available to identify which individual aromatase inhibitor has the greatest efficacy.

Gonadotrophin-releasing hormone (GnRH) analogues

Downregulation of the gonadotrophin-releasing hormone (GnRH) receptors in the pituitary is achieved by the application of continuous secretion of gonadotrophin-releasing hormone analogues. These analogues of the naturally occurring hypothalamic luteinizing hormone-releasing hormone (LHRH) initially cause a transient surge of gonadotrophin (LH) secretion, 'tumour flare'. However, with continuous exposure to these analogues, the LHRH receptors in the pituitary become desensitized, resulting in reduction in the secretion of gonadotrophins. They therefore cause a 'medical oophorectomy' in women and a 'medical orchidectomy' in men. The advantage of this medical suppression of gonad function with GnRH analogues is that the process is reversible.

Goserelin is the most commonly used agent and is about 100 times more potent than naturally occurring GnRH. It is given as a subcutaneously injected capsule on either a monthly or 3-monthly basis for prostate cancer or premenopausal breast cancer. Obviously, the symptoms are what would be expected from sex hormone withdrawal, with menopausal symptoms in women and lack of libido in men. Gynaecomastia is uncommon. However, in general, they are very well tolerated.

Antiandrogens

Flutamide is a non-steroidal antiandrogen and is a pure androgen antagonist used in men with prostate cancer. One of its important metabolites, hydroxyflutamide, is thought to be responsible for its cellular action. It blocks the binding of dihydrotestosterone to its receptor, so inhibiting the action of androgen. It is often used in combination with GnRH analogues. The side effects include gynaecomastia and/or breast tenderness, nausea and diarrhoea and tiredness. Bicalutamide is another non-steroidal antiandrogen that binds to androgen receptors and therefore inhibits androgen stimulation. Again, it is used in prostate cancer, usually in conjunction with a GnRH analogue.

Cyproterone acetate is a progestogenic antiandrogen and has two actions. First, it reduces the production of testosterone in the testis by inhibiting the secretion of the pituitary gonadotrophins. Secondly, it competes with androgen receptors, from which it displaces testosterone. It is used in prostate cancer to suppress the tumour flare with initial GnRH analogue therapy; and when GnRH analogues are contraindicated or poorly tolerated. Side effects include liver dysfunction, impotence, and fluid retention. There has been much interest in the new hormonal agent abiaterone. CYP171A is a member of the cytochrome P450 family and is responsible for the conversion of pregnelonone and progesterone to their 17α metabolites. In addition it can convert 17α-hydroxypregnelonone and 17α-hydroxyprogesterone to the androgens androstenedione and dihydroepiandrostenedione. Abiaterone binds CYP17A1 irreversibly and prevents the formation of androgens in the adrenal gland and peripheral tissues of castrate and noncastrate men. Studies suggest that the drug has activity in advanced prostate cancer following chemotherapy and androgen deprivation failure.

Female hormones (oestrogens and progestogens)

Synthetic rather than naturally occurring oestrogens (these are metabolized in the liver), such as diethylstilbestrol, are sometimes used in the treatment of prostate cancer. The side effects from these agents are significant, in particular, risk of cardiovascular disease and nausea and vomiting. With the advent of the antiandrogens, the use of these hormones is now declining.

Progestogens, such as medroxyprogesterone and megestrol, are occasionally used in the treatment of advanced breast cancer and also in endometrial cancer. Their mechanism of action is not completely understood but probably the most important effect is the antiestrogenic action and less important the direct cytotoxic action. Side effects include weight gain, fluid retention, increased blood clotting and risk of thrombosis and vaginal bleeding.

Targeted therapies

The real highlight in oncological research over the last few years has been the incorporation of targeted therapies into clinical practice. There has been a phenomenal increase in the understanding of the cellular and molecular events in carcinogenesis. By focusing on the differences between normal and malignant tissue, we can target pathways and receptors unique to cancer cells, thus avoiding the blunderbuss, universal killing of dividing cells of conventional cytotoxics. Molecular events that distinguish malignant from normal cells are activation of oncogenes (e.g. ras, erbB2), inactivation of tumour suppressor genes (e.g. p53), and activation of immortality genes (e.g. telomerase). At the cellular level, for a tumour cell to grow and divide it needs its own blood supply (angiogenesis), and the ability to migrate through local tissue (tumour invasion and migration).

Nearly all patients (90%) with chronic myeloid leukaemia have a specific genetic abnormality called the Philadelphia chromosome. This is a genetic mutation where reciprocal translocation between chromosomes 9 and 22 result in the production of the oncogene Bcr-Abl. Investigators have developed the agent imatinib mesylate (STI571) which specifically inhibits the receptor kinase of BCR-ABL. The results of the clinical trials are truly impressive; complete haematological responses have been seen in patients with chronic myeloid leukaemia who failed to respond to conventional agents. Moreover, not only is imatinib an oral drug, the patients had mild side effects, particularly when compared to their previous cytotoxic-induced toxicity. Results of this kind are really unprecedented in oncology and warranted the accelerated approval of imatinib for clinical use. The development of imatinib therefore represents a paradigm for the development of targeted therapies. Currently there are eight kinase inhibitors which have been approved for cancer therapy and over 100 in development. Key processes which have been targeted include

- Epidermal Growth Factor Receptor (EGFR) signalling pathway
- RAS-RAF-ERK (MAPK) and PI3 kinase pathway
- Vascular Endothelial Growth Factor (VEGF) signalling pathway
- Protease inhibitors.

Epidermal Growth Factor Receptor (EGFR) signalling pathway

EGFR (ERBB1) and ERBB2 (HER2) are overexpressed or amplified in many malignancies including non-small cell lung, breast, head and neck, pancreas and colorectal cancers. Licensed anti-EGFR therapies include monoclonal antibodies (cetuximab, panitumumab and trastuzumab) and oral small molecule inhibitors of the TK activity (gefitinib, erlotinib and lapatinib).

Trastuzumab (Herceptin) is a humanized anti-HER-2 (ERBB2) monoclonal antibody that has been approved for mono- or combination therapy (with paclitaxel) for women with HER-2 over expressing breast cancer. Recently it has also been licensed for HER-2 positive gastric cancer. Cetuximab (Erbitux) is a chimeric IgG1 antibody and is licensed for use in combination with irinotecan containing chemotherapy in patients with metastatic colorectal cancer with wild-type K-RAS mutation status. This treatment is complicated by a unique rash which is acneiform – indeed there is a suggestion that the rash may actually be a predictive biomarker of response to cetuximab. Other side effects include diarrhoea and infusion reactions. Panitumumab (Vectibix) is a fully human IgG2 monoclonal antibody that binds to the ectodomain of EGFR. It is also licensed for use in K-RAS wild type colorectal cancer.

Gefitinib (Iressa) is a Tyrosine Kinase Inhibitor (TKI) which blocks the binding of the adenosine triphosphate to the intracellular domain of EGFR. Only patients with activating EGFR mutations respond well to the drug and therefore gefitinib is only approved for use in metastatic non small cell lung cancer with activating mutations of the EGFR-TK. The most common side effects seen with gefitinib are rash, diarrhoea and fatigue. Erlotinib (Tarceva) is another EGFR TKI and is licensed for use in non small cell lung cancer and pancreas cancer. Lapatinib (Tykerb) is a dual specific TKI targeting both EGFR and HER-2. It is licensed for use in combination with capecitabine chemotherapy in patients with metastatic breast cancer who have progressed after trastuzumab and other chemotherapy therapy.

Signalling through RAS-RAF-ERK (MAPK) and PI3K-AKT:

Both these pathways are major downstream signals for the EGFR family members and RAS-regulated pathways interact at multiple points, including with the PI3K-AKT-mTOR pathway, and with c-MYC. The PI3K-Akt-mTOR pathway is activated in many cancers and is not surprisingly increasingly being targeted by new therapies. Temsirolimus is the first in class mTOR inhibitor licensed for use in metastatic renal cancer.

Vascular Endothelial Growth Factor (VEGF) signalling pathway

Angiogenesis is known to be pivotal in tumour progression and metastasis and as VEGF is the driving force behind angiogenesis, it is not surprising that it has been the target of many approaches. Agents have been developed that target the VEGF ligand, blocking its interaction with the VEGF receptors (Bevacizumab) and agents that directly block the receptor (tyrosine kinase inhibitors such as sunitinib). Bevacizumab (Avastin) is a recombinant humanized monoclonal antibody to VEGF-A. It is licensed for use in metastatic colorectal, breast, non-small cell lung and renal cancer. The side effect profile of bevacizumab includes hypertension, a class effect of VEGF inhibitors, thromboembolic events (both arterial and venous) and gastrointestinal perforation.

Since VEGF mediates its angiogenic effect through several tyrosine kinase receptors, many VEGF TKIs have been tested. Sorafenib (Nexavar) is licensed for use in renal cell, and hepatocellular cancer and Sunitinib (Sutent) is licensed for use in renal cell cancer and GIST. Numerous other TKIs are in clinical studies. Some are highly selective, targeting only specific VEGF receptors whereas others are more 'promiscuous' and target other kinases such as PDGF, EGFR. Despite being 'targeted' therapies, these drugs do have significant side effects including neutropenia, fatigue, rashes, diarrhoea, and stomatitis.

Proteasome inhibitors

These drugs, exemplified by Velcade (bortezomib, formerly known as PS341), prevent degradation of various proteins in the proteasome. Velcade is the first selective proteasome inhibitor and is licensed in patients with refractory or relapsed multiple myeloma. It is believed to be effective in myeloma by interfering with normal function of the NFkB signalling pathway, thus reducing tumour cell replication and angiogenesis and promoting apoptosis.

Immunotherapy

Essentially the main premise of immunotherapy approaches in cancer treatment is to stimulate the patient's immune system to attack the tumour. This can be either be achieved by immunizing the patient with a cancer vaccine or administrating therapeutic antibodies. To date there has been greater success with the latter approach and approximately nine monoclonal antibodies have been approved for the treatment of cancer.

Rituximab (Mabthera) is a chimeric monoclonal antibody targeting the CD20 antigen found on normal B cells and B cell lymphomas. It is licensed for use for follicular lymphoma, diffuse large B cell lymphoma and chronic lymphocytic leukaemia and has remarkably improved the outlook for these patients. It can be administered either as monotherapy or in combination with chemotherapy such as the 'CHOP' regimen. Iodine 131 tositumomab (Bexaar) and 90Y ibritumomab tiuxetan (Zevalin) are both radiolabelled CD20 targeted antibodies. They are licensed for use in some refractory lymphomas but their costs are prohibitive.

Alemtuzumab (previously known as CAMPATH) is a humanised monoclonal antibody targeting the CD52 antigen found on B lymphocytes. It has been licensed for use for patients with B-cell chronic lymphocytic leukaemia who are unable to receive the chemotherapy drug fludarabine. It is associated with significant haematological toxicity especially neutropenia.

Lenolidamide is an immunomodulating drug that is licensed for patients with advanced multiple myeloma (MM). It is a potent analogue of thalidomide and works in a number of ways: inhibiting proliferation of certain haematopoietic tumour cells (including MM plasma tumour cells and those with deletions of chromosome 5), enhancing T cell- and Natural Killer (NK) cell-mediated immunity, inhibiting angiogenesis, and inhibiting production of proinflammatory cytokines (e.g., TNF-α and IL6) by monocytes. In studies the most concerning side effects of treatment were venous thromboembolic events and myelosuppression. Not surprising there is also a significant risk of teratogenicity and therefore patients or their partners must not get pregnant while on treatment.

FURTHER READING

Bergh J. Quo Vadis with targeted drugs in the 21st century. J Clin Oncol 2009;27(1):2–5.

Campoli M, Ferris R, Ferrone S, Wang X. Immunotherapy of malignant disease with tumor antigen-specific monoclonal antibodies. Clin Cancer Res 2010;16(1):11–20.

Chanan-Khan AA, Cheson BD. Lenalidomide for the treatment of B-cell malignancies. J Clin Oncol 2008;26(9):1544–52.

Devita VT, Lawrence TS, Rosenberg SA, Depinho RA, Weinberg RA. Cancer principles and practice of oncology. 9th ed. Philadelphia: Lippincott Williams & Wilkins; 2011.

Gibson L, Lawrence D, Dawson C, Bliss J. Aromatase inhibitors for treatment of advanced breast cancer in postmenopausal women (Review). The Cochrane Library 2009;4:1–124.

Grothey A, Galanis E. Targeting angiogenesis: progress with anti-VEGF treatment with large molecules. Nat Rev Clin Oncol 2009;6:507–18.

Jordan VC, O'Malley BWO. Selective estrogen-receptor modulators and antihormonal resistance in breast cancer. J Clin Oncol 2007;25(36):5815–24.

Lurje G, Lenz H. EGFR signalling and drug discovery. Oncology 2009;77:400–10.

Perry MC. The chemotherapy source book. 4th ed. Philadelphia: Lippincott Williams & Wilkins; 2007.

Pezaro CJ, Mukherji D, De-Bono JS. (2011) Abiaterone acetate: redefining hormone treatment for advanced prostate cancer. Drug Discov today, Dec 19 [Epub ahead of print].

Quintas-Cardama A, Wierda W, O'Brien S. Investigational immunotherapeutics for B-cell malignancies. J Clin Oncol 2010;28(5):884–92.

Stavridi F, Karapanagiotou EM, Syrigos KN. Targeted therapeutic approaches for hormone-refractory prostate cancer. Cancer Treat Rev 2010;36:122–30.

Chapter | 20 |

Skin and lip cancer

Charles Kelly, Trevor Roberts, Cliff Lawrence

INTRODUCTION

Skin cancer is the most common human cancer. It can be divided broadly into two types. These are melanoma and non-melanoma. Keratinocyte-derived skin cancers are a group made up of squamous and basal cell carcinoma. A further group of much less common skin tumours, arising from the skin appendages, are primary cutaneous lymphoma, Kaposi's sarcoma and Merkel cell tumours.

Keratinocyte skin tumours and basal cell carcinoma, in particular, are the most common skin cancers. Their true numbers are often underreported as they do not have to be counted as new cancers in many cancer registries.

Basal cell carcinomas are very common and relatively benign. However, melanomas and squamous cell carcinoma of the skin carry a significant mortality, as do much less common Merkel cell tumours, skin lymphomas and Kaposi's sarcoma. In 2008, approximately 2000 people died from melanoma in the UK. By comparison, approximately 500 died from non-melanomatous skin cancer (NMSC).

The incidence of both melanoma and keratinocyte skin cancers is increasing decade on decade, and further increases can be expected as the population ages.

KERATINOCYTE SKIN TUMOURS

These are the most common form of skin cancer and develop from epidermal keratinocytes. The incidence of both squamous cell carcinoma (SCC) and basal cell carcinoma (BCC) is related to increased life-time sun exposure.

Aetiology

The following factors can all be involved in the development of keratinocyte skin tumours, but these skin cancers are all more common in white skin. Skin pigmentation protects from the development of these tumours, so that, at one extreme, albinos have a much increased risk of skin cancer, whereas NMSC is rare in people with black skin.

Ultraviolet radiation

Excessive exposure to ultraviolet B from sunlight and ultraviolet A (UVA) from sunbeds have been implicated as an aetiological factor. In the UK, a cohort who commonly presented with these tumours were those World War II soldiers who had served in the Mediterranean or the Middle or Far East. At that time, the importance of sun avoidance was not recognized and sun blocks were not available.

Premalignant skin lesions

Lesions such as actinic keratosis (Figure 20.1) or Bowen's disease (Figure 20.2), are known for their potential to develop into SCC. These lesions are found on sun-exposed parts of the body. Bowen's disease is squamous carcinoma in situ and, in about 5% of cases, develops into invasive squamous cancer. Actinic keratoses do carry an increased risk of developing SCC but only a small minority, approximately 1 in 1000, go on to become skin cancers.

Topical carcinogens

Direct skin contact with chemicals such as tar, pitch or non-solvent refined mineral oils, are a potential cause of squamous cell carcinoma.

Ingested carcinogens

These are becoming less common but, previously, it was relatively common to include arsenic in proprietary 'tonics'. Arsenic can cause multiple skin tumours, both squamous cell carcinomas and basal cell, as well as premalignant skin changes (Figure 20.3).

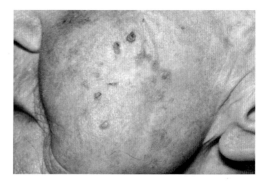

Figure 20.1 Actinic keratosis with a background of sun-damaged skin.

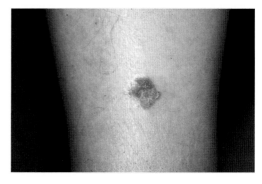

Figure 20.2 Bowen's disease on a limb. Note the colour and how superficial the lesion is.

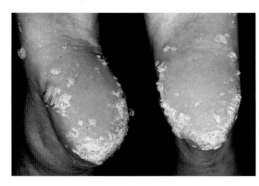

Figure 20.3 These thick keratoses developed following the ingestion of arsenic as a constituent of a 'tonic'.

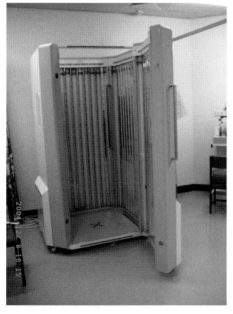

Figure 20.4 This is a typical ultraviolet A generating machine used in PUVA treatments. Note the tubes used to produce the UVA.

PUVA treatment for psoriasis (Figure 20.4)

This is an effective treatment for psoriasis, where a drug (a psoralen) is given before exposing the patient to UVA. However, this treatment does increase the chance of development of a keratinocyte origin tumour, particularly a squamous cancer. Risk increases with the cumulative dose of UVA.

Immunosuppression

This is most commonly seen now in patients who have had organ transplants, and the normal ratio of SCC to BCC is reversed, with squamous cell carcinoma becoming more common than BCC.

Basal cell naevus syndrome (Gorlin's syndrome)

This is an uncommon autosomal dominant genetic abnormality giving a familial syndrome, with patients at increased risk of developing multiple BCCs at a relatively young age. There are also other skeletal and skin abnormalities, such as tiny pinpoint lesions on the palms known as palmar pitting (Figure 20.5), dental cysts, frontal bossing, bifid ribs and calcification of the falx. These other abnormalities may well be picked up by chance when the patient is being investigated for other problems. Radiotherapy is contraindicated in patients with the syndrome, as it is thought that giving radiotherapy can initiate the development of BCCs. Medulloblastoma is also more common in patients with basal cell naevus syndrome (BCNS). It is important to exclude BCNS before radiotherapy is given to children with medulloblastoma because of the risk of radiation-induced multiple BCCs at the treatment site.

Xeroderma pigmentosa (Figure 20.6)

This is a very rare, autosomal recessive genetic condition where there is defective repair of DNA after damage by UV exposure. These patients can develop SCC or BCC of the skin, or Bowen's disease in childhood, after minimal sun exposure. Although very uncommon, this condition has provided great insight into the mechanism of skin cancer development.

Chronic trauma

Forms of chronic ulceration (Figure 20.7), direct thermal damage, or previous burn scars can all predispose to the development of squamous cell carcinoma of skin.

Age

These skin cancers are essentially a disease of the elderly. As the population ages the incidence of skin cancer is steadily increasing.

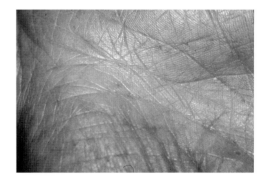

Figure 20.5 This shows the very subtle palmar pitting found in Gorlin's syndrome.

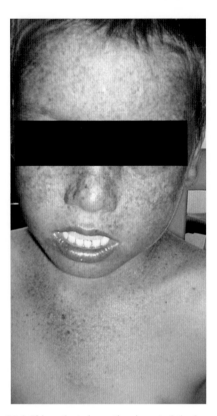

Figure 20.6 This patient shows the characteristic signs of skin damage at an early age, found in xeroderma pigmentosa. There are also cataracts present, which can also be found in this condition.

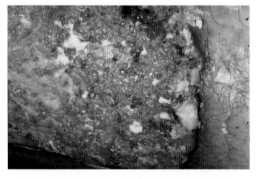

Figure 20.7 Marjolin's ulcer. Here a carcinoma has developed in a long-standing area of damaged skin on the leg.

Ionizing radiation

In the early days of radiotherapy, a variety of benign skin diseases were treated by ionizing radiation. Many years after treatment, basal cell or squamous lesions appeared in the irradiated skin. The maximum effects were seen in children treated for ringworm.

Basal cell carcinoma

This is the most common skin cancer in white populations, being three to four times as common as SCC of the skin. As the name suggests, these tumours arise from cells in the basal cell layer of the epidermis. They are more common in the elderly. As the main cause of these tumours is UV exposure, they are more common on sun-exposed sites (Figure 20.8A).

There are several clinical subtypes, the most characteristic being nodular basal cell carcinoma (see Figure 20.8B). This presents as a characteristic pearly papule or nodule, classically with the rolled translucent edge and telangiectasia. The centre of this lesion often ulcerates and becomes crusted. The lesion may appear as if it is about to heal, but then can progress into further cycles of growth, breakdown, crusting and regression. These lesions will not, however, disappear without active treatment.

There are other clinical subtypes as well as the classical nodular BCC including: superficial, micronodular, sclerosing, infiltrating and pigmented variants. Diagnosis of these variants may be difficult without a biopsy. It is rare for a BCC to metastasize but it can occur and is more frequent with longstanding, large lesions, which have often been neglected for years.

The commonest site for BCC is in a butterfly distribution in the central face. Elsewhere, tumours are more common on sun-exposed areas of skin. If untreated, tumours invade deep tissues, including bone, leading to extensive ulceration and deformity over several years in patients who have not sought medical help (see Figure 20.8C–E).

A typical example of a BCC at the left nasolabial fold before and 6 weeks after being treated with radiotherapy is shown in Figure 20.8F and G.

Squamous cell carcinoma of the skin

This is the second most common skin cancer after BCC and the incidence of this tumour is rising due to increased exposure to ultraviolet radiation, as there seems to be a direct association between development of these tumours and hours of sun exposure. These tumours can enlarge and cause local destruction and metastasize, initially to regional nodes, which should be checked clinically when the patient first presents.

Well-differentiated SCC produce keratin and the presence of keratin on the surface of a tumour is the characteristic feature of SCC. The best example of this is SCC producing a keratin horn, although these can also result from a benign cause, such as actinic keratosis or viral wart. Poorly differentiated, and hence more aggressive SCC are often less distinctive and present as a nodule or ulcer (Figure 20.9A). SCC may develop within Bowen's disease or actinic keratosis.

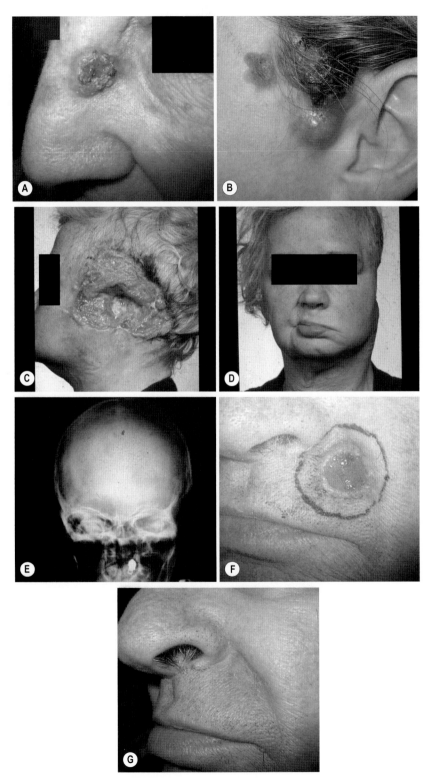

Figure 20.8 (A) This is a typical basal cell carcinoma, with a pearly appearance to the edge, and central ulceration. (B) Nodular basal cell carcinoma. (C–E) This is an advanced BCC. Note the local soft tissue destruction (C), the left 7th nerve palsy (D) and the bone loss due to erosion by this tumour (E). (F, G) A typical example of a BCC at the left nasolabial fold before and 6 weeks after being treated with radiotherapy.

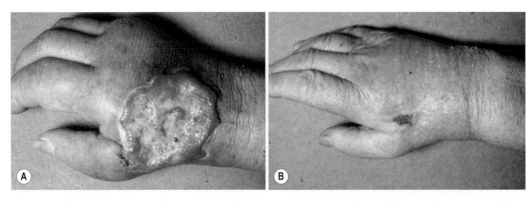

Figure 20.9 (A, B) This shows an extensive squamous cell carcinoma of the back of the hand before radiotherapy and four weeks after radiotherapy treatment.

A typical SCC before and 4 weeks after radiotherapy is shown in Figure 20.9A and B.

Cancer of the lip

Cancer of the lip is predominantly a malignancy affecting elderly males. The lower lip is affected more frequently than the upper lip by a factor of 10. Almost all lower lip cancers are squamous cell carcinomas. It is rare to find a basal cell carcinoma on the lip vermilion, but they can arise from skin immediately adjacent. Basal cell carcinoma develops most commonly on the skin close to the upper rather than the lower lip.

These malignancies are more common in fair skinned, weather-beaten outdoor workers. Sun exposure is one important factor but there may be others, such as pipe smoking, as cumulative UV exposure does not always correlate with some of the higher risk occupational groups prone to developing this cancer. As with squamous carcinoma of the skin, transplant patients are at a higher risk of developing lip SCC.

Clinically, premalignant changes leading to carcinoma of the lip may precede the development of a mass or ulcer within the lip. This then enlarges, involving more of the lip. Spread to the submental or submandibular nodes is possible, especially with larger or more poorly differentiated lesions, but spread to other neck nodes early on is uncommon. Classically, 5% of lip cancers have palpable nodes at diagnosis and 5% subsequently develop nodal metastases after successful treatment of the primary.

Management of cancer of the lip

Initially, a pathological diagnosis needs to be made with an incisional biopsy. The treatment options can be discussed with the patient. For early tumours involving only the vermilion of the lip, this can be removed with a lip shave and the oral mucosa advanced to replace the area removed. Superficial early tumours may be associated with other

areas of premalignant change. This technique allows for these areas of premalignant change to be removed at the same time and sent for histological evaluation to exclude other areas of carcinoma in situ or frank invasive change. With larger lesions, the tumour can be removed surgically using a 'V' or 'W' incision. Here, the amount of functional tissue loss may make radiotherapy more appropriate.

Radiotherapy is given using either an iridium implant or electron beam, using wax and lead behind the lip to protect the rest of the mouth and take advantage of the back scatter effect. Dose/fractionation regimens used include 55 Gy in 20 fractions or 66 Gy in 33 fractions. The cosmetic result is usually very good, as the lip has an excellent blood supply and healing usually occurs quickly and completely. As electron treatments are highly effective, iridium implantation is now rarely indicated.

Keratoacanthoma

These are benign but can be very difficult to distinguish from squamous cell carcinoma of the skin. They present as a rapidly growing nodule with a central keratin plug. The central plug detaches, and the residual lesion resolves (Figure 20.10A, B). They are problematic in that they cannot be differentiated from squamous cell carcinoma of skin by biopsy alone and, in the growth phase, the pathologist will usually call them a squamous cell carcinoma. As a result, although benign, they are often excised, in order to avoid missing a rapidly growing squamous cell cancer.

Treatment of non-melanoma skin cancer

As can be seen from the list below, there are several ways to treat these keratinocyte skin tumours.

There have been few randomized studies of different treatment modalities for BCC and SCC primary treatment, but Mohs' micrographic surgery (MMS) gives the lowest

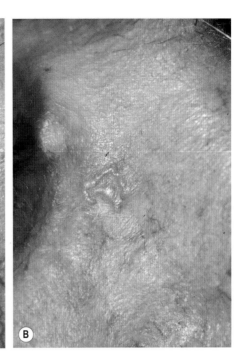

Figure 20.10 (A) Keratoacanthoma in its rapidly developing stage. The central keratin plug is obvious. This lesion has developed in a matter of a few weeks. (B) Keratoacanthoma in its healing stage. This is the same lesion as in Figure 20.9, three months later. The keratin plug was discharged spontaneously and complete healing rapidly ensued.

short- and long-term recurrence rate for BCC and probably for SCC. One of the few randomized control trials in the treatment of skin cancer, which was carried out in The Netherlands, has shown a lower, but not statistically significant, rate of recurrence after Mohs' surgery compared to conventional excision. Operative costs were higher for Mohs' methodology.

Patients with these tumours should be seen in the multidisciplinary skin cancer clinic where a treatment plan can be formulated for the individual patient. Often, the decision as to which treatment is given is based not on the historical evidence of the efficacy of that particular treatment, but on the size and site of the skin lesion, the age, fitness and wishes of the patient, and the local resources and distances from the local hospital and cancer centre. In general, surgery or radiotherapy are equally effective in eradicating these tumours. Radiotherapy is often avoided in younger patients on the basis that long-term cosmesis is usually better with surgery. As time passes, the surgical scar becomes less obvious, whereas the hypopigmentation produced by radiotherapy can become more prominent.

Curettage and electrolysis

This is the simplest approach, but is usually only suitable for small, previously untreated, well-defined BCCs less than 10 millimetres in diameter on non-critical sites (Figure 20.11A–D).

Cryosurgery with liquid nitrogen

This is used more for BCCs than SCCs. For 2–3 days after treatment there can be oedema, blister formation, sloughing and crust formation. It has the advantage of being able to be done in the outpatient clinic and can be useful in the frail elderly patient, where surgery is best avoided, and when the patient does not wish to travel to their local radiotherapy centre (Figure 20.12).

Surgical excision

Pathological evidence of complete removal is the main advantage, but for some morpheic BCCs this may give a false reassurance with subsequent recurrence. For these tumours, Mohs' micrographic surgery gives a higher rate of complete excision. The main disadvantage of surgical excision is that, in some sites, primary skin closure may be impossible and flap closure or skin grafting is required. The cosmetic results may be poor, especially in areas such as the tip of the nose.

Laser ablation

This is rarely if ever used. It is in effect using the laser as a cutting tool to remove the tissue similar to surgical excision. The defect left is usually allowed to heal by secondary

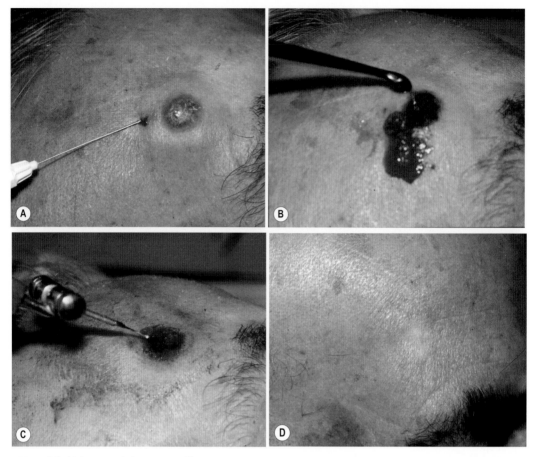

Figure 20.11 (A) This is an area being prepared for curettage, with local anaesthetic being given. (B) The tumour is then curetted out. (C) Further curettage is then performed at the tumour's base. (D) This shows the result at two years, following curettage.

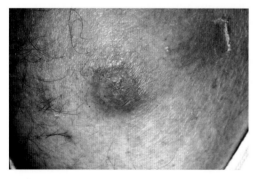

Figure 20.12 This is the appearance of an area of skin, one week after cryosurgery.

intention. Confirmation of complete excision may be more difficult with this technique than surgical excision because of the tissue distortion produced by the heat artifact at the excision margins.

Photodynamic therapy

A cream containing a porphyrin precursor is placed on the skin. This is metabolized by the tumour to porphyrin. The porphyrin is then activated by exposure to red light and, in the process, free radicals are produced which destroy the tumour. It is partially effective and still being developed. It is mainly reserved for large superficial truncal BCCs.

Mohs' micrographic surgery

This technique uses repeated excisions at the tumour site until there is no histological evidence of any remaining tumour. It gives the highest cure rate, but is also resource intensive. The interval between excisions depends on whether frozen sections or fixed tissue are examined by the pathologist. Frozen sections enable the surgeon to do several excision stages in one day. Inevitably, the time taken to fix and examine paraffin embedded sections results in the excision stages being spread over several days (Figure 20.13A–G).

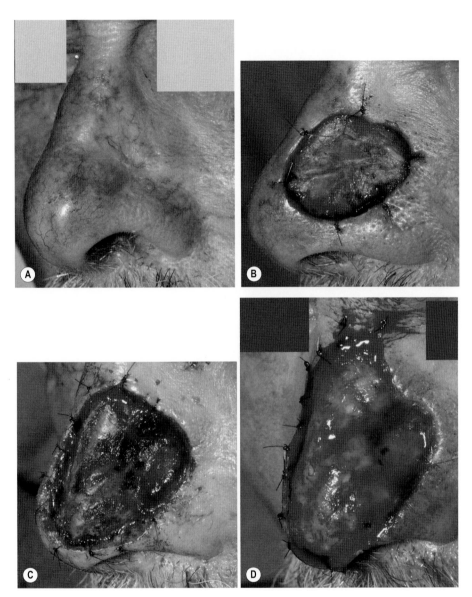

Figure 20.13 (A–G) This series of clinical photographs shows Moh's micrographic surgery, with the initial incision, the further wider excisions, and the final result.

Continued

Imiquimod

This can be considered an experimental treatment at present. It is now licensed for the treatment of superficial BCCs, and works through immunomodulation by the topical preparation causing release of interferons into the skin. It can be used for superficial BCC; early studies suggest a 20% 2-year recurrence rate.

Radiotherapy for keratinocyte skin cancers

Radiotherapy is particularly useful in treating tumours of the central face, around the nose and eyes, where surgical treatment may give a relatively poor cosmetic result or more loss of function than with radiotherapy. There is a relative contra-indication for giving radiotherapy to certain sites, such as the

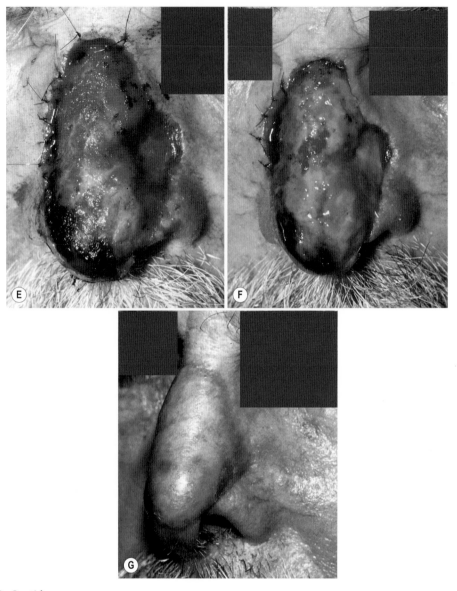

Figure 20.13, Cont'd

pinna, with its underlying cartilage; the back of the hand with its tendons lying superficially and the anterior shin where there is a relative lack of underlying subcutaneous tissue. Even these sites can be treated in appropriate patients if due consideration is given to the skin condition, site of treatment and treatment volume, total dose and fractionation.

In giving radiotherapy around the eye, treating the lateral upper eyelid may cause damage to the lacrimal gland and ducts leading to a permanently dry eye and, in treating lesions at the medial canthus, the lacrimal drainage system can be occluded. However, if the lacrimal duct is

uninvolved by cancer and is patent before radiotherapy begins, it is more likely than not to remain patent after radiotherapy.

The radiotherapy dose used for treating skin malignancies varies from centre to centre and dose/fractionation schedules have developed empirically over the years. In general, the more fractions used the better the late cosmetic result (Table 20.1). As well as efficacy in curing the tumour, other factors, such as the late cosmetic effects and convenience to the patient are important. Some elderly, frail patients will trade off the cosmetic outcome against

Table 20.1 Examples of superficial radiotherapy fractionation regimens for treating basal cell & squamous cell carcinoma of the skin

TOTAL DOSE (Gy)	NUMBER OF FRACTIONS	FRACTION INTERVAL
18	1	-
28	2	7 weeks apart
35	5	daily (if <4 cm field size)
45	10	daily (if >4 cm field size)

convenience if they can visit the radiotherapy treatment centre for fewer visits, without compromising the probability of cure.

Radiotherapy can be given to these skin cancers using either superficial x-ray beams, usually in the range 50–120 kV, or with electron beams. The latter are used where rapid fall-off of the depth dose is required to spare underlying normal tissue. If the skin tumour overlies cartilage or bone, low voltage x-rays are absorbed disproportionately owing to the high atomic number of bone compared to soft tissue, and the risk of radionecrosis is much greater than following treatment with electrons.

Electron beam treatment

Sites where the use of electron therapy beams may be indicated in preference to superficial x-ray beams include the pinna, nasolabial fold or the back of the hand. In the latter site, the use of an electron beam may reduce damage to the underlying tendon sheaths.

Electron beams are also used to irradiate larger areas of skin, either treating larger single epithelial skin tumours or when treating skin lymphomas. As can be seen in

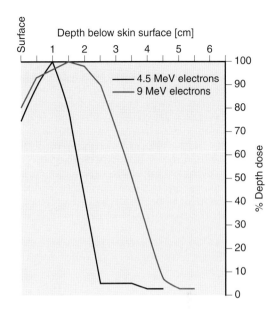

Figure 20.15 This diagram shows how two electron beams of different energies interact with matter, delivering different doses at depth, depending on their energy.

Figures 20.14 and 20.15, superficial x-ray beams lose energy exponentially through matter (Figure 20.14) and electron beams reach a peak (at a depth proportional to the energy of the beam) and then fall off rapidly, delivering very little radiation at depth (Figure 20.15).

With superficial tumours, using an electron beam the aim is to have the tumour within the 85% isodose (Figure 20.15) and to achieve this for some tumours, bolus may be needed to increase surface dose. Electron beams have a larger penumbra and have a different beam profile to superficial x-ray beams. Low energy electron beams as used in treating skin tumours show isodoses coming together at depth and this requires that a larger margin of normal tissue is included at set-up, for example 1.5 cm instead of 1 cm.

Electron backscatter (Figure 20.16A)

Electron beams also have the advantage of being able to use the physical phenomenon of backscatter. If electrons encounter lead, a proportion will be scattered back towards the direction of the incident beam, and by placing wax in front of the lead, some of the backscatter electrons will be absorbed in the wax. By choosing the thickness of the lead and the wax carefully, the degree of backscatter can be modified. This allows greater homogeneity within the treated area. However, the amount of backscatter is difficult to measure and its contribution to irradiating the tumour volume changes with every individual patient set-up. Electrons are scattered in many directions, not just at 180° to

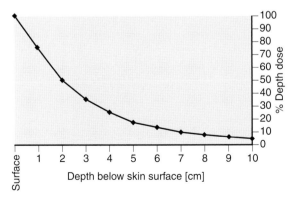

Figure 20.14 This shows the exponential fall-off of dose at depth as a superficial x-ray beam penetrates tissue.

the incident beam, and may contribute to dose outside the treatment volume and so by placing wax in front of the lead, some of these backscattered electrons will be absorbed in the wax. Backscatter therefore has both positive and negative potential effects (Figure 20.16B–F illustrate an SCC of pinna treated by electrons).

One of the most common treatment sites for the use of backscatter to clinical advantage is when a cancer of the lower lip is treated with electrons. Wax and lead are put behind the lip. The lead helps to protect the oral cavity from the electron radiation beam. By varying the thickness of the wax for each individual patient, depending on how thick the lip and tumour are and, consequently, how wide the target volume needs to be, the degree of backscatter can be modified, giving greater homogeneity in dose across the tumour.

Figure 20.16 G–L shows a wax and lead block being used for a lower lip cancer with the area to be treated marked out in Figure 20.16I.

Superficial x-ray treatment

Most small BCCs on the face can easily be treated using x-ray energies of 90–120 kV. A lead cut-out is placed around the lesion with a margin of 5 mm if a BCC, and 10 mm if an SCC (Figure 20.17A, B). If the lesion is an irregular shape, then a lead cut-out may need to be specifically made, tracing the area to be treated with adequate margin onto a piece of lead, which is then cut out. If the treated site is close to the eyes, then an external or internal eye-shield is used to keep radiation dose to the eye to a minimum (Figure 20.18).

Each fraction takes only a few minutes to deliver and the patient should be warned that the reaction will start with erythema, followed by ulceration, over which a crust forms. Healing takes place underneath this crust, which detaches a few weeks after treatment. If it is detached prematurely, or is inadvertently knocked off, a second or even a third crust can form.

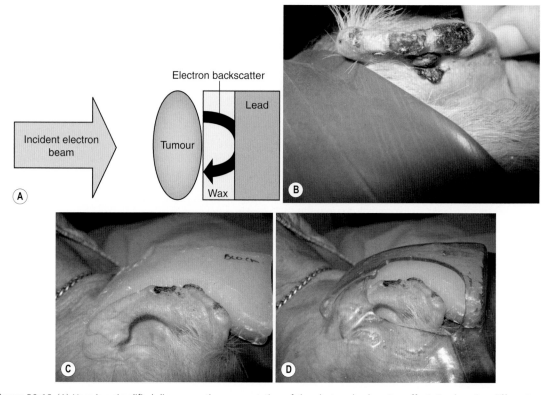

Figure 20.16 (A) Here is a simplified diagrammatic representation of the electron backscatter effect. By choosing different thicknesses of the lead and wax used, both the amount of backscatter, and how many backscatter electrons are absorbed by the wax, can be controlled, improving the homogeneity of dose over the tumour volume. (B–F) Here, use is made of the electron backscatter effect in treating a squamous cell carcinoma on the pinna of the ear. (B) The lesion. (C) Wax and lead are then placed behind the ear, in the thicknesses required for maximal affect. (D) A Perspex cut-out is then placed over the ear, giving the treated electron field and an alloy cut-out is then placed over this.

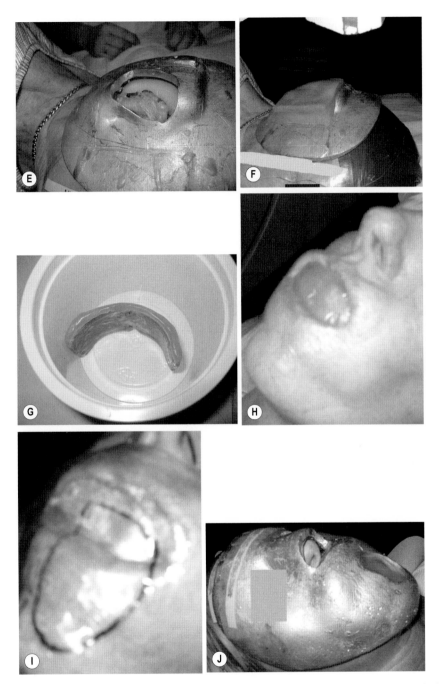

Figure 20-16, Cont'd (E) to tailor the electron beam to the treatment volume. (F) Finally, more wax bolus is applied to increase the percentage depth dose, at the skin surface. (G–L) The process of treating a lower lip cancer with electrons. A wax and lead insert is first made, the treatment volume marked out with it inserted and then a Perspex mask fitted over this. An alloy cut-out is then placed on top. In this case, it is large, not to protect the whole face, but because it is less likely to fall off during treatment. Further wax is used to increase the surface electron dose at the lip. Finally, the treatment reaction on the last day of treatment after 55 Gy in 20 fractions is shown.

Continued

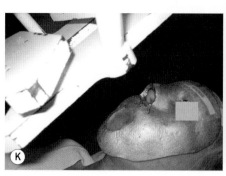

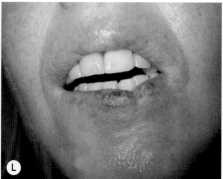

Figure 20-16, Cont'd

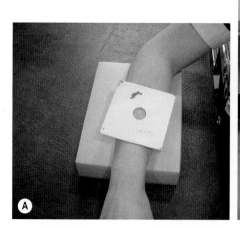

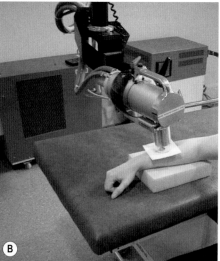

Figure 20.17 (A) This is a typical example of a lead cut-out used in treating small skin tumours with a superficial x-ray machine. (B) This shows a superficial x-ray machine being set up with a volunteer.

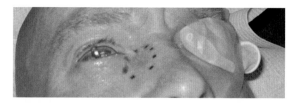

Figure 20.18 If eye-shields are required, either an external shield as shown covering this patient's left eye, or an internal gold shield can be inserted under the eyelid after anaesthetizing the conjunctiva with local anaesthetic, as shown with the right eye.

After the acute reaction has settled down, late changes may develop with the possibility of hypopigmentation and telangiectasia.

Moulds

Skin lesions can also be treated by the use of the an applied mould containing a radioactive source which the patient wears in apposition to the tumour for a set number of hours per day until the dose prescribed is delivered. This method of treatment is not commonly used in the UK today, although there is some interest in its reintroduction.

MELANOMA

The incidence of melanoma is rising worldwide, but successful public education programmes have reduced mortality in countries such as Australia.

Aetiology

Melanoma is much more common in white races and is related to UV radiation exposure. There is evidence that episodes of sunburn before the age of 15 increase the risk of developing melanoma.

Approximately 50% of melanomas arise in pre-existing moles and 50% on otherwise normal skin.

Subtypes of melanoma

As with other skin tumours, there are several types of melanoma.

Superficial spreading (Figure 20.19)

Superficial spreading is the most common representing 60–70%. It appears as a flat, pigmented lesion which may be related to a naevus. As the name implies, it initially grows outwards before invading downwards. Consequently, patients may present with a better prognosis if they seek help while the lesion is still in its horizontal or 'radial' growth phase, which may last for many months or even years.

Nodular melanoma (Figure 20.20)

Nodular melanoma is less common, making up 15–20 %. It appears clinically as a papule or nodule, usually pigmented, which represents the malignancy in vertical growth phase from early in its natural history. This gives a worse prognosis at presentation. The clinical course is more rapid than with superficial spreading lesions.

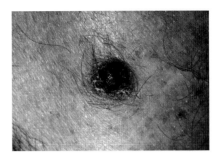

Figure 20.20 Nodular melanoma.

Lentigo maligna melanoma (Figure 20.21)

This makes up 5–15 % of melanomas. It is most commonly found in the skin of the nose or the cheek in the elderly and develops within a premalignant pigmented lesion known as lentigo melanoma (Figure 20.22), which can be present for several years. This lesion eventually enlarges, undergoes malignant change and may develop a central pigmented nodule.

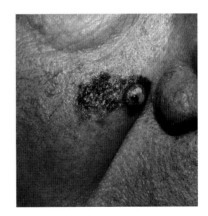

Figure 20.21 Lentigo maligna melanoma.

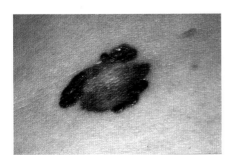

Figure 20.19 Superficial spreading melanoma.

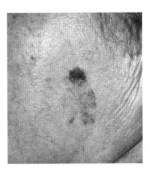

Figure 20.22 Lentigo maligna, from which lentigo maligna melanoma can develop.

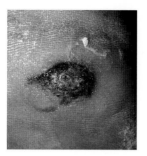

Figure 20.23 Acral melanoma on the heel.

Acral lentiginous melanoma (Figure 20.23)

Acral lentiginous melanoma is much less common, only 5–10% of melanomas, and seen more frequently in pigmented skin. It can occur on the palms, sole of foot, or characteristically beneath nails. There may be a relatively long radial growth phase. In some cases of subungual melanoma, suspicion may be raised by extension of the pigmentation onto the skin of the proximal nail fold (Hutchinson's sign).

Note that not all melanoma presents as pigmented lesions and a non-pigmented 'amelanotic melanoma' (Figure 20.24A) can cause diagnostic confusion until it is biopsied.

Diagnosis

Clinically, there should be suspicion that a melanoma may be developing. There are three cardinal features to look out for when considering the possibility of malignant change in an existing mole:

- increase in diameter
- change of colour
- change in shape, i.e. becoming asymmetrical or developing border irregularity.

This is the basis of the ABCD method: Asymmetry, Border, Colour, Diameter.

Moles greater than 6 mm are more likely to be malignant. Dermatoscopic examination using an amplified illuminated image is a helpful adjunct to clinical examination.

Melanoma TNM staging

The TNM classification for melanoma changed considerably with the publication of the TNM classification of malignant tumours, 6th edition 2002, compared to the previous 5th edition of 1997. The 6th edition has now been superseded by the 7th edition, 2009 which also changed this classification. One of the major classification changes introduced, is that Clark level (Table 20.2) is no longer included in the classification. There is now

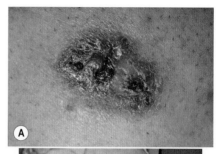

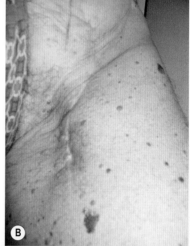

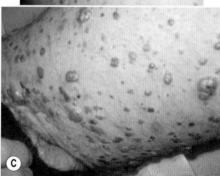

Figure 20.24 (A) This shows an amelanotic melanoma, which is not markedly pigmented. (B) Malignant melanoma in transit metastases. (C) The same patient 4 months later.

recognition of ulceration as a prognostic factor. Breslow thickness, which is the depth between the epidermal granular layer and the deepest melanoma cells measured in millimetres, is usually regarded as the most accurate method of measuring invasion, although Breslow thickness can occasionally underestimate invasion if there has been regression of the primary tumour, as uncommonly occurs with melanoma. Less importance is now accorded to Clark level and it is not now included in the TNM classification (Tables 20.2 and 20.3).

Table 20.2 Depth of skin invasion described by Clark level

CLARK LEVEL	
I	Melanoma confined to epidermis
II	Papillary dermis invaded
III	Invasion to the papillary-reticular dermis junction
IV	Reticular dermis invaded
V	Subcutaneous fat invaded

Table 20.3 The 2009 7th edition TNM staging system for malignant melanoma

pT1a	< or equal to 1.0 mm, without ulceration & mitosis <1/mm^2
pT1b	< or equal to 1.0 mm, with ulceration or mitosis =/> 1/mm^2
pT2a	1.01-2.0 mm, no ulceration present
pT2b	1.01-2.0 mm, ulceration present
pT3a	2.01-4.0 mm, no ulceration present
pT3b	2.01-4.0 mm, ulceration present
pT4a	>4 mm, no ulceration present
pT4b	>4 mm, ulceration present
N1a	1 node involved, microscopically positive
N1b	1 node involved, macroscopically positive
N2a	2–3 nodes involved, microscopically positive
N2b	2–3 nodes involved, macroscopically positive
N2c	satellite lesions or in-transit metastases *without* nodal involvement
N3	> 4 nodes involved or matted node mass or satellite lesions or in-transit metastases *with* nodal involvement
M1a	Skin, subcutaneous tissue, lymph nodes beyond the regional lymph nodes
M1b	Lung metastases
M1c	Any other site or any metastasis with elevated lactic dehydrogenase (LDH)

These classifications can be gathered together into stage groupings, so that each stage can bring together several TNM classes (Table 20.4).

Stage and prognosis

In summary, the stage and subsequent prognosis depend on tumour thickness and the presence or absence of ulceration. The finding of nodal spread shows the melanoma has already metastasized and ultimate survival depends on the number of nodes involved by melanoma and the quantity of tumour in the lymph nodes (macroscopic or microscopic). Distant spread to liver, lungs or brain carries a grave prognosis with average survival times of 3–12 months depending on the metastatic site. Patients with metastases confined to the skin can often have a surprisingly long survival time.

An approximate measure of prognosis against stage at presentation would be as in Table 20.5. More detailed prognostic data can be found in Balch et al (see Further reading).

Table 20.4 Clinical & pathological staging prognostic groups

Stage IA	T1a
Stage IB	T1b/T2a
Stage IIA	T2b/T3a
Stage IIB	T3b/T4a
Stage IIC	T4b
All of the above are N0	
Stage IIIA	T1a-4a + N1a/2a
Stage IIIB	T1a-4a + N1b/2b/2c *or* T1b-4b + N1a/N2a/N2c
Stage IIIC	T1b-4b + N1b/2b/2c or Any T + N3
Stage IV	Any T or any N + M1

Table 20.5 Five-year survival rates for stage groups

STAGE AT PRESENTATION	5-YEAR SURVIVAL (%)
I	95
II	75
III	60
IV	15

Management of melanoma

It is important to have a high level of suspicion if there is any change in a pigmented skin lesion. Change in size or shape, degree or homogeneity of pigmentation, ulceration or bleeding in a pigmented lesion should lead to referral to the local melanoma screening clinic.

A suspicious mole should be excised with a margin of 2 mm. 'Shaving' a suspected melanoma is contraindicated because this will not allow the true Breslow thickness to be measured and results in incomplete excision. The pathology report should give the depth of invasion in millimetres (the Breslow thickness) and state whether ulceration and/or regression are present or not and whether excision is complete. These are all prognostic factors. If regression is present then this may obscure the dermo-epidermal junction and the given Breslow depth may be an underestimate.

If melanoma is discovered, the patient should then undergo a definitive wider local excision. If the tumour was 1 mm Breslow thickness or less, another lateral excision margin of 1 cm is taken, down to the deep fascia. Tumours greater than 1.0 mm thick are normally excised with a 2 cm lateral margin down to deep fascia.

Thicker, more advanced melanomas carry a higher risk of occult positive lymph nodes. Prophylactic node dissection to identify those with occult metastases has not improved survival and is associated with a high potential complication rate, including wound infection and lymphoedema. Patients who require node dissection can be identified by the sentinel biopsy technique. Trials are being performed of the technique of sentinel node biopsy, where the first node that drains the area of the primary tumour is identified by injecting both a blue dye and a radioactive marker close to the site of the primary tumour bed. The theory that underlies the concept of sentinel node biopsy suggests that these markers are then taken up by the local lymphatics, and identify the first or 'sentinel' draining node. This node is then sampled surgically and, if tumour free, then it is thought that it is unlikely that there is tumour in further nodes and the patient will therefore not require a nodal block dissection. If the sentinel node is positive, then block dissection is required. No survival advantage has been shown so far for sentinel node biopsy compared to removing nodes if and when they are found by clinical examination. Even sentinel node biopsy is associated with some surgical complications. Currently, standard of care in the UK is observation of potential node bearing areas and surgery if required.

Adjuvant treatment for melanoma

At present, there is some evidence that the adjuvant use of high-dose interferon may improve survival in deeper melanomas (>4 mm Breslow depth) or in early node-positive disease at presentation. Not all authorities in Europe accept this evidence, but high-dose interferon is widely used in the adjuvant setting in North America.

At present there is no agreed adjuvant treatment for melanoma, in the UK but in some centres adjuvant radiotherapy is considered for the postoperative treatment of nodal drainage areas in the neck, axillae or groins if patients have been shown to have had large, multiple nodes or extracapsular spread, to attempt to improve local control. This is based on trials performed by the Australian Trans Tasman Radiation Oncology Group (TROG). Patients at high risk of metastatic recurrence should be offered the opportunity to enter clinical trials of adjuvant treatment. Several trials are ongoing using immune modulators or targeted drugs such as Bevacizumab, a monoclonal antibody which acts by blocking angiogenesis, blocking Vascular Endothelial Growth Factor A (VEGF-A).

Management of recurrent or metastatic melanoma

Any evidence of further local, regional or metastatic melanoma requires that the patient be restaged to define the extent of the recurrence. If there is only local recurrence at the primary site, further surgery should be considered. This may be appropriate even if there is other locoregional or metastatic disease present in order to achieve local control.

If regional lymph nodes are involved, a nodal block dissection may be indicated, depending on the extent and fixity of the nodal disease, the extent of other disease and patient factors such as performance status, frailty, co-morbidities present and the potential functional loss and changes in quality of life (both positive and negative) that extensive surgery may bring. In selected cases, adjuvant radiotherapy may improve local control after surgery as after nodal dissection for primary disease.

In-transit metastasis may present in a limb (see Figure 20.24B, C). These represent disease in cutaneous lymphatics between the primary site and local draining nodes. They can erupt and involve widespread areas of skin as small erythematous or pigmented macules and nodules. In-transit metastases can be very problematic and distressing to the patient, especially if they break down or coalesce into larger masses. Patients who develop this condition can be referred to one of a few specialized units around the country which offer isolated limb perfusion (ILP): a technique in which the circulation in a limb is isolated and chemotherapy is given to the limb alone, without significant amounts of drug entering the general circulation. This technique can give considerable palliative benefit and, in some patients, a complete response may be achieved with all the nodules and papules disappearing. If in-transit metastasis affects the skin of the trunk, then the area cannot be isolated and systemic chemotherapy is required.

Patients may develop blood-borne metastasis, most commonly in the liver, lungs, brain or bone. Radiotherapy is useful for brain and bone and cutaneous metastases. Malignant melanoma is often said to be 'radioresistant' and it is true that melanoma cells can sustain more sublethal damage than other cancer cell lines, but this can be countered by using regimens utilizing a higher dose per fraction and treating less frequently, e.g. treating three times per week rather than five times per week. Cutaneous metastasis can be treated by relatively small electron fields, restricting both field size on the skin and the depth treated.

Chemotherapy using DTIC (dimethyl triazeno imidazol carboxamide – also known as dacarbazine) has been the standard treatment for visceral soft-tissue metastasis, although the response rate is only about 15%. Combination chemotherapy regimens may produce an increased overall response rate but at the cost of much greater morbidity. There is no evidence that combination chemotherapy results in improved survival compared with single-agent DTIC. DTIC was previously given over several days because of its emetogenic potential. However, with modern antiemetic regimens, it can there be given as a single dose of 800–1000 mg/m^2 every 3 weeks. Two or three cycles are given and the patient is reassessed.

If there has been a positive response to chemotherapy, DTIC is continued for six cycles. If there has been disease progression it should be stopped. Recently, further chemotherapy options have been developed for patients with metastatic melanoma, with the introduction of two new treatments which act in entirely different ways. Ipilimumab is an antibody which blocks cytotoxic T-lymphocyte associated antigen 4, present on cytotoxic T lymphocytes and results in an active immune response to melanoma cells. Vemurafenib is a B-raf enzyme inhibitor which can cause cell death in melanomas which show a V600E B-raf mutation. This mutation is characterised by glutamic acid replacing valine at position 600 on the B raf protein. Vemurafenib is only effective in melanomas with this mutation. Other drugs with similar mechanisms of action are also being developed.

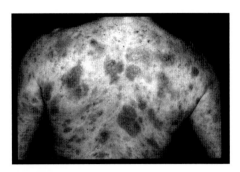

Figure 20.25 Mycosis fungoides, with patches, plaques and nodules.

development of large abnormal circulating T cells, the so-called Sézary cells, in the peripheral blood in association with lymphadenopathy and erythroderma is diagnostic of Sézary syndrome. Patients with this condition are also at greater risk of developing other squamous cell carcinomas of the skin and internal malignancies, especially lung cancer.

There is a wide range of treatments for cutaneous T-cell lymphomas. Topical chemotherapy with nitrogen mustard, carmustine or PUVA, all have high response rates for early disease. For thicker plaques, total skin electron therapy is effective (Figure 20.26A–E). Systemic chemotherapy is indicated for more advanced disease. There are studies in progress evaluating immunotherapy with interferon or interleukin, monoclonal antibody therapy, photopheresis and new combination chemotherapy regimens.

Primary cutaneous B-cell lymphomas are rare and include a wide variety of subtypes including, for example, primary cutaneous follicular centre cell lymphoma and marginal zone B-cell lymphoma. In general, these lymphomas have a more indolent course. They are more likely to be managed by local radiotherapy presenting as a solitary mass, or systemic chemotherapy if they have spread. Secondary cutaneous lymphomas may also affect the skin.

CUTANEOUS LYMPHOMAS

Primary cutaneous lymphomas are uncommon tumours. The majority are T-cell lymphomas with less than 25% being B cell. They are more common in males. At present, their aetiology is unknown, but a viral association has been suggested.

Within the primary cutaneous T-cell lymphomas, mycosis fungoides is the most common type and usually presents in men over 60. There is a range of clinical presentation varying from erythematous cutaneous patches, which may show very slow progression to thickened plaques or nodular tumours, over several years (Figure 20.25).

The development of lymphadenopathy or visceral organ involvement worsens prognosis markedly and the

MERKEL CELL TUMOURS

These tumours represent neuroendocrine carcinoma of the skin. They tend to affect the elderly, often presenting as a painless nodule in the head and neck or on a limb. They may respond well to initial treatment, but go on to recur locally or to develop metastatic spread. They are treated with wide local excision where possible, with post-operative radiotherapy, or radiotherapy alone, if inoperable. Chemotherapy is used for advanced local or recurrent disease, using agents similar to those used in small cell lung cancer, such as cisplatin and etoposide. Initially, tumours may respond to chemotherapy but almost inevitably recur. The main differential diagnosis of Merkel cell tumours is small cell carcinoma, which has metastasized

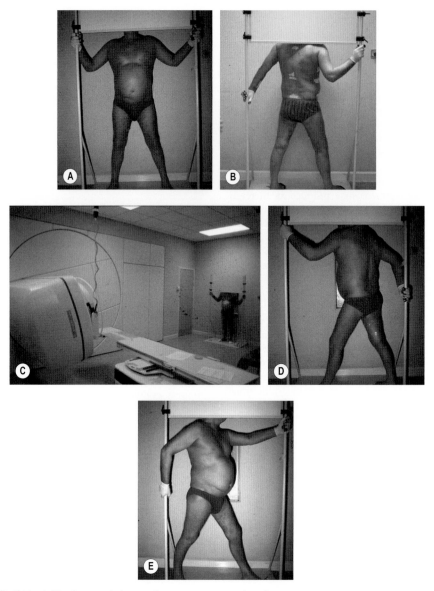

Figure 20.26 (A–E) Total skin electrons being used to treat cutaneous lymphoma.

to the skin. Cytokeratin 20 is useful in differentiating between these two possibilities histologically.

SKIN SARCOMA

Primary sarcomas of the structures of the skin or subcutaneous tissues are uncommon but may present as a diagnostic problem. They often have no defining clinical characteristics and most often present as a skin or subcutaneous nodule. These tumours can arise from a range of

connective tissue cell precursors, including vascular nerve and muscle tissues with a wide arange of pathological types and subtypes, often not easy to diagnose even with adequate histological material.

The most important pathological diagnosis is to decide if the tumour is benign or malignant, with the potential to recur or metastasize. If the tumour is benign and has been excised completely then no further intervention is required.

True malignant sarcomas affecting the skin, for example angiosarcoma, can carry a poor prognosis. These vascular malignancies (Figure 20.27A) present with an erythematous

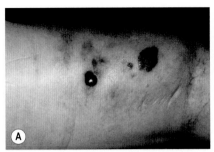 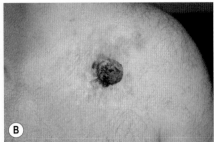

Figure 20.27 (A) Angiosarcoma. (B) Dermatofibromasarcoma protuberans.

or vascular nodule, which can then ulcerate or go on to form several other nodules. They can metastasize early and wide surgical excision is the treatment of choice. They are also associated with developing in areas of post-mastectomy lymphoedema, either in the chest wall or arm, often a decade after initial surgery. This phenomenon is known as the Stewart Treaves syndrome.

Other malignant variants of sarcoma which can develop from skin structures, include malignant fibrous histiocytoma, malignant peripheral nerve sheath tumours and clear cell sarcoma, which is a malignancy derived from melanocytes. These are all uncommon and initial treatment for all is wide surgical excision.

As well as the skin sarcomas with true metastatic potential, there are also connective tissue tumours that can affect the skin, showing local invasion and having the potential for local recurrence if inadequately excised. Metastases are very rare. The most common example in this group would be dermatofibrosarcoma protuberans (see Figure 20.27B). These tumours can be difficult to diagnose pathologically, especially in their early stages, when histologically they may appear to be benign. They have a long natural history, with local recurrences stretching over years. The can dedifferentiate and become more aggressive clinically and histologically more malignant. If this occurs, there is a greater risk of metastasis.

KAPOSI'S SARCOMA

This is a particular form of vascular sarcoma which is derived from endothelial cells. It has become much more prevalent with the increased incidence of AIDS. Kaposi's sarcoma (KS) has several variants including: classical KS, and epidemic KS, both associated with human herpes virus type 8. There are also types associated with immunosuppressive treatment and African KS.

Before the AIDS epidemic, classical KS was a rare disease, affecting elderly males, usually of Italian or East European Jewish descent, who developed the pigmented patches and nodules around the lower leg or ankle (Figure 20.28A–C). These tumours develop slowly, but patients are at risk of developing a second malignancy, often non-Hodgkin's lymphoma. Most patients are treated with relatively low doses of radiotherapy, such as 8 Gy in a single fraction, which may be repeated.

Epidemic KS develops in approximately 20–25% of patients with AIDS, although there was a much higher incidence in AIDS patients when the epidemic first started. Since the introduction of highly active antiretroviral treatment (HAART), the incidence of age-related Kaposi's sarcoma has reduced. Patients with this variant are more likely to develop disseminated disease. Chemotherapy is used to treat Kaposi's sarcoma using agents such as liposomal doxorubicin or a taxane. These tumours can be exquisitely sensitive to radiotherapy: great care must be taken in treating sites such as the oral mucosa or considerable morbidity can be caused. There have been a variety of dose schedules used, all giving relatively low total doses for the management of this condition, such as a single 6 Gy fraction, using a low energy electron beam, for single or a few cutaneous lesions, or 12 Gy in three fractions. There is a suggestion that using slightly higher fractionated doses, such as 20–30 Gy in 10–15 fractions may produce a longer lasting response for individual lesions.

SKIN APPENDAGE TUMOURS

These are also known as adnexal tumours. They arise from skin structures including the hair follicle, sebaceous glands or sweat glands. There is a wide range of benign skin appendage tumours which occasionally undergo malignant transformation. They most often appear as smooth non-distinctive masses which are diagnosed not by their clinical appearance, but on biopsy histopathology. There are multiple pathological subtypes (Figure 20.29A, B).

Sebaceous carcinoma is an example of an uncommon potentially metastatic skin appendage tumour. These classically occur on the eyelid, diagnosed on biopsy. Surgery is the treatment of choice. Sweat gland carcinoma gives a similar indistinct clinical picture. These tumours usually present as an odd-looking BCC or SCC, with the diagnosis again

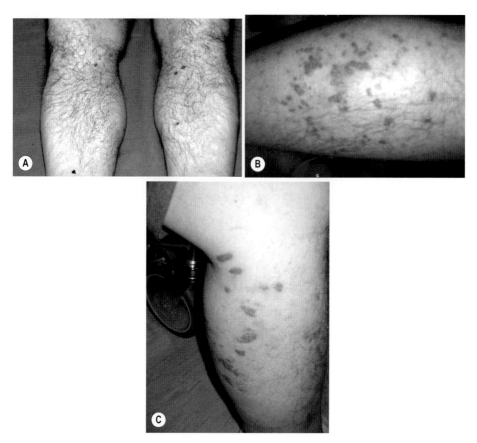

Figure 20.28 (A–C) Kaposi's sarcoma.

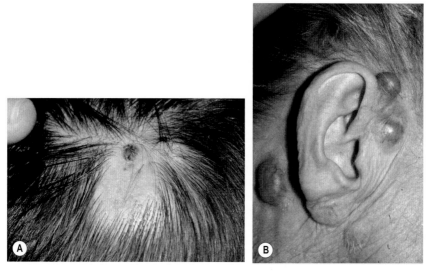

Figure 20.29 Skin appendage tumours. (A) A sebaceous naevus with an associated basal cell carcinoma. (B) A multiple cylindroma, with a typically non-characteristic appearance.

not been made until excision biopsy has been done. Surgery is again the treatment of choice.

Paget's disease can occur outwith the breast; extra mammary Paget's disease. The most common site is the vulva. This condition, thought to arise from epithelial cells in an apocrine duct, looks like eczema. It can give rise to pruritus and ulceration and may spread to locoregional nodes and even metastasize systemically.

FURTHER READING

Locke J, Karimpour S, Young G, et al. Radiotherapy for epithelial skin cancer. Int J Radiat Oncol Biol Phys 2001;51:748–55.

Petit JY, Avril MF, Margulis A, et al. Evaluation of cosmetic results of a randomized trial comparing surgery and radiotherapy in the treatment of basal cell carcinoma of the face. Plast Reconstr Surg 2000;105:2544–51.

Bishop JN, Bataille V, Gavin A, et al. The prevention, diagnosis, referral and management of melanoma of the skin: concise guidelines. Clin Med 2007;7:283–90.

Balch CM, Buzaid AC, Soong SJ, et al. Final version of the America Joint Committee on Cancer staging system for cutaneous melanoma. J Clin Oncol 2001;18:3635–48.

Tsao H, Atkins MB, Sober AJ. Management of cutaneous melanoma. N Engl J Med 2004;351:998–1012.

Thompson JF, Scolyer RA, Kefford RF. Cutaneous melanoma. Lancet 2005;365:687–701.

Morrison WH, Garden AS, Ang KK. Radiation therapy for non melanoma skin carcinomas. Clin Plast Surg 1997;24:718–29.

Ott MJ, Tanabe KK, Gadd MA, et al. Multimodality treatment of Merkel cell carcinoma. Arch Surg 1999;134:388–93.

Stelzer KJ, Griffin TW. A randomised prospective trial of radiation therapy for AIDS-associated Kaposi's sarcoma. Int J Radiat Oncol Biol Phys 1993;27:1057–61.

Hersh E, Weber J, Powderly J, et al. Long-term survival of patients (pts) with advanced melanoma treated with ipilimumab with or without dacarbazine. J Clin Oncol 2009; 27:15s (suppl; abstr 9038).

Hodi FS, O'Day SJ, McDermott DF, et al. Improved Survival with Ipilimumab in Patients with Metastatic Melanoma. N Engl J Med 2010;363:711–722.

Chapman PB, Hauschild A, Robert C, Improved Survival with Vemurafenib in Melanoma with BRAF V600E Mutation. N Engl J Med 2011; 364:2507–2516.

Burmeister BH, Mark Smithers B, Burmeister E, et al. A prospective phase II study of adjuvant postoperative radiation therapy following nodal surgery in malignant melanoma: Trans Tasman Radiation Oncology Group (TROG) study 96.06. Radiother Oncol. 2006;812:136–142.

Chapter | 21 |

Head and neck cancer – general principles

Christopher D. Scrase

CHAPTER CONTENTS

INTRODUCTION

'Head and neck cancer' is a rather inaccurate term for describing cancers of the upper aerodigestive tract – tumours of the facial skin and the brain are not conventionally included. They are a diverse group, comprising oral cancers, as well as those of the oropharynx, larynx, nasopharynx and hypopharynx; also the paranasal sinuses, salivary glands and ear. The overall incidence is approximately 11 cases per 100 000 per year in England and Wales, although there are regional variations. The incidence is increasing at present (see the 'aetiology' section of this chapter). Although the treatment for these areas is often highly specialized, they also have many features in common with regard to investigation, diagnosis and management. Perhaps more than any other anatomical site, the concept of multidisciplinary team working is paramount in head and neck cancer and it is essential that the team members are involved as early as possible to provide the best outcome in terms of tumour control, maintaining function and acceptable cosmesis. Radiotherapy, and to an increasing extent chemotherapy, are now widely used, either as primary therapy or post-operative treatments.

DEMOGRAPHICS

Head and neck cancers make up 4–5% of all new cancers. The incidence is higher in males than females, although the ratio is different for specific cancers: oral cavity (2:1), larynx (4:1), but these numbers are changing due to an increasing incidence of smoking in women. The majority of head and neck cancers present beyond the fifth decade with an average age of onset of 60 years. Cancers of the head and neck are more commonly found in people from the lower social classes and this is multifactorial with higher incidences of smoking and alcoholism, late presentation, poor oral hygiene, inadequate diet etc. It is linked to delayed diagnosis and worse outcome.

AETIOLOGY

The most important risk factor in the development of head and neck cancers is tobacco. Smoking or chewing tobacco is associated with 85–90% of head and neck malignancies. Alcohol intake has also been shown to cause an increase in this group of cancers. There is also a synergistic effect of combining alcohol and tobacco with regard to developing cancers in this site. There is also a clear increase in the incidence of second malignancy of the head and neck and other sites (lung, oesophagus) in persistent smokers.

Other risk factors in head and neck cancers have been suggested including poor oral hygiene, dental disease and trauma from badly fitted dentures, though direct causation has not been demonstrated. Viral infections have also been investigated for a role in the aetiology of head and neck cancers. There is a very strong association with Epstein-Barr virus infection and nasopharyngeal cancer. There is an increasing incidence of human papilloma virus (HPV) associated oropharyngeal and oral tumours, particularly in the USA. Such tumours develop in younger patients and have a distinctive pathological appearance – basaloid and predominantly poorly differentiated carcinoma. Immunosuppression is known to be a risk factor for malignancy and this includes cancers of the head and neck. Tertiary syphilis is another predisposing factor, although the authors have never knowingly seen a patient – but this rare disease is increasing in frequency again, and needs to be remembered.

Pre-malignant conditions also exist which predispose for the development of head and neck cancers. These are most commonly seen in the oral cavity and include leukoplakia (white patches) which carry an approximately 5% risk of progressing to invasive malignancy and, more sinisterly, erythroplakia. Regular specialist follow up is therefore essential. Lichen planus with dysplastic features can also become malignant and requires monitoring.

Radiation exposure is also a risk factor for developing head and neck cancers. A previous history of radiotherapy treatment should be sought in newly diagnosed patients. It will also have an impact on any future radiotherapy treatment options.

PREVENTION AND EARLY DIAGNOSIS

When diagnosed early, head and neck cancer has quite good chances for cure, but at present there is no established screening programme. It has been shown that targeted education in the primary sector with general practitioners and dentists has had some impact on early referral for oral cancers. This is important as patients presenting with advanced disease have a poorer prognosis.

Tobacco cessation is also an important factor in preventing head and neck cancers. The prevalence of cigarette smoking has fallen by over 20% in men over the last 20 years (Figure 21.1). Aggressive treatment of pre-malignant conditions is important in reducing the incidence of invasive cancer.

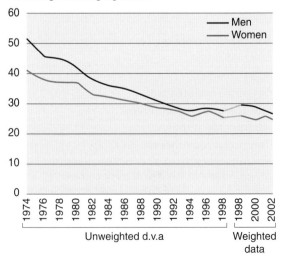

Figure 21.1 Prevalence of smoking 1974–2002.

TUMOUR TYPES

The majority (over 90%) of cancers of the head and neck are squamous cell carcinomas (SCC) arising from mucosal cells. They are usually graded into well-, moderate- or poorly-differentiated on the basis of their histological assessment (mitoses, pleomorphism). Poorly-differentiated tumours tend to metastasize to lymph nodes more frequently than well-differentiated lesions. The remainder are made up of small numbers of adenocarcinoma, lymphoma (these are treated by a different team in most institutions), sarcoma, melanoma and various salivary gland tumours (muco-epidermoid, adenoid cystic, acinic tumours). It is essential that a histological diagnosis is confirmed before treatment to ensure the correct management and a specialist head and neck pathologist must be part of the multidisciplinary team.

PRESENTATION

The majority of cases of head and neck cancer present symptomatically. The symptoms therefore depend on the primary site and the adjacent structures that may be involved. This may be a visible lesion in the oral cavity – leucoplakia, erythroplakia or non-healing ulcer – or may relate to a swelling or mass in the oropharynx, hypo-pharynx or larynx. There may be hoarseness, difficulty swallowing, discomfort or pain on eating, referred aural pain, trismus or cranial nerve palsies. The onset of these symptoms is an indication for urgent referral to a head and neck department. More non-specific symptoms of weight loss, anorexia or generalized discomfort can also be seen in this group of patients.

A common presentation of head and neck cancer is with lymph node metastases in the neck. The histology may be confirmed by FNA (fine needle aspiration) or biopsy. A thorough search for a potential primary tumour is required. However, in a number of patients, this remains occult and treatment must then be planned to cover potential sites of origin.

INVESTIGATION

Patients presenting with possible head and neck cancer should be referred urgently to a specialist head and neck oncology team. The work-up requires confirmation of the histological diagnosis and full examination under anaesthetic of the aerodigestive tract for accurate staging and to exclude second primary lesions. Cross-sectional imaging with computed tomography (CT) or magnetic resonance imaging (MRI) with contrast enhancement is also essential for staging purposes detailing anatomical extent of the primary lesion and any nodal involvement. Imaging of the chest with chest x-ray or CT is required to exclude pulmonary metastases or a synchronous lung primary. There may be a synchronous primary in up to 10% of head and neck cancer patients and these are often tobacco related. The incidence of distant metastases is reported between 5 and 30% and the majority is in the lung, although very occasionally bone or liver secondaries are found. The occurrence of metastases correlates with increasing stage of the primary tumour and the number, size and bilaterality of lymph node involvement at presentation. Positron emission tomography (PET) is increasingly used in staging head and neck cancer, and offers possibly exciting opportunities, but its exact role remains to be defined. It offers potential for patients with cervical lymphadenopathy and an occult primary but, perhaps, at present, its main use is assessment following radiotherapy to look for residual or persisting disease.

All head and neck cancer patients should be discussed in a multidisciplinary meeting at the time of diagnosis and staging to determine the optimum treatment. The choice is usually between radical surgery ± postoperative radiotherapy (or chemoradiotherapy) or primary radical radiotherapy (or concurrent chemoradiation) with possible neck dissection for residual disease. The decision is usually determined by the site of the primary tumour, the size of the primary tumour, evidence of lymph node involvement and patients' co-morbidity or individual preference. Before embarking on any radical treatment options, there are a number of preparatory steps that need to be assessed.

NUTRITION

Head and neck cancer patients have many reasons to be malnourished prior to diagnosis of their malignancy. Many have a background of excessive alcohol intake, the tumour may have resulted in impaired swallowing function or caused oral discomfort. The success of any radical treatment is compromised by inadequate nutrition and morbidity is also increased. It is essential that all head and neck cancer patients have assessment by a specialist dietician prior to any treatment. They may require enteral feeding prior to treatment and will certainly need it following surgery. Patients receiving radical radiotherapy will usually have a course of treatment over many weeks and will develop mucositis and dysphagia in the acute phase. Naso-gastric tube or percutaneous gastrostomy should be actively considered in all patients, especially those with large treatment fields and are essential for patients being considered for concurrent chemoradiation where the acute toxicity is usually increased. It is also important for the dietetic input to continue regularly throughout the treatment course – patients need to be weighed weekly, outcome data show ongoing weight loss to be a negative prognostic factor – and in the recovery phase following treatment which may last many weeks. Close monitoring should therefore continue during the follow-up period until tube feeding is no longer required and patients have returned to sufficient oral intake and proven maintained weight.

DENTITION

Patients receiving radical radiotherapy for head and neck cancers will often have treatment fields involving part or all of the mandible and the salivary glands. Following radiotherapy, these patients are often left with xerostomia. Saliva has a protective role in neutralizing oral acids and reducing dental caries. Tooth decay and dental problems can be increased post-radiotherapy. Patients need to have a full dental assessment prior to radiotherapy. The ideal is for review by a restorative dentist or maxillofacial team to remove teeth if required. Any problem teeth should be removed and, as this typical patient population has often neglected their oral hygiene, many end up with a dental clearance. Dental extractions should be done a minimum of 2 weeks before commencing radiotherapy. Edentulous patients should be reviewed to ensure dentures are well fitting and will not aggravate their radiotherapy reaction by movement.

When taking consent from patients for radiotherapy, they must be counselled about the risks of dental problems following the treatment and, in particular, osteoradionecrosis of the mandible which can develop spontaneously but is more likely after dental procedures, particularly extractions (Figure 21.2). Patients need to be encouraged to use fluoride mouthwash or gel daily and to have regular dental check-ups – and if dental work is considered necessary it should be performed by specialist hospital dental teams in view of the high risk of complications.

INDICATIONS FOR RADIOTHERAPY

Definitive radiotherapy

The chief aim in using radiotherapy in head and neck cancer is organ preservation. In early laryngeal cancer, equivalent cure rates are attainable with radical radiotherapy and laryngectomy, but the former has the clear advantage of normal voice preservation. In some sites, radiotherapy is the only option or preferred option due to the inaccessible nature of the primary, e.g. nasopharyngeal cancer.

Postoperative radiotherapy

The purpose of postoperative radiotherapy is to improve locoregional control. It has recently been estimated that cancer-specific and overall survival at 5 years might be improved by about 10% with postoperative radiotherapy.

There are a number of indications for postoperative radiotherapy (Table 21.1). In some cases, postoperative radiotherapy is mandatory, in other situations the real benefit to the patient is less clear.

Postoperative radiotherapy should ideally commence within 6 weeks of surgery as evidence suggests an inferior outcome if started later than this.

Palliative radiotherapy

As a general rule, radiotherapy should be used with curative intent and with standard curative doses. On occasions, however, patients will not be fit to undergo any form of radical radiotherapy and radiotherapy can provide useful symptom relief.

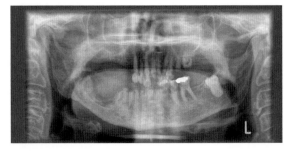

Figure 21.2 Orthopantomogram (OPT) of mandible showing osteoradionecrosis on right side.

Table 21.1 Indications for postoperative radiotherapy
Positive (involved) resection margins
Extracapsular lymph node spread
Close resection margins, i.e. <5 mm
Invasion of soft tissues
≥2 nodes involved
>1 positive nodal group (i.e. level)
Involved node >3 cm in diameter
Vascular invasion
Perineural invasion
Poor differentiation
Stage III/IV
Multicentric primary
Oral cavity/oropharynx tumours with involved nodes at level IV/V
Carcinoma in situ/dysplasia at resection margin/'field changes'
Guidelines for cervical nodal irradiation in squamous cell carcinoma of the head and neck. Reproduced with kind permission of Dr M. Henk and the CHART steering committee

RADIOTHERAPY PLANNING

Once radiotherapy has been decided as the treatment modality for head and neck patients, there are a number of steps required prior to commencing. Patients need to be informed of all possible side effects (see Toxicity of treatment) and to give consent.

Immobilization

The next step is to consider immobilization. Tumours in the head and neck may be relatively small compared to other anatomical sites and they are also often adjacent to several critical normal structures. It is therefore essential for accurate treatment delivery that patients have good quality reproducible immobilization. In general, this involves an individual shell to cover the head, neck and, sometimes, the shoulders. These shells are commonly either thermoplastic or rigid Perspex and are created specifically for the patient during the planning phase. The patient then has subsequent imaging in the mask. Although the thermoplastic shells sometimes appear more flexible, they can still provide an accurate set-up. Occasionally, stereotactic frames or relocatable devices may be used but these are not usually required for most head and neck patients. Mould room staff who make the shell also require information about the patient's position (usually supine) and the orientation of the neck. This is important and is determined by the site one intends to irradiate and needs consideration of the intended beam arrangement: an extended neck position would be required for treatment of the parotid bed and middle/inner ear to facilitate the exiting posterior oblique field below the contralateral eye. It is also necessary to consider whether the patient requires a mouth bite or tongue depressor. A mouth bite is used to push the tongue *out* of the treatment volume, e.g. maxillary antral tumours. A tongue depressor is used to push the tongue *into* the treatment volume, e.g. oral tongue tumours.

The most important issue of any immobilization device is to know what the reproducibility of set-up is for any particular patient. All centres should know the accuracy of their set-up for a particular device as this is the information required for determining the margin from clinical target volume (CTV) to planning target volume (PTV). In practice, an accuracy of 3–5 mm can be expected with existing devices.

TARGET VOLUMES

Definitive radiotherapy

When radiotherapy (with or without chemotherapy) is the definitive treatment, a gross tumour volume (GTV) is present and a planning CT scan will allow it to be delineated combined with information from the examination under anaesthesia (EUA), histology and other diagnostic imaging. Help from a specialist radiologist is recommended. The CTV is to account for microscopic spread. Overtly involved nodes should be included in that CTV. Occult lymph node metastases occur in up to 20–30% of the N0 neck patients, so prophylactic irradiation is required for many head and neck tumours and is delineated as a separate CTV. The sites where this is not considered are early glottic or subglottic cancers (T1/T2 disease) (Table 21.2). The likelihood of nodal involvement has been widely studied and it is clear that the probability increases with site of primary, size of primary and differentiation.

The regions of the neck have been divided into levels to allow international consensus on the lymph node anatomy (Figure 21.3):

- level I contains the submental and submandibular lymph nodes
- level II contains the upper jugular lymph nodes, which are above the hyoid bone
- level III contains the mid-jugular lymph nodes, which are between the hyoid bone and the cricoid cartilage
- level IV contains the lower jugular lymph nodes beginning below the cricoid
- level V contains the lymph nodes of the posterior triangle
- level VI contains the pretracheal lymph nodes.

The levels that are included in the treatment of any particular primary site depend on the anatomical drainage and knowledge of patterns of lymph node spread. Lymph node maps for the N0 neck have been compiled to aid the planning of radiotherapy. In unilateral structures (parotid, buccal mucosa, lateral floor of mouth), it is possible to treat the primary site and ipsilateral neck nodes but, in midline structures, bilateral treatment is required because the lymph drainage may be to either side of the neck. With conventional radiotherapy techniques, the decision to treat unilaterally and thus spare the contralateral parotid gland is a major benefit for the many cured patients who are spared xerostomia. With intensity modulated radiotherapy (IMRT), it is possible to treat the neck bilaterally and spare at least one parotid gland. There is now level one data to support this approach.

Postoperative radiotherapy

The principles discussed in the previous section on definitive radiotherapy are applicable in the postoperative setting, but there are some important additional points to note.

As a general rule, the whole surgical bed where the tumour was located should be included in the postoperative irradiated volume, at least to an intermediate dose (discussed later). By CT planning, it often becomes apparent that changes within the subcutaneous tissues will give volumes at risk that are bigger than anticipated.

Table 21.2 Indications for nodal irradiation by tumour site

INDICATIONS	IRRADIATION
Oral cavity	
T2N0 with well-lateralized primary	Levels I and II on the same side
T2N1 with well-lateralized primary	Levels I to V on the same side
T2N0 with primary approaching midline, all T3N0 and T4N0	Levels I, II and III bilaterally
All others	Levels I to V bilaterally
Oropharynx	
T2N0 tonsil	Levels I and II on the same side
T2N1 tonsil	Levels I to V on the same side
T2N0 other sites	Levels I, II and III bilaterally
All others	Levels I to V bilaterally
Nasopharynx	
Squamous cell carcinoma T1 – T4 N0	Level II, retropharyngeal and upper posterior triangle
All undiferentiated carcinoma and squamous carcinoma with node involvement	Levels I to V
Hypopharynx	
All	Levels 1 to V bilaterally
Paranasal sinuses	**Retropharyngeal nodes**
Squamous carcinoma	Lateral pharyngeal nodes only
Squamous carcinoma N+ and undifferentiated carcinoma	Levels 1 to V on the same side
Larynx	
T1–2N0 glottic	No nodal irradiation
T3–4N0 glottic	Levels II and III bilaterally
T2N0 supraglottic	Levels II and III bilaterally
All others	Levels 1 to V bilaterally

Lymph node levels are defined as follows: level 1, submandibular; level II, upper deep cervical; level III, middle deep cervical; level IV, lower deep cervical; level V, posterior triangle

Consideration of the risk-benefit is then required dependent in part on the irradiation technique.

Unless there is gross residual disease or where radiotherapy is planned for the primary site following a neck dissection, a GTV will not be apparent on the planning CT scan. It is often helpful to co-register any diagnostic scans with the planning CT scan in determining more precisely the pre-operative GTVs CTV.

Debate continues on whether to irradiate the neck postoperatively when it is planned to irradiate the primary site and there is no nodal disease identified in the neck dissection specimen. The additional morbidity of irradiating the lower neck to intermediate prophylactic doses is relatively low compared to the rest of the neck, while recurrence in those not irradiated is difficult if not impossible to salvage. The decision must rest with the treating clinician, but a

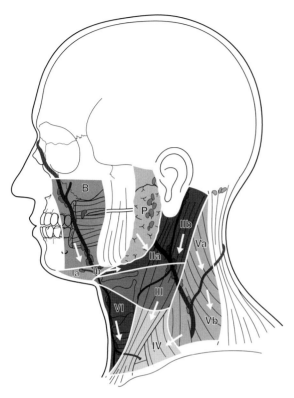

Figure 21.3 Lymph node levels in the neck.

factor in that decision-making process will be the adequacy of the neck dissection.

The retropharyngeal nodes are not routinely sampled in a neck dissection. Dependent on the tumour site (and hence risk of involvement), these should be included if the rest of the neck is to be irradiated postoperatively.

RADIOTHERAPY TECHNIQUE

Conformal radiotherapy (3DCRT)

In the past, conventional planning for head and neck radiotherapy has involved orthogonal films taken in the simulator with fields defined directly. With developments in radiotherapy planning, it has become possible to shape beams to shield normal structures and thereby reduce toxicity. A CT scan with the patient located in the immobilization device is a prequisite to the process. The GTV and CTV(s) are defined directly on the CT. Structures to be avoided, including the spinal cord, are outlined separately. The volumes are then used for planning purposes. In practice, a parallel-opposed field arrangement may still be utilized, especially when the neck is to be irradiated bilaterally, but the process allows for some conformality and thus normal tissue sparing.

Intensity modulated and image guided radiotherapy in head and neck cancers

Developments in computer and the multileaf collimator (MLC) technology have facilitated the emergence of IMRT. It has significant potential in the many subsites within the head and neck territory because of the high degree of conformality that may be achieved. This section will elaborate on the principles of IMRT and their application to head and neck tumours. The reader should be aware that IMRT may be utilized in other body sites and the principles as discussed here may be applicable elsewhere.

Image guided radiotherapy (IGRT) is distinct from IMRT. The technique of IGRT is intended to ensure the target volume as defined at the outset of treatment is treated consistently throughout the course of radiotherapy. Organs move and patients move, though immobilization techniques should ensure that patient movement is less than 3 mm in the head and neck region. IGRT then has as its purpose to correct for motion and set-up errors by imaging the treatment area on a daily basis. IGRT clearly may be utilized with conventional head and neck techniques, but it is potentially more valuable with IMRT in view of the high degree of conformality that can be achieved here.

What is intensity modulated radiotherapy?

Any radical radiotherapy technique aims to treat tumour tissue while minimizing the exposure of healthy adjacent normal tissue. In the head and neck region, it is self-evident that there are many normal tissues that potentially need not be treated. The clinical target volume is often complex with structures nearby which, if damaged, could result in catastrophic sequelae, e.g. binocular blindness and myelopathy. Conventional techniques, as described previously, use parallel-opposed fields to minimize these risks by the 'shrinking-field' technique (Figure 21.4).

Computer tomographic delineation of target volumes facilitates the use of 3-dimensional conformal radiotherapy (3DCRT). By defining a CTV and a margin for set-up error to give the planning target volume (PTV), the resulting field with blocks or MLCs will achieve improved conformality and potentially reduced normal tissue dose (Figure *evolve* 21.5 🖱).

Wedges, partial transmission blocks and compensators modulate the beam as it exits the linear accelerator and are established techniques in improving the dose distribution within the patient with head and neck cancers. They are in essence a form of beam intensity modulation. However, they have an inability to address the complex often concave target volumes encountered in the head and neck region.

Intensity modulated radiotherapy uses the computer control of the MLC to produce either a finite or 'infinite' number of subfields within each field to improve target volume coverage. In essence, in a single 'beam's-eye-view', the

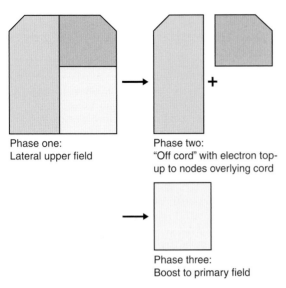

Phase one:
Lateral upper field

Phase two:
"Off cord" with electron top-up to nodes overlying cord

Phase three:
Boost to primary field

Figure 21.4 Three-phase 'shrinking field' treatment.

target volume is seen as a three-dimensional structure and treated as such. Photographers will be able to relate this to the concept of depth of field. The net effect of such complex beam modulation (Figure 21.6) is the ability to treat concave target volumes with normal tissues in the concavity.

How is intensity modulated radiotherapy achieved?

Beam modulation then may be achieved by a number of ways. There are two major approaches that have been adopted by linear accelerator vendors to facilitate intensity

modulated radiotherapy. Both techniques use the MLC in variable but fixed gantry positions during treatment.

'Step and shoot' technique

Here a finite number of subfields or segments are applied at each specified gantry angle. The sum of these multiple segments gives the beam modulation required (Figure evolve 21.7 🖱).

'Sliding window' technique

In this situation, the MLC leaves move continuously at each gantry angle. The leading and trailing leaves move at variable speeds resulting in 'dynamic' beam modulation (Figure evolve 21.8 🖱).

Tomotherapy or literally 'slice by slice' therapy is another approach to achieve beam modulation. IMRT techniques originated with 'bolt-on' mini-MLCs. Currently dedicated tomotherapy machines exist with a rotating beam and a treatment couch that moves during treatment rather like a spiral CT.

Treatment planning in IMRT

Assuming a technique of IMRT along the lines of the previous section, it is apparent that conventional ('forward') planning techniques cannot be used (Figure 21.9). In other words, it is not possible to define a target volume and expect the planner to work out the modulation of each beam (or beam profile) to achieve the desired conformality. Instead, computer technology has assumed that role 'driven' by the planner aided by various inputted parameters (or planning constraints). Planning then when using IMRT requires a different approach: instead of a plan being arrived at by a

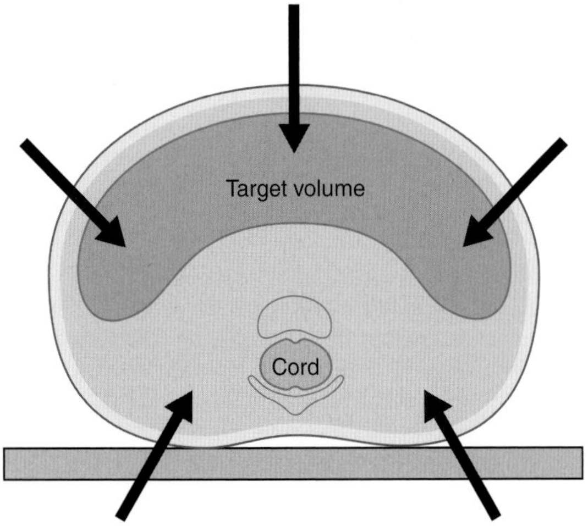

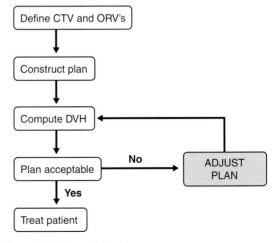

Figure 21.6 Treating a target volume with normal tissue in the concavity.

FORWARD PLANNING

Figure 21.9 Forward planning.

manual iterative process (often itself reliant on the experience of the planner), parameters including the intended target volume dose to a specified volume *and* maximum and median/mean doses allowed to normal tissues are specified at the outset. This is a process known as 'inverse' planning.

It is evident that the process of inverse planning requires absolute clarity of target volume definition (Figure 21.10). This is not a minor issue as arriving at definitions, particularly in the head and neck area, is through a process of integration of all planning data. This will include any pretreatment visual inspection and imaging, operative findings, pathology results, postoperative and planning scans and knowledge of patterns of spread. Clearly, this approach should be applied to all radiotherapy where accurate target volume definition is necessary, i.e. curative radiotherapy, but the ability of IMRT to achieve a high degree of conformality makes this crucial. International guidelines now exist for the definition of the nodes in the cervical chain which should lead to some uniformity between centres, but none exist thus far for the primary tumour.

The process of inverse planning requires as much clarity on normal tissue volume definition as that of the clinical target volume. In the head and neck region, these organs at risk (OARs) would include the spinal cord, brainstem, brain, optic pathway, cochlea and salivary tissues. Failure to delineate these accurately could mean that they are irradiated unintentionally beyond conventional tolerance limits as IMRT achieves its goal of improved conformality in simple terms by moving dose elsewhere. Secondly, normal tissues, once delineated, require a specification of dose. These constraints may be specified in terms of maximum doses (e.g. spinal cord) or dose-volume constraints (e.g. parotid glands) and will be determined on the functional unit arrangement (i.e. parallel versus series).

INVERSE PLANNING

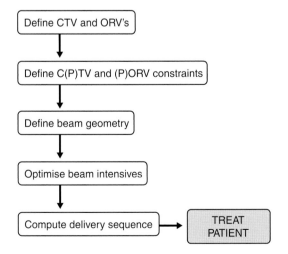

Figure 21.10 Inverse planning.

It is because IMRT achieves its goal through 'shifting dose' that some structures that would not have been irradiated using conventional techniques need delineation. For example, in the treatment of oropharyngeal tumours, the oral cavity will receive modest doses of radiation. By specifying a limit of dose there, it is possible to minimize the impact of irradiation on the oral mucosa. In addition, it is helpful to treat the patient in such circumstances in an extended neck position to move the oral cavity out of the primary portals. Fictitious structures ('dummy' organs) might need to be drawn to keep dose out of areas that would never normally be irradiated and/or to try to improve conformality of target volume coverage. The end result is an array of volumes for the planner to utilize (Figure *evolve* 21.11). This process is time-consuming but a prerequisite to successful IMRT. Software programs are under development that should speed this process through the use of stored templates of normal structures with built-in 'elasticity' to morph to the individual patient's anatomy and body profile.

Before IMRT be undertaken, there is a need to carry out a number of pretreatment checks. This process of individual pretreatment verification seeks to ensure that the treatment plan is being delivered by the linear accelerator. This is only a check however of the output of the linear accelerator. On-treatment verification would include geometrical checks of patient position, typically using orthogonal fields and verification of delivered dose (e.g. thermoluminescent dosimeters (TLDs) diodes or portal dosimetry).

The scope of IMRT in head and neck tumours

The improvement in conformality in head and neck tumours with IMRT has two important fundamental benefits. First, it facilitates the coverage of complex and especially concave target volumes. Secondly, it can achieve avoidance of dose-limiting normal tissues.

It is perhaps the 'avoidance' function that is more useful in head and neck tumours. The parallel-opposed technique does, as the name suggests, treat everything in its path. Mucosa and salivary glands that need not necessarily be treated can now be spared by this approach (Figure *evolve* 21.12). The net effect is the expectation of reduced toxicity. This has perhaps been best explored in relation to reducing xerostomia through sparing of one or both parotid glands. In addition, however, is the improved tolerability of some of the more intense schedules that are emerging as superior in the management of head and neck tumours, i.e. altered fractionation and concurrent chemoradiotherapy.

An improvement in conformality, however, also facilitates comprehensive coverage of the target volume as defined as well as dose escalation. With conventional even 3DCRT approaches some compromise in target volume coverage may be necessary if normal tissue tolerance has been reached. The obvious example is in the treatment of cervical nodes overlying the spinal cord. Typically, these would be treated with electrons of a specified energy. IMRT treats this concave volume to the specified dose (acknowledging that there will be some inhomogeneity) with sparing of the underlying cord without the need for electron applicators. In other sites, such as the paranasal territory, some of the target volume may be at risk of complete sparing because of the complex interrelationship of normal tissue and tumour volumes (Figures *evolve* 21.13 and 21.14). Dose escalation can be used at areas of greatest risk of recurrence, e.g. gross residual primary tumour and nodes with extracapsular spread.

Dose escalation with IMRT needs consideration of radiobiological principles. A single 'phase' technique is used throughout the whole volume (Figure *evolve* 21.15) with different doses specified according to areas of variable risk, e.g. gross disease, 'high-risk' (e.g. involved nodes post-excision) and 'low-risk' territories (e.g. elective nodes in contralateral neck). Not only is the total dose modified according to perceived risk but so is the *dose per fraction*. A higher than conventional dose per fraction will have a higher cell kill effect and is important in the area that is dose escalated. This approach is called the synchronous or simultaneous integrated boost technique (SIB) (Figure *evolve* 21.16) and is established as an approach in IMRT of the head and neck. Care is clearly required in the volume of normal tissue exposed to this as higher than expected morbidity may result because of the negating effect on normal tissue damage. In areas to receive prophylactic irradiation, the total dose may need to be modified upwards to compensate for the longer elective treatment (e.g. 54 Gy in 30 fractions rather than 50 Gy in 25 fractions – see later section) to compensate for repopulation.

Clearly, IMRT has real potential to improve the outcome of patients with head and neck cancer. Its implementation requires multiprofessional engagement.

Pitfalls to intensity modulated radiotherapy

Provided the treating clinician is confident in target volume definition, the risks of geographical miss are small. Parallel-opposed techniques 'work' because the degree of volume definition is not required. Indeed, conventional head and neck radiotherapy is still undertaken by many using fields defined by bony landmarks. It is useful to think of 3DCRT and IMRT as a volume-defining initial process with fields as part of the verification process. Thinking in terms of 'volumes' in all head and neck cases makes the transition to IMRT a much smoother process.

Secondly, there is a need to be quite specific on normal tissue tolerance. The landmark paper of Emami, from the pre-CT planning era was published in 1991 and is still widely used. The recently published QUANTEC data has revised or enhanced estimates of tolerance.

Thirdly, there remains the issue of low-moderate dose irradiation. The spreading of dose to achieve the desired

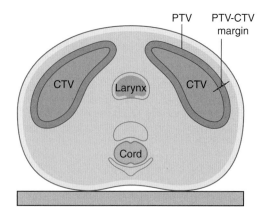

Figure 21.17 PTV–CTV margins.

conformality may have some undesirable effects. It is predicted that second malignancies may be increased as a consequence of this. Whether these risks, arrived through modeling, become a clinical reality remains to be seen. In addition, it is unknown what the effects of adding chemotherapy will have on these zones. Since chemotherapy is often utilized concurrently in head and neck cancers, this issue needs clarification.

IGRT

There is the need to revisit IGRT introduced earlier in this section. Patients with head and neck tumours need a high degree of reproducibility and this is generally achieved through good immobilization techniques. These immobilization devices cannot achieve complete immobility and it is for that reason that a CTV–PTV margin exists even in IMRT (Figure 21.17). IGRT seeks to reduce *this* margin by daily imaging of, in the case of head and neck tumours, bony and soft tissues, and repositioning of the isocentre. This 'on-line' approach of imaging and correction *before* the treatment itself then facilitates a reduction in that CTV–PTV margin. IMRT then seeks to achieve conformality of the CTV, IGRT a reduction in the PTV margin required (Figure 21.18).

DOSE AND FRACTIONATION

Definitive radiotherapy

The conventional schedule for radiotherapy to head and neck cancer involves the delivery of 66–70 Gy in 2 Gy fractions over 6.5 to 7 weeks treating 5 days per week. A BIR study looking at a short schedule (3–4 weeks) compared with the conventional schedule in larynx cancer did not show any significant differences – since this further centres have published data suggesting that this hypofractionated accelerated schedule is useful for small volume treatments – 50 Gy in

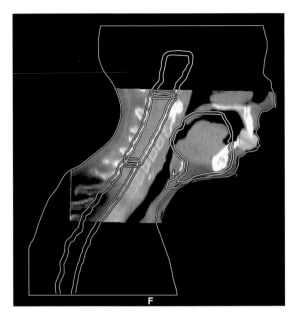

Figure 21.18 IGRT (in this case cone beam CT).

16 fractions over 3 weeks or 55 Gy in 20 fractions over 4 weeks.

The use of acceleration and hyperfractionation was tested in a trial of CHART (continuous hyperfractionated accelerated radiotherapy) versus conventional 2 Gy per fraction per day schedule. This showed no increase in overall survival and a non-significant increase in tumour control (but reduced nodal control) for a dose of 54 Gy given in three daily fractions over 12 days continuously. Subgroup analysis did show improved outcome in T3/4 larynx cancers and well-differentiated tumours. The overall feeling was that 54 Gy was insufficient. CHART has not been adopted as a schedule in the UK. However, the use of moderate acceleration with conventional fractionation has been shown to be beneficial. The DAHANCA group compared six fractions per week with the standard five (still using 2 Gy per fraction). In total 66–68 Gy was given in either 6.5 or 5.5 weeks. They showed improved 5-year local control in the moderately accelerated group of 68% versus 56% for standard therapy. The extra treatment was either given on Saturday or the patients were treated twice on the Friday (with ≥6 hour gap).

Other studies have looked at increasing dose or acceleration but with a split in the course of treatment to allow recovery of the acute toxicities. The evidence suggests that the repopulation occurring in the gap reduces any benefit from the dose escalation and the late toxicity is often increased.

A newer schedule is to use a concomitant boost to the primary site during the conventional radiotherapy. This treats the first phase of treatment (primary disease plus involved nodes and microscopic spread) in the morning and then later the same day a second smaller boost dose is given to the phase two volume involving the gross disease only. The dose is 1.8 Gy daily with a 1.5 Gy boost for the last 12 treatments – total dose 72 Gy in 42 fractions over 6 weeks. This accelerates the overall treatment time.

A recent meta-analysis of fractionation schedules has concluded that there is a survival benefit with altered fractionation. The largest survival benefit was evident with hyperfractionation not dissimilar to the benefits seen with concurrent chemoradiation. Accelerated schedules resulted in a lesser survival gain though such a schedule would be easier to implement in the clinic. Accelerated hypofractionated schedules (i.e. dose per fraction slightly higher than 2 Gy) are gaining acceptance in IMRT schedules as mentioned earlier.

One of the difficulties in interpreting the above findings and implementing them into routine practice is the additional role of chemotherapy. The role of chemoradiation with acceleration or changes in fractionation has not been fully established and there are concerns regarding additional toxicity with conventional techniques.

Postoperative radiotherapy

Doses to sites of gross residual disease, i.e. the primary and involved nodes, are treated to doses similar to the definitive setting, i.e. 66–70 Gy when using 2 Gy fractions with the remainder of that node station (i.e. level) treated to at least 60 Gy. The remainder of the operated neck can be treated to lower doses of around 50 Gy: it has been suggested that the operated neck requires a higher dose to sterilize microscopic residual disease than the unoperated neck. If it is intended to irradiate the contralateral neck then 46–50 Gy should suffice.

CHEMOTHERAPY IN HEAD AND NECK CANCER

There has been much work done looking into chemotherapy agents in head and neck cancer. Many drugs have been shown to have some response in squamous cell cancers of the head and neck, in particular, the platinum compounds, 5-fluorouracil, methotrexate, bleomycin, vinca alkaloids and, more recently, the taxanes. There is an increasing amount of data showing benefits of the addition of chemotherapy.

Concurrent chemotherapy and definitive radiotherapy

At present, the accepted standard treatment for radical non-surgical therapy is concurrent cisplatin chemotherapy with radical radiotherapy. The evidence for this comes from Pignon's meta-analysis (2000) which showed a small but significant survival advantage to the combined treatment but only if the chemotherapy was given concurrently. This benefit was not seen in induction or adjuvant schedules. The overall survival benefit for any chemoradiation schedule was approximately 4% but increased to 8% if cisplatin was the chemotherapy drug chosen. Concomitant chemotherapy is given simultaneously with radiation therapy to improve local and distant control. The mechanisms for action include the elimination of micrometastases and increased sensitivity to the radiotherapy.

The standard schedule for concurrent chemoradiotherapy for head and neck cancer involves cisplatin given intravenously on days 1, 22 and 43 of the radiotherapy at a dose of 100 mg/m^2. Alternatively (and increasingly in the UK), the cisplatin is being delivered using the weekly schedule of 40 mg/m^2 for 6 weeks – as utilized in the chemoradiation schedules for cervical carcinoma. There is anecdotal evidence that this regimen is better tolerated than the 3-weekly schedule, particularly in the head and neck cancer population. Patients require a satisfactory full blood count and adequate renal function. Nutritional support is essential and a feeding tube is advised in all patients undergoing combination treatment. Acute toxicity is usually more severe in these patients and should be looked for and managed aggressively.

Concurrent chemotherapy and postoperative radiotherapy

A previous section has outlined the range of indications for postoperative radiotherapy. Some situations would be considered particularly adverse for locoregional recurrence and, in these cases, consideration should be given to concurrent chemoradiation postoperatively. Two recent trials and a consensus view have suggested that such patients would be those with positive primary resection margins and those with pathologically involved nodes with extracapsular spread.

Induction chemotherapy

Neoadjuvant or induction chemotherapy is used to downstage a primary tumour before definitive surgery or radiotherapy and to decrease the incidence of distant metastases. In the Pignon meta-analysis of chemotherapy with radiotherapy in head and neck cancer, there was evidence that organ preservation was increased in patients receiving chemotherapy followed by radical radiotherapy compared with primary surgery for advanced but resectable laryngeal cancer. Although the original meta-analysis did not show any real survival benefit, a more recent review on updated data has shown that induction schedules may convey a survival advantage of up to 2–3%. The majority of these studies used the previous standard induction chemotherapy schedule of cisplatin and 5-fluorouracil. Two recent published studies have shown promising activity for the triplet schedule of docetaxel, cisplatin and 5-fluorouracil in terms of survival, re-igniting the debate of induction chemotherapy and its role in locally advanced head and neck cancer.

CHEMOTHERAPY IN THE PALLIATIVE SETTING

Chemotherapy is used for palliation in patients with recurrent or metastatic head and neck cancer. If patients have not received prior treatment with chemotherapy, then cisplatin and 5-fluorouracil will be considered as first-line treatment. Second-line chemotherapy agents have a minor response rate and the use of docetaxel, gemcitabine and others is still being evaluated. Methotrexate in a weekly schedule can be a well-tolerated second-line therapy for palliation of symptoms, particularly in older or frail patients. The dose of 40–50 mg/m^2 iv given each week with folinic acid 15 mg qds over 24 hours (commenced 24 hours after the methotrexate) is one suitable schedule. More recently, cetuximab, an antibody to epidermal growth factor receptor (EGFR), has demonstrated useful activity in the palliative setting. This approach is discussed later in the chapter.

TOXICITY OF TREATMENT

Radiotherapy for head and neck cancer has many side effects which must be effectively communicated to the patient before embarking on treatment. A detailed explanation is essential for informed consent but also to improve compliance with the full course of treatment to give the best chance of a successful outcome. As with radiotherapy to any part of the body, the side effects (apart from fatigue) relate to structures within the radiation field. They can be divided into acute (early) or late side effects. Reactions will to some extent be site specific and are discussed in more detail in the next chapter. However, it is useful to consider the principles here.

Acute toxicity

Mucositis will develop in the treatment field for all patients with head and neck cancer and can be severe and disabling. It may be mild (grade 1/2), but is often severe (grade 3) (Figure *evolve* 21.19🖰), especially in those receiving concurrent chemotherapy, which may lead to a break in treatment. Grade 4 mucositis (frank ulceration) should not be allowed to develop. Management includes analgesia using the pain ladder. Opiates may be required at some stage. Topical agents may be used initially and alongside systemic analgesia. Patients must have their weight monitored and nutritional supplements considered. The majority of patients will have a level of discomfort that requires opiate level analgesia. This can be administered in oral preparations (solutions, syrups etc.) or delivered via feeding tube if present. It can often become difficult for patients to tolerate oral medications, particularly in the latter stages of treatment, but the development of transdermal delivery systems for opiates can be an excellent alternative in head and neck cancer patients where swallowing is often difficult or uncomfortable and, in the main, these have avoided the need for subcutaneous infusions of opiate, which were occasionally required in the past for patients with severe symptoms.

Dysphagia secondary to mucositis, loss of taste, loss of appetite and thickened secretions lead to weight loss in head and neck cancer patients. This should be predicted prior to treatment and a feeding tube considered in all patients with large treatment fields, especially those to be treated by chemoradiotherapy. If patients without a tube are struggling and losing weight, a tube may need to be inserted during treatment – this will usually involve a radiologically placed gastrostomy. Prophylactic tube insertion is usually more satisfactory and allows early feeding to be initiated before the patient develops difficulties.

Thickened secretions can be alleviated with carbocisteine which has a systemic mode of action and acute xerostomia managed symptomatically.

A skin reaction is seen in any treated area and develops as the treatment progresses. The skin changes from mild redness (Figures *evolve* 21.20 and 21.21🖱) through brisk erythema to desquamation – initially, dry changes and peeling but progressing to moist desquamation (Figure *evolve* 21.22🖱). A skin care regimen should include washing with lukewarm water and unperfumed soap, avoiding shaving until treatment is completed and applying regular aqueous cream. Once skin is broken then a barrier product should be used. The optimal regimen is unclear and is often centre specific. Patients should be reviewed regularly post-treatment to monitor the resolution of skin and mucosal reactions.

Fatigue is seen in many patients receiving radical radiotherapy. It has been shown that maintaining a level of gentle activity is the best way to overcome the asthenia during therapy. In head and neck cancer patients, especially those receiving chemoradiotherapy, it is usual to monitor the haemoglobin during radiotherapy and transfusing patients as required to keep the level greater than 12 g/dl. There is evidence that radiotherapy is less effective in patients with anaemia, although no good evidence exists that correcting anaemia improves outcomes. Indeed, one randomized trial using erythropoietin to prevent anaemia, found a worse outcome in the treated group.

Late toxicity

Skin pigmentation/atrophy is seen in patients treated with head and neck radiotherapy due to the doses received by the skin. Skin sparing is achieved where possible due to the use of megavoltage radiotherapy and cutting out the immobilization shell in the treatment beam. This bolus effect can be used to advantage if there is evidence of skin involvement in a tumour.

Alopecia in the treated areas can be seen in the head and neck patient. Patients should be warned of the possibility – particularly if they have facial hair. If the area receives a dose exceeding 60 Gy then the alopecia may be permanent.

Xerostomia is a common late side effect of radiotherapy to the head and neck. It most commonly arises due to radiotherapy to the parotid gland, although the submandibular and sublingual glands can also be included. The risk of xerostomia increases with increasing dose. The initial symptom may become apparent from as early as the first week of therapy and irreversible damage to the gland will arise with modest doses. It can be a most distressing side effect for patients and efforts to minimize the dose to salivary glands should be considered during radiotherapy planning. Once it has developed, patients should be offered artificial saliva preparations and advised to use fluoride mouthwashes regularly. Dental check-ups are essential.

Osteoradionecrosis is the breakdown of bone in an area treated with radiotherapy. It is seen in the mandible most often in head and neck cancer patients and can be triggered by dental extractions. It may mimic local recurrence of tumour. It is difficult to manage as further surgery can exacerbate the problem. The best management is prevention, which means dental treatment prior to radiotherapy and aggressive dental hygiene post-radiation treatment. Patients must be educated about the risk of dental work after radiotherapy and seeking specialist advice for any treatment required. It should be performed under general anaesthetic and with antibiotic cover.

Myelitis secondary to radiotherapy is a rare but recognized side effect from head and neck radiotherapy. There is considerable debate over what constitutes a safe dose of radiation to the spinal cord. This is complicated due to many variables including volume treated, fraction size and total dose. Different series have described different maximal doses. The general consensus is that 44–46 Gy is a safe total dose, although many feel that up to 50 Gy in 2 Gy per fraction is acceptable. Higher doses may be achievable with careful planning if clinically indicated but, given the catastrophic nature of permanent damage to the spinal cord – particularly at the cervical level – a conservative approach is usual. To achieve these doses in head and neck treatments using conventional parallel-opposed lateral fields involves direct treatment with photon fields up to 44–46 Gy. The photon fields are then reduced to continue to treat the target and anterior neck and the posterior neck (overlying the spinal cord) has its remaining dose delivered using electrons at an energy to treat nodal disease but to spare the underlying cord. This results in a risk of less than 1% of permanent damage owing to myelitis. Some patients may develop Lhermitte's syndrome secondary to early transient myelitis. In Lhermitte's syndrome, patients complain of tingling or 'electric shocks' in the legs. This can be provoked by flexing the neck. These symptoms begin about 6 weeks following the radiotherapy and may last a few months. Progression to late damage is rare. IMRT can improve the coverage of nodes in this situation (as discussed earlier) though there have still been reports of Lhermitte's syndrome.

MOLECULAR ONCOLOGY – FUTURE DEVELOPMENTS

New therapeutic agents which exploit knowledge about the cell cycle and control of cancer growth are being used with increasing frequency in treatment of cancers. In head and neck cancer in the past, radiosensitizers were used to try to utilize the hypoxia seen in tumours and increase the benefit of the radiation. The original drugs unfortunately had significant neural toxicity and were therefore not adopted as standard treatments in the UK.

More recently, a monoclonal antibody to the epidermal growth factor receptor (EGFR) has been developed which shows a survival advantage when combined with radiotherapy compared with radiation alone. Another agent with activity against EGFR1 and HER2 (EGFR2) is currently under evaluation. It is hoped that knowledge of the molecular processes will lead to more 'designer' drugs. These may eventually replace the currently used and less specific conventional chemotherapy agents.

FURTHER READING

Ang KK, et al. Randomised trial of addressing risk features and time factors of surgery plus radiotherapy in advanced head-and-neck cancer. Int J Radiat Oncol Biol Phys 2001;51:571–8.

Bernier J, et al. Postoperative irradiation with or without concomitant chemotherapy for locally advanced head and neck cancer. N Engl J Med 2004;350:1945–52.

Bernier J, et al. Defining risk levels in locally advance head and neck cancers: a comparative analysis of concurrent postoperative radiation plus chemotherapy trials of the EORTC (#22931) and RTOG (#9501). Head Neck 2005;27:843–50.

Bonner JA, et al. Radiotherapy plus cetuximab for squamous-cell carcinoma of the head and neck. N Engl J Med 2006;23:1125–35.

Bourhis J, et al. Hyperfractionated or accelerated radiotherapy in head and neck cancer: a meta-analysis. Lancet 2006;368:844–54.

Budach W, et al. A meta-analysis of hyperfractionated and accelerated radiotherapy and combined chemotherapy and radiotherapy regimens in unresectable locally advanced squamous cell carcinoma of the head and neck. BMC Cancer 2006;6:28.

Cooper J, et al. Postoperative concurrent radiotherapy and chemotherapy for high-risk squamous-cell carcinoma of the head and neck. N Engl J Med 2004;350:1937–44.

Dische S, et al. A randomised multicentre trial of CHART versus conventional radiotherapy in head and neck cancer. Radiother Oncol 1997;44:123–36.

Fletcher GH. Elective irradiation of subclinical disease in cancers of the head and neck. Cancer 1972;29:1450–4.

Fu KK, et al. A radiation therapy oncology group (RTOG) phase III randomized study to compare hyperfractionation and two variants of accelerated fractionation to standard fractionation for head and neck squamous cell carcinomas: First report of RTOG 9003. Int J Radiat Oncol Biol Phys 2000;48:7–16.

Gregoire V, et al. Selection and delineation of lymph node target volumes in head and neck conformal radiotherapy. Proposal for standardizing terminology and procedure based on surgical experience. Radiother Oncol 2000;56:135–50.

Gregoire V, et al. CT-based delineation of lymph node levels and related CTVs in the node-negative neck: DAHANCA, EORTC, GORTEC, NCIC, RTOG consensus guidelines. Radiother Oncol 2003;69:227–36.

Gregoire V, et al. Proposal for the delineation of the nodal CTV in the node-positive and the post-operative neck. Radiother Oncol 2006;79:15–20.

Gupta NK, et al. A randomised clinical trial to contrast radiotherapy with radiotherapy and methotrexate given synchronously in head and neck cancer. Clin Radiol 1987;38:575–81.

Institute of Physics and Engineering in Medicine. Report 96 Guidance for the clinical implementation of intensity modulated radiation therapy. IPEM; 2008.

Jackson A, et al. The Lessons of QUANTEC: Recommendations for Reporting and gathering data on Dose-Volume Dependencies of Treatment Outcome. Int J Radiat Oncol Biol Phys 2010; 76 Issue 3 Supplement.

Lengelé B, et al. Anatomical bases for the radiological delineation of lymph node areas. Major collecting trunks, head and neck. Radiother Oncol 2007;85:146–55.

Moharti BK, et al. Short course palliative radiotherapy of 20Gy in 5 fractions for advanced and incurable head and neck cancer: AIIMS study. Radiother Oncol 2004;71:275–80.

Nutting CM, et al. Parotid-sparing intensity modulated versus conventional radiotherapy in head and neck cancer (PARSPORT): a phase 3 multicentre randomized controlled trial. The Lancet Oncology 2011;12:127–36.

Overgaard J, et al. Five compared with six fractions per week of conventional radiotherapy of squamous-cell carcinoma of head and neck: DAHANCA 6&7 randomised controlled trial. Lancet 2003;362:933–40.

Peters LJ, et al. Evaluation of the dose for postoperative radiation therapy of head and neck cancer: first report of a prospective randomized trial. Int J Radiat Oncol Biol Phys 1993;26:3–11.

Pignon JP, et al. Chemotherapy added to locoregional treatment for head and neck squamous-cell-carcinoma: Three meta-analyses of updated individual data. Lancet 2000;355:949–50.

Pignon JP, et al. Meta-analyses of chemotherapy in head and neck cancer (MACH-NC): an update. Int J Radiat Oncol Biol Phys 2007;69 (Suppl. 2):S112–4.

Posner MR, et al. (TAX324 Study Group). Cisplatin and fluorouracil alone or with docetaxel in head and neck cancer. N Engl J Med 2007;357:1705–15.

Vermorken JB, et al. (EORTC 24971/TAX 323) Study. Cisplatin, fluorouracil, and docetaxel in unresectable head and neck cancer. N Engl J Med 2007;357:1695–704.

Wiernik G, et al. Final report of the general clinical results of the British Institute of Radiology fractionation study of 3F/wk versus 5F/wk in radiotherapy of carcinoma of the laryngo-pharynx. Br J Radiol 1990;63:169–80.

EVOLVE CONTENTS (available online at: http://evolve.elsevier.com/Symonds/radiotherapy/)

Chapter | 22 |

Sino-Nasal, Oral, Larynx and Pharynx Cancers

Christopher D. Scrase, Paul Symonds

NASOPHARYNX

Anatomy

The nasopharynx is cuboidal in shape and comprises the most superior of the three pharyngeal structures. As such it has a direct communication with the nasal cavity anteriorly and oropharynx inferiorly (Figure 22.1).

Anterior wall

This comprises the posterior choanae and nasal cavity.

Posterior wall

This is formed by the tissues of the prevertebral space adjacent to the first and second cervical vertebrae.

Lateral walls

The pharygobasilar fascia forms this and the posterior wall. Within this is the opening of the eustachian tube and, more posteriorly, a deep recess called the fossa of Rosenmüller (lateral nasopharyngeal recess) (Figure 22.2).

Superior wall

Strictly, the roof slopes in an anterior to posterior direction abutting the base of skull. The sphenoid sinus lies superiorly and the superior component of Waldeyer's ring, most prominent in childhood, is located here. There is a depression in the mucosa in the midline known as the pharyngeal bursa which sometimes extends into the basi-occiput.

Inferior wall

This is, in reality, an imaginary horizontal running from the lower border of the soft palate to the posterior pharyngeal wall.

Incidence of nasopharyngeal tumours

Cancer of nasopharynx (NPC) is rare in the UK and USA with an annual incidence of <1 per 100 000. By contrast, NPC is

Figure 22.1 Section of the pharynx, from front to back.

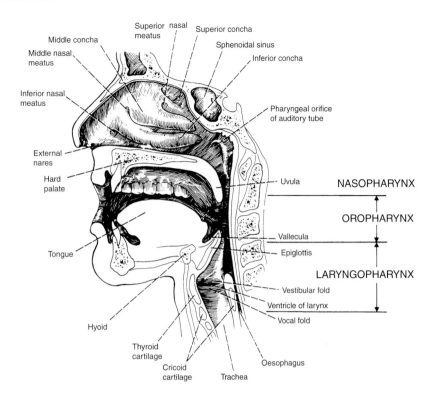

NASOPHARYNX

OROPHARYNX

LARYNGOPHARYNX

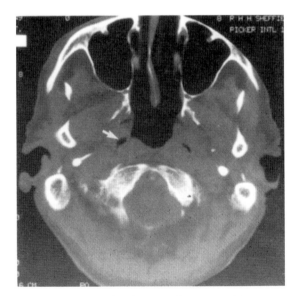

Figure 22.2 CT scan showing normal anatomy of the nasopharynx. The fossa of Rosenmü ller (pharyngeal recess) is arrowed.

(Courtesy of Dr R. Nakielny, Sheffield).

the fourth most common new malignancy in Hong Kong with an incidence of 21.4 and 8.3 per 100 000 per annum in men and women, respectively. It is common only in certain racial groups such as South Chinese (not Japanese), Inuit (Eskimos) and Maghrebian Arabs. The fact this disease is common only in some racial groups gives a clue to the aetiology of this disease (see below).

Staging system for nasopharyngeal tumours

The staging system follows the same general rule as other head and neck cancers with one important exception. The prognostic impact of regional nodes does not have the same implications as elsewhere. As such, the N component of the TNM classification is different.

T1	Tumour confined to the nasopharynx
T2A	Tumour extends to the oropharynx and/or nasal cavity without parapharyngeal extension
T2B	Tumour with parapharyngeal extension, i.e. infiltrates beyond the pharyngobasilar fascia
T3	Tumour that invades bony structures and/or paranasal sinuses
T4	Tumour with intracranial extension and/or involvement of cranial nerves, infratemporal fossa, hypopharynx, orbit or masticator space

N1   Unilateral (including midline) lymph node(s) ≤6 cm above the supraclavicular fossa
N2   Bilateral lymph node(s) ≤ 6 cm above the supraclavicular fossa
N3A   Any lymph node >6 cm
N3B   Any node that involves the supraclavicular fossa

Aetiology, pathology and lymphatic spread

Squamous cell carcinomas comprise the commonest histological type. They may be subdivided into well to poorly differentiated types, those with a heavy lymphatic infiltrate ('lymphoepithelioma'), transitional cell tumours and keratinizing and non-keratinizing types. The WHO usefully classifies nasopharyngeal tumours as follows:

Type 1   Well-differentiated keratinizing type
Type 2   Moderately-differentiated non-keratinizing type
Type 3   Undifferentiated type typically with an extensive lymphocytic infiltrate.

The presence of keratin (i.e. type 1) is associated with local infiltration while type 3 tumours tend to disseminate widely.

NPC is associated with infection with the Epstein-Barr virus (EBV). EBV DNA is incorporated into the tumour genome. Antibodies to EBV (IgG and IgA) precede tumour development by several years and the antibody titer is correlated with tumour burden, remission and recurrence. A practical point is the detection of EBV genomic material in the biopsies from neck lymph node metastases from an apparent unknown primary may point to the origin in the nasopharynx. Infection with EBV is common and is the cause of glandular fever. In Hong Kong, almost all children aged 10 years have been infected by the virus. Even in Hong Kong, only a small minority develop NPC. Genetic and dietary factors seem important in tumour development. Searches for genes conferring susceptibility to NPC have focused on human leukocytes antigen (HLA) genes. The genes encode proteins required for viral lysis.

Three HLA alleles have a consistent association with an increased risk of NPC in South Chinese and other Asian populations. They are HLA-A2, B46 and B17. Dietary factors are also important, including eating salt dried fish (containing carcinogenic nitrosamines) and lack of fresh fruit and vegetables (lack of antioxidants).

While squamous cell carcinomas form the majority of nasopharyngeal cancers, other pathologies are recognized in this region. These include adenocarcinoma, adenoid cystic carcinoma and lymphoma. Treatment may vary according to the tumour type according to the propensity for nodal spread and response to radiation, though the principles of technique as described here can still broadly be applied.

It is because of the rich lymphatic supply that these tumours commonly spread and, indeed, present with neck nodes. This spread may be bilateral but the distribution is dissimilar to other head and neck squamous cell carcinomas and is reflected in the TNM classification outlined earlier. Seventy to 90% of cases have nodes at some point. Levels 1A/B are rarely involved while levels 2 and 5 (the post-cervical chain) can be considered the first echelon nodes for this tumour site.

Nasopharyngeal cancers have a high propensity for distal haematogenous spread and, as a consequence, distal failure. This is generally unlike other head and neck squamous cell carcinomas where locoregional control is the barrier to success (though the more aggressive treatments are starting to alter this pattern).

Signs and symptoms

The first presenting symptom is often painless node enlargement confirmed on examination. These are often bilateral in their distribution and, as mentioned earlier, typically involve the posterior cervical chain.

Other common symptoms include nasal obstruction and epistaxis through expansion into the nasal cavity and auditory disturbances, especially unilateral deafness and recurrent otitis media. Examination findings may confirm a mass in the post-nasal space and cranial nerve palsies especially of II–VI through direct expansion through bone and via nerve foramina and IX–XII through compression from Rouviere's node. Rouviere's node is the most superior node of the retropharyngeal node chain and overlies the transverse process of C1.

Patients may report headaches though other symptoms or signs will usually be readily apparent.

Diagnosis and staging

The diagnosis may be strongly suspected on clinical grounds alone from the above findings especially on nasendoscopic examination, but histological confirmation of any nasopharyngeal mass will be required. A formal examination under anaesthesia will often be helpful in delineating the extent but further locoregional staging, best with magnetic resonance imaging (MRI), is mandatory. A computed tomography (CT) scan, while adequate, does not afford the same degree of information, particularly in the base of skull region.

In the context of neck nodes where a primary is not readily apparent, especially when they lie posteriorly in the upper neck, the finding of EBV genomic material using DNA amplification techniques (PCR) is usually indicative of a clinically inapparent nasopharyngeal primary and treatment should be along the lines of such tumours.

Since nasopharyngeal cancers have a high propensity for systemic spread, a work-up for distal disease is essential. As such, haematological and biochemical screens and a chest x-ray are an absolute minimum. More detailed imaging of the viscera (CT scan of chest and abdomen) and bones (isotope scan) are essential for more advanced disease and if basic screening tools are in any way suspicious. A positron emission tomography (PET)-CT may be useful in that regard.

Treatment

The relative inaccessible nature of the primary tumour and frequent involvement of Rouviere's node dictates that radiation therapy is the main modality for treatment. In addition and unlike other head and neck squamous cell carcinomas, the presence of substantial neck nodes should not lead to initial surgical excision as they generally respond well to radiation therapy. Any nodes that have failed to respond adequately or at recurrence can, provided the primary disease is controlled, then be managed by an appropriate neck dissection.

Prior to radiation therapy, a thorough dental assessment is mandatory with essential treatment performed as necessary.

Small tumours of the nasopharynx can be adequately treated with radiation alone. However, the majority should, co-morbidity permitting, be managed with concurrent chemoradiation. The nasopharynx is the one head and neck site where concurrent chemoradiation has been more readily adopted internationally due in part to the intergroup 0099 study. This study compared concurrent chemoradiation and adjuvant chemotherapy with radiotherapy alone and showed a significant advantage in survival with the combined modality approach. The control arm was particularly inferior, however, when compared with other studies. Further studies and a recent meta-analysis specifically of nasopharyngeal cancers have, however, supported the concurrent chemoradiation approach. Neoadjuvant chemotherapy may result in useful reduction of the primary and/or nodal disease. A major problem in delivering adjuvant chemotherapy is the poor compliance following definitive therapy. Research from Taiwan suggests that adjuvant treatment after concomitant chemoradiotherapy may only be necessary for patients with a high chance of developing metastatic disease. This includes patients with a single lymph node >6 cm, multiple nodes over >4 cm or supraclavicular nodes. The most frequently used regimen is cisplatin (100 mg/m^2 or 20 mg/m^2 for 5 days) plus 5-fluorouracil ($400–100 \text{ mg/m}^2$ daily by infusion for up to 4 days). This is repeated at 3–4 weekly intervals during radiotherapy.

Radiation technique (Figures *evolve* 22.3–22.8 🔊 for NPC section)

The technique of Ho forms the basis of the 2-dimensional approach to treating nasopharyngeal carcinoma. Treatment fields are precisely defined according to local staging. Determination of the primary clinical target volume is now very much individualized based on all clinical information available allowing for a more conformal 3-dimensional approach. The pattern of spread outlined earlier dictates that the whole cervical lymphatic chain should be outlined and treated as routine, though doses prescribed will be determined by whether they are overtly involved and proximal to the primary site or more distal and clinically uninvolved. In other words, even in early cases, at least prophylactic doses of radiation should be given to the nodes.

A full head and neck immobilization device is mandatory with the shoulders kept well down. A tongue depressor is frequently utilized but a drop in jaw position might negate the perceived benefits of this technique in sparing the oral cavity. A single shell is preferred throughout the treatment with the degree of neck extension optimized at the outset.

Except in the case of intensity modulated radiotherapy techniques, a multiple phase technique will be utilized to treat the primary disease and involved nodes using parallel-opposed fields. The lower cervical nodes will be treated by an anterior (or anterior-posterior (AP) depending on the location of nodes in the AP plane) field matched on preferably by the mono-isocentric technique. As a general rule, matching of fields should not occur at sites of gross disease but this may not be practical in nasopharyngeal cancers.

Where the primary tumour is relatively small (T1, T2), it might be practical to irradiate it as a final phase with a three-field technique thereby sparing some of the laterally placed normal structures from the maximum intended dose. Alternatively, and according to available expertise, intracavity, stereotactic radiosurgery or intensity modulated radiotherapy (IMRT) may facilitate dose escalation at the site of gross disease with improved local control.

Complications

The significant volumes of normal tissue ordinarily irradiated can give rise to a range of long-term sequelae.

Irradiation of major aspects of the salivary tissue will lead to chronic xerostomia. The technique of IMRT may facilitate less of an impact here, though care will need to be taken in underdosing any adjacent diseased lymph nodes. In practice, it may be prudent to spare only the superficial parotid glands bilaterally even using IMRT.

High doses of radiation may be delivered to a substantial component of the mandible, particularly when using the parallel-opposed technique and where there are involved nodes. As a consequence, treatment risks osteoradionecrosis (ORN) and preventive measures beyond meticulous radiation technique should be adopted. Moreover, the proximity of the pterygoid muscles to the primary target volume will give rise to trismus and jaw exercises should be encouraged to minimize this.

Endocrine failure due to irradiation of the pituitary and thyroid glands, though relatively easy to treat, is a not uncommon outcome in long-term survivors and should be actively sought through routine testing in the follow up of these patients.

Advanced tumours with extension into the skull base introduce additional tissues exposed to the high doses of radiation that will be necessary to achieve local control. Aspects of the temporal lobes, optic nerves and chiasm, middle and inner ear will be irradiated and, as a consequence, are at risk of late neurological damage. The addition of chemotherapy may add to this toxicity. In all cases, the brainstem and spinal cord are organs of risk and prescribed doses should not exceed an agreed tolerance dose. The complex interrelationship with such a range of normal tissues mandates a meticulous radiation technique to minimize these complications. The technique of IMRT lends itself to such a site but does not obviate the need for precise target volume delineation. Results using IMRT demonstrate superior coverage of advanced tumours and an improvement in disease control.

The undifferentiated type of nasopharyngeal cancer is rather more radiosensitive and, as such, slightly lower doses may be delivered with a consequent lessening effect on late sequelae.

Results

Small tumours of the nasopharynx are successfully treated in about 80–90% cases. More advanced tumours, when treated optimally, will result in 5-year survival rates of the order of 50–70%. Those patients with extensive nodes and/or involvement of the skull base with cranial nerve palsies fare particularly badly with 5-year survival rates

ranging from 0 to 20%, often succumbing to distal failure. Late recurrences are recognized suggesting that follow up beyond 5 years might be prudent and/or advising patients and primary care practitioners of this so that they can re-referred without delay. Recurrent disease may, on occasions, be amenable to re-irradiation as long as volumes to be treated are relatively small and the patient is prepared to accept the additional risks associated with such an approach.

NOSE AND NASAL CAVITY

Anatomy

The external nose is like the tip of an iceberg with a complex array of passageways and air cavities within it that form the nasal cavity and paranasal sinuses. The hair-bearing entrance that forms the vestibule and the mucociliary escalator provides an important initial defence against the inhalation of germs (Figure 22.9).

The nasal vestibule lies within the aperture of the nostril. It is bounded laterally by cartilage that forms the nasal ala, medially by cartilage that forms the columella and inferiorly by the most anterior portion of the floor of the nose. Importantly, this area is lined by squamous epithelium as an extension from the outside skin.

The nasal cavity or nasal fossa proper lies between the maxillary sinus inferiorly and the eyes and ethmoidal sinus superiorly. It is divided into two by a midline cartilaginous septum.

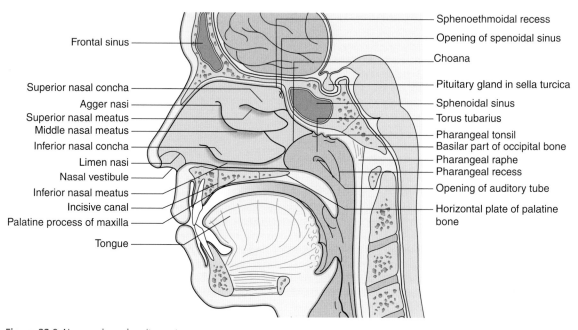

Figure 22.9 Nose and nasal cavity anatomy.

Superior wall

This is comprised of the cribriform plate of the ethmoidal sinus. The olfactory apparatus which lies here provides us with our sense of smell.

Inferior wall

Broader than the superior wall, this is formed from the hard palate.

Anterior wall

The nasal bones and cartilage that form the external nose give rise to the anterior wall.

Posterior wall

The posterior border of the hard palate and maxillary sinus gives an open passage into the nasopharynx.

Lateral wall

Three turbinates overlie the lateral wall which itself is formed from the medial walls of the maxillary sinus inferiorly and the ethmoid sinus superiorly.

Incidence

Many cancer registries combine nasal, paranasal and middle ear tumours together when reporting incidence, as all three types are rare. The incidence of all three types combined is 1:100 000 per annum. About two-thirds of all cases arise in the sinuses giving a true incidence of nasal cancer of about 0.3:100 000. The nasal vestibule is the most common site of origin. Men who have worked in the chromium industry (Glasgow/Teeside) or nickel refining (South Wales) are at increased risk of developing this rare cancer. Chromate-induced cancers are often accompanied by a septal perforation.

Staging system

The system used for the nasal cavity is identical to that for ethmoidal sinus tumours in view of the anatomical relationship of these two structures. The reader is referred to the later section on paranasal sinus tumours for fuller details, but the following summarizes the T classification as applicable here.

T1 Tumour restricted to one subsite of the nasal cavity
T2 Tumour involves two subsites in a single site or extends to involve an adjacent site within the nasoethmoidal complex
T3 As ethmoid sinus
T4A As ethmoid sinus
T4B As ethmoid sinus

Aetiology, pathology and lymphatic spread

The normal lining of the nasal cavity is pseudostratified columnar ciliated epithelium except for the vestibule, as mentioned earlier, that comprises squamous epithelium with sweat and sebaceous glands.

The aetiology of true nasal cavity tumours is not dissimilar to that of the paranasal sinuses with many environmental factors being implicated. Smoking is associated with the commonest histological subtype seen. Such squamous cell carcinomas arise most commonly at the lateral wall.

Other histologies comprise the remaining 20% and include adenocarcinoma, adenoid cystic carcinoma, melanoma, lymphoma, plasmacytoma and sarcoma. Inverted papillomas, themselves rare, can transform or coexist with squamous cell carcinoma. Olfactory neuroblastomas (aesthesioblastomas) arise from the olfactory tissue at the level of the cribriform plate. Basal cell carcinomas can arise in the vestibule.

The lymphatic drainage of the nasal cavity can be usefully divided into two. The main part of the nasal cavity drains via the nasopharynx to the retropharyngeal nodes and upper deep cervical nodes (levels 2A and 2B). The lower anterior portion drains to the submandibular (level 1B), parotid (preauricular) and jugulodigastric (level 2A) nodes. The nasal vestibule itself includes, additionally, the buccinator node as part of the facial lymphatic complex.

Signs and symptoms

Unlike paranasal sinus tumours, these tumours tend to present comparatively early with obstructive symptoms and epistaxis. However, symptoms of benign disease can blur the presence of malignancy and squamous cell carcinomas of the lateral wall may, on further investigation, be a late manifestation of maxillary sinus disease. Inspection of the nasal cavity will typically reveal a fleshy outgrowth.

Diagnosis and staging

Biopsy of the suspected lesion is required. A polypoidal lesion may be snared off and may give rise to an unsuspected tumour when examined pathologically. It may be necessary to perform a lateral rhinotomy to obtain adequate exposure and surgical evaluation of lesions within the nasal cavity.

Except for the small tumour of vestibule, which can usually be demarcated in the clinic, tumours of the nasal fossa proper require thorough staging with CT and/or MRI. Care must be taken in interpreting benign secretions from malignant infiltration of soft tissue and bone invasion as this may impact on the degree of surgery.

Certain tumour types, for example adenoid cystic as well as lymphoma, will require exclusion of distal involvement as this may dictate local management.

Treatment (see Figures *evolve* 22.10–22.14 🐭)

Small tumours of the vestibule can be managed by either surgery or radiotherapy. The choice will in part be based on the expected cosmetic outcome.

More advanced tumours of the vestibule or those of the nasal fossa proper will usually require surgical clearance often followed by radiotherapy, especially if it is a squamous cell carcinoma in view of the propensity for bone invasion. Lymphomas and plasmacytomas can be managed by primary radiotherapy at appropriate doses with or without the addition of chemotherapy.

Inoperable nasal cavity tumours should be managed by combined chemoradiation according to the co-morbidity of the patient.

Radiotherapy technique

Tumours of the vestibule and low anterior nasal fossa tumours may be treated by a direct anterior appositional electron beam, implantation with iridium wires, direct lateral photons or an anterior oblique wedged pair field arrangement (Figure *evolve* 22.15 🐭). The choice will be dictated by the extent of the clinical target volume (CTV) and the physical constraints of the particular modality as well as local expertise. The relatively superficial nature of these tumours and the shape that presents dosimetry problems usually dictates the need for some bolus material on the skin surface when using external beam treatment. The facial lymphatics may be included as a separate target volume and treated prophylactically using separate electron fields.

More advanced tumours and those within the nasal fossa proper frequently require an approach similar to that used for maxillary sinus tumours. Here, a midline anterior and two lateral photons are used to cover adequately the defined target volume or ideally IMRT. The reader is referred to this later section for more details.

CT planning for all but the most superficial tumours facilitates accurate tumour definition and normal tissue avoidance. The true CTV may extend much more posteriorly than initially envisaged and therefore needs to be delineated with precision.

As with all head and neck tumours, good immobilization is required. A mouthbite is used to move the tongue away from the treatment volume. For superficial tumours treated by electrons, this may also facilitate the placement of lead material for shielding and wax bolus for the anterior wedge photon technique.

Complications

Superficial tumours will inevitably manifest acute skin reactions that usually heal promptly. In the longer term, atrophy of the nasal cartilage may result in some loss of the original nasal profile.

Deeper tumours managed with techniques similar to that used for paranasal sinus tumours may be complicated by damage to the normal tissues in the vicinity. Atrophy of the nasal lining will result in dryness and a tendency towards the development of crusts. Regular use of a saline spray helps to address this. Epiphora will result if there is stenosis of the nasolacrimal duct.

Results

The diversity of pathologies at this site and the relative rarity even of squamous cell carcinoma of the nasal cavity give rise to only limited outcome data. Nonetheless, early squamous cell carcinoma of the vestibule can be expected to result in cure rates of the order of 80–90% at 5 years. More advanced tumours of the vestibule and fossa proper will give rise to cure rates of the order of 40–60%. Olfactory neuroblastomas carry a better prognosis, while patients with mucosal melanomas generally fare badly.

PARANASAL SINUS TUMOURS

Anatomy (Figure 22.16)

The paranasal sinuses comprise four pairs of linked hollow cavities within the anterior and mid-portions of the skull that link to the nasal cavity. They are named according to the bone within which they lie. The purpose of the paranasal sinuses is to lighten the bone and give resonance to the voice.

Maxillary sinuses

Lying under the eyes, these sinuses are pyramidal in shape. The base of the pyramid forms the lateral wall of the nasal

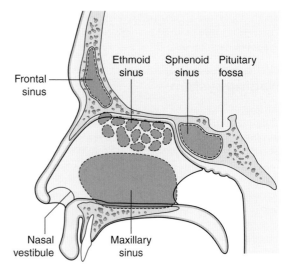

Figure 22.16 Paranasal sinus anatomy.

cavity with the apex extending towards the zygomatic process. The superior aspect comprises the floor of the orbit and the ethmoidal sinus while the inferior extent is that of the alveolar process and typically lies just below the floor of the nasal cavity. The infraorbital nerve traverses the roof of the sinus while the first and second molar teeth typically project into the sinus floor. The posterior wall abuts the infratemporal and pterygopalatine fossae. The maxillary sinus drains via the ostium maxillare beneath the middle concha.

Frontal sinus

Lying over the eyes in the frontal bones, these sinuses only reach full size after puberty. They drain into the nasal cavity through the middle meatus beneath the middle concha via the frontonasal duct.

Ethmoid sinus

Lying either side of the upper part of the nasal cavity and between the orbits, these sinuses are grouped into three portions: the anterior and middle drain into the nasal cavity via the middle meatus, the posterior via the superior meatus beneath the superior concha. A thin bony lamina (the lamina papyracea) separates the sinus from the orbital and nasal cavities. The optic nerve lies posterior to the sinus and the anterior cranial fossa superiorly.

Sphenoid sinus

Lying deep in the skull base beneath the pituitary gland, this sinus, which also develops mainly after puberty, drains into the nasal cavity via the sphenoethmoidal recess above the superior concha of the nasal cavity. The nasopharynx lies inferiorly and the nasal cavity anteriorly to the sinus while the optic nerve and cavernous sinuses lie laterally.

Incidence of paranasal sinus tumours

These tumours are rare with a crude incidence of <0.5/100 000. Most tumours arise in the maxillary sinus, less commonly the ethmoid sinus. Tumours arising de novo in the frontal and sphenoidal sinuses are especially rare. Frequently, multiple sinuses are involved at presentation.

Staging system for paranasal sinus tumours

The TNM system as described here is only applicable to maxillary sinus tumours. The ethmoidal sinuses are classified separately. There is no formal system that applies to tumours of the sphenoidal and frontal sinuses. The N component is as elsewhere for head and neck squamous cell carcinomas.

	Maxillary sinus	Ethmoidal sinus
T1	Mucosa only	One subsite
T2	Bone erosion/destruction (not posteriorly)	Two subsites
T3	Bone erosion/destruction (if posteriorly), involvement of the subcutaneous tissues floor and medial wall of the orbit, pterygoid fossa and ethmoid sinus	Involvement of the medial wall and floor of the orbit, maxillary sinus, cribriform plate
T4A	Involvement of the anterior orbital contents, skin of the cheek, pterygoid plates, infra-temporal fossa, cribriform plate, sphenoidal or frontal sinuses	As maxillary sinus
T4B	Involvement of the orbital apex, dura, brain, middle cranial fossa, cranial nerves (excluding the second division of the Vth cranial nerve), nasopharynx or clivus	As maxillary sinus

Though it does not form part of the TNM staging system, division of maxillary sinus lesions into those arising from the infrastructure, that is anteroinferiorly, from lesions arising from the suprastructure which lie supero-posteriorly is potentially useful. This division arises from a theoretical line drawn from the medial canthus to the angle of the mandible in a lateral plane (Ohngren's line) (Figure 22.17).

Aetiology, pathology and lymphatic spread

The healthy sinuses are lined with ciliated columnar epithelium. Squamous cell carcinomas comprise the commonest histological subtype and, as with other head and neck squamous cell carcinomas, are associated with smoking and, to a lesser extent, excess alcohol. Adenocarcinomas, particularly of the ethmoid sinus, occur and are associated with hard wood furniture manufacturers. Other tumour types include adenoid cystic carcinoma, melanoma and lymphoma.

The lymph system is remarkably sparse and, as such, tumours can be quite advanced without involved nodes. The corollary is that it is rare to present with neck nodes from an unsuspected primary located in the paranasal sinuses. Lymphatic drainage is typically towards the retropharyngeal (Rouviere's node) and upper deep cervical

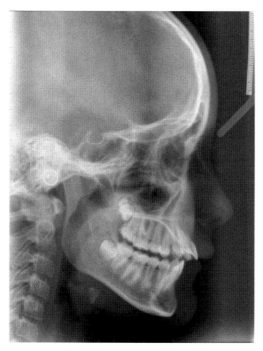

Figure 22.17 Radiograph illustrating Ohngren's line dividing the suprastructure and infrastructure of the paranasal sinuses.

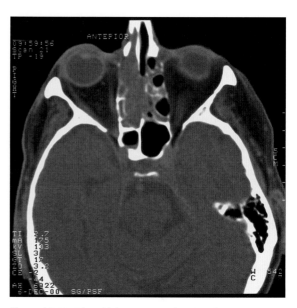

Figure 22.19 Ethmoid sinus tumour showing close proximity to optic nerve and chiasm.

nodes (level II) unless the tumour is particularly anteriorly placed when the buccinator, level I and IIA nodes are at risk.

Signs and symptoms

The complex anatomical relationship with neighboring structures is reflected in the diverse presenting features of these tumours. On the other hand, the air cavities permit substantial expansion and, as such, these tumours often present late, the early symptoms blurring with benign inflammatory disease.

Maxillary sinus tumours present with symptoms and signs related to the mode of expansion of the tumour: inferiorly, pain related to teeth and ulceration may manifest while inferoposteriorly, there is trismus (Figure *evolve* 22.18 🐭), superiorly, proptosis and diplopia; medially, nasal stuffiness with discharge which may not necessarily be bloody; anteriorly and laterally, a soft tissue mass may emerge in the cheek. If the infraorbital nerve is involved there will be numbness of the cheek and upper lip.

Ethmoidal sinus tumours frequently present with nasal obstruction. There may, in addition, be a discharge which again may not be blood-stained. Less commonly, there may be bone expansion overlying the superior aspect of the nose (Figure 22.19).

Bearing in mind the rarity of primary tumours of the sphenoidal sinus, these will typically present with deep-seated pain, often referred to the vertex of the skull, and there may be associated cranial nerve palsies. Frontal sinus tumours may simply present with bony swelling.

Diagnosis and staging

Initial assessment in the clinic should comprise a thorough examination including the use of a nasal speculum and upper airway endoscopy. The oral cavity must be inspected. A mass may be readily apparent and a sample taken for histological assessment. An examination under anaesthesia will invariably be required.

Plain x-rays may demonstrate bony erosion but an MRI scan will ultimately be required to define this more precisely as well as locoregional staging generally. Care must be exercised in the interpretation of signal changes on MRI which may reflect inflammatory disease (which often coexists). An orthopantomogram (OPG) will assist in the assessment of tooth preservation.

Treatment

As a general rule, surgery and postoperative radiotherapy will be indicated for tumours of the maxillary and ethmoidal sinuses except for the rare T1 lesion with complete clearance. Surgery will comprise a partial or total maxillectomy (depending on location and extent), ethmoidectomy and/ or sphenoidectomy. Surgery also facilitates drainage of the sinus ('fenestration') as obstruction is invariably associated with infection. This alone should be performed if the tumour is inoperable prior to radiotherapy with/without chemotherapy.

Where radiotherapy comprises definitive therapy, it may be given concurrently with chemotherapy and/or following neoadjuvant chemotherapy. On occasions, surgery may follow such therapy.

Radiotherapy when given postoperatively is delivered to the operative bed comprising the original location of the tumour and known and potential areas of spread. In the definitive setting, the volume irradiated will be determined by all staging information available to the clinician. When neoadjuvant chemotherapy has been used, the pretreatment volume will typically be used where it is safe to include it. In practice, routine coverage of the whole ipsilateral paranasal complex is indicated.

Radiotherapy technique (Figures
evolve 22.20–22.23 🖱)

An immobilization device should be used. Care should be taken in achieving the optimal head position. In practice, it is often best for the plane of the floor of the orbit to be perpendicular to the treatment couch. A tongue depressor facilitates movement of the tongue inferiorly *away* from the treatment volume. A full head and neck shell over the shoulders, even if the intention is not to irradiate the neck nodes, should give rise to smaller set-up errors and is preferred.

The volume definition has been outlined above. Volumes should be delineated on a contrast-enhanced planning CT scan. Rarely is it necessary to include the neck nodes as a clinical target volume but the retropharyngeal nodes should be included as routine. Co-registration of images is invaluable in the process of volume delineation. A typical conformal technique will comprise 6 MV photons using a two- or three-field arrangement. The contralateral beam supplements any fall off in dose at the posteromedial margin. Beam weighting will vary according to the target volume shape and body profile but, typically, will derive predominantly from the anterior beam. As such, there is a significant exiting dose. Beam arrangements for ethmoidal and sphenoidal sinus tumours are best derived following careful volume delineation.

The doses used will be determined by treatment intent. Gross disease postoperatively and when used in the definitive setting will demand a higher dose (see elsewhere) with consideration to irradiation of critical normal tissues.

Complications

The biggest risk with treatment of these tumours is lack of local control given the generally advanced nature at presentation. On the other hand, those patients who do survive long term or are cured are at risk of treatment-related sequelae.

Late sequelae following surgery relate to fibrosis within the operated bed potentially exacerbated by radiotherapy and issues related to any prosthesis used.

Radiotherapy with or without surgery will invariably result in some xerostomia due to the irradiation of the ipsilateral parotid gland with its usual sequlae. It is for that reason that any teeth remaining following resection should be in healthy condition. Trismus may result and should be actively managed with appropriate jaw exercises. Unless the orbit is frankly involved, the globe is spared but the lens and retina are at risk of damage and the exiting anterior beam gives a significant dose to the optic chiasm and brainstem. Binocular blindness is a rare but catastrophic complication of maxillary sinus irradiation. Pituitary failure may emerge in long-term survivors.

Given the complex relationship of tumour and normal tissues, particularly the optic chiasm, it is anticipated that the technique of intensity modulated radiotherapy will facilitate a reduction of such late sequelae by improved conformality and preliminary data support this view.

Results

Overall, paranasal sinus tumours lead to a 25–30% 5-year survival. Tumours within the infrastructure and where there is good clearance by surgery give rise to more favourable outcomes of the order of 50% 5-year survival.

LIP AND ORAL CAVITY CARCINOMA

Anatomy

Cancers of the lip arise from the vermilion (external) border.

The anatomical sites conventionally regarded as constituting the oral cavity are buccal mucosa, upper and lower alveolus, retromolar trigone, hard palate, tongue (anterior two thirds: anterior to the circumvallate papillae) and the floor of mouth.

Incidence of oral cavity carcinoma

The oral tongue and then the floor of mouth are the commonest subsites. Overall, they are still a rare group of cancers making up less than 1% of cancer deaths. The UK incidence of lip and oral cavity cancers in 2004 was just under 5000, or six cases per 100 000 population. The incidence remains higher in men than women, although the ratio has fallen from 5:1 to just over 2:1 with increasing prevalence of alcohol and tobacco use in women.

Staging system for oral cavity and lip carcinoma

T1   Tumour <2 cm
T2   Tumour 2–4 cm

T3   Tumour >4 cm

T4a   Tumour invades through cortical bone, inferior alveolar nerve, floor of mouth, or skin of chin or nose (lip) and cortical bone, into deep/extrinsic muscle of tongue, maxillary sinus, or skin of face (oral cavity)

T4b   Tumour invades masticator space, pterygoid plates, or skull base, or encases internal carotid artery

N1   Single ipselateral node ≤3 cm diameter

N2A   Single ipselateral node >3 cm ≤6 cm

N2B   Multiple ipselateral nodes ≤6 cm

N2C   Bilateral or contralateral nodes ≤6 cm

N3   Any node >6 cm

Aetiology, pathology and lymphatic spread

Whereas tumours that occur within the oral cavity share with the majority of other upper aerodigestive tract tumours the etiological factors of exposure to alcohol and tobacco, tumours of the lip tend to be seen in patients with much exposure to sunlight, particularly smokers. Alcohol seems to be less important in the aetiology of cancers of this site. Other risk factors for oral cavity cancers include local trauma (e.g. badly fitted dentures) and leukoplakia. There is an association with betel nut, chewed in many cultures and also with syphilis, which is still prevalent in some parts of the world.

Cancers of the lip are almost always squamous cell carcinomas and over 90% of the oral cavity cancers are too. A small proportion of oral cavity tumours are adenocarcinomas or arise from the minor salivary glands of the oral cavity.

Nodal involvement in cancers of the lip occurs rarely (<5% of all cases at presentation) but the incidence is higher with large, poorly differentiated tumours or those at the angle of the mouth (Figure 22.24). The neck nodes can be a site of potential relapse and therefore must be included in follow-up assessment. Nodal disease can be salvaged surgically and therefore prophylactic neck radiotherapy is usually not required in lip tumour management.

In oral cavity cancers, spread may be local to adjacent structures including the mandible. Nodal involvement is usually primarily to the submental and submandibular glands followed by the upper deep cervical nodes, i.e. levels 1A, 1B and 2, though disease can spread directly to levels 3 and 4, so-called 'skip' nodes (Figure 22.25). Midline tumours may develop bilateral nodal spread. Retropharyngeal nodes are rarely involved in this group of cancers.

Signs and symptoms

Lip cancers present in a similar manner to skin tumours with visible lesions over the lip. There may be a non-healing ulcer or persistent scabbing. The lesions may be ulcerative or exophytic. There can be discomfort or bleeding associated

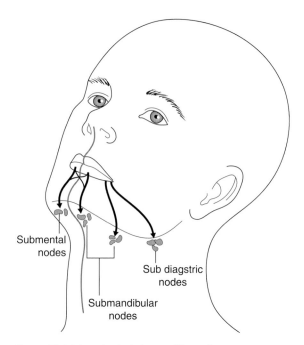

Figure 22.24 Lymphatic drainage of lower lip.

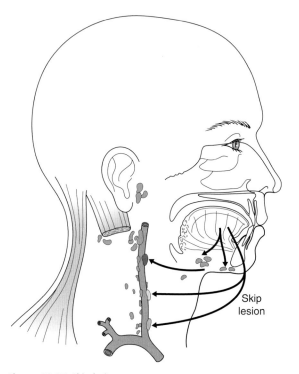

Figure 22.25 Skip lesion.

with the area and occasionally infiltration of adjacent skin or the underlying oral mucosa (Figure *evolve* 22.26 🖱).

Oral cavity cancers also commonly present with ulcerated lesions. They are often detected at dental check-up and can be associated with leukoplakia or erythroplakia. Local pain can be a symptom and, in more advanced tumours, may radiate to the ear on the involved side (Figures *evolve* 22.27 and 22.28 🖱).

Diagnosis and staging

Patients should be referred to a specialist head and neck team for full assessment. Local examination should be performed including full inspection of the oral cavity and nasendoscopy to examine the rest of the aerodigestive tract. Imaging is required for any tumours in the anterior part of the oral cavity to exclude mandibular involvement (Figures 22.29 and 22.30). It also assists in the assessment of dentition prior to any planned radiotherapy. For oral cavity tumours, CT or MRI of the primary site is required to determine depth of invasion or involvement of adjacent structures (Figures 22.31 and 22.32) and, as with any head and neck cancer, imaging of the neck nodes and chest is required to exclude distant spread.

A biopsy of the lesion is required and can be done in the clinic or as part of an examination under anaesthetic if more detailed information about tumour extent is required.

Treatment Lip cancers

Most lip cancers occur on the lower lip and, because of their conspicuous position, the majority of these tumours presents relatively early, and so are regularly curable. Both surgery and radiotherapy are treatment options, and the choice between the two often comes down to deciding which will give the better cosmetic/functional result. Very

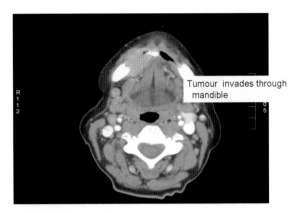

Figure 22.30 Carcinoma of lower alveolus.

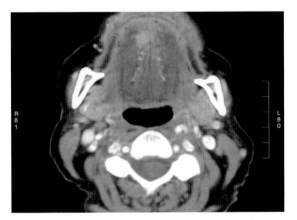

Figure 22.31 Carcinoma of anterior floor of mouth.

small superficial lesions can be treated by a 'lip shave', as long as an adequate deep margin is obtained. This will give a very good cosmetic result.

Larger lesions, if treated surgically, require a wedge excision and, in many cases, this will give a less satisfactory long-term outcome than treatment with radiotherapy which, as a result, is widely used in the treatment of these tumours.

Radiotherapy technique

The technique will be similar to that used for skin tumours. A margin of at least 1 cm is required around the disease as assessed by inspection and palpation to arrive at a suitable CTV.

An individualized lead cut-out, and an internal gum shield will usually be used. This arrangement facilitates appropriate sparing of the adjacent tissues including the unaffected (usually upper) lip and the deeper tissues of the oral cavity. These lesions are usually exophytic, so electrons will often be preferred to low energy x-rays and,

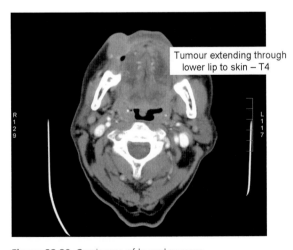

Figure 22.29 Carcinoma of buccal mucosa.

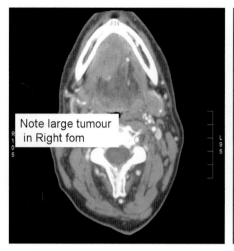
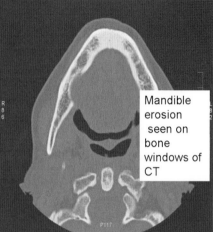

Figure 22.32 Advanced cancer of floor of mouth.

because the energy chosen is likely to be less than 12 MeV, a few millimetres of wax should be placed over the lesion to ensure maximum dose at the tumour surface. The gum shield will require wax on its anterior surface to absorb any backscatter electrons that could potentially enhance the dose to the treated volume. An alternative is to use orthovoltage photons ($\approx$250 kV) which may be more practical to administer in an elderly patient. Care will need to be exercised in the degree of underlying bone irradiated that cannot be shielded by the gum shield (Figures *evolve* 22.33–22.35 🐭).

Dose schedules for squamous cell carcinomas of the lip are similar to those for skin cancers and the reader is referred elsewhere. Longer fractionation schedules give better long-term cosmesis than a few large fractions and are preferred. Usual treatment regimens for these tumours range from 50 to 55 Gy in 15–20 fractions, treating daily.

Cancers of oral cavity

Whereas at many other head and neck sites primary radiotherapy (or, increasingly, chemoradiotherapy) is becoming more usual as first-line treatment, this is not so for oral cavity tumours, where primary surgery retains its place. High-level evidence to support the use of surgery here is scant, but other evidence does support this approach.

In general, survival after treatment for head and neck cancer in the UK has shown very little change over past decades. Oral cavity tumours are an exception. Recent data from the Scottish Cancer Registry show that 5-year survival for oral cancers has improved by about 50% since 1980. In the late 1970s/early 1980s, primary radiotherapy was widely employed in the UK for oral cancer. At about that time, the Canniesburn plastic surgeons began to persuade the rest of the head and neck oncology community that primary surgery with modern reconstructive techniques offered a relatively non-mutilating approach, and one that achieved excellent local control (often not achieved with primary radiotherapy). Over the next decade, this approach became almost universal around the UK (as in other parts of the world), and this seems the likeliest explanation for the improved survival figures that have been achieved.

The surgery for oral cavity cancers depends on the extent of the primary. Small T1 and T2 lesions may be suitable for simple excision which may be left to heal or closed with a split-skin graft or free flap. Larger lesions or those with more extensive invasion may require hemi-mandibulectomy with or without removal of part of the mandible and reconstruction with myocutaneous flaps (e.g. pectoralis major flap).

Radiotherapy remains an integral part of many patients' treatments, as postoperative adjuvant treatment has been established as an important part of the overall management of many of these tumours. In recent years, evidence has accumulated of the value of adding chemotherapy to radiotherapy schedules in high-risk patients.

Selection criteria for giving postoperative radiotherapy or chemoradiotherapy are widely agreed, even if the evidence level for some of these indications is not high. The reader is referred to the earlier chapter on these criteria.

Radiotherapy as definitive treatment is still an option for patients with early T1 or T2 tumours of the floor of mouth or lateral part of the mobile (anterior two-thirds) tongue. The results of surgery and radiotherapy for such tumours are very similar and much depends on local expertise.

The tumours that respond best to radiotherapy tend to be superficial and exophytic. Ulcerated tumours do less well and perhaps should be considered more carefully for surgical resection.

Brachytherapy for T1/T2 tongue tumours is still widely practised in continental Europe but expertise is lacking in many parts of the UK and only some centres offer this form of radiotherapy. Suitable lesions are less than 1 cm thick and no more than 2.5 cm in length situated on the lateral edge of the mobile part of the tongue (Figure *evolve* 22.36 🐭). Such lesions can be implanted with three or four iridium hairpins spaced 12 mm apart to cover the lesion plus a margin of 1 cm. A typical dosage is 65 Gy in 6–7 days. In France, brachytherapy treatment is often accompanied by a supra-hyoid neck dissection.

Significant involvement of the alveolar ridge by even a small floor of mouth tumour is a contraindication to radiotherapy. Involvement of the mandibular bone occurs early when tumour originates or spreads to the gingival mucosa. Tumour can spread rapidly through the marrow cavity. Involvement of the mandible is an indication for surgery followed by radiotherapy.

T3 or T4 tumours of the tongue or the oral cavity (Figures 22.37 and 22.38) are difficult to cure with radiation alone. Radiotherapy alone in patients with co-morbidity felt to be truly unsuitable for surgery gives cure

rates of 10–30% at best, but these outcomes may be enhanced with concurrent chemotherapy.

Tumours of the buccal mucosa are usually well differentiated and may originate from areas of leukoplakia. Small T1 verrucous tumours may be readily treated by surgical excision, but the functional and cosmetic results are better when larger T1 or T2 tumours are treated with radiotherapy: the control rates are similar for surgery or radiation treatment.

Radiotherapy technique

An immobilization device is used and should include fixation of the shoulders even if it is not intended to irradiate the neck nodes comprehensively. An intra-oral device is frequently used. For tongue tumours, it has as its purpose to move the tongue *into* the treatment volume and, as a consequence, achieve sparing of some of the palate. There is then sparing of some of the minor salivary tissue. For buccal tumours, its intention is different: here, it is helpful to move the tongue *away* from the irradiated mucosa and thereby lessen the toxicity.

Volumes should be defined on a planning CT scan. A fundamental decision is whether to treat the neck bilaterally. This decision should be based on the anticipated risk of contralateral spread and will vary according to tumour site within the oral cavity. For well-lateralized tumours, an ipsilateral approach will often suffice and has as its advantage sparing of the contralateral parotid gland. As a result, permanent xerostomia is reduced. Relapse in the contralateral neck can potentially be salvaged later.

Postoperatively, the surgical tumour bed and nodes are included even if node negative, though this is an area of debate (see earlier). For most oral cancers seen in UK practice, there is a low risk of involvement of the retropharyngeal nodes so they can be excluded from the CTV unless there is extensive node involvement pathologically. This has the benefit of sparing the temporomandibular joint and part of the parotid tissue. For large buccal mucosal or hard palate tumours, a different view might be considered. For anteriorly placed oral cavity tumours where the patient is node negative, it is reasonable to exclude level 5 (and 2B) making the delivery of radiotherapy simpler when using conventional techniques. Where there is involvement of the mandible, the whole of that hemimandible should be included in the initial CTV.

In the definitive setting, the primary site is treated with a 2–3 cm margin to give the primary CTV. The nodes treated will vary according to the primary site and the level of risk of involvement can be used to dictate an appropriate dose.

A typical field arrangement is to treat the upper neck, i.e. the oral cavity and level 1 and 2 nodes, with a parallel-opposed pair and the lower neck with an anterior field matched at approximately the level of the bottom of the hyoid bone using the mono-isocentric technique. There is midline shielding for the spinal cord and upper oesophagus in the lower neck field. The cord is spared in the lateral fields

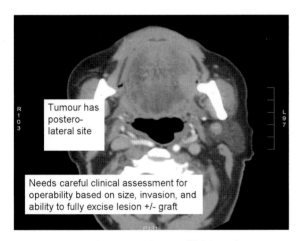

Tumour has postero-lateral site

Needs careful clinical assessment for operability based on size, invasion, and ability to fully excise lesion +/- graft

Figure 22.37 CT showing carcinoma of left lateral tongue.

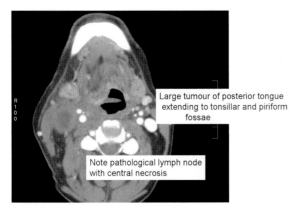

Large tumour of posterior tongue extending to tonsillar and piriform fossae

Note pathological lymph node with central necrosis

Figure 22.38 CT showing carcinoma of base of tongue.

before tolerance is reached and any additional dose required topped up with electrons. The IMRT approach discussed earlier in the chapter in many ways simplifies the delivery technique and enables useful salivary gland sparing.

The doses of radiation used will be dictated by the disease burden, i.e. gross residual disease or when radiotherapy is used as the definitive treatment and involved nodes require the highest doses. Actual doses used are discussed in the previous chapter. Doses to the upper neck will be specified at reference point typically midline; doses to the lower neck are often specified at a depth of 2.5–3.0 cm.

Complications

Acute reactions with radiotherapy to the oral cavity include the usual effects on the skin and mucosa but should be self-limiting. The effect on nutrition can be profound and should be managed aggressively if not proactively.

Late effects will be determined in part by the site of irradiation and the selection of dose. Some sparing of salivary tissue may be possible and, as such, complete xerostomia may not be inevitable. Taste and a heightened intra-oral sensitivity may result. Fibrosis of the neck may result though the relative impact of surgery and radiotherapy is poorly documented. Mucosal ulceration may occur but usually heals with conservative measures, i.e. antimicrobial mouthwashes. Osteoradionecrosis (see Figure 22.2) can be minimized by meticulous dental hygiene prior to and following radiotherapy. The least amount of mandible should be irradiated while ensuring complete coverage of the volume at risk. Hot spots in the treatment plan should be avoided, particularly overlying the mandible. Recent data have supported IMRT in that regard by optimizing dose homogeneity.

Results of treatment

Lip cancer

As mentioned previously, the majority of these tumours present relatively early and if treated with radical radiotherapy have an excellent chance of cure. T1 and T2 lesions would be cured in 90–100%. Larger or more advanced tumours have a worse prognosis.

Oral cavity cancers

The same rules apply for these cancers as others in the head and neck. Small, early cancers have a better prognosis than those with invasion into adjacent structures or nodal involvement. T1 and small T2 lesions of the oral cavity may be cured by surgery (or radiotherapy) alone and the overall survival is 85–95%. This can fall to as low as 50% for T4 tumours or those with extensive nodal disease. Survival figures at 5 years following implantation of tongue cancers are up to 90% for T1 tumours, falling to 50–75% for T2 lesions.

OROPHARYNGEAL CARCINOMA

Anatomy

The oropharynx comprises the tonsil, the base of tongue, otherwise known as the posterior one-third of the tongue, and the undersurface of the soft palate. It is continuous with the nasopharynx superiorly, the hypopharynx inferiorly and the oral cavity anteriorly. The major components of Waldeyer's ring lie within the oropharynx: only the superior component lies within the nasopharynx. The function of the oropharynx is multifactorial: swallowing and respiration, including protection of the airway, phonation, taste and immune surveillance.

Anterior wall

There is no true anterior wall as the oropharynx communicates directly with the oral cavity. The anterior tonsillar pillar divides the oral cavity from the oropharynx while the circumvillate papillae (sulcus terminalis) on the surface of the tongue divides the oral tongue from the base of tongue.

Posterior wall

This is formed by the tissues of the prevertebral space adjacent to C2 and C3 and constitutes the posterior pharyngeal wall.

Lateral wall

The palatoglossal (anterior pillar) and palatopharyngeal (posterior pillar) arches, the faucial tonsil ('the tonsil') and a small component of the pharyngeal wall constitute the lateral wall of the oropharynx. The parapharyngeal space lies more lateral still. The internal and external carotid arteries, internal jugular vein, superior cervical ganglion and retropharygeal nodes lie within this area.

Superior wall

The superior wall is composed anteriorly of the undersurface of the soft palate. Otherwise there is a direct opening into the nasopharynx.

Inferior wall

The hyoid bone constitutes the anatomical boundary between the oropharynx and hypopharynx. The valleculla, which is a trough that lies between the tongue base and the epiglottis, lies within this area. Lingual tonsillar tissue gives the inferior component of Waldeyer's ring.

Incidence of oropharyngeal tumours

Cancers of the oropharynx are uncommon with a worldwide incidence of 125 000 per year. In the UK, there were almost 900 new cases diagnosed in 2004 according to the CRUK database. These cancers mainly occur in the fifth to seventh decades and are approximately three to four times more common in men than women.

Of oropharyngeal cancers, the most common are tonsillar ($\approx 60\%$) followed by 25% in the base of tongue and 10% in the soft palate.

Staging system of oropharyngeal tumours

Tx	Primary tumour cannot be assessed
T0	No evidence of primary tumour
Tis	Carcinoma in situ
T1	Tumour ≤ 2 cm in greatest dimension
T2	Tumour >2 cm but 4 cm or smaller in greatest dimension
T3	Tumour >4 cm in greatest dimension
T4a	Tumour invades the larynx, deep/extrinsic muscle of tongue, medial pterygoid, hard palate or mandible
T4b	Tumour invades lateral pterygoid muscle, pterygoid plates, lateral nasopharynx, or skull base or encases the carotid artery
Nx	Regional lymph nodes cannot be assessed
N0	No regional lymph node metastasis
N1	Metastasis in a single ipsilateral lymph node, 3 cm or smaller in greatest dimension
N2a	Metastasis in a single ipsilateral lymph node larger than 3 cm but 6 cm or smaller in greatest dimension
N2b	Metastasis in multiple ipsilateral lymph nodes, 6 cm or smaller in greatest dimension
N2c	Metastasis in bilateral or contralateral lymph nodes, 6 cm or smaller in greatest dimension
N3	Metastasis in a lymph node larger than 6 cm in greatest dimension

Aetiology, pathology and lymphatic spread

As with other head and neck cancers, tobacco and alcohol consumption are the most significant risk factors for developing cancers in this region. There are no specific genetic risk factors for this type of tumour. There appears to be a specific group of oropharyngeal carcinomas in younger (often non-smoker) patients which are found to be associated with the human papilloma virus (HPV). Here, there appears to be distinct histopathological appearances with less differentiation and basaloid type cells. Review of the outcome of these specific tumours compared with the typical squamous cell carcinomas suggests an improved prognosis. It may also direct future treatment strategies given the recent developments of vaccines directed at cervical cancer prevention.

Histologically, almost all oropharyngeal carcinomas are the squamous cell cancers prevalent in the head and neck region. One variant of the SCC of the oropharynx is the lymphoepithelioma. Histologically, it is lymphocyte predominant and may mimic lymphoma. It may arise in the base of tongue, tonsils or nasopharynx. It is a very radiosensitive variant of squamous cell cancer. Other cancers in this area include minor salivary gland carcinomas and lymphoma. Mention has already been made of Waldeyers ring. It is a site of extra-nodal non-Hodgkin's lymphoma. Approximately one-quarter of tonsillar tumours are such lymphomas.

The oropharynx has a rich lymphatic supply; 60% of oropharyngeal cancers have nodal involvement at presentation. In tonsillar tumours, this is predominantly unilateral spread unless the primary crosses the midline and is important when determining volumes to irradiate. Tonsillar cancers drain to the adjacent jugulodigastric or subdigastric node (the so-called 'tonsillar node') and then the remainder of the deep cervical nodes of level 2 and 3. The remainder of oropharyngeal cancers are midline structures and therefore can drain to bilateral nodes. Tumours of the soft palate and posterior pharyngeal wall drain to the retropharyngeal nodes and upper deep cervical lymph nodes, i.e. level 2. Base of tongue tumours commonly spread to the mid and upper cervical nodes, i.e. levels 2 and 3.

Signs and symptoms

Cancers in this region commonly present with sore throat or painful swallowing. Tumours in the tonsillar region or posterior oropharynx may present with earache due to extension into the parapharyngeal space or the sensation of a 'lump in the throat'. Tumour or ulceration in the oropharynx can usually be visualized in the clinic via direct inspection or nasendoscopy. A fine needle aspiration (FNA) or biopsy can often be taken at the time.

As with many head and neck cancers, the presentation may be via a neck mass from secondary lymph nodes. In this case, the primary may be identified from tonsillectomy or blind biopsies of the tongue base at examination under anaesthesia (EUA) or endoscopy.

Diagnosis and staging

Patients with a history of persistent sore throat should be referred urgently to the ENT clinic. Patients may also be referred urgently for persistent tonsillar swelling or neck lymphadenopathy.

A full history should be undertaken. The importance of co-morbidities may affect whether patients are operable or can be treated with chemotherapy and/or radiotherapy. This is particularly the case in patients who are heavy smokers or have a history of alcohol intake.

A full ENT examination is performed in the clinic. This allows delineation of the primary. It should include

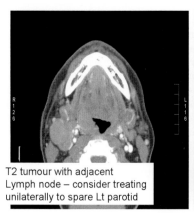

T2 tumour with adjacent
Lymph node – consider treating
unilaterally to spare Lt parotid

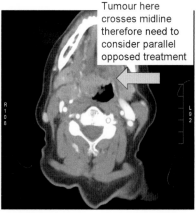

Tumour here
crosses midline
therefore need to
consider parallel
opposed treatment

Figure 22.40 CT scan showing
carcinoma of tonsil.

indirect laryngoscopy or fibreoptic examination to look for synchronous tumours. The neck should be clinically examined for palpable lymph nodes.

Patients should have an examination under anaesthesia and biopsy to confirm the tissue diagnosis (Figure *evolve* 22.39 🖱).

Radiological assessment of the primary is essential to complete the staging. This is usually a CT or MRI scan (Figure 22.40). This may also reveal pathological lymphadenopathy not identified clinically. Imaging of the chest is also essential for exclusion of metastatic spread or synchronous primary tumours of the lung.

Treatment

Currently, management of primary tumours of the oropharynx is largely non-surgical. Chemoradiation is the 'standard-of-care' for the younger and healthier patients, radiotherapy alone for the less robust, typically using an altered fractionation schedule. Management of neck disease is more complex, and the integration of surgical interventions with chemoradiation is subtle.

Control of even large primary cancers can now often be achieved without surgery, but significant nodal disease is still widely considered to be a more intractable problem, and neck dissection retains an important place, especially for more extensive neck disease. This meaning any 'N' stage above N1, i.e. multiple nodes or nodes >3 cm. Clinical N1 disease is usually well controlled by radiation, with or without chemotherapy.

Many patients with oropharyngeal cancer present with cervical lymphadenopathy and an asymptomatic primary tumour. A complex interaction between clinical oncologists and other members of the team must be initiated early, even before the suspected primary site has been confirmed. A positive cytological diagnosis from the node should be followed by examination under anaesthesia, biopsy of any suspicious areas, random biopsies of oropharynx, nasopharynx and

hypopharynx and, if no obvious primary site has been identified clinically, an ipsilateral tonsillectomy.

A neck dissection with biopsy of the suspected primary site ('biopsy' can mean 'tonsillectomy' here) is a reasonable first therapeutic gesture. The pathological detail can inform later radiotherapy planning especially with regards to dose. However, the increasing availability of PET-CT means that we can consider delaying neck surgery for use only in lesions that seem resistant to chemoradiation. Excellent regression of even large neck masses is not unusual after chemoradiation, but sometimes this clinical improvement is illusory, and then neck recurrence can be a harbinger of disaster.

Patients not treated with neck dissection initially should be examined closely during and after radiotherapeutic treatment. If there is residual nodal disease post-radiotherapy then the patient requires a neck dissection. There may be no remaining active disease but FNA or biopsy are not reliable and surgery is essential. There is increasing evidence that a PET-CT may be useful in node-positive patients who appear to have had a complete clinical response to chemoradiotherapy. The PET-CT should be done 10–12 weeks post-treatment to allow inflammatory changes to resolve. If the scan is negative then the patient can be followed up as per the usual protocol. If positive then a neck dissection should be considered. This is still an area requiring ongoing research.

Radiation technique
(Figures *evolve* 22.41–22.48 🖱)

Patients are treated in an immobilization device that includes the head and shoulders. The patient is treated supine. The neck will typically be in a 'neutral' position, unless the patient is treated with IMRT, when a more extended position is preferred as part of the oral cavity can then be excluded from the primary beam. A tongue depressor is not usually used.

A planning CT scan co-registered with diagnostic scans facilitates precise volume definition. The primary CTV must include reasonable margins to account for microscopic spread. This means inclusion of the parapharyngeal space that surrounds the oropharynx, in the case of tonsillar tumours, a component of the soft palate and tongue base even if not overtly involved and some of the oral tongue for tongue base tumours. The selection of lymph nodes is based on known pattern of spread of these tumours. A well-lateralized early tumour of the tonsil rarely spreads to the contralateral lymph nodes and, as such, affords useful sparing of the contralateral salivary tissues. Where a neck dissection has been carried out, this additional information allows for appropriate doses to be specified according to the risk of disease, i.e. nodes with extracapsular spread would be irradiated to a high dose.

Tonsillar tumours

Small ipsilateral primary tumours with a node-negative neck can be treated with a small volume treatment that includes the primary site and level 1B and 2A cervical lymph nodes. In practice, the CTV will extend superiorly to the level of the hard palate and inferiorly to at least the level of the hyoid bone. The medial margin, as discussed earlier, should include part of the soft palate and tongue base and, as such, extends to the midline. Anteriorly, the volume extends beyond palatoglossus to the middle of the tongue and, posteriorly, just anterior to the spinal cord to include level 2A (but not 2B) nodes.

The above treatment field can be treated with a wedged pair arrangement which allows coverage of the volume but has the advantage of sparing the contralateral parotid gland and thus avoiding permanent xerostomia.

The relatively small volumes of irradiation mean that shorter fractionation schedules, such as 55 Gy in 20 daily fractions, are reasonable.

Large tonsillar tumours and other oropharyngeal tumours

Larger tumours of the tonsil which approach or cross the midline, that have spread locally to the base of tongue or which are node positive should be treated with a volume which encompasses the primary and bilateral upper cervical neck nodes.

Other oropharyngeal tumours, i.e. base of tongue, post-pharyngeal wall and soft palate, usually require a similar bilateral approach due to the high risk of contralateral lymph node involvement.

A typical field arrangement to achieve coverage of these volumes, i.e. the primary and node levels 1 and 2, is with a pair of parallel-opposed lateral fields. The lower neck, i.e. node level 3 and 4, is treated with a matched anterior field with shielding for the central structures. Typically, the match point for these patients is at the level of the hyoid bone. If there is bulky lymphadenopathy, the match point should, wherever possible, be moved inferiorly so that overt disease lies above that point. In patients with tongue base tumours, the match point is typically slightly more inferior too at the level of the thyroid notch to encompass the primary CTV. Alternatively an IMRT approach can be used.

Fractionation schedules used in this situation are very much along the lines of that discussed in the previous chapter. Concurrent chemotherapy, certainly in younger fitter patients, forms an important component of this treatment. Indeed, the strongest evidence for concurrent chemoradiotherapy originates from oropharyngeal tumours.

Complications

Acute reactions in the oropharynx are predictable. Mucositis will compromise nutrition and should be managed aggressively. In practice, this often means that these patients have feeding tubes sited prior to therapy and opiate analgesia. Acute xerostomia and the often copious mucous production should be managed symptomatically. Skin reactions and reversible alopecia will occur in the irradiation portals.

Chronic xerostomia is a common side effect of wide-field radiotherapy as used here. There is now level one evidence that sparing of at least one parotid gland with IMRT techniques (either the contralateral gland or bilateral superficial glands) results in an improvement in the quality of life of these patients. Trismus may result from high dose radiotherapy to the pterygoid muscles. Active stretching exercises can help to alleviate this.

Results

For node-negative tumours, the 5-year survival for oropharyngeal tumours is ≈75%, but this almost halves for patients with involved nodes. Local control ranges from 75 to 95% for T1 tumours falling through the stages (80% for T2, 60% for T3) to approximately 10–35% for T4 disease. Five-year survival for the same groups is 60–80% for T1 but less than 30% for T4 disease.

LARYNX

Anatomy

The larynx is a cartilaginous frame held in position by intrinsic muscles and ligaments. The anterior and lateral part of this box is formed by the thyroid cartilage. The cricoid cartilage is below the thyroid cartilage forming a complete ring around the larynx just below the vocal cords.

The larynx is divided into three areas. The supraglottis, glottis and subglottis (Figure 22.49). The structures of the supraglottis are the epiglottis, the ariepiglottic folds, the aretinoids, the ventricular bands (often called the false

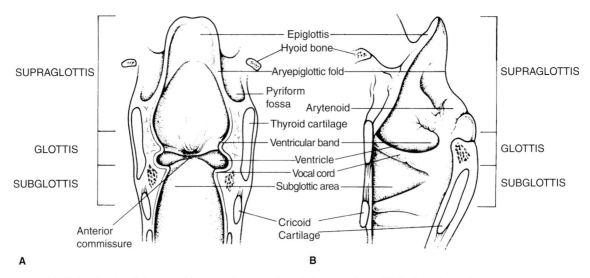

Figure 22.49 Landmarks of the normal larynx and pharynx from A the posterior and B the lateral aspect. *(Redrawn from Robinson, Surgery, Longmans)*

cords) and the ventricular cavities. The true glottis is the area by the vocal cords. The subglottic area is the area beneath the vocal cords, and above the trachea.

Incidence of laryngeal cancer

In the UK in 2000, there were 2407 cases of laryngeal cancer (4.1 per 100 000 per annum) which makes the larynx the most common site for head and neck cancer in the UK. In some parts of France, Spain and Italy, the incidence of laryngeal cancer can be up to six times more common. Unlike the UK, where true glottis is the most common site, the supraglottic area is the most common site for laryngeal tumours in southern Europe. In the West Midlands region of England, 60–70% of tumours begin in the glottis, 25% of cases are supraglottic, 2% only are true subglottic cancer and the remainder are transglottic tumours, where the precise site of origin cannot be determined.

Staging system for laryngeal cancer

See Table 22.1.

Aetiology, pathology and lymphatic spread

As with many head and neck cancers, laryngeal tumours tend to develop in smokers. Infection with HPV may be the aetiological agent in some non-smokers. The higher incidence of supraglottic cancer in parts of Europe may be due to the type of alcoholic drink consumed and the use of dark rather than blond tobacco. The true glottis

has a poor lymphatic supply and tumours arising from the true vocal cord are relatively slow to metastasize to regional lymph nodes. This is even true of T3 glottic cancers. But supraglottic carcinoma of larynx spreads far more readily to the lymph nodes within the neck. The incidence of lymph node spread from even T1 and T2 lesions ranges between 27 and 40% and for T3/T4 lesions the rate of lymph node metastasis is 55–65%.

Initially, lymphatic spread is upwards to the jugulodigastric lymph nodes immediately beneath the angle of the jaw. Tumours also commonly spread to the mid-jugular lymph nodes. Over 95% of laryngeal tumours are invasive squamous carcinoma. Usually well differentiated but some tumours, especially of the supraglottic region, can be poorly differentiated and more likely to spread to lymph nodes. A common variant of well-differentiated squamous cancer is a verrucous carcinoma. This tumour contains a large amount of keratin and has a heaped-up warty appearance. Sometimes, invasive cancer can be preceded by carcinoma in situ of the epithelium of the vocal cords. However, this usually transforms into invasive cancer within 1–2 years of detection.

Signs and symptoms

The first symptom in more than 90% of patients with true glottic cancer is hoarseness. Comparatively small tumours of the vocal cords can cause marked changes in the voice. Advanced tumours of the vocal cords may narrow the airway, especially if a vocal cord is paralyzed, leading to stridor. This is a whistling noise when the patient breathes and is an oncological emergency. Untreated, the patient will develop progressive dysponea and can suffocate. For this

Table 22.1 TMN clinical classification

T – PRIMARY TUMOUR		
Supraglottis		
T1	Tumour limited to one subsite of supraglottis with normal vocal cord mobility	
T2	Tumour invades mucosa of more than one adjacent subsite of supraglottis or glottis or region outside the supraglottis (e.g. mucosa of base of tongue, vallecula, medial wall of piriform sinus) without fixation of the larynx	
T3	Tumour limited to larynx with vocal cord fixation and/or invades any of the following: post-cricoid area, pre-epiglottic tissues, deep base of tongue	
T4	Tumour invades through thyroid cartilage and/or extends into soft tissues of the neck, thyroid and/or oesophagus	
Glottis		
T1	Tumour limited to vocal cord(s) (may involve anterior or posterior commissure) with normal mobility	
	T1a	Tumour limited to one vocal cord
	T1b	Tumour involves both vocal cords
T2	Tumour extends to supraglottis and/or subglottis and/or with impaired vocal cord mobility	
T3	Tumour limited to larynx with vocal cord fixation	
T4	Tumour invades through thyroid cartilage and/or extends to other tissues beyond the larynx, e.g. trachea, soft tissues of neck, thyroid, pharynx	
Subglottis		
T	Tumour limited to subglottis	
T2	Tumour extends to vocal cord(s) with normal or impaired mobility	
T3	Tumour limited to larynx with vocal cord fixation	
T4	Tumour invades through cricoid or thyroid cartilage and/or extends into other tissues beyond the larynx, e.g. trachea, soft tissues of neck, thyroid, oesophagus	
N – REGIONAL LYMPH NODES		
NX	Regional lymph nodes cannot be assessed	
N0	No regional lymph nodes	
N1	Metastasis in a single ipsilateral lymph node 3 cm or less in greatest dimension	
N2	Metastasis in a single ipsilateral lymph node more than 3 cm but not more than 6 cm in greatest dimension or in multiple ipsilateral lymph nodes none more than 6 cm in greatest dimension or in bilateral or contralateral lymph nodes none more than 6 cm in greatest dimension	
	N2a	Metastasis in a single ipsilateral lymph node more than 3 cm but not more than 6 cm in greatest dimension
	N2b	Metastasis in multiple ipsilateral lymph nodes none more than 6 cm in greatest dimesnion
	N2c	Metastasis in bilateral or contralateral lymph nodes none more than 6 cm in greatest dimension
N3	Metastasis in a lymph nodes more than 6 cm in greatest dimension	

reason, patients with stridor should be immediately referred for consideration of an emergency tracheostomy or urgent laser debulking.

Hoarseness is less common as a symptom for early supraglottic cancer. Most patients complain initially of either a sore throat or a foreign body-like sensation in the upper larynx which they often describe as either caused by a fish bone or a piece of silver paper. Hoarseness only develops when the tumour reaches the vocal cord. More advanced tumours may have pain referred to the ear and patients may occasionally cough up blood (haemoptysis).

Diagnosis and staging

In the UK, the National Institute of Clinical Excellence recommends that any patient with hoarseness persisting for more than 3 weeks and heavy smokers aged 50 or older, especially heavy smokers and drinkers, be referred to a head and neck cancer clinic to be seen within 2 weeks of referral. This is also true of patients with an unexplained persistent sore or painful throat. Many laryngeal cancers are visible in a mirror during indirect laryngoscopy or, these days, more likely during a flexible fibrooptic examination. As well as visualizing the larynx, the neck should be carefully palpated for lymph nodes, especially in the jugulodigastric area.

Patients should then have an examination under anaesthetic and a complete assessment of spread. The mobility of the vocal cords should be assessed with the patient conscious and anaesthetized. Paralysis of a vocal cord is a potentially grave sign and places the patient into stage T3. CT and MRI scanning may give further information about the degree of spread, as these imaging modalities may show small impalpable lymph nodes in the neck or subglottic spread (Figures 22.50 and 22.51).

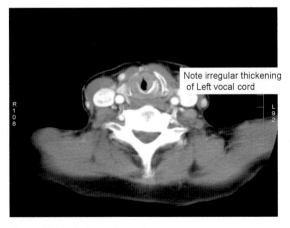

Figure 22.50 Early carcinoma larynx.

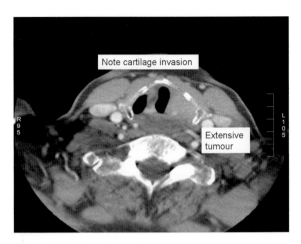

Figure 22.51 T4 carcinoma larynx.

Most patients with laryngeal cancer smoke. Smoking can affect the cardiovascular and respiratory systems. If the patient has chronic obstructive airways disease (COPD) or ischaemic heart disease, this may alter management decisions. Such patients may only be fit for less radical treatments and surgery or chemoradiotherapy may be contraindicated. Patients should have at least a chest x-ray to eliminate a synchronous carcinoma of bronchus. Advanced cases of laryngeal cancer should have a spiral CT scan of lung to exclude the possibility of pulmonary metastases.

Treatment

Early tumours (stage 1, stage 2)

In the USA and Europe, some early laryngeal cancers are treated by hemilaryngectomy, however, functional results are usually less satisfactory than radiotherapy with a poorer voice quality and a tendency for aspiration of fluids. Laser therapy is used increasingly for small tumours, especially on the middle third of the vocal cord. Voice quality may be poorer than following radiotherapy.

The majority of patients in the UK with early laryngeal cancer are treated by radical radiotherapy.

Glottic cancers (Figures *evolve* 22.52–22.56 🖱)

The larynx is a mobile structure and, although the vocal cord occupies about 1 cm only, the radiation volume should be at least 4 × 4 cm to allow for vocal cord movement during respiration and swallowing. The penumbra of many linear accelerators when treating small fields can be as large as 1.5 cm, therefore 6 cm fields are often used to treat a T1 glottic cancer (Figure *evolve* 22.57 🖱). A beam directing shell is used to reduce laryngeal and patient movement. The centre of the field (the vocal cords) is usually 1 cm below the thyroid cartilage promontory (the Adam's apple). The position of the vocal cords can be confirmed by screening the patient on a simulator during quiet respiration. Parallel opposed is the most commonly used field configuration. Anterior oblique fields are often useful in patients with short necks and offer a theoretical advantage of a lower dose to the carotid arteries and less subsequent radiation-induced vascular disease. The anterior commissure of the larynx may be close to the skin and in the megavoltage 'build up' area. If this area is involved by tumour, a 1 cm thick wax block has to be placed over the skin above the tumour to ensure the anterior part of the larynx receives a full dose. Dosage schemes in use nationally and internationally range from 50 Gy in 16 fractions to 66 Gy in 33 fractions. The British Institute of Radiology 'short versus long' trial compared a 3-week schedule against a 6-week schedule and showed that, if anything, the complication rate was higher among patients treated over 6 weeks. T2 glottic cancer is treated in a similar way to T1 tumours but often slightly larger fields are used (7 cm in length). Many centres give a slightly higher dose for T2 tumours (52.5 Gy in 16 fractions for T1, 55 Gy for T2 in 20 fractions or 60 Gy in 30 fractions for T1 carcinomas and 60 Gy in 25 fractions for T2 tumours).

Supraglottic carcinoma of larynx

Owing to the fact that supraglottic larynx tumours are more likely to spread to lymph nodes in the neck, some centres advocate prophylactic irradiation of the jugular chain even if there are no palpable lymph nodes or lymph nodes detectable on MRI scanning. Many oncologists incorporate at least the jugulodigastric lymph node within the irradiated volume for part or all of the treatment. This lymph node partially overlies the upper part of the supraglottis (the epiglottis) and it is comparatively easy to include this node within the treatment volume by increasing the length of the treatment field by 2 cm or so. Typical treatment volume for an early supraglottic larynx cancer would stretch from 1 cm beneath the vocal cords to 1 cm above the tip of the epiglottis. Somewhat higher doses are often given to treat supraglottic compared to glottic cancer. In the USA, doses of 70 Gy in 7 weeks are frequently prescribed. In the UK, schedules vary between 50 Gy in 16 fractions to 66 Gy in 33 fractions.

Complications of treatment for early laryngeal cancer

Most patients develop a brisk radiation mucositis towards the end of treatment but this usually resolves within a month. A small number of patients develop persisting laryngeal oedema. This is more common in supraglottic cancers where the incidence can be as high as 25% and more common among heavy smokers. Treatment is by advising cessation of smoking, antibiotics, if there is evidence of infection, and corticosteroids. Persistent severe laryngeal oedema may be a reason for tracheostomy.

Patients with persisting oedema should be carefully examined for persisting recurrent tumour. Laryngeal necrosis is rare with an incidence of <1%.

Advanced (T3 and T4) carcinoma of larynx (Figures *evolve* 22.58–22.64 🖱)

The management of T3 tumours is controversial (Figure *evolve* 22.65 🖱). Some ENT surgeons would say that all T3 cancers should be treated by laryngectomy. Many oncologists would reject this point of view as being too rigid. Patients who are likely to do well with a fixed vocal cord are those with a relatively small bulk of tumour, especially exophytic lesions. Tumours forming deep ulcers, especially bulky transglottic cancers, are best treated by surgery if the patient is fit for laryngectomy. However, some patients with tumours best treated by surgery are unfit for this radical treatment. The most common contraindication to surgery is chronic obstructive airways disease caused by smoking.

Total laryngectomy leads to loss of voice and a permanent tracheostomy. Patients' views with regard to survival and voice preservation differ. Some patients may prefer a trial of radiotherapy then a salvage laryngectomy if radiotherapy fails rather than proceeding to immediate surgery. The only randomized trial in which patients with T3 cancers were randomized to immediate total laryngectomy or radiotherapy followed by surgery yielded a similar 5-year survival of 60% in both arms and two-thirds of irradiated patients retained their larynx.

Unlike patients with T3 lesions, those with large T4 cancers are less likely to be suitable for salvage laryngectomy if radiotherapy fails. Surgery is the treatment of choice for such patients. Again, a minority of T4 patients may have to be treated with radiotherapy or chemoradiotherapy if they are unfit for surgery. Patients with T3 true glottic cancers may be treated with relatively small fields. However, patients with more extensive tumours are often treated in two phases. Phase one incorporates known disease plus possible areas of lymph node spread and phase two concentrates on known disease with a small margin (see Figures *evolve* 22.59–22.65 🖱). Patients are often treated to doses of 66–70 Gy in 6.5–7 weeks, often with concomitant chemotherapy (see below).

Postoperative radiotherapy

Incomplete excision of laryngeal tumour with positive surgical margins is an absolute indication for radiotherapy treatment. Laryngeal cancers can spread outwith the larynx either by infiltration through the thyroid cartilage or through the thyrocricoid membrane into the soft tissues of the neck. Such spread, again, is an indication for postoperative therapy as is extranodal spread. Many oncologists would offer postoperative radiotherapy if there is one lymph node containing metastatic cancer greater than 3 cm or two lymph nodes involved by tumour smaller than 3 cm. Techniques vary, the aim would be to include nodal drainage areas normally anterior to the spinal cord. If there is extensive lymph node involvement, occasionally the posterior triangle nodes need to be included within the treatment volume.

The tracheostomy opening is a potential site for recurrence, especially if the patient has had an emergency tracheostomy or if there is subglottic tumour. The tracheal stoma should be included in all or part of treatment. The radiation reaction though can be brisk around the tracheostomy with soreness, desquamation and occasionally bleeding after doses as low as 40 Gy in 20 fractions. Patients are usually treated with lateral parallel-opposed fields plus a single anterior field to take in the tracheostomy and the lower cervical lymph nodes or anterior and posterior fields. If anterior and posterior fields are used, the neck should be extended to take the parotid glands and oral cavity outwith the treated volume. Differential weightings, such as treating largely from an anterior field (4:1) weighting, are popular in the USA.

Chemotherapy

The vogue, especially in the USA, was to give patients two or three cycles of cisplatin and 5-fluorouracil prior to laryngectomy or radiotherapy. Objective response rates are seen in up to 70% of patients but this shrinkage is not shown in randomized trials to translate into improvement in survival. However, phase II and phase III trials have shown up to 8% improvement in survival of patients with advanced laryngeal cancer who are given concomitant cisplatin-based chemotherapy during radiotherapy. Such regimens are associated with brisk mucositis but, as yet, there is no evidence that they increase late complications.

Results of treatment

Early laryngeal cancers

Some centres report a 5-year survival greater than 90% for patients treated with T1 glottic cancers. Approximately 5% of patients require salvage laryngectomy, even among those with T1 lesions. The need for salvage laryngectomy increases to 10–15% for those with T2 lesions. The overall local control rate is in the order of 80% with 80–85% 5-year survival. Results tend to be slightly inferior for supraglottic lesions. Local control and 5-year survival tends to be 5–10% less than those reported for true glottic cancers.

Advanced laryngeal cancers

It is possible to get 65% 5-year survival with radiotherapy alone in selected T3 glottic cancers. In the past, more advanced transglottic T3 lesions had between a 40–50% survival if treated by radiotherapy alone rising to about 65% if treated by laryngectomy with postoperative radiotherapy

if required. The results of radiotherapy alone can be substantially improved by the administration of concomitant cisplatin chemotherapy.

HYPOPHARYNGEAL CARCINOMA

Anatomy (Figure 22.66)

The hypopharynx extends posterolaterally in relation to the larynx, at the level of the hyoid bone to about the lower level of the cricoid cartilage. The hypopharynx comprises the piriform fossa, the post-cricoid region and the posterior pharyngeal wall and, therefore, cancers of these three regions comprise the hypopharyngeal carcinomas. The piriform fossae (or sinuses) are pear-shaped channels that run alongside the larynx and are adjacent to the inner aspect of the thyroid cartilage. The post-cricoid region is behind the larynx and runs from the arytenoids to the inferior border of the cricoid cartilage. The posterior pharyngeal wall links the floor of the vallecula to the cricoid cartilage (Figure *evolve* 22.67 🖱).

Incidence of hypopharyngeal tumours

Cancers of the hypopharynx are uncommon. There were 450 new cases in the UK in 2004 (CRUK data). These tumours mainly occur in the fifth to seventh decades and are approximately three to four times more common in men than women.

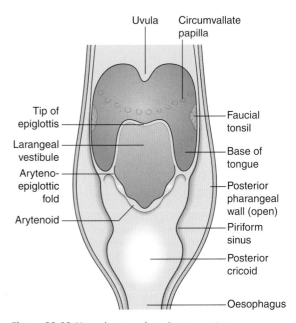

Figure 22.66 Hypopharyngeal carcinoma anatomy.

Staging system of hypopharyngeal tumours

T1   Tumour limited to one subsite and/or measuring ≤2 cm in greatest dimension

T2   Tumour involves more than one subsite of the hypopharynx or an adjacent site, does not fix the hemilarynx and/or measures >2 cm but not >4 cm in greatest dimension

T3   Tumour measures >4 cm in largest dimension or fixes the hemilarynx, or extends into oesophagus

T4a   Tumour invades thyroid/cricoid cartilage, hyoid bone, thyroid gland, oesophagus, central compartment soft tissue

T4b   Tumour invades prevertibral fascia, encases carotid artery, or invades mediastinal structures

Regional lymph nodes are staged as per other head and neck sites.

Aetiology, pathology and lymphatic spread

As with other head and neck cancers, tobacco and alcohol consumption are the most significant risk factors for developing cancers in this region. There are no specific genetic risk factors for this type of tumour. The postcricoid cancers may be associated with iron deficiency anaemia as part of the Plummer-Vinson syndrome.

Tumours of the hypopharynx are rare in the UK but commoner in parts of Europe. Piriform fossa tumours are more prevalent in the Mediterranean regions while postcricoid tumours are commoner in parts of Northern Europe.

Histologically, almost all hypopharyngeal carcinomas are the squamous cell cancers prevalent in the head and neck region.

The hypopharynx has an extensive lymphatic supply (Figure 22.68). The majority of piriform fossae cancers have nodal involvement at presentation. There is early spread to the upper and mid deep cervical nodes (level 2 and 3) but the drainage can include all levels including the supraclavicular nodes. Spread can be bilateral. The posterior pharyngeal wall drains to the retropharyngeal nodes and deep cervical lymph nodes. The post-cricoid region drains to levels 3 and 4 and the paratracheal nodes (level 6). The extensive nodal drainage generally needs to be considered in radiotherapy planning.

Signs and symptoms

Cancers in this region commonly present at an advanced state with sore throat which may radiate to the ear or with painful or difficulty swallowing. There may be hoarseness or haemoptysis. Tumour or ulceration in the hypopharynx can usually be visualized in the clinic via nasendoscopy and FNA or biopsy taken if required.

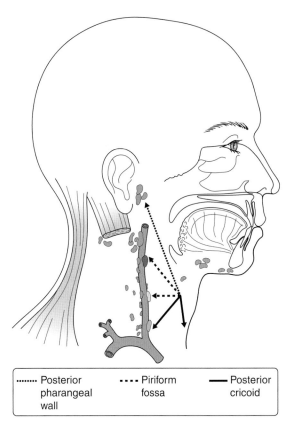

| ······· Posterior pharangeal wall | · · · · Piriform fossa | —— Posterior cricoid |

Figure 22.68 Hypopharynx lymphatic supply.

As with many head and neck cancers, the presentation may be via a neck mass from secondary lymph nodes. In this case, the primary may remain unidentified or visualized at examination under anaesthetic.

Diagnosis and staging

Patients with a history of persistent sore throat should be referred urgently to the ENT clinic. Patients may also be referred urgently for the other symptoms listed above or due to the presence of neck lymphadenopathy.

A full ENT examination is performed in the clinic. This allows delineation of the primary and facilitates exclusion of synchronous tumours. It should include indirect laryngoscopy or fibreoptic examination. The neck should be clinically examined for palpable lymph nodes. Patients should have an examination under anaesthesia and biopsy to confirm the tissue diagnosis. Radiological assessment of the primary is essential for full locoregional staging (Figure 22.69). This may also reveal pathological lymphadenopathy not identified clinically. Imaging of the chest is also essential for exclusion of metastatic spread or synchronous primary tumours of the lung.

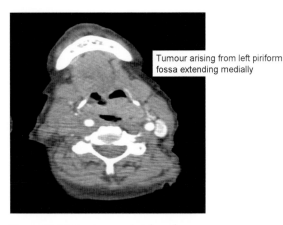

Tumour arising from left piriform fossa extending medially

Figure 22.69 Carcinoma of piriform fossa.

Treatment

Surgery is considered the optimal initial treatment for bulky or T4 tumours in this region and usually involves pharyngo-laryngectomy. In other instances, the aim of organ preservation via treatment with radiotherapy or concurrent chemoradiotherapy should be considered. Tumours of the piriform fossa have two very sinister aspects: they have a great propensity for extensive submucosal spread, and for lymphatic dissemination, and the latter can be bilateral. Postoperative or definitive radiotherapy therefore needs to be extensive and would ordinarily include the retropharyngeal nodes as these are not part of the standard neck dissection and the lower central structures routinely spared with conventional techniques. Patients with nodes managed without initial surgery should be monitored very closely following completion of treatment along the lines discussed for oropharyngeal tumours.

Radiotherapy technique

Patients are treated in supine position and immobilized in the usual fashion. The shell must extend over the shoulders. The shoulders should be held well down as the primary target volume sits relatively low in the neck and would be clipped by standard lateral fields.

A planning CT scan facilitates delineation of the primary tumour and nodes. The intimate relationship between areas of the hypopharynx means that primary CTVs are generally quite large themselves. The choice of nodes to include in the irradiation volume, i.e. the nodal CTV is based on the previous discussion though, in practice, all the nodes in the neck are irradiated. The exception would be small tumours of the piriform fossa, i.e. T1 and low volume T2 with no clinical or radiological evidence of node involvement. In this case, the primary site and immediate draining nodes, i.e. levels 2A and 3 alone, can be irradiated.

Piriform fossa

For small, node-negative T1/T2 tumours of the piriform fossa then the radiotherapy treatment involves treatment of the primary site with upper cervical nodes in an arrangement similar to that for supraglottic tumours, i.e. two lateral fields only. For all other piriform fossae tumours, the 'classical' three-field technique (two parallel-opposed fields to the pharynx and upper neck, with a single anterior field for the lower neck) is widely used.

When using the three-field technique, whereas for many other tumours of the head and neck region, the lower anterior field will conventionally use midline shielding to protect the larynx, hypopharynx, upper oesophagus and spinal cord, the situation is different here. The first three aforementioned are likely to be part of the CTV or to be unavoidable. The propensity of hypopharynx cancer to spread submucosally means that central shielding of the midline in the lower neck could lead to tumour sparing, so the midline shielding must be omitted. Care must now be taken with evaluating dose to the spinal cord. A widely-used convention is that dose from this field is prescribed at a depth of 3 cm. The spinal cord is not many centimetres beyond this, so caution is advised. Unless there is gross disease in the lower neck, it may be preferable to limit the dose from this field to 46 Gy at the 3 cm reference point. There is yet another consideration for cord dose. When no midline shielding is used, the junction of the upper edge of the lower neck anterior field with the lower edge of the laterals can potentially lead to an area of overlap if there is even minor imprecision in set-up. This could lead to a part of the spinal cord receiving far more than 50 Gy, with consequent risk of radiation myelopathy. To prevent this, a small shielding block (or one leaf of a multileaf collimator (MLC)) on the lower posterior corner of the lateral fields is frequently used unless there is gross disease there. This, of course, results in a small area of underdosing, but in a very low-risk area, even in node-positive patients.

Posterior pharyngeal wall tumours

The location of these tumours means that surgery is unlikely to result in complete clearance and is either completely avoided or is conducted in combination with radiotherapy. The volumes irradiated will be similar to piriform fossa tumours, though level 5 can be avoided if node negative simplifying to some extent the delivery technique.

Post-cricoid tumours

In node-negative cancers, treatment is given with radiotherapy to the primary tumour and adjacent nodal areas (levels 3, 4 and 6). The classical set-up is similar to that for subglottic tumours, i.e. two lateral double-wedged fields are used which are angled inferiorly to increase the dose to the lower neck and upper mediastinum. In node-positive patients, the target volumes do not lend themselves to optimal coverage with conventional techniques and surgery to the nodes would ordinarily be carried out in combination with postoperative radiotherapy.

Clearly, IMRT, as discussed in the previous chapter, has great potential at all of these tumour sites both in terms of simplifying delivery approaches and in delivering the full dose as intended to the CTV(s).

Radiotherapy prescriptions will follow the principles in the previous chapter. The large volumes characteristic of these tumour sites do not lend themselves to short fractionation schedules. Concurrent treatment with platinum will generally be an essential component of treatment.

Complications

Treatment results in a predictable acute reaction of mucositis which should be managed as discussed earlier. If patients have not undergone a pharyngolaryngectomy (and hence a stoma), they are at risk of aspiration pneumonia and this should be managed aggressively.

Late complications at this site will include xerostomia because of the need to extend the volume superiorly unless some sparing of the glands is possible by IMRT. Some patients have permanent dysphagia, either secondary to strictures or late damage to nerves and muscles leading to uncoordinated swallowing.

RESULTS

Overall, the prognosis with hypopharyngeal carcinoma is poor. The main reason for this is the advanced stage at diagnosis in the majority of cases. The presence of nodes gives rise to a particularly poor outcome. Most patients succumb to distal metastases, intercurrent illness, or second primaries if locoregional control has been attained. The outcome for tumours diagnosed at an earlier stage is predictably more favourable: treatment of T1 lesions can give rise to local control rates of greater than 85% but with T2 and T3 lesions the control falls to less than 60% translating into 5-year survival rates of about 35%.

For very advanced hypopharyngeal tumours, standard therapy is surgery and postoperative (chemo-) radiation, though the clinician may opt with the patient to manage the condition palliatively in the light of an anticipated poor outcome (10% 5-year survival) and the significant morbidity and mortality from treatment. An organ-preservation approach may be adopted in selected patients. Mature data from an EORTC study of induction chemotherapy followed by radical radiotherapy in responders give credence to this approach, although most patients in this series had T3 disease.

FURTHER READING

Alpert TE, et al. Radiotherapy for the clinically negative neck in supraglottic laryngeal cancer. Cancer Journal 2004;10:335–8.

Agulnik M, et al. State-of-the-art management of nasopharyngeal carcinoma: current and future directions. Br J Cancer 2005;92:799–806.

Al-Sarraf M, et al. Chemoradiotherapy versus radiotherapy in patients with advanced nasopharyngeal cancer: phase III randomized Intergroup study 0099. J Clin Oncol 1998;16:1310–7.

Baujat B, et al. Chemotherapy as an adjunct to radiotherapy in locally advanced nasopharyngeal carcinoma. Otolaryngol Head Neck Surg 2007;137:1–4.

Byers RM, et al. Selective neck dissections for squamous cell carcinoma of the upper aerodigestive tract: patterns of regional failure. Head Neck 1999;21:499–505.

Candela FC, et al. Patterns of cervical node metastases from squamous carcinoma of the oropharynx and

hypopharynx. Head Neck 1990;12:197–203.

Chen SW, et al. Hypopharyngeal cancer treatment based on definitive radiotherapy: who is suitable for laryngeal preservation? J Laryngol Otol Oct 2007;12:1–7.

Claus F, et al. An implementation strategy for IMRT of ethmoid sinus cancer with bilateral sparing of the optic pathways. Int J Radiat Oncol Biol Phys 2001;51:318–31.

Duthoy W, et al. Postoperative intensity-modulated radiotherapy in sinonasal carcinoma. Cancer 2005;104:71–82.

The Department of Veterans Affairs Laryngeal Cancer Study Group. Induction chemotherapy plus radiation compared with surgery plus radiation in patients with advanced laryngeal cancer. N Engl J Med 1991;324:1685–90.

Forastiere AA, et al. Concurrent chemotherapy and radiotherapy for organ preservation in advanced laryngeal cancer. N Engl J Med 2003;349:2091–8.

Garden AS, et al. Early squamous cell carcinoma of the hypopharynx: outcomes of treatment with radiation alone to the primary disease. Head Neck 1996;18:317–22.

Jackson SM, et al. Cancer of the tonsil: results of ipsilateral radiation treatment. Radiother Oncol 1999;51:123–8.

Jones AS, et al. The treatment of early laryngeal cancers (T1–T2N0): Surgery or irradiation? Head Neck 2004;26:127–35.

Lee MS, et al. Treatment results and prognostic factors in locally advanced hypopharyngeal cancer. Acta Otolaryngol 2007;22:1–7.

Kam M, et al. Treatment of nasopharyngeal carcinoma with intensity-modulated radiotherapy: the Hong Kong Experience. Int J Radiat Oncol Biol Phys 2004;60:1440–50.

Levendag PC, et al. Local tumour control in radiation therapy of cancers of the head and neck. Am J Clin Oncol 1996;19:469–77.

Lefebvre JL, et al. Larynx preservation in pyriform sinus cancer: preliminary results of a European Organisation for Research and Treatment of Cancer phase III trial. EORTC Head and Neck Cancer Cooperative Group. J Natl Cancer Inst 1996;88:890–9.

Mazeron JJ, et al. Iridium 192 implantation of T1 and T2 squamous cell carcinomas of the mobile tongue. Int J Radiat Oncol Biol Phys 1990;19:1369–76.

O'Sullivan B, et al. The benefits and pitfalls of ipsilateral radiotherapy in carcinoma of the tonsillar region. Int J Radiat Oncol Biol Phys 2001;51:332–43.

Orus C, et al. Initial treatment of the early stages (I,II) of supraglottic squamous cell carcinoma: partial laryngectomy versus radiotherapy. Eur Arch Otorhinologol 2000;257:512–6.

Parsons TJ, et al. Squamous cell carcinoma of the oropharynx: surgery, radiation therapy, or both. Cancer 2002;94:2967–80.

Scola B, et al. Management of cancer of the supraglottis. Otolaryngol Head Neck Surg 2001;124:195–8.

Shah JP, et al. The patterns of cervical lymph node metastases from squamous carcinoma of the oral cavity. Cancer 1990;66:109–13.

Varghese C, et al. Predictors of neck node control in radically irradiated squamous cell carcinoma of the oropharynx and laryngopharynx. Head Neck 1993;15:105–8.

Wendt CD, et al. Primary radiotherapy in the treatment of stage I and II tongue cancers: importance of the proportion therapy delivered with interstitial therapy. Int J Radiat Oncol Biol Phys 1990;18:1529–30.

EVOLVE CONTENTS (available online at: http://evolve.elsevier.com/Symonds/radiotherapy/)

Chapter | 23 |

Thyroid cancer

Ujjal Mallick, Joyce Wilkinson, Charles Kelly

INTRODUCTION AND EPIDEMIOLOGY

Thyroid cancer is a spectrum of tumours characterized by different biology and clinical behaviour. The presence of a micropapillary carcinoma of thyroid may have little impact on life expectancy, whereas anaplastic thyroid cancer is often lethal. While this disease is uncommon, representing only about 1% of all cancers, thyroid cancer is the most frequently occurring endocrine malignancy and incidence of Papillary thyroid cancer is increasing. It is the fastest rising cancer in men and women in the United states. In excess of 2100 new cases each year in the UK and over 48,000 in the United States. The incidence is increasing worldwide (213,000 new cases in 2008) including a 2.6-fold increase in the USA 1973–2006.

Differentiated thyroid cancer is highly curable (about 95% or more five year survival) and can also affect children, young adults. Thyroid cancer should be treated by a multi-disciplinary team of experts.

ANATOMY

The thyroid gland is situated in the anterior part of the neck just above the clavicle and sternum (Figure 23.1). The gland consists of a right and left lobe joined by an isthmus which crosses the trachea at the second and third cartilaginous rings. The average weight of the thyroid gland is 20 g. The parathyroid glands lie on the posterior surface of both thyroid lobes and the recurrent laryngeal nerves are in a cleft between the trachea and the oesophagus. Lymphatic drainage from the thyroid can be to nodes superior to

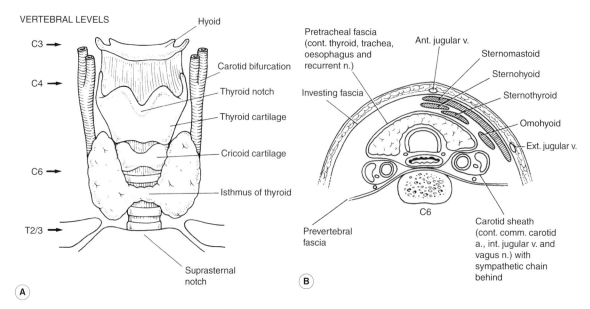

Figure 23.1 (A) Structures palpable on the anterior aspect of the neck, together with corresponding vertebral levels. *(Redrawn from Ellis, Clinical Anatomy, 5th edn, Blackwells, 1975)*. (B) Transverse section of the neck through C6 showing the relations of the thyroid gland. *(Reproduced with permission from Ellis, Clinical Anatomy, 5th edn, Blackwells, 1975)*.

the thyroid gland, lateral to the gland and to the paratracheal region.

ETIOLOGICAL FACTORS

Thyroid cancer shows two age-related peaks of incidence, one before the age of 40 and one after 60. The condition is approximately three times as common in women than men. Exposure to ionizing radiation in childhood, either therapeutic, such as radiotherapy for Hodgkin's disease, or associated with environmental exposure, increases the risk of developing thyroid cancer. There is, however, no proven relationship between the development of thyroid cancer and administration of iodine-131 for the treatment of hyperthyroidism.

Other medical conditions which affect the thyroid have also been linked with an increased risk in developing thyroid cancer, namely, endemic goiter, which occurs in areas where there is low natural iodine, Hashimoto's thyroiditis, a past history of thyroid adenoma or a family history of thyroid adenoma or cancer. Some genetic conditions which increase the risk of thyroid cancer include Gardener syndrome, Cowden's syndrome, familial adenomatous polyposis and the multiple endocrine neoplasia syndromes.

Thyroid cancer initiation and progression is supposed to be through accumulation of genetic and epigenetic events. It point mutations of BRAF (Predominantly Papillary) and RAS (N,H,K-Ras Predominantly Follicular) genes and Chromosomal rearrangements-RET/PTC-(Papillary particularly radiation induced), PAX8/PPARγ (Follicular); abnormal miRNAs' (microRNA) with gene methylation problems also play its part. All these are now being detected on Fine needle aspiration cytology. This will avoid diagnostic lobectomies for indeterminate and benign nodules in the future protecting patients from unnecessary surgery as well as allowing one-stage total thyroidectomy for cancer patients (instead of lobectomy followed by total thyroidectomy in Thy3 cases) and saving costs. P53 mutations are thought to be a late event in progression from differentiated to Anaplstic thyroid cancer in a high proportion of cases.

PRESENTATION, DIAGNOSIS AND PATIENT PATHWAY

The most common presenting feature is a painless, lower neck lump in the thyroid area which may or may not have been noted to have increased in size. In more advanced cases, patients may complain of a lump on the side of the neck due to spread to lymph nodes, hoarseness or change in voice suggesting recurrent laryngeal nerve involvement, stridor or, rarely, dysphagia. A rapid enlargement of the mass or a rapid development of symptoms, suggesting compression of other structures, may be due to a more rapidly growing anaplasic carcinoma or Lymphoma.

In the first instance, the patient should be referred to an ENT or general surgeon with a particular interest and experience in managing thyroid cancer. A history of the development of the mass, any relevant personal past history or family history of thyroid problems is important. Examination is undertaken to define whether the mass is solitary or multiple, whether it is tender, which might suggest a benign cause, and whether the mass is fixed to the skin or to underlying structures in the neck. Any enlarged lymph nodes within the neck are noted. Development of stridor is a medical emergency, demanding urgent hospital admission.

Ultrasound and Fine Needle Aspiration Cytology (FNAC) are essential for neck masses suspected of being a thyroid cancer. Ultrasound guidance may help in obtaining the aspiration cytology and can help to distinguish solid from cystic masses in the neck. It can differentiate between solitary and multiple nodules, helps to detect involved lymphnodes (if needed by guided FNAC) and can provide sonographic features suggesting probable malignancy in some cases.

Follicular cancers cannot be differentiated from adenomas on FNAC alone as evidence of invasion is required and lobectomy is usually necessary. If FNA cytology is not helpful, it should be repeated and, if this is still inconclusive, thyroid lobectomy should be performed to obtain enough tissue for diagnosis. There are no indications for an incisional biopsy of the thyroid, which might compromise future therapeutic interventions.

Radioactive iodine scans can rarely help differentiate non-functioning 'cold' nodules within the thyroid, which may represent a malignancy, from 'hot' nodules which rarely contain a cancer, but usually these scans are not helpful with diagnosis, and are much more useful in the postoperative period for diagnosing residual disease or early recurrence.

Computed tomography (CT) and magnetic resonance imaging (MRI) scans are not routinely required but can help show the local extent of spread, detailing involvement of lymph nodes and other neck structures.

Thyroid function tests, which are usually normal in patients with thyroid cancer, calcium, phosphate and thyroglobulin can be sampled for baseline measurement, but thyroglobulin level is not useful in the preoperative phase. If there is any suspicion that the thyroid tumour may be a medullary cancer, then the calcitonin level is checked.

Staging is performed using the TNM system which is summarized in Table 23.1. All anaplastic carcinomas are considered T4 tumours.

One major disadvantage of the TNM system is that the presence of positive nodes does not necessarily give a worse prognosis, consequently making this staging system less useful in the practical setting than at other cancer sites.

In addition to the TNM system, there are other risk categorisation systems. 'AMES', based on *a*ge, distant *m*etastasis, tumour *e*xtent and tumour *s*ize.

This system defines high-risk patients as:

- distant metastasis present
- men >40 or women >50 years with either extrathyroid capsule spread *or* tumour size >5 cm.

Table 23.1 TNM staging system

T1	Tumour <=2 cm, intrathyroidal
T1a	<=1 cm
T1b	1-2 cm
T2	Tumour >2-4 cm, intrathyroidal
T3	Tumour >4 cm on with minimal extra-thyroid extension
T4	Tumour extending beyond the thyroid capsule
T4a	Subcutaneous tissue, larynx, trachea, R L Nerve. Oesophagus
T4b	Prevertebral fascia, mediatinal vessels, carotid artery
N0	No regional lymph node involvement
N1	Regional lymph node involvement
N1a	Level VI
N1b	Other regional
M0	No distant metastasis
M1	Distant metastasis present

Low-risk patients are described as:

- men equal to or less than 40 years (women 50 years)
- if older, primary tumour <5 cm *and* confined to thyroid.

Another system which gives prognostic information is the MACIS scoring scheme developed at the Mayo Clinic (Table 23.2).

DIFFERENTIATED THYROID CANCER

These tumours are divided into papillary and follicular thyroid cancers and are distinguished by their behavior, as they are sensitive to thyroid stimulating hormone (TSH), take up iodine and can produce thyroglobulin. All three of these factors are used in their management. It should be remembered that, in general, differentiated thyroid cancer carries a very good prognosis, with 20-year survival of over 85% in those patients who do not develop distant metastasis.

Papillary thyroid cancer is the most common type of thyroid cancer, accounting for almost 80% of all cases and its incidence is increasing world wide. These tumours are also derived from the follicular cells of the thyroid, and may show psammoma bodies, small flecks of calcification, on microscopy. The distinctive feature of these tumours is that they have characteristic nuclei (Orphan-Annie appearance) and they seem to grow in branching stocks (the so-called papillae). These tumours are often multifocal and

Table 23.2 MACIS score (Mayo Clinic)	
M	Metastases
A	Age
C	Completeness of resection
I	Invasion
S	Size

MACIS SCORE			
3.1 (if aged ≤ 39) or 0.08 × age (if aged ≥ 40 years)			
0.3 × tumour size in centimeters			
		+	
+1 (if incompletely resected)			
		+	
+1 (if locally invasive)			
		+	
+3 (if distant metastasis present)			
With this scoring system the 20-year cause specific survival using the MACIS score is			
Score	<6	6–6.99	7–7.9a

they can show more local extension and cervical node involvement and less tendency to haematogenous spread when compared to follicular cancers. Papillary carcinoma is three times more common in women than men with a peak incidence in the third to fourth decade of life.

Follicular thyroid cancer makes up about 10% of thyroid malignancy. It generally affects a slightly older age group than papillary cancer and tends to involve the neck nodes less. Follicular carcinomas are often solitary within the thyroid gland, have a marked tendency to invade the vascular channels and to spread via the bloodstream to distant sites.

Management of differentiated thyroid cancer

The aims of treatment are the removal of all thyroid cancer and any remaining normal thyroid tissue by surgery and radio-iodine treatment and the suppression of TSH by

T3 (triiodothyronine) or T4 (thyroxine). Successful treatment should result in an undetectable thyroglobulin level and no clinical, radiological or radio-iodine uptake scan evidence of thyroid cancer.

Surgery

Surgery is required for all thyroid cancer, if operable (except Lymphoma). If differentiated thyroid carcinoma >1 cm in size is confirmed, total thyroidectomy or near total thyroidectomy, with preservation of the recurrent laryngeal nerves and at least some of the parathyroid glands, should be carried out depending on diagnostic findings. Total lobectomy alone is indicated rarely in <1 cm or very low risk tumours. Surgical should be individualised and based on clinical, sonographic, staging and cytology findings.

Nomenclature currently used for diagnostic categorization is the Thy 1, Thy 2 etc. system, and can be found in the 'Guidelines for the management of Thyroid Cancer in Adults' published by the British Thyroid Association and the Royal College of Physicians of London. This system can be summarized as shown in Table 23.3. Further refinements of this system into Thy3a (atypia) and Thy3f (Follicular lesion) have been proposed recently.

Total thyroidectomy or near total thyroidectomy is required for follicular or papillary carcinoma >1 cm, familial papillary microcancers, multifocal cancers and in patients who have had previous neck radiation. During this procedure, at least one parathyroid gland is left behind but, even then, approximately one-third of patients will develop temporary symptomatic hypocalcemia.

Indications for lobectomy alone are exceptional, including follicular or papillary carcinoma less than 1 cm, where total lobectomy with TSH suppression by thyroxine is adequate.

Table 23.3 British Thyroid Association coding system	
Thy1	Non-diagnostic; FNAC needs repeating
Thy2	Non-neoplastic; two diagnostic tests with benign results with 3–6 months apart are needed to exclude malignancy
Thy3	All follicular lesions; lobectomy required with completion thyroidectomy if malignant histology
Thy4	Abnormal, suspicious but not diagnostic of any histological form of thyroid cancer; Treatment required depending on histology
Thy5	Diagnostic of thyroid malignancy; surgery required for differentiated thyroid cancer, other management may be more appropriate if other forms of malignancy
FNAC: fine needle aspiration cytology	

If there is lateral cervical neck node involvement, then a selective radical neck dissection should be considered. Removal of single nodes is inadequate treatment. Central neck node removal (level VI nodes), can be considered with or near total thyroidectomy in appropriate cases.

Radio-iodine ablation

This is recommended following surgery in many as it helps monitoring by measuring thyroglobulin, and might reduce recurrence and improve survival in high and intermediate risk cases patients with differentiated thyroid cancer by destroying any remaining microscopic foci of thyroid carcinoma cells. It destroys any remaining normal thyroid tissue and any rise in serum thyroglobulin following ablation should only suggest tumour recurrence, thereby helping earlier detection and treatment of recurrent disease. If there is a large thyroid remnant remaining, further surgery may be appropriate.

In some centres, the patient undergoes a postoperative radio-iodine uptake scan using iodine-123 to show any thyroid-derived tissue remaining. Iodine-131 is generally avoided so as not to interfere with the later ablation dose. This is followed by radio-iodine remnant ablation where the patient is usually given a dose of 3700 MBq of ^{131}I in the first instance. Thyroxin (T4) or usually triiodothyronine (T3) are withdrawn before radio-iodine to ensure TSH levels are >30 mu/l to enhance the uptake of ^{131}I.

Patients are discharged home when total body radioactivity has fallen below the permitted levels. The dose rate from the patient in mSeiverts is measured at 1 meter on each day of their hospital stay following administration of radio-iodine, these points are plotted on a graph, and future levels over the next few days are extrapolated.

Typical permissible doses are as follows: patients are allowed home using private transport when the dose rate from the patient has fallen to 40 mSieverts/hour. Use of public transport is only permitted when the dose emitted by the patient has fallen to 20 mSieverts. Patients are advised to avoid public gatherings such as going to the cinema or church, close contact with family members or journeys on public transport lasting longer than an hour until a level of 7.5 mSieverts per hour has been reached. Patients should not have close contact with children, pregnant women or go to work until the extrapolated level is 1.5 mSieverts/hour.

All patients require thyroid hormone replacement and can recommence thyroid hormone replacement with either thyroxine (T4). Thyroxine (T4) has the advantage of being given as a once daily tablet and gives more optimal suppression of TSH. The initial dose of T4 is usually 200 µg daily, which is altered depending on TSH measurements. As the half-life of T3 is shorter than T4 (thyroxine), it is easier to stop and then restart while the patient is undergoing scanning or radio-iodine treatment. The aim of thyroid replacement is twofold. The first is to replace the natural hormone produced by the gland and the second is to suppress the patient's thyroid stimulating hormone (TSH). This is produced in the pituitary gland, and can stimulate well differentiated tumours as well as any thyroid remnant. The target TSH level for suppression is <0.1 mU/L.

The patient has a further radio-iodine diagnostic scan, 4–6 months after ablation and, if any residual thyroid tissue still remains, the patient may require further treatment doses. If the 6-month challenge scan shows no evidence of any remnant of thyroid tissue, the patient does not require further radio iodine diagnostic (RAIS) scans and can be monitored clinically and by thyroglobulin level. Regular RAIS are being replaced in low risk cancers by thyroglobulin assessment only after recombinant human TSH injections and neck ultrasound (+/− FNAC).

If radio-iodine uptake scans are required, the patient must discontinue thyroxine 4 weeks prior to the scan. T3 can then be substituted for 2 weeks and discontinued 2 weeks before the scan. Many patients understandably complain of lethargy and other symptoms of severe hypothyroidism during this period when their replacement thyroid hormone is removed. These symptoms can be countered by the use of 'Thyrogen' (recombinant human TSH), which does not interfere with the challenge scan and allows the patient to continue with T4 treatment.

^{131}I therapy can cause some discomfort and swelling in the neck. This can be treated by a short course of steroids. Sialoadenitis, (inflammation of the salivary glands) can occur because of the preferential iodine uptake by these glands. Radiation cystitis from excretion of radio-iodine is also possible but both these are uncommon. Replacement thyroxine is restarted 2 days after any radio-iodine diagnostic (if no further treatment is planned), remnant ablation or treatment scan. Before any radioactive iodine is given, pregnancy should be excluded and patients advised to avoid pregnancy for one year after ^{131}I ablation or treatment. The usual dose for ablation is 3.7 GBq.

There is a small dose-related risk of developing leukaemia following treatment with radio-iodine. This risk increases with cumulative doses greater than 18.5 GBq and if the patient also has external beam radiotherapy to the neck. Patients who receive cumulative injections of ^{131}I do have a higher risk of developing second malignancies, for example bladder and salivary gland, as a consequence of the treatment. The total dose should be kept to <40 GBq in any individual patient and, as with any radiation, the total cumulative dose should be kept as low as possible.

Thyroid ablation is considered for many patients with tumours greater than 1 cm. There is a minority school of thought, particularly in the USA, that argues that radio-iodine ablation is only advised in high-risk patients and that in the low-risk group, optimal surgery with full TSH suppression should be sufficient. In this context, high-risk patients would be defined as having a primary tumour greater than 5 cm or with extra thyroid spread, extensive nodal or presence of distant metastasis. Trials are being designed to address this.

Thyroglobulin

Monitoring serum thyroglobulin level after radio-iodine ablation is a sensitive marker for recurrence, especially if the level rises after thyroxine replacement is withdrawn or recombinant human TSH is used to raise the TSH level to above 30 mU/L. It is important to know if antibodies to thyroglobulin are present as this may compromise the test (upto 25% of patients). Thyroglobulin levels are considered unreliable within 3 months of thyroidectomy. During follow up, one difficult diagnostic situation that can arise is the patient who develops rising levels of serum thyroglobulin with no positive radioactive iodine scan. Further investigations with CT, MRI or positron emission tomography (PET-CT) scanning may show suspected recurrent disease which does not take up iodine but can be treated with surgery or radiotherapy or newer targeted treatment. Empirical treatment with ^{131}I followed by a scan a few days later may show disease not seen on a normal uptake scan and was not infrequently used in the past. If the thyroglobulin level is slightly elevated but not rising, a watch and wait policy can be undertaken as it can spontaneously disappear over time.

Management of hypocalcemia

Transient hypocalcemia is relatively common after thyroidectomy, with 30% of patients needing some form of calcium supplementation. This drops to only 2% of patients requiring supplements at 3 months. Calcium levels can be checked postoperatively and calcium supplements started and titrated, as required, with the addition of α-calcidol if no improvement in serum calcium level with calcium supplements alone. Patients need to continue to be monitored for serum calcium level until this has stabilized.

Management of Loco regional recurrence

Up to 20% of patients may develop locoregional recurrence, usually signaled by a rising thyroglobulin or clinically recurrent disease detectable on ultrasound (or rarely other cross sectional imaging) or palpable in the neck. These patients may remain curable, with appropriate intervention. If operable, surgery should be considered as the first salvage procedure offered. Postoperatively, or if the recurrence is inoperable, and a radio-iodine uptake scan is positive, further radio-iodine therapy is appropriate. These patients obviously require further close monitoring, with clinical examination, thyroglobulin levels, and further radio-iodine ultrasound or other scans. If the locoregional recurrence is inoperable, or salvage surgery has been incomplete and the recurrent tumour does not take up radio-iodine, then external beam radiotherapy is an option.

Metastatic disease

Ten percent of patients will develop metastatic disease, usually to the lungs or bones. These metastatic sites may show radio-iodine uptake and respond to radioactive iodine therapy doses. Usually, higher radio-iodine doses are given for metastatic disease than for initial ablation, e.g. 5000 MBq. Even with initial iodine uptake, these metastatic sites may become radio-iodine uptake negative. In recent years palliative molecular targeted therapy with Sorafenib, sunitinib etc have been shown to improve progression free survival in these iodine refractory cases and are preferred than toxic chemotherapy which is rarely effective. These small molecule drugs are simple tablets which inhibit Receptor Tyrosine and Serine Threonine Kinase and pathways inside the cell via specific cancer cell membrane receptors. This prevents tumour growth, invasion and spread and increases cell death or apoptosis. Further palliative treatment consists of local radiotherapy to sites of bony pain, with orthopedic intervention.

Overall, the prognosis in differentiated thyroid cancer is generally good with 10-year survival figures for papillary cancer being over 90% and for follicular tumours over 85%. Prognosis is worse in the elderly or in the very young patient and men have a worse prognosis than women. Extra-thyroid invasion, vascular invasion, metastases at diagnosis and large size of primary tumour are all bad prognostic features. Surprisingly, lymph node metastases in the neck at the time of diagnosis have less effect on long-term survival if completely resected.

Survival of patients with metastatic well-differentiated thyroid cancer can be surprisingly good. In one series from the Royal Marsden Hospital London, 54% of patients with disease confined to the lungs were alive and free of disease 10 years after radio-iodine treatment. No patients with bone involvement which is difficult to eradicate with radioiodine alone survived longer than 8 years. The group of patients with distant metastases who have the best prognosis, are those who are female, under 45 years of age and have small miliary metastasis in the lungs which take up radio-iodine. A French series reported a 15-year survival of 89% in the subgroup of patients.

MEDULLARY THYROID CANCER (MTC)

Derived from parafollicular C cells, which produce calcitonin, these cancers are part of a familial endocrine cancer syndrome in 25% of the patients who develop this form of thyroid cancer. MTC is sporadic, without a familial component in 75% of cases. Not all patients with the inherited form give a positive family history as the condition can skip generations. These familial syndromes can be broadly divided into three.

Familial medullary thyroid cancer can occur by itself and is inherited in an autosomal dominant pattern and is associated with a mutation in the RET proto-oncogene. If this mutation is present, then almost 100% of patients will develop medullary thyroid cancer. If it occurs by itself without other endocrine neoplasia, the thyroid cancer may behave in a more indolent manner than when it appears as a part of the multiple endocrine neoplasia syndromes (MEN). It is also a component of the familial syndromes, MEN 2A, (also known as Sipple syndrome) and MEN 2B. Patients may develop pheochromocytoma in both 2A and 2B, hyperparathyroidism in MEN 2A, and ganglioneuromatosis in MEN 2B. Medullary thyroid cancer may occur relatively early in MEN 2B and be more aggressive.

Patients with any of these syndromes should be offered prophylactic thyroidectomy while still young, before medullary thyroid cancer develops. As this condition is potentially inheritable, patients and family members should be offered genetic testing with the local clinical genetics service after appropriate counselling, detailing the implications of positive or negative test results, for them and their relatives.

Diagnosis in this type of thyroid cancer can be made with FNA cytology. An elevated serum calcitonin helps confirm the diagnosis. Patients presenting with these tumours require screening for the other potential components of these familial syndromes, with CT and/or MRI of the neck, chest and abdomen. These cases should be treated by specialist teams including a surgeon, endocrinologist, geneticist, oncologist etc. in cancer centres for their rarity.

In those patients who present with this thyroid cancer, the majority will have positive neck nodes at presentation and so require total thyroidectomy with selective radical neck dissection. Adjuvant radiotherapy is rarely indicated. Serum calcitonin levels are used postoperatively for monitoring potential recurrence. Monitoring can be improved by using a pentagastrin-stimulated calcitonin evaluation. Radioactive iodine has no effect in these tumours.

If recurrent medullary cancer presents, then further surgery should be used, if possible. If surgery is not possible, high dose external beam radiotherapy may be considered in selected cases. In recent years targeted therapy with Vandetanib and Sorafenib are showing some benefit in progression free survival. Palliative chemotherapy, using a variety of agents in combination, has also been tried but not very effective.

ANAPLASTIC THYROID CANCER

Anaplastic tumours are less common making up less than 5% of thyroid malignancy but carry a much worse prognosis than differentiated thyroid cancer. Anaplastic carcinoma develops from the follicular cells. This rare tumour occurs in older patients who present with a rapidly growing mass in the neck. The trachea and oesophagus are frequently involved at an early stage leading to dysphagia, dysponea and, later, stridor. The voice may be hoarse because of infiltration of the laryngeal nerves and subsequent vocal cord palsies. Neck node involvement and metastatic spread, usually to the lung, are relatively common. Diagnosis is done with FNAC, core biopsy or very rarely open biopsy.

Patients usually have advanced disease at presentation and tend to be older and more frail than other thyroid cancer patients. In a small minority, surgery with total thyroidectomy and radical neck dissection may be possible. In the majority, surgery is either impossible or inappropriate and management is with external beam radiotherapy with or without concurrent chemotherapy. Anaplastic thyroid cancers, however, can show a variable radio-sensitivity with some tumours continuing to enlarge, even while undergoing radiotherapy.

Palliative chemotherapy with Adriamycin with or without cisplatin is also used. Median survival for this condition is usually between 6 and 9 months from diagnosis.

THYROID LYMPHOMA

These are non-Hodgkin's B-cell lymphomas of varying grade and can be associated with Hashimoto's thyroiditis. They usually present as an enlarging thyroid mass. Core biopsy is often required in addition to FNA cytology to determine the grade and type of lymphoma. Majority are high grade diffuse large B-cell lymphomas although low grade tumours do occur. Once a diagnosis of lymphoma has been made, staging is as for other extra nodal sites for lymphoma, with CT scan covering all the potential nodal and extra-nodal lymphoma sites, and marrow examination. Treatment is usually postoperative chemotherapy and radiotherapy or radiotherapy only to the neck with excellent long term survival.

THYROID SARCOMA

These tumours are uncommon, but can be difficult to distinguish from anaplastic thyroid cancer or sarcomatoid variants of differentiated thyroid cancers. As they are radio-iodine insensitive, treatment is with surgery and external beam radiotherapy.

HURTHLE CELL CARCINOMA

These tumours consist of eosinophilic Hurthle cells and have been thought to be variant of follicular carcinoma and stage for stage behave as such; however, some believe it is more aggressive than the other differentiated forms, with a higher incidence of recurrence and metastatic spread and a reduced 5-year survival because it does not usually take up radio-iodine (10% of cases).

EXTERNAL BEAM RADIOTHERAPY FOR THYROID CANCER

External beam radiotherapy (EBRT), although not used frequently, does have a role in all histological types of thyroid cancer. Its main role is in Differentiated Thyroid cancer (DTC), Anaplastic thyroid cancer and lymphoma. In medullary thyroid cancer it has a limited but defined role. In DTC according to UK BTA (2007) Guidelines the indications are:

As adjuvant treatment:

 i gross evidence of local tumour invasion at surgery, presumed to have significant macro or microscopic residual disease, particularly if the residual tumour fails to concentrate sufficient amounts of radioiodine

 ii extensive pT4 disease in patients over 60 years of age with extensive extranodal spread after optimal surgery, even in the absence of evident residual disease.

High-dose external beam radiotherapy as part of primary treatment:

 i unresectable tumours that do not concentrate radioactive iodine

 ii unresectable bulky tumours in addition to radioactive iodine treatment.

Palliative high dose

High-dose palliative external beam radiotherapy for recurrent neck disease uncontrolled by surgery and ^{131}I therapy.

Low dose palliation

Spinal cord compression
Stridor
Superior vena caval obstruction
Cerebral metastases with or without surgery
Solitary or limited number of bone metastases along with surgery etc if appropriate
Dysphagia
Bleeding tumour etc.

If palliative high dose treatment is to be given, a polyfoam or orfit head support, or similar, can be made for patient immobilization, but if radical or adjuvant radiotherapy is required, a customized beam directional shell (BDS) is preferable. Localization and treatment plan generation are done with a planning CT scan, with the patient planned and treated in a supine position, with the cervical spine as straight as possible. For large anterior and posterior parallel-opposed fields, used

for phase I of radical/adjuvant treatment, or in palliative treatments, the fields may be defined on a conventional simulator or virtual simulator (Figure evolve 23.2🖰).

The anatomical boundaries for the planning treatment volume are:

- tip of the mastoid process, superiorly
- the carina, inferiorly
- laterally to include the supraclavicular fossae (Figures evolve 23.3 and 23.4🖰).

This volume includes the thyroid bed and adjacent relevant lymph node drainage areas. The length of cervical and upper thoracic spinal cord should be noted as an organ at risk. This technique is appropriate for many ATC with poor prognosis in frail patients with a typical dose of 30 Gy/10 fractions.

For radical or adjuvant treatment, specially for DTC and MTC conformal 3D CT-based planning to cover the thyroid bed and level II to level VII nodes are usually required for phase 1. Subsequently a phase II planning target volume (PTV) is defined, encompassing the thyroid bed and immediate lymph nodes, as well as areas of residual disease which should be included in the high dose volume with usually about a 2 cm margin. In appropriate cases, the superior margin could be at the hyoid bone and the inferior margin at the suprasternal notch to reduce side effects (Figures evolve 23.5 and 23.6🖰).

3-D conformal treatment fields are used in this situation, with the PTV extending posteriorly, on both sides of the cord, encompassing the whole of the thyroid bed and lymph nodes (Figure evolve 23.7🖰). CT-based localization and planning allow summation of both phases, showing overall dose to the PTV and the organs at risk, in this case the spinal cord.

The maximum acceptable spinal cord dose should not exceed 46 Gy in 23 fractions if more than 20 cm of spinal cord is included in the treatment field. Lung and mandible shielding is also used, with either customized blocks or multileaf collimators.

The dose given for phase I, using a photon beam of adequate megavoltage energy, is 40–44 gy in 20–22 fractions, treated daily × 5 fractions per week.

For phase II, the dose is 20–22 Gy in 10–11 fractions, treated daily × 5 fractions per week.

In all treatments, dose is prescribed at the isocentre (ICRU reference point).

If the PTV extends into the upper mediastinum, then oblique fields can be tilted caudally by use of couch rotation, so that the field enters superiorly to the shoulder region (Figure evolve 23.8🖰).

If both the neck and superior mediastinum are treated, then the patient contour can change significantly in the longitudinal plane, and may require compensation in the caudal-cephalic axis.

Problems in planning occur when the PTV extends posteriorly to include the thyroid bed and nodes producing a concave volume which surrounds the spinal cord (see Figure *evolve* 23.7 🖱). A forward planned technique using anterior and posterior oblique fields with differential wedging and beam weights can be used to conform to a concave volume, however, the dose to the spinal cord is close to cord tolerance. Figure *evolve* 23.9 🖱 shows a four-field technique, with the spinal cord receiving 78% dose.

IMRT (Intensity Modulated Radio Therapy) provides a solution where the PTV curves around an organ at risk such as spinal cord, producing the desired concave volume, and improving dose distributions for thyroid cancer (Figure *evolve* 23.10 🖱). It is now fairly standard in many large centres in the UK and else where for high dose radical or adjuvant therapy for DTC, MTC and some good performance status ATC.

IMRT can achieve steep dose gradients between high dose PTV and nearby normal tissues. This allows improved protection of Organs At Risk (OAR) such as Spinal cord and Parotids, Pharyngeal constrictors etc while achieving dose escalation to tumour bearing target volumes. The planning process is called is Inverse Planning. Here the primary high dose volume (e.g. CTV1 intended dose 60–66 Gy), Prophylactic dose volumes (e.g. CTV2, delineating microscopic lymph node areas according to published concensus guidelines-intended dose 54 Gys) and OARS (spinal cord dose constraint 46 Gy, Parotid Median <24 Gy etc) are outlined. The planning system then by several iterations find out the best acceptable plan to meet these constraints. This produces superior and more optimal dose distribution and less early and late side effects and better quality of life due to improved OAR sparing confirmed by published trials. On going studies are looking at potentially better local control and survival due to dose escalation.

IMRT is a complex technique which relies on trained staff and is also more time intensive. IMRT can also be used to create plans delivering a concomitant boost to specific areas for dose escalation without extending treatment time.

It is ideally suited for Head and Neck, Thyroid, Prostate cancers and others. (Figures *evolve* 23.11– 23.13 🖱).

In the past, there was a vogue for treating thyroid cancers with a single anterior high energy electron field (20–30 MeV). Appropriate bolus was attached to the anterior immobilization shell (Figure 23.14). The disadvantage with this technique is that the upper mediastinum cannot be adequately treated, the dose distribution is not optimal and cosmesis is poor due to the high skin electron dose.

A minority of patients suffering from anaplastic cancers with good performance status (0-2), no distant metastases and a higher life expectancy may be treated to 60–66 gy using techniques described above with or without concurrent chemotherapy as definitive or neoadjuvant and adjuvant treatments along with surgery. However, the majority are treated by simpler palliative techniques. Parallel-opposed anterior and posterior fields are used with doses of 30 Gy given in 10 fractions. The apices of the lungs are usually shielded by multileaf collimators or lead blocks.

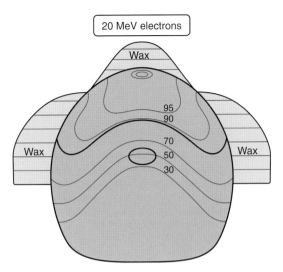

Figure 23.14 20 MeV electron field.

For palliation of symptoms for metastatic or recurrent cancers 30 Gy/10 F (fraction), OR 20 Gy/5 F or 8 Gy/1 F can be used depending on the situation.

Radiotherapy for thyroid lymphoma

This is usually given after four cycles of chemotherapy, using for example, the CHOP-Rituximab chemotherapy regimen. The anatomical PTV is as for other thyroid tumours, but nowadays only the volume on presentation with a margin (involved field) is usually preferred. The dose is usually about 30–40 Gys in 15–20 fractions for diffuse high grade lymphomas after chemotherapy. The lower dose is preferred for complete responders. Anterior and posterior, parallel-opposed fields are used. Rarely, where the lymphoma is low-grade, a midplane dose of 24–30 Gys are used in daily 2 grays/fractions without any chemotherapy 35 Gy in 20 fractions is used. The maximum acceptable spinal cord dose is no more than 40 Gy.

FOLLOW-UP POLICY FOR THYROID CANCER PATIENTS

It is now regarded as good practice to follow up patients who have developed differentiated thyroid cancer for life. This is because long-term survival is the rule, but patients are still at risk of developing late curable locoregional recurrence or treatable metastatic disease. These patients also require management of the TSH suppression (long term suppression can have cardiac effects and increased risk of osteoporosis), and potential calcium metabolism problems. They are also followed up because they have a small risk of developing second malignancies related to Radioiodine treatment. At each visit, patients are examined clinically, blood samples taken for thyroid function tests, thyroglobulin and Thyroglobulin antibody and a calcium screen if appropriate. Arrangements can be made for ultrasound, other imaging and radioiodine uptake scans.

FURTHER READING

Cooper DS, Doherty GM, Haugen BR, et al. Revised American Thyroid Association management guidelines for patients with thyroid nodules and differentiated thyroid cancer. Thyroid 2009;19:1167–214.

British Thyroid Association. Royal College of Physicians. Guidelines for the management of thyroid cancer. Second edition. 2007.

Powell C, Newbold K, Harrington KJ, Bhide SA, Nutting CM. External Beam Radiotherapy for Differentiated Thyroid Cancer. Special Issue Thyroid Cancer Clin Oncol 2010;22:456–463.

Tala H, Tuttle RM. Contemporary post surgical management of differentiated thyroid carcinoma. Special Issue Thyroid Cancer Clin Oncol 2010;22:419–429.

Clin Oncology 22(6) August 2010 Special Issue- Thyroid Cancer.

Hay ID, Bergstralh EJ, Goellner JR, et al. Predicting outcome in papillary thyroid carcinoma: Development of a reliable prognostic score in a cohort of 1779 patients treated surgically at one institution during 1940 through 1989. Surgery 1993;114:1050–8.

EVOLVE CONTENTS (available online at: http://evolve.elsevier.com/Symonds/radiotherapy/)

Gastrointestinal cancer

Ramesh Bulusu

CANCER OF THE OESOPHAGUS

Epidemiology

Oesophageal cancer is among the top ten commonly occurring cancers and has a distinctive epidemiologic pattern characterized by marked geographic variation. It is more common in China, Iran, Russia, South Africa, France and Switzerland. In the UK, in excess of 7000 new cases area diagnosed per year with an annual death rate of around 6900. Three to four decades ago, most esophageal cancers were squamous carcinomas. Over the last two decades, an increasing incidence of adenocarcinomas of the oesophagus and cardia has been observed. Within Europe there are significant differences in the incidence of esophageal cancer, the highest rates being in the UK with 4.2–8.9/100 000 cases and Holland with 4.2/100 000, the lowest being 0.7/100 000 in Poland and 0.5/100 000 in the Czech Republic.

Worldwide, males are more commonly affected than females. The male to female ratio in the USA ranges from 2.1:1 to 3.7:1. Both squamous and adenocarcinomas are rare before the age of 40 years and steadily increase with each decade of life. Racial and ethnic differences have been reported in high incidence areas and also in the USA. The black populations of North America and South Africa appear to be at increased risk of squamous cell carcinomas (rates in excess of 15 cases/100 000 person years).

Aetiology and pathology

The most common histological subtypes are squamous cell carcinoma and adenocarcinoma, accounting for more than 90% of tumours.

Risk factors for squamous cell carcinomas

Alcohol and tobacco make up the largest risk factors for oesophageal squamous cell carcinoma in the western world. The relative risk is reported as 6.2 for smokers who do not consume alcohol. Smokers who have significant intakes of alcohol have a 10–25 fold increased risk of squamous cell cancer. Equally, chewing tobacco and betel leaves as practised in southern Asia, contributes to the excess risk seen in these regions. Nitrosamines, N-nitroso compounds, aromatic amines, polycyclic hydrocarbons found in alcohol and tobacco, alone or in combination contribute to the carcinogenic effect.

Patients with iron deficiency anaemia and diet low in riboflavin – Plummer-Vinson/Paterson-Kelly Brown syndrome – are at a higher risk of upper digestive tract squamous cell carcinomas. Tylosis, a hereditary condition characterized by hyperkeratosis of the palms and soles and papilloma of the oesophagus, is associated with a one in three chance of developing oesophageal cancer below the age of 50 years. Long-standing achalasia cardia is associated with 5% risk of oesophageal squamous carcinoma. Patients with a history of previous cancer of the aerodigestive tract have a 2–4% incidence of esophageal cancer. A higher incidence of squamous cell carcinomas was observed in individuals exposed to ionizing radiation.

Risk factors for adenocarcinoma

Gastroesophageal reflux disease (GORD or GERD)

Acid and bile reflux result in intestinal metaplasia of the esophageal squamous epithelium. The area of metaplastic change looks red on endoscopy, whereas the normal oesophagus has a pearly appearance. This change is called Barrett's oesophagus. Obesity and smoking contribute to these changes. The probable morphological sequence is metaplasia→dysplasia→carcinoma, accompanied by a series of genetic events resulting in invasive cancer. The incidence of adenocarcinoma developing in Barrett's oesophagus is 0.5–1% per year.

Obesity

Risk of adenocarcinoma of the oesophagus increases with increasing body mass index with up to threefold increases reported in the very obese cohorts.

Alcohol and tobacco

The association between alcohol and tobacco and esophageal adenocarcinoma is less robust than for squamous cancer, but several large studies show that there is a moderate increased risk of adenocarcinoma of the oesophagus and the cardia of the stomach.

Anatomy (Figure 24.1)

The oesophagus is a flattened muscular tube of 18–26 cm in length with diameters varying from 1.6 to 2.5 cm. The oesophagus starts at the pharyngoesophageal junction at the level of C5–6 vertebral interspace and ends at the esophagogastric junction at the level of T1 vertebra. It is traditionally divided into three segments, cervical, thoracic and abdominal. The cervical segment is about 4–5 cm long and extends from the pharyngoesophageal junction to the thoracic inlet. The thoracic oesophagus extends from the thoracic inlet to the diaphragmatic opening. The abdominal segment is short varying from 1 to 2.5 cm, extending from the hiatus to the esophagogastric junction. The esophageal hiatus in the diaphragm is at the level of T10 vertebra. The oesophagus moves a few millimeters during quiet respiration and by as much as 3–4 cm during swallowing.

The lymphatic drainage is of importance to the surgeon and the oncologist. A dense lymphatic network is found in the submucosa, which travels a variable distance longitudinally before penetrating the muscle layer and draining into the periesophageal lymph nodes. This may explain the extensive intramural spread of the cancer beneath an intact mucosa and tumour-free margins may not necessarily mean complete tumour resection. The lymphatic drainage of the proximal oesophagus is towards the deep cervical chain and thoracic duct. The distal oesophagus drains into the lower mediastinal, left gastric and coeliac axis nodes.

The esophageal wall is composed of four layers: the innermost non-keratinized squamous epithelium – the mucosa, submucosal connective tissue, muscularis propria

Figure 24.1 Relations of the oesophagus and lymph node drainage.
(Reproduced with permission of Arnold from Jane Dobbs, Ann Barrett, Daniel Ash, Practical Radiotherapy Planning, 3rd edn, Arnold, 1999)

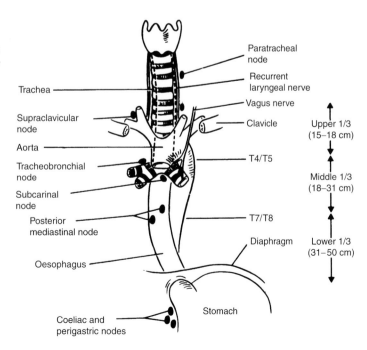

with inner circular and outer longitudinal layers and, finally, the adventitial layer. The myenteric or Auerbach plexus of nerves responsible for coordinating swallowing is located between the inner circular and outer longitudinal layers. The oesophagus has no mesentery or serosal lining which may explain the relatively easy spread of esophageal cancer into the surrounding tissues.

Clinical manifestations

Dysphagia and weight loss are the most common initial symptoms in over 90% of patients. Odynophagia (pain during swallowing) is seen in about 50% of patients. Epigastric pains, haematemesis, regurgitation of undigested food, aspiration pneumonia are less common but recognized symptoms. Cough from a tracheobronchial fistula, hoarse voice, superior vena caval obstruction and haemoptysis are less frequent. Pleural effusions and ascites and bone pain secondary to metastases can occur. Anorexia and right upper quadrant discomfort/pain may suggest liver metastases. Clinical examination should be directed at any presence of obvious metastatic disease, such as neck or supraclavicular lymph nodes, hepatomegaly, pleural effusions and ascites.

A thorough nutritional assessment by a specialist oncology dietician at baseline and at regular intervals while on treatment is mandatory.

Diagnostic evaluation (Tables 24.1–24.3)

Any patient who presents with recent onset dysphagia and weight loss should be investigated for a possible esophageal cancer. Many major centres have a fast track dysphagia endoscopy service available to minimize the delay in the diagnosis of the cancer.

In the majority of cases, upper GI endoscopy visualizes the tumour and its distance from the incisor teeth. The endoscopist should also define the lower extent of the tumour (if the lumen is traversable) and evaluate the esophagogastric junction. Multiple biopsies should be taken to maximize the yield. Any associated Barrett's segment, its length and relation to the invasive cancer should be noted.

In patients who are fit for curative treatment, the first step is a multislice computed tomography (CT) scan of the chest and abdomen to exclude obvious metastatic disease. CT has poor sensitivity in predicting the T or N stage. The sensitivity and specificity of CT for T4 disease are 25% and 94% respectively and for coeliac node involvement are 30% and 90% respectively.

In patients with localized disease, further evaluation of the T and N stage is best done by endoscopic ultrasound (EUS) by an experienced endoscopist. EUS has a high sensitivity and specificity in evaluating the T and N stage in esophageal cancer and has improved the preoperative

Table 24.1 Staging esophageal carcinoma

TNM staging system applies only for esophageal carcinomas

T: Primary tumour	
Tx	Primary tumour cannot be assessed
T0	No evidence of primary tumour
Tis	Carcinoma in situ
T1	Tumour invades the lamina propria or submucosa
T2	Tumour invades the muscularis propria
T3	Tumour invades the adventitia
T4	Tumour invades the adjacent structures

N: Regional nodes (see below)	
NX	Regional lymph nodes cannot be assessed
N0	No regional lymph node metastases
N1	Regional lymph node metastases

M: Distant metastases	
MX	Distant metastases cannot be assessed
M0	No distant metastases
M1	Distant metastases

For tumours of the upper thoracic oesophagus

M1a Metastases in cervical lymph nodes
M1b Other distant metastases

For tumours of the mid-thoracic oesophagus

M1a Not applicable
M1b Non-regional lymph nodes or other distant metastases

For tumours of the lower thoracic oesophagus

M1a Metastases in coeliac axis lymph nodes
M1b Other distant metastases
The regional lymph nodes depend on the anatomical subsite of the oesophagus (cervical or intrathoracic)

Cervical oesophagus

Scalene, internal jugular, upper and lower cervical, periesophageal and supraclavicular nodes

Intrathoracic oesophagus

Upper periesophageal (above the azygos vein), subcarinal, lower periesophageal (below the azygos vein), mediastinal, perigastric except coeliac axis nodes
pTNM Pathological classification

staging of esophageal cancer. The overall accuracy of EUS is 85% for T staging and 75% for N staging. EUS fine needle aspiration (FNA) enhances the accuracy of nodal staging and, in particular, is useful in confirming coeliac axis nodal status on cytology. EUS is less reliable in assessing T and N

Table 24.2 Stage grouping for esophageal cancer

STAGE 0	STAGE I	STAGE II	STAGE III	STAGE IV
Tis, N0, M0	T1,N0,M0	**IIA** T2/T3,N0,M0	T3,N1,M0	**IVA** Any T, any N, M1a
		IIB T1/T2N1,M0	T4,any N,M0	**IVB** Any T, any N, M1B

HISTOPATHOLOGICAL GRADING	
Gx	Grade of differentiation cannot be assessed
G1	Well differentiated
G2	Moderately well differentiated
G3	Poorly differentiated
G4	Undifferentiated

Table 24.3 Diagnostic evaluation of patients with esophageal cancer

Full blood count & renal & liver chemistry
CT scan of the chest & abdomen
Endoscopic ultrasound (EUS ± FNA)
Bronchoscopy (in selected cases)
FDG PET-CT
Isotope bone scan (if indicated)

stage following preoperative chemoradiation because it may not be able to differentiate between residual tumour and post-radiation inflammation/fibrosis.

In patients with hoarseness of voices or hemoptysis/unexplained cough, bronchoscopy is recommended to rule out recurrent laryngeal nerve involvement or tracheobronchial fistula.

The role of 2-fluorodeoxy-D-glucose positron emission tomography (FDG PET-CT) in the initial staging of potentially operable esophageal cancer has been the subject of numerous studies. In a recent systematic review, the pooled sensitivity and specificity of FDG PET for distant nodal and hematogenous metastases was 67% and 97%, respectively. The change in patient management as a result of FDG PET ranged from 3 to 20%. Preliminary data suggest that early FDG PET following neoadjuvant chemotherapy may predict pathologic response and overall survival and thus may define a subset of patients who are more likely to benefit from surgery.

Therapy

Surgery

Surgery remains the mainstay of treatment for all T stages of resectable esophageal cancer. The surgery involves resection of the primary tumour with an adequate margin along with regional lymph nodes. Two standard surgical techniques have been described for surgical resection of esophageal cancers – transthoracic (Ivor-Lewis technique) and trans-hiatal approach. The aim is complete resection. The margin status and the extent of nodal burden are powerful prognostic indicators for relapse-free survival.

Radiotherapy

External beam radiation alone or as part of combined modality treatment has been evaluated in both squamous cell and adenocarcinoma of the oesophagus. Primary radiation treatment alone for treatment of clinically localized esophageal cancer is not recommended in the curative setting. Both local and distant failure rates remain too high despite higher doses of radiation. Five-year survival is reported to be less than 5%. Preoperative radiation (i.e. without chemotherapy) has not shown any significant survival advantage. These two approaches are not recommended for patients fit for a potentially curative approach.

Definitive chemoradiation

Chemoradiation protocols typically use cisplatin and 5-fluorouracil (5FU) (recent studies have explored additional agents such as paclitaxel) with fractionated external beam radiation to a dose of 45–60 Gy. In two phase III trials in squamous cell carcinomas, definitive chemoradiation gave comparable median survival figures around 15–19 months with a 25–40% 2–year survival. Paclitaxel-based preoperative chemoradiation though has resulted in higher response rates; there is significant risk of postoperative complications, therefore, taxane-based chemotherapy with radiation has not become a standard of care.

Palliative radiotherapy can be recommended for local pain, bleeding or dysphagia; 8–10 Gy single fraction or 20–30 Gy in 5–10 fractions is given as a parallel-opposed pair. For patients with dysphagia, an esophageal stent may be more appropriate for providing good palliation.

Adjuvant radiation or chemoradiation

There are no prospective randomized trial data to support the routine use of adjuvant chemoradiation in resected esophageal cancer. Single institute series have shown some improvement in local control rates and progression-free survival but this could due to the inherent bias in the studies that the patients were fit enough to receive the adjuvant treatment.

Radiation therapy techniques

External beam radiation

Radiation planning using oral contrast (barium or gastrograffin) underestimates the tumour length. Three-dimensional conformal radiotherapy with CT planning is recommended. Joint planning with the endoscopist/radiologist to delineate the primary tumour based on the endoscopic ultrasound information will help to minimize the risk of a geographic miss. EUS can detect submucosal spread and gives a more accurate extent of the disease. Conventional margins above and below the tumour used to be 5 cm but, with modern imaging, this margin can be reduced to 3 cm and a 1.5–2 cm margin around the gross tumour volume (GTV) is adequate. A 3D conformal plan is generated with dose volume histograms defining the doses for the planned target volume, regions of interest including the spinal cord and lungs. A single phase three-field (anterior and two obliques) is the standard field arrangement to deliver a dose of 45–50 Gy in 1.8–2 Gy fractions. Chemoradiation patients will have concomitant intravenous 5-fluorouracil (5FU) or oral capecitabine and cisplatin during their radiation treatment. A widely used regimen is cisplatin 75 mg/m^2 day 1 plus 5-fluorouracil 1000 mg/m^2 infused over 24 hours on days 1–4 repeated every 3 weeks. Two to four cycles are given during radiotherapy. Weekly blood count and renal function monitoring is mandatory. Continuing dietary assessment prior to, during and after radiation, with nutritional support if necessary, is strongly recommended. Parallel-opposed fields (anterior/posterior) can be used for palliative radiotherapy.

Brachytherapy

Intracavitary treatment can be used for palliation of dysphagia and bleeding. Radiation dose can be delivered either through a low dose rate or a high dose rate technique. Doses of 5–20 Gy are delivered to a depth of 1 cm. Local control rates vary from 40 to 90%. The reported risk of stricture and/or fistula formation ranges from 2 to 38% and is known to be associated with the increasing brachytherapy fraction size. The role of intracavitary brachytherapy in the curative setting remains to be defined and has to be considered experimental.

Chemotherapy

Neoadjuvant chemotherapy

Preoperative chemotherapy with cisplatin and 5-FU (two cycles) has been the standard of care in the UK for patients with resectable esophageal cancer. Updated results from the MRC OE-2 trial of preoperative chemotherapy in patients undergoing curative surgery showed 5-year overall survival rates of 23% in the combined modality arm compared to 17% in the surgery alone arm. Newer agents and longer duration of therapy are being explored in clinical trials.

Trimodality therapy, i.e. preoperative chemoradiation followed by surgery has been evaluated in adenocarcinoma of oesophagus within the CALGB 9781 randomized trial. A significant survival advantage for the trimodality arm 39% (95% CI 21–57%) versus 16% (95% CI 5–33%) 5-year survival) was reported compared to surgery alone. This may be accepted as a new standard of care in North America. However, despite the expected accrual of 500 patients, the trial was closed due to poor accrual, after only 54 patients were recruited into this study.

Palliative chemotherapy

Platinum and 5FU/oral capecitabine based regimens are the accepted standard of care. Newer chemotherapy agents and targeted therapy with epidermal growth factor receptor/vascular endothelial growth factor (EGFR/VEGF) inhibitors will be explored in future trials.

Other treatments

Endoluminal techniques have been used for the treatment of Barrett's metaplasia and dysplasia. These include circumferential radiofrequency ablation, endoscopic mucosal resection (EMR) and photodynamic therapy. Endomucosal resection for early invasive mucosal lesions is fast gaining acceptance as a local curative treatment and is best performed in experienced centres. EMR is indicated for superficial lesions, i.e. high grade dysplasia and moderately to well differentiated carcinomas limited to lamina propria only.

Palliative treatment options are tailored to the individual patient and are best discussed in a multidisciplinary setting along with the palliative care team. Esophageal stenting provides palliation of dysphagia. Endoscopic laser treatment may be suitable for bulky endoluminal squamous tumours. Palliative radiation (external beam or brachytherapy) and chemotherapy are other alternative options for symptomatic benefit.

Esophagogastric junctional tumours

Adenocarcinomas of the esophagogastric junction have been divided into three subtypes as proposed by Siewert and Stein. Typ. 1 junctional tumours primarily arise from the distal oesophagus and involve the junction, typ. 2 junctional tumours straddle the junction and typ. 3 tumours are predominantly in the cardia of the stomach involving the junction. Typ. 1 junctional adenocarcinoma is treated using oesophagus protocols. Typ. 3 junctional tumours are thought to behave like gastric adenocarcinoma, therefore, are treated using gastric protocols.

Summary

Management of esophageal cancer has evolved over the past three decades. Treatment decisions should be made within a multidisciplinary team setting. Careful staging and selection of patients for curative treatments is vital and surgery should be performed in high volume specialist centres for best outcome. Combined modality treatments remain the standard of care in curative setting for all patients with oesophageal cancer except the very early tumours.

STOMACH

Anatomy

The stomach begins at the esophagogastric junction and ends at the pylorus. It is divided into three parts: cardia (fundus), body and pyloric antrum. The blood supply of the stomach is derived from the branches of the coeliac axis. The regional lymphatics drain into the coeliac axis nodes, splenic hilar, porta hepatis, gastroduodenal and suprapancreatic nodal groups. Venous drainage is primarily through the portal venous system into the liver.

Epidemiology

There is a considerable variation in the worldwide incidence of gastric cancer. The highest incidence is seen in Japan, South America and eastern Europe. The incidence in western Europe is in decline. However, the incidence of tumours of the cardia and esophagogastric junction has increased. The incidence of stomach cancer has been declining in the UK since 1930. CRUK (2004) reported 9660 cases in the UK with an incidence of 16.5 per 100 000 making this the sixth most common cancer in Britain.

Aetiology

Environmental and genetic factors play a role in the pathogenesis of gastric cancer. Carcinogens implicated in the aetiology include nitrates and nitrites in food, smoking and industrial dust exposure. The role of alcohol remains uncertain. Increased risk has been reported with a specific strain of *Helicobacter pylori* (CAG+ve) especially in non-cardia lesions. Pernicious anaemia and previous subtotal gastrectomy for benign conditions, and villous adenomas are thought to be associated with increased risk of gastric cancer after a long period of latency.

Genetic factors include mutations in specific genes, CDH1 and p53. CDH1 encodes for E-cadherin and mutations in this gene are associated with hereditary diffuse gastric cancer. Another familial gastric cancer syndrome is associated with p53 mutations. Gastric cancer is also a component of Li-Fraumeni syndrome, hereditary non-polyposis colorectal cancer (HNPCC), Peutz-Jegher polyposis, BRCA-2 mutations and juvenile polyposis.

Pathology

Adenocarcinoma constitutes 95% of the gastric cancers. They are classified into intestinal and diffuse types (Lauren's classification system). The intestinal type is more common in older patients, high-risk groups and men. The diffuse type is more commonly seen in women and younger patients and carries a poorer prognosis. Other histological types of gastric malignancies include carcinoids, lymphomas and gastrointestinal stromal tumours (GISTS). GISTS are the most common mesenchymal tumours of the gastrointestinal tract.

Clinical features

The most common presenting symptoms are anaemia, weight loss, anorexia, haematemesis, melena, upper abdominal pain/discomfort/mass, nausea/vomiting. Occult bleeding is more common than overt haematemesis. Possible clinical findings include anaemia, abdominal mass, left supraclavicular lymphadenopathy, and ascites.

Staging (Tables 24.4 and 24.5)

The initial investigations often include a barium meal/swallow and endoscopy. Gastroscopy and biopsy will confirm the diagnosis in the majority of patients. Multiple

Table 24.4 Stomach cancer TNM clinical classification

T: Primary tumour

TX	Primary tumour cannot be assessed
T0	No evidence of primary tumour
Tis	Carcinoma in situ: intraepithelial tumour without invasion of the lamina propria
T1	Tumour invades lamina propria or submucosa
T2	Tumour invades muscularis propria or subserosa
T3	Tumour penetrates serosa (visceral peritoneum) without invasion of adjacent structures
T4	Tumour invades adjacent structures

Notes:
1. A tumour may penetrate muscularis propria with extension into the gastro-perforation of the visceral peritoneum covering these structures. In this case, the tumour is classified as T2. If there is perforation of the visceral peritoneum covering the gastric ligaments or omentum, the tumour is classified as T3.
2. The adjacent structures of the stomach are the spleen, transverse colon, liver, diaphragm, pancreas, abdominal wall, adrenal gland, kidney, small intestine and retroperitoneum.
3. Intramural extension to the duodenum or oesophagus is classified by the depth of greatest invasion in any of these sites including stomach

N: Regional lymph nodes

NX	Regional lymph nodes cannot be assessed
N0	No regional lymph node metastasis
N1	Metastasis in 1 to 6 regional lymph nodes
N2	Metastasis in 7 to 15 regional lymph nodes
N3	Metastasis in more than 15 regional lymph nodes

M: Distant metastasis

MX	Distant metastasis cannot be accessed
M0	No distant metastasis
M1	Distant metastasis

Table 24.5 Stomach cancer stage grouping

Stage 0	Tis	N0	M0
Stage IA	T1	N0	M0
Stage IB	T1	N1	M0
	T2	N0	M0
Stage II	T1	N2	M0
	T2	N1	M0
	T3	N0	M0
	T4	N0	M0
Stage IIIB	T3	N2	M0
Stage IV	T4	N1,N2,N3	M0
	Any T	Any N	M1

Management

The optimal management of gastric cancer should take place within a multidisciplinary setting. The treatment options are surgery, neoadjuvant and adjuvant chemotherapy, adjuvant chemoradiation, palliative chemotherapy and radiation.

Surgery

The goal of surgery is complete resection. However, only 25–30% of patients with gastric cancer may be suitable for potentially curative surgery. A D1 gastrectomy involves removal of all regional nodal stations. More extensive radical lymphadenectomy has not shown to be of survival benefit. A randomized British Medical Research Council trial published in 1999 showed no survival advantage for more extensive D2 excision. Retrospective studies from Germany and from the surveillance epidemiology and end results database (SEER) in the USA found that survival was better if more than 10 lymph nodes were removed. There was increasing improvement in survival in patients as more nodes were found in the pathological specimen up to a maximum of 40. The German investigators found if patients had more than 25 nodes removed they had a better survival than those who had less than 25 lymph nodes removed. Surgery may be the only treatment needed for early lesions. However, in the majority of patients treated with a curative intent, a combined modality approach is necessary.

The most common sites of relapse following a curative resection are locoregional (lymph nodes, gastric bed and anastomosis) and metastatic (liver and peritoneal seeding).

Palliative gastrectomy can be offered for patients with obstructive symptoms such as bleeding and pain.

biopsies increase the sensitivity and yield. The TNM staging system is used for staging gastric cancer. Endoscopic ultrasound is of value in proximal cardia and junctional tumours. Cross-sectional imaging with a spiral CT is the first step to exclude overt metastatic disease. CT is not a sensitive tool for detecting peritoneal spread, therefore, laparoscopy is mandatory prior to surgery to detect any occult peritoneal spread. Laparoscopy may also help in identifying tumour in the lesser sac, on the surface of the liver and nodal disease. FDG-PET imaging may identify metastases not clearly seen on CT but 25–30% of primary gastric cancers are not FDG avid.

Perioperative (neoadjuvant and adjuvant) chemotherapy

The relapse rate is high for patients who have had gastrectomy for stages T2 and beyond. This is thought to be mainly due to the locoregional failure and micrometastatic disease present at diagnosis. Various adjuvant treatments have been explored to improve the survival. Perioperative chemotherapy with epirubicin/cisplatin/5-fluorouracil has been shown to improve the disease-free and overall survival in patients with resectable gastric cancer. The MRC UK MAGIC trial randomized over 500 patients to either surgery alone or three cycles of preoperative ECF (epirubicin 50 mg/m^2, cisplatin 60 mg/m^2 day 1 and infused 5-fluorouracil 200 mg/m^2 for 21 days) followed by surgery and then three more cycles of postoperative ECF. Both progression-free and overall survival were superior in the combined modality arm. Five-year survival rates were 23% in the surgery alone arm and 36% in the perioperative chemotherapy arm. In the UK, following the publication of this trial, perioperative chemotherapy has become the standard of care for patients with curable and resectable gastric cancers. Future directions explore the addition of targeted therapy (anti-VEGF – bevacizumab or anti-EGFR – cetuximab) to chemotherapy. In the current UK led international trial of perioperative chemotherapy (NCRI ST03), patients will be randomized to ECX (epirubicin, cisplatin and capecitabine) or the same plus the antivascular endothelial growth factor (VEGF) monoclonal antibody bevacizumab.

Adjuvant chemoradiation

In North America, adjuvant chemoradiation is offered for patients with resected gastric cancer based on the updated results of the Intergroup 0116 randomized trial comparing surgery alone to surgery followed by postoperative chemoradiation with 5-FU and folinic acid. The adjuvant chemoradiation improved the median progression-free survival (19 versus 30 months $P<0.001$) and overall survival (26 versus 35 months $P<0.006$). It is felt that a significant proportion of patients may have had suboptimal lymph node dissection and the postoperative chemoradiation may have compensated for the inadequate surgery. However, based on this pivotal study, adjuvant chemoradiation has become the new standard of care in North America.

Radiation techniques

The postoperative radiation target volumes are generated based on the tumour site in the stomach, known pattern of locoregional failure and need to be tailored to the individual patient's T stage and type of surgery. The clinical target volume includes the gastric/tumour bed, gastric remnant, nodal stations along the lesser and greater curvature of the stomach, coeliac axis, suprapancreatic, porta hepatis and splenic groups. Parallel pair anterior/posterior may adequately cover the volume but more complex techniques including oblique/lateral portals with 3D CT planning may help to optimize the dose and minimize the normal tissue dose. The standard dose fractionation is 45 Gy in 25 fractions over 5 weeks with concomitant intravenous 5-fluorouracil (425 mg/m^2, folinic acid 20 mg/m^2 for 5 days repeated every 4 weeks during radiotherapy and for two cycles after radiotherapy). The patient needs to be monitored carefully with weekly full blood counts, biochemistry, dietetic assessment including weight and adequate measures for gastrointestinal toxicity (nausea, vomiting, and diarrhoea).

Palliative treatments in advanced/metastatic gastric cancer

Palliative chemotherapy

Platinum- and fluoropyrimidine-based regimens are now considered to be the standard option for systemic chemotherapy for patients with advanced/metastatic gastric adenocarcinoma. CF, ECF and DCF are regimens with response rates of 35–45% and a median overall survival around 9 months. The REAL-2 study comparing cisplatin versus oxaliplatin and IV 5FU versus oral capecitabine showed that the four regimens are of similar efficacy. Docetaxel-based regimen, DCF (docetaxel, cisplatin and 5-fluorouracil) and irinotecan with cisplatin produce similar median survival figures of around 9 months. A recent meta-analysis based on aggregate data on the benefits of palliative chemotherapy confirmed the benefits of chemotherapy.

Recently, in the subpopulation of patients with HER-2 +ve gastric cancer, addition of Trastuzumab to cispaltin+ fluoropyrimidine chemotherapy has been shown to improve both overall and progression free survival. In the ToGA trial, the subgroup patients with HER-2 +ve (FISH +ve or IHC 3+ve) gastric cancers had a 4.2 months improvement in overall survival with the addition of trastuzumab to chemotherapy (16 months vs 11.8 months, HR 0.65 95% CI 0.51-0.83). This is considered as the new standard of care in HER-2 +ve metastatic gastric cancer.

Palliative radiotherapy

In selected patients, palliative radiotherapy (8–10 Gy in a single fraction or 20 Gy in five fractions) may help to palliate pain, bleeding, and obstructive symptoms.

Summary

Management of gastric cancer has improved over the last decade. Most patients with resectable gastric adenocarcinoma are likely to need a combined modality approach for best results. Future directions in systemic therapy include integrating the newer targeted molecules into existing protocols.

HEPATOCELLULAR CARCINOMA

Hepatocellular carcinoma is primary cancer of the liver cells. It is the fifth most common in the world and there are at least half a million cases annually. In the UK, it is much less common with an incidence of about 2500 cases annually making in the nineteenth most common cancer. There is a strong association with chronic viral hepatitis, especially hepatitis B, and the development of hepatocellular cancers. Common presenting features of primary hepatocellular carcinomas are abdominal pain, weight loss and the presence of hepatic mass sometimes with hepatic failure, ascites and other signs of chronic liver disease. Alpha-fetoprotein (afp) is elevated in 50–70% of such patients. The only hope of long-term survival of such patients is surgical resection of the tumour. This is only possible in less than 20% of cases. Tumours are not resectable if there is extrahepatic spread or extensive bilobar involvement. A patient with a normal liver can tolerate a resection of about three-quarters of the liver but if there is pre-existing liver disease, such major resections may not be possible.

Hepatectomy and transplantation is an option for some patients. However, the number of donor livers is limited and some patients become unfit for this treatment while waiting for a suitable organ. Other techniques such as radiofrequency ablation, cryosurgery and ethanol injection in skilled hands may offer the possibility of tumour destruction with limited damage to the liver.

This tumour is not particularly chemosensitive. Doxorubicin (Adriamycin) is the most widely used agent but response rates are only 10–20%. Sorafenib, an orally administered multityrosine kinase inhibitor has been shown to reduce the time to progression in advanced hepatocellular cancer compared to a placebo. Overall survival was 10.7 months for sorafenib against 7.9 months for a placebo. There is no role for radiotherapy in this condition. Overall 5-year survival for patients with this tumour is less than 5%. However, 5-year survival for patients with resectable disease is 30–50%.

Cholangiocarcinoma and Gallbladder cancer

Cholangiocarcinoma is a rare tumour arising from the ductal epithelium of the biliary tree. Chronic inflammation due to gallstones or parasites, such as liver flukes, has been implicated as cause for this condition. Patients tend to present with jaundice or weight loss and upper abdominal pain. The only curative treatment is surgical resection. This is usually rarely possible. Tumours that are largely extra-hepatic in nature are more likely to be resected, although a segment of liver normally needs to be resected as well. The vast majority of patients have irresectable disease. External beam radiotherapy along with extra-hepatic brachytherapy using iridium-192 has been shown to improve long-term survival compared to surgery alone in one Japanese series. Other studies have not confirmed the value of adjuvant radiotherapy. Most patients are treated by biliary stenting to relieve biliary obstruction as a palliative measure. The 5-year survival rate for patients with a cholangiocarcinoma is 5% or less.

Gallbladder cancer is rare and is associated with chronic infection and gallstones. Tumours are often asymptomatic until an advanced stage of the disease and may be masked by the signs and symptoms of gallstones and chronic inflammation. Surgical excision offers the best chance of cure. A portion of the liver, colon or duodenum may need to be resected along with the gallbladder and part of the biliary tree. In some small retrospective series, chemoradiotherapy to the excised tumour area has been shown to extend survival. A multivariate analysis of retrospective data has shown benefit for patients with either node positive or stage 2 disease or higher for postoperative chemoradiotherapy, but the value of this treatment needs to be tested in prospective clinical trials.

The majority of patients have irresectable disease and the aim of treatment is palliation. Such patients are often jaundiced, in pain and may suffer recurrent attacks of cholangitis. The best and simplest method of relieving jaundice and pain is intrabiliary stenting. The prognosis for most patients with gallbladder cancer is very poor with less than 5% 5-year survival.

ABC-02 trial compared cisplatin + gemcitabine combination with gemcitabine monotherapy in patients with inoperable/metastatic cholangiocarcinoma or gall bladder carcinoma. There was a 3.6 months overall survival advantage for the combination arm, (11.7 months vs 8.1 months, HR 0.64; 95% CI, 0.52 to 0.80; P<0.001). In addition, the tumour control rate in the combination arm was significantly better (81.4% vs. 71.8%, P=0.049). The combination of cisplatin + gemcitabine is now considered as the new standard of care in this rare cancer.

PANCREAS

Anatomy

The pancreas lies in the retroperitoneal space transversely along its long axis in the upper abdomen at the level of the first two lumbar vertebrae. It is divided into head, body and tail. The pancreas is closely related to the surrounding structures including the duodenum and jejunum, lesser sac, kidneys, transverse colon, spleen and superior mesenteric vessels. Pancreatic cancer often locally infiltrates these structures. The pancreatic duct joins the bile duct to form the common bile duct which opens into the second part of the duodenum through the major papilla.

Pancreatic tumours originating from the head can compress the common bile duct resulting in obstructive jaundice. The pancreas has a complex and extensive lymphatic drainage into the superior and inferior pancreaticoduodenal, coeliac axis, superior mesenteric and porta hepatis nodes. The tumour cells can also spread along the perineural pathways.

Incidence and epidemiology

Cancer Research UK (2004) reports over 7000 new cases in the UK annually with a rate of 12.1 per 100 000 per annum. This makes the pancreas the tenth most common cancer in the UK. More than 30 000 new cases are diagnosed in the USA each year. There has been an increase in incidence since the 1930s which levelled off in the 1970s. The mortality rate mirrors the incidence because of the poor prognosis. The causes of this cancer are largely unknown. The only known association is with smoking though the association is much less than seen with lung cancer. There is a doubling of incidence of this cancer in cigarette smokers. Exposure to organic chemicals is thought to increase the risk. Hereditary pancreatic cancer syndromes account for <10% of the cancers and include hereditary pancreatitis, familial melanoma, BRCA-2, familial adenomatous polyposis (FAP), HNPCC, Peutz-Jegher's and ataxia telangiectasia syndromes.

Pathology

Ninety percent of tumours in the pancreas are adenocarcinoma; 65% arise from the head of the pancreas. Neuroendocrine tumours, cystadenomas and cystadenocarcinomas are uncommon and have a better prognosis. The tumour spread is through local invasion into adjacent organs, in particular, perineural invasion through splanchnic nerves causing back pain. Lymphatic spread is common into regional and para-aortic lymph nodes. Tumours often metastasize to the liver and peritoneum. More than 80% of the patients with pancreatic cancer present with either locally advanced or metastatic cancer which is not amenable for curative treatments.

TNM staging (Tables 24.6 and 24.7)

Clinical features

The majority of the early symptoms are non-specific, therefore, most patients present with advanced disease. The common presenting symptoms are obstructive jaundice, weight loss, anorexia, back pain and fatigue. Back pain may be present in >50% of patients due to deep perineural invasion. Classically, this pain is referred between the shoulder blades and is partially relieved by sitting up and leaning forward. Less commonly, patients can present with new onset diabetes as a result of pancreatic insufficiency.

Table 24.6 Stage grouping for pancreas cancer

Stage 0	Tis	N0	M0
Stage IA	T1	N0	M0
Stage IB	T2	N0	M0
Stage IIA	T3	N0	M0
Stage IIB	T1, T2, T3	N1	M0
Stage III	T4	Any N	M0
Stage IV	Any T	Any N	M1

Table 24.7 TNM clinical classification for pancreas cancer

T – PRIMARY TUMOUR	
TX	Primary tumour cannot be assessed
T0	No evidence of primary tumour
Tis	Carcinoma in situ*
T1	Tumour limited to pancreas, 2 cm or less in greatest dimension
T2	Tumour limited to pancreas, more than 2 cm in greatest dimension
T3	Tumour extends beyond pancreas, but without involvement of coeliac axis or superior mesenteric artery
T4	Tumour involves coeliac axis or superior mesenteric artery
N- REGIONAL LYMPH NODES	
NX	Regional lymph nodes cannot be assessed
N0	No regional lymph node metastasis
N1	Regional lymph node metastasis
M – DISTANT METASTASIS	
M0	No distant metastasis
M1	Distant metastasis

*Tis also includes the 'PanIN-III' classification

Rarely, the cancer may be found following a bout of acute pancreatitis.

Clinical examination may reveal jaundice, evidence of weight loss, palpable supraclavicular nodes, umbilical nodule (Sister Mary Joseph's nodule). Superficial thrombophlebitis is a paraneoplastic feature. The liver may be enlarged and there may be epigastric fullness/mass on palpation.

Diagnostic evaluation and imaging

A full blood count may reveal anaemia and biochemical tests confirm obstructive jaundice. CA19.9, a serum tumour marker, is raised in between 60 and 90% of patients with pancreatic cancer.

Endoscopic retrograde cholangiopancreatography (ERCP) is an extremely useful investigation for evaluating the ampulla, obtaining cytological specimens and also for biliary drainage. Multislice CT with 3D reconstruction is extremely useful to define the relationship of the tumour to the vessels and surrounding structures. Endoscopic ultrasound by an experienced endoscopist will help in detecting small lesions, any nodal involvement and, more importantly, venous involvement. Endoscopic ultrasound-guided fine needle aspiration (EUS FNA) may increase the diagnostic sensitivity to near 100% and has been shown to be reliable for presurgical work up. Laparoscopy is helpful in detecting unsuspected peritoneal disease since up to 30% of patients with locally advanced pancreatic cancer have occult microscopic peritoneal disease. FDG-PET is an additional imaging modality with varying degrees of specificity and sensitivity in detecting pancreatic cancer. A recent meta-analysis showed a sensitivity of 73–100% and specificity of 53–100% for the detection of pancreatic cancer. In selected patients, magnetic resonance imaging (MRI) may offer a better definition of vascular anatomy prior to surgery.

Therapy

Surgery

Less than 20% of patients have potentially surgically resectable lesions. Standard surgical treatment is pancreatico-duodenectomy pioneered by Whipple and his team in 1935. Distal body and tail of the pancreas tumours may require en bloc resection of the spleen along with the pancreas. The overall 5-year survival following surgical resection is 5–20%. For best results, surgery should be performed in high volume centres with specialist experience. In the absence of distant metastases, the features which make a tumour potentially unresectable are significant involvement/encasement of the superior mesenteric vein, portal vein or superior mesenteric artery by the tumour or invasion of adjacent organs (kidney, adrenal, and colon). Patterns of failure after surgical resection without any adjuvant therapy are well described; 50–85% of patients have local relapse, 25–35% have peritoneal recurrences and 25–90% have liver metastases. Tumour stage, grade and resection margin status are the best predictors for survival after potentially curative surgery.

Chemoradiotherapy in locally advanced pancreatic cancer

Combined modality treatment with chemoradiation using fluoropyrimidines (5FU or capecitabine) is considered a standard approach for locally advanced pancreatic cancer in North America. 3-D conformal radiotherapy and intensity modulated radiotherapy (IMRT) techniques may optimize the tumour dose and minimize the radiation dose to the normal tissue. Dose escalation to 60 Gy or above has not shown to improve the survival in locally advanced pancreatic cancer. Median overall survival in these studies ranged between 7 and 12 months for the chemoradiation group. The structures around the pancreas, i.e. duodenum, kidneys, spinal cord, stomach etc., limit the radiation dose.

Intraoperative radiotherapy (IORT) and stereotactic radiotherapy remain investigational. IORT with electrons has been used to boost the dose to the primary tumour following external beam radiation or in patients who have had resection of their primary tumour. A dose of 15–30 Gy has been recommended. Local tumour control seems to have improved but with no major impact on the overall survival.

Preoperative chemoradiation in potentially resectable cancers may provide better local control and some survival benefit has been demonstrated in single institute retrospective series on par with adjuvant therapy. However, it is difficult to compare these studies because of small numbers and inconsistent criteria for patient selection and resectability. Down staging an initially unresectable tumour to enable resection with a neoadjuvant approach is rare. These approaches should be part of well-designed randomized clinical trials.

External beam radiation techniques

In patients with locally advanced pancreatic cancer, the target volumes are defined using the information from the imaging studies (EUS, CT). Multiple field (four to six) fractionated high energy photon beam techniques are used to deliver 45–50 Gy in 1.8 Gy fractions. The clinical target volume (CTV) includes the primary tumour, adjacent nodal groups (suprapancreatic, coeliac axis, and pancreaticoduodenal) and the duodenal wall for head of pancreas lesions. The superior extent of CTV should cover the coeliac axis with 1.5–2 cm margin and inferiorly the volume extends to include the superior mesenteric lymph nodes. The posterior margin of the CTV is crucial and should extend to at least 1.5 cm beyond the anterior margin of the vertebral body. This is to ensure that the splanchnic nerves and plexus are included in the CTV (note the risk of perineural spread). The anterior margin extends up to 1.5–2 cm from the GTV. All the organs at risk, i.e. stomach, duodenum, liver, both kidneys, spinal cord and surrounding small bowel should be outlined. One has to remember that pancreas, despite being a retroperitoneal organ, moves vertically up to 1.5–2 cm with respiration. This has to be taken into account in defining the CTV→planning target volume (PTV) margin in the vertical plane.

CT-based treatment planning and 3D-conformal radiation or IMRT techniques permit the generation of treatment plans that optimize the radiation dose to the PTV but minimize the dose to the critical organs at risk. Dose volume histograms for each of the organs at risk should be critically evaluated before accepting the final plan, in particular, the dose to the kidneys should be kept to a minimum. Some radiation centres recommend assessment of individual kidney function prior to starting radiation treatment. Postoperative adjuvant radiation fields are designed on the basis of the preoperative CT data on primary tumour site and extent, known nodal spread and operative clip placement.

Future strategies in combining radiation and systemic agents are likely to explore novel chemotherapeutic agents, targeted therapy with trastuzumab (HER-2neu antibody), cetuximab (EGFR antibody), erlotinib, sunitinib (tyrosine kinase inhibitors) etc.

Adjuvant therapy

The standard of care in North America is postoperative adjuvant chemoradiation with 5FU. This was based on one randomized study by the GITSG in the 1980s and subsequent non-randomized single institute prospective studies. Compared to historical controls, there seems to be a survival benefit with adjuvant chemoradiation, the overall median survival improved from 11–15 months to around 18–23 months.

Subsequent European studies did not support the use of adjuvant chemoradiation in resected pancreatic cancer. A recent ESPAC-1 study confirmed the benefits of adjuvant 5FU/folinic acid for six cycles. ESPAC-3 trial showed that both 5FU/FA and gemcitabine in the adjuvant setting have similar outcomes. ESPAC-4 trial is evaluating the addition of capecitabine to gemcitabine in the adjuvant setting in patients with resected pancreatic cancer.

Palliative chemotherapy

Single agent gemcitabine has been the standard of care for patients with inoperable or metastatic pancreatic adenocarcinoma. The pivotal phase III study compared what was then standard treatment, 5FU/folinic acid with single agent gemcitabine. Clinical benefit response (improvement in pain, performance status and appetite) was significantly better (24% versus 5%) as were median survival (5.7 versus 4.4 months) and 1-year survival rate (18% versus 2%) with gemcitabine. Subsequently, a large open label compassionate study involving over 3000 patients, showed a median survival of 4.8 months and 15% 1-year survival rate. Until recently, none of the combination regimens with gemcitabine showed any survival advantage, though platinum and gemcitabine combinations have showed some promise.

Gemcitabine + capecitabine and gemcitabine + erlotinib have shown a modest increase in the survival.

Supportive care for symptom palliation

Endoscopic biliary stenting of a resectable pancreatic tumour for the release of jaundice is as good as surgical bypass to relieve jaundice. The duodenal obstruction can be relieved by expandable stents. Pain relief is important for the palliation of pancreatic cancer. Severe pain can be caused by infiltration of the coeliac plexus and this can be relieved by destruction of the plexus by an injection of alcohol which can be carried out either under x-ray control or CT guidance.

Future directions in pancreatic cancer research hope for a better understanding of the molecular events, in particular, K-Ras and the downstream signaling pathways which may represent attractive therapeutic targets.

COLON AND RECTUM

Epidemiology

Malignancies of the colon and rectum constitute the third commonest form of cancer in the UK with an annual incidence of 34 000 new cases per year. The male to female ratio is 1.27 to 1 for rectal cancer, and 0.82 to 1 for colon cancer. The age specific incidence rises markedly over the age of 60 years, while less than 1% of all cases occur in patients under the age of 40.

Aetiology

Compelling data from the European Prospective Investigation into Cancer and Nutrition (EPIC) study suggest that dietary factors are important in the pathogenesis of colorectal cancer. The study shows a positive correlation between colorectal cancer and meat intake, and a strong inverse correlation with fiber intake. This correlates with finding of very low incidence rates of colorectal cancer in Africa, where the typical diet is associated with high fiber content. In addition, excessive smoking and alcohol consumption are thought to increase the risk of malignancy. There is an increased incidence of rectal cancer in southern Germany, which is thought to be due to the increased intake of dark beer.

Patients with chronic inflammatory bowel disease, such as ulcerative colitis and Crohn's disease, are at increased risk of developing colorectal cancer, and the risk is most marked in patients who have had active disease for more than 10 years. With active surveillance programs, the risk of malignancy in these patients can be reduced to the same level as the background population.

Colorectal cancer was one of the first sites where a model for stepwise progression from normal epithelium to dysplasia, neoplasia and invasive malignancy was formulated.

This is borne out clinically as early dysplastic polyps that are not excised have a risk of malignant transformation of about 5–10% at 10 years. Larger polyps, and multiple polyps increase the risk of malignant transformation.

Patients with a family history of bowel malignancy, or who have themselves had a previous bowel malignancy, are at increased risk of developing colorectal cancer. Two specific cancer syndromes, namely familial adenomatous polyposis (FAP) and hereditary non-polyposis colon cancer (HNPCC: Table 24.8), have generated much interest. Both are autosomal dominant mutations with high penetrance. The genetic mutations associated with these cancer predisposition syndromes have been isolated, and genetic screening can now be offered to families thought to be at risk. HNPCC is the most common hereditary syndrome accounting for 2–7% of the total. The diagnosis is based on strict clinical and molecular criteria. FAP accounts for 1% of all colorectal cancers. In this syndrome, multiple adenomas progress to invasive cancers in nearly 100% of patients by 40–50 years of age. Prophylactic surgery is recommended at age 16–21.

Histopathology and clinical features

The vast majority of colorectal cancers are adenocarcinomas. Macroscopically, they present as exophytic masses. They typically show glandular differentiation, mucin formation, and stain positively for carcinoembryonic antigen (CEA). Small cell carcinomas, lymphomas, melanomas and adenosquamous carcinomas have been reported.

Usually, patients will present with symptoms of rectal bleeding, altered bowel habit, or weight loss. The diagnosis is usually made by characteristic filling defects on barium enema ('apple core lesions') or at colonoscopy. Bulky lesions may present with overt bowel obstruction.

Occasionally, patients will present with liver metastases and no obvious primary tumour on barium enema or colonoscopy. In such cases, morphological features on light microscopy, CEA staining, and differential staining cytokeratins CK 7 and CK 20, can be helpful in confirming the tissue of origin. Tumours of the lower gastrointestinal tract are typically CK 7 negative and CK 20 positive.

Table 24.8 Revised Amsterdam criteria for suspected hereditary non-polyposis colon cancer (HNPCC)

3 relatives with an HNPCC-related cancer, one of whom should be a first degree relative of the other two
2 generations should be involved
1 case diagnosed under age 50
Familial adenomatous polyposis must be excluded
HNPCC cancers include colon and rectum, endometrium, small bowel, ureter and renal pelvis

Staging systems

The simplest staging of large bowel cancer is the Duke's staging scheme in which tumours are staged A to C. Stage A is tumour involving the mucosa or penetration into the submucosa, Stage B is penetration through the muscularis propria but no lymphatic spread and Stage C is spread to lymph nodes. This staging scheme has been modified over the years and the modified Astler-Coller scheme is widely used in the USA. The staging schemes are listed in Table 24.9.

Use of the UICC TNM should be encouraged where possible as it offers more accurate information on primary tumour and nodal status and, in the Royal College of Pathologists minimum data set for the reporting of colorectal cancer, use of the TNM classification is mandatory.

Colon cancer – treatment principles

Surgery

Surgery is still the main treatment modality. The aim of surgery is excision of the primary tumour with wide excision margins. The tumour spreads to the lymph nodes located in the mesentery close to the vascular supply for that portion of colon. This portion of node-bearing mesentery is excised along with the bowel. Continuity of the bowel is usually re-established by a direct anastomosis, either between excised segments of colon or the colon and the terminal ileum.

Adjuvant chemotherapy

Adjuvant chemotherapy is of proven benefit for patients with node positive (Duke's C) colon cancer. Six months of 5-fluorouracil and folinic acid chemotherapy given to such patients is estimated to reduce the risk of death by 30% which translates into a 10–13 % absolute improvement in survival. Two randomized controlled trials have confirmed that the addition of oxaliplatin to 5-fluorouracil and folinic acid improves 3-year survival by an additional 7%. Patients with Duke's B tumours have derived less benefit from adjuvant chemotherapy. Trials, such as the British QUASAR trial, have shown only a 3.6% increase in 5-year survival in this group of patients. However, Duke's B is a heterogeneous group of patients and multivariate analysis of patterns of relapse has shown that patients with T4 tumours, tumour perforation, lymphovascular invasion and poor differentiation are most likely to derive benefit from chemotherapy. The X-ACT trial has shown that oral capecitabine is at least as effective as 5-fluorouracil and folinic acid. Orally administered capecitabine is an alternative treatment for patients who may not be able to tolerate oxaliplatin-based regimens. Currently, irinotecan-based regimens have not been shown to give an advantage in an adjuvant setting therefore are not currently recommended.

Table 24.9 Staging schemes for colorectal cancer

DUKES	ASTLER-COLLER	MODIFIED ASTLER-COLLER	TNM	DESCRIPTION
A	A	A	T1N0	Nodes negative, limited to mucosa
	B1	B1	T2N0	Nodes negative; penetration into submucosa but not through muscularis propria
B	B2	B2	T3N0	Nodes negative; penetration through muscularis propria
		B3	T4N0	Nodes negative; penetration through muscularis propria with adherence to or invasion of surrounding organs or structures
C		C1	T1/T2 N1–N3	Nodes positive limited to bowel wall
C		C1	T1/T2 N1–N3	Nodes positive limited to bowel wall
	C1	C2	T3N1–3	Nodes positive penetration through muscularis propria
	C2	C3	T4 N1–3	Nodes positive; penetration through muscularis propria and adherence to or invasion of surrounding organs or structures

STAGE GROUPING

TNM				DUKES
Stage 0	Tis	N0	M0	
Stage 1	T1	N0	M0	A
	T2	N0	M0	A
Stage II	T3	N0	M0	B
	T4	N0	M0	B
Stage III	Any T	N1	M0	C
	Any T	N2	M0	C
Stage IV	Any T	Any N	M1	D

Chemotherapy for advanced disease

For nearly 40 years, 5-fluorouracil has been the mainstay of treatment for advanced colorectal cancer. It is typically given with folinic acid to increase efficacy as an inhibitor of thymidilate synthetase. The response rate for 5FU and folinic acid based regimens is of the order of 20%. A number of regimens exist for administering 5FU, as outlined in Table 24.10. Many centres favor the Lokich regimen of continous venous infusion, due to the favorable toxicity profile, and ease of administration.

In the last decade, novel agents have become available with activity in colorectal cancer. The DNA topoisomerase 1 inhibitor irinotecan, used in combination with 5FU and folinic acid, yields a significantly higher response rate of 39%, with a survival benefit of 15.9 months. The novel platinum-based compound oxaliplatin shows similar response rates of 51%, when used in combination with 5FU and folinic acid. Both agents have activity in disease that has become resistant to 5FU, albeit with lower response rates than seen when used in first line therapy. Oxaliplatin and irinotecan regimens are listed in Table 24.11.

The development of oral fluoropyrimidines, such as capecitabine, provides another option for treatment, especially in elderly patients. Capecitabine is a pro-drug, which is selectively activated by thymidine phosphorylase to fluorouracil. Thymidine phosphorylase is expressed in much

Table 24.10 Typical 5FU regimens

Lokich regimen: 5FU 300 mg/m^2 per 24 hours as continuous venous infusion

Weekly regimen: 5FU 370 mg/m^2 iv bolus & folinic acid 20 mg/m^2 iv bolus weekly

Modified de Gramont regimen: Folinic acid 175 mg iv infusion, 5FU 400 mg/m^2 bolus, followed by 5FU 2800 mg/m^2 as a 46-hour ambulatory infusion

Table 24.11 Irinotecan and oxaliplatin regimens for metastatic colon cancer

FOLFOX

Oxaliplatin 85 mg/m^2 infused over 2 hours

Folinic acid 350 mg over 2 hours

Fluorouracil 400 mg/m^2 bolus and

Fluorouracil 2400 mg/m^2 infused over 46 hours

FOLFIRI

Irinotecan 180 mg/m^2 over 30–90 minutes

Folinic acid 350 mg over 2 hours

5-fluorouracil 400 mg/m^2 bolus then

5-fluorouracil 2400 mg/m^2 as a 46-hour infusion

Table 24.12 Prognosis of colon cancer by modified Duke's staging

STAGE	EXTENT OF TUMOUR	5-YEAR SURVIVAL
A	No deeper than submucosa	>90%
B1	Not through bowel wall	80–85%
B2	Through bowel wall	70–75%
C1	Not through bowel wall: lymph node metastases	50–65%
C2	Through bowel wall: lymph node metastases	25–45%

higher levels in tumour cells compared to normal tissue. Thus, concentrations of the active compound are higher in tumour cells than in normal tissue. Trials show that capecitabine has similar response rates to standard 5FU-based regimens.

Newer targeted therapies

Epidermal growth factor receptor (EGFR) antibodies represent a promising new option for patients with metastatic disease that has relapsed after standard chemotherapy. Cetuximab is a novel EGFR monoclonal antibody which, when used in conjunction with irinotecan, produced a 23% response rate in patients whose disease had previously progressed while receiving irinotecan-based chemotherapy. Anti-angiogenic agents including bevacizumab have been shown to be active in the advanced setting when added to combination chemotherapy.

The median survival for patients with metastatic colorectal cancer has improved over the past two decades (Table 24.12). Combination chemotherapy with targeted therapy is expected to improve the median survival to near 2 years. Patients with resectable liver metastases have an overall 5-year survival of 25–30% following hepatic resection and perioperative chemotherapy.

Radiotherapy and colon cancer

Unlike rectal cancer, there are no randomized controlled trials that show that radiotherapy decreases either local recurrence or improves survival in advanced colon cancer. However, there are a number of series that show radiotherapy can reduce local recurrence rates in colon cancer. Several retrospective studies suggest a subset of patients with high-risk factors for local recurrence, such as adherence or invasion of surrounding structures, may benefit from radiotherapy to the resected tumour bed. Either a single fraction of 8 Gy or up to 30 Gy in 10 fractions may be used as a palliative procedure in colon cancer to stop bleeding and help reduce pain.

Follow up

Follow-up protocols for patients with colonic cancer vary across institutions but, in all cases, the patient will undergo endoscopic examination to rule out any local recurrence or new primary lesions. Patients should also have imaging of the liver, either by CT or ultrasound scanning, as part of their follow-up protocol.

Rectal cancer – treatment principles

The quality of primary surgery for rectal cancer is of key importance in reducing local recurrence rates. Historically, 5-year local recurrence rates of 20% were common, which led to an interest in offering neoadjuvant radiotherapy to reduce the risk of local recurrence. Initial studies using preoperative radiotherapy to large pelvic fields produced a reduction in local recurrence rates, but at the cost of a fourfold increase in perioperative mortality. However, more recent studies using a short course of preoperative radiotherapy have produced better results. A dose of 25 Gy in five fractions, using smaller pelvic fields, yielded a reduction in local recurrence rates from 21% to 10%. A 10% improvement in overall survival was also observed, with no significant increase in perioperative mortality.

Specialist colorectal surgeons have been trained in the technique of total mesorectal excision (TME). This technique involves removal of the entire rectum and associated mesorectal fat, and reduces the risk of local recurrence at 5 years from 20% to 6%. It has also been shown that the single most important factor for predicting disease recurrence is the circumferential resection margin. The circumferential resection margin is said to be clear if there is no evidence of tumour from either the primary site, or in an associated lymph node, that extends to within 1 mm of the inked resection margin around the circumference of the excision specimen. Patients at high risk of local recurrence are typically offered long course postoperative radiotherapy, typically a dose of 45 Gy in 25 fractions over 5 weeks.

As TME surgery is now the gold standard for surgical excision, and recurrence rates have fallen to 5–6%, the role of preoperative radiotherapy has been brought into question. A recent Dutch study reported after a median follow up of just over 2 years, that the local recurrence rate was 2.4% for patients who received preoperative radiotherapy prior to TME surgery, compared to an 8.2% recurrence rate in patients receiving no preoperative radiotherapy. The MRC CR07 study was a large prospective study in which patients with operable rectal cancers are randomized to either receive short course preoperative radiotherapy, or primary surgery followed by long course postoperative radiotherapy if the circumferential resection margin is positive. Local recurrence after short course radiotherapy was 4.4% at 3-years compared to 10.6% (p<0.0001) for postoperative chemoradiotherapy.

Advances in pelvic imaging, specifically endoscopic ultrasound and magnetic resonance imaging of the pelvis, can provide excellent soft tissue definition in perirectal tissues, and visualize tumour penetration through the mesorectal fascia. Such patients may then be suitable for long course preoperative radiotherapy, to downstage the tumour prior to surgery.

Patients who are offered long course radiotherapy receive concomitant chemotherapy with either infusional 5FU at 200 mg/m^2/day continuous schedule OR oral capecitabine 825 mg/m^2 bid for the duration of radiotherapy. In more locally advanced tumours, neoadjuvant chemotherapy with oxaliplatin and capecitabine for 12 weeks, concomitant chemoradiation with oral capecitabine and another 12 weeks of adjuvant oxaliplatin and oral capecitabine is recommended.

Palliative radiotherapy can be very helpful in patients with advanced rectal tumours, with symptoms of bleeding or intractable pelvic pain. A short course of treatment (20–30 Gy in 5–10 fractions) is often used for such patients.

Radiotherapy technique

Technique

The patient is immobilized in the prone position using stocks to immobilize the legs. Ideally, the bladder should be comfortably full at the time of simulation. For conventional simulation, barium contrast is introduced into the rectum, and the lowest extent of disease is marked with a wire, together with an anal marker. AP and lateral simulator films are taken for volume definition. For CT planning, the patient is scanned from mid-femur to the umbilicus. Typically, the patient is treated with a three-field technique (8 MV or higher energies, using posterior and two lateral fields) or a four-field 'brick' for 6 MV machines.

Target volume

For primary radiotherapy treatment, the target volume includes the rectum and surrounding mesorectal fat, including the entire presacral space, together with local lymphatics. This includes the perirectal, obturator, and internal iliac nodes.

For conventional planning on orthogonal films, the volume is defined as follows:

Superior: L5/S1 interspace to encompass nodes in the true pelvis
Inferior: 3 cm below the lowest extent of the tumour, sparing the sphincter complex if at all possible
Lateral: 1 cm lateral to the pelvic sidewall, to cover the internal iliac nodes
Anterior: a margin should be allowed from the most anterior part of the rectum. A sagittal MRI image can be very helpful in determining this distance. Typically, the volume extends to the middle of the femoral heads
Posterior: the volume extends to the back of the sacrum, to encompass the entire presacral space.

Very extensive tumours with involvement of the bladder, or tumours that are being treated with palliative intent, are often treated with an anterior and posterior parallel-opposed pair of fields.

Radiotherapy planning using CT planning technique

Rectal tumours are ideal for CT planned conformal radiotherapy, as even small reductions in target volume can significantly reduce the volume of irradiated small bowel.

Patient set up: prone if patient can tolerate otherwise supine. Oral contrast to outline small bowel. Intravenous contrast to highlight vessels is strongly recommended.

Scan from L5 to 4 cm below the anal marker, recommended slice thickness is 3 mm.

The target volume definitions are given below:

GTV: primary tumour, extramural spread, nodes and any intervening normal rectal wall. Outlined on each CT slice.
CTVA: GTV with 1 cm margin in all directions.
CTVB: includes the mesorectal nodes within the mesorectum, presacral and internal iliac nodes.
CTVF (Final CTV): combination of CTVA and CTVB, modified at the clinician's discretion.
PTV: CTVF + 1 cm margin in all directions.

The anatomical boundaries for the CTVB are as follows:

Superior limit: S⅔ interspace for mid and lower third rectal cancers. There should be a 2 cm margin above the most superior limit of the GTV. CTVB margin may have to extend above S⅔ to achieve this 2 cm margin from the GTV
Inferior limit: CTVB inferior limit is 1 cm inferior to CTVA or the puborectalis muscle if there is no involvement of puborectalis (whichever is inferior). If there is involvement of puborectalis or sphincter or levator ani, then the lower limit for CTVB would be the ischiorectal fossa.
Lateral limit: No internal iliac node involvement—medial aspect of the obturator internus Internal iliac node involvement present—limit is bony pelvic sidewall
Anterior limit: 1 cm anterior to the anterior mesorectal fascia or 7 mm anterior to the internal iliac artery (whichever is anterior).
Posterior limit: anterior margin of the sacrum.

Dose and energy

Short course preoperative radiotherapy: 25 Gy in 5 fractions over 1 week (6–8 MV photons)

Long course preoperative radiotherapy: 45 Gy in 25 fractions over 5 weeks (6–8 MV photons) with concurrent intravenous infusional 5FU or oral capecitabine chemotherapy

Long course postoperative radiotherapy: 45 Gy in 25 fractions over 5 weeks (6–8 MV photons) with concurrent intravenous infusional 5FU or oral capecitabine chemotherapy

Palliative radiotherapy: 20–30 Gy in 5–10 fractions (6–8 MV photons)

Treatment toxicity

During treatment, patients may experience cystitis, proctitis and lethargy. The dose-limiting structure for long-term toxicity is the small bowel, with the associated risk of fibrosis, stricturing and obstruction. The risk of small bowel toxicity is directly related to the volume of irradiated small bowel. With careful planning, the risk of significant small bowel toxicity is reduced to around 5%. Other long-term toxicities that need to be considered are impotence in male patients and the increased risk of femoral neck fractures when lateral fields are used.

Chemotherapy

The experience of chemotherapy treatment for colon cancer has been applied to rectal cancers, as both have a propensity for nodal metastases and spread to the liver. Patients are offered adjuvant chemotherapy for high-risk Duke's B tumours and Duke's C tumours. The same chemotherapy regimens used in advanced colonic cancer are used in advanced rectal cancer.

Follow up

Patients with rectal cancer require regular endoscopic follow up to look for local recurrence, and the development of new tumours. In most protocols, the liver is imaged by CT or ultrasound scanning.

ANAL CANCER

Epidemiology and aetiology

Anal cancer constitutes 1% of all malignancies of the bowel, with 250–300 new cases being diagnosed each year in the UK. In most patients, no obvious predisposing factor can be found, though the incidence is higher in homosexual men, due to the association with human papilloma virus type 16 (HPV16) infections. HPV16 DNA is found in the tumour cell genome in 80–90% of tumours, in both men and women. The detection of HPV in the tumour is not a prognostic factor. Tumours are more common in immunosuppressed patients (HIV infection or systemic immunosuppression). Other infectious agents linked include herpes simplex virus, gonorrhea and chlamydia. Smoking has been shown to increase the risk of anal cancer. Tumours in the anal canal are more common in women, while anal margin tumours occur more commonly in men. Anal intraepithelial neoplasia (AIN) is associated with HPV infections and is thought to be a precursor for invasive carcinomas, though the natural history is not as clearly defined as in cervical intraepithelial neoplasia.

Anatomy

The anus is defined as extending from the rectum to the skin of the perianal region. The superior margin is the palpable upper border of anal sphincter and puborectalis muscle. Inferiorly, it extends to skin within a 5 cm radius of the anal verge (Figure 24.2).

There is a transition in the histological type of epithelium lining the anus. Perianal skin is squamous epithelium, which turns to a transitional type epithelium at the dentate line, and then into the glandular mucosal lining of the rectum.

The anus has a dense lymphatic supply via three main routes. The upper canal drains to perirectal and superior hemorrhoidal nodes. The area round the dentate line drains to hypogastric and obturator nodes. The anal verge and perianal skin drains to superficial inguinal nodes.

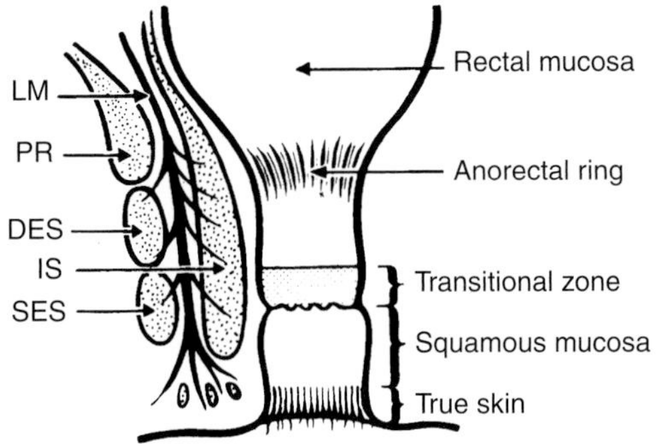

LM —

PR —

DES —

IS —

SES —

— Rectal mucosa

— Anorectal ring

— Transitional zone

— Squamous mucosa

— True skin

Figure 24.2 Anatomy of the anal canal. LM = longitudinal muscle, PR = puborectalis, DES = deep part of the external sphincter, IS = internal sphincter, SES = Superficial part of the anal sphincter.
(Reproduced with permission from Scott, An Aid to Clinical Surgery, 1977, Churchill Livingstone, Elsevier Ltd)

Histopathology

Approximately 80% of anal tumours are squamous cell carcinomas (Figure 24.3). The recognized subtypes are keratinizing large cell, non-keratinizing (transitional cell) and basaloid. Adenocarcinomas occur in 10% of cases, and tend to arise from the glandular mucosa of the upper anal canal. Other tumour types include lymphomas, melanomas, small cell carcinomas and sarcomas.

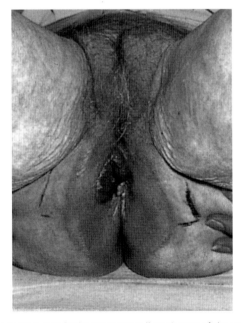

Figure 24.3 Exophytic squamous cell carcinoma of the anal margin.

Clinical features

The symptoms often are non-specific and common symptoms include anal pain and bleeding, pruritus, a mass in the anal region, or discharge. Occasionally, tumours may affect the sphincter mechanism and cause incontinence. On examination, patients may present with ulcerated or exophytic lesions, and inguinal lymphadenopathy may be present. Associated features, such as anal warts or leukoplakia, may be present. Inguinal lymph node metastases are noted in 15% of patients and surgical series show that pelvic nodal spread is present in about 30% of patients at presentation. Systemic metastatic spread is observed in less than 5% of patients at the time of initial diagnosis. Increasing tumour size and depth of penetration into the anal wall increase the risk of nodal metastases.

Staging

The UICC TNM 2002 classification is most commonly used. The staging classification differs for tumours of the anal canal and anal margin (Tables 24.13 and 24.14).

Diagnostic work up and staging

Full history and physical examination including risk factor assessment is followed by an examination under anesthetic to assess the extent of the tumour and to obtain a biopsy for histological confirmation of the diagnosis. One-third of patients present with enlarged inguinal lymph nodes. These should always be biopsied, as 50% of enlarged lymph nodes are reactive, usually due to infection associated with the primary tumour. The patient should also have a chest radiograph, and CT scan of the abdomen and pelvis to

Table 24.13
ANAL CANAL STAGING CLASSIFICATION
T1 Primary tumour ≤2 cm
T2 Primary tumour 2–5 cm
T3 Primary tumour >5 cm
T4 Tumour invades adjacent organs, e.g. vagina, urethra, bladder
N1 Perirectal node involvement
N2 Unilateral inguinal or internal iliac node involvement
N3 Perirectal and inguinal nodes, or bilateral inguinal/ internal iliac node involvement
M0 No distant metastasis
M1 Distant metastasis

Table 24.14
ANAL MARGIN STAGING CLASSIFICATION
T1 Primary tumour ≤2 cm
T2 Primary tumour 2–5 cm
T3 Primary tumour >5 cm
T4 Tumour invades deep extradermal structures, i.e. cartilage, skeletal muscle or bone
N0 No regional lymph node involvement
N1 Regional lymph node metastasis
M0 No distant metastasis
M1 Distant metastasis

complete staging. MRI of the pelvis provides improved soft tissue definition of the primary tumour, and pelvic lymph nodes. It may also be appropriate to perform HIV testing on patients, as patients with undiagnosed HIV and low CD4 counts tend to tolerate chemoradiation poorly.

Treatment

Surgery

In the past, abdomino-perineal excision was the treatment of choice for anal cancers, except for small lesions below the dentate line that could be treated with an implant. Surgery was typically associated with 50–70% 5-year survival rates, but with significant morbidity and the necessity for a permanent colostomy. Locoregional failure rates were around 25–35%. Patients with inguinal nodal disease at presentation have a poor outcome with surgery alone with only a 10–20% 5-year survival rate. Several trials reported favorable results with chemoradiation, producing long-term disease control, and preservation of normal sphincter function. Surgery can then be used to salvage patients with residual or recurrent disease after radiotherapy.

Definitive chemoradiation

Nigro et al, in 1974, first reported the benefits of concurrent chemoradiation for squamous cell carcinoma of the anal canal. Three major randomized clinical trials compared radiation alone to chemoradiation (chemotherapy consists of 5FU and mitomycin-C). Locoregional control, disease-specific and overall survivals were superior in the chemoradiation arm.

The UKCCCR ACT trial of chemoradiation with 5-fluorouracil and mitomycin-C showed that local control rates improved from 39% at 3 years with radiotherapy alone, to 61% with chemoradiation. Overall survival was also improved with chemotherapy, but failed to reach statistical significance. The treatment regimen from the ACT study

became standard practice in the UK. ACT II study evaluates the addition of cisplatin to the 5FU and mitomycin-C.

Radiotherapy treatment principles

Small tumours (T1N0 and T2N0) below the dentate line can be treated with a brachytherapy implant alone. Such tumours should not involve more than a 50% circumference of the anus, and should be less than 1 cm in depth.

Larger tumours and node-positive tumours should be treated with chemoradiation, followed by either in interstitial implant or a boost to the tumour bed.

Target volume – external beam radiotherapy

The clinical target volume includes the primary tumour, first station nodes (pararectal, hypogastric and obturator nodes), presacral and internal iliac nodes. In patients with positive inguinal nodes, the inguinal nodal areas must also be included in the treatment field.

Set-up – conventional planning

The patient is immobilized prone, with the bladder comfortably full to displace small bowel from the treatment field. A marker is placed at the anal verge and barium is instilled to opacify the rectum. Any enlarged inguinal nodes are marked with wire. The volume is treated with an anterior and posterior parallel pair arrangement. The field is defined as follows:

Superior: 2 cm above bottom of sacroiliac joints
Inferior: 3 cm below the anal marker, or 3 cm below the lowest extent of disease
Lateral: 1 cm lateral to the pelvic sidewall. If inguinal nodes are involved, the field needs to be extended laterally to include the affected inguinal nodes.

The first phase is treated to a dose of 45 Gy in 25 fractions over 5 weeks, with concomitant 5-fluorouracil and mitomycin-C given during weeks 1 and 5 of external beam radiotherapy. After a 6-week gap, the patient is then treated with an interstitial implant to a dose of 25 Gy, or a 15 Gy boost to the primary tumour.

Set-up – ACT II protocol

Again, patients are immobilized prone with a full bladder and a marker at the anal verge. Any enlarged nodes are marked with wire.

Phase 1 is treated using a parallel pair technique. The field is defined as follows:

Superior: 2 cm above bottom of sacroiliac joints
Inferior: 3 cm below lowest extent of disease
Lateral: Medial border of greater trochanter.

The phase 2 volume depends on the nodal status of the disease. For node-negative disease, a CT planned volume is used, with a 3 cm margin from GTV to PTV. For node-positive disease, treatment is continued with a parallel pair, using a 3 cm margin round the primary tumour and any enlarged nodes.

Phase 1 is treated to a dose of 30.6 Gy in 17 fractions, and phase 2 to a dose of 19.8 Gy in 11 fractions. Chemotherapy is given during weeks 1 and 5 of radiotherapy and, in the maintenance chemotherapy arm, again at weeks 10 and 14.

Treatment-related toxicity

Patients may experience nausea and vomiting with platinum-based chemotherapy, and may need to be admitted to the ward during the first and fifth weeks of treatment. Patients also develop diarrhea and cystitis during treatment. It is important to ensure that patients remain adequately hydrated during this period. Brisk skin reactions can occur during treatment, and this constitutes the main treatment-related morbidity for patients.

Follow up

Often an examination under anesthetic is repeated 6–8 weeks after completion of radiotherapy to assess the response to treatment. Magnetic resonance imaging can be of considerable benefit in detecting pelvic recurrence of these tumours. Patients who relapse locally after chemoradiation may be salvaged by surgical excision.

Salvage treatment

Patients with local failure without distant metastases after definitive chemoradiation may be considered for salvage abdominoperineal resection.

Palliative treatment

Ten to 20% of patients may develop metastatic disease after locoregional treatment. The most common site for spread is liver; lung, bone, lymph nodes and skin metastases have been reported. Cisplatin- and fluoropyrimidine-based chemotherapy produces response rates of around 50% with a median survival of 12 months. Palliative radiotherapy can be offered for patients with symptomatic nodal, bone or skin metastases.

Prognosis

The tumour size and the depth of invasion are important prognostic factors. Anal margin tumours tend to have a better outcome compared to the anal canal tumours. The overall survival at 5 years for anal canal tumours is 60–80% for chemoradiation patients and for anal margin tumours 5-year survival rates vary from 65 to 100%. Locoregional recurrence is associated with poor prognosis. Salvage surgery may prolong survival in a selected small proportion of patients.

Gastrointestinal Stromal Tumours (GISTS)

Gastro intestinal stromal tumours (GISTS) are the most common mesenchymal tumours of the gastro intestinal tract. However, they are rare tumours and account for <3% of all GI tumours and 5% of all soft tissue sarcomas. GISTS are defined as C KIT positive mesenchymal tumours arising from anywhere in the GI tract or abdomen. The median age at presentation is around 60 years. GISTS are uncommon before the age of 40 and extremely rare in children. They occur equally in both males and females. The most common site is stomach (60-70%) followed by small bowel (20-30%). GISTS are thought to arise from the precursors of the interstitial cells of Cajal (ICC), the pacemaker cells which initiate and control peristalsis. Mutations within the KIT and PDGFRA genes are common and have prognostic and predictive value.

GISTS can present as incidental masses in the abdomen. The common presenting complaints include gastrointestinal bleeding (50%), abdominal pain (20-50%) and feeling of a mass. The most frequent sites of metastases are liver (65%) and omentum (often without ascites) (21%). Risk stratification for relapse is assessed using tumour site, size and mitotic index.

In view of the rarity of GISTS, they should be managed by an experienced multidisciplinary team within a specialist cancer centre. Surgery remains the primary treatment for operable tumours. The response rates to chemotherapy are very low. The systemic treatment has been revolutionized by the discovery of KIT tyrosine kinase inhibitor, imatinib, which is effective in 85% of the patients with metastatic GISTS. Sunitinib, another multi targeted tyrosine kinase inhibitor is licensed for second line use in patients who have progressed or intolerant to imatinib. Recently Imatinib has been shown to improve both the progression free and overall survival in the adjuvant setting in resected high risk GISTS.

FURTHER READING

Esophagus

Herskovic A, Martz K, Al-Sarraf M, et al. Combined chemotherapy and radiotherapy compared with radiotherapy alone in patients with cancer of the esophagus. N Engl J Med 1992;326:1593–8.

Kelsen DP, Ginsberg R, Pajak TF, et al. Chemotherapy followed by surgery compared with surgery alone for localized esophageal cancer. N Engl J Med 1998;339:1979–84.

Allum WH. Medical Research Council Oesophageal Cancer Working Party: Surgical resection with or without preoperative chemotherapy in oesophageal cancer: a randomised controlled trial. Lancet 2002;359:1727–33.

Stomach

Cuscheri A, Weeden S, Fielding J, et al.
Patient survival after D1 and D2
resections for gastric cancer: long term
results of the MRC randomised
surgical trial. Br J Cancer
1999;79:1522–30.

Macdonald JS, Smalley SR, Benedetti J,
et al. Chemoradiotherapy after
surgery compared with surgery
alone for adenocarcinoma of the
stomach or gastroesophageal
junction. N Engl J Med
2001;345:725–30.

Cunningham D, Allum WH, Stenning SP,
et al. Perioperative chemotherapy
versus surgery alone for resectable
gastroesophageal cancer. N Engl J Med
2006;355:11–20.

Bang Y-J, Custem EV, Feyereislova A, et al.
Trastuzumab in combination with
chemotherapy versus chemotherapy
alone for treatment of HER2-positive
advanced gastric or gastro-
oesophageal junction cancer (ToGA):
a phase 3, open-label, randomised
controlled trial. The Lancet
2010;376:687–97.

Pancreas

Butturini G, Stocken DD, Wente MH,
et al. Influence of resection
margins and treatment on survival
in patients with pancreatic cancer:
meta-analysis of randomised
controlled trials. Arch Surg
2008;143:75–83.

Boeck S, Ankerst DP, Heineman V. The
role of adjuvant chemotherapy for
patients with resected pancreatic
cancer: systematic review of
randomised controlled trials and
meta-analysis. Oncology
2007;72:314–21.

Hepatobilary

Simmons DT, Baron TH, Petersen BT,
et al. A novel endoscopic approach to
brachytherapy in the management of
hilar cholangiocarcinoma.
Am J Gastroenterol 2006;101:1792–6.

Wang JS, Fuller D, Kim JS, et al. Prediction
model for estimating the survival
benefit of adjuvant radiotherapy for
gallbladder cancer. J Clin Oncol
2008;26:2112–7.

Valle J, Wasan H, Palmer DH, et al.
Cisplatin plus gemcitabine versus
gemcitabine for biliary tract
cancer. N Engl J Med
2010;362:1273–81.

Colon and rectum

Andre T, Boni C, Mouhedu-Boudiaf L,
et al. Oxaliplatin, fluorouracil and
leucovorin as adjuvant treatment for
colon cancer. N Engl J Med
2004;350:2343–51.

Wolpin BM, Meyerhardt JA, Harvey J,
et al. Adjuvant treatment for colorectal cancer. CA Cancer J Clin
2007;57:168–85.

Fearon ER, Vogelstein B. A genetic model
for colorectal tumourigenesis. Cell
1990;61:759–67.

Swedish Rectal Cancer Group.
Improved survival with preoperative
radiotherapy in resectable rectal
cancer. N Engl J Med 1997;336:980–7.

Kapiteijn E, Marijinen CA, Nagtengaal ID,
et al. for the Dutch colorectal cancer
group. Preoperative radiotherapy
combined with total mesorectal
excision for resectable rectal
cancer. N Engl J Med
2001;345:638–46.

Wolpin BM, Mayer RJ. Systemic treatment
of colorectal cancer. Gastroenterology
2008;134:1296–310.

Bingham SA, Day NE, Luben R, et al.
European prospective investigation
into cancer and nutrition. Dietary
fibre in food and protection against
colorectal cancer in the European
Prospective Investigation into Cancer
and Nutrition (EPIC): an
observational study. Lancet
2003;361:1496–501.

Anal

United Kingdom Coordinating
Committee for Cancer Research
Working Party. Epidermoid
anal cancer: results from the UKCCCR
randomised trial of radiotherapy
alone vs. radiotherapy, 5FU and
mitomycin. Lancet
1996;348:1049–54.

Bartelink H, Roelofsen F, Eschwege F,
et al. Concomitant radiotherapy and
chemotherapy is superior to
radiotherapy alone in the treatment of
locally advanced anal cancer: results of
a phase III randomised trial of
EORTC. J Clin Oncol
1997;15:2040–9.

Glynne-Jones R, Maudsley S. Anal cancer:
the end of the road for neoadjuvant
chemotherapy. J Clin Oncol
2008;26:3669–71.

Sebag-Montefiore D, Stephens RJ,
Steele R, et al. Preoperative
radiotherapy versus selective
postoperative chemoradiotherapy in
patients with rectal cancer (MRC
CR07 and NCIC-CTG C1016): a
multicentre, randomised trial. Lancet
2009;373:811–20.

Rectal Cancer

Gwynne S, Mukherjee S, Webster R, et al.
Imaging for target volume delineation
in rectal cancer radiotherapy — A
Systematic review. Clin Oncol
2012;24:52–63.

Chapter | 25 |

Tumours of the thorax

Alison Armour

LUNG CANCER

Lung cancer remains the second most common cancer and is fatal in 85–90% of cases. This was a rare disease at the beginning of the twentieth century but, due to the explosion of smoking around the World War II, the incidence dramatically increased. By 1950, 80% of men and 40% of women smoked. During the early 1960s, the danger of tobacco was identified and, since the 1970s, the rates of smoking in men have reduced.

Unfortunately, due to a lag period until the development of cancer, the incidence of lung cancer today reflects smoking habits of the population 20 years previously. The incidence of lung cancer in men has been falling since 1990 but this is not the case in eastern European countries, in undeveloped countries or in women. Unfortunately, the incidence of female lung cancer is expected to increase until 2015 when it will almost equal rates in men.

Cigarette smoking accounts for 85–90% of cases. However, only 10–15% of smokers eventually develop lung cancer. There is probably interplay between genetic susceptibility of the disease and environmental factors such as air pollution and radon.

Pathology

Non-small cell lung cancer accounts for the majority of cases; 35–70% are squamous; 9–29% adenocarcinoma and 3–16% large cell. The incidence of small cell is decreasing and is currently 15–20% of tumours. Unfortunately, mesothelioma, which was previously rare, is rapidly increasing in incidence.

Symptoms

Primary

Ninety percent of patients are symptomatic on presentation. Central tumours produce symptoms of cough, pain and hemoptysis. Obstructive infective symptoms or lobar collapse may cause dysponea. If the mediastinum is directly invaded or mediastinal glands are present, hoarseness (secondary to recurrent laryngeal nerve involvement), dysphagia, superior vena caval obstruction and pericardial irritation or effusion develop.

Peripheral tumours may grow to a larger size before causing symptoms. Dysponea may be the presenting sign of a pleural effusion. Direct extension into the rib or brachial plexus causes Pancoast's syndrome. This results in pain or sensory loss of the C7/8 T1 dermatomes and wasting of the small muscles of the hand. If the sympathetic plexus, which lies on the carotid artery, is affected Horner's syndrome is also seen. This is characterized by miosis, ptosis, enophthalmus and ipsilateral anhydrosis.

Secondary

Invasion of the lymphatic system often occurs early. Hilar, mediastinal, neck and even axillary lymphadenopathy is possible. Once the basement epithelium is broken, the patient is at risk of hematogenous spread. Secondary involvement of the liver, adrenals, brain and bones is common.

Paraneoplastic syndromes

Tumours may produce proteins or hormones such as excess adrenocorticotrophic hormone (ACTH) leading to Cushing's syndrome. Depending on the functionality of the protein, endocrine effects may be seen. Antigens expressed by the tumour may lead to cross tissue reactivity and syndromes suggestive of autoimmune disease.

Diagnosis

Patients presenting with the above symptoms require a chest x-ray. A lateral view may be helpful. A computed tomography (CT) scan of the chest and upper abdomen is recommended before bronchoscopy as peripheral tumours will not be reached by bronchoscopy and, in these cases, a CT-guided biopsy is required for histological diagnosis. Magnetic resonance imaging (MRI) can be used to determine if there are direct invasion structures contraindicating surgery but is not superior to CT in the detection of mediastinal disease (Table 25.1).

PET scanning

Positron emission tomography (PET scanning) is not currently widely used in the diagnosis and follow up of

Table 25.1 Assessment of patients with lung cancer

History and examination including performance status and weight loss
FBC, U&E, glucose, calcium, LFT
Chest x-ray and lateral
Bronchoscopy for histological/cytological diagnosis and to assess extent of the lesion
CT of chest and upper abdomen
Additional tests are required depending on symptoms and the results of the above

Additional staging if considering surgery:
Pulmonary function tests
Arterial blood gases
Coagulation screen
CT of chest, abdomen and brain
Mediastinoscopy to sample mediastinal lymph nodes
MRI scanning may have a role if direct invasion of other structures may contraindicate surgery

patients with lung cancer. The basis of PET scanning is the increased metabolic activity of cancer which avidly takes up glucose. Following administration of 18 fluorodeoxy-D-glucose (^{18}F-FDG) there is emission of positrons from tumour-bearing areas. PET scanning is a high resolution, whole body technique which can demonstrate the extent of tumour spread. It is also useful in differentiating between benign and malignant pulmonary nodules. PET can detect lymph node spread more accurately than even spiral CT scanning.

One disadvantage of PET scanning is the rather limited anatomical information provided and a supplementary CT scan must be performed with image overlay to relate increased metabolic activity to anatomical sites. Moreover, it is possible to have a false positive scan.

Increased glucose metabolism may also be seen in a variety of inflammatory conditions including active tuberculosis, sarcoidosis abscesses and pneumonia.

Non-small cell lung cancer (NSCLC)

Staging

The NSCLC Staging system (Table 25.2) is based on the TNM (tumour, node, metastases) method of staging and divides patients into prognostic groups for treatment.

The staging and survival of NSCLC (Table 25.3) illustrates the prognostic importance of the current staging system.

The management of NSCLC

Surgery

Surgery offers the best chance of cure. Patients must be carefully selected, as incomplete excision is of no benefit. Patients must undergo extensive staging and, in practice,

Table 25.2 The staging system of NSCLC

T STAGE	DISEASE EXTENT
T_0	No evidence of tumour
T_{is}	Carcinoma in situ
T_x	Tumour cells obtained from sputum, no site of primary found on bronchoscopy
T_1	Tumour <3 cm surrounded by visceral pleura or lung tissue
T_2	Tumour larger than 3 cm but more than 2 cm from the carina. Involves the visceral pleura or causes atelectasis or obstructive pneumonitis of less than one lung
T_3	Tumour less than 2 cm from the carina but not involving it. Tumour invades chest wall; diaphragm; mediastinal pleura; parietal pericardium or causes atelectasis or obstructive pneumonitis of the whole lung
T_4	Tumour invades heart; great vessels; trachea; oesophagus; vertebral body; pleural effusion or satellite tumour nodules within the same lobe
N_x	The nodal status cannot be determined
N_0	No regional lymph node involvement
N_1	Ipsilateral peribronchial and/or hilar lymphnode involvement
N_2	Ipsilateral mediastinal and/or subcarinal lymphnodes
N_3	Contralateral mediastinal or hilar lymphnodes. Supraclavicular lymphnodes
M_x	Distant metastases cannot be determined
M_0	Distant metastases absent
M_1	Distant metastases present

only those with stage I and II tumours and good cardiopulmonary function are suitable for surgery (Table 25.4).

Occasionally, patients may have surgically resectable disease but are unable to tolerate a surgical procedure due to medical co-morbidity. These patients may be considered for radical radiotherapy.

Radical radiotherapy

Thoracic radiotherapy is particularly challenging as the tumour is a moving target within an area surrounded by critical and radiosensitive tissues, such as lung parenchyma and spinal cord. In addition, the characteristics of the beam are altered as the beam passes through lung tissue. Careful planning is required to take these challenges into account (Table 25.5).

Technique

Patients should be CT planned, lying supine in an immobilization device. The patient is instructed to breathe normally. The normal treatment position is 'arms up, elbows flexed' but, for apical tumours, it may be better to have the arms down (Figure 25.1).

A CT scan is performed from the level of the larynx to the bottom of L2. This is to enable accurate delineation of the target and the lungs, spinal cord and other critical structures so that dose calculations to these structures are possible.

Target volume

Traditionally, 'elective nodal irradiation' was suggested for early stage NSCLC. Using this technique, the field extends from 5 to 8 cm below the carina, includes the entire mediastinum and bilateral hilar and extends superiorly to include the bilateral supraclavicular fossae. Such fields result in significant toxicity that limits the total dose deliverable. There is no evidence that this technique is superior to 'involved field only' techniques. The regional nodal recurrence with both is low, local recurrence more likely and the adoption of 'involved field only' treatment allows the possibility of dose escalation.

The 'involved field only' technique requires the treatment to be CT planned. The gross tumour volume (GTV) should be defined as all radiologically demonstrable tumour and any nodes over 1 cm in size. A planning target volume of GTV plus 1.5 cm in the lateral dimension and 2 cm vertical margin should be applied.

The type of plan created depends on the site of the tumour, whether central or peripheral. If the patient has undergone pneumonectomy, surgical clips may define the clinical target volume. It is important to ensure that beams pass through the resected space and spare the remaining contralateral lung (Figure *evolve*s 25.2 and 25.3 🖱).

Usually, three fields are required for optimum dose distribution but, occasionally, if there is a small peripheral tumour, wedged opposed oblique fields may be used (Figure *evolve* 25.4 🖱).

Depth dose tables estimating the dose at each point in tissue have been derived from experiments in solid tissue. Since air is much less dense, there is less scatter of the beam on traversing lung. As a result, the dose is 3% greater for every centimetre of lung traversed. Therefore, on calculating the dose to the tumour, the lung correction factor must be applied (Figure *evolve*s 25.5 and 25.6 🖱).

Tolerances

It is hard to specify patient factors that predict the development of pneumonitis, but the mean lung dose and V_{20} (the volume of both lungs receiving more than 20 Gy) can help identify those particularly at risk.

Table 25.3 Staging and survival of NSCLC

STAGE	TNM SUBSET	5-YEAR SURVIVAL CLINICAL STAGE (%)	5-YEAR SURVIVAL PATHOLOGICAL STAGE (%)	MANAGEMENT
0	Ca in situ			
IA	T1N0	61	67	Surgery or radical radiotherapy
IB	T2N0	38	57	
IIA	T1N1	34	55	
IIB	T2N1 T3N0	24	39	
IIIA	T3N1 T1–3N2	13	23	Contentious Radiotherapy/chemotherapy/palliation
IIIB	Any T N3 T4 any N	5		
IV	Any M1	1		Palliative

Table 25.4 Contraindications for surgery in NSCLC

OPERABLE	CONTRAINDICATIONS
FEV1 > 1.5 Stage I and II NSCLC	Poor lung function Phrenic nerve palsy (elevated diaphragm) Recurrent laryngeal nerve palsy (hoarseness) Invasion of trachea, aorta, heart, superior vena cava, oesophagus Distant metastases Metastatic SCLC Malignant pleural effusion

Table 25.5 Indications for radical radiotherapy

Stage 1&2 NSCLC – medically inoperable
Tumour volume approximately 5 cm
FEV>1; FVC>1.5
Weight loss <10%
Positive margins postoperatively
Heavy N2 disease postoperatively (individual patient basis)
Wedge resection
Stage 3 disease sufficiently downstaged to be included in a radical volume

A mean lung dose of 18–21 Gy is thought to give a low risk of development of pneumonitis, whereas 24–26 Gy patients are more likely to develop acute pneumonitis. V_{20}, the volume of both lungs receiving more than 20 Gy, is probably the most reliable predictor at present and it is suggested that this value be less than 32% to avoid grade 3 or more pneumonitis.

The spinal cord should receive no more than 40–44 Gy depending on fraction size. Twelve centimeters of

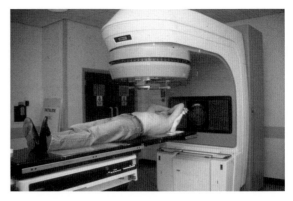

Figure 25.1 The treatment position for radical radiotherapy.

oesophagus should receive no more than 50 Gy. Heart doses at present are hard to define. They may not be reported routinely but the whole heart should receive less than 40 Gy and two thirds of it less than 55 Gy (Figure *evolve* 25.7 🖱).

Doses

Suggested radiation doses are given in Table 25.6.

Table 25.6 Suggested radiation doses for NSCLC

INDICATION	SUGGESTED DOSE REGIMENS
Radical postoperative dose	50 Gy 20–23 fractions given in 4–5 weeks
Radical radiotherapy	55 Gy 20 fractions given in 4 weeks 60 Gy 30 fractions given in 6 weeks

Acute reactions

General fatigue and oesophagitis are common. Oeophagitis should respond to simple analgesics and antacids and should settle within 4 weeks of treatment.

Late reactions

Acute pneumonitis occurs in 10% of cases and is the most common and serious complication of radical treatment. Patients present with dry cough, fever and shortness of breath. A chest x-ray may show a hazy appearance, usually in the treated area. Therapy should be oxygen, antibiotics and high dose steroids (prednisolone 60 mg per day). Occasionally Lhermitte's sign (an electric shock sensation when flexing the neck) is seen. Pulmonary fibrosis, esophageal stricture and pericardial effusion are seen in the longer term.

Palliative radiotherapy

The volume of a treatment field is determined by the site of the tumour and disease extent but the dose for palliative treatment was established by a series of MRC trials published between 1991 and 1996.

Table 25.7 demonstrates the effectiveness of palliative radiotherapy for the common symptoms of lung cancer.

Palliative treatments should be simple and effective. The treatment field should include the gross tumour volume and drainage nodal groups. Contralateral paratracheal nodal involvement has been found in 25–45% of tumours. Treatment is a parallel pair (average size 10 × 12 cm) (Figure 25.8).

Good performance status patients not suitable for neoadjuvant chemotherapy may benefit from 39 Gy in 13 fractions. This dose exceeds cord tolerance so many centres apply cord shielding to the posterior field once cord tolerance is reached.

Bone metastases

Bone pain and pathological fracture are common complications of lung cancer. Pain can be controlled by an 8 Gy single fraction delivered in a parallel pair or direct field.

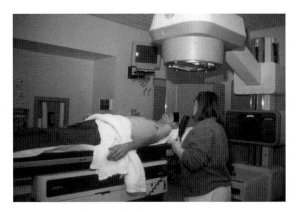

Figure 25.8 Palliative radiotherapy.

Brain metastases

Patients aged less than 60, with good performance status and controlled extracranial disease should receive whole brain radiotherapy, 20 Gy in five fractions.

Patients with isolated, accessible, single brain metastases and controlled extracranial disease should be considered for surgical resection or radiosurgery on an individual patient basis. This is usually followed by whole brain radiotherapy (30 Gy in 10 fractions) (Figure 25.9).

Chest retreatment

Retreatment of patients having had palliative radiotherapy can be considered on an individual patient basis if the patient has had a previous response to radiotherapy and it is more than 6 months from the initial treatment (Table 25.8).

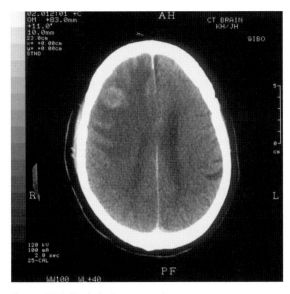

Figure 25.9 Single brain metastasis.

Table 25.7 Symptoms control rates: MRC studies of palliative radiotherapy			
	1991	1992	1996
Hemoptysis	81%	73%	92%
Cough	65%	52%	52%
Pain		65%	57%

Table 25.8 Suggested regimens for retreatment of palliative radiotherapy

PREVIOUS	RETREATMENT	COMMENT
8 Gy single	8 Gy single	
10 Gy single	20 Gy 5 fractions	If feel life expectancy short but patient worth treating
10 Gy single	20 Gy 10 fractions	If feel patient has reasonable life expectancy. Shield cord posteriorly
17 Gy 2 fractions	20 Gy 10 fractions	Shield cord posteriorly

Chemotherapy for non small cell lung cancer (NSCLC)

The quality of life of patients with metastatic NSCLC may be improved by the judicious use of platinum-based two drug combinations (doublets). A meta-analysis has shown a modest increase in survival of 1.5 months with platinum doublets compared to best supportive care. Doublets of cisplatin combined with gemcitabine, paclitaxel, docetaxel or vinorelbine give similar response rates of 20-30% and a similar median survival of 8-10 months. The average 1 year survival is 30-40%. The addition of a third drug did not increase response rates or survival. A meta-analysis showed cisplatin doublets produced a statistically significant better response rate and better survival when compared to carboplatin-based combinations. However, given the palliative nature of this type of chemotherapy the modest survival advantage offered by cisplatin compared to carboplatin has to be balanced against the greater toxicity, particularly nausea and vomiting associated with cisplatin. A combination of cisplatin (75 mg/m^2) and the anti-folate drug pemetrexed (500 mg/m^2) given 3 weekly is associated with fewer adverse side-effects than other combinations and is being used more frequently in the UK. A commonly used alternative regimen is carboplatin (AUC5) 3 weekly plus gemcitabine (1250 mg/m^2) day 1 and 8.

New trends in the radiation treatment of NSCLC

Stereotactic body radiation therapy (SBRT) is a method for delivery of high biologically effective doses to lung tumours while minimising normal tissue toxicity. Multiple beam angles are used to achieve sharp dose gradients. Tumour motion owing to breathing needs to be countered by techniques such as respiratory gating. Accurate tumour location

and verification of treatment by devices such as a cone beam CT scanner incorporated into the linear accelerator are vital. Treatment is usually given in a few large fractions such as 60 Gy in 3 fractions (RTOG) or 70 Gy in 10 fractions (MD Anderson). Early results seem as good as surgery for patients with inoperable stage I and II disease.

Small cell lung cancer (SCLC)

Natural history

There is a tendency for the disease to disseminate widely and rapidly resulting in 80% of patients having metastatic disease at presentation despite having symptoms for a short period, often weeks. Spread is local, via the lymphatics and hematogenous systems (Table 25.9). There is a high incidence of paraneoplastic conditions.

Staging and diagnosis

The following investigations are required fully to assess and stage the patient:

- history and exam (including performance status and weight loss)
- full blood count (FBC), full biochemistry screen including lactate dehydrogenase (LDH)
- chest x-ray
- CT chest and upper abdomen
- bronchoscopy for histological/cytological diagnosis
- other imaging and investigations determined by results of the above.

The staging classification for SCLC is currently under review.

Patients can be staged according to the TNM classification but patients are, at present, classified as having limited stage disease if the disease is confined to one hemithorax and as 'extensive stage' if the disease is more extensive.

The disadvantage of this system is that it excludes patients with contralateral mediastinal nodes that can be treated with consolidation radiotherapy and includes, at present, patients with pleural effusion not amenable to radiation treatment.

Table 25.9 Metastatic sites of SCLC

SITE	% METASTASES
Liver	62
Adrenal	39
Bone	38
Brain	50
Abdominal nodes	57

Table 25.10 Prognostic factors for SCLC

PATIENT	DISEASE
Performance status (<2 poor)	Stage of disease (limited, v. extensive)
Weight loss (>10% poor)	Serum bicarbonate <24
<70 years old	Serum sodium <132
	LDH or alkaline phosphatase (>1.5×normal)

Poor prognostic factors are listed in Table 25.10. Patients with more than one of these would not be considered for intensive treatment.

Management

Chemotherapy

Combination chemotherapy is necessary in this disease to improve quality of life and survival. With no systemic treatment, the survival of these patients is short, approximately 3 months.

Several regimens exist and most are equivalent (Table 25.11).

Chemotherapy can induce remission in 80% of limited stage patients and prolongs median survival to 14 months. Even 25% of patients with extensive stage disease can

Table 25.11 Suggested regimens for SCLC

REGIMEN	DRUG	DOSES	SCHEDULE
CAVE	Cyclophosphamide	750 mg/m^2	IV day1
	Adriamycin	40 mg/m^2	IV day1
	Vincristine	1.4 mg/m^2	IV day1
	Etoposide	75 mg/m^2	IV day 1
	Etoposide	150 mg/m^2	PO days 2&3
ICE (3 weekly)	Ifosfamide	5 g/m^2	IV day 1
	MESNA	5 g/m^2	IV day
	Carboplatin	300 mg/m^2	IV day1
	Etoposide	120 mg/m^2	IV days 1+2
	Etoposide	240 mg/m^2	po day 3
PE (3 weekly)	Cisplatin	75 mg/m^2	IV day 1
	Etoposide	100–120 mg/m^2	IV day 1–3
CE (3/4 weekly)	Carboplatin	AUC=5/6	IV day 1
	Etoposide	100–120 mg/m^2	IV day 1–3

achieve a complete response and a median survival of 8 months is expected (Table 25.12).

PE was originally developed as salvage therapy for relapsed or resistant small cell where response rates were 50%. However, it soon became established as first-line therapy because of its tolerability and ease of combination with radiation. Carboplatin can be substituted for cisplatin if renal clearance is inadequate and has the advantage of outpatient administration. Usually four to six cycles of chemotherapy are sufficient. There is no evidence that a more prolonged alternating regimen or dose intensive chemotherapy is of additional benefit as, for most patients, chemotherapy is essentially palliative treatment. A recent MRC trial suggested that for the good performance, limited stage patient, intensive chemotherapy may produce a small survival benefit.

More than 25% of patients are over 70 years and this is a group of patients who are under-represented in clinical trials and optimal therapy remains contentious.

Increased co-morbidity and reduced functional organ reserve lead some to suggest that patients over 70 years are at risk of compromised dose and increased toxicity. Treatment decisions should be based on clinical fitness, performance status and the disease extent. Fit patients should receive standard regimens. Frail patients may be better treated with single agent such as carboplatin, etoposide, or newer third-line agents such as taxanes, gemcitabine and vinorelbine.

Retreatment with chemotherapy on relapse can be considered if the patient remains of good performance status. Traditionally, CAV after PE results in low response rates (10%) but retreatment with the same regimen or newer agents, such as topotecan, may be considered where response rates of 40% have been reported. Responses, however, are of short duration. Unfortunately, patients who do not respond to first-line therapy or if relapse occurs within 3 months of treatment are unlikely to respond to further chemotherapy.

Radiotherapy

In 1992, two meta-analyses indicated that the addition of thoracic radiotherapy enhanced local control and gave a 5% improvement in survival at 3 years. The benefit of chest consolidation radiotherapy was demonstrated in patients achieving a good response to chemotherapy. It is therefore not appropriate for patients with a poor response to chemotherapy, extensive disease or patients with a pleural effusion, as the volume of the whole hemithorax is too large to treat safely.

The field is based on the extent of disease before chemotherapy, if possible. The mediastinum is usually included but, if it is a small peripheral tumour, it may be practical to treat the primary site only. Doses vary but most centres use between 40 and 50 Gy delivered in 15–25 fractions.

Techniques to cover the volume vary. The most frequently used is a parallel pair with lead shielding of the spinal cord (posterior field only) for the last three to five fractions.

Table 25.12 Chemotherapy response rates for SCLC

STAGE	RESPONSE RATE (%)	COMPLETE RESPONSE (%)	MEDIAN SURVIVAL (MONTHS)	2-YEAR SURVIVAL (%)
Limited	80	60	14	20
Extensive	60	23	8	<5

Table 25.13 Advantages and disadvantages of concurrent chemoradiotherapy

ADVANTAGES	DISADVANTAGES
Additional cell kill by radiation	Treat everyone not just those having good response
Synergistic effect of cisplatin and radiation	Toxicity more severe
Reduces the chance of chemoresistant clones being able to metastasize	Toxicity may compromise the systemic treatment
	Combining both modalities may compromise the dose of each

With the introduction of non-anthracycline chemotherapy regimens, the combination of radiation and chemotherapy became possible. Several issues remain, however, over volume, dosage and fractionation inconcurrent schedules (Table 25.13). Prophylactic cranial irradiation (PCI), however, is never combined with chemotherapy, instead being deferred to the end of chemotherapy treatment.

Concurrent chemoradiation

A recent meta-analysis suggested that, if radiotherapy is added to chemotherapy before or during the third cycle of chemotherapy, results are better.

In concurrent treatment, however, the volume size remains contentious. Early large randomized controlled trials used large volumes where the primary tumour, entire mediastinum and often supraclavicular fossa were included. More recently, an 'involved field only' approach is used where the field is determined by the pre-chemotherapy gross tumour volume.

CT planned volumes are mandatory for 'an involved field only' approach. In this situation, a CT generated three-field plan, with lung corrections, as described for NSCLC, is probably optimal for balancing both lung doses and cord doses.

The clinical target volume includes gross tumour volume and any nodes larger than 10 mm. A margin of 2 cm is added in the vertical margins and 1.5 cm in the lateral dimension. Mean lung dose should not exceed 35 Gy. Cord dose should be less than 45 Gy. No more than 12 cm of oesophagus should be included in the radical dose volume.

Doses ranging between 40 and 50 Gy are associated with a 40–50% local relapse rate. The maximum tolerated dose at present is considered to be 70 Gy given in 35 daily fractions (3% local relapse).

A dose relationship exists between total dose and local control but the doubling time of small cell is so short, sometimes days, that the overall treatment time becomes important.

Turrissi pioneered twice-daily fractionation where 45 Gy was given over 30 treatments in 15 days compared to 45 Gy given over 25 treatments in 5 weeks. There was a reduction in local (36 versus 52%) and systemic relapse (6 versus 23%). There was an improvement in 5-year survival (26% versus 6%). This is at present considered the maximum tolerated dose for twice daily fractionation.

Early concurrent chemoradiation and hyperfraction at present appear to be the treatment of choice in those patients fit enough to tolerate it, but local control remains a significant problem. Studies are therefore underway to investigate the role of dose escalation while keeping the overall treatment time short.

Prophylactic cranial irradiation (PCI)

Brain metastases are common. At diagnosis, 20% of patients have brain metastases which rises to 50% at 2 years and 80% at post-mortem. If chemotherapy alone is used, half of those patients who achieve complete response (CR) will relapse with brain secondaries within 2 years. The addition of radiotherapy reduces this incidence of brain metastases from 58% to 33% In addition, there is a small improvement in survival (5%)

The rationale of irradiating a sanctuary site was taken directly from the paediatric population where PCI had been found to reduce the site of brain relapse in childhood leukaemia.

Two large studies therefore confirmed the safety and effectiveness in PCI at reducing local relapse. But its influence on overall survival was more contentious and only suggested by the large meta-analysis.

Method

The patient's head is immobilized in the supine position. A parallel pair technique is used comprising of two opposed lateral fields. An anatomical line (from the outer margin of the orbit, outer canthus and through the lower tragus) can be used to set up the fields. Simulation is essential to check the temporal lobes and cribiform plate are included in the treated volume. Both fields are irradiated daily. The dose is prescribed to the midpoint intersection of both beams (ICRU 50).

Dose

The optimum dose of PCI is not known. Evidence suggests that a dose–response relationship probably does exist. The UK/EORTC trial compared three arms, no PCI versus 24 Gy versus 36 Gy. Three hundred and fourteen patients were recruited from 1987 t0 1995. No difference in local control rates was found between those patients that received no PCI or only 24 Gy. There was, however, a difference between the no treatment group and those that received 36 Gy; 24 Gy in 2 Gy fractions is probably insufficient but 24 Gy given in 3 Gy fractions is more effective. It is possible that higher doses per fraction produce better local control. However, retrospective studies suggest that CNS damage will occur with doses greater than 30 Gy given in fractions of 3 Gy or greater. Therefore, doses greater than 30 Gy should be given in fractions less than 3 Gy.

Toxicity

Common acute side effects are headache, tiredness, nausea, and reversible alopecia. These can be treated with steroids or other antiemetics. About 8–10 weeks post-irradiation, somnolence is common and anorexia, sleepiness and lethargy are common complaints. These are self-limiting, however, and do not predict late neurotoxicity. Patients with SCLC have a limited life span so the true incidence of late neurological damage is not known.

Timing of PCI

The optimum timing of PCI is unknown. Radiotherapy may cause disruption of the blood–brain barrier and can potentiate the neurotoxic effects of chemotherapy drugs. Most clinicians now administer this *after* chemotherapy. PCI must be completed within 6 months of diagnosis to be of benefit.

Safety

Small retrospective studies led to concern about the incidence of neuropsychological sequelae in patients treated with both chemotherapy and PCI.

However, two large trials incorporated an assessment of neurological function as part of follow up and found no difference between those patients who received PCI and those that did not.

These studies have shown no loss of neurocognitive function or neurological deficit following PCI. However, 40% of patients had some degree of cognitive impairment after chemotherapy but this was not worsened by PCI.

The role of surgery

Less than 10% of patients have stage one (T1, T2) disease and, occasionally, these patients have surgical resection to remove an undiagnosed pulmonary nodule. Small retrospective studies suggest that these patients may do well if standard chemotherapy and radiotherapy follow treatment. There is no evidence that patients with more advanced disease, T3 or N2 benefit from surgical treatment.

Mesothelioma

Mesothelioma is a malignant tumour of the pleura and the majority of cases are caused by exposure to asbestos.

There are two main types of asbestos fibres: serpentiles (white asbestos) and amphiboles (blue asbestos). White asbestos fibres are pliable, curly and easily broken down in the lung releasing magnesium, iron and silica. About 90% of industry used this type and, fortunately, it is rarely associated with mesothelioma. Blue asbestos fibres, however, are rigid and non-pliable. Lung phagocytes repeatedly attempt to breakdown these fibres and eliminate them. It is thought that this chronic inflammatory response leads to eventual mesothelial cell proliferation, mutation and malignancy. This may explain the long latency period of 20–40 years from first exposure to asbestos and development of this tumour. It may also explain why even a short period of exposure can result in mesothelioma.

Asbestos was commonly used for insulation in buildings and homes, building ships, and car parts. It is estimated that the risk of development of this disease is greatest in men born around 1945–50, of whom, it is anticipated that 1 in 150 will die of mesothelioma.

In Turkey, there is a high incidence of mesothelioma. At first this was thought to be due to asbestos like mineral fibres in the soil. However, these non-asbestos related tumours are hereditary in nature and have been found to be associated with carriage of an autosomal dominant gene.

Natural history

Clinically, it is a very heterogeneous disease, but the majority of patients will progress rapidly and succumb to their illness within 8 months but others may remain stable for some time without any clinical intervention.

Patients initially present with a pleural effusion but, in the later stages of the illness, the tumour encases, constricts and focally invades the underlying lung causing increasing pain and dysponea (Figure 25.10). Despite this, symptoms of superior vena cava obstruction and dysphagia are uncommon. Similarly, metastases are common at post-mortem but rarely clinically relevant unless surgery or a prolonged natural history alters the natural history of the disease.

Prognostic groups are based on the following factors: patient age, sex, weight loss and performance status, tumour histology and clinical stage, values of haemoglobin, leukocyte ($>8.3 \times 10^9$/L) and platelet count ($>400 \times 10^9$/L) at presentation.

Computed tomography with magnetic resonance imaging in selected cases often allows a fair approximation of clinical stage and PET scanning may prove to be of additional value.

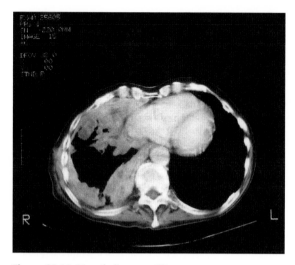

Figure 25.10 Mesothelioma on CT.

Several different staging systems exist with no general consensus on use. The Butchart staging system is the simplest (Table 25.14). The IMIG staging system is more detailed, based on TNM (Table 25.15). The disadvantage of these systems is that they are surgically based requiring information about surgical resection margins and lymph node involvement when the majority of patients are technically irresectable (Table 25.16).

Radiotherapy

Indications for the role of radiotherapy in mesothelioma are:

- prophylaxis drain site recurrence
- palliation of pain and shrinkage of chest wall masses
- postoperative in combined modality.

Mesothelioma has the ability to track out from the chest wall resulting in painful subcutaneous nodules. If radiotherapy is applied to the drain site area within 4 weeks, it alters the capillaries and stroma in this area making an unfavorable environment for tumour cells to embed and proliferate.

This practice therefore reduces the incidence of drain site recurrence from 40% to 0% in the original publications.

Two different beams can be used. Electrons can be applied in a direct field covering the wound and drain sites. Bolus is usually used to ensure 100% dose at the surface. The energy of the beam must be carefully chosen to cover this plus the required depth of the chest wall and thickened pleura.

Some institutions favour a kilovoltage field if electrons are not available. This could be applied in a direct field as long as the doses at depth are adequate for the particular patient. A dose of 21 Gy delivered over three fractions is a commonly used regimen.

Palliative radiotherapy

Radiation therapy is also performed to control pain. Irradiation is effective when pain is caused by a direct extension of the tumour into the chest wall and ribs. Conversely, it is not effective and may even be harmful if pain originates from compression of the intercostal nerve as a result of retraction of the chest wall. Post-radiation fibrosis can aggravate pain in these cases.

Postoperative adjuvant radiotherapy

At present, this treatment should not be considered outwith the context of a clinical trial. The challenges are multiple. The clinical target volume involves the entire hemithorax and mediastinum. It includes the full thickness of the chest wall at the incision sites. This area is surrounded by radiosensitive critical normal structures, e.g. the remaining contralateral lung, spinal cord, liver, spleen, kidney and intestine. The challenges of delivering a radical dose around an empty air-filled cavity and the need for correction factors should also be considered.

Usually, a mixture of photon beams and electrons is used to deliver a dose of 50–55 Gy to the resected area plus a margin to include other areas that may include tumour. Occasionally, small sites are boosted to 60 Gy. This treatment is still experimental, intensity modulated radiotherapy (IMRT) techniques are being developed and each plan should be carefully tailored to the individual clinical situation.

STAGE	DESCRIPTION	CATEGORY	PROGNOSIS
	Table 25.14 The Butchart staging system		
1	Tumour confined within the parietal pleura: ipsilateral pleura, lung, pericardium or diaphragm	Localized	16 months
2	Tumour invades chest wall, mediastinal structures plus N1 or N2 nodes	Advanced	5 months
3	Extension of disease through diaphragm to peritoneum or opposite pleura. N3 nodes. That is nodes outwith chest	Advanced	
4	Hematogenous spread	Advanced	

Table 25.15 The International Mesothelioma Interest Group staging system

TUMOUR (T)	DESCRIPTION
T1a	Tumour limited to ipsilateral parietal pleura. No involvement of visceral pleura
T1b	T1a but scattered foci of tumour involving the visceral pleura
T2	Tumour involving ipsilateral pleura (parietal, mediastinal, diaphragmatic and visceral) with at least one of the following features: • involvement of the diaphragmatic muscle • confluent visceral pleural tumour (including the fissures) or • extension of tumour from visceral pleura into the underlying pulmonary parenchyma
T3	Locally advanced but potentially resectable tumour. Tumour involving all of the ipsilateral pleural surfaces with at least one of the following: • involvement of endothoracic fascia • extension into mediastinal fat • solitary, completely resectable focus of tumour extending into soft tissues of the chest wall, non-transmural involvement of the pericardium
T4	Locally advanced technically unresectable tumour. Involves all the ipsilateral pleural surfaces with at least one of the following: • diffuse extension or multifocal masses of tumour in the chest wall with or without associated rib destruction • direct trans-diaphragmatic extension of tumour to the peritoneum • through to the contralateral pleura • direct extension of tumour to one or more mediastinal organs • direct extension of tumour into the spine • tumour extending through to the internal surface of the pericardium with or without a pericardial effusion or tumour involving the myocardium
Nx	Regional nodes cannot be assessed
N1	Positive ipsilateral bronchopulmonary or hilar lymph nodes
N2	Subcarinal or ipsilateral mediastinal lymph nodes including the ipsilateral internal mammary nodes
N3	Positive contralateral mediastinal, contralateral internal mammary, ipsilateral or contralateral supraclavicular lymph nodes
M0	No distant metastases
M1	Distant metetastases present

Table 25.16 Summary of TNM stage for mesothelioma

Stage 1a	T1a
Stage 1b	T1b
Stage II	T2
Stage III	Any T3, N1 or N2
Stage IV	Any T4, N3, M1

Chemotherapy

The role of chemotherapy in mesothelioma remains contentious. Single agent and combination regimens give response rates between 10 and 20%.

More recently, a newer agent, a multitargeted antifolate (Alimta-pemetrexed) has shown 40% response rates and a tolerable toxicity profile if patients are adequately replaced with vitamin B12 and folate.

Neuroendocrine tumours

Pulmonary carcinoid tumours are rare, accounting for only 1% of all lung tumours but the lung is the primary site of 25% of all carcinoid tumours. The biological aggressiveness of carcinoid tumours is variable but the majority are well differentiated and rarely metastasize. These tumours are found in main, lobar or segmented bronchi and present with cough, haemoptysis or local obstructive symptoms. Such tumours ideally should be treated by surgery and 5-year survival rates of 87–100% have been reported.

By contrast, patients with histologically atypical carcinoids (poorly differentiated, pleomorphic cells, increased mitosis and necrotic areas) have a poorer survival (5-year survival 25–69%). Such patients are more likely to develop metastatic spread to liver, bones, adrenals and central nervous system. Carcinoids may produce excess catecholamines and kinin production leading to the carcinoid syndrome. This is categorized by facial flushing often provoked by stress, excitement or alcohol, diarrhoea and, in the long term, fibrosis and incompetence of the right-sided heart valves.

Such patients have raised levels of catecholamine metabolites in urine such as 3-methoxy-4-hydroxy mandelic acid (UMA) and hydroxyindole acetic acid (HIAA). As well as conventional imaging, such as CT scanning, radiolabeled octreotide (octreoscans) can be useful in establishing the extent of disease.

Some series suggest up to 80% of tumours respond to radiotherapy and this is particularly useful in the treatment of bone metastases.

No chemotherapy combination has clearly been shown to be beneficial in this disease. Streptozotocin, 5-fluorouracil, cyclophosphamide, dacarbazine or doxorubicin alone or in combination have objective responses of 20–40% often of short duration.

Treatment for the majority of patients with systemic disease is usually symptomatic. The disease often follows an indolent course and somatostatin analogues, such as octreotide, usually markedly reduce the symptoms due to serotonin release from the tumour. Interferon is less effective in foregut carcinoids than at other sites, but a trial of interferon may be indicated in patients with progressive disease.

Thymoma

Thymoma presents as a mediastinal mass. It is well known for associated paraneoplastic syndromes. It has an unpredictable clinical behavior, which does not correlate with the pathological findings and may recur after many years.

Symptoms

Thymoma can present as an incidental finding on x-ray but, most commonly, presents in middle-aged females with symptoms secondary to compression or invasion of mediastinal structures. Spread occurs via the lymphatics or by

Table 25.17 Suggested investigations for thymoma

Hematology and biochemical profile
Chest x-ray
CT
MRI
PET

the haematogenous route. Thymoma is associated commonly with autoimmune-mediated paraneoplastic syndromes of myasthenia gravis, red cell aplasia, pure white blood aplasia, Cushing's syndrome and gammaglobulinaemia. Unfortunately, these do not always resolve with treatment of the underlying tumour.

Diagnosis

Investigations should concentrate on identifying the extent of disease in the anterior mediastinal and possible areas of spread followed by biopsy (Table 25.17).

Pathology and natural history

Thymomas can be classified as epithelial or lymphocytic. Mixed and spindle forms also exist. The tumour can behave unpredictably regardless of the pathological appearance. Differentiation between benign and malignant disease is determined by the presence of gross invasion of adjacent structures, metastasis, or microscopic evidence of capsular invasion.

Management

Surgical resection is the treatment of choice. Locally invasive, unresectable tumours or tumours greater than 5 cm should be treated with multimodality therapy.

Cisplatin-based regimens give good response rates of 70–100%. This should therefore be followed with surgery and postoperative radiotherapy (50 Gy). Aggressive resection is justified, as complete resection is an important prognostic factor (Table 25.18). Local recurrence may occur late where further surgical resection is indicated. In view of the propensity for late recurrence, 10-year survival figures are considered more reliable.

CONCLUSION

Radiation therapy remains an effective modality in the treatment of thoracic tumours. Radical treatment can be delivered to surgically inaccessible sites, delivered postoperatively or as

Table 25.18 Stage and survival figures for thymoma

STAGE	DESCRIPTION	SUGGESTED MANAGEMENT	5-YEAR SURVIVAL (%)	10-YEAR SURVIVAL (%)
I	Tumour is well-encapsulated without evidence of gross or microscopic capsular invasion	Surgical management	93	76
II	Tumour exhibits pericapsular growth into adjacent fat or mediastinal pleura, or microscopic invasion of the thymic capsule	Combination therapy	78	65
III	Tumour invades adjacent organs	Combination therapy	60	45
IVa	Intrathoracic metastatic spread occurs	Cisplatin-based chemotherapy	50	20
IVb	Extrathoracic metastatic spread (rare)	Cisplatin-based chemotherapy		

part of multimodality therapy. In addition, the technical problem of treating an often-moving target surrounded by radiosensitive critical normal tissues remains challenging for the clinical oncologist in the 21st century.

For many patients, however, radiation provides effective palliation from the symptoms of advanced cancers and, for the majority of patients, it will be the only cancer therapy they receive.

FURTHER READING

Mountain CF. Revisions in the international system for staging lung cancer. Chest 1997;111:1710–7.

Medical Research Council Lung Cancer Working Party. Inoperable non-small cell (NSCLC): a Medical Research Council randomised trial of palliative radiotherapy with two fractions or ten fractions. Br J Cancer 1991;63:265–70.

Medical Research Council Lung Cancer Working Party. A Medical Research Council (MRC) randomised trial of palliative radiotherapy with two fractions or a single fraction in patients with inoperable non-small cell lung cancer (NSCLC) and poor performance status. Br J Cancer 1992;65:934–54.

Medical Research Council Lung Cancer Working Party . Randomised trial of palliative two-fraction versus more intensive 13-fraction radiotherapy for patients with inoperable non-small cell

lung cancer and good performance status. Clin Oncol 1996;8:167–75.

Pignon JP, Arriagada R, Ihde DC, et al. Effect of thoracic radiotherapy on mortality in limited small cell lung cancer. A meta-analysis of 13 randomised trials among 2,140 patients. N Engl J Med 1992;327:1618–24.

Turrisi A, Sherman CA. The treatment of limited small cell lung cancer: a report of the progress made and future prospects. Eur J Cancer 2002;38:279–91.

Auperin A, Arriagada R, Pignon J-P, et al. Prophylactic cranial irradiation for patients with small-cell lung cancer in complete remission. N Engl J Med 1999;341:476–84.

Arriagada R, Le Chevalier T, Borie F, et al. Prophylactic cranial irradiation for patients with small cell lung cancer in complete remission. J Natl Cancer Inst 1995;87:183–90.

Gregor A, Cull A, Stephens R, et al. Prophylactic cranial irradiation is indicated following complete response to induction therapy in small cell lung cancer: results of a multicentre randomised trial. Eur J Cancer 1997;33:1752–8.

PORT Meta-analysis Trialists Group. Post operative radiotherapy for radically resected N2 non-small cell lung cancer: systematic review and meta-analysis of individual patient data from nine randomised controlled trails. Lancet 1998;352:257–63.

Wiggins J. Statement on malignant mesothelioma in the United Kingdom. Thorax 2001;56:250–65.

Ramalingham S, Belani C. Systemic chemotherapy for advanced non-small cell lung cancer: recent advances and future directions. The Oncologist 2008;(Suppl):5–13.

EVOLVE CONTENTS (available online at: http://evolve.elsevier.com/Symonds/radiotherapy/)

Chapter | 26 |

Breast cancer

Ian Kunkler

CHAPTER CONTENTS

ANATOMY

Most of the breast tissue extends from the edge of the sternum to the anterior axillary line and from the second or third to the sixth or seventh costal edge. It overlies the second to the sixth ribs. Breast tissue can be found beyond these areas as high as the clavicle and laterally to the edge of the latissimus dorsi muscle.

Lymphatic drainage

The principal lymphatic drainage of the breast (Figure 26.1) is to the axillary nodes lying between the second and third intercostal spaces. Additional drainage occurs to the supra-clavicular nodes through the pectoralis major and to the internal mammary chain adjacent to the sternum.

PATHOLOGY

Epidemiology

Worldwide, breast cancer is the commonest form of malignancy in women. It accounts for 12% of all cancers, 18% of all female cancers, 10% of all cancer deaths and 20–25% of all female cancer deaths. In England, there are 41 000 new cases per year and, in the UK, over 12 000 women die of the disease per year. The incidence is highest in developed

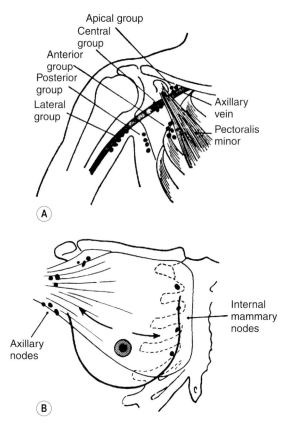

Figure 26.1 (A) The lymph nodes of the axilla. (B) Diagram of the principal pathways of lymphatic drainage of the breast. These follow the venous drainage of the breast – to the axilla and to the internal mammary chain.

(Reproduced with permission from Ellis, Clinical Anatomy, 5th edn, Blackwells, 1975)

countries and low but rising in less developed countries and in Japan. The risk of a woman developing the disease at some stage of her life is 1 in 12. The UK has the highest age standardized incidence and mortality for breast cancer in the world.

Female breast cancer is rare below the age of 30. The incidence rises rapidly during the reproductive years. After the age of 50, the incidence rises at a lower rate. The cumulative incidence in women in Europe and North America is approximately 2.7% by the age of 55, 5% by the age of 65 and 7.7% by the age of 75. Male breast cancer is rare, accounting for only 1% of breast cancer.

Encouragingly, the mortality of breast cancer is declining in the UK and USA and in much of western Europe. However, the mortality from breast cancer in central and eastern Europe and SE Asia continues to climb.

Aetiology

The aetiology of breast cancer is not fully understood, but a number of predisposing factors have been identified.

Genetic factors

High-risk mutations

It is estimated that up to 10% of breast cancers have a genetic basis. The sisters and daughters of a woman with breast cancer have a threefold increased risk of developing the disease. The risk of breast cancer for a woman whose sister is affected is doubled. Women who have a first-degree relative with premenopausal or bilateral breast cancer are at particularly high risk. At least five germline mutations predispose to breast cancer. These include mutations in BRCA1, BRCA2, p53, PTEN and ATM. BRCA1 and BRCA2 mutations confer the highest level of risk of breast cancer and also predispose to ovarian cancer. Germline mutations in p53 give rise to the Li Fraumeni syndrome (childhood sarcomas, brain tumours and early onset breast cancer) and mutations in PTEN to Cowden's disease.

The mode of inheritance is usually autosomal dominant with incomplete penetrance. It is important to note that the genetic susceptibility can be passed on by both males and females. Most cases of breast cancer with a genetic basis will have occurred by the age of 65. Those at substantial risk include women with:

- three first- or second-degree relatives with breast or ovarian cancer
- one first-degree relative with bilateral breast cancer
- two first- or second-degree relatives with breast cancer diagnosed under the age of 60 or ovarian cancer at any age on the same side of the family.

(First-degree relatives are mother, sister or daughter. Second-degree relatives are grandmother, granddaughter, aunt or niece.)

Low risk polymorphisms

Much of the risk of breast cancer may be conferred by low risk polymorphisms. Most of the polymorphisms relate to the alteration of the metabolism of steroid hormones or carcinogenic compounds.

Acquired

Benign breast disease

A number of benign conditions (e.g. fibroadenomas, palpable cysts) in the breast increase the risk of breast cancer, although the effect is small. Overall, the risk of breast cancer is raised by a factor of 1.5–3 for women with previous benign breast disease.

Menstruation

The epithelium of the breast proliferates during ovulatory cycles. This may be due to the stimulus of either progesterone or oestrogen. This causes temporary growth of the milk-secreting glandular tissue in preparation for possible pregnancy. If the menarche starts before the age of 12, the risk of breast cancer is nearly double that of women who begin to menstruate after the age of 13.

If menstruation continues above the age of 55, the risk of breast cancer is doubled compared with a normal menopause at 45 years. Early menarche and late menopause almost certainly confer an increased risk of breast cancer by prolonging the period in which both breasts are exposed to high levels of oestradiol (and possibly progesterone).

Oral contraceptive pill and hormonal replacement therapy

The role of the ovarian oestrogens in the genesis of breast cancer is strongly suspected. Oral contraceptives suppress the production of oestradiol and progesterone. Reductions in oestrogen levels may protect against breast cancer. Oral oestrogens, either as the contraceptive pill or as hormone replacement therapy, may accelerate the development of breast cancer.

Pregnancy

The risk of breast cancer in a woman rises with her age at first pregnancy. It is three times higher in women who have their first baby over the age of 30, compared with those under the age of 18.

Lactation

Women who have breast-fed their children are slightly less prone to breast cancer.

Age at first full-term pregnancy

Pregnancy itself seems to have a protective role. Women who first become pregnant before the age of 30 have a lower risk of breast cancer than women who first give birth after the age of 30.

Diet and life style

Nutrition and lifestyle may be principally responsible for large variations in breast cancer between countries and marked changes in these rates between migrating populations. Asian women, for example, experience much higher rates of breast cancer after moving to the USA.

The diet in the western hemisphere is dominated by fried or grilled food whereas in the East boiled and steamed foods predominate. Dietary fat, whose effects are mediated by oestrogens, is thought to be a key risk factor for breast cancer. An increased intake of calories, sugar, alcohol and saturated fats increases the risk of developing breast cancer.

Alcohol is known to increase the permeability of cell membranes, so assisting the transport of carcinogens. It also induces the proliferation of mammary epithelia in animal models. This results in higher serum concentrations of estradiol in premenopausal women.

Vitamins and selenium

Derivatives of vitamins A (alpha-carotene, beta-carotene, retinol), B and E (tocopherol) and selenium are thought to act as free radical scavengers. They protect lipids from peroxidation by free radicals and are involved in DNA repair. However, prospective studies have not shown that these substances reduce the risk of developing breast cancer.

Physical exercise

Physical exercise also appears to have a protective effect against breast cancer. This is probably due to non-specific immune stimulation and reduced oestrogen levels during recovery. A reduction in risk has been found in women between the ages of 30 and 35. However, the effect only becomes significant with at least 6 hours a week of moderate exercise. The reduction in risk is about 30% in such women compared to no exercise.

Smoking

Most studies of smoking and the incidence of breast cancer show no strong association between these factors.

Metabolic factors

In premenopausal women, epidemiological studies have shown that the risk of breast cancer is associated with high levels of insulin-like growth factor (IGF-1), with high levels of testosterone and with luteal insufficiency (i.e. low progesterone levels). Some studies suggest an association of breast cancer with high blood levels of insulin, glucose and triglycerides.

Ionizing radiation

The breast is one of the tissues most sensitive to the induction of malignancy by ionizing radiation. Exposure to ionizing radiation increases the risk of breast cancer. This is true of women who underwent low-dose breast irradiation for benign mastitis. There is a linear relationship between dose and incidence of breast cancer up to 4 Gy. Beyond this the incidence plateaus. It has been calculated that one extra cancer per year after 10 years may be caused by radiation from a single mammogram among 2 million women over the age of 50. The risk of breast cancer is well validated for women irradiated under the age of 40 with a relative risk of 1.1–2.7 at 1 Gy. Women irradiated in their teenage years by mantle radiotherapy for Hodgkin's disease, where the mediastinal fields commonly treat the medial part of both breasts, have an increased risk of breast cancer by a factor of 1 in 7 if aged 20–29 when treated by mantle radiotherapy rising to 50% at the age of 50 for girls treated before 20.

Children irradiated by the atomic bombs dropped on Nagasaki and Hiroshima showed an increased risk of breast cancer with dose.

Ductal and lobular carcinoma-in-situ

Premalignant in situ carcinoma may occur confined to the lobules (lobular carcinoma-in-situ (LCIS)) or ducts (ductal carcinoma-in-situ (DCIS)) without evidence of penetration on light microscopy of the basement membrane. DCIS occurs in 25% of breast cancers. With the advent of breast screening, the diagnosis of DCIS has increased three to four times and now accounts for 15% of cases detected by mammography. Ninety percent of DCIS is confined to one segment of the breast. DCIS is a heterogeneous disease based on histology, genetic alterations and clinical course. Inactivation of the tumour suppression gene, e-cadherin, is associated with the development of LCIS. Loss of the tumour suppressor gene, p53, is associated with the development of poorly differentiated DCIS. Most of the genetic alterations seen in DCIS are also seen in invasive cancer which often accompanies DCIS. Progression from DCIS to invasive is associated with the same degree of differentiation (i.e. poorly differentiated DCIS tends to progress to poorly differentiated invasive cancer).

Most cases present with non-palpable calcifications. Although mammography may detect over 80% of cases of DCIS, it commonly underestimates the extent of the disease. Magnetic resonance imaging (MRI) is more effective at detecting multifocality. Core biopsy is able to establish a diagnosis in 90% of screen-detected cases. DCIS is associated with a substantial risk of progression to invasive carcinoma, with a mean delay of about 7 years. There are two principal histological groups: comedo and non-comedo type. The most common non-comedo types are solid, cribriform, papillary and micropapillary.

LCIS is associated with an increased risk of tumour in both breasts, particularly infiltrating ductal carcinoma.

Histology

A lump in the breast may be benign or malignant. Benign lesions include cysts, fibroadenomas and papillomas. Malignant tumours mainly arise from the glandular epithelium (adenocarcinomas). Breast cancers are classified as of no

Table 26.1 Classification of invasive breast cancer
1. No special type
2. Special type
a. Tubular
b. Mucoid
c. Cribriform
d. Papillary
e. Medullary
f. Classic lobular

special type or of special type. The majority (80%) are of no special type. The histological types of breast cancer are shown in Table 26.1.

Invasive cancers have traditionally been classified by their microscopic appearance and by histological grade. Grading is based on nuclear pleomorphism, degree of glandular formation and frequency of mitoses. Grading yields useful prognostic information; both disease-free survival and overall survival are shorter for high-grade cancers.

If in excess of 25% of the main tumour mass contains non-invasive (in situ) disease and in situ disease is present in the adjacent breast tissue, the tumour is described as having an *extensive in situ component*. Such patients are at risk of developing invasive cancer elsewhere in the breast and are not suitable for breast conservation.

Lymphatic or vascular invasion within the tumour confers an increased risk of local and distant recurrence.

Inflammatory carcinomas are typified by an enlarged warm breast, often associated with an ill-defined underlying mass. Histologically, there is infiltration of the subdermal lymphatics. Prognosis is poor. In contrast, medullary carcinoma is slow growing and has a much better prognosis.

Lobular invasive carcinomas are often bilateral (40%) and multicentric. Paget's disease of the nipple is commonly associated with an underlying ductal adenocarcinoma.

DIAGNOSIS

The patient may notice a lump herself on routine or casual self-examination. Sometimes it is detected by her general examination as part of clinical examination for other reasons or as a result of routine examination in hospital. With the introduction of the breast-screening programme in the UK, asymptomatic breast cancer is being more frequently diagnosed among women routinely screened for breast cancer between the ages of 50 and 69. In 1998, 75% of women (1.2 million) aged 50–64 were screened, detecting 7000 cancers, a yield of 0.6% (6 per 1000). With the extension of the breast-screening program to older women up to the age of 69, the number of breast cancers detected through breast screening is likely to rise. Patients should be referred to a specialist breast unit with multidisciplinary management from surgeon, oncologist, radiologist, pathologist and breast care nurse.

Clinical assessment

A full history is required, including details of breast-related symptoms, particularly breast pain, nipple discharge, changes noted in the skin (erythema, dimpling) or shape of the breast, indrawing or distortion of the nipple, axillary lumps and systemic symptoms of weight loss, anorexia, nausea, vomiting, bone pain, breathlessness, headache or motor or sensory disturbance. A full menstrual history should be taken including onset of menarche, menopause, parity, age of first pregnancy, breast/bottle feeding and use of the contraceptive pill and hormone replacement therapy.

Mammography

Breast screening by mammography (Figure 26.2) in the UK is recommended to women between the ages of 50 and 69 every 3 years. In the UK, two views of the breast are obtained. In the countries where it has been widely applied (e.g. in Sweden), its use has been shown to reduce the mortality of breast cancer by 30%.

Features suggestive of malignancy are small microcalcifications, stellate opacities with 'legs' extending into the surrounding tissues (Figures 26.3 and 26.4) or distortion of architecture. Mammography may also show enlarged nodes in the axilla. About 15% of cancers are not detected by mammography and nearly 4% are neither palpable nor visible on mammography.

MRI scanning (Figure 26.4) may have an important role in the assessment of (a) the local extent of the primary tumour and of multifocality in younger women where the density of the breast is often a limiting factor to the resolution of

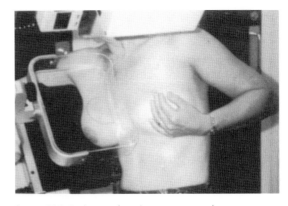

Figure 26.2 Patient undergoing mammography.
(Courtesy of the Rotherham Breast Screening service)

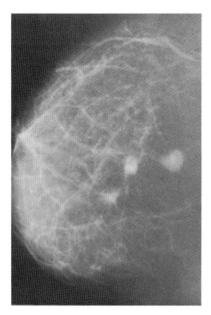

Figure 26.3 Mammogram showing three spiculated tumours in the breast.
(Courtesy of Dr R. Peck, Sheffield)

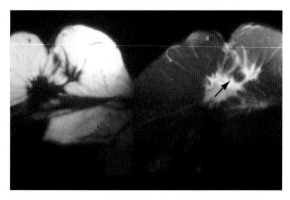

Figure 26.4 MRI scan showing recurrent cancer in the breast.
(Courtesy of Mr M. Dixon, Edinburgh Breast Unit)

mammography and (b) recurrent disease in the irradiated breast 18 months or more after radiotherapy has been completed. MRI may show 10–30% additional invasive cancer in patients presenting with a unifocal lesion. However, MRI may lead to the overestimate of the size of lesions, potentially resulting in unnecessary mastectomies.

Breast ultrasound

Ultrasound of the breast has an important role in helping to distinguish benign from malignant lesions, particularly when mammography is normal or equivocal. Malignant tumours tend to show an abnormal echo pattern

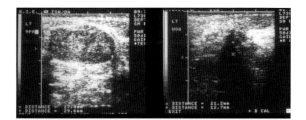

Figure 26.5 Ultrasound of the breast showing indistinct outline of carcinoma (right) compared to well-defined margins of benign fibroadenoma (left).
(Courtesy of Professor M. Dixon, Edinburgh Breast Unit)

(Figure 26.5). Colour Doppler ultrasound may show changes caused by increased tumour vasculature both in primary tumours and in lymph nodes.

Obtaining a histological diagnosis

It is important to obtain a histological diagnosis of breast cancer to confirm suspicious clinical or radiological features. If the tumour is palpable (usually 1 cm or larger), fine needle aspiration cytology (FNAC) is recommended as the initial method of confirming the diagnosis.

Core biopsy under local anaesthetic for palpable lesions or stereotactic image-guided core biopsy for impalpable lesions is becoming increasingly popular as an adjunct to FNAC.

STAGING

Staging is important to assess the local, regional and metastatic spread of breast cancer since management may differ significantly depending on the extent of the disease. Staging involves clinical, radiological and laboratory assessment. The simplest staging system which is still in use is shown in Table 26.2. However, the TNM classification of the

Table 26.2 Clinical staging of breast cancer

STAGE	CLINICAL FINDINGS
I	Freely movable (on underlying muscle). No suspicious nodes
II	As stage I but mobile axillary node(s) on the same side
III	Primary more extensive than stage I, e.g. skin invaded wide of the primary mass or fixation to muscle. Axillary nodes, if present, are fixed; or supraclavicular nodes involved
IV	Extension beyond the ipsilateral chest wall area, e.g. opposite breast or axilla; or distant metastases

Table 26.3 TNM classification of breast cancer

STAGE	CLINICAL FINDINGS
Primary tumour	
Tis	Carcinoma-in-situ
T0	No demonstrable tumour in the breast
T1	Tumour less than 2 cm in greatest dimension confined to the breast
T1a	Tumour 0.5 cm or less in maximum dimension
T1b	Tumour more than 0.5 cm but not more than 1 cm in greatest dimension
T1c	Tumour more than 1 cm but not more than 2 cm in greatest dimension
T2	Tumour more than 2 cm but less than 5 cm in greatest dimension
T3	Tumour more than 5 cm in its greatest dimension
T4	Tumour of any size with direct extension to chest wall or skin
T4a	Fixation to chest wall
T4b	Oedema, infiltration or ulceration of the skin of the breast
T4c	Both of above
Regional lymph nodes	
N0	No palpable nodes
N1	Mobile ipsilateral nodes
N2	Fixed ipsilateral nodes, fixed to each other or to other structures
N3	Ipsilateral internal mammary nodes
Distant metastases	
M0	No distant metastases
M1	Distant metastases including skin involvement beyond the breast area and supraclavicular nodes

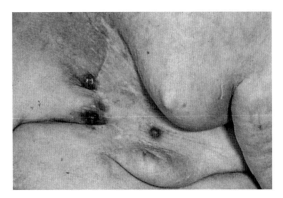

Figure 26.6 Nodular local recurrence on the skin flaps of a mastectomy scar.

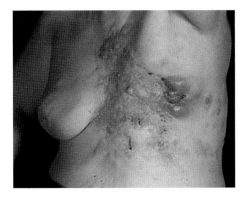

Figure 26.7 Widespread nodular recurrence over left chest wall following mastectomy, extending to the other breast.

(c) T0–2N0 disease with symptoms which could be due to metastatic disease (e.g. unexplained bone pain or weight loss), a liver ultrasound and a bone scan are recommended.

All patients with locally recurrent disease following mastectomy (Figures 26.6 and 26.7) or breast-conserving therapy, regional or metastatic recurrence require bone scan and liver ultrasound in addition to full blood count, liver function tests and chest radiograph.

TREATMENT OF DUCTAL CARCINOMA-IN-SITU

With adequate therapy, 99% of patients will survive following treatment. Where the prognosis is good, the morbidities associated with particular treatments (particularly from radiotherapy) need to be carefully weighed against the benefits of treatment.

The Van Nuys Prognostic Index takes account of three factors which influence the risk of local recurrence (margin width, tumour size and pathological subtype). For each

International Union Against Cancer (Table 26.3) has gained widespread acceptance.

Staging investigations

For patients with T1–2, N0, M0 disease, a full blood count, liver biochemistry and chest radiograph are recommended. For patients with (a) T3 or T4 tumours, (b) N1–3 or MI, or factor there is an assigned score of 1 to 3. The size categories are: ≤1.5 cm, 1.6–4 cm and ≥4.1 cm. The margin categories are: ≤1 mm, 1–9 mm and >10 mm. The pathological categories are: low grade without necrosis, low grade with necrosis, and high grade with or without necrosis. Following conservative surgery and radiotherapy, the 10-year actuarial disease-free survival is 100% for a score of 3–4, 77% for score 5–7 and 37% for a score of 8–9.

The rationale for mastectomy or whole breast irradiation as treatment for DCIS is related to the potential for multicentric disease and/or the presence of occult invasive cancer. Multifocal disease in the same quadrant is not unusual in patients with DCIS. Following wide excision and negative margins, 24–43% of patients will have residual DCIS in the same quadrant. Mastectomy remains the treatment of choice for multicentric DCIS and for large unicentric lesions. Recurrence rates after mastectomy are less than 1%. Regular mammography of the contralateral breast should be carried out, since there is an increased rate of contralateral breast cancer of approximately 7 per 1000. If the extent of the lesion is not more than 3–4 cm, then an attempt at conservative surgery may be made, aiming to achieve complete excision. The margins of clearance should be at least 1 cm. For patients with high-grade DCIS, postoperative whole-breast irradiation should be given, since it reduces the risk of local recurrence and of invasive cancer. The National Surgical Adjuvant Breast Project B-17 trial showed after 12 years of follow up that the incidence of both recurrent DCIS and invasive recurrence was reduced to 16% in patients treated by postoperative radiotherapy (50 Gy in 25 fractions over 5 weeks) compared to wide excision alone. For low or intermediate-grade DCIS, the role of radiotherapy is less clear and still the subject of investigation. There is no indication for axillary dissection or irradiation of the peripheral lymphatics in DCIS since the risk of positive axillary nodes is 4% or less. The overall prognosis of DCIS is excellent with in excess of 97% of patients alive and disease free 10 or more years following diagnosis.

Prognostic factors

While there are a large number of biological prognostic factors for breast cancer, none has surpassed the value of assessing the number of histologically involved nodes and tumour size. There is a direct correlation between number of involved nodes and survival (Figure 26.8). Ten-year survival is about 40–65% with one to three positive nodes, and 20–42% for those with 10 or more positive nodes. Ten-year survival is about 65–70% in women with negative nodes. By contrast, in excess of 50% of all women who are axillary node positive die within 10 years despite treatment.

Within any category of nodal status, tumour size is an independent prognostic factor. The decline in survival with increasing size of the primary tumour is shown in Figure 26.9. Less than 30% of patients with stage IIIb disease (T4) are alive at 10 years. Similarly, survival declines

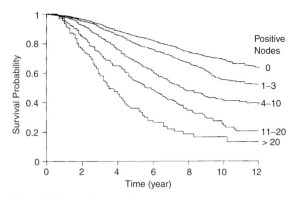

Figure 26.8 Survival by axillary node status.
(Reproduced with permission from Veronesi U (ed.) Baillière's Clinical Oncology, 1988)

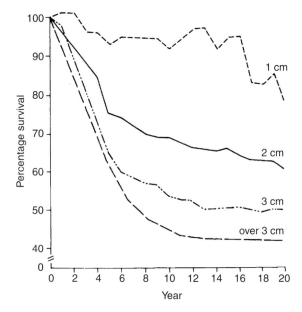

Figure 26.9 Age-corrected survival rates by tumour size for patients treated for breast cancer apparently confined to the breast.
(Reproduced from Halnan, Treatment of Cancer, Chapman & Hall, 1982)

with increasing tumour grade. Five-year survival falls from 80% for grade 1 to 25% for grade 3.

Endocrine therapy is based on blocking the effects of oestrogen which stimulates tumour growth or inhibiting its production. Oestrogen passes through the cell membrane and binds the oestrogen receptor (ER). ER alpha, one of the two species of ER binding to ligand, leads to phosphorylation and transcription. Most of the oestrogen is sited in the nucleus but some probably exists in the cell membrane where it may interact with growth factors. Activation of membrane ER by either oestrogen or tamoxifen and the ensuing activation of growth factor signalling may be a cause of tamoxifen resistance in certain patients which overexpress HER2. It is possible that a combination of ER-targeted therapy and growth factor receptor-targeted therapy might reverse tamoxifen resistance. The strategy is being tested in clinical trials. Cross-talk between growth factor receptor pathways and ER might elucidate the relationship between progesterone receptor (PR) expression and response to a variety of hormonal therapies. As a result of an active growth factor kinase cascade, the transcription of the PR gene may be inhibited. Hence, in some tumours, PR negativity may be a surrogate for active growth factor signalling. This would suggest that ER-positive, PR-negative tumours would respond better to aromatase inhibition than to selective oestrogen receptor modulators (SERMs), as in HER2-positive tumours. Indeed, the ATAC trial showed better outcomes in PR-negative tumours with anastrozole than tamoxifen. There is accumulating data that ER-positive, PR-negative tumours are a discrete subset with a tendency to higher growth factor receptor activity, relative resistance to SERMs and greater sensitivity to aromatase inhibitors, such as anastrazole and letrozole.

Oestrogen receptor status is predictive for disease-free and overall survival. Irrespective of stage, ER positivity predicts for longer disease-free (Figure 26.10) and overall survival. Higher recurrence and lower survival rates are found in ER-negative patients. About 60% of ER-positive patients will respond to hormonal manipulation. Progesterone receptor (PgR) status may also help. Oestrogen stimulates PgR production in normal reproductive tissue and in human breast cancer cell lines. The highest response and disease-free survival rate is seen in ER+/PgR+ tumours. Very few tumours are ER−/PgR+, consistent with the production of progesterone receptors being dependent on oestrogen synthesis. Lowest response and disease-free survival rates are seen in ER−/PgR− tumours (Figure 26.11).

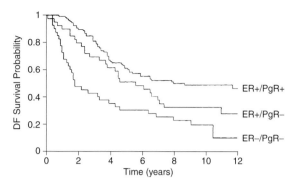

Figure 26.11 Disease-free survival by oestrogen and progesterone receptor status in pathological stage II patients. *(Reproduced with permission from Baillière's Clinical Oncology, International Practice and Research, 1988)*

Of the biological markers of prognosis including p53, cathepsin D, epidermal growth factor receptor and HER2/neu, HER2/neu is the most reproducible. Patients overexpressing HER2/neu have a higher risk of recurrence and shorter survival. There is evidence that tumours that overexpress HER2/neu are relatively resistant to chemotherapy with cyclophosphamide, methotrexate and 5-fluorouracil (5-FU) (CMF) and have greater responsiveness to anthracyclines. In addition, different gene profiles may be found for ER-positive and ER-negative patients.

Gene profiling

More recently, microarray based gene profiling has enabled thousands of genes to be studied in a one tumour. A microarray consists of known and unknown DNA samples on a solid slide (Figure 26.12). The probes may be cDNAs or oligonucleotides of varying length. The sequence hybridized to probes on the array can be fluorescently labelled. Expression signatures based on the expression level of large numbers of genes can be determined reflecting the properties of the cells studied. There is now preliminary evidence that DNA microarrays may be able to discriminate patients at higher or lower risk of systemic relapse among conventionally 'low risk' node-negative patients treated by breast conserving therapy. These findings will have to be validated prospectively in larger data sets before they can be used to determine management for individual patients.

TREATMENT OF EARLY BREAST CANCER

Mastectomy or breast conservation

The decision as to whether to perform a mastectomy or breast-conserving surgery should be discussed preoperatively in a multidisciplinary clinic by surgeon and oncologist, once

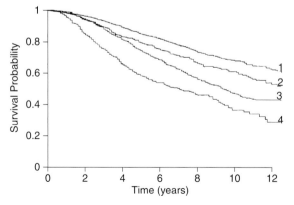

Figure 26.10 Survival by axillary node status and oestrogen receptor status in 854 patients: 1 = negative nodes ER+; 2 = negative nodes, ER−; 3 = positive nodes, ER+; 4 = positive nodes ER−.

(Reproduced with permission from Baillière's Clinical Oncology, International Practice and Research, 1988)

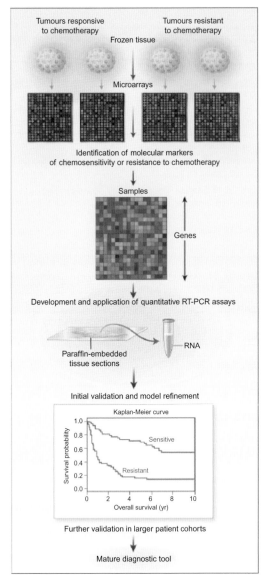

Tumours responsive to chemotherapy

Tumours resistant to chemotherapy

Frozen tissue

Microarrays

Identification of molecular markers of chemosensitivity or resistance to chemotherapy

Samples

Genes

Development and application of quantitative RT-PCR assays

Paraffin-embedded tissue sections

RNA

Initial validation and model refinement

Kaplan-Meier curve

Sensitive

Resistant

Overall survival (yr)

Survival probability

Further validation in larger patient cohorts

Mature diagnostic tool

Figure 26.12 Development of microarray based diagnostic tests for cancer. Primary or metastatic tumours are resected from patients; DNA microarray profiling is used to obtain gene-expression profiles of the tumours. Next, genome-computational and statistical analyses are used to identify gene-expression markers of responsiveness or resistance to chemotherapy; multiplex quantitative reverse transcriptase-polymerase chain reaction (RT-PCR) assays are developed for the best markers, and these assays are applied retrospectively or prospectively to formalin-fixed, paraffin-embedded tissue sections. On the basis of the results, researchers develop diagnostic and predictive models that can be validated in large cohorts of patients, resulting in a mature diagnostic tool.
(Reproduced with permission of the New England Journal of Medicine)

the results of staging investigations are available. A joint decision should be taken. In making this decision, due weight should be given to the patient's own preference.

The technical feasibility of local surgery, suitability for radiotherapy, cosmesis and locoregional morbidity all need to be taken into consideration. In considering the possibility of breast-conserving surgery, the tumour size, the size of the breast and the mammographic appearance or histology from excision or core biopsy are important. As a general rule, most tumours in excess of 3 cm are unsuitable for breast-conserving therapy unless the breast size is sufficiently large not to result in a marked tissue defect marring cosmesis. Greater flexibility in offering breast conservation is possible with the availability of newer surgical techniques to fill the tissue defect from local excision by a graft. Tumours of 3 cm or greater, judged clinically or radiologically, are generally best treated by mastectomy and axillary node clearance. Patients who have clinical or radiological evidence of multifocal disease or have an extensive intraduct component (EIC) are not suitable for breast conservation. About 25–30% of patients who undergo conservative surgery with clear margins will have residual tumour at the time of re-excision or mastectomy.

There is evidence that local recurrence rates following breast-conserving surgery are higher in younger women. Women under the age of 35 have a two- to fourfold higher risk of local recurrence after breast-conserving surgery and radiotherapy. This may in part be due to the difficulty of identifying cancers by mammography in younger women who tend to have more radiodense breasts or the more aggressive biology of the disease in younger women.

Lobular cancer

Some histological forms of breast cancer, typically lobular cancer, are commonly multifocal but poorly imaged by mammography. If a core or excision biopsy of an apparently localized tumour shows lobular carcinoma, an initial wide local excision may be carried out. If the margins are involved with invasive cancer or there is evidence of multifocal disease histologically, then breast conservation is not safe and mastectomy is advised.

Reconstruction after mastectomy

Mastectomy is a mutilating operation but much can be achieved in remodeling the breast by a variety of reconstructive techniques. Most patients should be offered the possibility of immediate breast construction.

Conservation therapy (limited surgery and postoperative radiotherapy)

In patients with T1 and small T2 tumours (up to 3 cm), some form of local surgery should be considered. The most popular choice is a wide local excision to obtain clear histological margins. This involves excision of the tumour with a margin of 1–2 cm. If the margins are found to be involved, a re-excision to clear the margins is recommended. If re-excision of the margins still shows tumour at the margin, breast conservation is not appropriate and a mastectomy is advised.

Alternatively, a more extensive local excision of the whole quadrant affected in the breast (quadrantectomy) may be carried out. The advantage of quadrantectomy is that local recurrence rates (about 1% at 5 years when combined with postoperative radiotherapy) are lower than after wide local excision and radiotherapy (about 5% at 5 years). The disadvantage is that the cosmetic result is generally poorer because of the asymmetry caused by the greater volume of tissue removed. Quadrantectomy or a very wide local excision may be considered in patients refusing or not fit for mastectomy or breast radiotherapy. This may be advisable in some older patients where co-morbidity may compromise suitability for mastectomy. Criteria for breast conservation are summarized in Table 26.4.

Local recurrence after breast-conserving therapy

The treatment of choice of local recurrence after radical radiotherapy is a mastectomy.

Management of the axilla

Some form of surgical procedure to obtain nodal histology is advised in all women with operable breast cancer. The surgical management of the axilla remains controversial and practice varies. For tumours 2 cm or less in diameter where the risk of axillary nodal involvement is lower than in larger tumours, a lower axillary node sample (of a minimum of four nodes) or sentinel node biopsy is advised.

Sentinel node biopsy avoids the morbidity of axilllary dissection. The sentinel node is the node most likely to drain the primary tumour. It is identified first by the injection of a vital blue dye or a radioactive tracer, or a combination of both. The combination of both techniques

Table 26.4 Criteria for breast-conserving therapy
1. Tumours up to 3 cm
2. Satisfactory cosmetic result anticipated
3. Postoperative whole breast radiotherapy technically feasible
4. Medically fit for surgery
5. Clear histological margins at primary excision or re-excision
6. Able to attend for regular clinical and mammographic follow up

is the most accurate. In most patients, the sentinel node is in the axilla but, in a few medially placed tumours, it may be in the internal mammary chain. The axilla is normally explored to identify the sentinel node either by the blue colour of the dye within it or by the high radioactivity scintillation count over it. If the sentinel node biopsy is positive, the surgeon may proceed to a complete axillary dissection or refer the patient for axillary irradiation. In specialist centres, sentinel node biopsy has 97% accuracy.

For patients with tumours >2 cm or with ipsilateral palpable nodes (N1), a level III axillary clearance up to the level of the medial end of the first rib is recommended. Normally, there should be at least 10 axillary nodes in a level III clearance and commonly 20–30. The local control in the axilla from a level III clearance is similar to a selective policy of axillary radiotherapy in patients with one or more involved nodes on a four node lower axillary sample. With either policy the axillary recurrence rate is similar, 5% at 5 years.

Morbidity of axillary treatment

Side effects of an axillary clearance include postoperative seroma and numbness in the upper limb. Lymphoedema occurs in 7–8% of cases. If axillary radiotherapy is added to the dissection, the risk of lymphoedema is substantially higher (between 30 and 40%).

After conventionally fractionated radiotherapy (e.g. 45–50 Gy in 20–25 fractions) to the axilla, the risk of lymphoedema is about 3–5%, i.e. lower than after axillary dissection. However, there is an increased risk of long-term restriction of shoulder movement and a small risk of brachial plexopathy (1% or less). This is a rare but serious complication and is usually irreversible. Very careful attention to radiotherapy technique with avoidance of overlap between axillary and breast/chest wall fields or moving the patient between the treatment of these fields is essential.

Postoperative radiotherapy

After breast-conserving surgery

In general, postoperative whole-breast irradiation should be delivered following wide local excision or quadrantectomy as part of breast-conserving therapy. A number of randomized trials comparing wide excision alone with appropriate systemic therapy have shown overall a fourfold reduction in local recurrence from the addition of whole breast irradiation (Table 26.5). There is much less randomized data on the role of postoperative radiotherapy in older patients, particularly over the age of 65, receiving adjuvant endocrine therapy. This is currently being evaluated by the PRIME trial.

Despite the evidence from clinical trials of a reduction in local recurrence after postoperative radiotherapy after quadrantectomy or wide local excision, there is no evidence from published trials of a survival advantage from the addition of radiotherapy.

Table 26.5 Results of randomized trials of breast-conserving surgery (BCS) with or without radiotherapy (RT)

LOCAL RECURRENCE (%)		MEDIAN FOLLOW UP	ANALYSIS	
	BCS alone	BCS + RT	(months)	
NSABP B-06	10	10	144	12 years actuarial
Canadian 1	35	11	91	8 years crude
Scottish	25	6	68	5 years actuarial
Swedish	18	2	64	5 years actuarial
Milan III	18	2	52	5 years actuarial
Canadian II	8	1	67	5 years actuarial

Modified from Wong J S and Harris J R 2001 Lancet Oncology 2: 11–17

Following mastectomy

More than half of the locoregional recurrences following mastectomy occur on the chest wall. The mastectomy scar is the commonest site of recurrence.

The role of adjuvant radiotherapy following mastectomy remains controversial. In 2000, a meta-analysis by the Early Breast Cancer Trialists' Group of 36 trials conducted pre-1985 found that in the first 10–20 years of follow up there was small increased risk of non-breast cancer deaths (2%) counterbalancing a small reduction in breast cancer deaths. The non-breast cancer deaths were largely due to vascular mortality. This is likely to have been due to irradiation of the heart or great vessels.

In 1997, two landmark randomized trials conducted in Denmark and Canada showed a 9–10% survival benefit from the addition of locoregional radiotherapy following mastectomy to adjuvant CMF (cyclophosphamide, methotrexate and 5-fluorouracil) chemotherapy. The much larger Danish trial (Figure 26.13) of over 3000 patients showed that a significant advantage accrued to patients receiving adjuvant irradiation (10-year survival 54% versus 45%). A trial from the same trial group (Figure 26.14) shows a similar 9% survival (45% versus 36%) benefit in high-risk

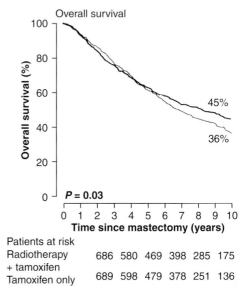

Patients at risk

| Radiotherapy + tamoxifen | 686 | 580 | 469 | 398 | 285 | 175 |
| Tamoxifen only | 689 | 598 | 479 | 378 | 251 | 136 |

Figure 26.14 Survival in Danish Cooperative Group trials of locoregional radiotherapy after adjuvant tamoxifen in high-risk postmenopausal women.
(Reproduced with permission from Elsevier Ltd from The Lancet, 1999; 353: 1642)

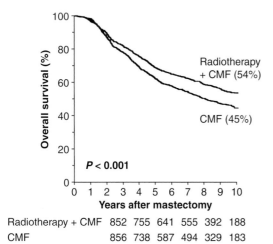

Radiotherapy + CMF 852 755 641 555 392 188
CMF   856 738 587 494 329 183

Figure 26.13 Survival in Danish Cooperative Group trials of locoregional radiotherapy after adjuvant CMF in high-risk premenopausal women.
(Reproduced with permission of the Editor from Overgaard et al., 1997; New England Journal of Medicine, 337: 949–955)

postmenopausal women receiving locoregional regional irradiation in addition to adjuvant tamoxifen. However, the survival advantage of the benefits of radiotherapy only emerged late (i.e. at 10 years). In both the Danish and Canadian trials, all of the peripheral lymphatics (axilla, supraclavicular and internal mammary chain) were irradiated. It is not clear whether irradiation of all of these areas, particularly the internal mammary chain is essential. A trial of the EORTC (European Organisation for Research and Treatment of Cancer) is evaluating the role of internal mammary irradiation. The radiotherapy technique in the Danish trial (see Figure 26.14) differed from the use of a pair of tangential fields in most UK centres to treat the chest wall. A combination of electron beam with limited penetration beyond the chest wall was used to treat the medial part of the chest wall and matched with a photon field to treat the lateral half of the chest wall. Ten-year follow-up data showed no excess of cardiac morbidity or mortality in the radiotherapy + systemic therapy group compared to those receiving systemic therapy alone. The results of the Danish trial emphasize the importance of good radiotherapy technique in minimizing the dose to the heart.

Indications for postmastectomy radiotherapy

International consensus supports the routine use of post-mastectomy radiotherapy for patients who have a 20% or more risk of locoregional recurrence:

1. tumours greater than 5 cm in diameter
2. four or more histologically involved axillary nodes.

In addition radiotherapy is indicated for:

3. close or involved surgical margins
4. chest wall recurrence following mastectomy.

Cumulatively, greater probability of local recurrence is conferred with the following risk factors:

1. axillary nodal involvement
2. grade 3 histology
3. lymphatic/vascular invasion.

How these factors should be weighted in the selection of patients for postmastectomy radiotherapy is not clear. It is known that the risk of local recurrence increases with the cumulative number of risk factors (high tumour grade, nodal involvment and lymphovascular invasion). In the absence of definitive data, a reasonable policy is to offer radiotherapy to patients with two or more of these factors. The role of postmastectomy radiotherapy in the group with one to three involved axillary nodes or negative with other risk factors, such grade 3 histology and lymphovascular invasion, is unclear and is being evaluated by the international SUPREMO trial (BIG 2-04).

Target volume and techniques for locoregional irradiation

In choosing a technique, guiding principles should be homogeneous irradiation of the target areas, avoidance of overlap of chest wall/breast with fields to the peripheral lymphatics, and minimizing dosage to critical structures (lung, heart and the brachial plexus).

This is not an easy task because of the variation in shape and thickness of the chest wall and breast in the craniocaudal and transverse planes. In addition, the sternum slopes when the patient is lying flat. The proximity of the lung to the target volume means that some lung is commonly irradiated. As a result, with conventional wedged tangential fields, it is difficult to reduce the variation in dose distribution across the volume to the ±5% that is achievable by radical radiotherapy at other tumour sites. Dose variation across the target volume may vary by up to 20%. Dose inhomogeneity is exacerbated by lung effects due to scatter and lung transmission. The aim should be to achieve a variation between the maximum and minimum dose of better than 15%.

CT simulation

Conventionally, in UK centres, most adjuvant irradiation has been planned without the benefit of CT planning or with only a single or limited number of CT slices.

Full CT scanning of the breast allows better selection of beam arrangements to minimize cardiac and pulmonary irradiation. This may require the patient to be planned with the ipsilateral arm abducted behind the head or with both hands holding a bar in front of the patient in order to fit into the bore of most CT scanners.

More recently, intensity modulated radiotherapy (IMRT) has become available to provide a more even distribution of radiation dose across the breast/chest wall while reducing unwanted irradiation of critical organs such as the lung and heart. IMRT allows the fluence intensity to be varied across the beam. Virtual simulation, which incorporates a laser positioning system and a CT scanner and treatment planning system, has replaced simulation in many centres. Constraints may be put on doses to critical organs and to the breast and chest wall. It has been shown that IMRT can reduce by 3–5% the dose to the top and bottom of the breast, where hot spots commonly occur with conventional wedged fields using 2D planning. Despite the better target coverage and reduced cardiac dosage from 3-dimensional planning over 2-D planning, the normal tissue complication probability (NTCP) for lung may increase.

Respiratory gated radiotherapy

One of the most promising techniques to reduce cardiac and lung irradiation is active breathing control in which there is computer controlled temporary suspension of breathing in a reproducible cycle.

Following respiratory training, the patient is positioned in a CT scanner without immobilization (Figure 26.15). Radiotherapy is delivered in maximal deep inspiration when the heart is maximally displaced posteriorly away from the treatment beams (Figure 26.16). The lung volume irradiated is also reduced.

443

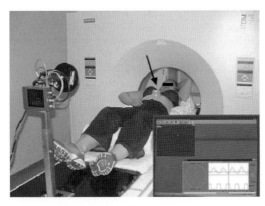

Figure 26.15 The Varian RPM™ system displayed in the CT-scanner facility. A passive, infrared light reflecting marker (indicated by an arrow) is placed on the patient's chest wall over the xiphoid process. The vertical motion of the marker is tracked by an infrared sensitive video-camera and the input projected to a computer screen breathing curve. The insert shows the gating computer screen, with the video-camera view and the breathing curve.

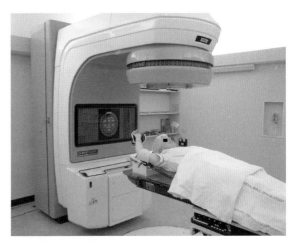

Figure 26.17 Patient lying on inclined breast board for adjuvant postoperative radiotherapy planning.
(courtesy of Mrs J Cameron, Edinburgh Cancer Centre)

Immobilization

Some form of immobilization is essential to provide a reproducible treatment set-up. A variety of devices are in use. These may include a breast board see (Figure 26.17) that fits onto the simulator and treatment couch, a custom-made foam mould from the head to the knees. The patient is treated supine with the arm abducted to 90 degrees. The breast

board can be inclined to a range of angles to flatten the chest wall/breast.

This technique simplifies matching and avoids the need for rotating the collimator. The disadvantage is that it increases the volume of lung irradiated in the shoulder field. Alternatively, the patient can lie supine with the arm abducted to 90 degrees. Rotation of the collimator is needed to keep the posterior beam edge parallel to the slope of the contour. The disadvantage is difficulty in matching the chest wall to the shoulder field.

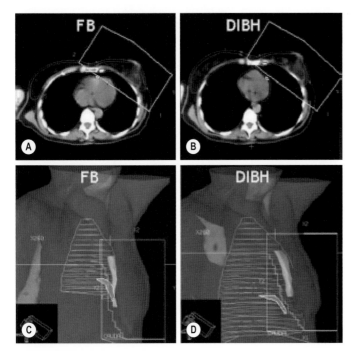

Figure 26.16 The tangential fields for different respiratory patterns, and the volume delineation principles. The transverse view at the same couch position for a sample patient in treatment position during (A) free breathing (FB) (B) deep inspiration breath-hold (DIDH) mode are displayed. In addition, beam's eye views of the medial field during (C) FB and (D) DIBH are shown. Note the difference in lung inflation, and in cardiac/LACDA (white encircled) position.
(Reproduced with permission from Elsevier Ltd.: Radiotherapy and Oncology, 2004, 72: 53–60)

For the large or very mobile breast, some additional form of immobilization (shell or sling) is needed. The very mobile breast tends to fall laterally, moving the posterior beam edge further back than the midaxillary point and increasing the volume of lung irradiated. The immobilizing device will bring the breast medially and reduce the volume of lung irradiated.

Separate fields (Figure 26.18) are planned to cover: (1) supraclavicular fossa, axilla and, if desired, the upper internal mammary chain and (2) chest wall/breast. Whether it is necessary to irradiate the internal mammary chain is still controversial and most UK oncologists do not attempt to include it in the target volume. If the internal mammary nodes are to be irradiated, it is best to use a direct anterior field using a mixture of photons and electrons of appropriate energy to cover them. Individualized CT planning is needed to ensure adequate coverage while limiting transmitted dosage to the underlying heart and lungs. Trying to include the internal mammary nodes within tangential fields is not recommended because of the greater risks of pneumonitis from the larger volume of lung irradiated and the uncertainty of adequate coverage. A computer plan of the dose distribution over the breast or chest wall should be derived from a CT-derived outline through the central plane. Three-dimensional treatment planning, which gives a greater appreciation of dose delivered to the heart and lung, is to be encouraged. In addition, it gives a greater appreciation of the extent of breast tissue, often extending beyond anatomical landmarks used for 2-dimensional planning.

Shoulder field

A direct anterior megavoltage field (see Figure 26.18) covers the supraclavicular fossa and axilla. The upper margin should be at the level of the thyrohyoid groove. The lateral margin should encompass the lateral border of the axilla. The length of the shoulder field should rarely exceed 10 cm, since the volume of lung irradiated rises as the lower edge of the treatment volume is extended inferiorly. This increases the risk of pneumonitis.

The shoulder joint and the part of the larynx within the field should be shielded by lead blocks. Some centres angle the shoulder field 15 degrees to exclude the spinal cord, although this is not essential as long as the dosage and fractionation are within cord tolerance. The lower border of the shoulder field should be non-divergent to avoid overlap with the tangential fields.

The axillary and supraclavicular nodes are commonly at the same depth and, therefore, a single anterior field may suffice. Some centres use a small direct posterior field (posterior axillary boost) to supplement the dose to the axillary nodes. The given dose to the posterior axilla is calculated to bring the mid-axilla to the prescribed dose. With 6 MV photons, roughly 80% of the prescribed midaxillary dose is delivered from the anterior field and 20% from the posterior field. The posterior field is often treated on alternate days unless the mid-axillary separation exceeds 20 cm.

Supraclavicular field

Where the axillary clearance shows the nodes to be involved, irradiation of the ipsilateral supraclavicular nodes should be considered. A threshold of at least four involved nodes is commonly adopted for medial supraclavicular irradiation. If the axilla is to be cleared, the surgeon should be asked to place metal clips up to the medial extent of the axillary dissection to ensure that the lateral margin of the supraclavicular field abuts on, but does not overlap, the field of the axillary clearance. The superior border of the supraclavicular field is the cricothyroid notch. The inferior border is the lower border of the clavicular head.

Chest wall and breast

The chest wall or breast is treated isocentrically and can normally be encompassed in a pair of wedged tangential fields (Figure 26.19) keeping the posterior beam edges parallel to minimize divergence into the lung. This should cover the scar of local excision or of the mastectomy. It normally extends from the level of the second costal cartilage down to 1–2 cm below the inframammary fold. The medial margin is the midline. The lateral margin is normally the mid-axillary line. Occasionally, the lateral margin may be slightly more

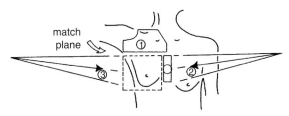

Figure 26.18 Diagram showing fields to the chest wall/breast, axilla, supraclavicular fossa and internal mammary chain.
(Reproduced with permission of the Editor of the British Journal of Radiology, 1984; 57: 736)

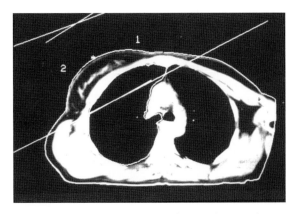

Figure 26.19 Two tangential breast fields. By keeping the posterior beam edges parallel, irradiation of the lung is reduced.

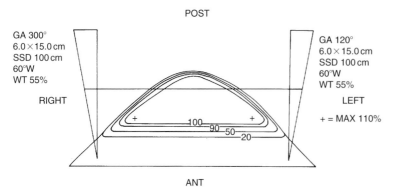

Figure 26.20 Isodoses of a pair of wedged tangential breast fields shown in Figure 26.19.

posterior in the conserved breast for a laterally placed tumour or if the mastectomy scar extends beyond this point. Some compromise is necessary in defining these field margins, balancing adequate coverage of the target volume with the need to avoid excessive lung irradiation. A typical dose distribution in the breast is shown in Figure 26.20.

Internal mammary node irradiation

The internal mammary chain (IMC) lies deep to the midline and about 2–3 cm to each side of the midline. If the internal mammary nodes are to be irradiated, a separate direct electron internal mammary field should be used. This will need to cross the midline. It will result in a cold spot beneath the match line with the photon field. Rotation of the electron beam so that it lies parallel to the photon beam to eliminate the area of underdosage should be avoided So doing will increase the volume of lung irradiated and risk of pneumonitis significantly.

Limitation of lung volume irradiated

At the time of simulation, the thickness of lung encompassed in the tangential fields should be measured (the central lung distance perpendicularly from the inner aspect of the chest wall to the posterior beam edge). The central lung distance should not exceed 3 cm. If it exceeds 3 cm, consideration should be given to bringing the medial and/or lateral margins of the fields inwards, as long as this does not involve skimping on the coverage of the wide excision or mastectomy scars. To avoid divergence into the lung, the posterior beam edges should be kept parallel.

Skin bolus

To overcome the skin-sparing effect of megavoltage skin bolus (0.5–1 cm depending on the energy of photons) should be applied to the chest wall to ensure full skin dosage in patients where the skin is involved by tumour. Practice varies in the use of bolus for postmastectomy radiotherapy when the skin is not involved. Some centres apply bolus to a limited area above and below the scar (where recurrences are commonest) or to the whole of

the chest wall, either for the whole or part of the course of radiotherapy. It is not clear which approach is optimal.

Field matching

One of the main challenges in breast/chest wall planning is to match the tangential fields to the shoulder field. Immobilization should minimize movement between the treatment of fields to avoid the risk of overdosage or underdosage at the junction. Fields may be matched using the light beam and lasers by eye using couch rotation (usually 5–6 degrees) and some collimator rotation. Alternatively, one can use:

1. a half beam block (Figure 26.21A) to counteract beam divergence, allowing the field edges to be abutted. Asymmetric jaws facilitate this. The match plane can be vertical (Figure 26.21B) or angled (Figure 26.21C)
2. a vertical hanging block
3. a single isocentre with blocks, avoiding the need for couch movement between fields.

Dosimetry

Planning is normally on a single CT slice. However, multislice CT scanning of the breast gives a better appreciation of the volume of lung and heart irradiated. 6 MV photons are adequate for most patients. Wedges are needed to compensate for missing tissue. Lung transmission increases the dose to the posterior breast. A correction factor of 10% may be needed. Variations in depth dose across the breast may be ±20%, particularly in larger breasts. Build-up to 100% is 5–10 mm from the skin surface for 6 MV photons.

Dose, energy and fractionation

Megavoltage irradiation (6 MV photons) is used for the tangential field to the chest wall or breast. The commonest regimens are 40 Gy in 15 daily fractions over 4 weeks, 45 Gy in 20 fractions over 4 weeks and 50 Gy in 25 fractions over 5 weeks. The latter is the standard in the USA and most of continental Europe.

Many of the current fractionation regimens have developed empirically. In the USA, 2 Gy fractions were widely

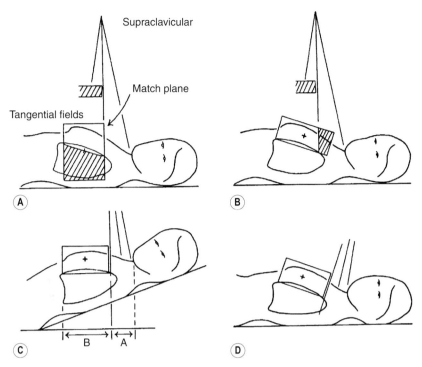

Figure 26.21 Matching fields in a breast treatment. (A) Using a rotated half beam block to counteract beam divergence between cervico-axillary and breast fields. (B) Lead block to trim superior edge of the tangential fields to form a vertical match plane. (C) Match plane vertical on an inclined breast board. (D) Match plane angled in supine position.
(Reproduced with permission of the Editor of the British Journal of Radiology, 1984, 57: 737)

adopted under the influence of Professor Gilbert Fletcher of the MD Anderson Hospital in Texas. For much of North America and continental Europe, 50 Gy in 25 fractions over 5 weeks is the international standard for postoperative locoregional radiotherapy. In the UK, shorter regimens with fraction sizes of 2.25–2.67 Gy were used delivering 45 Gy in 20 daily fractions over a month or 40 Gy in 15 fractions over 3 weeks.

Clinical trials, Table 26.6 such as the UK START trial based on radiobiological modeling, have compared the impact of

Table 26.6 Local control rates in randomized trials of accelerated radiotherapy					
TRIAL	**NO. PATIENTS**	**SURGERY**	**RADIATION SCHEDULE**	**LR(%)**	**MED FU (years)**
OCOG	1234	Lumpectomy	50 Gy/25fr/5 wks	3.2	5.8
			42.5 Gy/16 fr/3 wks		2.8
START	1410	Lumpectomy	50 Gy/25fr/5 wks N/A	4.5	
St Thomas	411	Mastectomy	37–45 Gy/12fr/5.5 wk	13	10
			30–32 Gy/6fr/2.5 wks		7
Necker	230	Lumpectomy	45 Gy/25fr/5 wks	7	5.5
		or mastectomy	23 Gy/4fr/2.5 wks		5
LR%: **local recurrence**; Med FU: median follow up					

shorter (so called hypofractionated regimens) on tumour control and acute and late morbidity in the conserved breast or after mastectomy. The Royal Marsden Hospital/Gloucestershire Oncology Centre fractionation trial compared 50 Gy in 25 daily fractions over 5 weeks with a hypofractionated regimen of 39 Gy in 13 daily fractions. Based on 142 events, the fractionation sensitivity for tumour was calculated as 4.1. Morbidity seems to be similar but data on local control are not yet available. In the Ontario fractionation trial, 50 Gy in 25 fractions over 5 weeks was compared to 42.5 Gy in 16 fractions of 2.67 Gy. There were no differences in local control. Shorter fractionation regimens would be more convenient for patients and less costly. Long-term follow up will be needed to assess the impact of hypofractionated regimens on locoregional control, morbidity and survival.

Conservation therapy

Boost to the tumour

Some form of boost of irradiation to the primary tumour is desirable to bring the tumour dose to 60 Gy in women under the age of 50. This is either given by electrons or by an iridium-192 implant (Figure 26.22). Either form of boost will give comparable local control. However, the higher surface dose of electrons will cause telangiectasia on the treated skin. For implants, telangiectasia at the skin entry and exit points of the iridium wire can be avoided if the sources lie just beneath the skin surface. In general, the breast tissue tends to be thinner in the more medial and lateral parts of the breast. In these sites, there may be inadequate tissue for an implant and electrons are preferable.

An iridium implant does enable a higher dose to be delivered than electrons for a similar level of morbidity. However, there is no compelling evidence that electrons are inferior to an implant in terms of local control in conservation therapy.

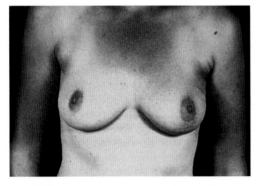

Figure 26.22 Excellent cosmetic result of postoperative radiotherapy and iridium implant following lumpectomy for early carcinoma of the left breast.
(Courtesy of Dr D Ash, Leeds)

Multifield

a. Shoulder field (supraclavicular + axilla)
   45 Gy maximum dose in 20 daily fractions over 4 weeks (6 MV photons)
   (with posterior axillary boost brings mid-axillary dose to 45 Gy treating alternate days)
b. Medial supraclavicular fossa
   45 Gy maximum dose in 20 fractions over 4 weeks (6 MV photons)
c. Breast or chest wall
   45 Gy target absorbed dose (TAD) in 20 fractions (6 MV photons)

Boost to the primary

It has been conventional to boost the site of tumour excision either with electrons of appropriate energy or temporary interstitial implantation using iridium-192. A large EORTC trial (Table 26.7) of over 5500 patients showed an overall 40% reduction in the risk of local recurrence with the use of the boost. Patients with clear margins after wide local excision were treated with whole breast irradiation (50 Gy in 25 fractions over 5 weeks) and randomized to either a boost (electrons 10 Gy) or implant. Age was an independent risk factor for recurrence. In women under the age of 40, the local recurrence with the boost was 10% compared to 20% without the boost. The absolute reduction in recurrence was smaller in women over the age of 40, but still statistically significant up to the age of 50. Radiation morbidity was increased in women receiving a boost. On this basis, for patients with clear excision margins, a boost is not recommended in women who are 50 or older. In patients for whom re-excision of positive margins is not possible, an electron or iridium-192 implant boost would still be indicated. Implantation can be carried out intraoperatively or postoperatively.

Electrons

The appropriate electron energy, usually 9–12 MeV, is chosen according to the depth of the breast tissue at the site of the tumour-bearing area. This is often judged clinically but is more accurately measured by ultrasound or CT postoperatively. In order to avoid transmission of unwanted irradiation to the underlying lung, a Perspex degrader of appropriate thickness can be interposed between the electron applicator and the skin to attenuate the beam. The boosted volume should cover the tumour-bearing area with a margin of 1–2 cm (to take account of the inbowing of electron isodoses at depth) judged from clinical, mammographic and perioperative findings. Surgeons should be encouraged to place metal clips at the site of the excision, which assist the clinical oncologist in the identification of the tumour bed.

Electron boost dose

15 Gy maximum dose in 5 daily fractions over 1 week.

Table 26.7 Local control and overall survival in randomized trials of boost irradiation after whole breast radiotherapy

TRIAL	NO. PATIENTS	RT SCHEDULE	LR (%)	OS (%)	MEDIAN FU (years)
EORTC	5318	50 Gy/25fr/ 5 wks	7.3	91	5.1
	22881	50 Gy/25fr/5 wks	4.3	91	
		+ boost 16 Gy/8fr/1.5 wks			
Lyon	1024	50 Gy/25fr/5 wks	4.5	90	3.3
		50 Gy/2t5fr/5 wks			
		+ boost 10 Gy/5fr/1 wk	3.6	91	
Nice	664	50 Gy/25fr/5 wks	6.8	NA	6.1
		50 Gy/25fr/5 wks	4.3	NA	
		+ boost 10 Gy/5fr/1 wk			

LR: **local recurrence**; OS: overall survival; FU: follow up

Partial breast irradiation

There is increasing research interest in partial breast irradiation as an alternative to whole breast irradiation. Postoperative radiotherapy may not always be carried out because of associated co-morbidity. At the same time, in some 'low-risk' patients, the probability of recurrence outside the quadrant harbouring the primary tumour may be low. Partial breast irradiation can be delivered with low or high dose rate brachytherapy and intraoperative or external beam radiotherapy. A main advantage is a reduction in the length of postoperative treatment while taking account of the risk of subclinical disease in the tumour bed.

Low dose brachytherapy

Implantation of needles or plastic tube into the tumour bed can be carried out during surgery. The clinical target volume is defined with a 2 cm safety margin. Loading with radioactive sources (iridium-192) is performed on the fifth postoperative day after the postoperative histology report is available. A dose rate of about 0.60 Gy /hour is used. This allows completion of treatment in 3–4 days.

High dose brachyherapy

The technique of implantation is similar to low dose brachytherapy; 3.4–5.2 Gy are delivered with at least 6 hours between fractions to total dose of 32–37.2 Gy. Assuming an alpha/beta ratio of 3 Gy for late reacting tissues and a dose per fraction of 3.4 Gy, 34 Gy in HDR

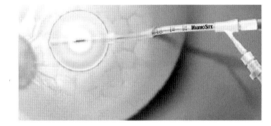

Figure 26.23 Breast brachytherapy with Mammosite.

brachytherapy is equivalent to 43.5 Gy conventionally fractionated. The Mammosite HDR system has a catheter comprising a multilumen tube with balloon assembly, (Figure 26.23). The balloon is inflated to fit the size of the excision cavity. An Ir-192 source is inserted into the balloon to deliver the required dose. On completion of therapy, the balloon is deflated and the catheter removed. Compared to interstitial brachytherapy, the dose distribution may be less uniform.

External beam radiotherapy

A clinical trial at the Christie Hospital in Manchester compared whole breast irradiation with electron beam therapy to the site of excision. The actuarial breast recurrence rate for invasive ductal cancer was 15% for partial breast irradiation compared to 11% for whole breast radiotherapy at a median follow up of 65 months ($P = 0.01$ $Chi^2 = 9.1$ with 1df).

Intraoperative radiotherapy (IORT)

Intraoperative radiotherapy (IORT) can be delivered by photons or electrons. A mobile linear accelerator can be used in the operating theatre to deliver electrons (ELIOT (electron intraoperative radiotherapy)) directly into the tumour excision cavity. The skin margins are pulled out of the treatment field. Doses ranging from 10 to 21 Gy have been given. This extends the duration of surgery by 15–20 minutes. A trial in Milan is evaluating the role of intraoperative electrons as a perioperative single fraction of electrons. This has potential advantages in countries where accessibility of patients to radiotherapy centres is difficult or expensive. Long periods of radiotherapy may impact adversely on quality of life and are a heavy drain on limited healthcare resources.

A photon radiosurgery system delivering 50 kV x-rays has been used to deliver doses of 5–20 Gy into the operative site. The system used a range of spherical applicators of different sizes (Figure 26.24). A dose of 15 Gy prescribed at 2 mm from a 3.5 cm diameter applicator delivers 7.5 Gy at a depth of 5 mm.

There are no uniformly agreed criteria for eligibility for partial breast irradiation. Suggested criteria include tumour < 3 cm, unifocal, without an extensive intraduct component, close or negative margins and zero to three involved nodes.

It should be emphasized that large randomized studies will be needed to assess the clinical and economic effectiveness of partial breast irradiation techniques.

Local recurrence after mastectomy

If local recurrence occurs on the chest wall, 'spot' recurrence should be locally excised if feasible. Sixty to 70% of patients

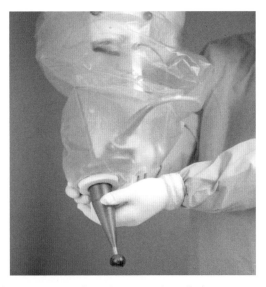

Figure 26.24 Intra beam intra-operative radiotherapy.

treated by local excision alone will develop a second local recurrence. For multiple 'spot' recurrences this is unlikely to be practical. Radical radiotherapy (40–50 Gy conventionally fractionated) to the chest wall and the supraclavicular fossa is recommended. If irradiation of the supraclavicular fossa is omitted, recurrence rates at this site may be as high as 28%.

For an isolated axillary recurrence, a level III clearance should be considered. Axillary irradiation is only considered if there is macroscopic disease remaining after a clearance or a previous clearance has been undertaken. Most of the available evidence does not support the use of axillary irradiation for patients with extracapsular spread in patients who have undergone a level III axillary clearance.

General care

During treatment

If the margins of the treatment fields are marked by a small number of tattoos, the patient can wash the treatment area during a course of radiotherapy. Shoulder exercises to keep the joint supple should be taught by a physiotherapist and practised by the patient during and after treatment.

After treatment

Apply an emollient cream, such as oilatum or aqueous cream, to areas of dry desquamation and antibiotic ointment (e.g. graneodin) or flamazine to areas of moist desquamation.

Morbidity of radical radiotherapy

Intact breast

1. Breast oedema is common, particularly in the first year after radiotherapy. It is commoner in patients who have had an axillary clearance.
2. Subcutaneous fibrosis is common and may give rise to progressive shrinkage of the irradiated breast over a period of years.

Postmastectomy

1. Skin – telangiectasia.
2. Lymphoedema of the ipsilateral arm.
3. Rib fractures. These occur in 1–2% of patients
4. Pneumonitis and lung fibrosis. Occasionally, transient cough occurs during radiotherapy but usually settles within a few weeks. Some degree of fibrosis is observed on chest radiograph. The features of clinical pneumonitis are dry cough, dysponea and fever 6–12 weeks after completion of radiotherapy. The risk increases with the number of fields treated and the use of chemotherapy. For patients treated by tangential fields alone without systemic therapy the risk is less than 1%.

5. Fibrosis of the shoulder joint can occur if the axilla is irradiated, restricting shoulder movement.
6. Cardiac morbidity. Patients, particularly if irradiated over the age of 60, are at increased risk of coronary artery disease and potentially of disease of other cardiac structures.
7. Radiation-induced sarcoma. This is an extremely rare complication with a mean latency of 13 years from the time of radiotherapy. Prognosis is very poor. Mean survival is 15 months.
8. Hypothyroidism may occur because of inclusion of the thyroid gland in the shoulder or medial supraclavicular field.

ADJUVANT HORMONAL AND CYTOTOXIC THERAPY

Rationale

It is generally accepted that a substantial number of patients with apparently localized breast cancer harbor systemic micrometastases. These are currently beyond the detection of the conventional staging.

All patients should be considered for some form of adjuvant systemic therapy to try to eradicate micrometastases.

Recommendations based on prognostic factors are summarized in Table 26.8

Who benefits?

The Early Breast Cancer Trialists' Group has provided a series of 5-yearly meta-analyses of over 75 000 women with early breast cancer. The overview shows clearly that both hormonal (tamoxifen or oophorectomy) and cytotoxic therapy (CMF or anthracycline-containing combination chemotherapy) reduce the relative risk of relapse or death by up to 30% at 10 years. The overall survival benefits are more modest, with a 4–12% gain in overall survival. The benefits in overall survival are greater in premenopausal than postmenopausal women. In women over the age of 70, there are few data on the benefit of adjuvant chemotherapy and some evidence that the degree of benefit falls with increasing age.

Following polychemotherapy, women aged 50–59 gain a 14% reduction in risk of death compared to 8% in women aged 60–69. The survival gains in the under 50 and 50–69 age groups are shown in Figure 26.25. Life expectancy is likely to be prolonged on average by 4 years for women under the age of 50 and by 1–3 years in women over the age of 50. Adjuvant chemotherapy reduces 10-year breast cancer mortality by 27%. For a woman who has a 50% chance of dying from breast cancer under the age of 50, the approximate reduction in risk of death is 13.5%. For a woman with a 10% risk of death at 10 years, the risk of death is about 8%.

Table 26.8 Recommendations for adjuvant systemic therapy based on prognostic factors		
LOW RISK	**INTERMEDIATE RISK**	**HIGH RISK**
	Prognostic factors	
Premenopausal/postmenopausal	Premenopausal	Premenopausal or postmenopausal
Tumour size <2 cm	Tumour size >2 cm	Any tumour size
Grade 1 or II	Grade III	Any grade
Axillary node negative	Axillary node negative	
ER positive	Axillary positive (1–3N+)	>4 axillary nodes positive
	ER negative	ER positive or negative
HER2 negative	HER 2 positive	HER2 postive/negative
Treatment		
Tamoxifen for 5 years (grade 1)	4 cycles of Epirubciin	Bonnadonna (4 cycles of
Tamxoifen for 5 years and OS	+ 4 cycles of CMF	Adriamycin +8 cycles of CMF
(goserelin for 2 years or oophorectomy) (if premenopausal and grade II)	Tam 5 yr if ER+	Tam 5 yr if ER+

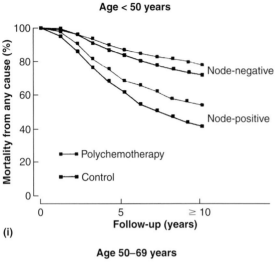

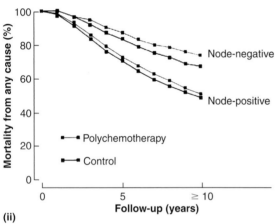

(i)

(ii)

Figure 26.25 Survival with and without adjuvant polychemotherapy in early breast cancer in women under the age of 50 years and 50–69 years.
(Reproduced from Parmar M K B, Adjuvant Therapy, Medicine 1999; 27:12: 32–34 by kind permission of The Medicine Publishing Company)

There is evidence that anthracyline-containing regimens increase the probability of survival compared to non-anthracycline-containing regimens such as CMF but at the cost of greater toxicity, particularly myelosuppression. Taxanes have been widely adopted in the adjuvant setting in the USA for high-risk younger woman. To date there is no published evidence of the superiority of taxane-containing regimens over anthracycline-containing regimens.

Adjuvant tamoxifen

Adjuvant tamoxifen (20 mg orally daily) reduces the risk of death by about 15%. The survival benefits of adjuvant tamoxifen are shown in Figure 26.26. Women with

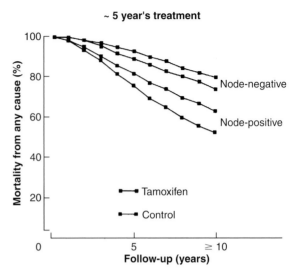

Figure 26.26 Survival with and without 5 years of adjuvant tamoxifen in early breast cancer.
(Reproduced from Parmar M K B, Adjuvant Therapy, Medicine 1999; 27:12: 32–34 by kind permission of The Medicine Publishing Company)

oestrogen receptor (ER)-rich tumours have 3–10 times the benefits of ER-poor patients. Life expectancy is increased by 2–3 years in women on tamoxifen for 2–3 years. If tamoxifen is added to chemotherapy in ER-rich tumours, additional benefit accrues, as also happens when chemotherapy is added to tamoxifen. In addition, tamoxifen reduces the risk of contralateral breast cancer.

The optimal duration of administration of tamoxifen is not clear, but most of the current evidence suggests that 5 years is probably optimal.

Aromatase inhibitors

The role of aromatase inhibitors as an alternative to tamoxifen or in combination with it was explored in the ATAC trial. The trial of over 9000 postmenopausal node-negative and predominantly oestrogen receptor-positive patients showed a statistically significant 2.4% gain in recurrence-free survival at 4 years in the anastrazole alone group over tamoxifen alone. In addition, there was a highly significant reduction in risk of contralateral breast cancer in the anastrazole alone group. In addition, the incidence of endometrial cancer, vaginal bleeding and discharge, venous thromboembolism and cerebrovascular accidents was reduced in the anastrazole treated group (Table 26.9). However, musculoskeletal symptoms and bone fractures were more common with anastrazole At 5 years, there was still a better disease-free survival with anastrazole compared to tamoxifen. However, there was no difference in breast cancer-specific survival. It is uncertain whether the findings can be extrapolated to node-positive patients.

Table 26.9 Toxicities in ATAC trial comparing adjuvant tamoxifen (T) and anastrazole (A)

TYPE OF TOXICITY	HAZARD RATIO	A%/T%
Endometrial ca	0.29	0.2/0.8
Vaginal bleeding	0.50	5.4/10.2
Arthralgia	1.32	35.6/29.4
Fracture	1.49	11/7.7
Ischaemic (cardiac)	1.23	4.1/3.4
Ischaemic (cerebral)	0.70	2/2.8
Thromboembolism	0.61	2.8/4.5

In the BIG 1-198 trial, 8028 postmenopausal patients with endocrine sensitive breast cancer were randomized to 5 years of tamoxifen (20 mg daily), 5 years of letrozole (25 mg daily), 2 years of tamoxifen followed by 3 years of letrozole or 2 years of letrozole followed by 3 years of tamoxifen. Analysis of the comparison of the tamoxifen (5 years) and letrozole (5 years) with a median follow up of 35.5 months showed a significant advantage in disease-free survival of letrozole over tamoxifen (Table 26.10). Patients on tamoxifen had significantly more thromboembolic events. Patients on letrozole had significantly more bone fractures and deaths from cardiac or cerebrovascular causes.

Adjuvant hormonal therapy after 5 years of tamoxifen

There is an emerging body of data to suggest that additional adjuvant hormonal therapy with the more recent and more potent aromatase inhibitors, such as letrozole and exemestane, may reduce the risk of recurrent breast cancer in patients treated initially with tamoxifen.

In the National Cancer Institute MA17 trial, over 5000 postmenopausal patients, mainly ER positive, were randomized after 5 years of adjuvant tamoxifen to either 2.5 mg of letrozole or placebo. The disease-free survival was superior in the letrozole group with a 4-year disease-free survival of 93% compared to 87% with placebo which was highly statistically significant. Overall survival was improved by 2% in the letrozole group (96% versus 94%) but was not statistically significant. In the Intergroup exemestane trial, patients were randomized after 2–3 years of tamoxifen to either a further 2–3 years of tamoxifen or the aromatase inhibitor, exemestane 25 mg orally for a further 2–3 years. There was an absolute benefit in disease-free survival of 4.7% which was statistically significant and led to early closure of the trial. Overall survival was not significantly different.

Tamoxifen confers a similar reduction in risk of death in node-positive and node-negative women. However, the absolute reduction in risk is greater in node-positive women. The absolute gain in 10-year survival between 5 years of tamoxifen and no tamoxifen is 6% for node-negative and 11% in node-positive women. It confers benefit in both premenopausal and postmenopausal ER-positive women.

Table 26.10 Trials of adjuvant endocrine therapy

	ATAC	BIG-198	IES	ABSCG/ARNO	MA-17
Rx	Postop	Postop	2–3 yr T	2 yr T	5 yr T
	A,T,AT	Let	Exem	A	Let
Patient nos	8028	1319	4742	?312	5187
Med age (y)	64	61	64	63	62
% N+	34	41	50	27	46
%HR+	84	99.8	81	100	100
% CT	21	25	32	?	100
Med FU (months)	33	26	30.6	26	28
HR DFS	0.83	0.81	0.68	0.59	0.57
P value	?0.01	0.003	0.0005	?	?

Rx: treatment; A: arimidex; T: tamoxifen; Let: letrozole; Exem: exemestane; N+: node positive; HR+: hormone receptor positive

Beyond 5 years the reduction in risk by tamoxifen is thought to decline and has to be balanced against the small risk of tamoxifen-induced endometrial cancer. Adding tamoxifen to chemotherapy in ER-positive patients confers additional benefit. All patients who are ER positive regardless of their menopausal or nodal status should be considered for adjuvant endocrine therapy for 5 years.

Toxicity of tamoxifen

Postmenopausal symptoms of hot flushes, vaginal dryness and sexual dysfunction are experienced by 20–40% of patients. Cognitive deficits also occur (as they do after cytotoxic chemotherapy). These symptoms can significantly interfere with a patient's quality of life. Transient thrombocytopenia occurs in 5–10% and vaginal bleeding in 5%. Tamoxifen increases the development of benign endometrial changes, such as hyperplasia. The risk of endometrial cancer, particularly in women who have been on tamoxifen for 5 years or more, is increased three- to fourfold, although the risk remains very small. The risk of endometrial cancer is 0.02%.

Care should be taken to avoid giving tamoxifen concurrently with chemotherapy since it increases the risk of a stroke. Tamoxifen should therefore only be started once chemotherapy has been completed.

Tamoxifen plus chemotherapy

Treatment with both tamoxifen and chemotherapy gives added benefit in patients with ER-positive disease in both node-positive and node-negative women. This also applies to postmenopausal ER-positive patients. However, in ER-negative, node-negative women, the NSABP B-23 trial showed no benefit of the addition of tamoxifen to chemotherapy.

Adjuvant ovarian suppression

Suppression of ovarian function is one of the longest established of adjuvant therapies. It was Sir George Beatson, a surgeon in Glasgow who, in 1895, first showed that oophorectomy could reduce the activity of breast cancer. A small randomized trial conducted in Edinburgh comparing patients with operable breast cancer treated by adjuvant oophorectomy or CMF chemotherapy showed that oophorectomy had a significant advantage over CMF in ER-positive patients and CMF over oophorectomy in ER-negative patients. The Oxford overview showed a highly significant increase in recurrence-free survival (25%) in premenopausal women under the age of 50 treated by oophorectomy.

For node-positive premenopausal women the gains in recurrence-free and overall survival at 15 years were 10.5% and 13% respectively. Much smaller but still statistically significant benefits in both these parameters were seen in premenopausal node-negative women.

Medical ovarian suppression by goserelin (3.6 mg given subcutaneously monthly) provides a reversible means of stopping ovarian function. Goserelin is commonly given for 2 years. It has the advantage that, if the patient finds the premenopausal symptoms intolerable (e.g. flushing and sweating), it can be stopped. If after 6 months of goserelin, menopausal symptoms are found still to be tolerable, the alternatives are to stay on goserelin or to proceed to an oophorectomy. If the patient prefers to stay on goserelin, it can be stopped after 2 years to check whether the patient is menopausal (raised LH and FSH with reduced estradiol levels).

Ovarian suppression and chemotherapy

Most trials show no difference in disease-free survival between ovarian suppression and chemotherapy in ER-positive premenopausal patients.

Adjuvant combination chemotherapy (polychemotherapy)

The 2000 Oxford overview shows no significant reduction in recurrence or risk of death comparing prolonged single-agent chemotherapy versus no chemotherapy. Prolonged combination chemotherapy (typically CMF) shows highly significant reductions in recurrence and death in women under the age of 50 and those aged 50–69. The reduction in risk of recurrence emerged in the first 4 years following treatment and the advantage in survival persists up to 15 years. The age-specific benefits do not appear to be influenced by the ER status of the primary tumour, menopausal status or the administration of adjuvant tamoxifen. The proportional reductions in risk were similar in node-positive and node-negative patients. The absolute differences in 10-year survival are 11–12% for node-positive patients and 4–5% for node-negative disease. For the 50–59 and 60–69 age groups, combination chemotherapy improved 10-year survival by 4% and 2% respectively.

More recently, the use of anthracycline-based chemotherapy (e.g. containing doxorubicin or epirubicin) has increased. The Oxford overview shows highly significant additional reductions in recurrence or death from anthracycline-containing regimens compared to CMF. The proportional reduction in risk did not appear to be affected by the age at diagnosis or by axillary nodal status. There were absolute gains of approximately 4% in survival, which persisted to 10 years.

Advances in adjuvant chemotherapy focus on (i) the introduction of non-cross resistant cytotoxic drugs, manipulation of the size of dose, dose density and total cumulative dose of the most active agents, (ii) the development of molecular markers predictive of response, and (iii) identification of women most likely to benefit from therapy.

To date trials of high dose chemotherapy with haematopoietic stem cell support have shown no advantage of adjuvant chemotherapy at conventional doses.

In the USA but not yet in Europe, taxanes are considered as a standard component of adjuvant chemotherapy. The CALGB 9344 trial and the BCIRG 001 trial show a long-term gain in survival (3–7% at 5 years) from a combination of adriamycin plus cyclophosphamide followed by paclitaxel or concomitant TAC (docetaxel, Adriamycin and cyclophosphamide) over Adriamycin plus cyclophoshamide (AC) or fluorouracil, Adriamycin and cyclophosphamide (FAC). In Europe, epirubicin-containing regimens are the standard at present. Current trials, such as the NSABP B-30, are evaluating the optimal combination and sequencing of anthracyclines and taxanes and the incorporation of new agents with efficacy in the metastatic setting (e.g. gemcitabine in the TANGO trial). The ECOG 1199 trial is comparing paclitaxel versus docetaxel and weekly versus three-weekly administration of taxanes. It is likely the success of trastuzumab (herceptin) in the metastatic setting will in time lead to its incorporation into adjuvant chemotherapy regimens. Four major randomized trials (NSABP B31, Intergroup N9831, BCIRG 006 and the Hera trial) are assessing the role of trastuzumab in the adjuvant setting. The role of the incorporating anti-angiogenic agents, such bevacuzimab, in the neoaduvant and adjuvant setting is also under evaluation. Metronomic chemotherapy is a relatively new concept. It refers to the frequent delivery of low doses of chemotherapy often over prolonged periods (e.g. 2 years). Metronomic AC (Adriamycin, cyclophosphamide) and weekly paclitaxel are under evaluation in a North American trial. In addition, the concept of low dose metronomic consolidation chemotherapy with oral cyclophosphamide and methotrexate after completion of standard chemotherapy is being evaluated in the IBSCG -22-00 trial.

To date, there are no predictive markers of response to chemotherapy. The EORTC p53 trial in high risk ER negative with high grade tumours is exploring the hypothesis that the benefit of the taxanes is mainly limited to the subgroup of patients with p53 mutated tumours. The MINDACT trial will test the hypothesis that microarray-based gene expression profiling is superior to traditional clinical and prognostic factors. Hopefully, it may identify patients currently receiving chemotherapy who do not need it.

Choice of drugs

For low-risk, older or unfit patients, six cycles of CMF are suggested (Table 26.11). For patients at intermediate risk of recurrence (one to three nodes positive), EPI-CMF (four cycles of of epirubicin followed by four cycles of CMF are recommended (Table 26.12B). With four or more positive axillary nodes, the anthracycline-containing regimen is more intensive with four cycles of doxorubicin followed by eight cycles of CMF chemotherapy (Table 26.12A).

Table 26.11 Adjuvant CMF regimens

CLASSICAL		
Cyclophosphamide	100 mg/m^2 orally	Days 1–14
Methotrexate	40 mg/m^2 i.v. bolus	Days 1 and 8
5-Fluorouracil	600 mg/m^2 i.v. bolus	Days 1 and 8
Repeated every 28 days		
ALTERNATIVE		
Cyclophosphamide	750 mg/m^2 i.v.	3-weekly
Methotrexate	50 mg/m^2 i.v.	3-weekly
5-Fluorouracil	600 mg/m^2 i.v.	3-weekly

Table 26.12 (a) Doxorubicin + CMF (Bonnadonna) adjuvant regimen; (b) epirubicin + CMF

A. DOXORUBICIN + CMF
Doxorubicin 75 mg/m^2 i.v.
Repeated every 21 days for 4 courses
Followed by 8 cycles of CMF
Repeated every 21 days
B. EPIRUBICIN + CMF
Epirubicin 100 mg/m^2 on day 1
Repeated every 21 days for 4 cycles
Followed by 4 cycles of CMF

Morbidity

The morbidity of adjuvant cytotoxic therapy may be both physical and psychological. For CMF chemotherapy, acute toxicity includes nausea and vomiting, temporary alopecia, lassitude, and soreness of the eyes (the latter due to secretion of methotrexate into the tears). Neutropenia-related infection is less common with CMF than with more intensive anthracycline-based chemotherapy. The anthracyclines (doxorubicin and epirubicin) cause complete, although reversible, alopecia. They are also potentially cardiotoxic, and cardiac function, judged clinically by electrocardiogram and cardiac ejection fraction, should be adequate before use. The risk of symptomatic cardiac dysfunction, for example, using a combination fluorouracil, epirubicin (at a dose of 100 mg/m^2) and cyclophosphamide (FEC 100) is 2% at 8 years. The risk of cardiac death is less than 1% if guidelines on maximum cumulative dose are respected. There appears to be no added risk of cardiotoxicity from combining taxanes with anthracyclines. With cumulative doses of anthracyclines, the long-term risk of inducing leukaemia increases. However, if a total dose of 720 mg of epirubicin is not exceeded, there is no increased risk of leukaemogenesis. More recently, cognitive dysfunction has been recognized as a complication of chemotherapy caused by damage to the frontal cortex. The risk factors for this are unknown.

Primary systemic therapy

The rationale for the use of preoperative chemotherapy in locally advanced breast cancer is that, in animal models, resection of the primary tumour accelerates metastatic growth. The application of preoperative systemic therapy might reduce or sterilize metastatic disease. Other benefits include increased resectability of the tumour either by mastectomy or breast conserving surgery and improving locoregional control. Pathological response is usually based on the response of the primary tumour and not the nodes. If a pathological complete response can be obtained, it confers the best prognosis. Nonetheless, it has yet to be proven that pathologic response or measures of cell division reliably predict patient outcomes.

To date six randomized trials have compared primary systemic therapy to adjuvant chemotherapy (Table 26.13) in patients with operable breast cancer. The findings of these trials are the basis of primary systemic therapy in both operable and inoperable breast cancer to achieve downstaging. The largest, conducted by the NSABP (National Adjuvant Breast and Bowel Project (NSABP)), B-18 trial randomized 1523 patients with T0–3,N0–1 operable breast cancer to either four cycles of Adriamycin and cyclophosphamide before or after primary surgery. For primary systemic therapy, the clinical response rate was 80% with a complete response rate of 36%. In the primary systemic therapy arm, there were significantly fewer patients found to have pathologically involved axillary nodes (41% versus 57%). However, there was no difference in overall or disease-free survival. In subset analysis, patients who were younger (≤49 years) had significantly better disease-free and overall survival (55% versus 46% and 71% versus 65% respectively). An important additional finding was that a pathological complete response conferred a better prognosis. Patients with a pathological complete response had a significantly better 5-year survival. The disease-free

Table 26.13 Randomized trials of primary systemic therapy versus adjuvant chemotherapy for breast cancer

TRIAL	STAGE	NO. PATIENTS ASSESSABLE	PST AND ADJUVANT THERAPY	cCR (%)	pCR (%)	DFS (%)	OS (%)
Semiglasov	IIB/IIIA	137	TMF-RT-TMF	12.4	29	81	86
		134	RT-S-TMF	5.9	19	72	78
Mauriac	T>3 cm	134	EVM-MTV-RT	33	NR	50	73
		138	S-EMV-+ MTV			50	72
Scholl	IIB/IIIA	191	FAC + RT-S	30	NR	59	86
			RT-S-FAC	41	NR	55	78
Powles	T1–2,N0–N1	105	MT-RT-MT	19	10	NR	NR
Van der Hage	T1c–T4b	350	FEC-S-RT	6.6	3	82	65
	N0–N1	348	S-FEC			84	70
NSABP	B-18T1–3	763	AC-S	36	13	55	70
		760	S-AC			53	69

PST: Primary systemic therapy; cCR: complete clinical response; pCR: complete pathological response; DFS: disease-free survival; OS: overall survival; S: surgery; RT: radiotherapy; TMF: thiotepa, methotrexate, fluorouracil; EVM: epirubicin, vincristine, methotrexate; MTV: mitomycin, thiotepa, vinblastine; FAC: 5-fluorouracil, doxorubicin, cyclophosphamide; MT: mitoxantrone, mitomycin, methotrexate, tamoxifen; FEC: 5-fluorouracil, epirubicin, cyclophosphamide; C: doxorubicin, cyclophosphamide; NR: not recorded
From Hutcheon A W and Heyes S ASCO, 2004

and overall survival for such patients at 9 years were 85% and 75% respectively.

MANAGEMENT OF LOCALLY ADVANCED BREAST CANCER (LABC)

Locally advanced breast cancer (LABC), or stage III breast cancer, refers to tumours >5 cm in diameter (T3) or associated with involvement of the skin or chest wall (T4) or with fixed axillary nodes or ipsilateral supraclavicular nodes. LABC still presents a major challenge in management. It accounts for between 5% and 30% of patients presenting to the breast clinic. A typical example in shown in Figure 26.27. These are a very heterogeneous group of tumours with widely differing natural histories. Results with surgery and radiotherapy were disappointing with high levels of locoregional and systemic failure. Substantial improvements have been achieved with the addition of systemic therapy. Nonetheless, long-term survival is only about 50%. The evidence base is much weaker than for early breast cancer. Much of the published literature is based on case series, with mixed populations of patients some including patients with inflammatory breast cancer and others not. Often, in studies of systemic therapy, locoregional therapy is not well defined. However, long-term survival remains poor at about 50% and systemic failure remains a major problem.

Clinical features

The main features of LABC are skin nodules, peau d'orange (T4b), inflammatory changes (T4d), ulceration and fixity to the chest wall (T4a), fixed axillary nodes (N2) or lymphoedema (N3). Local pain, bleeding, ulceration and infection are common symptomatic problems. The natural history of locally advanced disease varies widely. In some patients, distant metastatic disease will rapidly supervene, in others the disease remains locoregional and relatively indolent.

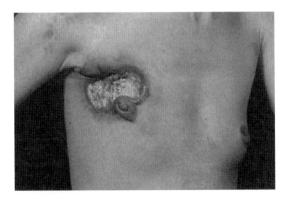

Figure 26.27 Locally advanced and inoperable carcinoma of the right breast (T4).

Principles of management

The management of LABC should be multidisciplinary. Surgery, radiotherapy and systemic therapy in different combinations need to be tailored to the clinical features of the patient's cancer to maximize locoregional control and reduce the risk of distant metastases.

For patients with operable IIIA disease, the choice is between modified radical mastectomy followed by adjuvant systemic therapy and radiotherapy or preoperative chemotherapy followed by surgery and radiotherapy.

Role of surgery

Surgery has a limited role in the management of locally advanced disease. It encompasses: (i) initial core biopsy for diagnosis and ER status; (ii) mastectomy and axillary clearance in operable patients; (iii) mastectomy (ideally with myocutaneous flap reconstruction) for residual masses after chemotherapy and radical radiotherapy; and (iv) palliative debriding of infected and/or necrotic areas to reduce odour. For inflammatory breast cancer (T4d), only patients with complete clinical resolution of inflammatory changes following chemotherapy should be considered for mastectomy. Mastectomy as the primary procedure or when inflammatory changes persist after neoadjuvant systemic therapy is likely to be followed rapidly by recurrence in the skin flaps.

Trials of adjuvant chemotherapy in patients with stage III disease are rare. The Oxford overview of randomized trials of adjuvant systemic therapy does contain some patients with large operable cancer. It showed that all patients gained from adjuvant chemotherapy irrespective of tumour size. On this basis, it is reasonable to extrapolate the results of the overview to patients with operable stage IIIA disease.

Primary chemotherapy followed by surgery

There are a limited number of case studies and randomized trials which have compared preoperative chemotherapy to postoperative chemotherapy. These were predominantly in stage I and II disease but did include some patients with T3 tumours. While preoperative chemotherapy did downstage some patients sufficiently for their cancer to be managed by breast conserving surgery rather than mastectomy, there was no difference in disease-free or overall survival. Indeed, some trials showed downstaging followed by conservative surgery resulted in a higher risk of local recurrence and survival was poorer.

Choice of systemic therapy

Data on the optimum chemotherapy for LABC are similarly sparse. The few trials that have been conducted had small numbers of patients. Two trials have shown an advantage of anthracycline-containing chemotherapy over no systemic therapy. One trial showed no difference in disease-free or overall survival between a combination of CMF with epirubicin and vincristine to CMF alone. The recommendations for anthracycline-based chemotherapy for LABC are largely extrapolated from studies of node-positive, metastatic breast cancer.

Based on trials of adjuvant chemotherapy, six cycles of cyclophosphamide, Adriamycin (CAF) or cyclophosphamide, epirubicin and 5-fluorouracil (CEF) is probably better than six cycles of CMF. In a trial of women with LABC randomized to CEF or epirubicin plus cyclophosphamide, there was no difference in survival at a median follow up 5.5 years (53% and 51% respectively). It is important to confirm continuing response up to six cycles of chemotherapy. In non-responders, chemotherapy should be stopped to avoid further toxicity. If sufficient tumour debulking has been achieved for surgery, this should be followed by postoperative radiotherapy. If there is no response and the tumour remains inoperable, radical radiotherapy should follow.

Taxane-containing regimens are under evaluation and there is some evidence that an anthracycline-containing regimen followed by a taxane may improve clinical and pathological response in LABC. One study comparing a combination of a taxane (doxetaxel) to FAC, showed superior disease-free survival and overall survival with TAC. It is, however, premature to provide definitive guidance on the use of taxanes in this setting.

Hormonal therapy

Patients with LABC who are oestrogen and/or progesterone positive should receive tamoxifen at the end of chemotherapy. For patients who are not suitable for chemotherapy and are hormone receptor positive, primary treatment with tamoxifen (20 mg daily) or the aromatase inhibitor letrazole (2.5 mg) is recommended. Responses to hormonal therapy may take 6–8 weeks to occur. Patients who are premenopausal and hormone receptor positive and are not suitable for chemotherapy should receive a luteinizing hormone releasing hormone agonist (goserelin, 3.6 mg subcutaneously monthly).

Locoregional therapy

If erythema of inflammatory changes or peau d'orange resolve with chemotherapy, mastectomy and axillary clearance should follow. Postoperative radiotherapy is given to the chest wall and, if there are four or more involved axillary nodes, to the medial supraclavicular fossa. There is no good evidence to determine whether or not the internal mammary nodes should be irradiated. Breast conserving therapy for LABC is not standard therapy. However, there are some patients where the degree of debulking achieved by chemotherapy does make breast conserving therapy

possible. In addition, there are selected patients with very small tumours which involve the skin early due to their proximity to the inframammary fold where the amount of breast tissue is small.

There is limited information on the role of breast reconstruction at the time of mastectomy. Reconstruction is generally best delayed until after the completion of chemotherapy and radiotherapy. If undertaken at the time of mastectomy, complications may delay chemotherapy and radiotherapy.

Target volume

The target volume should include the chest wall or breast (in the case of conservative surgery) and, if the axilla has not been cleared, the peripheral lymphatics.

Technique

The principles of radical radiotherapy for early breast cancer apply also to locally advanced disease, both for the intact breast or following mastectomy. The only difference is that 0.5–1 cm of skin bolus should be applied to the breast or chest wall to ensure that the skin receives a full dose (to overcome the skin-sparing effect of megavoltage radiotherapy). Axillary surgery is not normally carried out at staging and, therefore, the peripheral lymphatics will normally be irradiated. If mastectomy and a level III axillary clearance have been carried out, the axilla should not be irradiated. Where there is macroscopic disease which would cross the conventional breast/shoulder field junction, it is best to use an 'en bloc' technique, treating both the breast and the peripheral lymphatics in a perspex jig (see Figure 26.15).

Dosage and fractionation

While there is evidence of a dose response effect in locally advanced disease, escalating dosage beyond 60–70 Gy is associated with an increased risk of major complications. Hyperfractionated radiotherapy may have advantages in reducing repopulation during radiotherapy. The long-term results of studies of hyperfractionated radiotherapy are awaited. Until there is convincing evidence of improved local control, conventional dosage and fractionation are recommended.

1. Post-mastectomy
40 Gy in 15 fractions over 3 weeks or 45 Gy TAD in 20 fractions over 4 weeks or 50 Gy in 25 fractions over 5 weeks (6 MV photons) (applying skin bolus)
2. Intact breast
40 Gy in 15 fractions over 3 weeks 45 Gy TAD in 20 fractions over 4 weeks or 50 Gy in 25 fractions over 5 weeks (6 MV photons) (applying skin bolus)

Boost

Ten to 15 Gy maximum dose in five daily fractions over 1 week with electrons of appropriate energy. To judge the appropriate choice of energy of electrons, an ultrasound scan should be carried out towards the end of the radical course of breast irradiation and the distance from the skin surface over the tumour to the maximum depth of the tumour measured. The other dimensions of the tumour should also be measured to help the selection of the appropriate electron field size.

Palliative radiotherapy

In some patients, radical radiotherapy is not advised either because of poor medical condition, advanced age or evidence of metastatic disease elsewhere. Palliative radiotherapy can be very effective for symptomatic relief of local bleeding, ulceration, pain from axillary involvement and secondary upper limb lymphoedema. Responses are usually only partial but may be prolonged. However, even some shrinkage can be worthwhile, improving the morale of the patient where chemotherapy or hormonal therapy has been unsuccessful.

Technique

This should be simple, either with parallel-opposed or tangential fields at megavoltage confined to the macroscopic area of tumour using a small Perspex jig or, for flat limited areas of tumour, by a single electron field using a Perspex degrader to bring up the skin to full dose.

Dose

The dose is 20 Gy in five daily fractions over 1 week (electrons or 4–6 MV photons).

BONE METASTASES

Approximately 20–30% of patients present with bone metastases as the first site of metastatic disease. Sixty to 70% will develop bone metastases at some stage in the course of their disease. Bone metastases cause significant morbidity due to pain, pathological fractures, hypercalcaemia or spinal cord compression. Patients with bony metastases should be considered for up to 2 years of bisphosphonate therapy. The optimum duration for bisphosphonate therapy is uncertain. There is evidence that benefit diminishes after 2 years of therapy so that 2 years of therapy seems reasonable. Two large double-blind placebo-controlled randomized trials have shown significant reductions (50%) in skeletally-related events with 90 mg intravenous pamidronate in patients with lytic bone metastases. Time to first skeletal event was prolonged by 50%. Zolendronate

has been shown to be more effective than pamidronate in the treatment of hypercalcaemia and has largely replaced pamidronate for the treatment of hypercalcaemia and the prevention (4 mg monthly intravenous infusion over 15 minutes) of skeletal-related events. Ibandronate is a newer bisphosphonate which may be given orally or by intravenous infusion with similar efficacy. Oral clodronate (1600 mg day) is an alternative but its bioavailability is limited and gastrointestinal intolerance is common. In future, biochemical markers (such as telopeptide) of bone resorption may provide a better guide to the optimum duration of treatment and to response. Such markers might identify which patients might benefit from higher bisphosphonate dose or more prolonged duration of treatment.

Patients at risk of pathological fracture should be referred to an orthopaedic surgeon for consideration of mechanical stabilization (Figure 26.28) followed by postoperative palliative radiotherapy.

Technique

Single or parallel-opposed fields are used. Single fields suffice for the thoracic, lumbar spine and sacroiliac joints. The cervical spine can be treated by a single posterior field but this will cause a sore throat due to the exit dose through the mouth. Lateral opposed fields reduce the dose to the mouth and resulting mucositis.

Dose

Single fractions of 8 Gy are recommended at megavoltage. Following surgical stabilization, fractionated radiotherapy is given: 20 Gy in five fractions over 1 week at megavoltage.

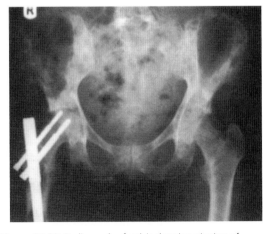

Figure 26.28 Radiograph of pelvis showing pinning of pathological fracture of right hip due to extensive mixed and sclerotic disease from breast cancer.

Palliative surgery

Where there is extensive ulceration and secondary infection causing distressing and offensive odour, surgical debridement of the affected area is often helpful in improving these symptoms. This can be repeated if necessary.

Medical management of metastatic disease

Although about 90% of patients present with localized disease, about 50% of patients with involved nodes and 10% of those who are node negative will relapse within 5 years. There is no curative treatment for metastatic disease. Treatment is still essentially palliative since the average life expectancy from the time of diagnosis of metastatic disease is of the order of 18 months to 2 years. Nonetheless, durable and clinically useful disease control can be obtained by hormonal, and/or cytotoxic therapy. In addition, therapy with bisphosphonates can be useful in reducing the risk of complications of bony metastases. Aims of treatment are principally relief of cancer-related symptoms, improvement in quality of life and prolongation of life. Prognosis is governed by a complex interaction of factors including number and site of metastases, disease-free interval, hormonal sensitivity and expression of the epidermal growth factor, HER-2. Better prognosis is associated with hormone sensitive, HER-2-negative tumours, a long disease-free interval (>1 year), absence of visceral involvement and a limited number of sites of metastases.

Principles of management

The choice of treatment must take into account the age and general medical condition of the patient, menopausal status, oestrogen receptor (ER) status, sites of metastatic involvement, the tempo of the disease and expression of HER-2. It is important that all centres should have access to ER status, since ER-negative tumours are non-responsive to endocrine therapy. In addition, there should be access to human epidermal growth factor receptor-2 (known as HER-2) status. An elevated serum level of HER-2 in ER-positive women with metastatic disease correlates with an inferior and shorter response to endocrine therapy. There are two general forms of systemic therapy: hormonal and cytotoxic. In addition, in patients whose tumour over-express HER2 (defined as score of 3+ on immunohisto-chemistry (IHC) or 2+ on IHC with a positive FISH (fluorescent in situ hybridization) test) may benefit from herceptin as single agent or in combination with chemotherapy. In general, hormonal therapy is better tolerated than cytotoxic therapy and, in the absence of immediately life-threatening aggressive disease, is the preferred first line of treatment in ER-positive disease. For ER-negative disease and disease progressing on endocrine therapy, chemotherapy is the treatment of choice in fit patients. The general schema of systemic therapy for metastatic cancer is shown in Table 26.14.

Menopausal status and hormone receptor status

In general, more postmenopausal than premenopausal patients are oestrogen receptor positive. Premenopausal patients tend to have more aggressive disease and are more commonly ER negative, especially under the age of 40. Patients with aggressive and/or ER-negative disease require chemotherapy.

Oestrogen and progesterone (PgR) receptor status is a useful guide to clinical response. ER+/PgR+ tumours have a response rate of 77%, ER+/PgR− of 27%, ER−/PgR+ of 46% and ER−/PgR− of 11%. In premenopausal ER-positive patients, options include ovarian suppression by medical means (goserelin 3.6 mg monthly subcutaneously), oophorectomy, radiation-induced menopause and tamoxifen. There is evidence in advanced disease that goserelin and tamoxifen have synergistic effects with a higher response rate (but no additional survival benefit) and are best prescribed together.

The advantage of goserelin is that it is reversible once withdrawn. This has particular advantages in women who tolerate poorly the menopausal symptoms that it induces and wish to stop the treatment and continue tamoxifen alone. Oophorectomy is usually performed as a laparoscopic procedure.

In general, response to one hormonal agent predicts response to subsequent hormonal therapy. Overall, 50–60% of ER-positive patients will respond. The duration of disease control by first-line hormonal therapy is usually about 18 months. About 25% of patients who respond to first-line hormonal agent will respond to second-line hormonal therapy. However, only 15% of patients who fail to respond to first-line therapy will respond to second-line hormone therapy.

For first-line therapy in premenopausal ER-positive women in the absence of visceral life-threatening disease, a combination of tamoxifen (20 mg orally daily) and ovarian suppression with goserelin (3.6 mg subcutaneously monthly) is suggested; for second-line therapy, anastrazole, an aromatase inhibitor, can be substituted for tamoxifen while continuing ovarian suppression with goserelin. If second-line hormonal therapy fails, cytotoxic chemotherapy should be considered.

For first-line therapy for recurrent disease in postmenopausal women the choice is between tamoxifen (20 mg per day), an aromatase inhibitor (anastrazole; 1 mg orally daily) or letrozole (2.5 mg orally daily); for second-line therapy, exemestane, an aromatase inhibitor (25 mg orally daily), is recommended; for third line therapy a progestogen, megestrol acetate (160 mg orally daily), is suggested. Anastrazole commonly causes joint stiffness due to its musculoskeletal effects. Megestrol acetate causes weight gain and should be avoided in patients with cardiac disease and/or thromboembolism.

Table 26.14 Schema of systemic therapy for metastatic breast cancer

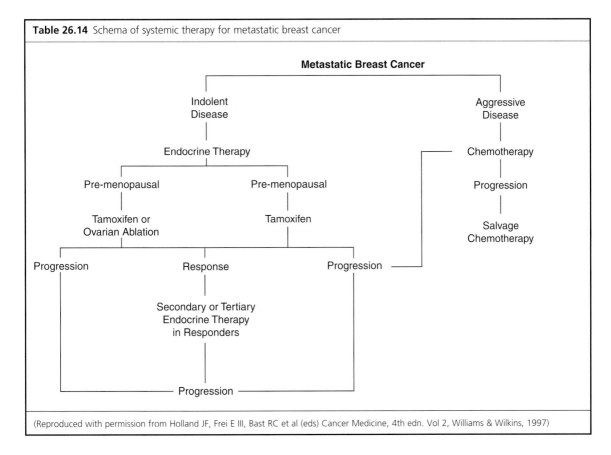

(Reproduced with permission from Holland JF, Frei E III, Bast RC et al (eds) Cancer Medicine, 4th edn. Vol 2, Williams & Wilkins, 1997)

Patients who are most likely to benefit from hormonal therapy for relapsed disease have one or more of the following characteristics:

- disease-free survival over 2 years
- soft tissue or bone disease
- older postmenopausal.

Sites of metastases and impact on management

Visceral metastases (e.g. liver disease) tends to respond less well to hormonal therapy and better to cytotoxic therapy. However, durable responses to hormonal therapy are occasionally seen with ER-positive liver metastases.

Cytotoxic therapy

Breast cancer is moderately sensitive to chemotherapy. In general, combination chemotherapy has a higher overall response rate and slight advantage in survival over monotherapy. Commonly used agents are doxorubicin, taxanes (doxetacel and paclitaxel), epirubicin, methotrexate and 5-fluorouracil. Newer agents include herceptin and capecitabine.

Herceptin

Herceptin is a monoclonal antibody to the HER2-*neu* c-erb2 oncogene. When amplified, the *HER2* gene stimulates tumour growth. A transmembrane tyrosine kinase receptor is encoded by HER2-*neu* which is very similar to the epidermal growth factor receptor. Inactive receptor monomers are bound together to form active dimers. Once dimerization has occurred, intracellular tyrosine kinase is activated and leads to signals which result in changes in gene expression and tumour growth. Herceptin is suitable for the 30% of patients who overexpress the cell surface antigen. Herceptin has a 13–16% response rate in heavily pretreated patients. It can be used in combination with cisplatin or paclitaxel. The addition of herceptin to anthracyclines or to a taxane (paclitaxel) increases median time to progression. The greatest addition to response rate came from combining herceptin with paclitaxel. The most serious side effect of herceptin is cardiotoxicity. It may precipitate cardiac failure. Pretreatment ventricular function tested by echocardiography or isotope ventriculography must be normal and must be repeated every 6 weeks during therapy. If ventricular functions or cardiac symptoms develop, treatment should be stopped. The rate of cardiac dysfunction is similar with herceptin as single agent as anthracycline-containing chemotherapy. Some degree of cardiotoxicity occurs in 7%

Table 26.15 Treatment schedule for herceptin

Loading dose 4 mg/kg i.v. by infusion over 90 minutes
If loading dose is tolerated, subsequent weekly doses of 2 mg/kg i.v. by infusion over 30 minutes

of patients and severe cardiotoxicity in 5%. However, when herceptin is combined with an anthracycline, the rate of cardiotoxicity increases to 28% (of which 19% are severe). As a rule combining herceptin with anthracyclines should be avoided.

While it has cytotoxic activity when used alone (Table 26.15), its maximum effects are delivered in conjunction with conventional chemotherapy in terms of overall survival, progression-free survival and overall response rates. HER2 testing is by immunohistochemistry or fluorescence in situ hybridization (FISH).

Side effects include allergic reactions and cardiac failure. Caution in the use of herceptin should be exercised in patients with a history of cardiac disease. Cardiac function should be monitored by radio-isotope ventriculography ever 6 weeks. If the cardiac ejection fraction falls below the normal range, development of cardiac symptoms and/or signs, treatment with herceptin should be stopped.

Capecitabine is an oral fluoropyrimidine with a slow release of 5-FU. The usual dose is 1250 mg/m^2 b.d. for 14 days. Gastrointestinal or renal toxicity may be dose limiting. The combination of capecitabine and docetaxel improves time to progress, overall survival and response rates in women whose disease has progressed on or after anthracycline therapy.

Combination chemotherapy

Median time to response varies from 6 to 14 weeks. Median duration of response is 6–12 months. Response rates to second-line combination chemotherapy are generally much lower (about 20%) and to third-line therapy. 5% or less. In only about 15–20% of patients is a complete response obtained. There are wide variations in the combinations of chemotherapy used in metastatic breast cancer. For fitter patients, particularly in patients with visceral disease, an anthacycline (Adriamycin 60 mg/m^2 iv 3 weekly) combined with cyclophosphamide (600 mg/m^2 iv 3 weekly) is an appropriate first line combination. For patients whose disease has progressed on an anthracycline-containing regimen, a taxane (Table 26.17) (combined with herceptin in HER-2 positive patients) is recommended. The optimal duration of chemotherapy is unclear. For most agents, administration of two initial courses to test responsiveness of the tumour followed by up to four additional courses if there is continuing response with acceptable toxicity is common practice. Decisions about the continuation or cessation of treatment should taken by patient and doctor taking

account of symptoms, signs, toxicity, quality of life and patient preference.

There is a wide range of palliative regimens of combination chemotherapy in use. For first-line treatment for relapse in patients who are fit for anthracycline therapy, doxorubicin/epirubicin and cyclophosphamide (Table 26.16) are suggested. If liver function is impaired, weekly epirubicin 20–30 mg/m^2 for 12–18 weeks can be tried. If patients are unfit for anthraclyines, then cyclophosphamide, methotrexate and 5-fluorouracil are recommended (Table 26.17). The response rate to CMF is 40–50%.

For second-line therapy, patients who have progressed on anthracyclines should be considered for a taxane, e.g. docetaxel or paclitaxel (Table 26.18). A reduction in dose or withdrawal of therapy may be needed in patients with impaired liver function. Alternative second-line regimens are mitomycin-C and infusional 5FU, mitomycin-C + methotrexate + mitoxantrone (MMM) or classical CMF. The MMM regimen may be suitable for frailer patients owing to its limited toxicity. In older patients, an oral anthracycline (idarubicin) should be considered.

Capecitabine is an orally active prodrug of 5FU with an objective response rate of 36%. It is given in a dose of 2500 mg/m^2 over 14 days. Response rates are similar to taxanes in patients previously treated by anthracyclines. Hand-foot syndrome and gastrointestinal toxicity are common and

Table 26.16 Palliative doxorubicin/epirubicin and cyclophosphamide

Doxorubicin 60 mg/m^2 or epirubicin 75 mg/m^2
Cyclophosphamide 600 mg/m^2
Given every 3 weeks

Table 26.17 Palliative CMF regimen

Cyclophosphamide	600 mg/m^2 i.v. bolus	Day 1
Methotrexate	40 mg/m^2 i.v. bolus	Day 1
5-fluorouracil	600 mg/m^2 i.v. bolus	Day 1
Repeated every 21 days for up to 6 courses		

Table 26.18 Palliative single therapy with docetaxel

Docetaxel 85–100 mg/m^2
Repeated every 21 days for up to 6 courses
Dose reduction to 75 mg/m^2 if liver function disturbed or toxicity

commonly require reductions in dose (e.g. to 2000 mg/m^2) or occasionally cessation of therapy. There is a synergistic cytotoxic effect if capecitabine is combined with docetaxel. The combination of docetaxel with capecitabine has a higher response rate (42% versus 30%) when compared to docetaxel alone. Median survival with the combination was 14 months compared to 11 months with docetaxel alone. Gemcitabine has a first line response rate of between 23 and 37% (Table 26.19). There are synergistic effects when it is combined with either cisplatin or paclitaxel.

Bone marrow involvement

Bone marrow involvement complicates the delivery of cytotoxic therapy since the associated leukopenia and thrombocytopaenia due to impaired marrow function may compromise the delivery of full-dose chemotherapy. Doses of chemotherapy have to be reduced to 50% or less of standard dosage. Weekly low dose intravenous epirubicin (20 mg/m2) is generally well tolerated. If chemotherapy is successful, haemoglobin, white count and platelet levels should eventually rise. Bone marrow involvement is not an absolute indication for cytotoxic therapy since responses are seen in ER-positive patients. However, rapidly evolving bone marrow infiltration will require chemotherapy.

Growth factor support

For patients who are experiencing treatment delays due to febrile leukopenia, treatment with granulocyte colony-stimulating factor (GCSF) is recommended. GCSF is given daily by subcutaneous injection, starting not less than 24 hours after chemotherapy and continuing until the predicated neutrophil nadir has passed and recovered into the normal range. Duration of treatment is normally up to 14 days depending on the drug regimen, dosage and scheduling. Common side effects include pain and redness at the injection site and bone pain.

Table 26.19 Single agent chemotherapy first line responses rates in metastatic breast cancer	
Paclitaxel/docetaxel	36–68%
Doxorubicin and epirubicin	40%
Cyclophosphamide	36%
Mitoxantrone (mitozantrone)	27%
Methotrexate	26%
5-Fluorouracil	28%
Vinorelbine	40–52%
Gemcitabine	23–37%

OVERALL SURVIVAL IN BREAST CANCER

As seen in Figure 26.29, the mortality of breast cancer exceeds that of the unaffected women, even up to 30 years or more after initial treatment.

Overall survival from the time of diagnosis of metastatic disease is about 18 months. The tempo of metastatic disease varies widely. It may be relatively indolent in bone with disease controlled for many years. However, the tempo of visceral disease is often more aggressive with survival often of 6 months or less.

FOLLOW UP

The main goals of follow-up are:

1. detection of locoregional or metastastic recurrence, second primary tumour and contralateral breast cancer
2. assessment and treatment of complications of treatment
3. encourage compliance with therapy
4. psychosocial support
5. maintain and monitor response to treatment and treatment-induced morbidity and facilitate rehabilitation.

Clinical trials have failed to show an improvement in patient outcomes from more intensive versus less intensive follow up for systemic recurrence. There is no evidence that the early detection of asymptomatic disease at distant sites improves survival or quality of life. Routine imaging apart from mammography is not recommended as part of follow-up care.

From the patient's perspective, reassurance that there is no evidence of recurrence or of progressive disease is probably the most important. Most of the evidence suggests, at least for women treated for operable breast cancer, that most recurrences whether after breast conservation or mastectomy present symptomatically. It is probable that a policy of annual mammography to detect local recurrence in the conserved or contralateral breast and rapid access to the breast/oncology clinic for women with new symptoms would be much more cost-effective.

Follow-up after breast-conserving therapy

For patients managed by breast-conserving therapy, the priorities are the detection of local recurrence which can be treated by mastectomy and of contralateral breast cancer. The risk of contralateral breast cancer is three to five times that of the normal population.

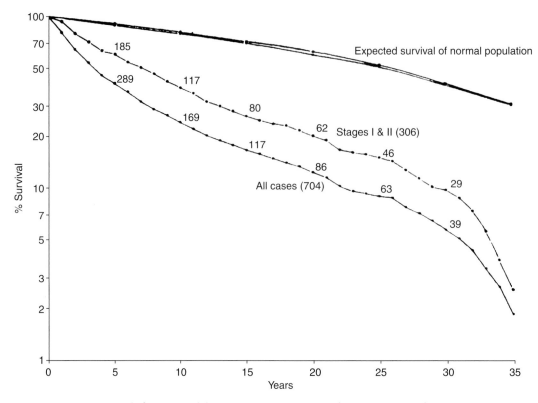

Figure 26.29 Long-term survival of women with breast cancer. Survival curves for all patients and for stages I and II only. *(Reproduced with permission from The Lancet, 1984)*

Recurrence rates within the treated breast remain constant at 1% per year up to 15 years. This argues that the frequency of follow up does not need to be any more frequent in the early years after completion of treatment than in later years. Most studies of follow up after breast-conserving therapy have been with annual mammography. Optimum duration of follow up is unclear. However, annual follow up to 10 years seems reasonable. At this point, women who still lie within the UK screening age group (i.e. up to 69 years) should be returned to the 3-yearly breast-screening programme. For women 70 years or older, further follow up should be decided on an individual basis between the patient and their surgeon/oncologist.

Follow-up after mastectomy

Local recurrences on the chest wall are commonest in the first 2 years after mastectomy and 80% of chest wall and axillary recurrences occur within the first 5 years. The evidence-based guidelines of the American Society of Clinical Oncology recommend a careful history and clinical examination every 3–6 months for 3 years, then visits every 6–12 months for 2 years, and then annually thereafter. Optimum duration of follow up is uncertain. However,

10 years seems reasonable. Beyond 10 years the guidelines are as for patients managed by breast conservation.

BREAST CANCER IN PREGNANCY

The diagnosis of breast cancer in pregnancy is uncommon but presents difficult decisions for patient, oncologist and obstetrician. Close liaison between oncologist and obstetrician is essential. The interests of both mother and child need to be taken into account.

Most tumours are high grade and lymphovascular invasion is common. Lymph node involvement is reported to be as high as 79%. Most tumours (over 70%) are oestrogen-receptor negative. On average, delay in diagnosis of breast cancer is 8.2 months during pregnancy compared to 1.9 months in non-pregnant women. Management will be influenced by the stage of pregnancy, the preference of the patient and the stage of the disease. However, it should follow as far as possible the protocol for non-pregnant patients. A subsequent pregnancy after the diagnosis of breast cancer does not adversely affect prognosis. Indeed, there is some evidence that it may have a favourable effect on survival.

With adequate shielding of the fetus, mammography should not be harmful. However, the increased density of the breast during pregnancy may obscure the radiological signs of malignancy. In the first trimester, termination is normally advised and followed by standard treatment.

Surgery can be safely performed during pregnancy. In general, this is delayed until at least the 12th week of gestation since, before this point, the risk of spontaneous abortion is highest. Breast conserving surgery should be considered if possible with axillary lymph node dissection but not sentinel node biopsy using a radioactive tracer. No adjuvant radiotherapy or adjuvant systemic therapy is given until the delivery of the baby.

In the second trimester, the choice is between conservative surgery or mastectomy or termination of pregnancy followed by standard adjuvant therapy.

In the third trimester of pregnancy, the breast becomes more vascular. Small tumours may be treated with wide local excision followed after delivery by postoperative radiotherapy. For larger tumours, simple mastectomy with axillary node clearance is recommended. Elective induction or caesarean section at 36 weeks is followed, if indicated, by postoperative radiotherapy (same criteria as in the non-pregnant patient).

Adjuvant radiotherapy is not given during pregnancy since with a total dose of 50 Gy conventionally fractionated, the fetus will receive 2 Gy (i.e. excess of the 0.05 Gy safe limit). Radiotherapy can be safely delayed up to 6 months after surgery.

Anthracyclines and cyclophosphamide can be safely delivered during pregnancy. The combination of 5-fluorouracil, epirubicin and cyclophosphamide can be delivered without adverse effect on the infant. The last cycle of chemotherapy should be delivered around the 34th week of pregnancy.

Delivery between days 1 and 14 of the chemotherapy cycle should be avoided. Platelet count should be $\geq 80\times10^9/L$. Hormonal therapy, if indicated, should be started after delivery and after chemotherapy has been completed.

BREAST CANCER IN MALES

Breast cancer in men is rare, only representing 1% of breast cancer. Most cases occur in an older age group than in women, typically occurring over the age of 60. In some cases, there is a genetic predisposition. A variable proportion of cases (3–20%) carry a mutation of the *BRCA2* gene. A family history of male breast cancer is a major predisposing factor to female breast cancer. In addition, *BRCA2* mutations are associated with an increased risk of other cancers such lymphomas, laryngeal and kidney cancer.

Presentation is typically with locally advanced disease often affecting the nipple. Fixation to the chest wall is common. The advanced state of the local disease is in part probably due to the limited amount of breast tissue that the tumour has to invade and the lack of awareness among men that they can develop breast cancer.

Treatment where the disease is operable is by simple mastectomy and axillary node clearance. Postoperative radiotherapy is often needed because of skin infiltration. Although the rarity of the tumour means that there are no trials of adjuvant therapy, the same principles should apply as in female breast cancer. For ER-positive patients, tamoxifen is advised and for ER-negative disease, CMF chemotherapy. The outcome of the disease is usually poor with 5-year survival of about 40% reflecting the commonly advanced nature of the disease at presentation.

FURTHER READING

Early Breast Cancer Triallists' Collaborative Group. Polychemotherapy for early breast cancer: an overview of the randomised trials. Lancet 1998;352:930–42.

Early Breast Cancer Triallists' Collaborative Group. Favourable and unfavourable effects on long-term survival of radiotherapy for early breast cancer: an overview of the randomised trials. Lancet 2000;355:1757–70.

Whelan TJ, Julian J, Wright J, et al. Does locoregional radiation therapy improve survival in breast cancer? A meta-analysis. J Clin Oncol 2000;18:1220–9.

Hannoun-Levi JM, Courdi A, Marsiglia M, et al. Breast cancer in elderly women: is partial breast irradiation a good alternative? Breast Cancer Res Treat 2000;81:243–51.

Overgaard M, Hansen PA, Overgaard J, et al. Postoperative radiotherapy in high-risk premenopausal women who receive adjuvant chemotherapy. N Engl J Med 1997;337:949–55.

Overgaard M, Jensen MB, Overgaard J, et al. Postoperative radiotherapy in high-risk postmenopausal breast cancer patients who receive adjuvant chemotherapy. Lancet 1999;353:1641–8.

van der Vijver MJ, He YD, Van't Veer LJ, et al. A gene-expression signature as a predictor of survival in breast cancer. N Engl J Med 2002;347:1999–2009.

Clinical practice guidelines for the care and treatment of breast cancer: 15. Treatment for women with stage III or locally advanced breast cancer. CMAJ 2004;170:983–94.

Chetty U, Jack W, Prescott RJ, et al. Management of the axilla in operable breast cancer treated by breast conservation: a randomized clinical Trial. Edinburgh Breast Unit. Br J Surg 2000;87:163–9.

Howell A, Cuzick J, Baum M, et al. ATAC Trialists' Group. Results of the ATAC (Arimidex, Tamoxifen, Alone or in Combination) trial after completion of 5 years' adjuvant treatment for breast cancer. Lancet 2005;365:60–2.

Fossati R, Confalonieri C, Torri V, et al. Cytotoxic and hormonal treatment for metastatic breast cancer: a systematic review of published randomized trials involving 31,510 women. J Clin Oncol 1998;16:3439–60.

O'Shaughnessy J, Miles D, Vukelja S, et al. Superior survival with capecitabine plus docetaxel combination therapy in anthracycline-pretreated patients with advanced breast cancer: phase III trial results. J Clin Oncol 2002;20:2812–23.

Chapter | 27 |

Gynaecological cancer

Paul Symonds

ANATOMY

The female reproductive organs lie within the pelvis and are the vulva, vagina, uterus and fallopian tubes. These are represented in Figures 27.1 and 27.2.

INCIDENCE OF GYNAECOLOGICAL CANCER

The incidence of gynaecological cancer in England in 2007 is shown in Table 27.1. The incidence of cervical cancer has declined markedly over the last 40 years. This falling trend has been accelerated by the success of the cervical screening programme (Figure 27.3). However,

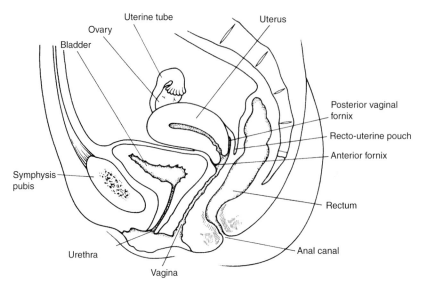

Figure 27.1 Sagittal section of the uterus and its relations.
(Redrawn from Ellis, Clinical Anatomy, 5th edn, Blackwells, 1975).

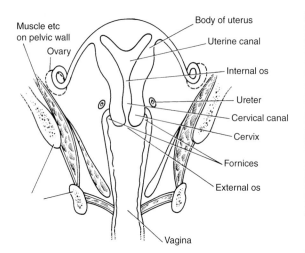

Figure 27.2 Coronal section of the uterus and vagina. Note the important relationship of the ureter to the cervix.

Table 27.1 Incidence of gynaecological cancer in UK in 2007 (CRUK)		
SITE	**NUMBER OF CASES**	**INCIDENCE PER 100 000**
	PER ANNUM	**WOMEN**
Vulva	1120	3.6
Cervix	2828	9.1
Body of Uterus	7214	23.2
Ovary	6537	20.9

cervical cancer is the most important female cancer in much of the developing world including south Asia, sub-Saharan Africa and South America. In some parts of the USA and Canada, the incidence of carcinoma of body of uterus is more than double that seen in the UK. This may be associated with the epidemic of obesity in North America.

Ovarian cancer is now the most common gynaecological cancer in Britain. It is also the most difficult to cure.

CARCINOMA OF CERVIX

Causes of cervical neoplasia

In virtually all cases of cancer of cervix, there is evidence that the tumour is associated with infection with the human papilloma virus (HPV), particularly types 16 and 18. The human papilloma virus produces proteins that bind to the products of two important tumour suppressor genes, p53 and Rb1.

Risk factors associated with cervical cancer are those that promote sexually transmitted disease. These are particularly the age of first intercourse and number of sexual

Figure 27.3 Lymphatic drainage of the cervix: (a) obturator; (b) internal, external and common iliac; (c) lateral sacral; and (d) para-aortic.
(Reproduced from Souhami and Tobias, Cancer and its Management, Blackwells, 1986).

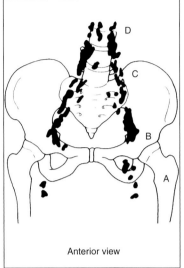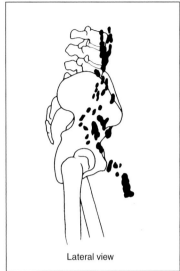

Anterior view

Lateral view

partners. There is a lower incidence of cervical carcinoma in women using barrier methods of contraception. Male behaviour is also important. Partners of men in certain occupations, such as seamen, deep-sea fishermen and long distance lorry drivers, have a higher incidence of cervical cancer. So do those partners of men whose previous partners have developed cervix cancer. Smoking and immunosuppression are also associated with cervical cancer. Cervical neoplasia is more common in women who are HIV positive.

Pathology of cervical cancer

Viral infection of the cervix may lead to premalignant change which is called dysplasia. This can be detected in exfoliated cells removed during a cervical smear. Cervical dysplasia is graded mild, moderate or severe. The terms CIN1, CIN2 and CIN3 are histological terms used to describe increasing degrees of dysplasia, mild, moderate and severe in biopsy material. In some women, there is a progression from mild to severe dysplasia and then invasive cancer. This often takes many years to develop and can be detected during cervical screening. Treatment of premalignant disease is highly effective. Patients with moderate or severe dysplasia are offered ablative treatment using large loop excision, laser vaporization or cryotherapy. However, in most cases, dysplasia is self-limiting. Even the most severe form of dysplasia, CIN3 (previously called carcinoma in situ), will only progress to invasive cancer in between 20 and 40% of women if left untreated. Between 85 and 95% of cases of invasive cancer of cervix are squamous carcinomas. The remainder are adenocarcinoma or adenosquamous tumours. There is some evidence that the incidence of adenocarcinoma is increasing among younger women. Some authorities feel adenocarcinoma of cervix has a worse prognosis than squamous cancer when treated by radiotherapy.

Carcinoma of cervix spreads predominantly by direct invasion and through the lymphatic system. Initially, the tumour spreads into the uterus or vagina and parametrium (the tissues around the uterus). Later, it can infiltrate bladder or rectum. The tumour spreads to the iliac and then para-aortic lymph nodes (Figure 27.4) Blood-borne spread is less common and this may lead to liver, lung and bone metastases.

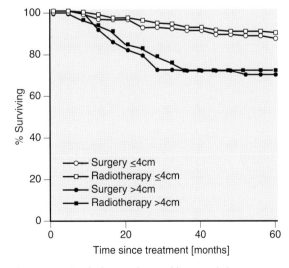

Figure 27.4 Survival stage 1b operable ca cervix in a randomized trial of 343 patients treated by surgery or radiotherapy.

469

Symptoms and investigations of cervical cancer

Premalignant changes are usually asymptomatic. The cardinal symptom of invasive cervix cancer is irregular vaginal bleeding. This may be bleeding after intercourse or bleeding in between periods. Sometimes, the women will have a brown vaginal discharge. Pain is usually a symptom of advanced disease and suggests spread to adjacent organs around the cervix. Backache may be associated with para-aortic lymph node spread.

Patients with cervical cancer are staged clinically according to the FIGO staging system (Table 27.2). Accurate staging of cervical cancer is essential so that appropriate treatment can be planned. The cornerstone to staging is an examination under anaesthesia (EUA). The cervix and

Table 27.2 FIGO 2009 staging: carcinoma of the cervix uteri		
Stage I	The carcinoma is strictly confined to the cervix (extension to the corpus would be disregarded)	
	Ia	Invasive carcinoma which can be diagnosed only by microscopy. All macroscopically visible lesions, even with superficial invasion, are allotted to Stage Ib carcinomas. Invasion is limited to a measured stromal invasion with a maximal depth of 5.0 mm and a horizontal extension of not >7.0 mm. Depth of invasion should not be >5.0 mm taken from the base of the epithelium of the original tissue, superficial or glandular. The involvement of vascular spaces, venous or lymphatic, should not change the stage allotment
	Ia1	Measured stromal invasion of not >3.0 mm in depth and extension of not >7.0 mm
	Ia2	Measured stromal invasion of >3.0 mm and not >5.0 mm with an extension of not >7.0 mm
	Ib	Clinically visible lesions limited to the cervix uteri or preclinical cancers greater than stage 1a
	Ib1	Clinically visible lesions not >4.0 cm
	Ib2 (Figures 27.5 and 27.6)	Clinically visible lesions >4.0 cm
Stage II	Cervical carcinoma invades beyond the uterus, but not to the pelvic wall or to the lower third of the vagina	
	IIa	No obvious parametrial involvement
	IIa1	Clinically visible lesion ≤4.0 cm in greatest dimension
	IIa2	Clinically visible lesion >4 cm in greatest dimension
	IIb (Figures 27.7 and 27.8)	Obvious parametrial involvement
Stage III	The carcinoma has extended to the pelvic wall. On rectal examination, there is no cancer-free space between the tumour and the pelvic wall. The tumour involves the lower-third of the vagina. All cases with hydronephrosis or non-functioning kidney are included, unless they are known to be due to other causes	
	IIIa	Tumour involves lower-third of the vagina, with no extension to the pelvic wall
	IIIb (Figures 27.9 and 27.10)	Extension to the pelvic wall and/or hydronephrosis or non-functioning kidney

Table 27.2 FIGO 2009 staging: carcinoma of the cervix uteri—cont'd	
Stage IV	The carcinoma has extended beyond the true pelvis, or has involved (biopsy-proven) the mucosa of the bladder or rectum. A bullous oedema, as such, does not permit a case to be allotted to stage IV
IVa (Figure 27.11 and Figure *evolve* 27.12🖱)	Spread of the growth to adjacent organs
IVb (Figure 27.13)	Spread to distant organs

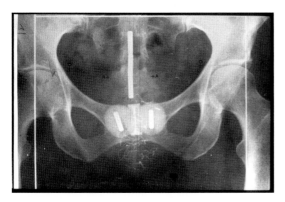

Figure 27.5 Manual insertion of a long central tube and ovoids containing cesium.

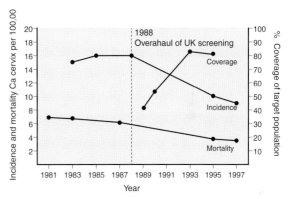

Figure 27.7 Impact of 1988 overhaul of UK cervical screening programme on incidence and mortality of cervical cancer in UK.

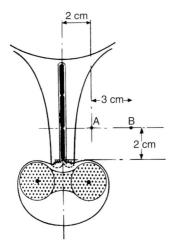

Figure 27.6 Diagrammatic uterus and vagina, showing intrauterine tube, cross-sections of ovoids in lateral fornices, separated by spacer, and points A and B.
(Reproduced with permission of Arnold from Ralston Paterson, Treatment of Malignant disease, 2nd edn, Edward Arnold, 1943).

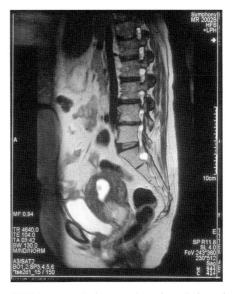

Figure 27.8 Large cervical tumour in endocervical canal.

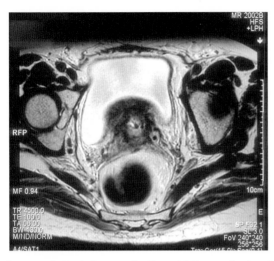

Figure 27.9 Cervical tumour (as Figure 27.8) extending into R parametrium.

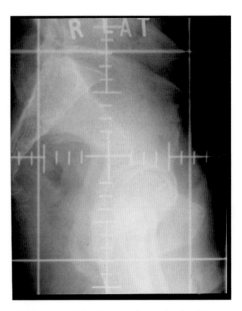

Figure 27.11 Lateral simulator radiograph of pelvis (stage IIb ca cervix as Figures 27.8 and 27.9).

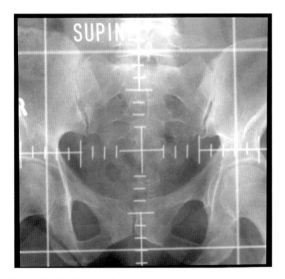

Figure 27.10 AP simulator radiograph of pelvis (stage IIb ca cervix – as Figures 27.8 and 27.9).

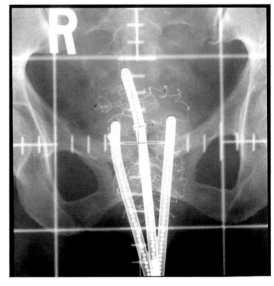

Figure 27.13 A-P view Selectron insertion stage IIb ca cervix (as Figures 27.8 and 27.9).

vagina are inspected and palpated for evidence of tumour. Rectal examination is essential to assess the degree of parametrial spread and to find if the tumour is fixed to the pelvic sidewall. This is usually accompanied by a cystoscopy and, if necessary, a proctoscopy and sigmoidoscopy. Patients usually have a computed tomography (CT) or magnetic resonance imaging (MRI) scan of the abdomen and pelvis looking for nodal spread and urinary obstruction. MRI scanning is a more effective method for imaging the primary tumour, although spiral CT scanning and MRI are probably equally effective in the evaluation of lymph node metastasis.

Treatment

Stage is the most important factor related to outcome. However, tumour size is also an important prognostic feature. It is noteworthy that the survival figures in Table 27.3 relate to patients treated by radical surgery or radiotherapy rather

Table 27.3 Carcinoma of the cervix. Patients treated in 1990–92. Survival by FIGO stage (n = 11 945)

STAGE	PATIENTS (N)	OVERALL 5-YEAR SURVIVAL (%)
Ia1	518	95.1
Ib2	384	94.9
Ib	4657	80.1
IIa	813	66.3
IIb	2251	63.5
IIIa	180	33.3
IIIb	2350	38.7
IVa	294	17.1
IVb	198	9.4

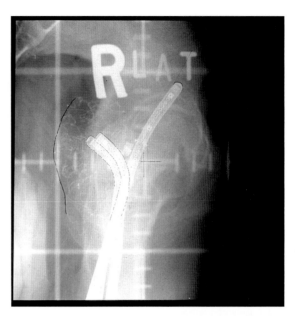

Figure 27.14 Lateral view Selectron insertion stage IIb ca cervix (as Figures 27.8 and 27.9).

than chemoradiotherapy, as combination treatment has only been given on a wide scale after 1999.

Treatment of stage I disease

Stage I tumours are subdivided into stage Ia and stage Ib. They are further subdivided according to tumour size. Stage Ia cases are those that are treated by less than radical means. The prognosis is excellent for stage Ia1 patients and the problem is to avoid overtreatment. A cone biopsy or simple hysterectomy offers many of these patients a virtual 100% change of cure. The outlook is almost as good for stage Ia2 patients. The optimum management of this group has not been clearly defined. The management options vary from cone biopsy to simple or modified radical hysterectomy.

Stage Ib is divided into patients with tumours confined to the cervix and uterus less (stage Ib1) or greater than 4 cm (stage Ib2). Patients with stage Ib1 tumour may be treated by radical hysterectomy. Usually, such patients are relatively slim, fit and often premenopausal. In a radical hysterectomy (a Wertheim's hysterectomy), the ureter is mobilized to allow wide excision of the uterus and cervix with removal of the cardinal ligaments and a wide cuff of vagina. The pelvic lymph nodes are also usually removed.

Stage Ib2 patients are usually treated by radiotherapy as these tumours have often spread to pelvic lymph nodes. If treated by surgery such patients usually require postoperative radiotherapy.

The only large randomized trial of radiotherapy and surgery in operable cervical cancer showed equally good results for both modalities (Figure 27.14). The number of serious complications was higher in the surgical arm.

However, complications of surgery are usually easier to rectify than the complications of radiotherapy.

Postoperative radiotherapy

Radiotherapy is given after surgery if there is an increased risk of local recurrence. Radiotherapy is mandatory if a stage Ib tumour is inadvertently treated by simple hysterectomy, as retrospective studies have shown 5-year survival figures of only 50% in this situation without radiotherapy. Indications after radical surgery include positive surgical excision margins and lymph nodes involved by tumour. Treatment may be external beam radiotherapy with or without brachytherapy (intracavity treatment) to the upper one-third of vagina. Concomitant chemotherapy may improve long-term survival.

Treatment of stage II–IVa

A few patients with stage IIa disease with early involvement of the vaginal vault are suitable for treatment by radical hysterectomy. Most are treated by radiotherapy which remains the mainstay of treatment of patients with stages IIb– IVa.

Carcinoma of cervix is usually treated by a combination of both external beam and intracavity (brachytherapy) treatment. Occasionally, patients with stage 1b tumours less than 4 cm are treated by brachytherapy alone. The target volume for external beam therapy is normally the cervical tumour plus the internal and external iliac lymph nodes. If there is significant involvement to the vagina by treatment, often the whole vagina is included within the treatment volume. Patients are irradiated with 6–25 MV x-rays using a four-field technique if possible. Anterior, posterior and two lateral fields are used. Typical anatomical boundaries of the volumes are as follows. The superior limit of the treated volume may be at the sacral promontory or at the L4–5 junction to incorporate the whole of the common iliac chain of lymph nodes. The bottom of the obturator foramen is often taken as the inferior margin but, if there is significant vaginal involvement, the inferior margin may need to be at the introitus. The lateral margins are usually 1 cm beyond the bony margin of the true pelvis. The lateral posterior treatment volume limit is often at the S2/S3 junction in the sacrum. The lateral field anterior treatment volume margin is halfway through the symphysis pubis. These margins may have to be adjusted to take into account EUA or MRI scan finding (Figures 27.15–27.20). Thin patients or those with very bulky disease may need to be treated with parallel-opposed fields.

Increasingly, CT or MRI scanning shows small volume lymph node metastasis in the para-aortic region. Such patients may need to be treated using extended spade-shaped parallel-opposed fields. The handle of the spade covers the para-aortic region and the blade covers the pelvis.

The dose that can be given by external beam radiotherapy is limited by the radiation tolerance of the small bowel. Doses of up to 50 Gy can be given to the pelvis in 2 or 1.8 Gy fractions. If the para-aortic nodes are irradiated in continuity with the pelvis, the dose must be limited to 45 Gy given in 1.8 Gy fractions (Figures 27.21–27.24).

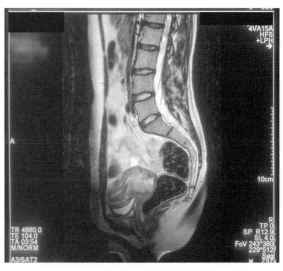

Figure 27.16 Large stage Ib2 cervical tumour before treatment.

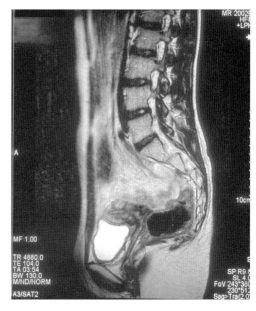

Figure 27.17 Complete regression after chemoradiotherapy (cf Figure 27.16).

Intracavity brachytherapy

The cervix was one of the first tumours to be successfully treated by radium. A number of systems were developed, in particular the Stockholm, Paris and Manchester methods. Many of the modern afterloading techniques owe their origin to the Manchester technique in which a tube containing radium (latterly cesium) was placed within the uterus and two rubber ellipses (ovoids) were placed against the cervix

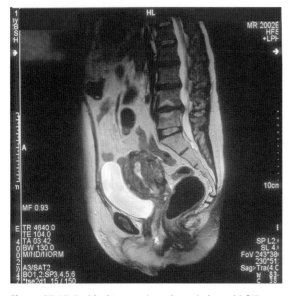

Figure 27.15 Residual tumour in endocervical canal (cf Figures 27.8 and 27.9).

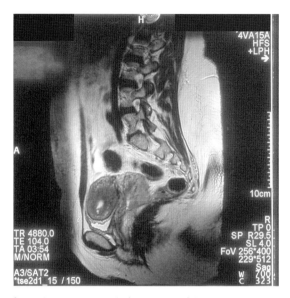

Figure 27.18 Large cervical tumour involving rectum stage IVa before treatment.

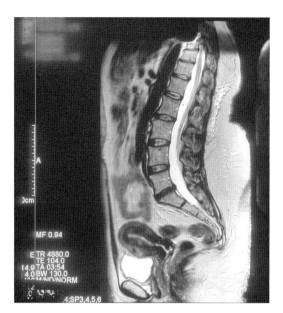

Figure 27.20 Complete response after treatment without a recto-vaginal fistula.

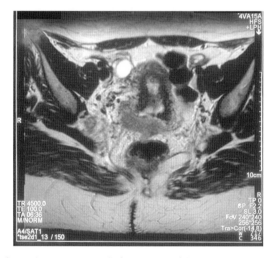

Figure 27.19 Large cervical tumour involving rectum stage IVa before treatment.

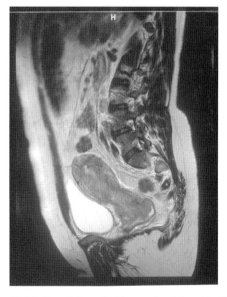

Figure 27.21 Stage IVb cervical tumour involving virtually the whole of the uterus plus upper vagina with para-aortic node metastases.

(Figure *evolve* 27.25🖱). Gauze packing was used to secure the applicators and reduce the dose received by the rectum. Treatment was prescribed to point A which was a geometric point 2 cm superior and 2 cm lateral from the cervical os (Figure 27.26). Typical doses given to point A using low dose rate (0.5 Gy per hour) cesium sources after external beam radiotherapy are 25–30 Gy.

Excellent results can be achieved using manually inserted cesium. The disadvantage with inserting 'live' cesium sources is high doses received by theatre staff and nurses looking after the patient. Consequently, most centres in the western world have adopted afterloading techniques. Hollow applicators are placed within the uterus and vagina, the position of the applicators are checked using fluoroscopy and check radiographs and then radioactive sources are inserted by remote control (Figure 27.27). For the last 15 years, one

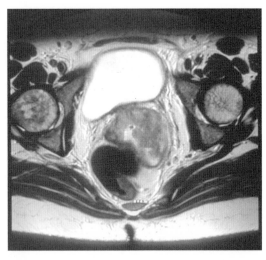

Figure 27.22 Same tumour as Figure 27.21 extending around rectum.

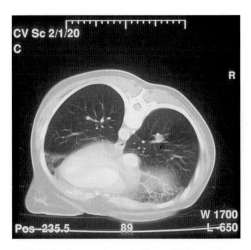

Figure 27.24 Patient as shown in Figure 27.21 – pulmonary metastases and lymphangitis.

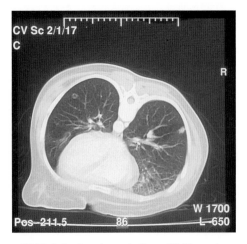

Figure 27.23 Patient as shown in Figure 27.21 – pulmonary metastases and lymphangitis.

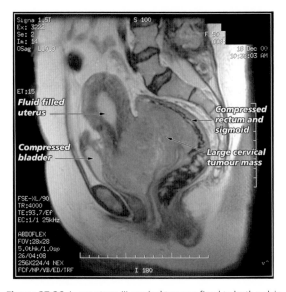

Figure 27.26 Large stage III cervical tumour fixed to both pelvic sidewalls and involving the vagina. The tumour is compressing on both bladder and rectum.

of the most popular afterloading devices was the medium dose-rate Selectron. Many departments are now converting to high dose-rate (HDR) machines using high intensity iridium sources. Treatment is completed in a matter of a few minutes. Typical A point dose rates during medium dose rate Selectron treatments are 1.8 Gy/h compared to 0.5 Gy/h using manually inserted sources. To allow for dose rate effect, overall doses to point A from the Selectron are reduced by about 10–20% compared to manually inserted cesium dosage. High dose-rate treatments are usually fractionated. Fraction sizes should not exceed 7 Gy to point A per treatment. Further information is given in the brachytherapy chapter (see Chapter 11).

Chemoradiotherapy

The addition of chemotherapy to radiotherapy in the treatment of carcinoma of cervix appears to improve prognosis. A meta-analysis of 19 published and unpublished trials comparing patients given concomitant chemotherapy plus radiotherapy to radiotherapy alone showed that the addition of chemotherapy reduced the odds of death by 29%. The absolute survival benefit for a typical patient with stage III disease who would have had a 40% chance of cure with radiotherapy alone is improved by 12% to 52%

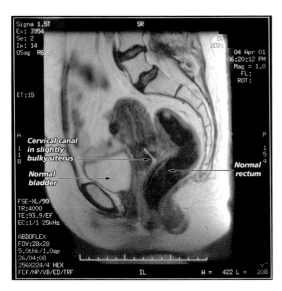

Figure 27.27 Large stage III tumour 3 months after chemoradiotherapy. Complete response. This patient was discharged from the clinic in 2007, 7 years after treatment.

(Figures 27.26 and 27.27). As well as improving local control, the addition of chemotherapy also seems to reduce significantly the incidence of distant metastases. Cisplatin given weekly (40 mg/m^2) is the current regimen of choice. This gives as good results as more toxic regimens.

Complications of treatment

Radiotherapy for cervical cancer gives some of the highest complications of treatment. Patients may develop bladder or rectal fistulae (Figure 27.28). Endarteritis of small blood vessels and fibrosis may result in stenosis of small or large bowel leading to intestinal obstruction. However, the overall incidence of late effects should not exceed 6%. There is no

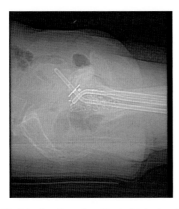

Figure 27.28 Selection insertion. Central tube in uterus, ovoids against cervix, pack under ovoids to reduce close to bladder.

evidence currently that giving chemotherapy along with radiotherapy increases the frequency of late effects.

Future trends

The irradiation of vulnerable tissue may be reduced further by the increased use of conformal techniques and intensity modulated radiotherapy (IMRT). As many departments adopt HDR brachytherapy they also move to CT and MRI imaging in order to plan brachytherapy. There is also a move away from prescribing to point A and to calculate the total dose delivered by external beam and brachytherapy to the tumour plus vulnerable organs such as bladder and rectum. In Vienna, they aim to deliver 85 Gy to 90% isodose line (D90) enclosing the tumour (including external beam and brachytherapy dosage) as long as a volume of 2 cc of bladder or rectum does not receive doses of 76 and 63 Gy respectively. Drugs such as gemcitabine or capecitabine in addition to cisplatin when given along with radiotherapy may further improve survival figures.

CARCINOMA OF ENDOMETRIUM

The causes of endometrial cancer are unknown. There is no evidence of a genetic basis. However, environmental factors, particularly oestrogen, are important. Physiological conditions and diseases that expose the endometrium to high levels of oestrogen are important in the development of this condition. These include early menarche, late menopause, nulliparaty, polycystic ovarian disease and, rarely, oestrogen producing ovarian tumours. Patients who are obese have a greater risk of endometrial cancer as adrenal steroids are metabolized to oestrone and oestrogen in adipose tissue. Both oestrogen only hormone replacement therapy (HRT) and tamoxifen (used in the treatment of breast cancer) can lead to endometrial hyperplasia and endometrial cancer.

Pathology

The majority of tumours are adenocarcinoma of endometrioid type. Atypical types such as clear cell or serous papillary tumours carry a worse prognosis. Tumour grade and spread into the myometrium are useful predictors of pelvic node spread. Patients with poorly-differentiated tumours are at higher risk of developing both vaginal vault recurrence and spread to pelvic lymph nodes than patients with well-differentiated tumours. Survival tends to fall with increasing depth of myometrial invasion as the extent of myometrium invasion correlates with involvement of pelvic and para-aortic lymph nodes by tumour. This is especially true of poorly-differentiated tumours.

Routes of spread

Tumour may extend beyond the endometrial cavity to involve the cervix or vagina. Parametrial spread is extremely uncommon. Distant spread is first to iliac lymph nodes or occasionally directly to para-aortic nodes without iliac involvement. Blood stream spread is unusual. Staging takes into account pathological features and the pattern of spread. The current FIGO staging is shown in Table 27.4. Over 80% of patients have stage I tumours.

Treatment

The mainstay of treatment is simple hysterectomy. The prognostic effect of removal of pelvic lymph nodes (lymphadenectomy) is the subject of current clinical trials. Patients with well- or moderately well-differentiated tumours confined to the inner half of the myometrium require no further treatment.

Radiotherapy

Radiotherapy may be given as an alternative to surgery, as postoperative adjuvant treatment or to treat pelvic or vault recurrence. Patients who are treated primarily by local radiotherapy are often extremely obese or have serious intercurrent disease which are both contraindications for surgery. Five-year survival of 72% has been reported in this group of patients treated by two interuterine cesium insertions in Manchester. Patients who require external beam radiotherapy prior to an interuterine insertion can be selected by MRI scanning which is good at showing myometrial invasion by tumour. Doses used are similar to those used to treat carcinoma of cervix.

Postoperative radiotherapy

Both the Dutch PORTEC trial and the Medical Research Council (MRC) ASTEC trials showed no survival advantage for routine postoperative radiotherapy for patients with immediate risk (grade I FIGO Ib, G2 Ib, G3 Ia) tumours. There was a statistically significant decrease in pelvic recurrence compared to observation alone after surgery but no overall survival benefit.

Patients with more aggressive tumours may benefit from postoperative radiotherapy. A meta-analysis and systematic review by Johnson and Cornes showed postoperative radiotherapy increased survival by 10% for patients with poorly differentiated tumour penetrating more than half way through the myometrium (stage Ib G3). When planning radiotherapy, the target volume should include the internal and external iliac lymph nodes plus the upper two-thirds of the vagina. Field arrangements and volume irradiated are very similar to those used in the treatment of cervical cancer. Doses of 40–45 Gy are given in 1.8 or 2 Gy fractions (Figure 27.29).

Radiotherapy can be used with curative intent if previously unirradiated patients develop an isolated pelvic recurrence. Five-year survival rates of 50–80% have been reported in patients with isolated vaginal vault recurrence, although this falls to about 20% in patients with pelvic side-wall disease.

Table 27.4 FIGO 2009 staging: carcinoma of the endometrium	
Stage I	Tumour confined to the corpus uteri
Ia	No or less than half myometrial invasion
Ib	Invasion equal to or more than half of the myometrium
Stage II	Tumour invades cervical stroma, but does not extend beyond the uterus
Stage III	Local and/or regional spread of the tumour
IIIa	Tumour invades the serosa of the corpus uteri and/or adenxae
IIIb	Vaginal and/or parametrial involvement
IIIc	Metastases to pelvic and/or para-aortic lymph nodes
IIIc1	Positive pelvic nodes
IIIc2	Positive para-aortic lymph nodes with or without positive pelvic lymph nodes
Stage IV	Tumour invades bladder and/or bowel mucosa, and/or distant metastases
IVa	Tumour invasion of bladder and/or bowel mucosa
IVb	Distant metastases, including intra-abdominal metastases and/or inguinal lymph nodes

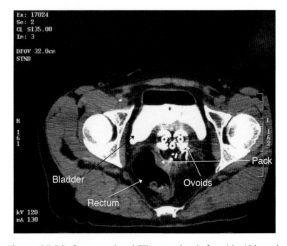

Figure 27.29 Cross-sectional CT scan at level of ovoids. Although the pack under the ovoids reduces the dose to the central part of the rectum; the rectum is displaced to the right. Owing to abnormal anatomy, the rectum is close to the ovoids with a risk of late damage. The bladder also prolapses downwards, especially on the right and is also at risk of late effects.

Brachytherapy

Brachytherapy (usually ovoids) in addition to external beam radiotherapy reduces the risk of vaginal recurrence and improves survival in patients with stage II (involvement of cervix) tumours.

The major use for vaginal brachytherapy is to treat patients with intermediate-risk tumours rather then external beam radiotherapy. The Dutch PORTEC-2 study showed an identical survival and very similar local recurrence rates at 3 years after treatment, but brachytherapy patients had radiation-induced side effects and a better quality of life. Brachytherapy is easy to administer via a vaginal cylinder that can be inserted without an anaesthetic.

Other treatment modalities

Some endometrial cancers exhibit progesterone and/or oestrogen receptors. About a third of patients with endometrial cancer will show an objective response to progesterogenic hormones such as megestrol acetate (160 mg daily). Response rates tend to be higher in patients with well-differentiated tumours especially those who are progesterogen receptor positive. Chemotherapy is of limited value in the treatment of endometrial cancer. Doxorubicin is the best single agent with a 20–40% response rate. Response rates greater than 50% have been reported with doxorubicin and cisplatin combinations. Recently, paclitaxel has also been used in combination with carboplatin with response rates of up to 70%. However, there is little evidence of improved survival for combination chemotherapy compared to single agent doxorubicin. Responses tend to be of short duration and survival tends to be about 9 months in patients with metastatic disease. Response rate to carboplatin is between 25 and 35% and may be the drug of choice for elderly unfit patients.

Results of treatment

The majority of patients suffer from stage I cancers. Five-year survival for patients with stage Ia disease is over 90%. This falls to about 70% for patients with stage Ic disease. Reported 5-year survival for patients with stage II disease is between 85 and 60% and stage III disease between 75 and 40%, depending on the treatment modality and degree of histological differentiation of the tumour.

Future trends

About 20% of patients with endometrial cancer will die, usually from distant metastases rather than pelvic recurrence. A trial conducted by the Nordic Society of Gynaecological Oncology (NSGO) showed an 8% improvement in 5-year progression-free survival after chemotherapy and postoperative radiotherapy (82%) compared to 74% (radiotherapy only) in 'high risk' (G3 Ib–III) patients.

Combined chemoradiotherapy is being tested further in the Anglo-Dutch PORTEC-3 trial.

SARCOMAS OF THE UTERUS

Sarcomas of the uterus are rare. They arise from the supporting tissues of the uterus and are classified as stromal sarcomas, leiomyosarcomas and carcinosarcomas (previously called mixed mesodermal sarcomas). They tend to spread via the blood stream, particularly to the lungs. Carcinosarcomas also tend to spread via the lymphatic system. There is also a high frequency of both local recurrence and metastases within the peritoneal cavity.

The primary treatment of these tumours is by surgery. Radiotherapy has been shown to decrease local recurrence. There have been claims that postoperative radiotherapy improves survival and this was tested in an EORTC randomized trial of 240 patients. This showed improved local control with radiotherapy but no overall survival advantage.

Radiotherapy is sometimes useful in inoperable cases. Carcinosarcomas tend to be more radiosensitive than leiomyosarcomas. There is no proven role for adjuvant cytotoxic chemotherapy but chemotherapy may provide palliation for patients with systemic spread. Doxorubicin is probably the most effective agent. This may be combined along with cisplatin in patients with carcinosarcomas. However, leiomyosarcomas are usually resistant to cisplatin. Paclitaxel has been used recently in the treatment of uterine sarcomas. The response rates of single agent or combination treatment are 30–40% with a response duration of 6–9 months. The overall 5-year survival of this group of patients is about 30%.

CANCER OF THE OVARY

Aetiology

In the majority of cases, the cause of ovarian cancer is unknown. However, epithelial ovarian cancer is more common in women who have never been pregnant or had an early menarche or late menopause. Conversely, the incidence of ovarian cancer is reduced in women who have had multiple births and there is good evidence that oral contraceptives reduce the incidence of this disease. The protective effect of birth parity and oral contraceptives is probably through suppression of ovulation. About 5% of ovarian cancers are familial. The most important hereditary syndromes are associated with carriage of the BRCA1 complex on chromosome 17 and the BRCA2 complex on chromosome 13. The BRCA 1 + 2 genes are also associated with breast cancer and sometimes colon and endometrial cancer. Familial tumours tend to develop at a younger age than sporadic cancers. Women with two or more first degree relatives who have developed ovarian cancer or one who has developed breast cancer and one other relative who has developed ovarian cancer before the age of 50 may be offered genetic counselling and, if possible, testing for the BRCA1 and 2 genes. These patients may also be offered screening for ovarian and breast cancer. Prophylactic oophorectomy may also be recommended in certain cases.

Pathology

Benign or malignant ovarian tumours may be solid or cystic. Some benign ovarian cysts may exceed 30 cm in diameter and weigh many kilograms. About 10% of ovarian tumours may be classified as borderline. These are tumours that have some histological features of malignancy but lack stromal invasion.

Malignant ovarian tumours are subdivided into epithelial, germ cell and sex cord. Eighty-five percent of ovarian tumours are classified as of epithelial origin and develop from the surface epithelium of the ovary. Some histological subtypes are more aggressive than others and have a worse prognosis. Undifferentiated and clear cell tumours tend to have the worse prognosis. Mucinous tumours tend to present with earlier stage disease and have a better outlook.

Method of spread

Ovarian cancer tends to be a disease of the abdominal cavity and rapidly spreads across the peritoneal cavity to involve the omentum, a fatty apron close to spleen and left kidney. There may be also multiple peritoneal deposits, particularly in the subdiaphragmatic areas. These peritoneal deposits may produce large volumes of ascitic fluid. A potentially fatal consequence of peritoneal disease is intestinal obstruction. The cancer may also spread to pelvic and para-aortic lymph nodes, the liver and pleural cavity of the chest by direct spread across the peritoneum or via the blood stream. Involvement of lung parenchyma is less common. Metastasis to other sites, particularly bone and brain, is exceedingly rare.

Clinical features

Late stage diagnosis is the rule rather than the exception and, justifiably, ovarian cancer has the nickname the 'silent killer'. There are no typical symptoms. Women may complain of abdominal bloating or non-specific gastrointestinal symptoms. One of the first signs may be the discovery of a large pelvic mass or ascites.

Investigations and staging

Investigations in most cases are for a pelvic mass with or without ascites. The tumour marker CA125 is elevated (above 35 international units per litre (iu/L)) in about 50% of patients with early stage and 80% of patients with more advanced stage disease. CT scanning of the abdomen is excellent for demonstrating primary tumour with significant peritoneal spread and involvement of the omentum. CT scanning can also show the degree of spread to adjacent organs and is useful for predicting operability. As many as 60–70% of patients have spread beyond the pelvis at diagnosis and are placed in stages III or IV. FIGO staging of this disease is listed in Table 27.5.

Needle biopsy under CT control from the primary tumour or omental metastases can confirm the diagnosis in inoperable cases. Ascites may have to be drained to relieve discomfort and shortness of breath. Ascitic fluid should always be examined cytologically for the presence of malignant cells.

Treatment

Surgery

The role of surgery is both diagnostic and therapeutic. At laparotomy, the full extent of peritoneal spread must be assessed, particularly the subdiaphragmatic areas and the paracolic gutters (the areas adjacent to the large bowel). The aim of surgery is to remove as much tumour as possible. If possible, both ovaries and the uterus should be removed along with the omentum. All macroscopic disease should be removed if possible. If not, residual peritoneal disease should be debulked to leave individual residual tumours of less than 1 cm. There are numerous non-randomized studies which indicate that optimal debulking improves prognosis but there have been no randomized controlled trials comparing aggressive debulking against more conservative surgery.

Chemotherapy

Following surgery, the mainstay of treatment is chemotherapy. Primary debulking surgery is only possible in 40–50% of women. A large number of patients have bulk residual disease after surgery. Patients with stage III or IV disease even after optimal surgery will rapidly relapse without further treatment but, fortunately, epithelial ovarian cancer is fairly chemosensitive. Regimens such as carboplatin and paclitaxel or carboplatin alone will give response rates of 60–70% in advanced disease. Currently, there is considerable controversy over which is the best chemotherapeutic regimen in this disease. In the USA and Germany, a combination of paclitaxel and carboplatin is favoured. The Medical Research Council ICON3 study, which recruited over 2000 patients mainly from the UK and Italy, showed that optimal dose carboplatin gave as good results as carboplatin and paclitaxel. Median survival was approximately 3 years in both arms of the study. Recently, randomized controlled trials have shown an improvement of almost 9% 5-year survival by the use of adjuvant chemotherapy in stage I disease and there is now a case for treating patients with early stage disease, especially those with adverse features, such as poorly-differentiated histology, with adjuvant chemotherapy.

Table 27.5 FIGO 2009 staging: carcinoma of the ovary

Stage I	Growth limited to the ovaries		
		Ia	Growth limited to one ovary; no ascites present containing malignant cells. No tumour on the external surface; capsule intact
		Ib	Growth limited to both ovaries; no ascites present containing malignant cells. No tumour on the external surfaces; capsules intact
		Ic	Tumour either stage Ia or Ib, but with tumour on surface of one or both ovaries, or with capsule ruptured, or with ascites present containing malignant cells, or with positive peritoneal washings
Stage II	Growth involving one or both ovaries with pelvic extension		
		IIa	Extension and/or metastases to the uterus and/or tubes
		IIb	Extension to other pelvic tissues
		IIc	Tumour either stage IIa or IIb, but with tumour on surface of one or both ovaries; or with capsule(s) ruptured; or with ascites present containing malignant cells or with positive peritoneal washings
Stage III	Tumour involving one or both ovaries with histologically confirmed peritoneal implants outside the pelvis and/or positive retroperitoneal or inguinal nodes. Superficial liver metastases equals stage III. Tumour is limited to the true pelvis, but with histologically proven malignant extension to small bowel or omentum		
		IIIa	Tumour grossly limited to the true pelvis, with negative nodes, but with histologically confirmed microscopic seeding of abdominal peritoneal surface, or histologically proven extension to small bowel or mesentery
		IIIb	Tumour of one or both ovaries with histologically confirmed implants, peritoneal metastasis of abdominal peritoneal surfaces, none exceeding 2 cm in diameter; nodes are negative
		IIIc	Peritoneal metastasis beyond the pelvis >2 cm in diameter and/or positive retroperitoneal or inguinal nodes
Stage IV	Growth involving one or both ovaries with distant metastases. If pleural effusion is present, there must be positive cytology to allot a case to stage IV. Parenchymal liver metastasis equals stage IV		

Radiotherapy

Whole abdominal radiotherapy in the radical treatment of ovarian cancer administered either using large fields or the so-called moving strip technique must be counted as obsolete. Radiotherapy is largely palliative and is used to shrink symptomatic ovarian masses, especially tumours causing pain or bleeding. Doses of 20–30 Gy in 5–10 fractions are usually given using parallel-opposed fields.

Results of treatment of epithelial tumours

In the past, the 5-year survival associated with stage I disease was about 65%. This may have reflected rather poor staging. Recently, trials of adjuvant chemotherapy have demonstrated 5-year survivals of up to 90% in this group of women. The 5-year survival for stage II disease is 40–60%. True stage II cases are relatively uncommon. The bulk of women have stage III disease which carries a 30–40% 5-year survival. The 5-year survival for stage IV disease is about 5–10%.

RARE TUMOURS OF THE OVARY

Sex-cord tumours

The most common of the sex-cord tumours are granulosa cell tumours. These display a spectrum of aggressiveness. Some may behave in benign fashion and others extremely aggressively. They are found predominantly in post-menopausal women but can occur at any age including before puberty. These tumours often produce steroid hormones, particularly oestrogens, which can cause post-menopausal bleeding in older women and precocious puberty in young girls. Over 80% of patients present with stage I disease. Treatment is predominantly by surgery. Bilateral disease occurs in up to 25% of patients. Usually, both ovaries are removed along with the uterus. A single ovary may be removed in young women with stage I disease preserving fertility. Granulosa cell tumours can recur up to 30 years after initial surgery. The site of recurrence is usually within the abdominal cavity or the liver. Metastases from granulosa cell tumour can be hemorrhagic leading to internal bleeding. Because of the rarity of this tumour there have been few comparative studies of chemotherapy in this disease but cisplatin-based regimens, such as the BEP regimen (bleomycin, etoposide and cisplatin) or CAP (cyclophosphamide, Adriamycin, cisplatin), can offer very useful palliation.

Most of the radiotherapy literature comes from the 1960s, but this tumour is more radiosensitive than the commoner epithelial cancers. Pelvic radiotherapy is sometimes used as an adjuvant after surgery or in the palliation of advanced disease. Pelvic fields are treated with doses of 45–50 Gy in 20–25 fractions depending on the size of treated volume. Overall, the prognosis is good in the short term with a 5-year survival of over 80%.

Leydig-Sertoli cell tumours are rare. More than half of these tumours produce male hormones that can cause virilization. The majority of these tumours behave in a benign fashion and present with stage I disease. Malignant lesions are exceedingly rare.

Germ cell tumours

Dysgerminomas account for 2–5% of all ovarian tumours and usually occur in women under 30 years old. Histologically, they are similar to seminoma of the testes in men and tend to spread in a similar way via the pelvic and para-aortic lymph nodes. The majority of tumours present with stage I disease, although up to 15% of tumours can be present in both ovaries. Surgery is usually aimed at conservation of fertility with removal of only one ovary, but such patients

need very close follow up owing to the risks of developing a further tumour in the remaining ovary.

This tumour is extremely chemosensitive. The BEP regimen (bleomycin, etoposide and cisplatin) is effective if patients relapse after surgery with a 5-year survival of about 85%. The tumour is quite radiosensitive and, in the past, patients have been treated with wide-field radiotherapy with doses between 20 and 40 Gy in 2–4 weeks. Good long-term survival has been reported following wide-field radiotherapy. However, my experience is that chemotherapy gives better results than radiotherapy. An added advantage is that fertility is more likely to be preserved following chemotherapy than radiotherapy.

More than 98% of ovarian teratomas are benign, most commonly cystic teratomas or dermoid cysts. Malignant teratomas are rare and have a similar histological appearance to those arising in the testes. The same chemotherapy regimens used to treat the more common testicular teratomas in males are also used in ovarian disease, particularly the BEP regimen. The outlook for such patients is not as good as male testicular teratoma patients with a 5-year survival of about 50%.

TUMOURS OF THE VAGINA AND VULVA

There were only 243 new cases of vaginal cancer in the UK in 2007. This may be because the FIGO rules state that if the cervix or the vulva is involved the tumour should be assigned to either site. The staging of vaginal cancer is listed in Table 27.6.

The majority of tumours are squamous and tend to occur in women over 60. Surgery as a primary treatment has a limited role and the majority of patients are treated in a similar fashion to cervical cancer. Usually, such patients receive

Table 27.6 FIGO 2009 staging: carcinoma of the vagina

Stage 0	Carcinoma in situ, intraepithelial neoplasia Grade III
Stage I	The carcinoma is limited to the vaginal wall
Stage II	The carcinoma has involved the subvaginal tissue but has not extended to the pelvic wall
Stage III	The carcinoma has extended to the pelvic wall
Stage IV	The carcinoma has extended beyond the true pelvis or has involved the mucosa of the bladder or rectum; bullous oedema as such does not permit a case to be allotted to stage IV
IVa	Tumour invades bladder and/or rectal mucosa and/or direct extension beyond the true pelvis
IVb	Spread to distant organs

Table 27.7 FIGO 2009 staging: carcinoma of the vulva

Stage I	Tumour confined to the vulva
Ia	Lesions ≤2 cm in size, confined to the vulva or perineum and with stromal invasion ≤1.0 mm, no nodal metastasis
Ib	Lesions >2 cm in size or with stromal invasion >1.0 mm, confined to the vulva or perineum with negative nodes
Stage II	Tumour of any size with extension to adjacent perineal structures (1/3 lower urethra, 1/3 lower vagina, anus) with negative nodes
Stage III	Tumour of any size with or without extension to adjacent perineal structures (1/3 lower urethra, 1/3 lower vagina, anus) with positive inguino-femoral lymph nodes
IIIa	(i) With 1 lymph node metastasis (≥5 mm) or (ii) 1–2 lymph node metastasis(es) (<5 mm)
IIIb	(i) With 2 or more lymph node metastases (≥5 mm) or (ii) 3 or more lymph node metastases (<5 mm)
IIIc	With positive nodes with extracapsular spread
Stage IV	Tumour invades other regional (2/3 upper urethra, 2/3 upper vagina) or distant structures
IVa	Tumour invades any of the following: (i) Upper urethral and/or vaginal mucosa, bladder mucosa, rectal mucosa or fixed to pelvic bone or (ii) Fixed or ulcerated inguinofemoral lymph nodes
IVb	Any distant metastasis including pelvic lymph nodes

pelvic radiotherapy, the target volume being the whole vagina and the pelvic lymph nodes. If the patient is fit enough, cisplatin should be given along with external beam radiotherapy. This would be followed by an intracavity insertion for tumours in the upper half of the vagina or iridium implantation for tumours in the lower half of this structure. Results of treatment tend to be somewhat worse than in cervical cancer with about a 75% 5-year survival for stage I, 60% for stage II, 30% for stage II and 15% for stage IV.

Vulval cancer tends to be a disease in elderly women with a mean age of diagnosis of approximately 70 years. Seventy-five percent of vulval cancers are squamous carcinoma and they predominantly metastasize via the lymphatic system to the groins. Staging takes into account the tumour size and whether lymph node metastases are present (Table 27.7). The primary treatment of vulval carcinoma is surgery using the triple incision technique, a bilateral groin node dissection and radical vulvectomy. As many of the women with this disease are elderly and have intercurrent disease, some are not suitable for this treatment. However, there is difficulty in administering radiotherapy to this region. The folds of the groin and vulva lead to loss of skin sparing when megavoltage radiotherapy is administered to this region and patients develop a risk of radiation reactions with moist desquamation after relatively modest doses of radiotherapy such as 45 Gy in 25 fractions. This limits the scope of radiotherapy in this disease. Radiotherapy has been shown to reduce pelvic and groin recurrences when given postoperatively in patients with one or more positive lymph nodes. There is also an improvement in 5-year survival.

Chemoradiotherapy is being used increasingly in patients who have initially inoperable disease. Drugs such as cisplatin, 5-fluorouracil and mitomycin have been given along with radiation therapy. A review of published data has shown that the complete response rate is 60% following chemoradiotherapy but the complication rate for this treatment can be high with up to a 10% death rate, particularly secondary to neutropenic sepsis. Chemoradiotherapy can shrink inoperable tumours and make such lesions operable. However, wound healing may be impaired.

The most important factor in vulval cancer is the presence of inguinal nodal metastases. Patients without nodal involvement have a 70–80% 5-year survival. Survival falls to 30–50% for those with involved inguinal lymph nodes (one to more than four positive lymph nodes).

FURTHER READING

[1] Pecorelli S. Revised FIGO staging for carcinoma of the vulva, cervix and endometrium. Int J Gynaecol Obstet 2009;105:103–4.

[2] Landoni F, Maneo A, Columbo A, et al. Randomised study of radical surgery versus radiotherapy for Stage Ib-IIa cervical cancer. Lancet 1997;350:28–33.

[3] Green J, Kirwan J, Tierney J, et al. Survival and recurrence after

concomitant chemotherapy and radiotherapy for cancer of the uterine cervix: a systematic review and meta-analysis. Lancet 2001;358:781–6.

[4] Vale CL, Tierney JF, Davidson SE, Drinkwater KJ, Symonds P. Substantial improvements in UK cervical cancer survival with chemoradiotherapy: results of a Royal College of Radiologists Audit. Clin Oncol 2010;22: 590–601.

[5] Faust G, Davies Q, Symonds P. Changes in the treatment of endometrial cancer. Br J Obstet Gynaecol 2010;117:1043–6.

[6] Creutzberg CL. Surgery and post operative radiotherapy versus surgery alone for patients with stage I endometrial carcinoma: multi-centre randomised trial. PORTEC study group. Post operative radiation therapy in endometrial carcinoma. Lancet 2000;355:1404–11.

[7] International Collaborative Ovarian Neoplasm Trial 1 and Adjuvant Chemotherapy in Ovarian Neoplasm. Two parallel randomised phase III trials of adjuvant chemotherapy in patients with early stage ovarian carcinoma. J Natl Cancer Inst 2003;95:105–12.

[8] International Collaborative Ovarian Neoplasm (ICON) Group. Paclitaxel plus carboplatin versus standard chemotherapy with either single agent carboplatin or cyclophosphamide doxorubicin and cisplatin: in women with ovarian cancer: the ICON 3 randomised trial. Lancet 2002;360:505–12.

[9] McGuire WP, Hoskins WJ, Brady MT, et al. Cyclophosphamide and cisplatin compared with paclitaxel and cisplatin in patients with stage III and stage IV ovarian cancer. N. Engl. J. Med. 1996;334:1–6.

[10] Homesley H, Bundy BN, Sedilis A, Adcock L. Radiation therapy versus pelvic node dissection for carcinoma of the vulva with positive groin nodes. Obstet Gynecol 1986;68:733–40.

EVOLVE CONTENTS (available online at: http://evolve.elsevier.com/Symonds/radiotherapy/)

Chapter | 28 |

Kidney, Bladder, Prostate, Testis, Urethra, Penis

Duncan B. McLaren

KIDNEY

Anatomy

The kidneys lie retroperitoneally on the posterior abdominal wall. They are approximately 11 cm long and 6 cm wide in adults. The left kidney is 1 cm higher than the right. The right kidney is related in front to the liver, the second part of the duodenum and the ascending colon. In front of the left kidney are the stomach, the pancreas, descending colon and the spleen. On the top of each kidney lies an adrenal gland. Behind the kidneys lie the diaphragm and the 12th rib. On the medial side of the kidney there is an opening, the hilum, through which pass the renal artery and vein, and the ureter. The renal vein drains into the inferior vena cava. The lymphatic drainage is to the para-aortic nodes. The anatomical relationships are shown in Figure 28.1.

Pathology

The three principal malignant tumours of the kidney are Wilms' tumour (nephroblastoma) in children (described in Chapter 33), renal cell adenocarcinoma (also called clear cell carcinoma, hypernephroma and Grawitz's tumour) and transitional cell carcinoma of the renal pelvis. Adenocarcinoma arising from the renal tubules accounts for 80% of tumours. Macroscopically, the tumour appears as a yellowish vascular mass. Microscopically, the tumour cells are large with a foamy or clear appearance to the cytoplasm. The nucleus is small, central and densely staining.

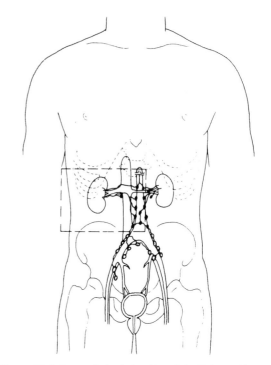

Figure 28.1 Anatomical relationships of the kidney with lymphatic drainage pathways and typical treatment volume when irradiating the renal bed.
(Reproduced with permission from Souhami & Tobias, Cancer and its Management, Blackwells, 1986)

Renal cancer is uncommon, accounting for 3% of all cancers and 1.5% of cancer deaths. Over the last 10 years, the incidence has risen by 23% in men and 29% in women within the UK, a pattern reflected throughout the world. Overall there is a 2:1 male to female ratio in incidence and the disease occurs mainly in the 5th–7th decades of life. The aetiology of renal cell carcinoma is unknown, though smoking and obesity are risk factors. Thirty percent of patients present with metastatic disease.

Spread

There is direct spread through the renal substance and into the perinephric fat of the renal bed. The characteristic mode of spread is permeation along the renal vein and into the inferior vena cava. Tumour may rarely extend up to the right side of the heart, completely blocking the inferior vena cava. Lymphatic spread to local renal hilar and para-aortic lymph nodes and hematogenous metastatic spread to lung, bone and brain are common. The tempo of metastatic disease may be unpredictable; however, <10% remain alive at 5 years from diagnosis. Rarely, spontaneous regression of metastases may occur following nephrectomy.

Clinical features

Presentation is usually with local symptoms. Painless hematuria is the commonest or colicky pain secondary to clots of blood. Other symptoms are aching or a mass in the loin which may be noticed by the patient. A coincidental finding following radiological imaging of the abdomen is an increasingly common presentation. Distant metastasis may be the first presentation, such as pathological bone fracture, haemoptysis from pulmonary metastases or symptoms of raised intracranial pressure from cerebral deposits. Systemic features such as anaemia, loss of weight and unexplained fever may occur. The kidney may be palpably enlarged.

Investigation and staging

The urine may contain frank or microscopic evidence of blood. Urine cytology may show malignant cells. The most important investigation is an intravenous urogram (IVU), which may show distortion of the calyces (the channels that drain urine to the renal pelvis and are outlined by the contrast medium) by the tumour. Calcification within the tumour may be visible on plain radiographs. Ultrasound and computed tomography (CT) scanning (Figure 28.2) are helpful in distinguishing between solid and cystic renal masses. Ultrasound may show extension of tumour into the renal vein or inferior vena cava. CT scanning of the chest, abdomen and pelvis may show direct tumour spread, venous and lymph node involvement and soft tissue metastases in liver and lung. Angiography is an invasive procedure and its use is diminishing. It still has a role in demonstrating the renal artery and new vessel formation when the kidney is to be

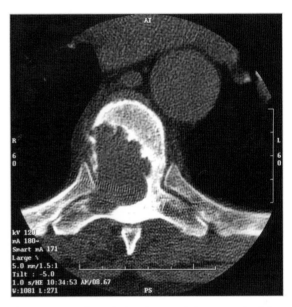

Figure 28.3 Radiograph showing osteolytic metastasis of the vertebral body from renal cell carcinoma.

embolized (i.e. material introduced into the renal arterial to cut off its blood supply and cause death of part or the whole of the kidney). Bone metastases are typically osteolytic (Figure 28.3).

No staging system for renal cell cancer has universal acceptance. The UICC 1997 TNM classification is shown in Table 28.1.

Treatment

Surgery is the main treatment for localized renal cell cancer. Radiotherapy and embolization have more limited roles. Chemotherapy is of unproven value. Immunotherapy has been superseded by oral tyrosine kinase inhibitors (TKIs) as first-line therapy for metastatic disease.

Surgery

Nephrectomy is indicated for tumours confined to the kidney and/or regional nodes. Extension into the inferior vena cava is not necessarily a contraindication to surgery. There is debate as to the role of nephrectomy in the presence of metastatic disease. Bulky, symptomatic tumours with small volume metastases should still be considered for nephrectomy prior to starting TKI's at subsequent radiological progression. In selected patients, aggressive surgical removal of the primary tumour together with solitary metastases, particularly in lung and bone, may be followed by up to 35% 5-year survival. Palliative removal of the kidney may be required to control pain or haemorrhage or if a painful syndrome following embolization occurs.

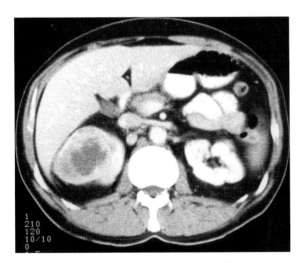

Figure 28.2 CT scan showing a typical renal cell carcinoma in the right kidney.

Table 28.1 TNM staging of primary renal tumours

STAGE	CLINICAL FINDINGS
Tumour	
T0	No tumour
T1	Tumour 7.0 cm or less in greatest dimension, limited to the kidney
T2	Tumour more than 7.0 cm in greatest dimension, limited to the kidney
T3	Tumour extends into major veins or invades adrenal gland or perinephric tissues but not beyond Gerota's fascia
T3a	Tumour invades adrenal gland or perinephric tissues but not beyond Gerota's fascia
T3b	Tumour grossly extends into renal vein(s) or vena cava below diaphragm
T3c	Tumour grossly extends into vena cava above diaphragm
T4	Tumour extends beyond Gerota's fascia
Tx	Primary tumour cannot be assessed
Nodes	
N0	No regional lymph node metastasis
N1	Metastasis in single regional lymph node
N2	Metastasis in more than one regional lymph node
Nx	Regional lymph nodes cannot be assessed
Metastases	
M0	No distant metastases
M1	Distant metastases
Mx	Distant metastases cannot be assessed
Histological grading	
G1	Well differentiated
G2	Moderately differentiated
G3–4	Poorly differentiated/undifferentiated
Gx	Grade of differentiation cannot be assessed

Embolization

Embolization of the kidney via a catheter inserted into the renal artery may be useful in both operable and inoperable cases. In operable cases, embolization is indicated where there is concern about blood loss at nephrectomy, e.g. in patients who refuse blood transfusion on religious grounds. In inoperable cases, it is effective in controlling renal pain and hematuria. A postembolization syndrome with pain, ileus, and infection may complicate embolization.

Radiotherapy

Renal cell carcinoma is relatively resistant to radiation. Pre- or postoperative radiotherapy does not reduce local recurrence where the tumour has spread locally outside the kidney. Its role is palliative to relieve symptoms from the primary tumour or from distant metastases.

Kidney

Target volume

The whole of the kidney and the regional nodes should be included (see Figure 28.1).

Technique

A parallel-opposed anterior and posterior pair of fields is used.

Dose and energy

30 Gy in 10 daily fractions over 2 weeks (6–8 MV photons) or single 8-10 Gy for haematuria

Distant metastases

Brain and bone metastases are treated by palliative radiotherapy, as described on pages 553 and 581, respectively.

Chemotherapy

Chemotherapy has little value in renal cancer. Single agent vinblastine with <10% response rate is most extensively used. Oral progestogens such as Provera have been claimed to benefit 20% of patients, however, in randomized clinical trials, this has fallen below 10%. Their major use is in the palliation of systemic symptoms such as anorexia.

Immunotherapy

The observation that spontaneous regression of metastases may occasionally occur stimulated interest in immunotherapy. Interferon-alpha and interleukin-2 (IL-2) stimulate the body's immunological attack on tumours. Toxicity is marked with a profound flu-like illness with fever, rigors, anorexia, weight loss, myalgia and fatigue. IL-2 may lead to a capillary leak syndrome when administered intravenously, subcutaenous administration, however, is better tolerated. In those patients who respond, a few long-term remissions have been observed. The MRC Trial RE04 compared the relative merits of single agent interferon versus combination interferon, IL-2 and 5-fluorouracil (5FU) for metastatic disease. Survival was equivalent for each regimen at 18 months with similar poor objective response rates of less than 20%.

Tyrosine kinase inhibitors (TKIs)

The most exciting agents in the treatment of renal cancer are the oral tyrosine kinase inhibitors, sunitinib and pazopanib which are now used as first line therapy. TKIs inhibit a number of tumour cell proliferations and angiogenesis pathways, particularly vascular endometrial growth factor receptor (VEGFR), platelet derived growth factor receptor (PDGFR) and the stem cell receptor c-kit. Sunitinib has been shown to give a longer median progression-free survival (11.9 months versus 5 months) than alpha interferon in a large randomized trial of previously untreated patients with metastatic renal cancer plus a higher objective response rate (31% versus 6%). Diarrhea, skin marks (hand–foot syndrome) and hypertension are the most common adverse effects. At progression second line agents both TKI's and mTor inhibitors appear to offer potential further survival benefit.

Results of treatment

The outlook depends on the stage at diagnosis. For tumours confined to the kidney, 5-year survival varies from 50 to 80%. Extrarenal or renal vein invasion, lymph node and blood-borne metastases all confer a poor prognosis. Patients with metastatic disease at presentation have a median survival of only 12 months, with 20% remaining alive 2 years from diagnosis.

BLADDER

Anatomy

The bladder is related anteriorly to the pubic symphysis, superiorly to the small intestine and sigmoid colon, laterally to the levator ani muscle, inferiorly to the prostate gland and posteriorly to the rectum, vas deferens and seminal vesicles (see Figure 28.7) in the male and to the vagina and cervix in the female. At cystoscopy, the bladder mucosa and ureteric orifices can be inspected. Lymphatic drainage is to the iliac and para-aortic nodes.

Pathology

The bladder, ureters and renal pelvis are lined by transitional cell epithelium (urothelium). The same type of tumours may arise anywhere along the urinary tract but cancers in the renal pelvis and ureter are rare compared with those in the bladder. Prostatic adenocarcinoma and other pelvic tumours also sometimes secondarily involve the bladder.

Aetiology

In the majority of cases of bladder cancer, the aetiology is unknown. However, as discussed in Chapter 14, occupational exposure to certain carcinogens has accounted for some cases. The production of aniline dyes and processing of rubber are associated with 2-naphthylamine, now recognized as a procarcinogen. Workers in these industries are now offered regular cytological examination of urine to detect abnormalities or tumours at an early stage.

Smoking is perhaps the commonest factor that predisposes to bladder cancer. Bladder cancer is up to six times commoner in smokers than non-smokers and increases in frequency with the number of cigarettes smoked. Phenacetin, formerly used as an analgesic drug, and the cytotoxic alkylating agent cyclophosphamide may give rise to urothelial tumours. Squamous carcinoma tends to complicate chronic irritation of the bladder including a parasitic disease, schistosomiasis (formerly known as bilharziasis), which is common in Egypt and Central Africa. Adenocarcinoma occurs on the dome of the bladder in relation to embryological remnants of the urachus, and also from the trigone at the bladder base.

Genetic alterations in bladder cancer are common. Deletion of markers on chromosome 9 is an early event. Subsequent mutation in *p53* allows cells with DNA damage to proceed through the cell cycle, replicating genetic errors. Loss of the pRb (retinoblastoma) gene product disrupts cell cycling and increases the mitotic index. Patients with both mutations have higher-grade more advanced disease and a poor response to treatment.

Epidemiology

Bladder cancer is common and accounts for 4.4% of all cancers and 3.4% of cancer deaths. The male to female ratio is 3.8:1 and it has a peak incidence at the age of 65. The impact of smoking in women has seen a greater rise in incidence in this group over the last 10 years compared to men. It is twice as common in Caucasians as in Blacks. Over 90% are transitional cell carcinomas.

Macroscopic appearance

The chief types on inspection of the bladder are (1) papillary and (2) solid. Multiple growths are common.

Papillary carcinoma has a base with surface fronds. The tumours tend to be multiple and to appear in crops. Confined at first to the mucosa and submucosa, they eventually invade the submucosa, muscle coat and then outside the bladder.

Solid carcinoma is nodular, often ulcerated, grows more rapidly and infiltrates early.

From the point of prognosis, a division can be made between superficial (papillary) and invasive (solid) bladder cancer. Superficial bladder tumours are the commonest (80%) and become invasive in 10–20% of cases. By contrast, invasive cancer, untreated, carries a very poor prognosis. The degree of invasion correlates with the risk of metastatic disease. Invasion of the lamina propria (the layer of tissue between the epithelium and the muscle layer of the bladder), superficial and deep muscle is associated with 20%, 30% and 60% incidence of lymphatic invasion.

Microscopic appearance

Benign tumours of the bladder are very uncommon. However, low-grade transitional cell malignant tumours are often erroneously referred to as papillomas.

Malignant tumours of the bladder include:

- transitional cell carcinoma; papillary and solid variants
- adenocarcinoma (uncommon)
- squamous carcinoma (rare in the UK)
- sarcomas (all very rare).

Transitional carcinoma accounts for 90% of bladder cancer and is classified histologically into grades 1–3 corresponding to well-, moderately- and poorly-differentiated tumours. The degree of differentiation is important. High-grade tumours grow faster and infiltrate sooner.

After muscle has been invaded, lymphatic spread is to the pelvic and then para-aortic nodes. Blood-borne metastases are common to lung, liver and bone.

Clinical features

The presenting symptom is usually painless frank hematuria. Occasionally, clots of blood are passed and are even more suggestive of the diagnosis. Papillomatous types grow slowly and may cause no other symptoms for a long time. When aggressive carcinomas invade muscle, there may be urinary frequency, dysuria and pain, especially when there is extravesical (i.e. outside the bladder) spread into the pelvic soft tissues. Bacterial cystitis may be associated with the tumour and may aggravate symptoms.

Obstruction of one or both ureters can occur at any time, with no symptoms at first. Later, there may be upper urinary tract infection, pain in the flank(s) and eventual renal failure from backpressure. In localized bladder disease, clinical examination is usually unremarkable.

Investigation and staging

Urine

The urine should be examined for red cells, pus cells and bacteria as well as undergoing cytology for malignant cells. Urine cytology is a valuable screening method for industrial workers at risk. Malignant cells are present in the urine of 60% of cases of bladder cancer, particularly the higher-grade tumours. However, negative cytology does not exclude malignancy.

Biochemistry

Serum urea, creatinine and electrolytes are measured for evidence of renal impairment.

Radiology

Radiology is important in the diagnosis and staging of bladder cancer. An intravenous urogram will determine the site of the tumour in the bladder and exclude a lesion higher up in the renal tract. Obstruction at the lower end of the ureter(s) will be shown by dilatation of the ureter and renal pelvis (hydroureter and hydronephrosis). Filling defects in the bladder can also be shown. A CT scan of the abdomen and pelvis may demonstrate extravesical spread or lymphadenopathy. Magnetic resonance imaging (MRI) scanning is the more effective modality to demonstrate deep muscle invasion and spread to pelvis lymph nodes.

Cystourethroscopy

This is the most important investigation of all. Under general anesthesia, the urethra and the whole of the bladder are inspected. The number, site, size and character of the tumours are noted and a biopsy taken. While the patient is relaxed under the anesthetic, a bimanual examination of the pelvis is made, with a finger in the rectum and the other hand on the lower abdomen. In this way, the tumour may be palpated and any extravesical spread assessed.

Clinical staging of bladder cancer is according to the TNM classification (Figure 28.4 and Table 28.2).

Treatment

Treatment will depend on the stage, histology, size and multiplicity of tumours and the age and general medical condition of the patient.

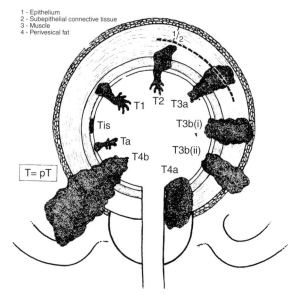

Figure 28.4 T staging of bladder cancer – UICC classification. *(Reproduced with permission from Hermanek P, Hutter R V P and Sobin L H (eds) 1997 International Union Against Cancer TNM Atlas. Illustrated guide to the TNM classification of malignant tumours, 4th edn, Springer-Verlag)*

Table 28.2 TNM staging of bladder cancer

STAGE	CLINICAL FINDINGS
Tumour	
Tis	Carcinoma in situ
Ta	Papillary non-invasive carcinoma
T1	Invasion into submucosa but not beyond the lamina propria
T2a	Invasion into superficial detrusor muscle
T2b	Invasion into deep detrusor muscle
T3a	Invasion into perivesicular tissues microscopically
T3b	Invasion into perivesicular tissues macroscopically
T4a	Invasion of prostate or vagina
T4b	Invasion of pelvic side-wall or abdominal wall
Nodes	
N0	No evidence of nodal involvement
N1	Single node <2 cm diameter
N2	Single nodal metastasis 2–5 cm diameter or multiple nodes none exceeding 5 cm
N3	Node >5 cm
Metastases	
M0	No metastases
M1	Distant metastases

Superficial Ta and T1 tumours

Superficial tumours are biopsied and removed by transurethral resection (TUR) or diathermy at the time of cytoscopy. Random biopsies of the bladder are carried out to exclude carcinoma in situ. In the majority of patients, these tumours tend to recur rather than invade (up to 60% recurrence rate). For this reason, cystoscopic follow up needs to be life long.

If recurrences are multiple or high grade, intravesical chemotherapy or BCG should be used to reduce the recurrence rate to 40%. Intravesical BCG may reduce the recurrence rates for carcinoma in situ from 80% to 40% and may also delay the rates of progression. Cystectomy is indicated if these measures fail.

Superficial tumours do respond completely to radical radiotherapy in over 75% of cases, but there is recurrence in more than 50%. For this reason, radical radiotherapy is rarely used in T1 lesions.

Invasive bladder cancer (T2 and T3)

Surgery and radiotherapy are the standard treatments for invasive bladder cancer.

T2 tumours

Endoscopic resection (TURBT) alone is inadequate to control these tumours. Additional radical treatment with either cystoprostourethrectomy (removal of the bladder and prostate with diversion of the ureters onto the abdominal wall) or radical radiotherapy is required. Local practice will determine treatment. Europe and America have favored cystoprostourethrectomy as the treatment of choice. In the UK, radical radiotherapy with salvage cystectomy for those patients with persistent or recurrent tumour remains a valid option. This policy has the advantage that the patient has a better chance of tumour control with the bladder intact. If radiotherapy fails, there is a 30% chance of successful salvage by cystectomy. By contrast, if primary cystectomy fails, radical radiotherapy is rarely successful for recurrent disease. Each policy carries a similar 5-year survival of about 50–60%.

T3 tumours

If bimanual palpation and/or radiological imaging have demonstrated macroscopic extension of disease outside the bladder, cure rates fall to around 40% at 5 years. Such patients are more commonly treated with radical radiotherapy than with surgery. Combined modality treatment with concurrent chemotherapy (5FU and mitomycin C or nicotinamide and carbogen) and radiotherapy appears to improve local control at 2 years in comparison to standard conformal radiotherapy alone in patients with T2-T3 disease.

T4 tumours

A distinction must be made between T4a and T4b tumours. T4a means tumour penetration into the prostate or vagina. T4a includes both aggressive deeply invasive tumours infiltrating the prostate and less aggressive superficial tumours extending into the prostatic urethra and/or ducts. The latter has a much better prognosis than the former. T4a tumours should be treated radically. T4b tumours are fixed to neighboring structures, are inoperable and should be treated with palliative radiotherapy.

Adenocarcinoma and squamous carcinoma of the bladder

Neither of these is very radiosensitive and they are better treated by cystectomy.

Neoadjuvant chemotherapy

Combination cisplatin-based chemotherapy for two to four cycles prior to radical therapy improves survival for muscle invasive transitional cell carcinoma (TCC) by 5%.

A complete response at cystoscopic re-evaluation predicts for better survival and organ preservation should be considered. Cystectomy and pelvic nodal clearance is indicated for a poor response. To date, adjuvant chemotherapy following cystectomy has only improved time to treatment failure rather than survival, although studies are ongoing. Concerns over delaying definitive treatment and chemotherapy-related toxicity exist. Appropriate patient selection for neoadjuvant chemotherapy is important.

Radical radiotherapy

The following are criteria for accepting patients for radical radiotherapy:

- age <80 years (unless particularly fit)
- adequate general medical condition
- no inflammatory bowel disease or symptomatic adhesions
- good bladder function
- minimal or no CIS
- transitional cell carcinoma
- single tumour <7 cm maximum diameter
- recurrent T1G3, T2–T4a
- no metastases.

Target volume

The treatment volume is 1–2 cm around the tumour, judged by bimanual examination and CT scanning. The bladder is emptied before CT planning and before each treatment.

Radiation planning technique

The tumour is localized by a CT planning scan and has replaced using a cystogram (Figure 28.5).

CT planning allows greater definition of the planning target volume (PTV). The patient is planned in the same position on the CT scanner as on the simulator and treatment couches (supine with feet in foot stocks and hands by the side). On the planning computer, the width of the target volume to encompass the tumour with a 1–2 cm margin is chosen. The superior and inferior target volume being 1 cm above and below the upper and lower limits of the bladder. It is common practice to cover the prostatic urethra in the PTV in view of the risk of local recurrence. The position of the rectum and femoral heads are marked on the computer and translated to the treatment plan. An open anterior and two lateral wedged or posterior oblique wedged fields are used, treating isocentrically (Figure 28.6). A direct lateral field is preferred at our institution to reduce rectal doses in view of the sharp fall-off of the field. With high-energy photon beams such as 15 MV, femoral-head doses are kept below 50% of the tumour dose. The use of conformal therapy techniques is routine and improves treatment-related morbidity in addition to possible dose escalation in the future. IMRT is increasingly being used

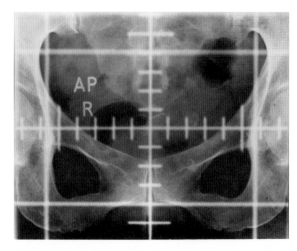

Figure 28.5 Simulator radiograph showing anterior treatment volume for radical radiotherapy of a transitional cell carcinoma of the bladder.

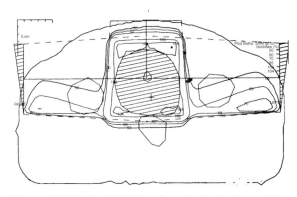

Figure 28.6 Isodose distribution for radical radiotherapy of the bladder using anterior and two lateral fields.

to treat patients at risk of pelvic lymph-node involvement in addition; whether this improves survival however is unproven.

Dose and energy

55 Gy in 20 daily fractions over 4 weeks (9–16 MV photons) or

64 Gy in 32 daily fractions over 6.5 weeks (9–16 MV photons).

Concurrent chemotherapy and radiotherapy (chemo-rt) should be considered for all patients fit enough to receive it and can be given safely after neoadjuvant chemotherapy or on its own... BC2001 reported improved local control at 2 years to 71% after concurrent chemo-rt with 5FU and mitomycin C over RT alone. Similarly, in an attempt to overcome tumour hypoxia in the bladder, nicotinamide and carbogen in combination with radiotherapy within the BCON study has improved local control and survival in comparison to RT alone.

Radiation reaction

Before radiation begins, attention is paid to the patient's general condition and nutrition. The patient's hemoglobin level should be maintained over 12 g/dL, by blood transfusion if necessary, since anaemia will reduce the amount of oxygen available to the tumour. It is known that reduced oxygenation in parts of the tumour contributes to resistance to radiation. Urinary infection should be treated with antibiotics. The urine should be made sterile if possible before radiation begins, since inflammation has adverse effects on radiation response. However, with an ulcerated mass this may not be possible until the tumour has shrunk in response to radiation.

Acute reactions

1. Frequency and urgency, from radiation cystitis during and after the course, are common but not usually serious unless bacterial infection is gross. Painful spasm may require an antispasmodic drug. Fluid intake must be strongly encouraged. The patient should be warned that he or she might pass fragments in the urine (blood clot and tumour) and a little fresh blood.
2. Bowel reactions are also to be expected in almost every case – usually mild diarrhea and tenesmus. If they are severe, treatment may have to be suspended or dosage reduced.

Late reactions

1. Fibrosis of the bladder. The bladder wall may be so contracted by fibrosis and the bladder volume so reduced that uncontrollable frequency may make life intolerable. Ureteric diversion may be required.
2. Telangiectasia on the bladder lining may develop, with repeated bleeding. It may be possible to seal them off with the diathermy point at cystoscopy. If they are uncontrolled by this means, cystectomy may be required.
3. Late bowel reactions are similar to those after the irradiation of cancer of the cervix (p. 470), though less common (<5%). Loops of bowel trapped in the pelvis by adhesions after previous surgery or inflammatory disease are especially at risk. There may be bleeding from telangiectasia on the bowel mucosa, ulceration, even necrosis and perforation. If conservative measures, e.g. steroid enemas, fail, a defunctioning colostomy may be required.

Palliative radiotherapy

Palliative radiotherapy should be considered in the following circumstances: age (>80 years) or poor general condition with either significant local symptoms (e.g. hematuria) or symptomatic metastases, e.g. bone and skin.

Technique

A parallel-opposed anterior and posterior pair of fields are used. A cystogram is recommended for bladder localization preferably or virtual simulation if available. The treatment volume includes the bladder with a 2 cm margin or bladder and pelvic nodes if involved.

Dose and energy

30 Gy in 10 daily fractions over 2 weeks (9–16 MV) or 21 Gy in 3 fractions over 1 week (9–16 MV).

Chemotherapy

Response rates of greater than 50% have been reported using cisplatin-based regimens, such as cisplatin, methotrexate and vinblastine (CMV), methotrexate, vinblastine, doxorubicin and cisplatin (MVAC) or gemcitabine and cisplatin (GC) for metastatic disease. Median survival following chemotherapy depends on sites of disease. Nodal disease carries a relatively good prognosis with a median survival of 24 months, in comparison, median survival for disease in organs such as the liver, remains disappointing at <12 months.

Results of treatment

The 5-year survival for radical radiotherapy is 80% for T1, 55–60% for T2, 40–45% for T3 and 25–30% T4 tumours.

PROSTATE

Anatomy

The prostate gland lies just below the base of the bladder and in front of the rectum (Figure 28.7). It resembles a chestnut in size and shape. Through it passes the prostatic urethra. Into the urethra empty the ejaculatory ducts, which carry sperm from the seminal vesicles, which lie behind and to each side of the prostate gland. The prostate is divided into two lobes by a median groove. From a functional point of view, it is divided into a peripheral zone, central zone and transitional zone. It is surrounded by a thin layer of fibrous tissue (true capsule) and a layer of fascia continuous with that surrounding the bladder (false capsule). Between these two layers lies the prostatic venous plexus. Part of the venous drainage is to a plexus of veins lying in front of the vertebral bodies. This may account for the tendency of prostate cancer to spread to the vertebrae.

Pathology

Cancer of the prostate gland is the second commonest malignancy in men in the UK. In total, 37051 new cases and 10168 deaths were recorded in 2008. There has been

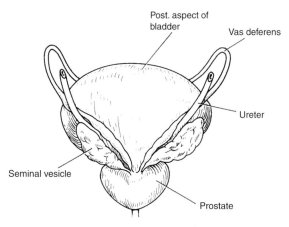

Figure 28.7 Prostate, seminal vesicles and vas deferens in a posterior view of the bladder.
(Redrawn from Ellis, Clinical Anatomy, 5th edn, Blackwells, 1975)

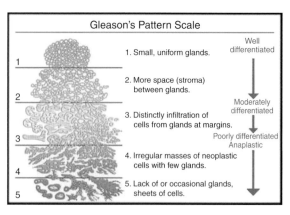

Figure 28.8 Gleason grading system for carcinoma of the prostate.
(Reproduced with permission from Kirby R S, Brawer M K and Denis L J (eds) 2001 Prostate Cancer Fast Facts, 3rd edn, Health Press)

a significant rise in the incidence of prostate cancer in the last twenty years due to a combination of increased awareness, PSA testing and an ageing population with the opportunity to develop the disease.

The exact aetiology of prostatic cancer is unknown. It is commonest in the seventh and eighth decades and rare under the age of 40. Marked worldwide variations in incidence exist. In particular, Japan has rates considerably lower than in the USA. A correlation with diet and, in particular, high fat consumption is directly implicated. Genetic factors have a role; siblings are at increased risk with a positive family history and USA Blacks have higher levels of disease noted compared to USA Whites. Environmental factors include exposure to radiation, heavy metals and chemical fertilizers, although no definitive link has been determined.

Over 95% are adenocarcinomas, 70% arising from the peripheral part of the gland. The differentiation of prostate cancer is graded according to the Gleason grading system. It is based on the extent to which the tumour cells are arranged into recognizable glandular structures, grade 1 tumours forming almost normal glands while grade 5 tumours consist of sheets of cells (Figure 28.8). Because of the heterogeneity in prostate cancer, the two most common grades seen are added together to give a Gleason score.

Before the advent of PSA testing and greater patient awareness, in 75% of cases the tumour had spread beyond the gland at the time of presentation, and 50% had distant metastases. The introduction of PSA screening in countries such as the USA, however, has dramatically reduced the numbers of patients presenting with advanced disease.

Prostate cancer may spread directly to the bladder, seminal vesicles and rectum. Lymphatic spread is to the obturator, presacral, internal and external iliac nodes. Further spread is to the common iliac and para-aortic nodes. It readily invades the pelvic veins and thence the pelvic bones and vertebrae. Bone secondaries are typically of sclerotic type, showing as an increased density on the radiograph because they induce new bone formation.

The natural history of the disease is very variable. It may be indolent in the elderly patient with a well-differentiated tumour and an incidental finding at post-mortem. The disease tends to run a more aggressive course in younger men, particularly with poorly-differentiated tumours.

Hormonal sensitivity

The prostate has analogies with the breast and is under hormonal control. Removal of male hormones by orchidectomy, or administration of female hormones (oestrogens), causes shrinkage of the normal gland, and of 80% of tumours.

PSA and screening

Prostate-specific antigen is a glycoprotein that liquefies semen. Approximately 20% of men with PSA levels above the normal range of 4 ng/mL have prostate cancer, and this risk increases to more than 60% in men with a PSA level above 10 ng/mL. PSA levels increase in proportion to the volume of disease and can be used to monitor the response to treatment and development of metastatic disease. PSA has largely superseded the use of an enzyme, acid phosphatase, secreted by normal and malignant prostate tissue, in the diagnosis and assessment of response to treatment.

The benefits of screening for prostate cancer are as yet unproven. The results of two large screening randomized controlled trials (RCTs) were conflicting. The European study improved prostate cancer survival by 20% but at the expense of significant over treatment. Forty nine men required a prostatectomy to save the life of one additional man. The American PLCO study did not show a survival advantage, however many men in the control arm had PSA screening performed outside of the study and so reduced any potential benefit to the screening arm. At present there are no plans to introduce a UK mass prostate screening program however, increased case detection through PSA testing will continue.

Clinical features

The prostate often undergoes benign enlargement, and the early symptoms of cancer may be similar, i.e. increased frequency and difficulty of micturition. Hematuria and urinary obstruction can occur. Bone pain or pathological fracture may be the first presenting symptom. Back pressure on the kidneys may cause renal impairment. Sacral, sciatic or perineal pain may occur from infiltration of nerves in the pelvis. Clinical evidence of disease is rare under the age of 45.

Diagnosis and staging

The presence of a hard irregular gland on rectal examination suggests the diagnosis. This should be confirmed by a biopsy of the prostate. Usually, 10 to 12 biopsies of the prostate (five or six from each lobe) are conducted under transrectal ultrasound guidance. Prostatic carcinoma is staged using the TNM classification (Table 28.3) the local stage of the disease is mainly based on rectal examination. This may be supplemented by ultrasound, CT or MRI scanning. MRI scanning in particular is helpful in showing extracapsular spread, enlarged pelvic nodes and local invasion of the bladder, seminal vesicles and rectal wall. Surgical dissection of the pelvic nodes to assess pelvic node involvement has not gained wide acceptance in the UK since it does not improve survival. A bone scan is recommended in view of the high incidence of bone metastases if the PSA is greater than 10 or the Gleason score is 7 or above.

Treatment

Clinically localized disease T1–2N0M0

There are no randomized controlled trials to determine the optimum treatment for early prostate cancer. The PROTECT study randomized patients to either active monitoring, radical prostatectomy or radical radiotherapy and may help address the relative roles of these treatments for localized early prostate cancer in due course.

The clinical behavior of the disease is unpredictable, a situation made worse by the lack of accurate prognostic indicators of disease behavior. Aggressive treatment of indolent disease exposes patients to the toxicity of treatment, whereas undertreatment may lead to potentially curable disease causing significant morbidity or cancer-related death. Balancing these issues requires time and experience.

Treatment options include:

- active surveillance (radical treatment still offered at progression)
- watchful waiting (non curative hormonal therapy offered at progression)
- radical radiotherapy
- prostate brachytherapy
- radical prostatectomy.

Table 28.3 TNM staging of prostate cancer

STAGE	CLINICAL FINDINGS
Tumour	
T1	Clinically inapparent tumour not palpable or visible by imaging
T1a	Tumour incidental finding in 5% or less of tissue resected
T1b	Tumour incidental finding in more than 5% of tissue resected
T1c	Tumour identified by needle biopsy (e.g. due to elevated PSA)
T2	Palpable tumour confined to the gland
T2a	Tumour involves half a lobe or less
T2b	Tumour involves more than half a lobe
T2c	Tumour involves both lobes
T3	Tumour extending beyond the capsule
T3a	Extracapsular extension (unilateral or bilateral)
T3b	Tumour invades seminal vesicle(s)
T4	Tumour fixed or invading adjacent structures
Nodes	
N0	No nodes involved
N1	Regional lymph nodes involved
Metastases	
M0	No distant metastases
M1a	Non regional lymph node(s)
M1b	Bone(s)
M1c	Other sites

Factors that should influence the choice are the age and general condition of the patient, the likelihood of progression to symptomatic disease and the morbidity of treatment, particularly on sexual function. In general, patients should have a life expectancy of greater than 10 years before being treated radically. This is because untreated, it may take several years for there to be any symptoms from their disease, and several years beyond that before death ensues. Generally, the higher the PSA, Gleason score and T stage, the higher the chance of tumour progression and the need for radical treatment. Elderly, medically unfit men with less-aggressive histological features may be managed by watchful waiting (with deferred hormonal therapy and/or palliative radiotherapy for symptomatic progression). Younger fitter men with low risk prostate cancer may be treated with active monitoring initially with radical treatment offered on progression of disease based on an increase in gleason grade on repeat biopsy or significant rise in PSA. The philosophy behind this approach is to spare treatment related toxicity in men who may have indolent disease.

There is evidence that radical therapy can cure localized prostate cancer, with survival curves flattening off between 10 and 15 years from treatment. The chance of local control with radiotherapy decreases with increasing PSA, grade and stage of disease. Neoadjuvant hormonal therapy for 3 months before radiotherapy has demonstrated improved local control and survival for Gleason 3+3 tumours over radiotherapy alone. The hormonal treatment reduces the size of the prostate by 30% and hence the treatment volume. It also reduces the number of tumour cells to irradiate, possibly through synergistic apoptotic mechanisms.

Dose escalation

Single institution data suggest that dose escalated radiotherapy improves local control and PSA relapse-free survival (a surrogate for actual survival). The RTO1 trial has recently provided randomized phase III evidence of the safety and efficacy of increasing dose from 64 Gy to 74 Gy in UK institutions. At 5 years, biochemical progression-free survival was significantly improved to 71% versus 60% in favor of 74 Gy. This improved local control, however, came at a cost with 33% patients in the dose escalated arm versus 24% patients in the standard arm reporting late bowel toxicity at 5 years. A Dutch study comparing 68 Gy versus 78 Gy has also shown better progression-free survival at 5 years (64% versus 54%) but no difference in overall survival. The low alpha/beta ratio of prostate cancer suggests that prolonged fractionated schedules may not be radiobiologically as efficient as hypofractionation. The CHHiP study is addressing the merits of doses such as 60 Gy in 20 fractions versus 57 Gy in 19 fractions versus 74 Gy in 37 fractions. It is also unclear whether there is any extra benefit to dose escalation in combination with neoadjuvant hormonal therapy versus dose escalation alone.

Intensity modulated radiotherapy (IMRT) may offer even greater gains. The ability of intensity modulated radiotherapy tightly to sculpt dose to the prostate, particularly at the prostate–rectal interface is of particular value. Doses in excess of 80 Gy have already safely been administered with excellent PSA relapse-free survival without additional neoadjuvant hormonal therapy.

In order for these radiation doses to be delivered, tight treatment margins are required which in turn requires accurate tumour localization. Using online portal imaging to localize bony anatomy ensures accurate field set-up only. The prostate is a mobile organ, the position of which is influenced by changes in rectal and bladder filling. The two most popular methods of image guided radiotherapy to ensure accurate treatment delivery are daily mv or kv imaging of fiducial markers placed within the prostate via transrectal ultrasound or the use of weekly cone beam CT.

Radical radiotherapy

Target volume

If the tumour staging demonstrates that the tumour is confined to the prostate and there is no obvious involvement of the pelvic nodes, the target volume is confined to the tumour and any local extension (e.g. seminal vesicles), with a 1 cm margin of normal tissue around it. At the rectal–prostate interface a margin of 0.6 cm is satisfactory. The role of additional pelvic radiotherapy is unclear, however, an increasing number of protocols treat the pelvis if there is a risk of nodal involvement of at least 15%.

Technique

A three-field technique is used, either with one anterior and two posterior oblique fields at 120 degrees to each other or one anterior and two wedged lateral fields. We tend to favor the latter in view of the sharp rectal cut-off in dose. The patient lies supine, feet in foot stocks. Localization is done with a CT planning scan. The bladder should be full to displace the dome of the bladder and small bowel out of the field. CT cuts of 3–5 mm are taken through the pelvis. The CTV (clinical target volume) of prostate ± seminal vesicles is outlined. Difficulty in localization of the prostatic apex and extension into the bladder are common areas of fault. The decision to include the seminal vesicles in the CTV is based on imaging and the following equation:

Low risk of SV involvement

T1/T2a with $(PSA + [Gleason\ score - 6] \times 10] < 15$

Moderate risk SV involvement

T2b or T1/T2a with $(PSA + [Gleason\ score - 6] \times 10] \geq 15$

A planning target volume with 1 cm margin around the prostate (0.6 cm at the rectum) is created. The rectal outline from anus to rectosigmoid junction, bladder and femoral heads are marked and a plan produced. With conformal treatment, the volume is shaped to follow the prostate and, in so doing, shield as much of the normal tissues such as the rectum as possible (Figure 28.9). A typical isodose distribution is shown in Figure 28.10. Dose escalation requires a two- phase technique. The PTV is shrunk to treat the prostate and base of seminal vesicles with a 5 mm margin after 56 Gy in 28 fractions if treating to 74 Gy. Dose volume histograms are used to limit the dose to critical structures such as rectum and bladder.

Typical dose volume constrainsts are outlined below.

For rectum:

- Up to 3% to receive ≥74 Gy i.e 100%
- <25% to receive ≥70 Gy i.e 95%

- <30% to receive ≥67 Gy i.e 90%
- <50% to receive ≥55.5 Gy i.e 75%
- remainder to receive up to 44 Gy, i.e 60%

It is recommended that the 60% isodose should not cross the posterior rectal wall.

For bladder:

- <25% to receive ≥74 Gy, i.e 100%
- <50% to receive ≥67 Gy, i.e 90%

Dose and energy

Hypofractionation 55 Gy in 20 daily fractions over 4 weeks (9–16 MV photons)

or

57 Gy-60 Gy in 19 to 20 daily fractions within the CHHiP trial

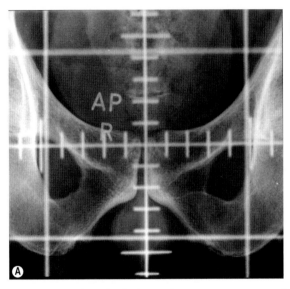
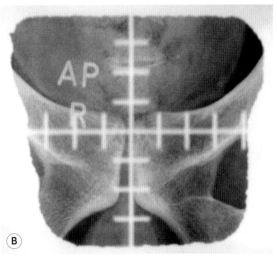

Figure 28.9 Conformal radiotherapy for prostate cancer, anterior field without blocks (A) and with blocks (B).

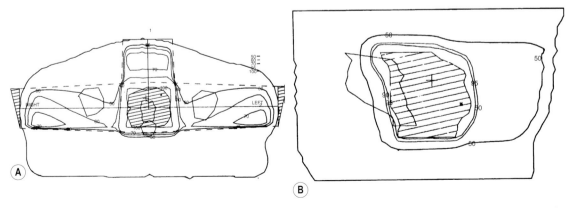

Figure 28.10 Isodose distribution for radical radiotherapy of the prostate using anterior and two lateral fields. (A) Transverse section; (B) sagittal section.

Dose escalation: 74 Gy in 37 daily fractions over 7.5 weeks (9–16 MV photons).

Acute reactions

About half way through a radical 4-week course, urinary frequency and, occasionally, dysuria occur. These can often be relieved an anti-inflammatory agent, such as Froben 50 mg t.d.s. and normally settle within 4 weeks of the end of treatment. Diarrhea and tenesmus from acute proctitis have a similar time course and are treated with a low-residue diet, Fybogel and, on occasion, steroid suppositories.

Late reactions

Significant late reactions may occur in 3–5% patients. The main late urinary effects are chronic cystitis, urethral stricture or incontinence. Loss of sexual potency also occurs. At 2 years from completion of combined neoadjuvant hormonal therapy and radical radiotherapy, 50% of previously potent men will be impotent. Bowel morbidity includes rectal ulceration or stricture and small bowel obstruction. Symptoms are tenesmus, rectal bleeding or incontinence. Proctitis may respond to steroid (Predsol) enemas but, ultimately, a defunctioning colostomy is required in exceptional circumstances.

Results of radical radiotherapy

The 5-year survival for T1 is 90%, T2 is 78% and, for T3, 59%.

Pelvic lymph node irradiation

The treatment of pelvic lymph nodes remains controversial but is increasingly being adopted for high risk patients within the UK. A Radiation Therapy Oncology Group (RTOG) trial has shown better progression-free survival when pelvic irradiation (45 Gy in 25 fractions) is combined with definitive irradiation to the prostate (72.2 Gy). Many centres offer whole pelvic radiotherapy if the risk of nodal metastases exceeds 15%. The risk of pelvic lymph node involvement is calculated by the following formula:

$$2/3 \text{ PSA} + (\text{Gleason score} - 6 \times 10)$$
$$= \text{percentage risk of nodal spread.}$$

Ideally, the pelvic nodes and the prostate should be treated using an IMRT technique.

Prostate brachytherapy–Low Dose rate Seeds

Prostate brachytherapy is now an accepted treatment modality for early prostate cancer. In the traditional preplan technique, the treatment is delivered in two phases. In the first phase, a volume study is performed with the patient in an extended dorsal lithotomy position, usually under a general anesthetic. A transrectal ultrasound probe mounted on a stepping unit scans the prostate from base to apex in 5 mm slices. On each slice, the prostate is outlined and the volume calculated. Prostate volumes above 50 ml

may lead to pubic arch interference at the time of implantation. In these cases, a volume of up to 70 ml may be reduced by 30% and so be suitable for subsequent implantation after 3 months of androgen deprivation therapy.

Once the volume study has been performed, the images are transferred to the planning computer. The exact seed location and number of needles required to deliver the implant is then determined using 3–D planning. The x and y coordinates are provided by the template grid against the perineum and the z coordinate set by the transrectal probe position in relation to the base of the prostate. Dose constraints to the rectum and urethra are built into the plan.

The second phase of the procedure is the implant itself. The patient is repositioned as for the volume study and the prostate position is checked. The brachytherapist guides the implant needles directly into the prostate through a closed transperineal approach (Figure 28.11). Each needle is loaded with either iodine-125 or palladium-103 seeds. It has been suggested that palladium should be used for higher grade tumours owing to its greater dose rate. In practice, however, there are no data to demonstrate any difference in PSA relapse-free survival using either isotope. In the UK, the majority of centres use iodine-125. A dose of 145 Gy to a PTV of the prostate capsule plus 3 mm is delivered. The inverse square law determines that the dose to the rectum, bladder and neurovascular bundles is very low, with resultant decreased toxicity in comparison to external beam and surgery. The procedure takes approximately one hour and the patient is discharged the next day with rapid resumption of normal activity.

An alternative and increasingly popular approach to the two-phase technique is intraoperative planning. With this technique, the whole treatment is delivered in a single visit. The patient is positioned in theater as before. The brachytherapist places the needles under transrectal ultrasound control into the prostate, usually adopting a modified

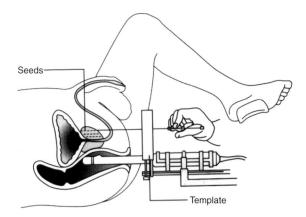

Figure 28.11 Brachytherapy for early prostate cancer.
(Reproduced with permission from Kirby R S, Brawer M K and Denis L J (eds) 2001 Prostate Cancer Fast Facts, 3rd edn, Health Press)

peripheral loading pattern. A plan is produced based around the needle position. Optimization of the plan via adjustment of the needle position is performed prior to loading as an afterloading technique. Whichever technique is adopted, the aim is to deliver a dose of 145 Gy to at least 90% of the prostate (D90) on post-treatment dosimetry.

Appropriate selection criteria are listed below:

- life expectancy of 10 years
- organ confined disease T1–T2b on MRI
- PSA less than 20
- Gleason score ≤7
- international prostate symptom score (IPSS) <20 (a high score indicates marked irritative or obstructive symptoms and predicts for post-treatment urinary retention and significant urinary toxicity)
- Q Max >10 cc/s (if below 10 cc/s then greater risk of post-treatment urinary retention)
- no previous TURP, (seeds fall into cavity and affect doseimetry)
- prostate volume ≤50cc (above this the risk of pubic arch interference increases).

The major toxicity is radiation-induced urethritis that may last some months. Frequency, dysuria and mild obstructive symptoms are common. Urinary retention and proctitis may be seen in 5% of patients. Patients are routinely placed on an alpha blocker for 3–6 months and encouraged to have a high fluid intake. Proctitis is treated as for external beam radiotherapy. In carefully selected patients, outcomes appear very good with PSA relapse-free survival of greater than 90% at 10 years of follow up in good prognosis patients. Clinical trials comparing radical prostatectomy to prostate brachytherapy have so far not been undertaken.

Prostate Brachytherapy–High Dose Rate HDR

High dose rate brachytherapy is increasingly being adopted as a treatment for men with high risk prostate cancer in combination with external beam radiotherapy. A single high dose 15 Gy HDR boost dose followed by 35.75 Gy in13 fractions of external beam to the prostate and seminal vesicles two weeks later has been commonly used. For those Centre's wishing to treat pelvic nodes in addition then 46 Gy in 23 fractions following the implant are required. HDR can deliver very high biologically effective radiation doses in a shortened overall treatment time to the tumour while the rapid fall off in dose limits surrounding normal tissue toxicity.

Radical prostatectomy

Patients who are medically fit with organ-confined disease are suitable for surgery. A nerve-sparing radical prostatectomy has improved potency rates post-procedure. Severe incontinence is noted in <5%, but a higher proportion may have mild stress incontinence. Positive surgical margins in at least 30% of carefully staged patients are common. Laproscopic prostatectomy is gaining popularity due to improved surgical visualization of the urethral anastomosis and neurovascular bundles and potentially shorter inpatient postoperative stay. The use of robotic assisted laparoscopic prostatectomy can shorten the surgical learning curve and is now available in a number of UK urology centres.

Locally advanced T3N0M0, T4aN0M0

These patients have a greater risk of metastatic disease. The combination of radiotherapy and hormonal therapy improves outcome. It is now accepted that for men with locally advanced prostate cancer (T3/4 Gleason Score 8-10), longer term hormonal therapy of at least 2 years improves survival over shorter 6 month therapy. It is important that hormonal therapy is given concurrently with the radiotherapy. In our institution, we offer 3 months of neoadjuvant and concurrent hormonal therapy before stopping the adjuvant hormonal therapy after 2 years if the PSA is 0.1 or less. PR07 has confirmed that the addition of radiotherapy to locally advanced disease improves survival over hormone therapy alone and is now the accepted standard of care. The definition of treatment failure following radical radiotherapy is the nadir PSA value post treatment + 2ng/ml as per the Houston definition.

Metastatic disease

Hormonal therapy

Most prostatic tumours contain elements sensitive to the androgenic hormone testosterone. Hormonal treatment is designed to reduce levels of testosterone circulating in the blood. This may be achieved in a number of different ways:

1. removal of the testes, which secrete testosterone (orchidectomy)
2. oral oestrogens, e.g. diethylstilbestrol
3. chemical compounds, similar to luteinizing hormone-releasing hormone (LHRH analogues), which diminish the pituitary production of luteinizing hormone (LH) and thus reduce testosterone production – these are administered by monthly or 3-monthly depot injection
4. oral agents which block the cellular action of androgens (e.g. cyproterone acetate, biclutamide).

About 80% of patients will respond to hormonal therapy. The median duration of response is 18–24 months. Early intervention with hormonal therapy reduces complications of the disease, such as pathological fractures; however, it does not appear to improve survival. Median survival once patients become hormone refractory is 6 months. Maximum androgen blockade does offer a small survival advantage in the order of 2.5% at 5 years but at greater cost and toxicity. For this reason, it has not gained uniform acceptance. Intermittent hormonal therapy is still under investigation.

Cytotoxic chemotherapy

There is renewed interest in cytotoxic chemotherapy in hormone refractory patients. Recent randomized trial data comparing docetaxel (Taxotere) chemotherapy versus mitoxantrone has for the first time demonstrated a survival benefit of nearly 3 months for the Taxotere arm. Taxotere 75 mg/m^2 q21 with prednisolone 5 mg bd continuously over six to 10 cycles would now be considered the gold standard regimen. Introduction of chemotherapy at early stages of disease is an area of ongoing research. Second line treatment with Cabazitaxel chemotherapy and oral targeted hormonal Cyp17 blockers such as Aberaterone Acetate have further extended survival in men post Taxotere chemotherapy.

Palliative radiotherapy

Radiotherapy has a useful role in relieving pain from bone metastases. It can also shrink advanced local disease causing symptoms of outflow obstruction and pelvic nodes causing lymphedema and nerve compression.

Technique

Parallel-opposed field or single fields.

Dose and energy

1. *Prostate*: 30 Gy in 10 daily fractions over 2 weeks (9–10 MV photons)
2. *Bone metastases confined to a limited area, e.g. lumbar spine*: single fraction of 8 Gy or 20 Gy in five daily fractions (4–6 MV photons)

Widespread

Hemibody irradiation. Where there are widespread painful bony metastases, hemibody irradiation may be considered to encompass all the painful areas. Improvement in pain control tends to be prompt and may last the few months until death. Treatment of the lower half of the body is better tolerated because the side effects are minimal.

Preparation. The patient is given intravenous fluids and fasted before treatment. Regular antiemetics are given before and after treatment.

Treatment volume. For the lower half, the field usually extends from the umbilicus to the knees and for the upper half from the top of the head to the umbilicus. Overlap with the lower field is avoided.

Acute reaction. Nausea and vomiting occur at the end of treatment and last for up to 6 hours. Lethargy is common. If the upper half is treated, hair loss starts at about 10 days. The mouth becomes dry and taste sensation is altered. The blood count reaches its low point at 10–14 days. Hemoglobin, white blood cell and platelet counts are all reduced (pancytopenia) and remain so for up to 8 weeks. Cough and shortness of breath occurring at 6 weeks are usually indicative of radiation pneumonitis. If both halves of the body are treated, an interval of at least 6 weeks is left after the first hemibody irradiation to allow the systemic effects to settle and the blood count to recover.

Technique. The patient is treated supine. Parallel-opposed anterior and posterior fields are used at extended focus skin distance (FSD) (140 cm).

Dose and energy. Lower half of body
8 Gy midplane dose in a single fraction (9–10 MV photons)
Upper half
6 Gy midplane dose in a single fraction (9–10 MV photons)

Strontium-89. Strontium-89 is a pure beta emitter with a half-life of 50 days. It is selectively taken up by bone metastases. After a 150 MBq dose, relief of bone pain may occur in 60–70% of patients, with little hematological toxicity. It is best avoided in those with a 'super-scan', as little benefit can be expected. If used early in the metastatic process, strontium can delay the onset of symptoms in new sites of bone disease. Alpharadin or radium^{223} is an alpha emitter that gives high dose irradiation to the bone and has shown a survival advantage for men with hormone refractory disease over best supportive care in a recent randomized controlled trial. Biphosphonate therapy has been demonstrated to reduce bone pain and risk of pathological fractures in men with hormone refractory disease.

TESTIS

Anatomy

Each testis (the diminutive form 'testicle' is also in common use, with its adjective testicular) lies within a fibrous capsule (tunica albuginea) within the scrotum (Figure 28.12). In the

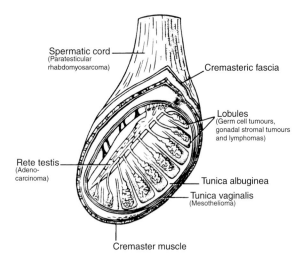

Figure 28.12 Diagram of testis and spermatic cord indicating sites of tumour origin. Paratesticular rhabdomyosarcoma may arise from connective tissue of the cord or of adjacent structures. *(From Textbook of Uncommon Cancers, Williams C J, Krikorian J G & Green M R, 1988, © John Wiley & Sons Limited. Reproduced with permission)*

embryo, the testes arise on the posterior abdominal wall and migrate downwards through the inguinal canal to the scrotum.

The testis is divided into 200–300 lobules. Each of these contains one to three seminiferous tubules. These drain into the epididymis, which lies on the posterior border of the testis. The lymphatic drainage of the testis is to the para-aortic nodes. It is important to note that the skin of the scrotum drains to the inguinal nodes. To avoid surgical contamination of the scrotal skin, the testis is surgically removed through an inguinal incision.

Pathology

Aetiology

The main factor predisposing to the development of germ cell tumours of the testis is an undescended testis. This accounts for 10% of cases. The risk is increased fivefold if one testis is maldescended and 12-fold if both are maldescended. However, even if one testis is maldescended, there is an increased risk of testicular cancer in the normally descended testis on the other side. Intratubular germ cell neoplasia or carcinoma in situ is a premalignant condition which gives rise to malignancy in 50% of patients within 5 years.

Testicular cancer is the commonest form of malignancy in men between the ages of 20 and 40. The incidence is rising, possibly through increased exposure to environmental oestrogens. Currently, there are about 2005 new cases per year in the UK (year 2000 figures). It accounts for 0.1% of deaths from cancer. The types of common (germ cell tumours) and rarer tumours and their sites of origin in the testis are illustrated in Figure 28.12.

Germ cell tumours

There are two main tumour types that arise from the germ cells: seminoma and teratoma. Teratoma occurs mainly between the ages of 20 and 35, and seminoma between 25 and 40 years. Over the age of 50, tumours are more likely to be non-germ-cell tumours. These are non-Hodgkin's lymphomas and tumours arising from other structures of the testis (Sertoli and Leydig cell tumours). Paratesticular rhabdomyosarcoma (see Figure 28.12) occurs in infancy and in young adult life.

Seminoma

Seminoma is the commonest type (60%). It arises from the cells of the seminiferous tubules. It is solid with a pale cut surface like a potato. There are two principal types: *classical* and *spermatocytic*. The characteristic histological feature of classical seminoma is its uniform appearance. The cells are rounded with a central nucleus and clear cytoplasm. The tumour is divided into lobules by a fibrous stroma, associated with a variable infiltration of lymphocytes.

Spread of seminoma may be local to the epididymis and to the spermatic cord, but lymphatic spread is more important. The first group of nodes to be invaded is the upper para-aortic, at the level of the renal hilum. Further lymphatic spread may be upward to the mediastinum and even the supraclavicular nodes through the thoracic duct, or downward to the lower para-aortic and pelvic nodes. If extratesticular tissues of the scrotum are invaded, including the scrotal skin, their draining inguinal lymph nodes may be invaded. Blood-borne spread is much less common.

Spermatocytic seminoma is uncommon and generally seen in older men. The tumour cells show differentiation to spermatocytes, and their behavior is benign. Metastases are extremely rare.

Teratoma

Teratoma accounts for the remainder of germ cell tumours. Strictly speaking, a teratoma shows differentiation towards all three embryological germ cell layers of ectoderm (e.g. skin, neural tissue), endoderm (e.g. gut, bronchi) and mesoderm (e.g. fat, cartilage). In practice, the British classification applies the term more widely (while American terminology refers to this group as non-seminomatous germ cell tumours). Teratomas are subtyped according to their cell constituents as:

- teratoma differentiated
- malignant teratoma intermediate
- malignant teratoma undifferentiated
- malignant teratoma trophoblastic.

Teratoma differentiated (TD) shows cysts lined by various mature-looking epithelium surrounded by smooth muscle, with islands of cartilage and neural tissue. In infants, its behavior is benign but, in adults, it is rare and can give rise to metastases. *Malignant teratoma undifferentiated* (MTU), by contrast, has no recognizable differentiated structures, but has undifferentiated rather than carcinomatous tissue. It often has tissue resembling yolk sac (YST), and there are frequently syncytiotrophoblast giant cells. These account for secretion of alpha-fetoprotein (AFP) and human chorionic gonadotrophin (HCG), respectively, which can be measured in the blood and are invaluable as markers of tumour load. It has an aggressive clinical behavior with early metastasis via lymphatics to para-aortic lymph nodes, and blood-borne spread to the lungs. *Malignant teratoma intermediate* (MTI) has a mixture of differentiated and undifferentiated tissues. *Malignant teratoma trophoblastic* (MTT) has tissue resembling gestational choriocarcinoma (i.e. syncytiotrophoblast and cytotrophoblast), either throughout or in combination with features of other teratomas. Large amounts of HCG are secreted and the clinical course is very aggressive with widespread blood-borne metastases.

Tumour markers

The two tumour markers, alpha-fetoprotein (AFP) and human chorionic gonadotrophin (HCG) are helpful in

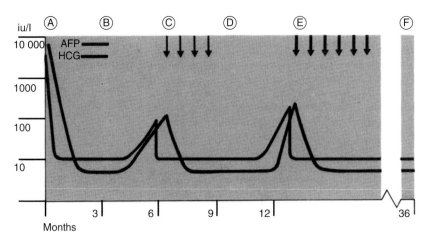

Figure 28.13 Tumour markers in the management of testicular cancer. (A) Both HCG and AFP are elevated before orchidectomy but fall following operation (HCG more rapidly because of its short half-life). (B) No evidence of recurrence, followed by a rise in marker levels. (C) Combination chemotherapy for recurrence is followed by a fall in levels to normal (D). (E) A further rise in marker levels is treated more intensively and the patient is disease free at 3 years (F).
(Reproduced with permission from Souhami & Moxham, Textbook of Medicine, Churchill Livingstone, 1990)

the diagnosis, staging and monitoring of response to treatment (Figure 28.13). AFP has a half-life of about 5 days. It is produced by yolk sac elements but is not specific to teratoma. Elevated levels occur in the presence of liver damage. HCG is mainly a marker of trophoblastic neoplasms; it can, however, occur in seminoma. The half-life of HCG is 24 hours and of the beta subunit 45 minutes. Markers for the presence of seminoma are much less reliable. Serum placental alkaline phosphatase (PLAP) is often raised in the presence of seminoma, particularly if there is bulky disease. However, false-positive and false-negative results for PLAP are common. Lactate dehydrogenase (LDH) is an important non-specific marker of disease volume and has been incorporated into the International Germ Cell Consensus Classification (Table 28.4).

Clinical features

The usual presentation is a gradually enlarging painless testicular swelling, although atrophy of a testis may occur. The tumour feels hard. A third of patients describe pain in the testis, a third a dragging sensation, 10% give a history of trauma. The first symptoms and signs may be of metastatic spread (hemoptysis from lung metastases, back pain from para-aortic metastases, loin pain from ureteric obstruction or neck lymphadenopathy). Malignant teratoma trophoblastic (choriocarcinoma) may produce gynaecomastia (breast enlargement).

Diagnosis and staging

The diagnosis is made by surgical removal of the testis through an inguinal incision (inguinal orchidectomy)

and histological examination. Immunocytochemical stains of the tumour for the presence of AFP and HCG may be positive. Blood levels of AFP and HCG are measured pre- and postoperatively. A chest radiograph is required (for overt lung metastases), together with a CT scan of the thorax (for small-volume lung and mediastinal metastases) and of the abdomen (abdominal nodal and liver metastases).

The Royal Marsden staging classification (Table 28.5), based on the extent of spread and bulk of disease, has been widely used for determining management. Although still useful for seminoma stage II nodal size subgrouping, it has been largely superseded by the IGCCC prognostic grouping.

Treatment

Seminoma – good prognosis

Stage I and IIa

Postoperative abdominal node irradiation should be considered. An alternative is a single cycle of carboplatin AUC5 which can reduce the risk of relapse on a par to radiotherapy. Surveillance with chemotherapy for relapse is also an option for selected men although the pattern of relapse is less predictable than with teratoma and long term follow up and scanning required.

Target volume

For stage I and IIa uncomplicated disease, postoperative radiotherapy to the para-aortic nodes alone is still frequently used. The 2–3% of patients who will relapse in the pelvis following irradiation can then be salvaged with chemotherapy. The upper margin of the para-aortic field is at the level of the junction of the 10th and 11th thoracic

Table 28.4 The IGCCC prognostic grouping

TERATOMA	SEMINOMA
Good prognosis with all of:	
Testis/retroperitoneal primary	Any primary site
No non-pulmonary visceral metastases	No non-pulmonary visceral metastases
AFP <1000 ng/ml	Normal AFP
HCG <5000 iu/l	Any HCG
LDH <1.5 upper limit of normal	Any LDH
56% of teratomas	90% of seminomas
5-year survival 92%	5-year survival 86%
Intermediate prognosis with all of:	
Testis/retroperitoneal primary	Any primary site
No non-pulmonary visceral metastases	Non-pulmonary visceral metastases
AFP ≥1000 and ≤10000 ng/ml or	Normal AFP
HCG ≥5000 and ≤50000 iu/l or	Any HCG
LDH ≥1.5 normal and ≤10 normal	Any LDH
28% of teratomas	10% of seminomas
5-year survival 80%	5-year survival 73%
Poor prognosis with any of:	
Mediastinal primary or non-pulmonary visceral metastases	No patients classified as poor prognosis
AFP >10000 ng/ml or	
HCG >50000 iu/l or	
LDH >10 normal	
16% of teratomas	
5-year survival 48%	

Table 28.5 The Royal Marsden Hospital staging classification of testicular tumours

STAGE	CLINICAL FINDINGS
Mk+	Rising serum markers with no other evidence of metastases
I	No evidence of metastases
II	Abdominal node involvement
a	<2 cm diameter
b	2–5 cm diameter
c	>5 cm diameter
III	Nodal involvement above the diaphragm
IV	Extralymphatic metastases
L1	Lung metastases three or less in number
L2	Lung metastases more than three in number (all 2 cm or less in diameter)
L3	Lung metastases more than three in number (more than 2 cm in diameter)

vertebrae. The lower limit is the junction of the 5th lumbar vertebra and the first sacral vertebra. Where there has been previous inguinoscrotal surgery, such as hernia repair, the field is extended to cover the ipsilateral pelvic and inguinal nodes (Figure 28.14). This 'dog leg'-shaped field is vertical in the para-aortic region and diverges at the level of the junction of the fourth and fifth lumbar vertebrae. The lower limit of the field is the bottom of the obturator foramina and should include the inguinal scar. Previous orchido-pexy, removal of the testis through the scrotum or exten-sion of tumour to the tunica vaginalis requires the ipsilateral scrotum to be irradiated in addition.

Technique: PA strip

An anterior and posterior pair of fields is used. The patient is simulated supine at normal FSD. The width of the para-aortic field is normally 8–10 cm. The field is off set to include the renal hilar nodes on the side of the orchidect-omy. The contralateral border is the lateral extent of the pedicle of the vertebral body. Care should be taken not to include more than one-third of the renal substance within the para-aortic fields on either side. An intravenous urogram (IVU) during simulation is essential to verify the position of the kidneys if virtual simulation is not available.

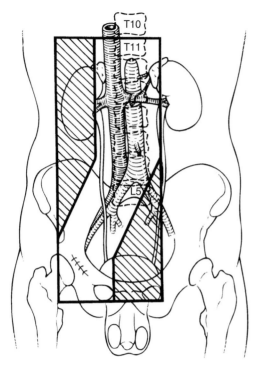

Figure 28.14 Treatment volume for ipsilateral pelvic and para-aortic ('dog leg') irradiation for testicular seminoma.

Technique: dog-leg

An anterior and posterior pair of fields is used. The patient is simulated supine throughout, if treatment under couch at an extended FSD (about 140 cm) can be achieved. Multi-leaf collimators (MLC) or customized MCP blocks protect tissue outside the treatment volume. Care should be taken not to include more than one-third of the renal substance within the para-aortic fields on either side. An IVU is used to verify the position of the kidneys if virtual simulation is not available. If there is involvement of the lower para-aortic nodes and risk of retrograde spread to the pelvic lymph nodes, then an 'inverted Y'-shaped field should be used to treat the para-aortic and pelvic nodes. If the hemiscrotum is to be treated, a direct electron field of appropriate energy or 300 kV x-rays may be used with shielding of the contralateral testis.

Dose and energy

Seminoma is one of the most radiosensitive of all cancers and can be cured with relatively modest doses. The present standard dose is:

20 Gy in 10 daily fractions over 4 weeks (9–16 MV photons).

Acute reaction. About 50% of patients will experience nausea lasting for 2–3 hours following treatment. Regular use of a 5-HT$_3$ antagonist is recommended.

Late reactions. Late side effects are rare. Dyspepsia occurs in 5%, occasionally with evidence of peptic ulceration. Using the radiation technique and dosage described, the dose to the contralateral testis is very low (less than 0.5 Gy). Nonetheless, this dose is sufficient to cause a moderate reduction in sperm count for 2–3 years, but it is not associated with permanent infertility. There are some concerns about the long-term complications of adjuvant radiotherapy such as second malignancy and hypertension. For stage 1a seminoma, a single infusion of carboplatin area under the curve (AUC) 7 may well be as effective as 2 weeks of radiotherapy in preventing disease relapse. Full trial publication is awaited, however, initial results look encouraging.

Stage IIb, IIc, III and IV

In stage IIb disease, radiotherapy for small-bulk disease can still be used, however, there is a greater chance of relapse. In addition, in stage IIb and stage IIc disease, increasingly bulky abdominal nodes make it difficult to avoid irradiating more than one-third of the renal substance on both sides. Four cycles of combination chemotherapy with bleomycin, etoposide and cisplatin (BEP) (Table 28.6) are recommended for these stages. In good-prognosis seminoma in men over 40 or in those with previous chest irradiation, EP may be used to decrease the risks of bleomycin lung.

Results of treatment

The results of treatment in early-stage seminoma are excellent, reflecting its radiosensitivity: 5-year survival rates by stage are 95% for stage I and 90% for stage IIa and IIb. For more advanced stages, cure rates have improved with the availability of effective combination chemotherapy: 5-year survival for stages IIc and III is 75% and for stage IV 65%.

Teratoma

Stage I

Teratoma has a higher incidence of extralymphatic spread. In the presence of extralymphatic metastases, irradiating the para-aortic nodes prophylactically may compromise the ability to deliver subsequent combination chemotherapy at desired dosage and frequency. About 30% of

Table 28.6 BEP chemotherapy regimen		
Bleomycin	30 mg i.v. bolus	Days 1, 8, 15
Etoposide	100 mg/m² i.v. infusion	Days 1–5
Cisplatin	20mg/m² i.v. infusion	Days 1–5
Repeated every 21 days		

patients with stage I disease following orchidectomy will have subclinical metastases and will relapse (80% of whom will relapse in the first 12 months). To avoid overtreatment of the majority of patients, a policy of close surveillance with treatment at relapse is recommended. Patients with lymphatic or vascular invasion are at greater risk of relapse (40%) and are not suitable for surveillance. Such patients are best treated by two cycles of adjuvant combination chemotherapy.

Surveillance

For patients for whom a surveillance policy is adopted, tumour markers, chest x-ray (CXR) and clinical examination are performed monthly in the first year with 3-monthly CT scans of chest and abdomen. In the second year, follow up should be 2-monthly with CT scans at 18 and 24 months. Subsequent follow up should be 3-monthly for the third year, 6-monthly to the fifth year and annually thereafter to 10 years.

Stages II–IV

These stages should be managed by combination chemotherapy (see below).

Cytotoxic chemotherapy

The development of curative combination chemotherapy for advanced testicular cancer in the 1980s has been one of the most important advances in oncology.

The combinations of drugs used for treating seminoma are the same for teratoma. The most effective regimens contain cisplatin. Cisplatin was successfully combined with vinblastine and bleomycin (PVB). Now vinblastine is replaced by etoposide, which is less myelotoxic, without loss of efficacy. This regime is known as BEP (see Table 28.6). An attempt to reduce toxicity by replacing cisplatin with carboplatin has proved to be less effective. Before each course of chemotherapy, a number of investigations are carried out to assess fitness to treat, and to modify dosage, if necessary, because of the toxicity of the agents. A full blood count is required because of the myelotoxicity of etoposide.

Cisplatin is toxic to the kidney and to hearing. Renal function tests (serum urea, electrolytes and creatinine, 24-hour urine creatinine clearance or formal EDTA GFR) and hearing (audiometry) should be measured before, during and after treatment.

Bleomycin can be toxic to the lung (see below). Full lung function tests (including gas transfer factor) are carried out before treatment and repeated if toxicity is suspected.

Sperm storage, if available, is desirable for men wishing to father children following chemotherapy since sterility is commonly induced. Normally, an initial sample is examined to count the number and motility of the sperm. If satisfactory, two additional samples are taken for sperm banking. However, chemotherapy, if urgently required, should not be delayed to await this procedure.

Dosage and scheduling. Normally four courses of BEP are given at 3-weekly intervals. Patients with good risk disease can be cured with just 3 cycles as demonstrated in the MRC TE20 trial without compromising the 90% overall survival. For those patients in the intermediate- or poor-risk IGCC groups, survival is 40–70%. Efforts to increase the efficacy of chemotherapy schedules through dose intensification and new combinations are ongoing. As yet, there has been no improvement over standard BEP.

Monitoring response to treatment. Clinical examination, chest radiograph, tumour markers, full blood count, and renal function tests are repeated before each cycle of treatment to monitor the response to and toxicity of treatment.

Following surgery, a fall in tumour marker levels in line with their half-lives usually indicates that there is no residual disease. A slower fall or rising levels suggest residual disease.

It may be necessary to delay the next cycle of chemotherapy or modify its dosage if blood count, renal function or hearing deteriorate below certain thresholds. Every effort should be made to deliver the chemotherapy on schedule and granulocyte colony-stimulating factor (GCSF) support may be required. Chemotherapy should not be given if the neutrophil count is below $1.0 \times 10^9/$ L. CT scan of chest and abdomen is repeated after three cycles to confirm that the disease is responding. Rapid resolution of disease is usual after the first course. Residual 2–4 cm masses may, however, persist for several years.

Management of residual abdominal masses

Resection of residual abdominal masses following chemotherapy is indicated for teratoma. Seminoma resection is difficult and usually not indicated due to a lack of tissue planes and tumour infiltration beyond resection margins. A policy of observation is usually recommended. Resection of residual masses after treatment for teratoma shows that most of them (44%) are due to differentiated (mature) teratoma or to fibrosis and necrosis (34%). Residual tumour is found in 22%. If recurrence occurs, as it does in 10–20% of patients, it is most likely to develop at a site of initial involvement. If surgical expertise is available, resection of residual masses is desirable. It serves both as a diagnostic and therapeutic procedure. Further chemotherapy is indicated if residual disease is found, but the outlook is poor, with less than 50% of such patients remaining free of disease.

Toxicity

In addition to renal damage and ototoxicity (impaired hearing), cisplatin causes severe nausea and vomiting and peripheral neuropathy. The 5-HT antagonists (ondansetron and granisetron) can reduce nausea and vomiting. Intravenous hydration is required 24 hours before cisplatin is given and for 24 hours afterwards to reduce the risk of renal damage. Nonetheless, the majority of patients will experience temporary renal damage. A 20–25% reduction in glomerular filtration rate is usual.

Etoposide causes alopecia and myelosuppression. The incidence of septicemia with etoposide is less than with vinblastine since it is less myelosuppressive.

Bleomycin may cause pneumonitis. Presentation is with progressive dysponea. This complication may occur after relatively modest doses (e.g. 200 mg). It can be progressive, is irreversible and carries a 1% mortality. Other side effects are fever, skin rashes, pigmentation and Raynaud's phenomenon.

Results of treatment

Ninety percent of patients with small-volume disease are cured following chemotherapy. For large-volume disease in extralymphatic sites, the probability of survival is reduced to 50–70%.

The 5-year survival is 90% for stages I and IIa, 70% for stages IIb and III, and 50–60% for stage IV.

TESTICULAR LYMPHOMA

Testicular lymphomas are rare (4% of testicular tumours). They are mainly non-Hodgkin's lymphomas. Clinical features that help to differentiate them from germ cell tumours are bilaterality (20% at presentation or subsequently), older age group (over 50 years), different pattern of metastases, absence of maldescent and of gynaecomastia. They are usually of high grade (diffuse large B cell). Stages IAE and IIAE are only cured in 50% of cases with three cycles of CHOP chemotherapy and radiotherapy to the scrotum (IA) and involved nodes (IIA). For this reason, six cycles of chemotherapy are recommended followed by radiotherapy. For stage III and IV disease, CNS chemoprophylaxis is required in addition to scrotal irradiation.

Dose and energy

35 Gy in 20 daily fractions over 4 weeks (6–10 MV photons)

Results of treatment

The prognosis is poor. Overall 5-year survival is 20%. For stage IAE and IIAE, it is 50%. Average survival with stage IV disease is about 8 months.

URETHRA

Tumours of the urethra are rare and are usually transitional carcinomas. Predisposing factors are as for bladder cancer (p. 489). Presenting symptoms and signs are pain and hematuria.

Female urethra

The tumour is twice as common in women as in men. In the proximal third, transitional carcinoma predominates and, in the distal two-thirds, squamous carcinoma predominates. The distal urethra drains to the inguinal nodes and the proximal urethra to the iliac nodes. Presenting features are offensive discharge, bleeding or a mass.

Treatment

Surgery in the form of a cystourethrectomy is perhaps the treatment of choice. In those who are unsuitable, then attempts at organ preservation can be considered. For superficial squamous carcinoma of the urethral orifice, three iridium hairpins are an alternative treatment. A dose of 60–65 Gy is given in 6–7 days. For more proximal lesions, radical external beam irradiation using an anterior and two lateral wedged fields is used. A dose of 55 Gy is given in 20 daily fractions over 4 weeks using megavoltage.

Results of treatment

The cure rates with surgery and radiotherapy are similar at about 50%.

PENIS

Cancer of the penis is a rare tumour responsible for 0.4% of all cancers and 0.1% of cancer deaths. It occurs in older men, typically between 50 and 70 years old. The disease is commoner in South-east Asia, China and Africa. In Uganda, penile carcinoma is the second commonest male cancer.

Pathology

Aetiology

The disease rarely occurs among peoples who practice circumcision. There is a high incidence in Hindus, who are never circumcised. Phimosis is present in up to 50% of cases. Poor penile hygiene is thought to be an important predisposing factor. There is a strong association with human papilloma virus infections. There are several premalignant conditions, including viral warts (condyloma acuminata) and erythroplasia of Queyrat. The primary tumours are squamous carcinomas, usually well differentiated. Secondary deposits are rare but can occur from prostate and bladder cancer.

Clinical features

These tumours occur as warty growths or, more commonly, as indurated ulcers on the glans or the sulcus at the base of the glans. Symptoms have often been present for a year or more before presentation. The first sign may be an infected or bloody discharge from beneath the prepuce. Growth is superficial at first, then by invasion of the penile shaft. If the lesion is visible, the diagnosis is usually obvious. If phimosis hides it, the glans must be exposed by incising and peeling back the prepuce (dorsal slit) or by complete circumcision, under anesthesia. A biopsy is taken at the same time.

Lymphatic spread occurs early to the inguinal nodes, though enlargement here may simply reflect infection. The nodes may eventually ulcerate. Blood-borne metastases are rare and late.

Staging

Both TNM and Jackson staging systems are in use (Table 28.7). If inguinal nodes are enlarged, fine needle aspiration of the node with cells sent for cytology can help

to distinguish tumour from infection. A CT scan of the pelvis may show the extent of abdominal lymphadenopathy.

Treatment

Surgery and radiotherapy are the main treatments for penile cancer. Factors which influence the choice of treatment, are the age and general condition of the patient, the extent of the disease, the desire to retain sexual function and the capacity to pass urine in the standing position for young males.

Surgery

Specialized surgical techniques are now available which can excise early invasive tumours and reconstruct the penis with a split skin graft for an excellent cosmetic and functional result. More advanced tumours involving the deeper corpora and urethra require amputation of part or the whole of the penis. Although curative if the inguinal nodes are not involved, the procedure is associated with considerable psychological morbidity, especially for young males.

Radiotherapy

Radical radiotherapy is still an effective treatment for early penile cancer since it permits the organ to be conserved. However, if there is deep invasion of the shaft, the chances of control by radiation are poor and surgery is preferable. Invasion of the urethra also favors surgery, since post-radiation fibrotic stricture is very liable to occur.

Treatment techniques and dosage

The choice of technique and energy will depend on the extent and site of the disease. For tumours confined to the glans or the prepuce, superficial, orthovoltage, electron beam or implants are possibilities. For infiltrating tumours or where the inguinal nodes are involved, megavoltage irradiation is required.

Implantation

A single or double plane implant with iridium-192 should include within the target volume a 2 cm margin around the tumour. Tumours greater than 4 cm in any dimension or invading the corpora cavernosa should not be implanted.

The implant (Figures 28.15–28.17) is carried out under a general anesthetic and following catheterization. The penis is held upright and away from the testicles and thighs by foam padding secured by adhesive tape to the thighs. The dose to the testis is usually up to 3 Gy. This can be reduced by interposing 2–3 mm of lead shielding if fertility needs to be conserved. The dose to the reference isodose using the Paris system should be 60–65 Gy. Duration of treatment is normally 6–7 days.

Table 28.7 TNM and Jackson staging systems for penile cancer

STAGE	CLINICAL FINDINGS
Tumour	
T1	Tumour invades subepithelial connective tissue
T2	Tumour invades corpus spongiosum or cavernosum
T3	Tumour invades urethra
T4	Tumour invades other structures
Nodes	
N0	No regional nodes
N1	Single inguinal node
N2	Multiple unilateral nodes or bilateral nodes
N3	Deep inguinal or pelvic nodes
Metastases	
M0	No distant metastases
M1	Distant metastases present
Jackson classification	
I	Tumour confined to the glans or prepuce
II	Tumour extending on to the shaft of the penis
III	Tumour with operable inguinal nodes
IV	Tumour with inoperable metastases

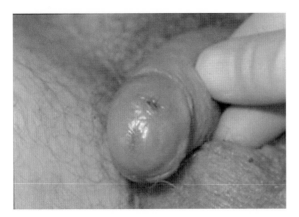

Figure 28.15 T1 Ca penis on glans.

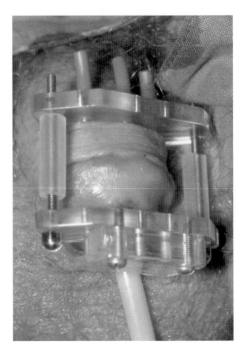

Figure 28.17 Afterloading rigid iridium wire implant of T1 penile cancer.

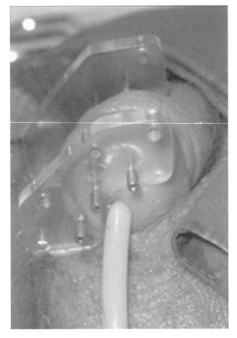

Figure 28.16 Afterloading rigid iridium wire implant of T1 penile cancer.

Superficial or orthovoltage therapy

For very small (T1) superficial tumours 100 kV or 250 kV x-ray therapy may suffice. A 0.5 cm margin of normal surrounding tissue is included in the treated volume. A dose of 50 Gy is given in 15 fractions over 3 weeks. Alternatively, low-energy (6 MeV) electrons can be used using an appropriate thickness of Perspex over the lesion to bring up the surface dose to 100%.

Megavoltage

Treatment volume. If there is evidence of spread on to the shaft of the penis, the whole of the penis should be treated.

Technique. A rectangular wax block with a central cylindrical cavity is made to encompass the penis and ensure homogeneous irradiation of the whole volume. The penis is treated en bloc by a parallel-opposed pair of lateral fields.

Dose and energy. 50–55 Gy in 20 daily fractions over 4 weeks at megavoltage (4–6 MV photons)
or 60 Gy in 30 daily fractions over 6 weeks at 4–6 MV photons.

Acute reactions

These are like skin reactions elsewhere but more marked and moist desquamation is commoner. The urethral reaction causes discomfort and dysuria. If very severe it may result in acute retention requiring catheterization.

Late reactions

These include telangiectasia, skin atrophy, urethral stricture and necrosis. Urethral dilatation is required for stricture. Necrosis occurs in less than 10% of cases.

Management of regional nodes

If inguinal nodes are found to be histologically involved at presentation, a block dissection of the groin should be carried out, followed by radical radiotherapy to the primary. There is no value in giving prophylactic groin node irradiation. The only role for radiotherapy in the treatment of groin nodes is for palliation. For fixed inoperable nodes neoadjuvant chemotherapy for downstaging prior to lymphadenectomy for locally advanced patients can be considered.

Palliative radiotherapy

Technique

A simple parallel-opposed pair of fields to the affected groin.

Dose and energy

30 Gy in 10 daily fractions over 2 weeks at megavoltage.

Palliative chemotherapy

Cisplatin-based chemotherapy can be considered for fit patients. Response rates of 30–40% have been reported.

Results of treatment

Early superficial tumours have a high cure rate: 5-year survival for stage I disease is about 90%. This falls to 60% in stage II and 30–40% in stage III.

FURTHER READING

Bolla M, Van Tienhoven G, Warde P, et al. External irradiation with or without long-term androgen suppression for prostate cancer with a high metastatic risk: 10-year results of an EORTC randomized study. Lancet Oncol 2010;11(11):1066–73. Epub 2010 Oct 7.

Bolla M, De Reijke TM, Van Tienhoven G, et al. Duration of androgen suppression in the treatment of prostate cancer. N Eng J Med 2009;360(24):2516–27.

Warde P, Mason M, Ding K, et al. Combined androgen deprivation therapy and radiation therapy for locally advanced prostate cancer: a randomized phase 3 trail. Lancet 2012;378(9809):2104–11. Epub 2011 Nov 2.

Schroder FH, Hugosson J, Roobol MJ, et al. Screening and prostate cancer mortality in a randomized European Study. N Engl J Med 2009;360(13):1320–8 Epub 2009 Mar18.

De Wit R, Roberts JT, Wilkinson PM, et al. Equivalence of three or four cycles of bleomycin, etoposide and cisplatin chemotherapy and of a 3- or 5-day schedule in good prognosis germ cell cancer; a randomized study of the EORTC and treatment of genitourinary tract cancer group and the MRC. J Clin Oncol 2001;19(6):1629–40.

Oliver RT, Mason MD, Mead GM, et al. Radiotherapy verses single dose carboplatin in adjuvant treatment of stage I seminoma; a randomised trial. Lancet 2005;366(9482):293–300.

Motzer RJ, Hutson E, Tomczak MD, et al. Overall survival and updated results for sunitinib compared with interferon alfa in patients with metastatic renal-cell carcinoma. J Clin Oncol 2009;27(22):3584–90. Epub 2009 Jun 1.

Rini BI, Escudier B, Tomczak P, et al. Comparative effectiveness of axitinib verses sorafenib in advanced renal cell carcinoma (AXIS): a randomised phase 3 trial. Lancet 2011;378(9807):1931–9. Epub 2011 Nov 4.

Sawhney R, Bourgeois D, Chauhary UB. Neo-adjuvant chemotherapy for muscle-invasive bladder cancer: a look ahead. Ann Oncol 2006;17:1360–9.

Mosconi AM, Roila F, Gatta G, Theodore C. Cancer of the penis. Crit Rev Oncol Hematol 2005;53:165–77.

Chapter | 29 |

Lymphoma and disease of bone marrow

Gillian D. Thomas, Matthew Ahearne, Martin J.S. Dyer

CHAPTER CONTENTS

INTRODUCTION

Lymphomas present as solid masses arising in lymph nodes or at extranodal sites anywhere in the body, while the leukaemias and multiple myeloma are diseases primarily of the bone marrow. They are chemo- and radiosensitive and, in contrast to the common 'solid' tumours, many are curable despite being widespread. Treatments range from simple oral chemotherapy and low-dose radiotherapy to high dose chemotherapy, total body irradiation and haemopoietic stem cell transplantation (HSCT). Immunotherapy now has an important role.

MALIGNANT LYMPHOMAS

The malignant cell is the lymphocyte, with 90% of B cell and 10% of T cell origin. Lymphomas are conventionally divided into Hodgkin's (HL) and non-Hodgkin's (NHL). The former, named after Thomas Hodgkin who described it in 1832, is highly curable, while NHL is a diverse group of conditions.

Aetiology and epidemiology

HL accounts for 0.7% of all cancers and 0.4% of cancer deaths. In the UK, the incidence is three per 100 000 population per year in men and 1.8 for women. There are two age peaks, from 15 to 35 and a smaller old-age peak. There is an association with the Epstein-Barr virus (EBV) and with higher social class.

NHL occurs in 11 per 100 000 and the median age is 55–60. Childhood incidence is very low but higher (particularly Burkitt's lymphoma) in developing countries. Overall, the male:female ratio is 1.5:1, although this varies between subtypes.

The causes of most NHL are unknown, but the risk is increased in immunodeficiency syndromes, immunosuppression following organ transplantation, AIDS, autoimmune disorders, and coeliac disease, and following certain infections or exposure to ionizing radiation and carcinogenic chemicals. Characteristic acquired chromosomal defects include the following translocations, involving the immunoglobulin genes on chromosome 14q32:

- t(14;18)(q32;q21) in about 80% of follicular lymphoma, involving the *BCL2* gene on chromosome 18q21
- t(11;14)(q13;q32) in all cases of mantle cell lymphoma, involving the *Cyclin D1* gene on chromosome 11q13
- t(8:14)(q24;q32) in Burkitt's lymphoma, involving the *MYC* gene on chromosome 8q24.

NHL can result from chronic antigenic stimulation of lymphocytes, as in marginal zone lymphoma of mucosa-associated lymphoid tissue (MALT) following *Helicobacter pylori* infection, usually in the stomach or, rarely, following *Chlamydia psittici* infection. Burkitt's lymphoma, originally described in East African children and classically in the jaw, is associated with the Epstein-Barr virus (EBV). A rare but very aggressive type of T-cell NHL is caused by infection with the human T-cell leukaemia virus type. 1 (HTLV-1).

Pathological characteristics

Prognosis and therapy depend on the maturity and subtype of the cell of origin. This is defined by:

1. morphology – appearance and arrangement of cells
2. immunophenotyping – cellular differentiation (CD) cell surface antigens identified by a panel of antibodies
3. cytogenetics – chromosome translocations
4. molecular biology – gene expression.

The WHO classification includes HL and NHL (Table 29.1). A specialist haematopathologist is essential for accurate categorization. Morphologically, aggressive NHL can resemble poorly differentiated carcinoma and indolent NHL may be confused with benign lymphadenopathy.

Hodgkin's lymphoma

Hodgkin's lymphoma is characterized by RS (Reed-Sternberg) cells, although these are only 2–4% of the cells present: the bulk of the tumour consists of normal, reactive lymphocytes, histiocytes, plasma cells, granulocytes and fibroblasts. RS cells are large and multinucleate with prominent eosinophilic nucleoli and express CD30 and CD15. Overall survival is excellent, around 80% at 5 years.

Table 29.1 Simplified WHO classification of tumours of haematopoietic and lymphoid tissues

CHRONIC MYELOPROLIFERATIVE DISEASES

CML
PRV
Myelofibrosis
Thrombocythemia

MYELODYSPLASTIC/MYELOPROLIFERATIVE DISEASES AND SYNDROMES

Acute myeloid leukaemias

AML with cytogenetic abnormalities or with prior dysplasia/therapy

PRECURSOR B-CELL NEOPLASM

Precursor B lymphoblastic leukaemia/lymphoma (ALL)

MATURE B-CELL NEOPLASMS

CLL/small lymphocytic lymphoma
Marginal zone lymphoma: splenic/nodal/MALT
Myeloma and plasmacytoma
Follicular lymphoma
Mantle cell lymphoma
Diffuse large B-cell lymphoma
Mediastinal large B-cell lymphoma
Burkitt's lymphoma

B-CELL PROLIFERATIONS OF UNCERTAIN MALIGNANT POTENTIAL

Post-transplant lymphoproliferative disorder

PRECURSOR T-CELL NEOPLASMS

Precursor T-lymphoblastic leukaemia/lymphoma (ALL)

MATURE T-CELL AND NK-CELL NEOPLASMS

T-cell and NK-cell leukaemias
NK/T-cell lymphoma
Peripheral T-cell lymphoma
Anaplastic large cell lymphoma and cutaneous ALCL
Mycosis fungoides and Sézary syndrome
Angioimmunoblastic T-cell lymphoma
Enteropathy-type T-cell lymphoma

HODGKIN'S LYMPHOMA

Nodular lymphocyte predominant HL

CLASSICAL HL

Nodular sclerosis
Lymphocyte-rich
Mixed cellularity
Lymphocyte-depleted

There are four histological subtypes termed classical HL (cHL), lymphocyte rich, nodular sclerosing grade 1 and 2, mixed cellularity and lymphocyte depleted, which is very rare but carries a poor 5-year survival of 20%. The most common is nodular sclerosing, with 'nodules' of cells within 'sclerosing' fibrous bands which often persist as a residual inactive mass after treatment. The fifth category of HL, lymphocyte predominant, differs histologically and clinically. It has an extremely long natural history with distant relapses, more like indolent NHL.

Non-Hodgkin's lymphoma

Follicular lymphoma and diffuse large B-cell lymphoma (DLBCL) together make up 80% of all NHL seen in the West. They may be described as indolent and aggressive respectively, and grouped with other NHL subtypes though each is quite distinct.

Aggressive NHL

DLBCL behaves aggressively but is curable in about 50%. Bone marrow is involved in 10–15%. It forms sheets of large cells, often multinucleate with prominent nucleoli. Adverse prognostic markers include expression of p53 and BCL2 proteins and MIB-1 (Ki67). High proliferation rates (100% MIB-1 staining) are associated with programmed cell death (apoptosis) as in Burkitt's lymphoma. Pale apoptotic cells in a uniform background of dark blue malignant lymphocytes appear as a 'starry sky'. Thus, at the aggressive end of the spectrum of DLBCL, it may appear and behave like Burkitt's or lymphoblastic lymphoma, which are the truly 'high grade' types which grow and spread most rapidly but are curable with aggressive treatment. Over the last decade, gene expression profiling of DLBCL cases have identified two major subtypes based on unique gene 'signatures': germinal centre B-cell like (GCB-DLBCL) and activated B-cell like (ABC-DLBCL). The latter is associated with greater resistance to conventional chemotherapy and worse clinical outcomes.

Mantle cell lymphoma, characterized by cyclin-D1 and CD5 expression, progresses slowly but has a poor prognosis (median survival 3–4 years) due to chemoresistance. Peripheral T-cell lymphoma also falls in this relatively poor prognostic category.

Indolent NHL

In follicular lymphoma, cells arise from lymph node germinal centres and form structures resembling normal follicles. Grade 3 behaves as DLBCL and grades 1 and 2 behave in a 'low grade' indolent way (median survival 7–9 years). It inevitably recurs, unless truly localized at diagnosis (15%). It can transform into DLBCL with a poor prognosis. Bone marrow involvement is common (>60%). Marginal zone lymphomas, presumed to arise from the small B cells of nodal or splenic marginal zones, also behave indolently.

Extranodal NHL

DLBCL is the usual type of NHL presenting in the head and neck (Waldeyer's ring, nasal sinuses, thyroid), bone, testis, breast and brain. In the stomach, orbit, salivary glands, lung and spleen, the marginal zone lymphoma predominates, while intestinal lymphoma is commonly of T-cell origin and associated with coeliac disease. NHL may arise in the skin from either B or T cells. Histological diagnosis is often difficult and clonality studies using *IG* or *TCR* rearrangements are needed to distinguish reactive conditions. Mycosis fungoides is a very slowly progressive epidermal tumour of T-cell origin which may develop a leukemic form (Sézary syndrome). Anaplastic large cell lymphoma (ALCL) is also of T-cell origin, may arise in skin or elsewhere, and has a good prognosis if CD30 and ALK antigens are expressed. Cutaneous B-cell NHL includes follicular, marginal zone, and DLBCL.

Clinical features

All lymphomatous nodes may spontaneously wax and wane. They have a rubbery consistency and tend to be smooth, multiple, discrete, mobile and painless. They can enlarge to 10 cm or more without fixation or skin involvement, in contrast to carcinomatous nodes which invade surrounding structures early. However, patients with aggressive lymphoma can deteriorate rapidly with dehydration, hypercalcemia, anaemia, infection and damage to critical organs.

HL usually presents with enlarged nodes in the neck (60%), axilla (20%) or groin (15%). The spleen (10%) or, rarely, liver may be enlarged. Mesenteric nodes, bone marrow and extranodal sites are rarely involved in HL but commonly in NHL. Spread of HL is contiguous, from one lymph node group to the next: in NHL it may not be, and only 10% are localized at presentation.

Three characteristic 'B' symptoms are associated with lymphoma and a worse prognosis: drenching night sweats, weight loss (>10% of body weight in previous 6 months) and fever (>38°C) which may be of a specific periodicity (Pel–Ebstein fever). The disease is staged as A (none of these) or B (any of these). Itching (pruritus) occurs in 12%, but is not classed as a B symptom. Pain felt in involved lymph nodes after drinking alcohol is a symptom peculiar to cHL.

In NHL, 20% have involvement of extranodal sites. In the head and neck there is swelling, proptosis or nasal blockage. Thyroid lymphoma presents as a mass with stridor from tracheal compression, and sometimes a history of Hashimoto's thyroiditis. Primary NHL of bone mainly affects proximal long bones, with pain, swelling and pathological fracture. Testicular NHL presents at age 60–80 with a painless smooth swelling. Bilateral involvement occurs in 20%. NHL of the breast presents with a mass often indistinguishable from carcinoma. Gastrointestinal lymphoma can present with pain, anaemia or bowel obstruction. Primary cerebral lymphoma presents with raised intracranial pressure or focal neurological deficits including siezures. In the skin, mycosis fungoides starts as erythematous, flat, slightly scaly itchy lesions on the buttocks, upper thighs or breasts. These develop into thicker plaques, and then to fungating tumours with nodal and visceral involvement. The whole skin may become involved resulting in generalized erythroderma or 'l'homme rouge'. B cell cutaneous lymphoma is more likely to present as a discrete fleshy nodular lump with a tendency to ulcerate. Cutaneous ALCL occasionally undergoes spontaneous remission.

Diagnosis and staging

A formal excision biopsy is essential and should be sent fresh to the laboratory. Fine needle aspiration is inadequate for accurate diagnosis of lymphoma. There is usually no need to debulk tumour surgically.

Staging establishes the extent of the disease, using the Ann Arbor classification (Table 29.2), clinical assessment and essential investigations:

1. blood tests – full blood count, plasma viscosity, serum urea and electrolytes, calcium, liver function tests, lactate dehydrogenase (LDH) and β2-microglobulin
2. chest x-ray as baseline for reference
3. computed tomography (CT) scan of chest, abdomen and pelvis with intravenous and oral contrast
4. a bone marrow aspirate and a small core of bone (trephine) are taken from the posterior iliac crest
5. lumbar puncture for high-risk groups (see below). At the time of the procedure, it is usual to inject methotrexate 12.5 mg
6. positron emission tomography (PET) shows uptake of fluorodeoxyglucose (FDG) into areas actively metabolizing glucose and representing viable tumour in most cases. FDG-PET can assess response where there is a residual mass on CT, which may be fibrous tissue or lymphoma. Ideally, a pretreatment scan would be available for comparison.

Table 29.2 Ann Arbor staging classification of lymphoma

I. Involvement of a single lymph node region (I) or of single extralymphatic organ or site (IE)

II. Involvement of two or more lymph node regions on the same side of the diaphragm (II) or localized involvement of an extralymphatic organ or site and one or more lymph node regions on the same side of the diaphragm (IIE)

III. Involvement of lymph node regions on both sides of the diaphragm (III) which may be accompanied by localized involvement of an extralymphatic organ or site (IIIE) or by involvement of the spleen (IIIS) or both (IIISE)

IV. Disseminated involvement of one or more extralymphatic organs or tissues with or without associated lymph node involvement

---

Clinical prognostic factors

Early HL is 'very favorable' if stage 1A, NS or LP type, age <40 and female, and 'unfavorable' if age over 50, four or more sites involved, raised ESR and a large mediastinal mass.

Advanced HL is 'unfavorable' if stage 4, age over 50, low lymphocyte count, eosinophilia, low hemoglobin, low serum albumin and male.

In NHL, the international prognostic index (IPI) is a widely accepted prognostic score from 0 to 5, with one point for each of the following features:

1. age $\geq$ 60
2. more than one extranodal site
3. stage III or IV disease
4. high LDH
5. WHO performance status 2–4.

There is an increased risk of CNS relapse in DLBCL of the testis, paranasal sinuses, breast, and orbit, and in patients with heavy bone marrow involvement or with a high IPI score, and in Burkitt's and lymphoblastic lymphomas.

Treatment

Initial management

It is important to avoid treatment before any biopsy. If awaiting results then steroids may be given (e.g. prednisolone 60 mg daily) to arrest clinical deterioration. In an emergency, such as airway obstruction, treatment may have to be given with radiotherapy. Urgent chemotherapy can rescue very ill patients despite toxicity. Rapid tumour breakdown can cause a 'tumour lysis' syndrome due to release of cytokines and intracellular products causing raised serum urate, phosphate and potassium, reduced calcium and impaired renal and, rarely, lung function. To prevent this, patients should start allopurinol (300 mg daily), ideally, at least 24 hours before chemotherapy, and be very well hydrated. Individuals deemed at very high risk of tumour lysis (very high tumour burden as in Burkitt's lymphoma) may receive Rasburicase, a synthetic enzyme that breaks down the damaging urate.

Men should be offered sperm storage, but there are problems in the storage of ova. Eggs which have been individually frozen cannot be successfully fertilized. It is currently necessary to store embryos, which might be attempted for instance between a first line and a consolidation therapy. Preservation of ovarian tissue is under study.

Hodgkin's lymphoma

Radiotherapy (RT) was the first curative treatment for stage I–III HL. Staging originally involved laparotomy with multiple biopsies and splenectomy, and then total nodal irradiation (TNI) was given using 'extended fields' – a 'mantle' field covered all supradiaphragmatic nodes and an 'inverted Y' field the infradiaphragmatic nodes and spleen or splenic pedicle. This exploited the tendency for HL to spread along node chains.

Chemotherapy was first used in HL for disease incurable with radiotherapy. Although side effects were severe with MOPP (mustine, vincristine, procarbazine and prednisolone), additional cures were achieved and six to eight cycles of chemotherapy plus extended field radiotherapy became routine. After 3–8 years up to 10% developed secondary acute myeloid leukaemia (AML) and from 8 to 20 years, other secondary malignancies particularly in irradiated areas. Heart disease was also increased. After 10–15 years, the risk of death from these causes was greater than from relapse of HL, with many patients rendered infertile. The most common second tumour is lung cancer, with an enhanced risk in smokers. In young women treated with mantle fields, the risk of breast cancer increases with age from 8 years after treatment up to as high as 50% in middle age for those treated in their early teens, or up to 25% if treated aged 20–29, and early screening is now offered. Thyroid cancer, colon cancer and sarcomas are also seen.

Cure rates have been maintained using less toxic chemotherapy to reduce leukaemia and infertility, and smaller radiation fields with lower doses to minimize second malignancies and cardiotoxicity. Chemotherapy is used in young patients for all stages except very favorable stage 1A, where it would be acceptable to use radiotherapy alone. ABVD (doxorubicin, bleomycin, vinblastine and dacarbazine) has become standard, although it causes acute myelotoxicity, a small risk of cardiomyopathy and a 1% risk of fatal bleomycin lung toxicity. Two to four cycles plus 'involved field' radiotherapy is used in stage 1A and 2A and six to eight cycles ± RT for others. PET scanning helps to define complete response and the need for RT. Current trials are focusing on the use of early PET imaging during treatment to stratify patients into good and poor risk. Good-risk patients may go on to receive less demanding chemotherapy while poor-risk patients are escalated to more intensive regimens, such as BEACOPP (bleomycin, etoposide, etoposide, doxorubicin, cyclophosphamide, vincristine, procarbazine, and prednisone).

Extended field radiotherapy is used after a partial response to chemotherapy with disease at several sites, or where chemotherapy has had to be curtailed, especially in patients who would be unsuitable for HSCT. For elderly and unfit patients with early disease, radiotherapy alone may be the treatment of choice.

The overall 5-year survival is 70–80%.

Relapsed cHL may be cured with HSCT or sometimes further conventional chemotherapy or radiotherapy. Anti-CD30 antibodies are a promising new treatment for relapsed/refractory disease. Brentuximab vedotin, a novel antibody-drug conjugate has shown promising results in early studies.

Non-Hodgkin's lymphoma

Aggressive NHL

For more than 20 years, six to eight cycles of CHOP-21 (cyclophosphamide, hydroxydaunorubicin, oncovin (vincristine) and prednisolone once every 3 weeks) was the best treatment for DLBCL despite many trials of more intensive regimens. The recent addition of an anti-CD20 human/mouse monoclonal antibody (rituximab) to each cycle (R-CHOP) has increased complete response rates from 63 to 76% and overall survival at 3 years from 51 to 62% with minimal toxicity, so is the new gold standard. R-CHOP-14 fortnightly treatment is under investigation, using granulocyte colony stimulating factor (GCSF) to avoid neutropenic sepsis. Newer generation anti-CD20 monoclonal antibodies are available (Ofatumumab and GA-101) and currently under investigation.

In high-risk groups, prophylactic CNS treatment is given concurrently as intrathecal or high-dose intravenous methotrexate. Radiotherapy to sites of bulk is conventional.

For stage IA or IIA DLBCL, including extranodal sites, radiotherapy alone is curative in about 50%, but adding three cycles of chemotherapy increases the cure rate to 80% in chemosensitive patients. Eight cycles of CHOP seemed as effective as CHOP × 3 plus RT in one pre-rituximab trial but others show an advantage for RT and the combination is preferred. Full-course chemotherapy should be given if there is bulky disease or B symptoms or a high IPI score, usually with RT afterwards. Only 40% of DLBCL are truly localized. In testicular DLBCL, the contralateral testis should be irradiated to reduce the risk of recurrence.

At relapse after full-course chemotherapy, HSCT can be curative if chemosensitivity can be shown with salvage regimens (IVE, ICE, ESHAP, DHAP). Time to relapse is the most important predictive factor with rituximab refractory disease showing the worst outcome. Alternatives are oral etoposide and palliative radiotherapy. Radiolabeled anti-CD20 antibody is under investigation for DLBCL.

Burkitt's lymphomas are treated with mores intensive regimens, such as the CODOX-M/IVAC regimen, now combined with rituximab, and can cure around 50% of patients.

In primary cerebral lymphoma, standard chemotherapy can cross the blood–brain barrier initially while there is oedema around the tumour. CNS-penetrating drugs (high-dose methotrexate, cytarabine) are also used. Steroids are effective. Radiotherapy may prolong remission but causes lethargy and also significant cognitive impairment. Optimal chemotherapy, and the role of radiotherapy, are under investigation; prognosis is poor.

The optimal treatment of mantle cell lymphoma remains controversial and unsatisfactory. The benefit of maintenance Rituximab is currently under investigation. High-risk younger patients may be considered for consolidation with HSCT. Rare patients with localized disease may be considered for radical radiotherapy. Newer agents currently being tested alone and in combination with chemotherapy include lenalidomide, bortezemib, and temsirolimus.

Peripheral T-cell NHL is treated as DLBCL without rituximab as T cells lack CD20. Etoposide may be added to the CHOP regimen (CHOEP).

Indolent NHL

Truly localized (15%) follicular NHL may be cured with radiotherapy alone. For palliation, low doses can achieve lasting control.

In widespread disease, a 'watch and wait' approach is acceptable for asymptomatic patients. Immediate treatment with rituximab is under study. On symptomatic progression, for elderly patients, oral chlorambucil (e.g. 10 mg daily for 2 weeks every 4 weeks for six cycles) is appropriate. Younger patients should avoid alkylating agents and anthracyclines as first-line therapy. Currently, R-COP (=R-CHOP without Adriamycin; also called R-CVP) is often used; rituximab prolongs remission, although there is no known survival benefit as yet. R-CHOP is appropriate for follicular grade 3 or very bulky disease.

There is now increasing evidence that following induction and second-line chemotherapy, maintenance rituximab (375 mg/m^2 every 2–3 months for up to 2 years) significantly improves progression-free survival. However, to date, survival benefits have not been shown.

At relapse, re-biopsy is advisable to detect high-grade transformation. Selection and timing of treatment depends on the disease-free interval, extent of relapse, age and general condition, and includes HSCT. Rituximab alone (375 mg/m^2 weekly for 4 weeks) gives a 50% response rate with 13–17 months median time to progression in heavily pretreated patients and can be repeated with equal effect. Fludarabine is an effective oral agent.

Anti-CD20 monoclonal antibodies radiolabeled with yttrium-90 (a pure beta-emitter) or iodine-131 (beta and energetic gamma) are very promising new agents for refractory and transformed indolent NHL, with response rates of around 80% and remissions of several years in some patients. Zevalin (90Y-ibritumomab tiuxetan) is the murine parent of rituximab attached by the chelating agent tiuxetan to the radiolabel. It is given over 10 minutes with no need for hospital admission. Bexxar (131I tositumomab) is also a mouse antibody and seems equally effective but with more radiation protection issues; further research will establish the relative roles and optimal timing of these. Side effects include hypersensitivity reactions, delayed immunosuppression and secondary AML/MDS in 6%, partly due to previous chemotherapy.

Marginal zone NHL are described as three types: splenic, nodal, and those of MALT (mucosa-associated lymphoid tissue) origin. Splenectomy is appropriate for the first, and the others respond to the same agents and general approach as follicular NHL. Although the pattern of disease is different with more extranodal sites, radiotherapy can still be curative for disease truly localized to e.g. the stomach or parotid. Anti-helicobacter therapy is potentially curative in gastric MALT NHL. Gastric MALT can be monitored by regular endoscopies.

Mycosis fungoides has a median survival of 10 years. In the early stages, topical steroids can be used, then often photochemotherapy using long-wave ultraviolet light with oral psoralens (PUVA). Radiotherapy can be local or to the whole skin surface using low-energy electrons. Systemic treatments include CAMPATH (anti-CD52 antibody) which targets T cells. Combination chemotherapy with a CHOP-type regimen is used in visceral disease but complete response rates are low (20–25%).

Special situations

Lymphoma in children

Radiotherapy in children causes growth retardation in the treated area and they are particularly susceptible to second malignancies, so chemotherapy is used alone wherever possible. Lower radiation doses have been shown to be adequate in paediatric Hodgkin's and extranodal presentations are rarer: lymphadenopathy is the presenting feature in 90%.

Lymphoma in pregnancy

HL is the most common diagnosis. Staging should avoid exposure to ionizing radiation, using magnetic resonance imaging (MRI) or ultrasound in preference to CT. Radiotherapy is potentially teratogenic during the first trimester. Above a dose of 0.1 Gy to the fetus there is a risk of inducing an abnormality. Chemotherapy has an unquantified risk of teratogenesis or carcinogenesis to the fetus.

Termination should be considered if treatment is essential before the early second trimester, if the fetal dose would exceed 0.1 Gy or chemotherapy is indicated. If the diagnosis is made late in the second or in the third trimester, it may be possible to postpone treatment until delivery is induced at 32–34 weeks. Localized radiotherapy above the diaphragm can be safely given, and single agent chemotherapy may control symptoms in HL for a few weeks but, if the disease is life threatening, then combination chemotherapy is best. With ABVD, the risk of carcinogenesis or infertility in the child should be low.

Patients who have been successfully treated for Hodgkin's disease should be advised to avoid pregnancy for 2 years after the end of treatment, because after this the risk of relapse falls markedly. Subsequent pregnancy does not increase the risk of relapse.

Lymphoma in HIV and post-transplant

HIV-associated lymphoma is usually aggressive, presenting with high IPI scores and often CNS disease. Patients are more prone to succumb to infective complications of treatment. NHL is an AIDS-defining illness but HL is not. Median survival is 7–18 months with standard chemotherapy. Highly active antiretroviral therapy (HAART) in combination with chemotherapy has improved complete response rates and early studies suggest that adding rituximab may improve 2-year survival further from less than 50 to around 60%. Lymphomas of the Burkitt type are associated with a poorer outcome.

Post-transplant lymphoproliferative disease (PTLD) is an often localized NHL presenting after organ transplantation. It usually remits on gradual withdrawal of immunosuppressive therapy but, if not, then options include infusion of HLA-matched cytotoxic T lymphocytes.

MULTIPLE MYELOMA

Multiple myeloma accounts for 0.9% of all cancers and 1.3% of cancer deaths. Its incidence is 3 per 100 000 per year with about 3000 new cases annually in the UK. The median age at diagnosis is 62 years and the male to female ratio is 1.5:1. The aetiology is unknown. Median survival is 3–4 years from diagnosis with wide variations.

Pathology

Myeloma is a tumour of plasma cells, which are immunoglobulin-producing B lymphocytes. Their bone marrow microenvironment is increasingly well understood and new molecular targets for treatment identified as a result. Myeloma cells potentiate osteoclast activity and inhibit differentiation of osteoblast precursors, uncoupling bone formation from resorption so multiple lytic bone lesions are characteristic. They also produce a specific immunoglobulin (Ig) or paraprotein, detectable by immunoelectrophoresis and useful for diagnosis and treatment monitoring. While an intact immunoglobulin molecule is too large to enter the renal tubules, free light chains (Bence Jones protein) may be produced and are found in the urine. Normal immunoglobulins are reduced resulting in recurrent infections (immune paresis). In 5%, there is no secreted protein and the disease is termed non-secretory. Bence Jones only is found in 20%, while Ig subtypes are found with frequencies reflecting normal levels, i.e. IgG in 50–60%, IgA 20–25%, IgD 2%, IgE and IgM <1%. Paraproteinemia is also found in lymphoma. IgM is associated with Waldenstrom's macroglobulinemia or marginal zone lymphoma. In the normal population, paraproteinemia is found in 1% aged over 25, 3% over 70 and 25% over 90 years old. This is monoclonal gammopathy of uncertain significance (MGUS) and carries an annual risk of 1% of progression to multiple myeloma. Asymptomatic early myeloma is termed 'smoldering'.

Clinical features

The commonest presenting feature is bone pain (70%) from a rib or vertebra. The destruction of cortical bone leads to pathological fractures in about 25% and hypercalcemia in 30%. Alkaline phosphatase is normal, and bone lesions lytic. Spinal cord compression is occasionally the presenting feature and is an emergency. Humoral and cell-mediated immunity are impaired and recurrent infections are common. Most patients have a cytokine-mediated anaemia; pancytopenia due to marrow replacement is uncommon at presentation. A third have reduced white cell count and/or platelets. ESR is raised. Renal failure occurs due to deposition of Bence Jones protein in the renal tubules, dehydration, infection and non-steroidal anti-inflammatory drugs.

If the paraprotein level is high enough, a hyperviscosity syndrome develops, characterized by visual impairment, lethargy and coma. This is most commonly associated with IgM subtype as these form larger structures in the blood. Amyloidosis, a deposition of abnormal protein in the kidneys, heart, nerves or other sites, is seen in about 10% of myeloma patients.

A plasmacytoma is a solitary plasma cell mass, usually arising in a rib or vertebra but also other bones and soft tissues, with or without a paraprotein. Progression to multiple myeloma is probable but not inevitable.

Diagnosis

There are three requirements:

1. serum or urine paraprotein
2. plasma cell numbers increased in the bone marrow (>10%) or biopsy of a mass
3. end-organ damage: hypercalcemia, renal impairment, anaemia, or bone lesions (CRAB).

Investigations

1. Full blood count
2. Serum urea, creatinine and electrolytes
3. Serum calcium
4. Serum electrophoresis
5. Urine electrophoresis.
6. Bone marrow examination
7. Skeletal survey (plain x-ray of whole skeleton to show lytic lesions, especially skull, ribs and vertebrae, or diffuse osteoporosis). Bone scans using technetium-labeled colloid are not helpful in myeloma as lytic lesions are not usually shown
8. MRI imaging of the spine if cord compression is suspected.

Prognostic factors

Poor prognosis is associated with:

1. increase in plasma-cell labeling index
2. increase in B2microglobulin level
3. low serum albumin
4. plasmablastic features in the bone marrow
5. circulating plasma cells
6. 17p and chromosome 13 deletions.
7. t(4;14) or t(14;16) translocation
8. increased density of bone marrow microvessels.

Treatment

Prophylactic continuous bisphosphonate therapy is standard for all patients, to inhibit bone resorption. Severe hyperviscosity is treated by plasmapheresis, in which some of the patient's plasma is replaced by an appropriate colloid solution (usually albumin) to reduce the level of paraprotein. Nephrotoxic agents should be avoided if possible. Dialysis may be required for renal failure. Control of pain and infection are important.

Chemotherapy is aimed at response defined by a reduction in paraprotein level to 50% or less, healing of radiological lesions, and more than 50% reduction in size of a plasmacytoma. Complete response is defined as the absence of detectable paraprotein or urinary light chains and normalization of the bone marrow with <5% plasma cells. Usually a plateau phase is reached where the disease is measurable but stable. It should be considered at an early stage whether each patient is a candidate for high dose therapy with HSCT. Survival is prolonged by using melphalan at 200 mg/m^2 followed by autologous transplantation. The oral regimen of cyclophosphamide, thalidomide, dexamethasone (CTD) is now the most widely used induction regimen. Thalidomide exerts an antiangiogenic and anti-inflammatory effect. Patients with a durable remission following first autograft often benefit from a repeat autograft. A mini-allograft (see HSCT under leukaemias) may be superior to a second autograft for a high-risk young patient with a sibling donor but carries significant transplant-related morbidity and mortality and therefore remains controversial.

For elderly patients and those not fit for HSCT, thalidomide-containing regimens remain first choice – an attenuated dose of CTD can be used or thalidomide combined with melphalan and steroid. Bortezumib, a proteosome inhibitor, and lenalidomide, a novel analogue of thalidomide, are often used in combination with dexamethasone in relapsed disease. Combinations of these two drugs with more established chemotherapy agents continue to be investigated for first line treatment in high-risk patients.

Radiotherapy in myeloma

Solitary plasmacytomata are treated radically with surgery and radiotherapy.

In diffuse disease, palliative radiotherapy relieves bone pain and is often used concomitantly with chemotherapy. Single fractions are usual. Hemibody treatments are effective for generalized pain in advanced disease: upper and lower fields can be used in sequence for refractory disease unless there is severe pancytopenia.

Spinal cord or cauda equina compression may occur at presentation or at any stage of the disease, and may be due to extradural disease or a collapsed vertebra. In diffuse disease, urgent radiotherapy (usually fractionated) is often preferable to surgery, but decompression and stabilization followed by radiotherapy is sometimes more appropriate so surgical consultation should be considered.

Total body irradiation (TBI) is sometimes used as part of HSCT.

LEUKAEMIA

Bone marrow (hemopoietic) stem cells develop into lymphocytes (lymphoid cell line) or red blood cells, platelets or granulocytes (myeloid cell line). Cells of all lineages at virtually any stage of differentiation may become malignant.

In acute leukaemia, the marrow fills with immature lymphoid or myeloid leukaemic cells which displace normal cells and enter the peripheral blood. Untreated, death rapidly results from anaemia, bleeding and immunosuppression.

In the chronic leukaemias, which arise from more mature cells, the disease can be stable with few symptoms for many years.

Leukaemia accounts for 2.1% of all cancers and 2.6% of cancer deaths and is more common in males. Described here are:

1. acute leukaemia
   a. lymphoblastic (ALL)
   b. myeloid (AML)
2. chronic leukaemia
   a. lymphocytic (CLL)
   b. myeloid (granulocytic) (CML).
3. other myeloproliferative disorders.

Acute leukaemia

ALL constitutes 80% of paediatric and AML 80% of adult cases.

AML increases with age (median 65). It may arise from myelodysplastic syndrome (MDS), a group of clonal stem cell disorders characterized by dysplasia in one or more lineages, ring sideroblasts and bone marrow blasts (if >20% this becomes AML). Radiation can cause AML evidenced by survivors of atomic bombs (20:1) and whole-spine irradiation for ankylosing spondylitis (10:1). The risk rises from about 3 years after exposure and peaks at 7–8 years.

Some cytotoxic drugs (alkylating agents, etoposide) can induce leukaemia. The risk after MOPP chemotherapy is 3%, and, if given with wide-field irradiation for HL, the relative risk is about 6:1. Industrial chemicals, mainly benzene, can also induce AML.

An inherited predisposition is evident in Down's syndrome (20:1). Ataxia telangiectasia and other DNA repair defect syndromes, such as Bloom's syndrome and Fanconi's anaemia, all predispose to either ALL or AML, but these are very rare. Infection is not the cause of leukaemia except in the rare adult T-cell leukaemia/lymphoma syndrome (HTLV1 virus).

Chromosomal abnormalities and translocations are numerous and useful in defining prognostic groups; their absence after treatment verifies remission.

Clinical features

The clinical features of ALL and AML are similar and are described elswhere along with the treatment of ALL.

Treatment of AML

Intensive combination chemotherapy is used to induce remission. Standard regimens involve cytarabine and daunorubicin, plus etoposide if younger, which can achieve results of about 80% remission in patients under 60 but, in older patients, it is only about 40%. Relapse is usual without further treatment, if possible with HSCT to obtain long-term remission/cure. There is a favorable 'good-risk' subgroup of whom two-thirds may be cured and where transplantation may be reserved for relapse, including those with promyelocytic disease where all-trans retinoic acid (ATRA) can induce blast cells to differentiate. New agents include antibody to CD33, found on the leukemic cell surface, which has been linked with a novel cytotoxic agent (gemtuzumab-ozogamicin, 'Mylotarg') and is currently being investigated in a large national UK trial. Such agents may improve complete response (CR) rates and it is therefore important that younger fitter patients are entered into national trials.

Long-term cure is possible in 30% of younger patients with HSCT, but cure is very unlikely in older patients or following relapse. Clofarabine, a purine analogue similar to fludarabine, is being trialled in older patients with AML to assess for improved response rates. In patients unfit for intensive chemotherapy, low-dose cytarabine or hydroxyurea is used to obtain some disease control. The prognosis is poor if AML has been preceded by MDS.

Chronic myeloid leukaemia

CML is a rare disease that occurs mainly in the fifth and sixth decades. The incidence in the UK is one in 100 000. There is a slight male predominance (1.4:1). In over 90% of cases, the *Philadelphia chromosome* is present, the result of a translocation from chromosome 22 to chromosome 9 resulting in a 'fusion' *BCR-ABL* gene whose protein product (p210 $^{\text{BCR-ABL}}$) is a tyrosine kinase enzyme essential for malignant transformation. The drug imatinib (Glivec) has been designed to inhibit this enzyme.

Clinical features

Presentation is with tiredness due to anaemia, or with splenomegaly which may be massive. The total white cell count is typically between 100 and 500 × 10^9/L, a mixture of myeloid cells at varying stages of differentation and less than 5% blasts, with this picture reflected in the marrow. The platelet count is normal or raised.

The natural history is of a chronic stable phase of 4–6 years, although this can be 1–20 years. A 6-month accelerated phase precedes the terminal blastic phase.

Treatment

In younger patients, the treatment of choice is allogeneic HSCT, the only curative option. Oral imatinib is highly effective at inducing both clinical and cytogenetic complete remission in chronic phase, in 95% and 70% of patients, repectively (less if in accelerated phase) and is the best non-transplant treatment. However, many patients relapse eventually due to the leukaemia cell developing resistance to the drug. Newer tyrosine kinase inhibitors (dasatinib, nilotinib) have been developed and have a role in imatinib resistance. Hydroxurea is useful to control high white cell counts during end-stage disease. After HSCT in chronic phase, 50% are disease free at 4 years, but if in accelerated phase, only 12%. Thus, treatment is aimed at controlling the disease until transplantation can be arranged. Timing can be very difficult and research is addressing ways to select high-risk patients for early HSCT.

Chronic lymphocytic leukaemia

CLL is the commonest form of leukaemia in the western world. Its incidence in the UK is five per 100 000. The male to female ratio is 2:1. It is usually seen in middle age, with the incidence increasing with age. About 5% of cases exhibit some family history of B-cell lymphoproliferative disease, but the nature of the involved gene(s) remains unknown. It is not linked to radiation or chemical exposure or chemotherapy.

Clinical features

Symptoms are mainly due to anaemia or infection though diagnosis is often made incidentally on a full blood count. The white cell count is usually between 30 and $300 \times 10^9/L$ and composed of small mature lymphocytes with condensed nuclei and scant cytoplasm. The bone marrow is hypercellular with an infiltrate composed of mature lymphocytes. Biopsy of enlarged nodes shows monotonous sheets of cells with characteristic proliferation centres.

Enlargement of lymph nodes of the neck and other peripheral sites, spleen and liver is common: staging systems are currently based on the number of these and on normal and abnormal cell counts into A, B and C. Adverse prognostic factors include stage B or C, male gender, age >60, lymphocyte doubling time <12 months, diffuse marrow infitration and >10% circulating prolymphocytes. Molecular markers of prognosis are p53 abnormalities, 11q23 deletions, high CD38/ZAP-70 expression and having an unmutated IgVH gene.

CLL is slowly progressive although, occasionally, notably with mutations of the p53 gene, resistant to all conventional therapy. In some patients, the disease is stable for over 20 years.

Treatment

Treatment is indicated for symptoms or if critical organs are threatened. Oral chlorambucil has historically been given first line, at doses of e.g. 10 mg daily for 2 weeks out of 4. Fludarabine induces more rapid responses and is given in combination with cyclophosphamide (with which it seems to synergize). Recently, the combination of fludarabine and cyclophosphamide with rituximab has been approved for first-line treatment. Sometimes, CLL can transform into a high-grade lymphoma (Richter's transformation) and is treated as for DLBCL.

The CD52 monoclonal antibody, alemtuzumab (CAMPATH), is effective though immunosuppressive. It is particularly useful in patients with certain molcular markers (p53 abnormalities), often in combination with steroids if bulky disease is present.

New therapies that interfere with the B-cell receptor signalling on the CLL cells are being developed including inhibitors of Bruton tyrosine kinase (BTK), Syk, and PI3 kinase.

With conventional treatment, the 5-year survival of CLL is about 60% overall.

MYELOPROLIFERATIVE DISORDERS

This is a related group of disorders including CML (above), polycythemia vera (PV), essential thrombocythemia (ET) and idiopathic myelofibrosis (IMF). They are slowly progressive with median survival of about 10 years. PV (excess red cells) and ET (excess platelets) can lead to myelofibrosis and to AML.

PV causes pruritus, splenomegaly and gout due to hyperuricemia, and PV and ET cause thromboses, particularly arterial, and less often hemorrhages.

Treatment is with antiplatelet drugs and hydroxyurea (a cytotoxic drug). Interferon is used less but has a role in selected patients unable to take hydroxyurea. Anagrelide is useful in ET as it prevents the maturation of platelets. Busulphan and radioactive phosphorus (P32) injections are effective but rarely used now because of the increased risk of leukaemia. Repeated venesection is used in PV to prevent the hemotocrit rising to dangerous levels.

In IMF, there is bone marrow fibrosis and failure with associated splenomegaly. It may due to stimulation of fibroblasts by abnormal megakaryocytes. Irradiation is effective at very low doses in shrinking the spleen.

It has recently been discovered that a mutation in another tyrosine kinase, JAK2, can be found in 90% of patients with PV and around 50% of ET and IMF. JAK2 inhibitors are now well developed and undergoing clinical trials. They may soon become standard care for these patients.

HEMOPOIETIC STEM CELL TRANSPLANTATION (HSCT)

This term is used to describe the collection and transplantation of HSC from bone marrow, peripheral blood or umbilical cord blood. It is essential to the delivery of high-dose treatments used increasingly in the haematological malignancies and will be referred to throughout this chapter.

Stem cells from the patient's own marrow are autologous and, if donated by another, HLA-matched person, allogeneic. Cells are transplanted by infusion through a central venous Hickman line and are then described as the 'graft'.

Autografting has a 1–2% mortality. Stem cells are harvested from the peripheral blood after stimulating them to proliferate by giving conventional chemotherapy and granulocyte-colony stimulating growth factors (GCSF), and they are reinfused after high-dose therapy which would otherwise be fatally myelosuppressive. It may not be possible to harvest cells following prior chemotherapy especially with alkylating agents and fludarabine and this problem has altered first-line treatments. Plerifixor inhibits a molecule in the bone marrow releasing stem cells into the peripheral blood and has shown to increase the success of harvesting procedures.

Allografting has about a 30% mortality, lower with a sibling than with a matched unrelated donor (MUD), but is the only curative option when there is residual disease in the marrow or where autografting has failed. High dose 'conditioning' therapy is given to eradicate the underlying disease and to immunosuppress the patient enough to prevent rejection of the transplant, e.g. cyclophosphamide 100 mg/kg over 2 days and total body irradiation (Cy/TBI). Chemotherapy may be used alone, e.g. cyclophosphamide and busulphan (Bu/Cy). Donor harvesting may be from peripheral blood or directly from bone (multiple punctures under general anesthesia) which gives a better yield of cells. Allografting has the beneficial effect of donor T lymphocytes recognizing residual malignant cells as foreign and destroying them.

Following chemoradiotherapy, the white cell and platelet counts drop within 10 days and recover after 3–6 weeks of intensive support with antibiotics, red cell and platelet transfusions. Graft-versus-host disease (GvHD) occurs when T cells from the donor react with antigenic targets on host cells. It may be acute (jaundice, skin rashes, diarrhea and weight loss) or chronic (arthritis, liver disease, malabsorption, oral mucositis and sicca syndrome, lung disease, pericardial and pleural effusions, scleroderma, skin rashes) and has a high mortality. The incidence is reduced by immunosuppression with cyclosporin A or tacrolimus and by depleting the donor T cells using monoclonal antibodies such as alemtuzumab (CAMPATH) and antithymocyte globulin (ATG). Blood products are irradiated to kill any T lymphocytes which may precipitate GvHD.

New treatments for GvHD include antibodies to tumour necrosis factor and interleukin-2, and extracorporeal photopheresis. Immunodeficiency due to defects of T-cell and B-cell functions occurs during the first 6 months and for longer in the presence of GvHD. Viral, bacterial and fungal infections may be fatal.

In the event of relapse after transplantation, donor T lymphocytes can be used therapeutically for their graft-versus-disease effect. This is exploited in 'mini-allografting' in patients unfit to undergo a myeloablative transplant: after reduced-intensity conditioning (no TBI), the host normal marrow survives and coexists with the donor marrow, and the donor T cells control the leukaemia.

RADIOTHERAPY DOSES, TECHNIQUES AND TOXICITIES

INRT: planned volume with the clinical target volume (CTV) = involved node/s with margin which follows node chains.

ISRT: planned volume with the CTV = the involved site (may be nodal as above) with defined margins.

IFRT: parallel-opposed beams covering the classical defined involved field, encompassing a node region.

EFRT: extended field encompassing all node regions on one side of the diaphragm: mantle (nodes above) and inverted Y (nodes below).

Megavoltage is used (4–10 MV photons). Palpable masses are outlined with wire; bolus may be needed to ensure an adequate dose to superficial nodes. Reference to pre-chemo PET-CT and contrast enhanced CT is essential.

Hodgkin's lymphoma

Following chemotherapy: 30 Gy in 15 fractions to involved node/site.

Young patients with stage 1A/2A good risk and PET negative after two cycles of chemo: 20 Gy in 10 fractions may be adequate.

Radiotherapy alone: 35 Gy in 20 fractions to extended field + 5 Gy in two fractions to site/s of bulk.

Palliative treatment: single fraction 5 Gy to small volume; 10–20 Gy in 5–10 fractions over 1–2 weeks for larger areas often adequate.

Non-Hodgkin's lymphoma

Diffuse large B cell lymphoma

Radical: post-chemo: 30 Gy in 15 daily fractions over 3 weeks to involved node/site.

Radiotherapy alone: 30 Gy in 15 fractions to extended field. Boost involved site to 40 Gy using a phase 2 volume.

Palliative: 20–30 Gy in 5–10 fractions is usual, to involved field. Large single fractions, e.g. 8 Gy may be appropriate for, e.g. bone.

Indolent lymphoma: follicular and marginal zone

Radical: generally radiotherapy alone: 30 Gy in 15 fractions over 3 weeks to involved field. If chemo has been given, treat involved site/nodes.

Palliative treatment: 4 Gy in two fractions can give prolonged remission in indolent NHL. Otherwise 24 Gy in 12 fractions is commonly used.

Extended fields – for nodal HL or NHL – no chemo/chemoresistance/palliation

Anterior and posterior at extended focus skin distance (FSD) (140 cm).

Mantle

Target volume: supradiaphragmatic nodes including occipital, submental and submandibular, but excluding preauricular/parotid nodes/Waldeyer's ring.

Position: supine with neck extended. Arms abducted and supported with hands on hips. (Figure *evolve* 29.1, 29.2 & 29.3 🖱).

Field borders

Superior: at tip of chin, positioned level with external occipital protuberance and mastoid process. Record distance from centre of top border on the chin to suprasternal notch.

Inferior: junction of 10th and 11th thoracic vertebrae.

Lateral: lateral to the humeral head to include the whole axilla.

Shielding

Lungs: superiorly shield from the lower posterior border of the fourth rib, to treat infraclavicular nodes, and laterally to 0.5 cm medial to the ribs down to T7/8, to treat lower axillary nodes. Between the lungs, the minimum field width is 7–8 cm at the inferior border, 9–10 cm at the hila and around any bulky nodes leaving a 2 cm lateral margin (from post-chemotherapy disease).

Spine: anteriorly a 2 cm strip from the centre of the superior border down to C5/6 shields the larynx, and a posterior strip down to C7 protects the cervical cord, adjusted if there is adjacent lymphadenopathy, to avoid underdosage. The rest of the spinal cord may be shielded from the posterior beam after 21 Gy unless there is (or was) central mediastinal adenopathy, in which case, limited shielding is added to within 4–5 cm of any enlarged nodes.

Shoulders: humeral heads and adjacent joint spaces are shielded from anterior and posterior beams throughout treatment unless there is an adjacent axillary node mass. Shielding can be done using multileaf collimators (MLCs) or partly with customized lead blocks.

Tattoos are placed to avoid rotation of the thorax.

Dose distribution

The axillae and neck receive 10–20% more than the inferior edge of the field. Shielding may be added over the relevant areas for one or two fractions, or compensators used throughout, unless inhomogeneity is effectively boosting residual disease.

Inverted Y

Target volume: all infradiaphragmatic nodes: para-aortic, pelvic, iliac and femoral. In conjunction with a mantle field and if extended to include the spleen or splenic pedicle this is TNI, while STNI omits the pelvic field from L5/S1.

Position: supine. Anterior and posterior fields are used at extended FSD (140 cm).

Field borders

Superior: junction of the 10th and 11th thoracic vertebrae or if matching to a mantle field, a gap (about 2 cm on skin) is calculated to have the 50% isodoses meet just posterior to the vertebral bodies on a lateral x-ray.

Inferior: the inferior margin of the obturator foramen, or covering involved nodes plus 5 cm.

Lateral: the greater trochanters of the femora.

Shielding

Abdominal cavity: lateral to the paraortic nodes (8–10 cm central strip or 2 cm beyond any node mass). The medial 1–2 cm of each kidney may be irradiated.

Bladder and genitalia: a midline block protects the bladder and urethra. Ovarian function is preserved by surgery (oophoropexy) to move them centrally for shielding, marking their position with clips. Lead cups over the testes can reduce their dose to <0.6 Gy.

Involved fields

Target volume: all pretreatment macroscopic and PET-positive disease and at least one anatomical node group such as the axilla or inguinal area, often two or three but less than mantle or inverted Y. Where a node mass with a well-defined edge has shrunk with chemotherapy away from an adjacent dose-limiting structure, such as lung, spinal cord or kidney, a 2 cm margin on residual disease is adequate laterally. There should be at least a 5 cm margin along the lymph node chain above and below the prechemotherapy disease, which may mean inclusion of part of the adjacent region, e.g. where the superior mediastinum was involved it is usual to treat both supraclavicular fossae.

Position: as for mantle or inverted Y fields: involved fields are subsets of these (Figures *evolve* 29.4–29.14 🖱).

Technique: parallel-opposed fields, with borders partly those of extended fields. The medial border of a neck field may be in the midline or at the edge of the spinal canal. CT planning may reduce normal tissue treated e.g. in the mediastinum.

Involved sites – ISRT (if nodal, may be referred to as INRT).

Volumes are irregular in shape and a good knowledge of anatomy is required to define them, with reference to standard atlases, radiological opinion, prechemotherapy PET scans and contrast enhanced CT scans for planning (Figure *evolve* 29.15 🖱).

A CTV is defined on the CT planning system. Where there is a residual node mass adjacent to another tissue, such as lung, the CTV may be at the edge of this mass in the axial plane, and does not need to encompass the original size. However, in the direction of the lymph node chain, the CTV is the pretreatment extent of abnormal nodes on PET-CT plus a 1.5 cm margin. This direction may not be directly superior-inferior, for instance, at the junction between node regions in the mediastinum/neck or abdomen/pelvis.

Where there is no residual mass, the volume describes the lymph node chain in the space bounded by other structures, such as muscle, large vessels, lung and bone.

A margin is added to the CTV to give the required PTV according to the site, set-up error, likely movement, and local departmental practice, and might vary from 5 mm to 1.5 cm.

ISRT for extranodal sites following chemotherapy is CT planned in a similar way to involved nodes. The CTV may define the whole organ, e.g. stomach, spleen, thyroid, where there were no adjacent nodes involved, or part of a node chain may need to be outlined in addition.

Extranodal involved fields

For radical treatment following response to chemotherapy, only involved sites need be treated as described above.

Head and neck

The patient is immobilized in a supine shell, and CT planning used for the whole treatment, for a second phase, or for matching of field edges (Figure *evolve* 29.16 🖱).

Waldeyer's ring

Fields extend from the base of the skull to the clavicles, including the cervical lymph node chains on both sides of the neck. A parallel pair of lateral fields cover the posterior nasopharynx, the adenoids, oropharynx and adjacent upper cervical nodes down to the thyroid cartilage. For extensive nodal involvement and/or partial response to chemotherapy, this can be extended anteriorly and posteriorly to cover submandibular and occipital nodes. A lower neck field is matched on using CT planning, avoiding junctions through sites of disease. Infraclavicular fossae are shielded (Figures *evolve* 29.17 & 29.18 🖱).

Thyroid

The thyroid gland and the cervical lymph node chains on both sides are included, with anteroposterior fields extending inferiorly into the superior mediastinum and superiorly to the submandibular nodes. CT planning can be used for a second phase to minimize spinal cord dose.

Orbit

The whole orbit is treated using CT planning. For small lateral and conjunctival indolent NHL, a single beam may suffice. Beams are angled to avoid the other eye (Figures *evolve* 29.19–29.24 🖱).

Nasal sinuses

Planning is as for carcinoma (Figures *evolve* 29.25–29.29 🖱).

Brain

The whole brain is treated with a parallel pair of lateral beams. As meningeal involvement is likely, the fields are extended down the neck to C2/3 and to cover the posterior orbit and facial nerve root as for ALL. Craniospinal treatment is only very occasionally indicated in relapsed NHL (see acute lymphoblastic leukaemia) (Figures *evolve* 29.30 & 29.31 🖱).

GI lymphoma

For gastric NHL, plan using barium and treat the stomach empty. Anteroposterior fields are often optimal, but CT planning may spare the kidneys or spinal cord especially for post-chemotherapy residual abdominal masses. Rectal lymphoma is planned as for carcinoma.

Bone

The whole of the affected bone should be included in the initial volume and a second phase used for the last 10 Gy. A parallel-opposed pair of fields is used, shielding soft tissues with a 2 cm margin.

Breast

The whole breast, axillary and supraclavicular nodes should be included and planned as for carcinoma.

Spleen

The CTV is the edge of the spleen. CT planning may help minimize the dose to the kidney. Palliative splenic RT is described below under leukaemia.

Toxicity

Acute side effects

All treatments cause tiredness and temporary hair loss and mucositis in the treated area, from 2 weeks into treatment and for about a month afterwards. Dry mouth and altered taste are usual where salivary tissue has to be treated, and may be lasting after bilateral high neck fields, with an increased risk of dental problems.

Late effects

The organs most subject to late effects are the thyroid, lung, heart and spinal cord. There is an increased risk of solid tumours in irradiated areas (see 000).

Thyroid

Up to 30% develop clinical or biochemical hypothyroidism several years after bilateral neck treatment, requiring thyroxine replacement therapy.

Lung

Lung function is minimally impaired in about one-third of patients undergoing mantle therapy. Symptoms, if any, are seen after about 6 weeks: dry cough and dysponea, which usually settle with steroids (prednisolone 40–60 mg/day).

Cardiac

Radiation-induced cardiac disease occurs in less than 5% of patients after mantle treatment and less with involved fields, although data are scarce. It can rarely present as transient pericarditis within a few months of treatment or much later as cardiomyopathy or premature coronary artery disease.

Neurological

Lhermitte's syndrome is a transient numbness, tingling (paresthesia) or an 'electric shock'-like sensation in the arms or legs following mantle or neck irradiation from 2 to 4 months afterwards. It may be due to transient demyelination of the spinal cord due to damage to oligodendrocytes but does not lead to permanent damage.

Bone

Avascular necrosis of the femoral head occurs in 2% of Hodgkin's patients, particularly following chemotherapy and steroid treatment, but radiotherapy including the hip is a contributory factor. Symptoms of hip pain develop on average about 2 years following the start of chemotherapy. Total hip replacement may be necessary. The humeral head may also be affected if it could not be shielded.

Fertility

Pelvic radiotherapy with lymphoma doses will cause infertility in most young people: for males sperm banking is effective but for women surgical oophoropexy and, if possible, cryopreservation of ovarian tissue are advised. HRT should be prescribed for premature menopause.

Growth

Growth retardation in children after radiotherapy includes limited height but also, for instance, thinning of the neck muscles and shortening of the clavicles from neck treatment.

Leukaemia

Cranial irradiation may be given as described elsewhere for ALL.

Total body irradiation (TBI)

14.4 Gy midplane dose in eight twice-daily fractions over 4 days (6 MV photons) or 12 Gy in six fractions over 3 days.

Technique

Techniques vary in detail from centre to centre, and some have machines dedicated to extended field treatment for TBI (Figures *evolve* 29.32–29.35 🖱).

Using a linear accelerator at extended FSD (about 4 meters), a lateral beam can treat the whole patient, who is then turned through 180° for the other side.

Thermoluminescent dosimeters (TLD) are positioned at regular intervals along each side of the body and tissue compensators can be conveniently attached to a rectangular Perspex screen placed alongside the patient. Typically, 1 mm, 8 mm and 6 mm brass compensators are placed over the head, neck and thorax respectively. Doses are measured at each fraction so as to adjust arm position and compensators, if necessary, to ensure dose homogeneity within ±5%.

Side effects

All are more common with single-fraction than with fractionated TBI.

1. Pneumonitis. Lungs are the dose-limiting organs. Since pneumonitis commonly occurs following bone marrow transplantation in the absence of radiation, the role of TBI in its causation is difficult to assess.
2. Cataract. The incidence of cataract is about 20% between 3 and 6 years.
3. Hepatic veno-occlusive disease. This is seen in up to 25% of patients but is usually mild. However, the mortality of established disease is high (30%).
4. Fertility. In females under 25, periods may return but in others permanent sterility is to be expected. Men are rendered azoospermic and should have sperm frozen.
5. Hypothyroidism. Hypothyroidism occurs in up to 30%.
6. Growth delay. Growth hormone secretion may be impaired, especially if previous cranial irradiation has been given.
7. Second malignancy.

Splenic radiotherapy

Used in myeloproliferative disorders, mainly CML and myelofibrosis, to shrink an uncomfortably large spleen and/or to improve blood counts by reducing splenic consumption: this is a delicate balance as counts will initially drop.

Dose

0.25 Gy per day, increasing by 0.25 Gy per day up to 1.5–2 Gy daily to a total dose of 3 Gy with 4–6 MV photons – if blood counts are very low.

Alternatively 0.5 Gy per day for 6–10 fractions, total dose 3–5 Gy.

Target volume

Irradiation of the whole of the spleen is not necessary to achieve shrinkage and symptomatic benefit. The kidney is dose-limiting but can tolerate 20 Gy so treatment can be repeated.

Field borders

The spleen can be outlined clinically or using CT or simulator screening.

Technique

Direct anterior or lateral fields (e.g. 15 × 10 cm) or a parallel pair can be used.

Myeloma

Radical treatment of solitary plasmacytoma: 40–50 Gy in 20–25 fractions. Rib deposits (Figures *evolve* 29.36 & 29.37 🖱).

Palliative treatment of multiple myeloma

Spinal deposits

8 Gy single fraction with a posterior beam using 250–300 kV or 4–10 MV photons to cover abnormal bone/s plus one vertebra on either side, about 8 cm width to include the transverse processes of the vertebrae, wider to include any paravertebral mass.

Soft tissue mass/spinal cord compression/ pathological fracture/severe pain

20 Gy in five fractions. Consider 30 Gy in 10 fractions for e.g. soft tissue with extensive bone destruction when disease is mainly in one area.

Rib deposits

8 Gy single fraction
Orthovoltage can be used to the painful area plus a margin of a few centimeters along the rib.

Hemibody radiotherapy for widespread deposits

This is now rarely used since systemic treatment options have increased.

If treating both in sequence, a gap of 6 weeks is necessary for recovery of blood counts.

Position

Supine with arms folded across the chest, hands on shoulders.
Upper half: 6 Gy single fraction
Lower half: 8 Gy single fraction

Field borders

Upper half: from chin to around umbilicus, and width to cover shoulders.
Lower half: from umbilicus to maximum field size inferiorly and width to cover iliac bones.

Technique

Extended FSD (140 cm), and anteroposterior parallel beams. The abdominal border is tattooed and a lateral film taken for matching of the other hemibody field (see under inverted Y).

Acute side effects

Nausea and vomiting, prevented with, e.g. granisetron 2 mg one hour before radiotherapy, dexamethasone 4 mg bd, plus metoclopramide 10 mg prn. Pneumonitis is rare at 6 Gy but has an increasing incidence above this dose to the whole lungs.

Diarrhea occurs in a third of patients 3–5 days after lower hemibody treatment, controllable with codeine or loperamide.

Pancytopenia is common and contributes to lethargy. Blood and platelet transfusions may be required.

Mycosis fungoides

Local

10 Gy in 5 daily fractions
80–100 kV for superficial lesions and 250–300 kV, or electrons of appropriate energy, for plaque or tumour stage.

Total body electron therapy (TBE)

This is a specialized treatment offered in regional centres, and techniques vary.
30 Gy in six fractions (once weekly) for 6 weeks.

Four fields can cover the whole body at extended source to surface distance (SSD) (120 cm) with the patient supine. Lead shielding is applied to protect the eyes and the finger nails. If the eyelids are involved, a lead internal eye shield is used. If 5 or 8 MeV electrons are used, Perspex is used to reduce the depth of penetration. Skin in folds (e.g. axilla and groin) is spared with this technique and may be marked for separate treatment when skin erythema develops. This can be minimized by positioning patients carefully.

Temporary alopecia and loss of nails are followed by permanent skin atrophy, oedema and radiodermatitis.

CHEMOTHERAPY REGIMENS AND TOXICITIES

All cause myelosuppression and the risk of fatal neutropenic sepsis, particularly the intravenous combination therapies, of which most cause total alopecia and the risk of infertility, particularly in men. The problems of nausea and vomiting (particularly due to anthracyclines, dacarbazine and mustine) have been transformed by new antiemetics in the HT3 blocker class (ondansetron, granisetron). Anthracyclines cause cardiomyopathy if a high cumulative dose has to be given but this is rarely a problem with first-line treatment. The vinca alkaloids (vincristine, vinblastine) cause peripheral neuropathy and constipation. Bleomycin can rarely cause pulmonary fibrosis which can be fatal. Oral chlorambucil alone is the least acutely toxic treatment used; it does not cause alopecia or much nausea but, like other alkylating agents (cyclophosphamide, melphalan, mustine), causes some irreversible toxicity to bone marrow and gonads.

Hodgkin's lymphoma

ABVD

Doxorubicin (Adriamycin) 25 mg/m^2 i.v.	Days 1 and 15
Bleomycin 10 000 units/m^2 i.v.	Days 1 and 15
Vinblastine 6 mg/m^2 i.v.	Days 1 and 15
Dacarbazine 375 mg/m^2 i.v.	Days 1 and 15
Repeated every 28 days	

Acute toxicity is marked (alopecia is usual, nausea, myelosuppression, constipation, painful veins, pulmonary fibrosis from bleomycin which is fatal in 1–30%, highest in elderly patients), but there is minimal risk of infertility or leukaemia with ABVD, so this is standard treatment.

ChlVPP

Chlorambucil 6 mg/m^2 (max. 10 mg) orally	Days 1–14
Vinblastine 6 mg/m^2 (max. 10 mg) i.v.	Days 1 and 8
Procarbazine 100 mg/m^2 orally	Days 1–14
Prednisolone 40 mg orally	Days 1–14
Repeated every 28 days	

This is well tolerated but with 3% risk of later leukemogenesis, and infertility is induced in men, but less likely in women. Only the vinblastine is intravenous and hair loss is unusual. Used less commonly but may be considered if ABVD is deemed unsuitable.

Stanford V

A multiple-drug, 12-week regimen with high control rates but radiotherapy to all masses >5 cm is mandatory.

BEACOPP

Intensive first-line treatment for high-risk patients.
Bleomycin
Etoposide
Adriamycin
Cyclophosphamide
Vincristine (Oncovin)
Procarbazine
Prednisolone

Non-Hodgkin's lymphoma

Follicular grade 1 and 2 and marginal zone

Oral chlorambucil: 10 mg daily for 14 days every 28 days × 6
Well tolerated with rare reports of serious toxicity but myelotoxic.

R-COP (also known as R-CVP)

As R-CHOP – see below, but without doxorubicin.

Mantle cell

FC

Fludarabine
Cyclophosphamide
Repeated every 28 days

Myelotoxic but well tolerated oral regimen without alopecia.

Diffuse large B-cell, T-cell-rich, B cell, follicular grade 3 (and for T-cell lymphomas)

Use CHOP alone without rituximab.

R-CHOP

Standard regimen; trials suggest adding etoposide or giving at 2-week rather then 3-week intervals, with GCSF. Alopecia, nausea, myelosuppression, peripheral neuropathy, antibody reaction, steroid effects, cardiomyopathy.

Rituximab 375 mg/m^2	Day 1
Cyclophosphamide 750 mg/m^2 i.v.	Day 1
Doxorubicin 50 mg/m^2 i.v.	Day 1
Vincristine 1.4 mg/m^2 (max. 2mg) i.v.	Day 1
Prednisolone 50 mg/m^2 orally	Days 1–5
Repeated every 21 days (minimum six courses)	

R-PMitCEBO

Equivalent outcome but weekly regimen; may be easier to tolerate for some patients.

Mitoxantrone	Day 1
Cyclophosphamide	Day 1
Etoposide	Day 1
Bleomycin	Day 8
Vincristine	Day 8
Rituximab 375 mg/m^2	Days 1, 21, 42, 63

Continued weekly, alternating days 1 and 8 for 12 –16 weeks

CNS prophylaxis

Methotrexate × 4 doses
1 g/m^2 iv on day 14
or 12.5 mg it on day 1 or 2
with each of 1st 4 cycles.

Burkitt type, lymphoblastic, (some DLBCL if 100% MIB-1 staining)

CODOX-M/IVAC

Intensive myelosuppressive regimen with CNS treatment.

Relapsed NHL

(R)IVE, (R)ICE

Rituximab
Ifosfamide
Etoposide (Vepesid) in IVE or carboplatin in ICE
Epirubicin
Reinduction regimens to minimize bulk and mobilize stem cells for harvesting.

BEAM

Busulphan
Etoposide

Cytosine arabinoside (Ara-C)
Melphalan

Myeloablative regimen

Oral etoposide: 50 mg bd po daily for 10 days q 3 – 4 weeks: palliative single agent.

Myeloma

CTD

Cyclophosphamide
Thalidomide
Dexamethasone

Generally well tolerated oral regimen. Specific side effects include pulmonary fibrosis (cyclophosphamide), neuropathy, thrombosis, teratogenesis, and thyroid dysfunction (thalidomide).

Bortezomib

A proteosome inhibitor with various sites of action. Main side effects include neuropathy and thrombocytopenia.

Lenalidomide

A novel analogue of thalidomide with similar side effects but neuropathy less likely.

Acute myeloid leukaemia

DA

Daunorubicin
Cytarabine (Ara C)

Significantly myelosuppressive. Commonly causes mucositis (oral ulcers, diarrhea) and, more rarely, conjunctivitis and cardiomyopathy.

FURTHER READING

Kyle RA, Rajkumar SV. Treatment of multiple myeloma: a comprehensive review. Clin Lymphoma Myeloma 2009;9:278–88.

Yahalom J. Radiation therapy after R-CHOP for diffuse large B cell lymphoma: the gain remains. J Clin Oncol 2010;28:4105–7.

Herbst C, Rehan FA, Brillant C, et al. Combined modality treatment improves tumour control and overall survival in patients with early stage Hodgkin's lymphoma: a systematic review. Haematologia (Budap) 2010;95:494–500.

Girinsky T, van der Maazen R, Specht L, et al. Involved-node radiotherapy (INRT) in patients with early Hodgkin lymphoma: concepts and guidelines. Radiother Oncol 2006;79:270–7.

Yahalom J, Mauch P. The involved field is back: issues in delineating the radiation field in Hodgkin's disease. Ann Oncol 2002;13(Suppl. 1):79–83.

Press OW. Radioimmunotherapy for non-Hodgkin's lymphomas: a historical perspective. Semin Oncol 2003;30(Suppl. 4):10–21.

Gustavsson A, Osterman B, Cavallin-Stahl E. A systematic overview of radiation therapy effects in Hodgkin's lymphoma. Acta Oncol 2003;42:589–604.

Kheng-Wei Y, Mikhaeel NG. Role of radiotherapy in modern treatment of Hodgkin's lymphoma. Adv Hematol 2011; Article ID 258797.

Ganem G, Cartron G, Girinsky T, et al. Localised low-dose radiotherapy for follicular lymphoma: history, clinical results, mechanisms of action, and future outlooks. Int J Radiat Oncol Biol Phys 2010;78:975–82.

Hoppe RT. The indolent extranodal lymphomas: what is the role of radiation therapy? Haematol Meet Rep 2009;3:10–4.

Strauchen JA. Immunophenotypic and molecular studies in the diagnosis and classification of malignant lymphoma. Cancer Invest 2004;22:138–48.

Coiffier B, et al. CHOP chemotherapy plus rituximab compared with CHOP alone in elderly patients with diffuse large B-cell lymphoma. N Engl J Med 2002;346:235–42.

Salles G, Seymour JF, Offner F, et al. Rituximab maintenance for 2 years in patients with high tumour burden follicular lymphoma responding to rituximab plus chemotherapy (PRIMA): a phase 3, randomised controlled trial. Lancet 2010;377:42–51.

Hallek M, Fischer K, Fingerle-Rowson G, et al. Addition of rituximab to fludarabine and cyclophosphamide in patients with chronic lymphocytic leukaemia: a randomised, open-label, phase 3 trial. Lancet 2010;376:1164–74.

The diagnosis and management of multiple myeloma, British Committee of Standards in Haematology; 2010. Available online: http://www.bcshguidelines.com/.

Armitage JO. Early stage Hodgkin's lymphoma. N Engl J Med 2010;363:653–62.

Barrett AJ, Savan BN. Stem cell transplantation with reduced-intensity conditioning regimens: a review of ten years experience with new transplant concepts and new therapeutic agents. Leukaemia 2006;20:1661–72.

Bruker B. Translation of the Philadelphia chromsosome into therapy for CML. Blood 2008;112:4808–17.

Younes et al. Brentuximab Vedotin (SGN-35) for Relapsed CD30-Positive Lymphomas. N Engl J Med 2010;363:1812–21.

Burger JA. Inhibiting B-Cell Receptor Signaling Pathways in Chronic Lymphocytic Leukaemia. Current hematologic malignancy reports. Curr Hematol Malig Rep 2011 Nov 22; [Epub ahead of print].

EVOLVE CONTENTS (available online at: http://evolve.elsevier.com/Symonds/radiotherapy/)

Chapter | 30 |

Tumours of the central nervous system

Neil G. Burnet, Kate E. Burton, Sarah J. Jefferies

INTRODUCTION

Primary tumours of the central nervous system (CNS) are relatively uncommon, accounting for only 2% of cancer deaths. However, the effect on the individual with a primary CNS tumour is frequently devastating, and brain tumours lead, on average, to a greater loss of life per patient than any other adult tumour. Primary CNS tumours affect patients of all ages, from childhood to old age, with a rising incidence from middle age onwards. In childhood, they are the commonest solid tumours (as opposed to leukaemias). The overall annual incidence is around 7 per 100 000 population, giving approximately 4400 people newly diagnosed with a brain tumour in the UK each year.

There is a huge range in outcome for patients with primary CNS tumours, from almost guaranteed cure in some conditions (e.g. germinoma) to almost guaranteed fatality in others (e.g. glioblastoma (GBM)). For patients with CNS tumours, a holistic approach is always required and, for many, involvement of the palliative care services is highly desirable. For many patients, driving is forbidden after the diagnosis of brain tumour (see below).

Tumour types

Overall, about 80% of CNS tumours are primary and 20% secondary. However, the proportions depend exactly on how the patient population is gathered. In our centre, approximately 200 new CNS cases are seen per year, and only 6% are due to metastases. The latter patients are generally seen and looked after by the site-specific specialist teams, based on the tissue of origin.

The major types of primary tumour are given in Table 30.1, and the percentages of these tumour types in our own practice are shown in Figure 30.1. The majority

Table 30.1 A simplified classification of the major categories of brain tumour

Intrinsic tumours (i.e. those arising within the brain substance)
Glial tumours
    Astrocytoma
    Oligodendroglioma
    Oligoastrocytoma
    Glioblastoma (GBM)
Ependymoma
Medulloblastoma
Germinoma / teratoma
Lymphoma (primary CNS lymphoma – PCNSL)

Extrinsic tumours of the brain covering
Meningioma

Other tumours
Pituitary adenoma and craniopharyngioma
Acoustic (vestibular) schwannoma
Skull base chordoma and chondrosarcoma

Cerebral metastases

Notes:
1. Glioblastoma used to be known as 'glioblastoma multiforme'
2. The glial tumours are divided into four grades: grade I and II together constitute low-grade gliomas (LGGs), while grade III and IV tumours together are the high-grade gliomas (HGGs). The term 'anaplastic' is equivalent to a grade of III. A grade IV glioma is a GBM.
3. Grade I tumours are rare in adults, though they do occur. They also appear in adult practice in patients treated as children who have outgrown the paediatric services.
4. A large number of other uncommon tumours also occur.
5. Medulloblastoma is predominantly a disease of childhood, but does occasionally occur in adults (i.e. patients over 16).

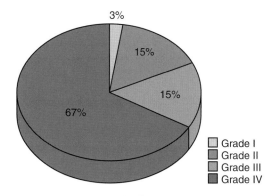

Figure 30.2 Percentages of different grades of glioma. Grade IV glioma is glioblastoma.

of tumours (58%) are gliomas (Figure 30.1). Of the gliomas, two-thirds are glioblastomas (Figure 30.2), making this the most common type of primary CNS tumour in adults. Gliomas in general, and glioblastomas, in particular, are devastating tumours, and therefore consume much of the energy and resources of the neuro-oncology unit. Although gliomas represent the major diagnosis of primary brain tumours, over a third of new referrals are for other tumour types, so appropriate attention also needs to be directed towards those.

Gliomas are graded according to the World Health Organization (WHO) 2000 classification, on a scale of I to IV, where IV is the most malignant. Grade I and grade II gliomas together are termed low-grade gliomas. Grade I tumours are more typical of childhood but occasionally occur in adults. Grade III and grade IV tumours together constitute high-grade gliomas. Grade III tumours may also be called 'anaplastic' and grade IV gliomas are known as 'glioblastomas'.

Gliomas arise from astrocytes and oligodendrocytes, cells which nourish and support neurons. Primary tumours of neurons alone are extremely uncommon, though they do exist (e.g. neurocytoma). There is a surprising large range of very rare tumours within the brain, but apart from those mentioned explicitly in Table 30.1, and described below, their overall management and outcome can generally be inferred from the grade of the tumour.

The male to female ratio for gliomas is 1.4 to 1. Meningiomas are commoner in females than males, in the ratio of 2:1, which is unusual in oncology. There are only two definite aetiological factors for the development of brain tumours: exposure to ionizing radiation and genetic predisposition. Genetic syndromes include Li-Fraumeni syndrome, neurofibromatosis types 1 and 2, Gorlin's syndrome and ataxia-telangiectasia. These syndromes may account for 1–2% of brain tumours. They are normally easily identifiable, and many of the cases present in childhood. Other genetic factors may play a part but as yet are ill understood. Mobile phones and electricity power lines

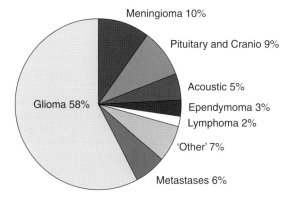

Figure 30.1 Frequency of the main tumour types in 1300 new adult neuro-oncology referrals. Metastases are few, accounting for only 6% in this specialized neuro-oncology practice.

have been proposed as predisposing factors, but good evidence exists that these do not influence risk.

Secondary CNS metastases may arise from primary tumours at almost any site. However, certain cancers have a propensity to metastasize to the brain. Lung cancer accounts for 60% of metastases, followed by breast (15%). Other tumours causing metastases include kidney, colon, melanoma, pancreas, and ovary. Metastases are usually multiple but occasionally can be solitary. The majority (85%) develops in the cerebrum.

Anatomy of the CNS

Anatomy is the key to understanding the presentation of neurological tumours, their spread, and concepts about treatment, particularly with radiotherapy and surgery.

Anatomy of the brain

Tissues of the brain

Within the brain substance itself, tissue is divided into grey and white matter. Grey matter covers the surface folds of the brain (gyri), and broadly is the location of active neurons. White matter lies below the gray matter and contains fibres which communicate with other parts of the brain and body, equivalent to electrical cabling. At a cellular level, the brain is composed of both neurons and cells designed to support the structure and function of those neurons, the glial supporting cells. Almost all tumours of the brain substance arise in the glial supporting cells (principally astrocytoma and oligodendroglioma). Primary tumours of neurons are very rare.

The major structures of the brain

Figure 30.3 shows the outside of the brain to explain the nomenclature of the principal lobes. In right-handed patients, the left hemisphere is almost invariably dominant.

The frontal lobe is very large, extending back to the central sulcus, which divides it from the parietal lobe. The motor cortex sits immediately in front of the central sulcus. More anteriorly, the frontal lobe is responsible for intellect, motivation and emotional response. Damage to the frontal lobes can affect intellectual performance, including reasoning, memory, the initiation of activity and insight. The medial frontal lobe is particularly important for these activities and damage to both medial frontal lobes is extremely destructive to the intellect. The motor speech centre (Broca's area) lies in the dominant frontal lobe (see Figure 30.3).

The parietal lobe extends from the central sulcus posteriorly onto the occipital lobe, and is also large. The parietal lobe has large areas which are silent, with no obvious functional activity. Immediately behind the central sulcus is the sensorimotor cortex, which deals predominantly with reception of sensory information. In reality, there are other areas adjacent to both motor and sensory cortices which support those functions.

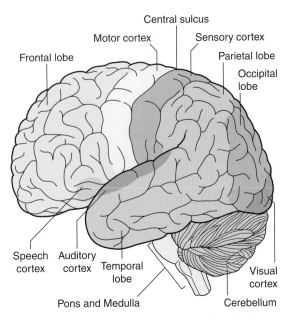

Figure 30.3 The major anatomical divisions of the brain.

At the most posterior part of the cerebral hemisphere is the occipital cortex, which deals with central processing of visual information. The optic radiation connects the optic tracts to the occipital cortex, and runs through the temporal and parietal lobes to arrive at its destination. Tumours lying along that pathway can therefore affect vision.

Inferiorly and laterally, with its tip in the middle cranial fossa, lies the temporal lobe. The medial part is involved in short-term memory. In the dominant hemisphere, the temporal lobe is the location for one of the speech centres, the auditory cortex.

The pons and medulla together form the brainstem. These have processing functions, important functional centres such as the respiratory centre, and also carry all motor and sensory information between the cerebral cortex and spinal cord (Figures 30.3 and 30.4). Even small lesions within the brainstem have very severe neurological effects. The function of the cerebellum is the subconscious control of movement. Damage to the cerebellum therefore leads to ataxia and other difficulties with coordinated movement.

The lobes of the brain communicate by extensive pathways made up of white matter. These run from front to back, side to side, and up and down through the brain. Tumours which spread through white matter tracts (especially the gliomas) therefore have access to pathways which can allow them to spread extensively. The corpus callosum (see Figure 30.4) is the major route of side to side communication between the two cerebral hemispheres. High-grade gliomas lying medially in the hemisphere often involve this structure, which allows spread into the opposite hemisphere.

Functional imaging, especially using magnetic resonance imaging (MRI), has demonstrated that damage to

Figure 30.4 Normal anatomy of the central nervous system. MR midline sagittal section.
(Courtesy Dr L Turnbull, MRI Unit, Sheffield)

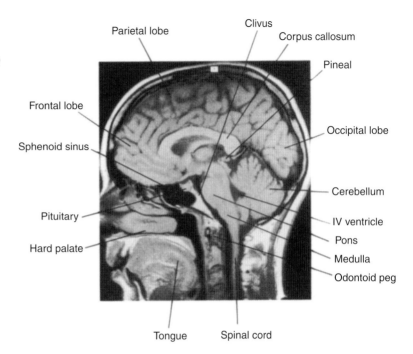

Parietal lobe

Clivus

Corpus callosum

Pineal

Frontal lobe

Sphenoid sinus

Occipital lobe

Cerebellum

Pituitary

IV ventricle

Pons

Hard palate

Medulla

Odontoid peg

Tongue   Spinal cord

particular areas of the brain, for example the motor cortex, can lead to some function being taken over by other areas, provided that the rate of damage is slow. In the adult, this can occur in only a modest way, but can explain why, in some circumstances, patients do not lose all the neurological function that would be expected.

Anatomy of the cerebrospinal fluid (CSF) pathways and hydrocephalus

The major cerebrospinal fluid (CSF) structures are shown in Figure 30.5. CSF is produced by the choroid plexus within the two lateral ventricles, and flows into the third ventricle anteriorly through the foramen of Munro (Figure 30.5). CSF exits the third ventricle posteriorly through the aqueduct, and flows into the fourth ventricle. From there, CSF leaves the fourth ventricle through three foramina (the foramina of Luschka laterally and the foramen of Magendie in the midline) to surround the outside of the brain. A small amount also passes down the central canal in the spinal cord. CSF is actively absorbed by the arachnoid granulations which protrude into the major venous sinuses, especially the superior sagittal sinus at the vertex of the skull. The CSF canals are lined by ependymal cells, from which ependymomas arise. These tumours are therefore related in space to the ventricular system.

Disturbance in the flow or absorption of CSF causes hydrocephalus. Obstruction of the flow before the exit foramina in the fourth ventricle leads to 'obstructive' hydrocephalus. Obstruction of the arachnoid granulations leads to 'communicating' hydrocephalus.

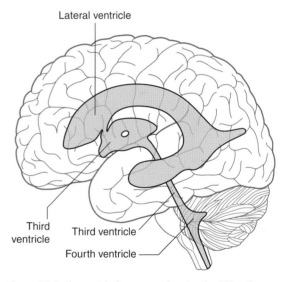

Lateral ventricle

Third ventricle

Third ventricle

Fourth ventricle

Figure 30.5 The ventricular system, showing the CSF pathways. See text for further details.

In neuro-oncology, tumours most commonly cause obstructive hydrocephalus. This is normally the result of obstruction in the fourth ventricle, by tumours growing in or around the ventricle (such as medulloblastoma or ependymoma), or within the cerebellum (most commonly metastases). The next most common location for obstruction is the aqueduct, from compression by tumour in adjacent brain or the pineal gland. More proximal obstruction can also occur at the foramen of Munro, usually from infiltrative high-grade glioma, causing hydrocephalus in one or both lateral ventricles.

Communicating hydrocephalus can be caused directly by tumour, when extensive meningeal involvement occurs. This is almost always metastatic (most commonly from breast cancer), and it is rare. A commoner cause of communicating hydrocephalus in neuro-oncology practice, is blood in the CSF, resulting from surgery or a spontaneous bleed directly from a tumour. Blood can occlude the pores in the arachnoid granulations. Often this resolves spontaneously but, occasionally, a CSF shunt (such as a ventriculoperitoneal (VP) shunt) must be inserted. Infection is also a cause, through the same mechanism.

Anatomy of the skull and meninges

The skull itself is divided into three fossae. The frontal fossa contains the frontal lobe; the middle cranial fossa contains the temporal lobe; the posterior cranial fossa contains the cerebellum. The cerebellum is divided from the rest of the cranial contents by the tentorium cerebelli ('tent'), except for an aperture through which the brainstem passes. The two cerebral hemispheres are divided by the falx cerebri. These two structures are composed of layers of tough meninges, and are designed to 'damp' movements of the brain which might otherwise be damaging to the delicate brain substance. They are relatively rigid. The falx and tentorium cannot be infiltrated by gliomas, and so present efficient barriers to their spread. Meningiomas, on the other hand, can spread along their surface, and their potential direction of spread can be appreciated by understanding this anatomy.

The meninges consist of three layers. The outer dura mater (usually known simply as dura) is a tough membrane, which acts like a periosteum; it is the part visible on imaging, and forms the falx and tent. Below and closely applied to the dura is the arachnoid mater. Below this lies the pia mater, a thin delicate layer which covers every surface and fold of the brain substance. In some places, there is a space (the subarachnoid space) between the arachnoid and pia, crossed by thin strands with a cobweb-like appearance (hence the origin of the name arachnoid). The dura lines the whole cranial cavity, including the skull base. In some areas, the dura splits to form venous channels, such as the superior sagittal sinus, and the cavernous sinuses. It also forms two important folds, the tentorium cerebelli and the falx cerebri, which are continuous with the dura covering the skull vault and skull base.

CLINICAL FEATURES – PRESENTATION OF BRAIN TUMOURS

Presenting symptoms and signs of CNS tumours are characteristic; patients may present with one or more classes of symptoms, as follows.

Specific focal neurological deficit

CNS tumours may make their presence known by local damage, leading to specific deficits dependent on the location of the tumour. For example, a meningioma affecting the motor cortex will produce weakness and stiffness typically in a limb, specifically depending on which part of the motor cortex is affected. A glioblastoma affecting the frontal lobe produces intellectual, motivational and memory problems. In this way, symptoms and signs indicate the site of the tumour, which can be confirmed with imaging. Tumours arising in eloquent areas typically present earlier than those in silent areas of the brain, simply because they produce symptoms when they are smaller. Tumours which grow slowly, for example meningioma, produce an insidious onset, with relatively mild symptoms and signs, despite often being surprisingly large when detected. Tumours which grow rapidly, and destructively, such as glioblastoma, produce symptoms and signs which often appear to commence abruptly.

Symptoms and signs relating to specific parts of the brain are as follows:

- frontal lobe – intellectual impairment and personality change.
- parietal lobe – sensory or visual inattention.
- fronto-temporo-parietal – speech disturbance, especially dysphasia
- occipital lobe – visual field defects.
- brainstem – cranial nerve defects, sensory or motor disturbance.
- cerebellum – loss of coordination of movement.

Epileptic seizure

Almost all CNS tumours can potentially cause epileptic seizures (as can craniotomy to treat them). These can take a number of forms, including generalized 'grand mal' seizures, 'Jacksonian' motor seizures, sensory seizures, and 'petit mal' absence attacks. Seizures are typically associated with slow-growing, low-grade gliomas, especially oligodendrogliomas. Seizures will often bring a tumour to light before other symptoms and signs and, for that reason, the presence of seizure is associated with a slightly improved survival in patients with high-grade glioma. Most patients are controlled with simple anticonvulsant medication, but where this is problematic, the advice of a neurologist is valuable.

Raised intracranial pressure

Raised intracranial pressure (ICP) typically produces a triad of symptoms: headaches, which are typically worse in the morning; nausea and vomiting; and papilloedema (oedema of the optic disk). Raised intracranial pressure most commonly arises as the result of obstructive hydrocephalus, and is therefore particularly associated with tumours in the posterior fossa. This can also be associated with drowsiness, mild confusion and sometimes with personality change.

Non-specific symptoms

Non-specific symptoms are common, and typical of CNS tumours. Such symptoms may be very difficult to identify as significant in the early phase of the illness. Headache, which may be local or generalized, but not related to raised ICP, occurs in some patients. The other characteristic symptom, particularly of high-grade glioma, is tiredness. Early symptoms may be frustratingly non-specific, and a patient who complains of vague headache, tiredness and feeling off color is not likely to be investigated for a primary CNS tumour.

PRINCIPLES OF MANAGEMENT

Although most patients come to oncology with a definitive diagnosis, it is important for oncologists to contribute to the multidisciplinary management of CNS patients.

Diagnosis – a combination of history, imaging and pathology

In neuro-oncology, perhaps more than any other area, it is helpful to combine information from the patient's history and examination findings, as well as imaging results and histology in determining the definitive diagnosis. The history and physical signs, especially the duration and any family history, may indicate a likely diagnosis or help to indicate whether the condition is a high-grade malignancy rather than a low-grade or benign tumour.

Typically, the diagnosis is suggested by computed tomography (CT) or magnetic resonance imaging (MRI). In some tumour types, such as vestibular schwannoma (acoustic neuroma), imaging is definitive; in other cases, imaging offers only a differential diagnosis. Classical difficulties arise in distinguishing glioma from primary cerebral lymphoma, and solitary metastasis from abscess or small glioma. Benign lesions can also have imaging appearances suggestive of malignancy. Therefore, biopsy is crucial for obtaining a definitive diagnosis.

Some CNS tumours, especially gliomas, are rather heterogeneous, and it is understood that biopsy material may not necessarily be representative of the whole tumour. Occasionally, it may contain necrotic material only. Thus, clinical history and imaging appearances must also be considered in defining the exact diagnosis.

Performance status in the treatment decision

Performance status is an important predictor of outcome, including survival, particularly for patients with glioma (Table 30.2). It also indicates how well the patient is likely to tolerate treatment. This is an important factor when

Table 30.2 WHO performance status and Glasgow coma scale (GCS).

The WHO Performance Status is useful in assessing patient capabilities, especially with respect to activities of daily living. The Glasgow Coma Scale (GCS) is a measure of conscious level.

WHO PERFORMANCE STATUS

0 = Able to carry out all normal activity without restriction
1 = Restricted in physically strenuous activity but ambulatory and able to carry out light work
2 = Ambulatory and capable of all self-care but unable to carry out any work; up and about >50% of waking hours
3 = Capable of only limited self-care; confined to bed or chair >50% of waking hours
4 = Completely disabled. Cannot carry out any self-care; totally confined to bed or chair

Glasgow Coma Scale (GCS)

Eyes open	Spontaneously	4
	To speech	3
	To stimulus	2
	None	1
Best verbal response	Orientated	5
	Confused	4
	Inappropriate words	3
	Incomprehensible	2
	None	1
Best motor response	Obeys commands	6
	Localize stimulus	5
	Flexion – withdrawal	4
	Flexion – abnormal	3
	Extension	2
	No response	1
Best score	**15**	
Worst	**3**	

recommending a treatment program. The choice can be between radical, palliative, or active supportive care. For patients with disabling neurology, especially those with GBM, supportive care may be the most appropriate option.

Principles of neurosurgery

The acquisition of histological material to define the diagnosis is extremely important. However, in many cases, there is also a role for a more extended procedure to debulk or remove the tumour, and relieve pressure effects (see sections on individual tumours). Surgical decompression improves symptoms quickly, allows reduced steroid doses, and facilitates radiotherapy, especially in patients with high-grade gliomas (HGGs).

Occasional HGGs grow with a cystic component to the tumour. If fluid reaccumulates, then a small catheter can be placed into the cyst and attached to a subcutaneous (Ommaya) reservoir. By inserting a needle through the skin, fluid can be aspirated without the need for a further surgical procedure.

Patients who present with, or develop, hydrocephalus may need a shunting procedure to redirect the flow of CSF. In adults, this is usually done with a ventriculoperitoneal (VP) shunt. Some patients with obstructive hydrocephalus can be successfully treated by a third ventriculostomy, avoiding the need for a shunt. In this procedure, a perforation is made in the floor of the third ventricle, allowing CSF to escape, and circumventing the obstruction.

Principles of radiotherapy planning for CNS tumours

The fundamental principles of radiotherapy (RT) planning and treatment delivery apply to CNS tumours. These include accurate and reproducible immobilization, high quality imaging to localize the tumour and critical normal structures, three-dimensional conformal or intensity modulated planning, and high precision treatment delivery.

Immobilization devices include Perspex or thermoplastic beam direction shells or, where a higher precision is required, a relocatable stereotactic head frame. The optimal position for the patient depends on the location of the tumour, and on the immobilization devices available. A supine position is more comfortable for the patient. Using couch extensions, such as an 'S' frame or a relocatable stereotactic radiotherapy (SRT) head frame, allows treatment of posterior lesions with the patient supine. With a Perspex or thermoplastic shell, patients with posterior lesions need to be treated prone, to allow appropriate beam directions without collision with the couch. The exception is for palliative RT, using parallel-opposed lateral fields, where the patient can be positioned supine. For craniospinal axis treatment, a prone treatment position allows palpation of the spine and accurate visualization of matching field junctions. There is no role for lateral shells, which are unstable and uncomfortable. Shells should be cut out to improve skin sparing.

Most planning is based on CT, because this delivers exact patient geometry and position without distortion, and because CT density is required for accurate dosimetry calculation. Preferably, intravenous contrast should be used because this enhances discrimination of the target. Although this changes the CT numbers slightly, dosimetry is affected by 1% or less. In most circumstances, tumours are less well demonstrated on CT than on MRI, and MRI should be considered an essential modality for planning. Typically, MRI does not have to be performed in the treatment position, provided suitable image coregistration software is available.

The correct choice of MRI sequence must be made, in order to optimize definition of the tumour. However, CT and MRI are complementary. While MRI is in general the better modality for showing tumour, CT is extremely useful to determine the extent of bone involvement, or the extent of a non-invasive tumour which is limited by bone. In the next few years, additional imaging is likely to be incorporated into planning, especially for gliomas. This includes newer MR sequences (such as diffusion weighted and diffusion tensor imaging), MR spectroscopy and PET (positron emission tomography) imaging. In some meningiomas that have been completely resected, coregistration with the preoperative MRI may be helpful in determining the location of the tumour and possible spread.

The definitions of gross tumour volume (GTV), clinical target volume (CTV) and planning target volume (PTV) as outlined in ICRU 83 should be used for planning purposes. Imaging shows the extent of the GTV; historical data are used to define a CTV margin around it, which is typically the same in all patients with the same condition. The PTV margin is designed to account for uncertainties in planning and treatment, and has systematic (i.e. 'treatment preparation') and random (i.e. 'treatment delivery') elements. The margin should be added based on the recipe formula outlined the British Institute of Radiology 2003 report 'Geometric Uncertainties in Radiotherapy', and incorporated into ICRU 83.

Conformal radiotherapy should be considered standard practice, because this limits dose to normal tissues. There is reasonable evidence that this in turn reduces complications in patients treated for CNS tumours, by reducing the volume of tissue, especially brain, receiving a high dose, or avoiding exposure to sensitive structures, such as the hypothalamus and pituitary gland (conformal avoidance). Eye lens doses should be estimated with thermoluminescent dosimetry (TLD) for future reference. On-treatment portal films or images should be used to confirm positioning for radical treatments.

Normal tissue tolerance to radiotherapy

Normal tissue tolerance is an important concept. It embodies both the risk of a complication and also the severity of its effect on the patient. The relevance also depends on the clinical setting: a higher risk of normal tissue damage might be accepted in a patient with a highly malignant tumour requiring a high RT dose who has only a low chance of long-term survival, than is reasonable in a patients with a benign tumour. The dose that is considered safe may therefore vary from one condition to another.

There is almost certainly a volume effect in normal tissue tolerance of CNS structures, as in other parts of the body. This means that the larger the volume irradiated, the lower the safe dose. The CNS is also particularly sensitive to the dose per fraction, and many of the dose-fractionation schedules used are designed to take advantage of this. Many of the data on tolerance in the CNS are based on literature reports which predate the use of modern imaging, especially MRI. Tolerance doses are thus far from absolute.

Tolerance of the brain itself (to avoid necrosis) is in the region of 54–60 Gy in approximately 30 fractions, depending on volume treated and dose per fraction. A volume effect also exists for intellectual damage. Using 3D conformal RT, intellectual damage in adults is uncommon with doses up to 54 Gy in 30 fractions. The brainstem is said to have a slightly lower tolerance than brain substance, approximately 54 Gy in 30 fractions (or 55 Gy in 33 fractions). The optic nerves and chiasm are also thought to be more sensitive than brain parenchyma. For benign tumours in this region, a dose of 45 Gy in 25 fractions to 50 Gy in 30 fractions should be safe, with a risk of blindness which is virtually zero.

The pituitary gland and hypothalamus have a much lower tolerance for hormonal dysfunction. There is probably little effect for doses under 20–24 Gy, but adults in whom these structures receive 40–60 Gy have a significant long-term risk of hypothalamic–pituitary axis dysfunction.

The lacrimal gland shows reduced tear output after doses over about 20 Gy (similar to salivary glands). The lens of the eye should not develop cataract after doses less than 5–6 Gy, spread out over 30 fractions. There is a 50% risk of cataract after a dose of 15 Gy. The middle and inner ears are also sensitive structures but in adults recover in most patients after doses up to 60 Gy. The risk of permanent alopecia depends on the dose to the hair follicles in the dermis. The risk is very low with doses below 10–15 Gy, but 50% of patients will develop permanent alopecia after 43 Gy (in 30 fractions) to the scalp. This dose is difficult to estimate routinely because the hair follicles normally fall within the build-up region.

The spinal cord has a tolerance of approximately 50 Gy in 30 fractions (equivalent to 46 Gy at 2 Gy per fraction). This may be a conservative (i.e. safe) estimate and, in some circumstances, higher doses may be appropriate, such as for GBM of the spinal cord.

Principles of steroid therapy

Steroids are used to treat oedema in the brain, caused by tumour or surgery, so many patients attend the neuro-oncology clinic already taking a steroid such as dexamethasone. A daily dose of dexamethasone (Dex) of 16 mg is considered the highest useful dose in most circumstances. This is a typical dose used perioperatively, and is usually reduced as quickly as possible. Patients on anticonvulsant drugs, which increase the metabolism of dexamethasone, occasionally benefit from higher doses in the palliative setting.

In patients requiring RT where significant intracranial pressure remains, steroid is needed, and may need to be increased during the course. However, there is no absolute indication for steroids during radiotherapy. In patients in

whom surgery has relieved intracranial pressure, none may be necessary. It is thus possible to reduce steroid doses during a course of RT.

Dexamethasone has important side effects, which can impact seriously on quality of life. These include increased appetite, weight gain, muscle weakness, gastric irritation, and diabetes. Rarely, it causes psychosis which is very distressing and difficult to manage. Patients should be managed with the minimum possible dose. For reduction, the dose must be tailed off slowly, and not stopped abruptly. Patients should also be issued with a steroid card.

Principles of additional supportive care

It is important to think holistically about patients with CNS tumours. This includes biological, psychological, social and cultural aspects of their care. This patient group is very diverse, with a wide range of diagnoses and prognosis, and the problems experienced by the patients therefore vary greatly. Even patients with benign tumours may experience major problems, even if these are not life threatening. For example, the seriousness of the condition is obvious in a patient with weakness due to GBM undertaking palliative treatment. However, hearing loss due to vestibular schwannoma can also have a distressing impact on a young patient who needs to hear for childcare or work.

Supportive input may be valuable to a patient throughout their journey. Needs vary according to tumour type, and may fluctuate throughout the patient's journey, with treatment or progression. Many patients benefit from practical and psychological support. The relevant support is often best developed by a specialist nurse, who will be part of most neuro-oncology teams. Key roles are liaison with the patient and family, other healthcare professionals and hospice services, and provision of information from local or general resources, such as Cancer BACUP (http://www.cancerbacup.org.uk/Home). For some patients, especially those with gliomas, financial benefits may be available.

Driving after a diagnosis of CNS tumour

Many patients with primary CNS tumours are not allowed to drive following the diagnosis. This is because there is a risk of seizure as the result of the tumour. There is also a small risk of seizure following craniotomy, whatever the underlying condition. In particular, patients with high-grade gliomas have their driving licenses revoked for 2 years, timed from the completion of treatment.

Decisions about licensing are made by the Driver and Vehicle Licensing Authority (DVLA), though with information provided from the clinical teams. In general, the DVLA will help patients to regain a license, and will provide an individualized decision in unusual circumstances. The DVLA provides information on the guidelines for return of licenses for medical practitioners which can be obtained from the DVLA website (www.DVLA.gov.uk). It is worth using this on-line facility, since the regulations do change from time to time.

Individual tumour types

HIGH-GRADE GLIOMAS

Pathology and clinical features

Glioblastoma (GBM) is the commonest primary CNS tumour in adults (see Figure 30.2). GBMs and grade III gliomas are collectively known as high-grade gliomas (HGGs). The major problems with high-grade gliomas are:

1. significant damage to neurological function
2. diffuse infiltration through the brain, often over quite large distances
3. resistance to treatment, including both RT and chemotherapy.

HGGs grow with an expanding, destructive process. Beyond the gross tumour, malignant cells infiltrate widely. The gross tumour is surrounded by a zone of extensive oedema. Steroid treatment reduces oedema, and may improve neurological function. However, there is no method to restore function which has been lost as a result of the destruction of neural tissue in the centre of the tumour.

HGGs, especially GBMs, are efficient at spreading through the brain, predominantly following white matter tracts (see above and Figure 30.4). Spread across the midline, principally through the corpus callosum, is a major route for invasion. This infiltration occurs at a microscopic level, and so currently cannot be imaged. The extent of invasion varies between individuals. Despite the wide infiltration, HGGs typically recur at the primary site. There is thus no survival advantage in irradiating the whole brain. HGGs very rarely metastasize outside the CNS.

Patients present as described above. On CT and MRI, HGGs can be seen as space-occupying lesions with surrounding oedema, causing mass effect. The gross tumour enhances with intravenous contrast. GBMs in particular have a heterogeneous enhancement in the gross tumour. This reflects their growth, with areas of necrosis within the tumour. The typical GBM is shown in Figure 30.6. In patients with pressure effects, surgical decompression may improve symptoms quickly, allowing reduced steroid doses, and facilitating radiotherapy.

Treatment

Management options may be radical (curative), palliative, or active supportive care only (Table 30.3). The decision depends on performance status, age and tumour location, as well as patient preference. Patients with poor neurological condition are unlikely to benefit from radical treatment, while older patients tolerate both the neurological effects of the tumour, and the treatment less well. For these patients

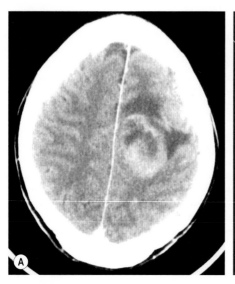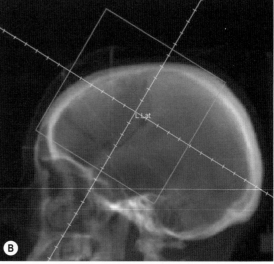

Figure 30.6 (A) CT with contrast of a patient with a GBM, showing a contrast-enhancing mass with central necrosis and surrounding oedema. (B) Lateral field, of a parallel-opposed pair of open laterals, for palliative RT for a patient with GBM. The GTV has been outlined, and a PTV has been grown with a margin of 1.5 + 0.5 cm. Finally, the fields have been added, with an additional 0.8 cm margin. The collimator has been rotated to follow approximately the radiological baseline, although the volume is above the eyes in this case. The craniotomy can be seen, and gives approximate confirmation of the correct target localization.

Table 30.3 Suggested criteria for choice of treatment in patients with HGG

Radical RT or chemo-RT	Age < 70 (younger in some centres)
	PS 0 or 1
	No significant neurological deficit remaining
Palliative RT	Age ≥ 70 and PS 0 or 1
	Age < 70, with a significant deficit
Supportive care	Severe residual deficit, e.g. hemiplegia Intellectual impairment

Note: the patient's choice should be considered in all cases. Where appropriate, agreement from the relatives is also valuable, especially for the supportive care option.

the option of shorter course, palliative treatment may be most suitable. For elderly patients, or those with very poor neurological function, quality of life is not improved by any available therapy. Referral for expert palliative and supportive care is therefore the most appropriate management.

Histological diagnosis is highly desirable provided further treatment will be given. For radical treatment, debulking surgery is to be preferred where possible. It extends survival but, equally importantly, it relieves mass effect. In turn, this improves neurological functioning, reduces steroid requirements and facilitates RT. For young, fit patients with GBM, the addition of chemotherapy with oral temozolomide has been shown to significantly extend survival.

The outcome of patients with HGG is surprisingly variable. The two most important prognostic factors for better outcome are younger age and better performance status. In terms of age, patients under 40 have the best outlook, those under 60 do less well, and those over 70 fare badly. The extent of surgical resection has prognostic value. Patients with brainstem HGG, in whom even biopsy is hazardous, do particularly badly. Presentation with epilepsy provides a small survival advantage, but this almost certainly is the result simply of making the patient present earlier in their illness pathway.

Radical treatment

Target volume

The patient should be immobilized in a beam direction shell, cut out to maximize skin sparing. Postoperative imaging is required to demonstrate the true extent and position of residual tumour after decompression. MRI produces superior definition of tumour, and should be coregistered to the planning CT. The gross tumour (GTV) is defined as the visible contrast-enhancing edge of tumour, shown most clearly on MRI, using T1W with gadolinium contrast.

The GTV is expanded isotropically to reach the CTV. Because of the infiltrative nature of HGGs, a large CTV margin is needed. Typically, a two-phase technique is used, with a 2.5 cm margin for phase 1 and 1.5 cm margin for phase 2. The CTV does not have to extend beyond the inner table of the skull, which is best shown on CT. Each CTV is expanded isotropically to its PTV with an appropriate margin, specific to the technique in each department. A margin of 0.5 cm is common. Outline critical normal structures, including the pituitary, eyes and lenses. It may be worth outlining the optic structures.

Technique

Conformal RT should be considered as standard. The use of non-coplanar beams, with field-in-field boosts is advantageous for most gliomas. The latter amounts to forward planned intensity modulated radiotherapy (IMRT). Thermoluminescent dosimetry (TLD) with lithium fluoride (LiF) is recommended to estimate doses to the eye, and portal imaging confirms patient positioning.

Dose and energy

For grade III (anaplastic) glioma:

> Phase 1: 45 Gy in 25 daily fractions over 5 weeks, with 6 MV photons
> Phase 2: 9 Gy in 5 daily fractions over 1 week, with 6 MV photons

For grade IV glioma (GBM):

> Phase 1: 40–50 Gy in 20–25 daily fractions over 4–5 weeks, with 6 MV photons
> Phase 2: 10–20 Gy in 5–10 daily fractions over 1–2 weeks, with 6 MV photons

This gives a total of 60 Gy in 30 fractions in 6 weeks.

Chemotherapy for radical treatment of GBM

Using the protocol from the EORTC trial, oral temozolomide is given in two blocks, the first concomitant with radical RT, and the second as an adjuvant treatment following RT.

Concurrent with RT: continuous daily dose of 75 mg/m^2 (i.e. 7 days per week), starting on the first day of RT, and finishing on the last day.

Adjuvant following RT: commencing 28 days after completion of RT, temozolomide daily for 5 days, at a dose of 150–200 mg/m^2. This is repeated 4-weekly for six cycles.

Side effects

Acute

Acute tiredness is almost invariable, though it is of variable severity. It appears to be related to the volume treated. It increases during the course, has a fluctuating pattern, and may be at its worst shortly after completion of radiotherapy. Early delayed somnolence is rare in adults.

Hair loss occurs in the entry portals and sometimes in the exit portals also, in about the third week after treatment starts. Hair washing has no effect on hair loss or scalp reactions, provided it is carried out carefully. Using conformal RT, scalp shielding can be used to protect some of the scalp, without compromise to the underlying target volume. With 54 Gy, hair regrowth is almost normal in most patients; with 60 Gy, at least some hair loss will be permanent. Erythema and soreness of skin can occur, particularly if the pinna is included in an entry port. Cutting the shell out reduces the skin dose, and minimizes skin reactions. If the external auditory canal is irradiated, this gets sore and crusted, and the wax becomes more viscid and difficult to remove. If the ear drum and middle ear are irradiated, then secretory otitis media (glue ear) may result, but this usually settles spontaneously. Inner ear damage is very uncommon.

In patients treated for HGG, headache and nausea are uncommon. Seizures occasionally worsen during radiotherapy. Dexamethasone is useful, and anticonvulsants should be reviewed.

Late

If the hypothalamus and pituitary have been irradiated, hormone failure may occur after a minimum of 1–2 years. Routine pituitary function tests are therefore appropriate in the few patients who are long-term survivors. Although the most important late effect in the brain is radionecrosis, this is extremely uncommon since the advent of 3-dimensional planning.

Deterioration during radiotherapy

Some patients deteriorate during radiotherapy. This is usually due to increased oedema, presumably resulting from tumour cell necrosis. It is usually treatable with an increase in dexamethasone dose. Occasionally, a cystic component can enlarge, and warrants neurosurgical intervention, such as aspiration and insertion of an Ommaya reservoir.

A few patients deteriorate during radiotherapy due to tumour progression. In these cases, it is appropriate to switch to palliative fractionation (see below), making an appropriate dose change according to the dose already delivered, or to stop RT altogether.

Results of treatment

The outlook is more favourable for grade III tumours, with 50% survival at 3 years, than for patients with GBM, for whom the figure is only 2–3%. Nevertheless, this small group of GBM patients is important. In a randomized trial of patients with GBM, the addition of oral temozolomide chemotherapy extended survival significantly: median survival was extended from 12 months to 14.5, and 2-year survival increased from 10% to 26%.

Palliative treatment

Target volume and technique

The patient should be immobilized in a beam direction shell. The intended beam arrangement is a parallel pair of lateral-opposing fields. CT is used for planning purposes, to outline the GTV; apply a slightly smaller margin of 1.5 + 0.5 cm for CTV + PTV margins; no editing of the CTV is necessary. The collimator should be rotated to follow approximately the radiological baseline, in order to avoid the eyes. If there is uncertainty in localizing the tumour, use a CTV margin of 2.5 cm, as for radical RT. An additional margin of around 0.8 cm is needed to allow for the field size to cover the PTV adequately (see Figure 30.6). Fields are placed using a virtual simulation tool.

Dose and energy

30 Gy in six fractions, treating three times per week, over 2 weeks, with megavoltage photons.

Side effects

Acute tiredness occurs with palliative RT, and hair loss is inevitable, though occurs after completion of RT. Although some regrowth occurs, hair does not return to normal. Erythema is mild, and headache and nausea are very uncommon. Due to the poor prognosis, late side effects are rarely relevant.

Results of treatment

The outlook for patients with HGG who receive palliative RT is poor, with a median survival of only 140 days (just under 5 months) from first presentation in oncology. However, a small number of patients survive for much longer, a few remaining alive for over 2 years. Those patients deemed unfit for palliative RT have a median survival of only 6 weeks.

LOW-GRADE GLIOMAS

Pathology and clinical features

Low-grade gliomas (LGGs) include those with WHO grade I and II. Grade I tumours are rare in adults. LGGs represent about 12% of the total number of cases referred to oncology (see Figures 30.1 and 30.2). Although LGGs present in similar ways to other primary tumours, seizure is a much more common presenting complaint than with other tumours. Oligodendrogliomas (of grade II) are particularly likely to present with epilepsy. Because of this tendency to cause seizure, many patients with LGG are followed up in neurology clinics. The course of the illness is extremely variable. Some LGGs appear never to progress, and others may take a decade or more to do so. However, some tumours show evidence of disease progression from the time of diagnosis. It is the patients with these tumours that are typically referred for an oncology opinion.

When these tumours progress, they may do so in their original form, but they may also undergo further genetic mutation causing transformation to a higher grade, grade III or even GBM. This occurs in about half the patients who progress, and is not itself caused or influenced by RT. The increase in grade changes the outlook.

Surgery has an important role in obtaining biopsy tissue to prove the diagnosis. It may also be helpful if there is substantial mass effect in the brain, because resection improves pressure symptoms. Beyond these indications, the role of surgery remains controversial. Surgical series typically contain younger patients with smaller tumours, and are therefore not directly comparable to radiotherapy or surveillance series.

Radiotherapy is indicated for patients with disease progression, demonstrated by worsening neurology, worsening epilepsy, or imaging. Pathological diagnosis from biopsy is recommended before radiotherapy is undertaken. In patients with progressive disease, RT almost certainly delays tumour progression and death, although incontrovertible proof for this is lacking. Whether RT actually cures some patients is not known. Radiotherapy improves epilepsy in about 50% of patients with low-grade glioma. In rare circumstances, it can be used to try to improve intractable epilepsy in a patient with LGG.

In patients without demonstrable progression, the timing of RT is less critical. There is excellent information that survival is unaffected by the timing of RT, whether it is given immediately or later when progression occurs. This is reassuring when counselling patients.

Currently, the role of chemotherapy as a first-line treatment is a matter for debate. It is effective in some patients, especially those with oligodendrogliomas with specific chromosomal translocations (specifically 1p to 19q), but the proportion of patients responding to radiotherapy is probably higher.

LGGs grow with diffuse infiltrative growth, without destruction of involved brain. Therefore, patients may have functioning brain within the tumour, even though tumours may be very large. This imposes a fundamental limitation on surgery for LGG. Neurological deficits caused by LGGs frequently improve following radiotherapy. It is therefore appropriate to consider patients for RT even if they have neurological deficits, which is entirely the opposite of HGGs.

In rare cases, LGG can be extremely extensive, affecting the whole of the hemisphere or almost the whole cerebrum. This is known as gliomatosis cerebri. Usually, this is not treated until progression of symptoms, but it does normally respond to RT. Although little normal brain can usually be spared, RT may be extremely worthwhile, improving neurological deficit in most patients and achieving long-term control in some.

On imaging with CT, tumours are typically large, with low density. Oligodendrogliomas often have areas of calcification, which give a characteristic speckled appearance, helpful in suggesting a preoperative diagnosis. On MRI, LGGs show low signal on T1W and absence of contrast

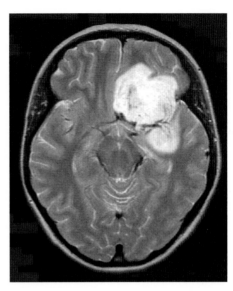

Figure 30.7 T2W MRI of a large grade II astrocytoma. Oedema within the tumour has a high signal (appears white). This region would be considered the GTV. CSF between the folds of the brain is also white. On CT, this area would be shown as a low-density region.

enhancement. The tumour is usually best delineated using a FLAIR or T2W sequence where CSF and oedema are appear white. This correlates with the low density seen on CT. A typical LGG is shown in Figure 30.7.

Radical treatment

Target volume

The patient should be immobilized in a beam direction shell, cut out to maximize skin sparing. If resection has been carried out, then postoperative imaging is required. Even if biopsy has been the only surgical procedure, current imaging is needed. MRI produces optimal localization of the tumour, especially the FLAIR or T2W sequences. This should be coregistered with the planning CT. The gross tumour (GTV) is defined as the visible high signal on FLAIR or T2W MRI, which equates to low density on CT. This volume is often very large. However, a CTV margin of approximately 1.5 cm can be used, smaller than for HGG, and treatment carried out in a single phase. The CTV does not have to extend beyond the inner table of the skull, which is best shown on CT. The CTV should be grown isotropically to its PTV, with an appropriate margin. A margin of 0.5 cm is common. Outline critical normal structures, including the pituitary, eyes and lenses. It may be worth outlining the optic structures.

Technique

Conformal RT should be standard, typically using three or four non-coplanar beams. A field-in-field boost may be needed to achieve dose homogeneity, especially for large target volumes. TLD is recommended to estimate doses to the lens, and portal imaging to verify treatment set-up.

Dose and energy

Single phase: 50.4–54 Gy in 28–30 daily fractions over 5.5–6 weeks, with 6 MV photons.

There is some evidence to suggest that a lower dose of 45 Gy in 20 fractions may be as effective. For patients with gliomatosis cerebri, a slightly smaller dose per fraction may be helpful, and a dose of 55 Gy in 33 fractions is suitable.

Side effects

Acute and late effects are similar to HGG, particularly grade III gliomas, for which the same dose is used. Seizures may worsen during radiotherapy. Dexamethasone is useful, and anticonvulsants should be reviewed. Late hypothalamus and pituitary dysfunction is an important issue in long-term follow up, particularly since the prognosis is much more favorable than HGG. Most studies of intellectual function suggest little or no detrimental effect from 54 Gy (in 30 fractions), over and above that already caused by the tumour (and surgery).

Results of treatment

The outcome of patients with LGG is very variable. However, younger age, smaller tumours, and lack of neurological deficit are prognostic for better outcome. In addition, the histological type also has an effect: oligodendroglioma histology has a better outlook than astrocytoma. Mixed tumours have an intermediate outlook.

Many patients with neurological deficits from tumour experience improvement, and this is a very important indication to undertake RT. This also applies to gliomatosis cerebri, despite the enormous volumes of brain affected. In half of patients who have epilepsy, the frequency and severity of seizures improves after radiotherapy.

In the large European trial which evaluated the timing of RT, early radiotherapy delayed progression of LGG by about 2 years. This increase in disease-free survival may be of value to patients. Median survival (i.e. 50% of patients alive) was around 7.5 years, irrespective of the timing of RT. Ten-year survival data from that trial are not available yet, but from other series the survival at 10 year is in the range 40–60%.

EPENDYMOMA (INTRACRANIAL)

Pathology and clinical features

Intracranial ependymoma is a rare primary tumour (see Figure 30.1), commoner in children than adults. It is thought to be derived from ependymal cells that line the ventricular system. It arises most often in the posterior fossa, though it can be supratentorial. Typically, posterior fossa lesions present as the result of obstructive hydrocephalus. Imaging demonstrates a contrast-enhancing tumour adjacent to the fourth ventricle but away from the midline. There is surrounding oedema, and typically enlarged ventricles above. Supratentorial ependymomas present in the same way as other cerebral primary tumours. On imaging, the appearances are very similar to HGG. Spread may occur in the CSF, so MR imaging of the spine is necessary to stage the patient.

Treatment

The maximum possible surgical resection is an advantage before radiotherapy. There is no definite role for adjuvant chemotherapy in adults. Although ependymoma can spread through the CSF, there is good evidence that prophylactic craniospinal RT confers no advantage.

Target volume

The patient should be immobilized in the conventional way, positioned either prone (in a two-piece shell), or supine in an 'S' frame, to allow for posterior beams. The shell should be cut out for treatment. For posterior fossa tumours, it is typical to consider the whole posterior fossa as the CTV, similar to the phase 2 treatment for medulloblastoma (Chapter 33). However, for lateralized tumours it may be acceptable to outline the GTV as enhancing tumour, and add a CTV margin of 1.5–2.5 cm. An appropriate PTV should be added. Supratentorial ependymomas should be treated along similar lines to HGG, using postoperative MRI to define the GTV. The CTV requires a margin of 1.5–2.5 cm, grown isotropically, which can be edited along the skull. An appropriate PTV should be added.

Technique

In adults, the posterior fossa is best treated with a plan, typically using three non-coplanar fields. The standard arrangement is with two posterior oblique and one posterior beam. This achieves the best conformation to the posterior fossa target volume. Supratentorial tumours require individualized beam arrangements, as per HGGs.

Dose and energy

Megavoltage x-rays of 6 MV or equivalent should be used. Single phase: 55 Gy in 33 daily fractions, over 6.5 weeks. An alternative is 54 Gy in 30 fractions, treating daily over 6 weeks.

Results of treatment

Ependymoma is curable in approximately 50% of cases.

PRIMARY CNS LYMPHOMA

Pathology and clinical features

Primary central nervous system lymphoma (PCNSL) is non-Hodgkin's lymphoma arising in the brain, typically of high-grade B-cell type. The incidence of PCNSL is increasing, but is still uncommon (see Figure 30.1). It affects patients of all ages, the incidence rising with age, and the majority are over 60. Myelosuppression predisposes to the development of PCNSL, and this was one of the early AIDS-defining diagnoses. Happily, this is now a rare complication of HIV.

Presentation is the same as other primary tumours arising within the brain substance, typically with headache, neurological deficit often including intellectual decline, or seizure. 'B' symptoms (see Chapter 29) are not a feature of PCNSL. On imaging, typical appearances are of a homogeneously-enhancing mass, often in a periventricular location (Figure 30.8). In approximately two-thirds of cases, PCNSL presents as a single mass; in one-third it is multifocal. The disease can spread within the brain, especially in the subependymal layer around the ventricular system, but it is rare for it to metastasize outside the CNS. Metastases to the brain from peripheral lymphoma are also rare.

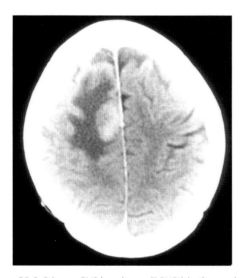

Figure 30.8 Primary CNS lymphoma (PCNSL) in the cerebral hemisphere, shown on CT. A homogeneously-enhancing mass can be seen. In approximately two-thirds of cases, PCNSL presents as a single mass; in one-third it is multifocal. A definitive diagnosis will require biopsy, to distinguish between high-grade glioma, metastasis and PCNSL. Note the similarity to Figure 30.6A.

Management principles

Biopsy is necessary to prove the diagnosis, but resection should not be undertaken if a diagnosis of PCNSL is suspected, because it does not improve the prognosis and carries a greater risk of neurological deficit. Steroids are cytotoxic to lymphomas (as with peripheral lymphomas). Therefore, if dexamethasone is given for symptom relief before a biopsy is performed, the lesion may disappear temporarily. The inclusion of lymphoma in the radiological differential diagnosis thus provides an important contribution to management.

Although treatment strategies have evolved, the optimum treatment remains unclear. Until about 20 years ago, radiotherapy was the mainstay of treatment. Treatment typically commenced with whole brain irradiation (e.g. to a dose of 45 Gy in 25 fractions), followed by a focal boost for localized disease (e.g. 9–10 Gy in five fractions). Treatment with radiotherapy alone is well tolerated but, in historical series, most patients recurred locally, with fatal consequences. Therefore, the addition of chemotherapy was investigated, a strategy that had proved effective in systemic non-Hodgkin's lymphoma. It became clear that combined chemoradiotherapy is superior to radiotherapy alone. However, a particular problem is late neurotoxicity associated with the combination of chemotherapy, especially methotrexate, with radiotherapy. This occurs commonly, especially in older people, and can be severely disabling or even fatal. Treatment schedules with very intensive chemotherapy alone were therefore developed, and can now be considered the mainstay of treatment. Overall, it appears that RT improves progression-free survival rates, but not overall survival. However, the neurotoxicity is worse with the combined treatment, affecting about half the patients receiving combined chemo-RT compared to a quarter treated with chemo alone. Since omitting RT does not compromise survival, and reduces serious toxicity, radiotherapy is now not recommended as part of the first line treatment for PCNSL. RT may be used as a salvage treatment.

Radical treatment – full dose radiotherapy

This is no longer considered conventional, but is included here in case of rare cases untreatable by chemotherapy.

Localized unifocal disease

Target volume and technique

The patient should be immobilized in a beam direction shell. For phase 1, the whole brain is irradiated, using a parallel pair of lateral-opposed fields. The 3D dose distribution should be computed and wedges or compensators can be used if dose homogeneity is outside ICRU recommended limits. Avoidance of high dose areas may reduce the risk and severity of late neurotoxicity.

For phase 2, a localized volume is treated, using a three-field plan, or equivalent. The GTV is the pre-chemotherapy enhancing disease seen on MRI. A margin of 1–2 cm should be allowed around this for the CTV, and the appropriate PTV margin added.

Dose and energy

Phase 1: 45 Gy in 25 daily fractions, over 5 weeks.
Phase 2: 9–10 Gy in 5 daily fractions, over 1 week.

Multifocal disease

Target volume and technique

Treat the whole brain with a single phase, as per phase 1.

Dose

Single phase: 45 Gy in 25 daily fractions, over 5 weeks.

Alternative lower dose single phase schedules have also been used by some groups, even for localised disease:

Single phase: 30.6–39.6 Gy in 17 – 22 fractions, over 3½–4½ weeks 45 Gy in 30 daily fractions, over 6 weeks

Palliative radiotherapy

This may be necessary for a few patients with poor performance status.

Target volume and technique

Immobilize and irradiate the whole brain with a single phase, as per palliative RT for metastases.

Dose

A variety of dose schedules can be utilized:

30 Gy in 10 fractions, treating daily, over 2 weeks
20 Gy in 5 fractions, treating daily, over 1 week
30 Gy in 6 fractions, treating on alternate days over 2 weeks (as for HGG).

Results of treatment

The major prognostic factors for better survival are younger age, especially less than 60, excellent performance status and chemotherapy. Suitability for chemotherapy is strongly determined by performance status. Localized disease, rather than a multifocal pattern, also carries a better prognosis. Long-term survival is poor, especially in patients over 60, who comprise the majority. In a series of unselected cases, the median survival was only 8 months, with a 5-year survival of 6%. However, in patients under 60 with good performance status who are treated intensively, the median survival should reach 3 years, and the 5-year survival 20–30%.

GERMINOMA

Clinical features and management principles

Germinomas are rare in adults, but present like other primary tumours. They frequently arise in the region of the pineal gland, close to the (CSF) aqueduct (see Figure 30.5) and, therefore, the symptoms and signs of hydrocephalus are common presenting features. They should be curable in almost every case.

Germinomas spread through the CSF, and therefore require RT to the whole craniospinal axis. The tumour has a curious predilection to form metastatic deposits on the optic chiasm. Different tumours show a wide range of growth rates, but a few grow extremely fast. This can lead to neurological deterioration taking place over days or even hours. If a patient has metastatic spread to the optic chiasm, rapid progression may threaten vision. Such deterioration warrants urgent treatment, with radiotherapy. This type of disease does not respond well to steroid treatment. Therefore, occasionally, a few fractions of emergency radiotherapy must be given urgently to treat neurological deterioration, while the full plan is prepared.

In adults, the standard treatment for intracranial germinoma should be radiotherapy. The total dose is modest, and the toxicity profile in adults is excellent, because growth is complete. There is therefore no advantage in considering an alternative strategy of reduced dose RT together with chemotherapy, at least at the present time.

Treatment

Target volume

Phase 1 should treat the whole craniospinal axis, and this is most effectively planned from CT. The technique is the same as for paediatric craniospinal RT (see Chapter 33), and requires careful attention to detail.

For phase 2, the primary site is treated to a higher dose. This should be localized using CT:MR coregistration, and the imaging must be carried out before RT starts, because the tumour is extremely radiosensitive and may disappear within a few days of starting RT. The GTV is the contrast-enhancing tumour. The CTV margin can be small, e.g. 1–2 cm, grown isotropically. The PTV should be grown from the CTV, with a standard margin, such as 0.5 cm.

Any sites of metastatic disease can also be boosted in this phase. Occasionally, the whole craniospinal axis must be treated to the phase 2 dose (see below).

Technique

Phase 1 as for paediatric craniospinal RT (see Chapter 33). For phase 2, use an appropriate beam arrangement, usually with three conformal fields.

Dose and energy

Phase 1: craniospinal axis: 25 Gy in 15 daily fractions in 3 weeks, using megavoltage x-rays.
Phase 2: 15 Gy in 9 fractions in 2 weeks, to boost the primary site and any sites of metastasis.

If necessary, in the case of extensive metastatic spread, it is possible to treat the whole craniospinal axis to 40 Gy in 24 fractions, provided that the full blood count is carefully monitored. If urgent RT is required while the craniospinal plan is being prepared, this can be done using a parallel pair of lateral fields. A few fractions (e.g. 5 Gy in three fractions) are normally sufficient to prevent clinical deterioration. It is probably best, in adults, simply to consider this as extra dose, added to the two phases described above.

Results of treatment

With good radiotherapy technique, the cure rate is almost 100%. This applies even if metastatic disease is present at diagnosis.

MEDULLOBLASTOMA

The management of medulloblastoma in adults follows the general principles of this disease in children. However, there is less need to reduce doses in adults who have mature brains and are fully grown. Exactly the same meticulous attention to detail of radiotherapy technique is needed. Survival advantage has been shown for the addition of chemotherapy in children. This issue needs to be addressed in adults.

The management of paediatric medulloblastoma is described in Chapter 33.

Dose and energy (adults)

Phase 1: craniospinal axis: 35 Gy in 21 daily fractions in 4 weeks, using megavoltage x-rays.
Phase 2: 20 Gy in 12 fractions in 2.5 weeks.

MENINGIOMA

Pathology and clinical features

Patients with meningioma present with a mixture of symptoms and signs. Headache is common. As with other primary tumours, meningiomas may also cause confusion and intellectual impairment, resulting from compression of the frontal lobes. Occasionally, patients may present with specific cranial nerve palsies, which is different from glial tumours.

The majority of meningiomas arise sporadically. However, they may be associated with previous radiation treatment, for example cranial RT used for childhood leukaemia. Unusually in oncology, they are commoner in women than men (2:1). Benign meningiomas normally express progesterone receptors (PR), but not oestrogen receptors (ER), and this may account for occasional reports of change during pregnancy or in patients using hormone replacement therapy. More malignant tumours typically become less well differentiated and lose this expression.

Meningiomas arise in the coverings of the brain, and so can occur at any intracranial site. However, the commonest two sites are the vertex of the skull, and the greater wing of the sphenoid bone. This is the ridge of bone which divides the anterior and middle cranial fossae. Tumours at the vertex can usually be fully resected. Those on the sphenoid wing are resectable if they lie laterally. Medial sphenoid wing tumours usually involve the cavernous sinus, which normally precludes complete resection.

In the first instance, management depends on whether surgical resection can be performed. In a neurosurgery practice, the majority of meningiomas are completely resectable and usually cured without the need for further treatment. In those which can only be partially resected, or are entirely unresectable, RT can be considered. Even if the whole meningioma cannot be removed, there may be advantage in debulking to reduce the tumour size, provided it is not at the cost of neurological damage. Some meningiomas grow so slowly that they appear to be static. These may be managed conservatively.

Optic nerve meningiomas cause visual deterioration. These tumours are normally diagnosed entirely on imaging. In these patients, surgery, including biopsy, can further damage vision. RT is effective in stabilizing the disease, and some patients experience an improvement in vision. RT is thus the treatment of choice for optic nerve meningioma.

The WHO grading of meningiomas is from grade I to III. Most tumours are of grade I and usually grow slowly. Grade II tumours, also known as 'atypical', may grow faster and have a higher tendency to recur. Grade III tumours, also known as 'malignant', are faster growing, more aggressive in their extension, and more difficult to eradicate. Although not as fast growing as HGGs, malignant meningiomas may still change over weeks to months. On average, malignant meningiomas occur in younger patients than the benign variety.

Meningiomas can infiltrate along the meninges, and this even applies to tumours known to be benign. They may also infiltrate through the foramina and fissures of the skull base, and these areas must be carefully reviewed when planning RT.

On imaging, tumours are of similar density to the surrounding brain. Sometimes they cause surrounding oedema. With contrast they normally enhance vigorously and homogeneously (Figure 30.9). It is typical to have meningeal enhancement extending away from the site of a meningioma, and this does not necessarily indicate tumour spread. Rather, this 'tail' is a useful diagnostic feature. Nevertheless, many patients referred for an oncology opinion have a tumour with a more invasive pattern of growth, with demonstrable extension along adjacent meningeal layers. A rule of thumb to distinguish the reactive 'tail' from infiltration is the thickness of

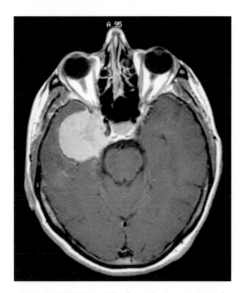

Figure 30.9 MRI (T1W + Gd) of meningioma arising from the medial wing of the sphenoid ridge. The cavernous sinus is involved. A small 'tail' of contrast enhancement can be seen in the meninges anteriorly in the middle fossa. The tumour was managed by subtotal resection and postoperative RT.

the meningeal layer: thickening of the meninges suggests tumour infiltration.

Treatment

Radiotherapy target volume

The patient should be immobilized in a beam direction shell, cut out to maximize skin sparing. For small lesions where high precision is desired, a relocatable stereotactic head frame can be used. If resection has been carried out, then postoperative imaging is required. A current MRI scan should be used for planning, coregistered with the planning CT. Both modalities are helpful for target volume delineation. MRI using a T1W sequence with gadolinium contrast produces optimal localization of the tumour. CT shows the limits of meningioma extension up to bone or, in uncommon cases where the tumour involves the bone, the extent of the invasion. CT also shows the foramina and fissures of the skull, through which meningiomas can spread.

The gross tumour (GTV) is defined as the visible edge of contrast enhancement on MRI, plus relevant skull boundaries. If resection has been carried out, coregistration with the preoperative MRI is very helpful. This shows the location of the tumour and therefore the meningeal surfaces into which spread might occur. There is very little hard evidence for the size of the CTV margin that should be used. For an individual tumour, its growth pattern suggests whether a small or large margin is needed. The most benign tumours grow as a slowly expanding mass, often relatively spherical in shape. In these cases, the CTV may be the same as the

GTV. However, many meningiomas show a more invasive pattern of growth, with extension along adjacent meningeal layers. Any such extension should be outlined in the GTV, and then an appropriate CTV margin should be added. Where histology is available, this can be incorporated into the margin decision. For grade II tumours, a CTV margin should certainly be added and, for grade III malignant meningiomas, an even larger CTV margin is appropriate. It is not necessary to expand the CTV isotropically. Meningiomas rarely invade the substance of the brain, so only a minimal margin is needed at the interface with the brain.

The following margins are general recommendations for the largest dimension of the CTV around the GTV. Where the GTV has been resected, the GTV can be localized from the preoperative imaging.

No histology, non-invasive growth	CTV = GTV
No histology, invasive pattern	CTV = GTV + 1.0–2.5 cm
Grade I, non-invasive growth	CTV = GTV
Grade I, invasive pattern	CTV = GTV + 1.0 cm
Grade II	CTV = GTV + 1.0 cm
Grade III	CTV = GTV + 1.5–2.5 cm

The CTV should be grown isotropically to its PTV, with an appropriate margin. It is helpful to outline critical normal structures, including the eyes and lenses, the pituitary, and optic nerves and chiasm.

Technique

Conformal RT or IMRT should be standard, typically using three or four non-coplanar beams. A field-in-field boost may be needed to achieve dose homogeneity, especially for large target volumes. TLD is recommended to estimate doses to the lens, and portal imaging to verify treatment set up.

Dose and energy

50–55 Gy in 30–33 daily fractions over 6–6.5 weeks, with 6 MV photons.

The dose may vary according to which critical structures are contained within the CTV and PTV. In some centres, a dose of 60 Gy is considered appropriate for malignant (grade III) tumours.

Side effects

Acute and late effects relate to the location irradiated. Tiredness does occur, even using small doses per fraction; it is, however, less marked than for patients treated for HGG. Hair loss occurs in about the third week after treatment starts. Hair washing has no effect on hair loss or scalp reactions, provided it is carried out carefully. Scalp shielding can be used to protect some of the scalp, without compromise to the underlying target volume. With 50 Gy, hair regrowth is almost always normal.

Erythema and soreness of skin are uncommon with 50 Gy in 30 fractions, though can occur with higher doses. Cutting the shell out reduces the skin dose, and hydrocortisone cream 1% applied topically reduces itching. The pinna and external auditory canal may be affected. If the external canal receives a significant dose, the wax becomes viscid and sticky. If the ear drum and middle ear are irradiated, then secretory otitis media (glue ear) may occur. This may cause noises in the ears, especially bubbling, reduction of hearing and, occasionally, difficulties with balance, but this is usually temporary and settles spontaneously. If the eustachian tube is treated, the same problem often occurs.

Occasional patients experience nausea, especially when the brainstem is irradiated. This is usually manageable with 5-HT3 antagonists. Patients occasionally require steroids during treatment for meningioma. Headache is also uncommon as an acute side effect.

In terms of late effects, if the hypothalamus and pituitary have been irradiated, hormone failure may occur after 1–2 years, so routine pituitary function tests are necessary during follow up. Intellectual function should not be affected, over and above changes already caused by the tumour (and surgery). In cases where high eye doses cannot be avoided, such as optic nerve meningiomas, cataracts may develop (see above).

Results of treatment

It is likely that RT improves the outcome in patients for whom surgery is either impossible or incomplete. The results of subtotal resection plus RT are equivalent to complete surgical excision, and may be safer for the patient. Meningiomas grow slowly, so that follow up needs to be carried out over a long period, at least 10–15 years.

Age does not appear to be prognostic, and should not be considered a bar to radical RT. Tumours which are larger, or of higher grade, have a higher chance of earlier relapse. In addition, it is likely that tumours with a high number of cells actively in the mitotic cycle have a higher probability of early relapse.

In general, meningiomas do not change in size after RT, although a few do shrink modestly. However, it is important for the patient to understand that no change after treatment represents a successful outcome. Neurological deficits, such as cranial nerve palsies do not usually improve. The exception is with optic nerve meningiomas: about one-third of patients experience some improvement in vision, even if there is no change in the size of the lesion on imaging.

Overall, control rates for patients with meningioma are good, though published results are quite variable. Survival after surgery and RT for benign meningiomas (i.e. grades I and II) is around 80–90% at 5 years, and 50–80% at 10 years. For patients with inoperable tumours treated with RT alone, control rates are probably on the low end of these ranges. Although these results are good, and much better than for patients with gliomas, there is room for improvement.

Patients with malignant meningiomas (i.e. grade III) have a worse outlook, with 5-year survival rates around 40%, that is about half the survival of patients with benign tumours.

Pituitary tumours and craniopharyngioma

PITUITARY TUMOURS

Pathology and clinical features

Pituitary tumours are virtually always primary adenomas of the anterior pituitary gland itself. Other primary tumours are exceedingly rare, and metastatic deposits involving the pituitary fossa, although well described, are uncommon.

Pituitary adenomas can be divided into secretory tumours that produce excess hormone and non-secretory ones that do not. Secretory adenomas most commonly produce an excess of a single hormone, usually growth hormone causing acromegaly, adrenocorticotrophic hormone (ACTH) which causes Cushing's disease, or prolactin leading to hyperprolactinemia. Other hormone production is very uncommon. Patients with secretory tumours usually present with the effects of the excess hormone production, and a small tumour confined to the pituitary fossa. In many cases, hormone levels can be controlled medically. However, surgery produces the quickest reduction of hormone levels in secreting tumours, and is often curative. Radiotherapy can reduce hormone levels, but often very slowly, over months or years, and is therefore not helpful as an acute treatment.

Non-secretory tumours typically present with symptoms and signs of optic chiasm compression. Occasionally, they present with pituitary failure, and are sometimes associated with headache. Surgical decompression results in immediate relief of pressure on the optic tract, and vision often improves by the time the patient wakes from the anaesthetic. Extension of tumour to the lateral walls of the pituitary fossa and cavernous sinus cannot be removed surgically, and is a frequent site for residual tumour.

After complete removal, radiotherapy is usually not required. However, a proportion do recur, so adequate follow up is essential. The indications for radiotherapy are relative, and patients are best managed through a multidisciplinary team. The decision regarding RT in an individual patient is the result of weighing the pros and cons of observation versus early RT. Indications in favor of radiotherapy include extensive residual tumour, invasion of the cavernous sinuses laterally, uncontrolled elevated hormone levels, and evidence of progression of tumour after surgery alone. Factors against radiotherapy include normal pituitary function, and young age, because of the risk of inducing a second tumour. Patient preference is also important. If recurrence does occur in a patient managed by surveillance, second operation may be desirable if the optic chiasm is compressed, before proceeding to RT.

In considering a patient for RT, it is important to ensure that the patient's hormone status is stable. It is useful to have pre-RT documentation of the visual fields. It is inadvisable to treat a patient with visual symptoms and signs which are unexplained, because any visual deterioration resulting from progression in the (unknown) pathology will be blamed on the radiotherapy. Postoperative MRI is useful both as a baseline before radiotherapy and to aid in the planning process (see below).

Treatment

Target volume

The patient should be immobilized in a beam direction shell; a comfortable, neutral position is recommended (see below). A relocatable stereotactic frame may also be used. Radiotherapy should be fully conformal. Although the pituitary fossa can be localized well on conventional simulator lateral radiographs, it is more difficult to be certain of the lateral extent of the target. Simulator radiographs do not show suprasellar extension in cases where this is present. Therefore, CT planning is preferred, with a current (postoperative) coregistered MRI (T1W+Gd). CT shows the bony anatomy well, especially inferiorly, where it may be difficult to distinguish tumour from bone marrow in the skull on MRI. MRI demonstrates involvement of the cavernous sinuses and suprasellar extension. MRI may be unnecessary for microadenomas confined to the sella, though such tumours rarely require RT.

The target is based on residual tumour bulk, which most commonly involves the cavernous sinuses. Very occasionally, tumours spread into the sphenoid sinus, although tissue seen in the sphenoid sinus postoperatively after transsphenoidal resection is most likely to be surgical packing. This does not have to be treated. Some tumours have residual suprasellar extension, even after surgery, and this must be included in the GTV. Reviewing the GTV on a coronal view can be helpful in confirming coverage, especially superiorly and inferiorly.

Pituitary adenomas do not infiltrate at a microscopic level, so no CTV margin is required for this. However, if there is uncertainty about the coregistration or outlining, then a small CTV margin may be added. The PTV should be grown isotropically with an appropriate margin.

Ideally, critical normal structures, especially the optic nerves, chiasm and tracts, should be outlined, so that the dose distribution and the dose-volume histograms (DVHs) for these can be reviewed. They can be outlined individually, or as a single unit. The expected DVH will differ according to which method is used. Alternatively, the dose plan must be reviewed on each CT slice to exclude 'hot spots' within these structures.

Technique

In general, a three-field conformal coplanar plan is ideal. Conventionally, this uses an anterior field, entering above the eyes (and preferably above the eye brows), and two opposed, wedged lateral fields. Other variations are possible, including posterior oblique rather than lateral fields, which do not require wedging. These reduce the temporal lobe dose, but a larger volume of normal tissue receives a low dose. Superior beams are not ideal because the beam exits through the whole body.

Thermoluminescent dosimetry measurements should be made to estimate the lens doses. Although they should be very low, the measurements prove that subsequent cataract or other visual problems are not the result of RT.

Dose and energy

45 Gy in 25 daily fractions over 5 weeks, with megavoltage x-rays. The prescription should be to the 100% dose point at the isocentre.

A slightly higher dose is sometimes recommended for Cushing's disease and for very large adenomas, such as 50 Gy in 30 fractions (as for craniopharyngioma).

Since these tumours are located centrally within the skull, there is a small advantage from using high energy (i.e. 10–15 MV) x-rays; in particular, this leads to slightly lower temporal lobe doses. However, if very small fields are required, dosimetry may be more secure with 6 MV x-rays.

Side effects

Hair loss over the temples occurs at 3 weeks, and will regrow. Mild erythema occasionally occurs in the anterior entry portal, but is seldom marked with high-energy beams. Some patients experience mild nausea and loss of appetite during RT, which is easily controlled with simple antiemetics. In some patients, ear symptoms occur as the result of acute irritation and blockage of the eustachian tube. Patients may report mildly reduced hearing, with bubbling in the ears and, sometimes, mild unsteadiness. These symptoms are due to fluid in the middle ear (secretory otitis media), which is unable to drain down the blocked eustachian tube, and settle spontaneously.

For patients already requiring hydrocortisone replacement, it is sensible to increase the dose, since a course of radiotherapy constitutes a stressful event. This should be the 'default' management. Typically, the dose can be increased by 50% or doubled. A few patients can be managed without this increase if they feel unperturbed about the impending treatment. Tiredness is a good measure of the dose of steroid required in this patient group. RT does increase the risk of hypothalamic–pituitary axis (HPA) dysfunction requiring hormone replacement. However, damage to the HPA is the result of the combination of tumour and surgery as well as RT. HPA dysfunction is dependent upon radiotherapy dose.

In all, half to three-quarters of patients require hormone replacement after surgery and RT.

The risk of late radiotherapy damage to the optic nerves should be negligible with a dose of 45 Gy in 25 fractions, prescribed to the isocentre. Therefore, if visual deterioration occurs after RT, it is important to look for a cause other than radiotherapy. Cataract should not occur with standard techniques.

Any radiotherapy treatment carries a risk of late second tumour causation. In patients treated for pituitary adenoma, the risk is roughly 1% per decade of follow up after treatment. Of the tumours caused, about half are benign, typically meningioma, and about half are malignant, for example glioblastoma or sarcoma. Because the risk is cumulative with time, this is especially important in younger patients.

Results of treatment

Postoperative radiotherapy produces very high rates of control. Overall, tumour control rates should be around 95% at 10 years and 90% at 20 years. However, control of hormone secretion is poorer, with only 60–80% achieving control of hypersecretion.

CRANIOPHARYNGIOMA

Pathology and clinical features

This is a rare tumour which predominates in children but can occur in adults. In adults, it typically presents with symptoms and signs related to raised intracranial pressure, compression of the optic chiasm and optic nerves, or reduction in pituitary hormone secretion. When these tumours are very extensive, pressure on the frontal lobes or involvement of the hypothalamus can cause behavioural disturbance. In children, it may present with other manifestations of damage to the hypothalamus, including precocious puberty.

Craniopharyngiomas are thought to arise from cells derived from the embryological structure known as Rathke's pouch, which extends from the embryonic pharynx to form the anterior pituitary gland. Craniopharyngiomas are normally cystic, with a thin wall, and may have some more solid components. The craniopharyngioma itself is lined by epithelium (reflecting its origin), which produces the cyst fluid. At both a macroscopic and a microscopic level, the wall of the cyst projects into spaces in the surface of the brain, to which it can be strongly adherent.

On CT, flecks of calcification are often seen. On MRI, the cyst has almost unique signal characteristics, being neither those of CSF nor brain; the cyst wall is normally well shown on the T1W sequence and enhances with gadolinium contrast. When opened surgically, thick viscous fluid is often seen, with the macroscopic appearances of machine oil and containing microscopic cholesterol crystals. This accounts for the MRI appearances of the cyst fluid.

Surgery achieves decompression and tissue for histological confirmation. Complete surgical removal is sometimes possible for very small lesions. More commonly, the tumours are large, complex and highly adherent to the brain, so that attempts to remove every finger-like projection of the cyst wall can produce very substantial traction injury to the brain. In general terms, decompression and subtotal resection plus radiotherapy produces similar local control rates to radical surgery, with much less neurological morbidity.

Radiotherapy is recommended for virtually all adult patients. Patients normally have panhypopituitarism already, so that this relative contraindication is absent. The recurrence rates following surgery alone, even after apparently complete removal, are high. Since the recurrence can increase neurological deficits, which are often found in patients with this disease already, the risk and consequences of recurrence greatly outweigh the risks from RT. In children, where delay of RT may in itself be an advantage, this balance is slightly different.

Treatment

Target volume

The patient should be immobilized in a beam direction shell, in a comfortable, neutral position. A relocatable stereotactic frame may also be used. CT planning should be used, with coregistered MRI (T1W+Gd). In some circumstances, coregistration with the preoperative MRI may also be helpful as a guide to the GTV.

RT for craniopharyngioma is more difficult to plan than for pituitary adenoma. The tumour is very adherent at both a macroscopic and microscopic level, and all parts of the brain with which the original tumour was in contact need to be irradiated. However, resection decompresses the tumour and reduces the mass effect, so shifting the anatomy. Thus, neither preoperative nor postoperative imaging exactly represents the location of the target, so that the internal anatomy of the brain must also be considered in the planning.

There are usually some solid or cystic remnants following surgery, which can be demonstrated with MRI; these represent the GTV. The CTV should contain the following: any postoperative gross tumour; the surface of the preoperative gross tumour; and a margin for any uncertainty in localizing either of these two volumes. It is reasonable for the CTV to 'follow' any shift of the brain following decompression, based on the anatomy. The PTV margin should be grown isotropically, depending on the immobilization method used.

As noted above, the optic nerves, chiasm and tracts, should be outlined, so that the dose distribution and the DVHs for these structures can be reviewed.

Technique

A three-field conformal plan is usual, as per pituitary adenoma. If the target is large or irregular, a non-coplanar plan may be useful. TLD measurements of the eye doses should be made.

Dose and energy

50–55 Gy in 30–33 daily fractions over 6 weeks, with megavoltage x-rays.

As noted above, there is a small advantage from using high energy (i.e. 10–15 MV) x-rays to reduce temporal lobe doses because these tumours are located centrally within the skull.

Side effects

Side effects are similar to those for pituitary adenoma. In the occasional patient with a very large craniopharyngioma, hair loss may be significant, but should regrow. Ear symptoms (as above) may occur, but this relates to the exactly how far posteriorly and inferiorly the PTV extends.

For patients already taking hydrocortisone replacement, it is sensible to increase the dose, as noted above. Most patients with craniopharyngioma already have complete loss of hypothalamic–pituitary axis hormones.

The major difference in side effects compared to pituitary adenoma is the small but important risk of visual deterioration during RT. The cystic component of a craniopharyngioma may refill with fluid at a variable period after surgery, and cause compression of the optic chiasm. Re-accumulation of cyst fluid is unrelated to RT itself, but may occur coincidentally during the postoperative phase when RT is being given. If visual deterioration occurs, urgent MRI is needed. If cyst recurrence is confirmed, urgent neurosurgical referral for operation should be made, to try to preserve vision.

The risk of late radiotherapy damage to the optic nerves should be very small with a dose of 50 Gy in 30 fractions, prescribed to the isocentre. The risk of second tumour formation is similar to patients with pituitary adenoma, but this risk is very much less than the risk of recurrence of the craniopharyngioma if RT is not given.

Results of treatment

Radiotherapy following surgery produces high rates of control, around 85–90% at 10 years, and 80% at 20 years. Limited surgery plus radiotherapy produces local control rates as good as those from radical surgery, with lower neurological morbidity.

VESTIBULAR (ACOUSTIC) SCHWANNOMA

Pathology and clinical features

Strictly speaking, the correct term for this tumour is vestibular schwannoma, though the older term, acoustic neuroma, is still commonly used. These tumours represent a small proportion of patients referred for an opinion regarding RT (Figure 30.10). They are a common cause of unilateral deafness, with a population incidence in the range 0.5–2 per 100 000 per year. Patients commonly experience tinnitus, despite losing hearing, and this is an additional presenting symptom. Rarely, a vestibular schwannoma can be large enough at presentation to compress the brainstem, causing disturbance of balance. Some are associated with the genetic condition of neurofibromatosis type 2 (NF-2), which often presents with bilateral vestibular schwannomas.

A multidisciplinary approach is desirable for the management of patients with vestibular schwannoma. This group of patients is almost unique in having a choice of treatment options, though the decision may not be simple. Patients with NF-2 may have other tumours in addition to bilateral schwannomas, and their care is extremely complex.

Small tumours can be managed with a 'watch, wait and rescan' policy, and some stabilize spontaneously for long periods of time. Active treatment is only required with disease progression. Small and medium-sized tumours

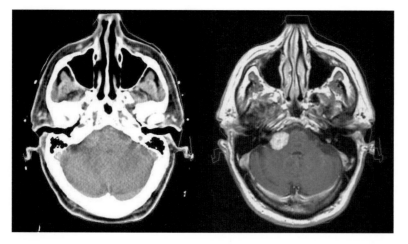

Figure 30.10 Planning CT and coregistered MRI of vestibular schwannoma (acoustic neuroma).

are well treated surgically, with very low rates of facial nerve damage. They are also well treated with both fractionated stereotactic radiotherapy (FSRT) and stereotactic radiosurgery (SRS). SRS can be performed using a Gamma Knife or linac-based 'X-knife'. Large tumours, with significant brainstem compression, usually require surgical resection. However, very large tumours may be too big to resect safely, and therefore are considered for radiotherapy. For these patients, FSRT is the appropriate technique.

Surgery is an excellent treatment, provided complete excision is achieved without undue disability. Most cases, though not all, are cured. Some surgical units prefer a 'translabyrinthine' approach, because it provides a safer approach for preservation of the facial nerve, but this is at the expense of irreversible hearing loss. It is therefore relatively more attractive to patients who are already deaf. For some patients, brainstem (cochlear) implants are possible.

Radiotherapy has excellent efficacy and low morbidity. Rates of local control appear similar for both surgery and RT, using either FSRT or SRS. Surgery has the attraction of removing the tumour and avoiding the small risk of radiotherapy-related second tumour risk, but has the disadvantages of a small operative mortality, protracted rehabilitation, a risk of facial nerve damage, and hearing loss depending on the surgical approach. Radiotherapy has the attraction of avoiding a major surgical procedure, has a lower rate of serious morbidity (and mortality) and probably a lower rate of facial nerve damage, at the expense of the tumour remaining in situ. Patient preference must be considered, and this group of patients is typically very well informed. Nevertheless, the decision may not be easy.

Treatment

Here, only the technique for FSRT will be described; SRS is a highly specialized technique, which should be studied in more specific texts.

Target volume

The patient should be immobilized in a beam direction shell or relocatable stereotactic frame. Radiotherapy should be fully conformal, based on CT planning with coregistered T1W+Gd MRI (see Figure 30.10). The tumour is not well shown on CT, but the internal auditory meatus (IAM) can be visualized. On MRI, the tumour is obvious, and extension into the IAM is obvious. Accuracy of the CT:MRI coregistration can be reviewed by comparing the bony canal of the IAM on CT with tumour extension into the canal on MRI. An accuracy of better than 1 mm should be achievable.

The GTV is the enhancing edge of the tumour seen on MRI. Provided the coregistration accuracy is high, no CTV margin is required. The PTV should be grown isotropically with an appropriate margin.

It is helpful to outline the pituitary so that a low dose can be confirmed. The cochlea is bound to lie within the PTV so that the dose is predictable without it being outlined. The eyes, specifically the lenses, should be outlined, to ensure that the tolerance dose is not exceeded, for example, by the exit dose from the posterior oblique beam. The ipsilateral parotid gland can also be outlined for the same reason.

Technique

A three-field conformal plan is usual, using anterior oblique and posterior oblique wedged fields and a lateral field, with coplanar or non-coplanar disposition depending on the exact target shape. Small volumes may also be treated with multiple arcs.

Dose and energy

50 Gy in 30 daily fractions over 6 weeks, with 6 MV photons.

Some centres have used higher doses, in the range 54–57.6 Gy, in 1.8 Gy fractions. Some hypofractionated schedules have also been designed, using lower doses in 12 fractions only. These doses exceed brainstem tolerance and are only suitable for small lesions. Preservation of cranial nerve function may be better with the slightly lower dose (50 Gy), but this needs to be formally evaluated. The variation in local control with dose also needs investigation.

Although the hearing preservation rate is lower in NF patients, a lower dose is not recommended lest the tumour control rates are reduced.

Side effects

Acute side effects include hair loss in the field entry portals, and there may be mild erythema of the skin. The skin within the external auditory meatus may also become irritated and, in the longer term, the wax may become thicker and more tenacious. Some patients experience mild nausea, which is easily controlled with simple antiemetics. A proportion of patients also experience some disturbance of balance, due to vestibulocochlear irritation. This resolves after RT, though this may take several weeks.

Important late effects include consideration of hearing preservation and cranial nerve function. Hearing preservation rates are in the region of 75% with both FSRT and SRS but also depend on tumour size in SRS series. Preservation of some useful hearing may be higher, and has been suggested to be as high as 90% in FSRT series. Patients with NF-2 have a higher risk of losing hearing, with a preservation rate of only 60%. Both FSRT and SRS series report facial neuropathy risks in around 1%, and trigeminal symptoms in 1–3% of patients. However, the risks are dose-related and may be lower than this with the suggested dose above.

There is a risk of late second tumour following RT, most relevant in younger patients. By analogy with the data from pituitary patients, and considering the small, lateralized volume, this is expected to be rather less than 1% per decade after treatment.

Results of treatment

Local control rates after fractionated stereotactic radiotherapy (FSRT) or stereotactic radiosurgery (SRS) are excellent, with approximately 95% tumour control at 5 years. This is equivalent to microsurgery results, though a direct comparison has never been attempted. Thus, radiotherapy has excellent efficacy as well as low morbidity.

CHORDOMA AND CHONDROSARCOMA OF THE SKULL BASE

Pathology and clinical features

These are rare tumours, but they present particular management problems. Chordomas and chondrosarcomas are distinct pathological entities. However, they share common features, and can be considered together. They are difficult to resect, and require very high doses of RT to achieve local control. Both types of tumour can metastasize.

Chordomas are twice as common as chondrosarcomas. They arise from remnants of the notochord, an embryological structure which elicits formation of the CNS. They may arise in the skull base, typically near but not in the midline, and along the whole length of the spine. The skull base, upper cervical spine and the sacrum are the most common locations. The distinction between a low skull base chordoma and an upper cervical tumour is often blurred. Chondrosarcomas also occur in the skull base, arising from bony or cartilaginous elements. These tumours usually present with pain, headache or cranial nerve palsies.

Treatment

Both tumour types require resection, which should aim to remove as much tumour as possible, and introduce space between tumour and brain stem. Because of their location, surgery is challenging and typically it is difficult to remove all tumour from the deep aspect. Radiotherapy should follow, but there is evidence that doses of at least 65 Gy are required. These have been treated very successfully outside the UK with proton or carbon ion radiotherapy. Since 2008

UK patients have been referred abroad under the proton Oversees Programme.

Target volume

The whole of the preoperative volume should be included in phase 1. For phase 2, a smaller volume should be boosted, corresponding to residual, imageable tumour or to the likely site of microscopic disease. Both pre- and postoperative imaging using CT and MRI are valuable. CT shows bone erosion, while MR demonstrates tumour itself.

If the brainstem and spinal cord are close by, then it is often appropriate to add a planning organ at risk volume (PRV) around these structures.

Technique

In order to minimize the PTV margin, and reduce dose to normal tissues, a relocatable stereotactic head frame is recommended, where possible. Patients whose tumours extend below the skull base require a beam direction shell. Individualized IMRT planning is required, in order to achieve high target doses without exceeding normal tissue tolerance, which might be life threatening. Each case should be considered individually.

Dose and energy

Chordoma
High doses are possible with image guided IMRT:

70 Gy in 39 fractions over 8 weeks
Sometimes a 2 phase approach can be used: 50–55 Gy followed by 15–20 Gy. Slightly higher doses can be used for residual extracranial disease

Chondrosarcoma

65 Gy in 39 fractions over 8 weeks

Even higher doses are given using protons (abroad).

Any plan needs to take into consideration the proximity of critical normal tissues.

Results of treatment

Excellent surgery has a profound effect on outcome. Thus, these cases are best treated in specialist centres including a skull base surgical team.

Local control is the most important problem. Chondrosarcomas can be controlled in over 80–90% of cases, and metastasize very rarely. Chordomas are less well controlled, with local control rates of only 40–80%. Of those chordomas that recur, local failure is the major problem, occurring in 95% of patients, but metastatic disease is found in 20%. This can be manifest as widespread dissemination, or involvement of regional lymph nodes. No effective treatment is available for patients who recur. The best results are reported following RT with protons or light ions.

SPINAL CORD TUMOURS – PRIMARY

Pathology and clinical features

The majority of these tumours are intrinsic, predominantly ependymomas or astrocytomas. Glioblastomas also occur, but thankfully are rare. Intrinsic tumours compress the spinal cord from within, and often produce some permanent neurological damage. They can usually be surgically debulked, which often improves the neurology, though it may not recover fully. Tumour removed at surgery provides the histological diagnosis. However, surgery is hazardous and, in some patients, neurological deficit worsens after operation. Often, subtotal resection, minimizing or avoiding neurological deterioration, is an appropriate strategy. Most intrinsic tumours of the cord require postoperative radiotherapy.

Low-grade (i.e. grade I) ependymomas of myxopapillary type are one of the most common primary tumours affecting the lower end of the spinal cord itself (the conus medullaris) and the lumbosacral nerve roots. Some of these tumours can be removed completely, perhaps over half, and may not require radiotherapy; in most, some residual tumour remains, and radiotherapy is highly effective in achieving long-term cure. In higher grade ependymomas, RT is necessary. Astrocytomas are usually high grade and require RT. Glioblastomas are usually irradiated, but have a bleak outlook. Temozolomide may be added.

Occasional extrinsic tumours also occur: meningiomas arise from the coverings of the cord; schwannomas and neurofibromas arise in nerve roots. These extrinsic tumours compress the spinal cord. Surgical removal relieves the compression, and the deficit often recovers. Surgery alone is usually curative.

Primary spinal cord tumours typically present with a mixture of sensory and motor impairment, related to the site of tumour involvement. Less commonly, they present with pain.

Treatment – radical

Target volume

The clinical target volume includes the whole spinal canal, anteriorly and laterally. Superiorly and inferiorly, a CTV margin of 2–3 cm is usual for the majority of intrinsic tumours. Around the CTV, the PTV should be grown isotropically, with a margin of 0.5–1 cm. The target is most appropriately localized from preoperative imaging, using vertebral levels. Postoperative MRI is useful to document the extent of residual disease.

In the past, ependymomas of the lumbosacral region have been treated to include the whole of the thecal sac below the tumour. Certainly, some of these tumours can be seen to have drop metastases or 'sugar-coating' disease at presentation. Historical series in which this extended target is favored largely predate the era of high quality MR imaging, and it is not clear if this is necessary in patients with no evidence of distal disease on MRI staging.

CT planning allows normal tissue structures to be delineated, such as the oesophagus and thyroid in patients with cervical tumours, the lungs and oesophagus in those with thoracic tumours, and the kidneys and possibly ovaries in patients with lumbosacral tumours.

Technique

The first decision is whether to position the patient prone or supine. A prone positioning has the advantage that set-up marks on the patient are directly related to the site to be treated, and the spine can be easily palpated by the radiographers. It also avoids the loss of skin sparing when beams pass through the treatment couch. However, it is less reproducible and less comfortable for patients. Patients who have significant neurological disability may be unable to adopt a prone position easily, and this may affect reproducibility of set-up. For patients with thoracic tumours who lie prone, there is the additional disadvantage that respiration moves the target volume anteroposteriorly, by up to 1.0 cm. Although this can be screened in the simulator, this movement must be included in the PTV margin, therefore increasing irradiation to normal tissue.

Cervical tumours are well treated in a prone positioning, and it is helpful to use a beam direction shell. If possible, the chin should be raised to avoid exit dose through the mouth. For thoracic tumours, a supine position is usually best, using a thoracic board, with the arms above the head. This allows lateral alignment tattoos to be placed in a reproducible position. Lumbar tumours are typically treated prone.

The optimum beam arrangement is almost always using a three-field plan, with two wedged posterior oblique beams and a direct posterior beam. The hinge angles for the posterior oblique beams are optimized to the shape of the target, and deeper normal tissue structures. In some patients, and especially those with lumbosacral tumours, a longitudinal wedge on the posterior field, or a field-in-field boost, can be effective in achieving dose homogeneity.

Dose and energy

50 Gy in 30 fractions, treating daily, over 6 weeks, with megavoltage photons.

This is a reasonable estimate of safe cord tolerance, in a patient with a spinal cord tumour. For patients with GBM of the spinal cord, a higher dose, such as 54 Gy in 30 fractions, should be considered.

Side effects

Side effects of treatment are usually very modest, and depend on the location of the tumour. It is unusual for neurological function to deteriorate and, if this does happen, it can be managed with increasing the steroid dose. Some esophagitis may occur in patients with cervical or upper thoracic tumours, but it is normally mild. Patients with lumbar or lumbosacral tumours may experience nausea or mild diarrhea, but these symptoms can be managed effectively with simple medication. Kidney doses should be low, and clinically unimportant. Spinal cord damage from RT should not occur with the dose noted above.

RT does not inhibit the normal recovery of neurological function which occurs after surgery, and may continue for up to a year following excision.

Treatment – palliative

A few patients require palliative treatment. This can be achieved with a simple beam arrangement, using the dose and fractionation as for palliative treatment of HGG.

Results of treatment

Ependymomas have a better prognosis than astrocytic tumours. Grade I lesions are cured in most patients, and grade II tumours in the region of 50% of patients. Higher grade ependymomas are rare, but as expected have a worse prognosis. Astrocytomas have a worse prognosis, grade for grade, than ependymomas. Glioblastomas of the cord have an appalling prognosis. Recurrence often occurs within a few weeks or months of treatment, and may include dissemination through the CSF.

CEREBRAL METASTASES

Clinical features and management principles

The majority of patients, approximately two-thirds, with cerebral metastases have multiple lesions (Figure 30.11). Around 80% occur in the cerebrum. Those in the cerebellum may cause hydrocephalus. Most patients also have active disease elsewhere. Occasionally, the first presentation is with metastasis, and biopsy may be important in establishing the diagnosis. Intra-axial metastases have similar presentation to primary tumours (see above).

Metastatic spread may also cause diffuse meningeal disease, infiltrating widely over the surface of the brain. This manifestation of disseminated disease may present with confusion, photophobia and neck stiffness, i.e. symptoms and signs associated with meningitis. It may also cause cranial nerve palsies, from involvement of meninges at the base of the brain. Metastatic disease may also affect the bones of the skull. Involvement of the skull base typically produces cranial nerve palsies, by compression of the nerves as they pass through the skull.

Patients with single or multiple cerebral metastases are almost always incurable. The treatment objective is therefore palliative, and additional supportive care should be instituted. Steroid treatment is normally appropriate to reduce surrounding oedema. Unless the patient is in the end stage of their disease, it is helpful for the patient to be restaged to assess the extent and aggressiveness of the

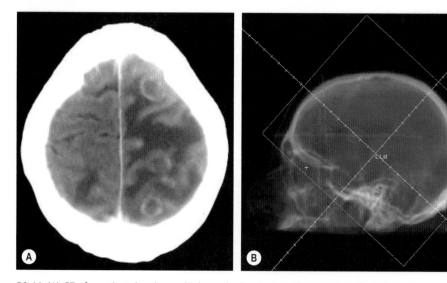

Figure 30.11 (A) CT of a patient showing multiple cerebral metastases from non-small cell lung cancer, surrounded by oedema. Three deposits are seen in the left hemisphere, and another single lesion is visible in the right cerebral hemisphere, posteriorly. Oedema is seen around each deposit. (B) Field for whole brain irradiation (WBI), showing adequate coverage around the skull, including at the skull base. The collimator angle allows sparing of dose to the eyes and pharynx.

disease, to guide systemic treatment, and inform prognosis. It is usually appropriate for the patient to be managed by the relevant site-specific team. As well as palliative radiotherapy, chemotherapy and hormonal therapy may be helpful.

A few patients have a solitary metastasis, are fit with no active disease outside the brain, and have a reasonable disease-free interval (e.g. 1 year) since completion of primary treatment. These patients may warrant more aggressive treatment, involving surgical resection or stereotactic radiosurgery (SRS). Both surgical resection and SRS improve local control within the brain. Both can be followed by whole brain irradiation (WBI), which treats micrometastatic disease and has been shown to improve control in the remainder of the brain. Surgical resection is particularly useful for patients with posterior fossa tumours causing hydrocephalus. Where SRS is to be used, it should be given before WBI, to ensure that the lesion is visible on imaging.

Some patients may be in sufficiently poor general condition that even simple palliative radiotherapy may not be of value. For meningeal disease, i.e. carcinomatous meningitis, in addition to palliative radiotherapy, intrathecal methotrexate may be of symptomatic benefit.

Treatment

Palliative radiotherapy treatment

Target volume and technique

Whole brain irradiation (WBI)

The patient should ideally be immobilized in a beam direction shell. At the least, the head should be immobilized using tape or bolus bags around the head. The whole brain should be treated, both cerebrum and cerebellum, since part of the objective is to treat micrometastases.

The standard beam arrangement is a parallel pair of lateral-opposing fields. These can be applied from simulator or CT imaging using a virtual simulator tool. The collimator should be rotated to follow approximately the radiological baseline, in order to avoid the eyes. Sufficient margin should be allowed, first for patient movement or day-to-day variation in positioning (i.e. a PTV margin) and, secondly, to allow an adequate field size to treat the whole brain effectively (see Figure 30.11).

If it is impossible to simulate, then simple landmarks can be used. The inferior border of the lateral field can follow a line between the lateral edge of the superior orbital ridge to the notch below the tragus of the ear. Clearance of the scalp by 1 cm at the other three edges will be sufficient.

Skull base irradiation

The beam arrangement is also a parallel pair of lateral-opposing fields, applied from simulator or CT. Under normal circumstances, when it is necessary to treat the bones through which the cranial nerves pass, the field should extend from the outer canthus down and back to the posterior edge of the foramen magnum. This will cover cranial nerves II–XII.

Dose and energy

Megavoltage x-rays are preferable. If orthovoltage x-rays must be used, then the head should be packed round with bolus material to approximate a tissue-equivalent cube, and a 10% dose reduction should be made to allow for the higher relative biological efficiency (RBE) of orthovoltage compared to megavoltage x-rays.

A variety of dose schedules is available:

> 30 Gy in 10 fractions, treating daily, over 2 weeks
> 20 Gy in 5 fractions, treating daily, over 1 week
> 12 Gy in 2 fractions, treating on consecutive days or up to 1 week apart.

Side effects

Side effects are the same as for palliative RT for HGG.

Palliative stereotactic radiosurgery (SRS)

Target volume and technique

SRS can be carried out using a skull fixation frame or a relocatable stereotactic head frame. To use a relocatable head frame successfully, the patient must have good teeth and normal neurological function. MRI demonstrates the tumour optimally, and should be electronically coregistered with the localization planning CT. The simplest systems use circular applicators, to treat spherical targets. Happily, metastases usually form an approximately spherical shape. The applicator with the appropriate diameter is chosen to cover the metastasis. Multiple non-coplanar, non-opposed arcs are normally used, starting and finishing to avoid entry or exit through the eyes. IMRT can also be used. An upper size limit of 3 cm diameter is usual.

The 'target' may be the edge of the gross tumour or an additional margin of 2–3 mm to allow for set-up inaccuracies. However, the patient position can be verified before treatment proceeds, and treating only the gross tumour minimizes acute side effects.

Dose and energy

The prescription is normally made to the 90% isodose line, which is placed around the edge of the target. Some centres prescribe to the 50% isodose.

Dose: 16–24 Gy in 1 fraction, at 90% isodose.

It is advisable to give steroids to cover the SRS, such as dexamethasone 16 mg starting 24 hours before treatment, for 24 hours after, then tailing off over 3–4 days.

In some centres, a higher WBI is used in patients with solitary metastases receiving SRS, such as 40 Gy in 20 fractions over 4 weeks.

Results of treatment

Provided patients are selected carefully, most of those who undergo treatment appear to benefit in terms of palliation of symptoms. Even so, survival of patients with cerebral deposits is generally poor, with survival after palliative radiotherapy of the order of a few months. This is normally dominated by the systemic illness. Some patients with solitary metastases, especially where systemic treatment can also be given, may live for 1 year or more. For patients with meningeal disease, the prognosis is much worse.

FURTHER READING

General management issues

Burnet NG, Bulusu VR, Jefferies SJ. Management of primary brain tumours. In: Booth S, Bruera E, editors. Palliative care consultations in primary and metastatic brain tumours. Oxford University Press; 2004.

Specifics of radiotherapy planning for CNS tumours

Burnet NG, Thomas SJ, Burton KE, Jefferies SJ. Defining the tumour and target volumes for radiotherapy. Cancer Imaging 2004;4:1–9.

Burnet NG, Jefferies SJ, Benson RJ, Hunt DP, Treasure FP. Years of life lost (YLL) from cancer is an important measure of population burden – and should be considered when allocating research funds. Br J Cancer 2005;92: 241–55.

Burton KE, Thomas SJ, Whitney D, Routsis DS, Benson RJ, Burnet NG. Accuracy of a relocatable stereotactic radiotherapy head frame evaluated by use of a depth helmet. Clin Oncol 2002;14:31–9.

Combs SE, Volk S, Schulz-Ertner D, Huber PE, Thilmann C, Debus J. Management of acoustic neuromas with fractionated stereotactic radiotherapy (FSRT): long-term results in 106 patients treated in a single institution. Int J Radiat Oncol Biol Phys 2005;63:75–81.

Hodson DJ, Bowles KM, Cooke LJ, et al. Primary central nervous system lymphoma: a single-centre experience of 55 unselected cases. Clin Oncol 2005;17:185–91.

Jansen EP, Dewit LG, van Herk M, Bartelink H. Target volumes in radiotherapy for high-grade malignant glioma of the brain. Radiother Oncol 2000;56: 151–6.

Stupp R, Hegi ME, Mason WP, van den Bent MJ, Taphoorn MJ, Janzer RC, Ludwin SK, Allgeier A, Fisher B, Belanger K, Hau P, Brandes AA, Gijtenbeek J, Marosi C, Vecht CJ, Mokhtari K, Wesseling P, Villa S, Eisenhauer E, Gorlia T, Weller M, Lacombe D, Cairncross JG, Mirimanoff RO. European Organisation for Research and Treatment of Cancer Brain Tumour and Radiation Oncology Groups; National Cancer Institute of Canada Clinical Trials Group. Effects of radiotherapy with concomitant and adjuvant temozolomide versus radiotherapy alone on survival in glioblastoma in a randomised phase III study: 5-year analysis of the EORTC-NCIC trial. Lancet Oncol 2009;10(5):459–66.

The Royal College of Radiologists . Imaging for oncology. BFCO(04)2. The Royal College of Radiologists; 2004.

van den Bent MJ, Afra D, de Witte O, et al. EORTC Radiotherapy and Brain Tumour Groups and the UK Medical Research Council. Long-term efficacy of early versus delayed radiotherapy for low-grade astrocytoma and oligodendroglioma in adults: the EORTC 22845 randomised trial. Lancet 2005;366:985–90.

Estall V, Treece SJ, Jena R, Jefferies SJ, Burton KE, Parker RA, Burnet NG. Pattern of relapse after fractionated external beam radiotherapy for meningioma: experience from Addenbrooke's Hospital. Clin Oncol 2009;21(10):745–52.

Minniti G, Amelio D, Amichetti M, Salvati M, Muni R, Bozzao A, Lanzetta G, Scarpino S, Arcella A, Enrici RM. Patterns of failure and comparison of different target volume delineations in patients with glioblastoma treated with conformal radiotherapy plus concomitant and adjuvant temozolomide. Radiother Oncol 2010;97(3):377–81.

Potluri S, Jefferies SJ, Jena R, Harris F, Burton KE, Prevost AT, Burnet NG. Residual post-operative tumour volume predicts outcome after high dose radiotherapy for Chordoma and Chondrosarcoma of the skull base and spine. Clin Oncol 2011;23 (3):199–208.

Thiel E, Korfel A, Martus P, Kanz L, Griesinger F, Rauch M, Röth A, Hertenstein B, von Toll T, Hundsberger T, Mergenthaler HG, Leithäuser M, Birnbaum T, Fischer L, Jahnke K, Herrlinger U, Plasswilm L, Nägele T, Pietsch T, Bamberg M, Weller M. High-dose methotrexate with or without whole brain radiotherapy for primary CNS lymphoma (G-PCNSL-SG-1): a phase 3, randomised, non-inferiority trial. Lancet Oncol 2010;11 (11):1036–47.

Chapter | 31 |

Eye and orbit

Adrian Harnett

CHAPTER CONTENTS

ANATOMY

The orbit is defined by bony margins and is conical in shape. It contains the eye, the optic nerve and the recti and oblique extraocular muscles. The optic nerve exits from just below the centre of the back of the eye and extends to the optic foramen at the apex of the orbit posteriorly. The globe is composed of three layers, an outer fibrous layer called the sclera, a middle layer which is vascular and is composed of the choroid, the ciliary body and the iris and an inner neural layer, the retina. The vascular choroid covers the inner surface of the sclera. The diameter of the eye is 2.4 cm and the lens is 0.5 cm from the anterior surface.

The movement of each eye is performed by six muscles, (four recti and two oblique muscles) and three cranial nerves, the IIIrd, IVth and VIth. The VIth cranial nerve supplies the lateral rectus muscle which moves the eyeball laterally. The medial, superior and inferior recti elevate, depress and move the eyeball inward, while the inferior oblique moves the eyeball upward and outward. All these four muscles are supplied by the IIIrd cranial nerve. The superior oblique which moves the eye downward and outward is supplied by the IVth cranial nerve.

The membrane lining the inner surface of the eyelids is the conjunctiva which courses over the anterior surface of the globe, extending to the corneoscleral junction. Tears are secreted by minor lacrimal glands situated on mainly the lower eyelid and can be supplemented by the lacrimal gland situated in the upper lateral part of the orbit. They drain into the nose through the nasolacrimal duct.

PATHOLOGY

Benign

Dysthyroid eye disease and reactive lymphoid hyperplasia

The pathology of both these conditions is poorly understood.

Malignant

Primary
Secondary/metastatic

Tumours can be classified as arising from the skin and adnexia, orbit or intraocularly. Basal cell carcinomas (BCC) and squamous cell carcinomas (SCCs) are skin tumours commonly arising on the face, especially around the eye and lower eye lid. In contrast, lacrimal gland and nasolacrimal duct tumours are rare, as are orbital tumours. Rhabdomyosarcoma of the orbit is a tumour of childhood. It is usually embryonal and is discussed in further detail in Chapter 33. Intraocular tumours are rare with retinoblastoma occurring in the very young and melanoma in adults. The choroid is the commonest site in the eye for metastatic disease.

Primary tumours of the eye and orbit are listed below:

1. Skin and adnexal
   a. Basal cell carcinoma (BCC)
   b. Squamous cell carcinoma (SCC)
   c. Lacrimal gland
   d. Nasolacrimal duct
   e. Miscellaneous
2. Orbital tumours
   a. Lymphoma
   b. Melanoma (conjunctival)
   c. Rhabdomyosarcoma
   d. Optic nerve glioma
3. Intraocular
   a. Melanoma (choroidal and iris)
   b. Retinoblastoma.

RADIATION AND OCULAR MORBIDITY

The lens

The eye contains structures that are both very radiosensitive and radioresistant. One of the most sensitive tissues in the body is the lens. Cataracts have been reported at doses as low as 2 Gy. However, it should be remembered that they invariably occur over the age of 70 and are associated with various common diseases, such as diabetes, and medications, such as steroids. The appearance and region of the cataract can help in deciding their causation. Radiation cataracts are caused by damage to cells in the anterior central area of the lens, which then start to form a cataract at the back of the lens centrally. The total dose, energy of radiation, volume of the lens, health of the eye and concomitant disease are all factors that play a part in cataract formation. When high doses are given with β-irradiation eye plaques, usually for treatment of posterior choroidal melanomas, cataracts often will not occur because of the rapid fall off of dose (as opposed to the historical use of cobalt plaques). After external beam radiotherapy, fractionated doses of over 10 Gy are likely to cause detectable lens opacities, usually occurring within 2–3 years of radiotherapy. Figure 31.1 shows a radiation cataract. Treatment of a cataract is by surgical removal, although if the eye is dry (most commonly as a result of radiotherapy), this may adversely affect the success of surgery.

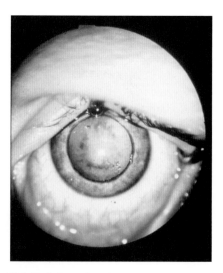

Figure 31.1 Radiation cataract.

The sclera and retina

The sclera, on the other hand, is radioresistant because it is avascular and can tolerate doses of up to 100 Gy by radioactive eye plaques to a small area. Above this dose there is a risk of necrosis. The retina can tolerate doses of 50 Gy but, above this, retinal damage is manifest by haemorrhages, exudates and atrophy. Radiation atrophy and post-subcapsular cataract are shown in Figures 31.2 and 31.3. The macula is the most sensitive area of the retina and doses here should be minimized or avoided if possible when using radioactive eye plaques. Similarly, as the dose increases above 50 Gy, there is an increasing likelihood of optic atrophy.

The cornea and lacrimal apparatus

These structures usually tolerate doses of up to 50 Gy well, depending on radiotherapy technique, energy, fractionation and attention to good eye care. It will result in erythema of both skin and conjunctiva, local irritation and lacrimation. If megavoltage radiotherapy is used, these reactions will be reduced due to build-up and skin sparing. Tear production is from the minor lacrimal glands mainly located on the lower eyelid and supplemented by the major lacrimal gland in the upper lateral part of the orbit anteriorly. This should be shielded in radiotherapy planning in an attempt to preserve tear production as much as possible. It is reduced above 30 Gy and patients may require hypomellose eye drops (artificial tears) above this dose and lacrilube. Doses of 50 Gy and above result in more serious problems.

Stenosis or occlusion of the nasolacrimal duct due to a tumour adjacent to the inner canthus will result in a weeping eye (epiphora). There is evidence that this does not happen due to radiotherapy alone if it is carefully fractionated and the tumour has not comprised the function of the duct already. A dose of 45 Gy in 10 fractions on a superficial unit (100 kV) is the minimum fractionation recommended. Figures 31.4 (before radiotherapy) and 31.5 (after radiotherapy) illustrate a basal cell carcinoma in this region treated with superficial radiotherapy.

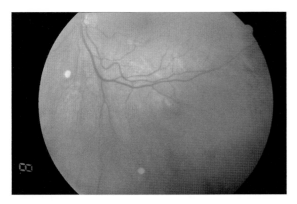

Figure 31.2 Radiation atrophy.

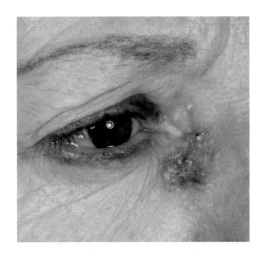

Figure 31.4 Basal cell carcinoma – pre-radiotherapy.

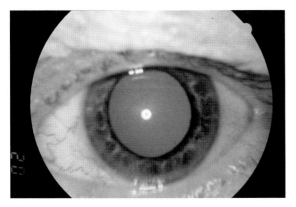

Figure 31.3 Radiation atrophy and postsubcapsular cataract.

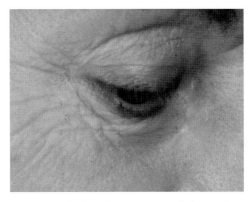

Figure 31.5 Basal cell carcinoma – post-radiotherapy 4 months later.

Developing a dry eye is not only very uncomfortable but may result in loss of vision. Corneal damage occurs, partly due to reduced sensation. Punctate keratitis and edema lead on to corneal ulceration, scarring, infection and impairment of vision. If high dose radiotherapy is given, the involvement of an ophthalmologist to give advice, eye protection and ensure good eye care is imperative during the course of radiotherapy. This will aid in achieving patient comfort, maximizing vision and minimizing late complications. Keratinization of the cornea is a late complication and occurs after doses in excess of 50 Gy. Rarely, it leads on to secondary revascularization.

PRINCIPLES OF IRRADIATION

These are governed by whether radical or palliative treatment is being given, the type of tumour, benign or malignant, radiosensitivity, its extent and patient factors, such as fitness and co-morbidity. The patient should have a comfortable set-up for radiotherapy, which is likely to make the treatment more reproducible, and appropriate immobilization. For palliative treatment, a simple device such as an orfit can be used but, for radical treatment, a full beam directional shell is usually necessary. It is often difficult to protect part of the eye (especially as it is a small structure), particularly the lens and cornea, although internal eye shields will achieve this when treating skin tumours around the eye. The major lacrimal gland can be shielded in some external beam radiotherapy plans.

Technique

For radical radiotherapy, patients are planned with the aid of a computed tomography (CT) scan. Paired wedged fields are usually most appropriate. A combination of three fields planned conformally may achieve a better isodose distribution for extensive tumours and reduce the dose to normal tissues (Figure *evolve* 31.6 🖱). A prescription to a dose of 54–60 Gy with 2 Gy daily treatments is commonly employed. Great attention should be paid to eye care and regular reviews should be performed by clinicians during the course of radiotherapy.

BENIGN CONDITIONS

Dysthyroid eye disease and reactive lymphoid hyperplasia

Pathology and clinical features

As already stated, the pathology of both these conditions is poorly understood. Thyrotoxicosis is often associated with marked eye signs, including exophthalmos, lid retraction and lid lag, corneal exposure and chemosis. This occurs

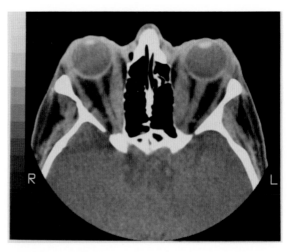

Figure 31.7 CT scan showing grossly enlarged medial recti in dysthyroid eye disease.

due to an infiltration of tissues in the orbital cone and, particularly, the extraocular muscles (Figure 31.7), although appearances on CT scans may be relatively normal. Medical treatment usually results in resolution of the eye problems but, occasionally, it can be more refractory or occurs (or recurs) when the patient is euthyroid or even hypothyroid.

Reactive lymphoid hyperplasia behaves as a low-grade lymphoma, again involving the orbital cone but usually more posteriorly. The commonest symptom is unilateral pain behind the eye and, less frequently, visual disturbance and exophthalmos. Due to difficulties in access and equivocal histology (an inflammatory infiltrate is often reported), the diagnosis is usually made clinically. CT is often normal or the inflammatory mass resolves very quickly after starting steroid therapy and therefore missed on imaging. However, relapse can occur on stopping or trying to reduce steroid therapy and, in this situation, radiotherapy is indicated.

Radiotherapy technique

For both conditions, patients are immobilized in a beam directional shell and CT planned. Although dysthyroid eye disease is occasionally unilateral, it is usually recommended to treat both eyes. Paired lateral radiation fields are used to encompass both orbits so that the 50% isodose is through the anterior pituitary (Figure 31.8). The fields are wedged and angled slightly posteriorly to accommodate for the tissue gap from the contour and to prevent divergence of the beam through the lens. This angulation posteriorly is usually of the order of 5° except where there is marked asymmetrical proptosis. As a result, the 10% isodose is parallel and through the posterior aspect of the lenses. Figure 31.9 shows moderately severe disease and

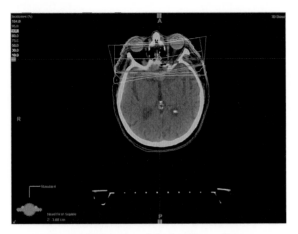

Figure 31.8 Dosimetric plan of dysthyroid eye disease.

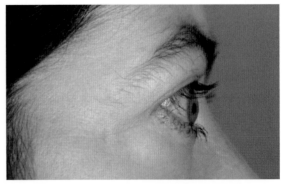

Figure 31.10 Ophthalmic Grave's disease – post-radiotherapy.

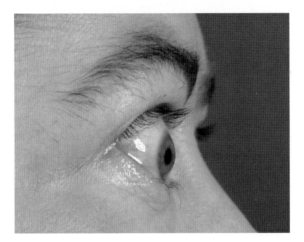

Figure 31.9 Ophthalmic Grave's disease – pre-radiotherapy.

Figure 31.10 is 9 months later following treatment with radiotherapy. The proptosis is much improved, the eyes are quiet and much more comfortable.

In the situation of reactive lymphoid hyperplasia, the disease is almost exclusively unilateral and so treatment is given on just the involved side. A pair of wedged megavoltage fields with an anterior and lateral are used. Megavoltage x-rays will allow some skin sparing to the anterior tissues, which will include the lens, but it is very difficult actually to add effective shielding for the lens.

Dose and energy

In dysthyroid eye disease, an initial fraction of 1 Gy prescribed to midline is given to ensure there is no increase in the inflammatory eyes signs and, particularly, any deterioration in vision. If this does occur, then the patient should be started on steroids, or the dose of steroids increased or radiotherapy suspended and urgent orbital decompression carried out. The daily dose should be increased after the first dose to 1.73 Gy per day to a total dose of 20 Gy in 12 fractions over 16 days. For reactive lymphoid hyperplasia, the standard dose is 30 Gy in 15 fractions over 19 days.

PRIMARY MALIGNANT TUMOURS

Skin and adnexia

Pathology and clinical features

Basal cell carcinomas are the commonest skin tumour and frequently occur on the face, especially around the eye. When they occur near the inner canthus, the nasolacrimal duct may be affected, causing the patient to complain of chemosis. They have a typical appearance, superficial, poorly demarcated and ulcerated (see Figure 31.4), as opposed to squamous cell carcinomas which have more of a pearly appearance. Nonetheless, biopsy should be performed to confirm the diagnosis. The incidence is higher in those who have a lot of sun exposure and so is related to outside occupations. They grow slowly and so may be neglected but, if left, will invade, ulcerate and destroy tissue locally (Figure 31.11). The ulcerating basal cell carcinoma in this case had extended into the orbit and frontal lobe.

Radiotherapy technique and dose

Local excision or radiotherapy can be used. In the latter case, this can be with superficial x-rays (SXR) or electrons. For BCCs, there should be a margin of 5 mm around the lesion and 10 mm for SCCs when using SXR (and slightly more for electrons). A cut out is made and a dose of 45 Gy in 10 fractions with 100 kV x-rays given. Figure 31.5 shows a good cosmetic result obtained 4 months after radiotherapy. A longer course of treatment should be used for larger lesions, giving 50 Gy in 15 fractions. Low-energy electrons can be used in preference to SXR, but protection of normal tissues is not as easy as with photons. Chemosis as a result of

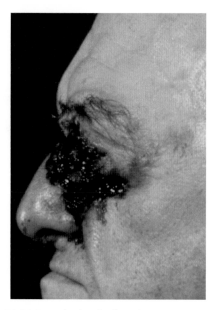

Figure 31.11 Extensive basal cell carcinoma.

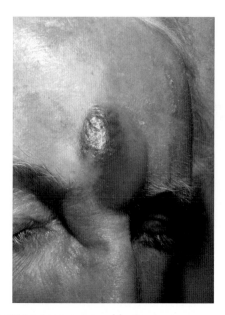

Figure 31.12 Angiosarcoma of forehead.

radiotherapy should not occur if it is reasonably fractionated and the nasolacrimal duct is not stenosed by the tumour. An internal eyeshield should be inserted for each treatment when the treated area is right next to the eye or involving the lower eyelid.

Lacrimal gland and nasolacrimal duct carcinomas are rare, locally invasive and difficult to treat. Involvement due to lymphoma must be excluded. Each case must be considered on its merits and discussed with the ophthalmic surgeon and oncologist in order that the most appropriate treatment is selected, either surgery or high dose radical radiotherapy.

As in other sites, rare primary tumours can occur around the eye. Figure 31.12 is one such example of an angiosarcoma arising on the forehead in an elderly retired fisherman. Note the characteristic appearance of a cystic red/purple lesion. They respond rapidly to radiotherapy but, despite high doses, also recur locally and regionally.

Tumours arising from adjacent structures

Other tumours can invade directly into the orbit and cause extensive destruction. One example is a maxillary sinus squamous carcinoma (see Figure *evolve* 31.6 🖱). Radiotherapy was planned with a three-field technique with fields one and two blocked medially for the contralateral eye and field three blocked posteriorly to shield the brain (Figure *evolve* 31.13 🖱). Bolus was used as shown and the red outline shows the GTV and light blue shows the PTV. Note the course of the contralateral optic nerve has been outlined. All fields were conformal, which is illustrated in Figure

evolve 31.14 🖱 for the right posterior olique field. A point dose for the left (contralateral) lens is shown.

Lymphoma

Pathology

Ocular lymphoma may be localized and the sole site of disease or a manifestation of widespread involvement. The former is more likely to be due to low-grade lymphoma and is very rarely bilateral, whereas high grade frequently involves other sites.

Clinical features

Presentation may be due to a typically discrete erythematous conjunctival lesion (Figure 31.15), minor eye discomfort, a mass most often involving the major lacrimal gland, ptyosis, chemosis, diplopia, exophthalmos and a red eye (Figure 31.16). Symptoms and signs of more widespread involvement can be present.

Diagnosis and investigation

A tissue diagnosis may have been obtained from either a lymph node biopsy if the patient has lymphadenopathy, occasionally from bone marrow examination or from the ocular site. Access to a posterior orbital mass is difficult even when the mass is relatively large. The usual staging procedures for lymphoma should be performed including

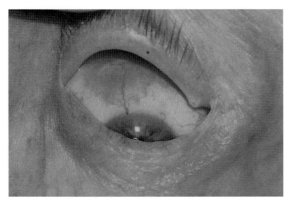

Figure 31.15 Conjunctival lymphoma – pre-radiotherapy.

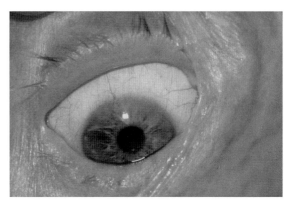

Figure 31.17 Conjunctival lymphoma – post-radiotherapy.

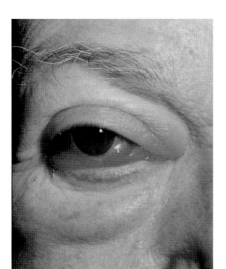

Figure 31.16 Conjunctival lymphoma – pre-radiotherapy.

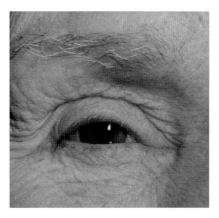

Figure 31.18 Conjunctival lymphoma – post-radiotherapy.

a whole body CT scan and bone marrow trephine. For what may appear to be localized conjunctival lymphoma, it is important to have a CT scan of the orbits as the tumour sometimes tracks around the globe and involves the orbital cone.

Treatment

Treatment will depend on the staging. For high-grade lymphoma and/or widespread involvement, chemotherapy is the first-line treatment, supplemented by radiotherapy when appropriate. The patient is set up and planned in the standard fashion with good immobilization as already described. For anteriorly placed low-grade lesions, a direct field with a small circular applicator or cut-out using superficial x-rays is usually appropriate. Figures 31.15 and 31.17 illustrate a typical case before and after radiotherapy. Low-energy electrons are an alternative. For more extensive or high-grade tumours after initial chemotherapy, megavoltage radiotherapy using paired wedged fields should be chosen or, occasionally, a direct field with photons or electrons. Again, response to radiotherapy treatment is shown in Figures 31.16 and 31.18.

A dose of 30 Gy in 15 fractions over 19 days is given for low-grade disease and 40–45 Gy in 15 fractions for high-grade disease.

Ocular melanoma

Melanoma is the commonest primary intraocular tumour. In adults, it most frequently affects the uveal tract, especially the choroid.

Clinical features and investigation

It is not uncommon for asymptomatic patients to be referred by an optician who, at a routine eye test, has detected a pigmented lesion in the fundus. Some of these lesions will be choroidal nevi but some will be melanomas (Figure 31.19). It may be difficult to distinguish between the two, particularly for a small melanoma, and so the patient may be initially managed conservatively with 6-monthly assessments. Other patients may present with visual loss which may be associated with retinal detachment. Pain does not often occur and may indicate a large tumour. Tumours arising from the iris and conjunctiva (Figures 31.20 and 31.21) are clearly visible and so are noticed by the patient or their family.

An expert ophthalmic assessment is mandatory by a clinician experienced in this field, and will include direct and/or indirect ophthalmoscopy (Figures 31.22 and 31.23), ocular ultrasound and fluorescein angiography. This may be supplemented by magnetic resonance imaging (MRI) for large tumours which may be considered for local resection. It may detect extraocular extension.

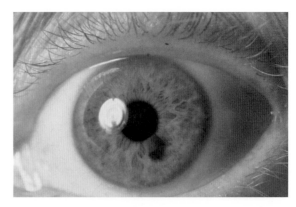

Figure 31.21 Melanoma of iris.

Natural history

Melanomas of the eye are often detected when they are very small and may measure under 5 mm at their base and

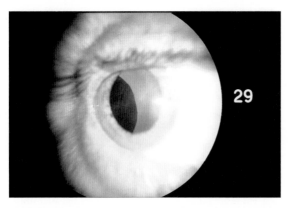

Figure 31.19 Choroidal melanoma – defined as large because it is easily visible on dilation.

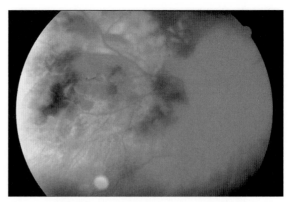

Figure 31.22 Choroidal melanoma – seen on indirect ophthalmoscopy.

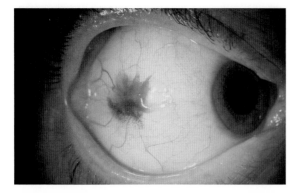

Figure 31.20 Conjunctival melanoma – visible as a poorly demarcated lesion.

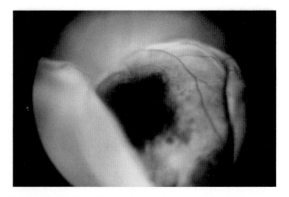

Figure 31.23 Choroidal melanoma – seen on indirect ophthalmoscopy.

1 mm in height. They grow slowly and so initial treatment may be observation in order to confirm the diagnosis. Some patients present with metastases, particularly involving the liver. Others develop metastatic disease up to 15 years later and, not surprisingly, the risk increases with the size of the ocular tumour at presentation. Patients with anterior placed tumours in the uveal tract are at higher risk than those with posterior choroidal melanomas.

Treatment

The mainstay of treatment of conjunctival and iris melanomas is local excision. Rarely, radioactive eye plaques are used as primary treatment or post-surgery. Due to the size of the tumour, enucleation may be the only option.

There are more treatment options for choroid and ciliary body tumours. Historically, enucleation has been the standard treatment but more conservative treatment using radioactive eye plaques, originally with cobalt-60 but now superseded by ruthinium or iodine, has been used for a long time. Studies have therefore shown that eye preservation has not adversely affected survival. Indeed, it was even considered by some to improve survival by possibly an immunoprotective mechanism.

It is unclear whether the dose to the base or apex of the tumour is important. Most centres prescribe a dose to the apex of 10 000 cGy (100 Gy). Retreatment has been carried out but it is advised that the total dose to the choroid does not exceed 100 000 cGy. Otherwise the risk of severe complications including vitreous hemorrhage and perforation of the globe becomes unacceptable.

For medium-sized tumours, local resection can be performed under hypotensive anesthesia. This is often supplemented with insertion of a radioactive plaque at the end of the procedure and removal several days later, depending on the activity of the plaque and the dose prescribed.

Unfortunately, very occasionally patients present with very extensive, neglected tumours (Figure *evolve* 31.24 🖱). Obviously, the treatment options in these situations are very limited. Radiotherapy has been used and, as in the figure, shows a response with regression of the extensive tumour. High fractionated doses have to be used, either with weekly fractions of 6 Gy or daily treatment to 60 Gy or more over 6 weeks, as employed in this patient.

Chemotherapy is not particularly active in metastatic uveal melanoma. The regimens employed are those similarly used in melanoma arising from the skin.

Retinoblastoma

Retinoblastoma is a rare tumour occurring in the very young, usually occurring in children under the age of 2. It arises from primitive cells in the retina and may occur as either an inherited or sporadic case. In the hereditary form, often both eyes are affected. It is due to an abnormal gene on chromosome 13, the Rb gene, which is a control on cell division and is thus referred to as a tumour suppressor gene. When it is lost from chromosome 13, it leads to uncontrolled cell replication and tumour formation.

Clinical features

Parents or family may notice a white reflex in the pupil, which usually indicates a large tumour, or a squint and difficulty in fixation. Extension into the orbit or perforation of the globe are very unusual but very serious with respect to prognosis as these patients are incurable. In advanced disease, rarely seen in patients in Europe at initial presentation, metastases may occur to the central nervous system and the bone marrow.

Diagnosis and investigation

Retinoblastoma is exceptional with respect to oncological management in that a biopsy for confirmation of the diagnosis is never performed and, indeed, contraindicated because of the high risk of spread of tumour cells outside the globe. Therefore, the diagnosis is a clinical one made in specialized centres with great expertise in retinoblastoma and characterized by appearances on bilateral indirect binocular ophthalmoscopy under general anesthetic. Even when enucleation is performed for a large tumour and/or a non-seeing eye, previous biopsy should not have been carried out.

Staging

The best known staging system is the Reese-Ellsworth classification. It is mainly based on tumour size, grouped into small (<4 disk diameters (DD)), medium (4–10 DD) and large (>10 DD). A disk diameter is just under one centimeter. Tumour height is important for decisions about mode of treatment but is usually governed by base diameter. The classification also takes into account whether the tumour is solitary or multiple, tumour location with respect to the macula, optic disk and anterior to the equator, vitreous seedling and retinal detachment. Late stage disease includes optic nerve and extrascleral extension.

Treatment

Treatment options are surgery, which includes local therapy including photocoagulation, cryotherapy, radioactive eye plaques and removal of the eye (enucleation), external beam radiotherapy and chemotherapy. Historically, enucleation was the treatment for retinoblastoma and still should be carried out for large tumours, tumours uncontrolled by more conservative measures and in eyes with little hope of vision. However, when both eyes are affected by a combination of large tumours and/or poor vision, an attempt is often made to try to preserve the less advanced eye and therefore some vision.

Small tumours can usually be treated by focal treatment with photocoagulation, cryotherapy or a combination of the two and useful vision preserved. Cryotherapy is a method of freezing the tumour but can only be used in more anteriorly placed tumours. Tumours that are larger or lie adjacent to the macula or optic disk are treated with a radioactive plaque, although some vision may be lost. Some plaques are designed with cut outs to reduce the dose on the margin next to the disk or optic nerve in order to preserve vision if possible. Historically, cobalt-60 plaques were used, but gamma radiation frequently caused ocular morbidity including cataract and radioprotection was a problem. It has therefore been replaced by ruthenium-106 and iodine-125 plaques, both of which are beta emitters and therefore not so penetrating. They are sutured onto the back of the globe overlying the tumour, its position outlined by transillumination. A dose of 40 Gy is given over 2–4 days, depending on the activity of the plaque at time of use, and prescribed to the apex of the tumour which has been measured by ultrasound. The maximum height of the tumour for treatment with radioactive eye plaque is 4 mm. The diameter of the plaque is most frequently 15 mm, although 20 mm plaques are occasionally used.

For larger tumours and multiple tumours, radiotherapy is no longer commonly used because of the risk of carcinogenesis. There are very accurate radiotherapy techniques employing a contact lens system on the front of the eye and acting as a reference point in order to bring in a lateral beam behind the front of the eye. This enables the whole of the retina to be treated but still avoids the radiosensitive anterior structures in the eye. A dose of 40 Gy in 20 fractions over 4 weeks is the standard dose, requiring a daily anesthetic for the child immobilized in a beam directional shell. Very occasionally, whole eye radiotherapy is required for large more anteriorly placed tumours or following enucleation for extrascleral extension.

Chemotherapy used to be employed only for palliation but, over the last 10 years, this has changed due to the appreciation of the risk of developing second primary tumours in hereditary retinoblastoma. External beam radiotherapy, previously often used as primary treatment, increases the risk of second malignancies further, particularly in children under the age of 1. As a result, chemotherapy has been moved forward and used in earlier stage disease with chemoreductive protocols using drugs such as carboplatin, etoposide and vincristine (CEV). The number of courses depends on the extent of disease and response, but chemoreduction will make many eyes amenable to local treatment with photocoagulation or cryotherapy. Indeed, the treatments may be used concurrently with chemotherapy.

Prognosis

The outlook for patients with retinoblastoma is excellent with over 95% cured. This prognosis should not be compromised by inexperienced management, either by biopsy of the tumour which may lead to disasterous sequelae, by performing conservative management with a large tumour (usually because it involves their better seeing eye) in an attempt to preserve vision in a young child, or thirdly, by using external beam radiotherapy and increasing the risk of second malignancy when alternative treatment would have been more appropriate. Patients with bilateral retinoblastoma have a 50% incidence of developing a second malignancy within 50 years of treatment of retinoblastoma.

It is therefore important in patients who present with no prospect of useful vision to sacrifice the eye and perform enucleation. Referral for prosthetic replacement should all be part of postoperative care and this will have to be ongoing as the young child grows.

Many posteriorly placed tumours can be controlled by conservative management and useful vision maintained, but this will depend on the size and position of the tumour (or tumours), and the treatment given. When tumour extends outside the eye, or there is metastatic disease, mortality is very high. Fortunately, these situations are uncommon.

Metastases

Pathology and clinical features

Secondary deposits to the eye via the blood stream are common but often not clinically evident or recognized. The most frequent site is the vascular choroid leading to retinal detachment. Therefore, presentation may be an oncological emergency due to sudden loss of vision. It usually occurs in patients known to have malignancy, especially from breast and lung cancer. Other tumours which less frequently metastasize are urogenital and upper gastrointestinal tumours. They usually indicate widespread metastatic disease and, consequently, a poor prognosis, except in some breast cancer patients. Patients may have brain metastases as well. If full fundal examination is carried out, asymptomatic metastases are not infrequently found, often involving the contralateral eye. Choroidal metastases have a characteristic appearance, with a yellow raised honeycomb lesion (Figure 31.25).

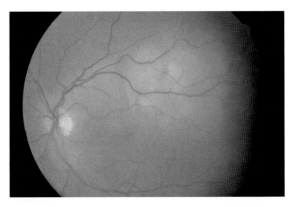

Figure 31.25 Choroidal metastasis from carcinoma of breast.

Radiotherapy should be given to try to preserve vision.

Rare ocular sites are eyelid metastases, as shown in Figure 31.26 from a breast carcinoma, and anterior chamber from a small cell lung carcinoma (Figure 31.27) which were treated with a short course of radiotherapy. Figure 31.28 shows regression of the deposit shortly after completing radiotherapy. Also, prostate cancer metastases can involve the orbit, usually due to expansion from a bone deposit resulting in visual disturbance or loss, diplopia, ptyosis or exophthalmos (see Figures 31.29 and 31.30).

Radiotherapy technique and dose

The patient lies prone on a head rest with the head supported and immobilized using a beam directional shell, flexifoam or an orfit. The target volume should include the whole eye.

Choroidal deposits can be treated by a single anterior megavoltage photon field or a lateral field angled 5–10° posteriorly. If an anterior field is used, the eye is treated open to take advantage of the skin-sparing effect of megavoltage to reduce the dose to the cornea and lens. In breast cancer, choroidal metastases are often multiple and/or

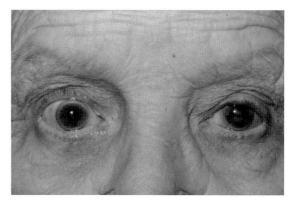

Figure 31.28 Anterior chamber metastasis from carcinoma of lung – post-radiotherapy.

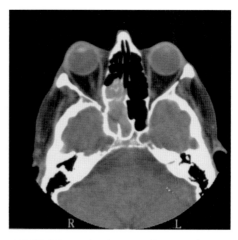

Figure 31.29 CT scan showing extensive prostatic metastatic deposit.

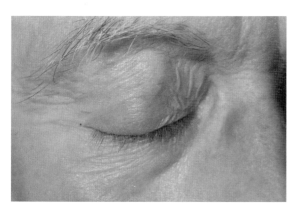

Figure 31.26 Eyelid metastasis from carcinoma of breast.

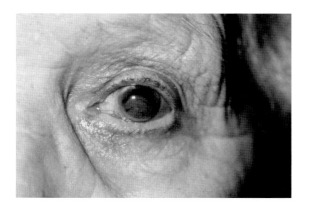

Figure 31.27 Anterior chamber metastasis from carcinoma of lung – pre-radiotherapy.

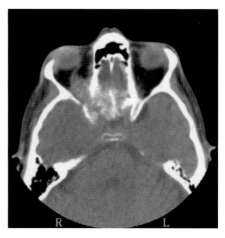

Figure 31.30 CT scan showing extensive prostatic metastatic deposit.

bilateral and so both eyes should be treated using parallel-opposed lateral fields. For more extensive lesions, field arrangements depend on the individual cases, but are usually single direct or parallel opposed. Occasionally, a pair of wedged fields is used, as shown in Figure *evolve* 31.31 🖱

which shows a dosimetric plan for a large renal metastasis. The globe was displaced medially.

A dose of 20 Gy in five daily fractions over one week with megavoltage radiotherapy is usually most appropriate.

FURTHER READING

Shields JA. Diagnosis and management of ocular tumours. Saunders and Co; 1988.

Harnett AN, Hungerford JL. Ocular morbidity to radiotherapy. In: Plowman PN, McElwain TJ, Meadows A, editor. Complications of cancer management.

Butterworth–Heineman; (1991). p. 361–78.

Pizzo P, et al. Principles and practice of paediatric oncology. 4th ed. Williams and Wilkins Lippincott; 2002.

Shields CL, Mashayekhi A, Demirci H, et al. Practical approach to

management of retinoblastoma. Arch Ophthal 2004;122:729–35.

Kingston JE, Hungerford JL, Madreperla SA, et al. Results of combined chemotherapy and radiotherapy for advanced intraocular retinoblastoma. Arch Ophthal 1996;114:1339–43.

EVOLVE CONTENTS (available online at: http://evolve.elsevier.com/Symonds/radiotherapy/)

Chapter | 32 |

Sarcomas

Martin Robinson, Paul Symonds, Mike Sokal

SOFT TISSUE SARCOMAS

Soft tissue sarcomas are malignant tumours arising from supporting connective tissues anywhere in the body. These structures (fibrous tissue, fat, blood vessels, smooth and skeletal muscle, tendons and cartilage) are derived embryologically from the mesoderm. Sarcomas of bone also occur and are discussed in this chapter under bone tumours. Tumours of peripheral nerves are generally included. Despite arising from a wide variety of tissues, they have many similarities in pathology, clinical findings and behavior.

Pathology

Soft tissue sarcomas are rare, representing 0.4% of all cancers and 0.3% of cancer deaths. The incidence is about 0.6 per 100 000 population per year. However, they constitute 6% of tumours in children under the age of 15. Most occur in the 40–70 age group. The sex ratio is virtually the same.

Their aetiology is largely unknown. In a minority of cases, genetic factors are involved. There is, for example, an increased incidence of the tumour in association with certain genetically transmitted diseases, e.g. Gardner's syndrome, tuberous sclerosis, Von Recklinghausen's disease and Li–Fraumeni syndrome. Rarely, soft tissue sarcomas may occur in the children of mothers with breast cancer of early onset.

Some sarcomas are radiation induced and occur within previously irradiated areas (especially for benign angiomas). The incidence of second sarcomas among young people who have been treated with both chemotherapy and radiotherapy for Ewing's sarcoma may reach 18%.

A large number of sarcomas have been found to have consistent chromosome abnormalities. The first demonstration of a specific gene abnormality associated with malignant transformation in man was the loss of the retinoblastoma (RB gene), a tumour supressor gene. There are alterations to the RB gene in up to 70% of soft tissue sarcomas. Chromosome translocations are the most common abnormality and are seen in virtually all cases of Ewing's sarcoma (primitive neuroectodermal tumours). 11:22 translocation is the most common, occurring in 85% of cases. In more than 90% of synovial sarcomas, there is a chromosome 18 translocation. Such cytogenetic abnormalities may be useful diagnostically and may be of prognostic significance. It is noteworthy that translocations tend to occur most commonly in high-grade tumours.

Rhabdomyosarcoma and soft tissue Ewing's sarcoma, although traditionally included in some lists of histological subtypes of soft tissue sarcomas, are quite different from the rest of the group, both in natural history and in being in general more chemo- and radiosensitive. Thus, the principles of treatment outlined below do not apply to these two histological types.

The World Health Organization (WHO) classification is the most commonly used, but this is extremely complex and a simplified version listing malignant tumours by their tissue of origin is presented in Table 32.1. From the point of view of management and prognosis, the histological subtype of management is generally less important than the histological grade and the size of the tumour. Grading may depend in part on the tumour subtype, but more often is assessed by scoring the degree of necrosis and mitotic index. The system described by Trojani is in regular use both in the UK and internationally. Low-grade tumours have a recognizable pattern of differentiation, relatively few mitoses, and no necrosis. High-grade tumours include all examples of certain subtypes (e.g. alveolar soft part), tumours with little or no apparent differentiation, and those with necrosis and a high mitotic rate. The tumour size is also important, and those over 5 cm are much more likely to recur locally or give rise to distant metastases.

Initial spread from the primary site is into adjacent tissue and along tissue planes between structures such as muscle bundles. Soft tissue sarcomas do not possess a true capsule but are often surrounded by a pseudocapsule of compressed surrounding tissues. This apparent encapsulation may tempt the surgeon to try to 'shell out' the tumour. Local recurrence from residual tumour at the periphery is then very likely (up to 90% within 2 years). Lymph

---

Table 32.1 Simplified version of the WHO classification of sarcomas

Fat
  Liposarcoma
Fibrous tissue
  Fibrosarcoma
  Myxofibrosarcoma
  Fibrous histocytoma
Smooth muscle
  Leiomyosarcoma
Skeletal muscle
  Embryonal rhadomyosarcoma
  Alveolar rhadomyosarcoma
  Pleomorphic rhadomyosarcoma
Blood vessels
  Angiosarcoma
Bone
  Osteogenic sarcoma
  Ewing's sarcoma
Nerve
  Malignant peripheral nerve sheath tumours
Sarcomas of uncertain differentiation
  Synovial sarcomas
  Epithelioid sarcomas
  Alveolar soft part sarcomas
  Haemangiopericytoma
  Gastrointestinal stromal tumours

node spread is infrequent, while blood-borne spread is common, giving rise to distant metastases, predominantly in the lungs.

Clinical features

Approximately 40% of soft tissue sarcomas occur in the upper and lower limbs. Of these, about 75% occur at or above the knee. Ten percent of sarcomas arise in the upper half of the body. Of the sarcomas of the trunk, 10% occur in the retroperitoneum and 20% in the chest or abdominal wall. Presentation with locally advanced disease is common, particularly with intra-abdominal sarcomas, which may reach a very large size.

The history is usually of a painless lump developing over a few weeks or months and occasionally over years. Pain may occur from pressure on local structures, e.g. nerves and joints. Occasionally, non-metastatic effects are seen (e.g. hypoglycaemia in malignant fibrous histiocytoma).

Diagnosis and staging

Important features of local examination for limb or truncal sarcomas is the position of the lesion superficial or deep to the fascia at the primary tumour site and any involvement of bone, vascular or neural invasion. Regional nodes, although uncommonly involved, should be palpated.

A biopsy is required. In 90% of cases, adequate histology can be achieved by needle core biopsy. Where an incisional biopsy is required, care should be taken to make the incision longitudinal so that any subsequent radical surgery or postoperative radiation fields can include it. This is particularly important where preservation of limb function is a major consideration. Appropriate siting of the biopsy is vital if the probability of local control is to be maximized. The biopsy should ideally be carried out by the surgeon who will undertake the definitive resection. There is otherwise the risk of tumour spillage, particularly after unplanned attempts to remove deep-seated lesions. If computed tomography (CT)-guided biopsy is needed, for example for impalpable deep-seated lesions, there is also potential for needle track contamination. Close liaison with the surgeon and clinical oncologist is needed to plan the best route of biopsy. Specialist pathology review is essential in view of the complexity of these tumours and the need for careful assessment of the tumour margins.

A full blood count, liver function tests, chest radiograph, plain radiographs of the tumour-bearing region (Figure 32.1) and liver ultrasound are the initial investigations. CT and magnetic resonance imaging (MRI) (Figures *evolve* 32.2–32.4🖱) scanning are important in defining the local extent and operability of the tumour. MRI is the imaging modality of choice for limb sarcomas since it provides good contrast between the tumour and adjoining normal tissues with particular regard to the tumour's relationship with the neurovascular bundle. It also provides

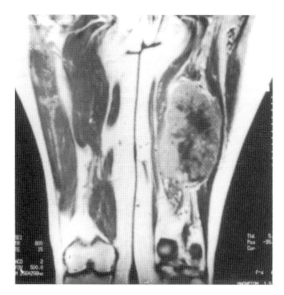

Figure 32.1 MRI scan showing soft tissue sarcoma with central necrosis in the hamstring compartment of the thigh.
(Courtesy of Dr L Turnbull, MRI Unit, Sheffield.)

better multiplanar versatility in planning surgery and radiotherapy. CT can be helpful in exclusion of cortical erosion of bone. CT and MRI are also useful in confirming any subsequent local recurrence, but are not currently used for routine follow up. CT of the thorax is advisable if chest radiography is normal and radical therapy is contemplated, since it may demonstrate small-volume lung metastases (Figure *evolve* 32.5🖱). The staging system commonly adopted includes grade, size, and presence/absence of metastases (Tables 32.2 & 32.3).

Management

A multidisciplinary approach (MDT) is required since surgery, radiotherapy and chemotherapy may all have a role to play, depending on the stage, site, grade and size of the tumour. A dedicated sarcoma MDT allows treatment to be carefully coordinated and minimizes the number of surgical procedures necessary. Correct procedures for biopsy, imaging and exclusion of metastatic disease are essential. Historically, amputation was the main treatment for limb sarcomas but, in the 1970s, it was appreciated that radiotherapy and less radical surgery could provide comparable results. Limb-sparing surgery with postoperative radiotherapy achieved the same survival as amputation, albeit with a slightly higher local recurrence rate. In the past, sarcomas were regarded as relatively radioresistant tumours. It is now known that they are relatively radiosensitive, comparable to breast cancer.

Local control while maximizing the probability of conserving limb function and long-term survival is of vital

Table 32.2 Stage grouping for soft sarcoma (UICC 2009) – taking into account histopathological grade

Stage IA	T1a	N0	M0	low grade
	T1b	N0	M0	low grade
Stage IB	T2a	N0	M0	low grade
	T2b	N0	M0	low grade
Stage IIA	T1a	N0	M0	high grade
	T1b	N0	M0	high grade
Stage IIB	T2a	N0	M0	high grade
Stage III	T2b	N0	M0	high grade
	Any T	N1	M0	any grade
Stage IV	Any T	Any N	M1	any grade

Table 32.3 Staging system for soft tissue sarcomas (UICC 2009)

T1	≤ 5 cms
T1a	Superficial
T1b	Deep
T2	>5 cms
T2a	Superficial
T2b	Deep
N0	No lymph node spread
N1	Involvement of regional lymph nodes
M0	No distant metastases
M1	Distant metastases

importance. For extremity limb sarcomas, 90% local control at 5 years should be the standard. The management of soft tissue sarcomas is controversial. In part, this reflects the limited number of randomized trials in this heterogeneous group of tumours. The relative rarity of non-extremity sarcomas makes the design of and recruitment to large randomized trials difficult. Few would dispute the primary role of radical surgery. If the surgical resection margins are clear, the 5-year local control for limb sarcomas is of the order of 90%. If the margins are involved, this falls to 60–80%. Involved margins are an independent risk factor for local recurrence. The extent

of the resection will depend upon the site of the tumour. The more distal the tumour in the limb, the more difficult a complete excision becomes. Radical excision surgery of retroperitoneal sarcomas is also rarely feasible. The primary tumour should be resected with one anatomical plane clear of the tumour at all stages. The aim of the surgery is to achieve a wide local excision (margin ≥2 cm where possible) (Figure 32.6). The resection should include all the skin and subcutaneous tissue near to the tumour, any previous excision or biopsy scars and areas containing blood clot from previous biopsies. The tumour itself should never be actively contacted during resection. Metallic clips at the margins of the excision are helpful in planning postoperative irradiation.

Amputation for extremity sarcomas is only indicated in the following situations:

1. when serious radiation-induced morbidity would result from attempting radical radiotherapy
2. in some distal limb sarcomas, where a below knee amputation may be more functional than a lower limb with the combined local morbidity of surgery and radiotherapy
3. when there is recurrent disease not suitable for limited resection or adjuvant radiotherapy.

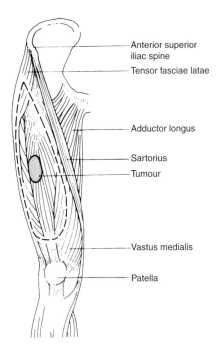

Figure 32.6 Compartmentectomy. The diagram illustrates the wide surgical excision of soft tissue situated, in this case, in the rectus femoris.
(Reproduced with permission from Souhami & Tobias, Cancer and its Management, Blackwells, 1986.)

Adjuvant therapy

For low-grade tumours less than 5 cm in size which have been widely excised with clear surgical margins, no further therapy is necessary in most cases. The same applies following an amputation. However, postoperative radiotherapy is indicated in the following circumstances to reduce the probability of local recurrence (see above):

- limb-conserving or limited surgery (see below)
- gross residual tumour or inadequate excision margins
- grade 2 or 3 histology
- tumours 5 cm or more in any dimension plus most tumours deep to the fascia
- virtually all tumours in the head and neck (because of the impossibility of adequate excision).
- after surgery for recurrent sarcoma if not previously irradiated.

Postoperative radiotherapy conventionally is with external beam (photons or electrons), although postoperative brachytherapy with iridium-192 (42–45 Gy over 4–6 days) had a high 5-year local control rate of 90% in a randomized trial compared to 65% for high- but not low-grade lesions. There are no randomized trials comparing brachytherapy with external beam irradiation. Brachytherapy should only be carried out in specialist units undertaking a substantial number of procedures. The reason for the ineffectiveness of brachytherapy in low-grade tumours is not clear. One possibility is that the long cell cycle in low-grade tumours may result in cells not entering the radiosensitive phase of the cell cycle during the period of brachytherapy. Retroperitoneal sarcomas require special mention. They are often huge, causing dramatic distortion of the patient's contour but rarely present as an emergency. Such cases should therefore always be discussed in the sarcoma MDT. The tumours are often dedifferentiated liposarcomas and as such have a very characteristic CT scan appearance. In these circumstances, preoperative biopsy may be eschewed, but if there is any radiological doubt, biopsy is mandated.

Surgery may require removal of many organs, spleen, one kidney, tail or body of pancreas or segments of large and/or small bowel. The placement of surgical clips around narrowly excised tumour areas can guide the clinical oncologist. The dose of post-operative radiotherapy is necessarily limited and >50 Gy is unlikely to be achievable. Recently, interest has been rekindled in the use of pre-operative RT, with very large fields being applied to a dose of 50 Gy in 1.8–2.0 Gy fractions. This has been made possible with the use of IMRT to spare radiosensitive organs such as kidney and spinal cord. An EORTC trial is recruiting now randomising to surgery alone or preoperative radiotherapy followed by radical resection 4–6 weeks later.

Protons are being used in clinical trials. Protons have a similar relative biological effectiveness (RBE) to photons. The advantage of protons is a reduction of dose to critical structures, such as the spinal cord or underlying bone. This can be done by varying the proton energy or by the use of wax compensators to alter the size of the Bragg peak and consequently the volume of tissue which is subsequently irradiated.

Not all sites are suitable for radical radiotherapy. Pelvic, thoracic or abdominal sarcomas present particular difficulties because of the morbidity that would be caused by wide-field irradiation, dose-limiting critical structures (e.g. the spinal cord). Placement of spacers in the abdominal cavity may be used to displace small bowel out of the high dose radiation field (Figures *evolve* 32.7 and 32.8🖱).

Limb-conserving surgery

If limb-conserving surgery is undertaken (i.e. removal of the tumour mass with narrower excision margins), postoperative radiotherapy is given to sterilize microscopic residual disease. In this way, a functional limb with a satisfactory cosmetic result can be achieved. Conservative surgery is contraindicated where high-dose radiotherapy is poorly tolerated (see below).

Timing of radiotherapy

Preoperative radiotherapy has the advantage that the tumour is well oxygenated and intact. It may also allow coverage by smaller radiation fields and use of lower doses without reducing local control. These advantages have to be balanced against the disadvantages of difficulties in interpreting pathology following irradiation and an increase in risk of wound complications. Retrospective series of preoperative radiotherapy are subject to selection bias but have suggested that preoperative radiotherapy may be of value in lesions >5 cm. A recent randomized Canadian trial comparing preoperative and postoperative radiotherapy was stopped because of increased wound complications in the preoperative arm. However, final limb function was still better in the preoperative group. Sites where preoperative radiotherapy may be considered within the constraints of normal tissue tolerance are the head and neck (paranasal sinuses, skull base, cheek and face), retroperitoneum, and extremity tumours.

Primary radical radiotherapy

Radical radiotherapy alone is indicated for patients unfit for surgery but otherwise in reasonable general condition, those who refuse surgery or where the anatomical site precludes it (e.g. retroperitoneum). Preoperative neoadjuvant radiotherapy is recommended for very large sarcomas.

Contraindications to radical radiotherapy

The high doses of radiotherapy required for sarcoma are poorly tolerated by highly stressed areas of the lower limb, e.g. Achilles tendon, or in the ribs where pathological fractures may occur. Radical radiotherapy to the Achilles tendon is inadvisable, especially in young and active patients, since rupture may occur.

Target volume

Definition of the target volume requires information from the surgeon, pathologist and radiologist. The surgeon should be encouraged to place radiopaque clips at the margins of the resection. The pathologist should comment on the adequacy of the resection. Very often, it is necessary to ask the surgeon to carry out a further excision before postoperative radiotherapy is undertaken. The radiotherapist needs to discuss with the radiologist the position of the tumour, local extent and any residual disease as seen on CT and MRI.

Most sarcomas tend to spread in the axial plane of the limb (major fascial planes, bone and interosseous membranes). For this reason, the margins of the radiation field must be generous in the craniocaudal directions. In the transverse plane, there can be greater confidence that local structures are not breached and field margins can be tighter. For non-extremity lesions, the orientation of the fields should follow the planes of the local musculature, while including the local fascial planes.

For the purposes of planning, the gross tumour volume (GTV) should be defined, with a margin around it to include the tissues at risk of microscopic involvement, to create the clinical tumour volume (CTV). In practice, the GTV is defined radiologically on CT or MRI. Whether or not the peritumoural oedema should be included in the GTV is unclear (it is not known if the oedema contains tumour cells). Including the peritumoural oedema will significantly increase the CTV in most cases. Until we know whether or not peritumoural oedema contains tumour cells, its inclusion within the CTV is not recommended.

In theory, the target volume should vary with the grade of the tumour. For well-differentiated (grade 1) tumours a 5 cm margin above and below the site of the original tumour is adequate. For moderately and poorly differentiated tumours (grades 2 and 3), a 10 cm margin maybe considered. However, in practice, the fields would be so large that radiotherapy may be considered inadvisable. The margins required are another uncertainty in sarcoma radiotherapy. The target volume has traditionally been reduced later in the treatment (see below) to include the length of the scar with a margin of security at either end of 2 cm for boosting with electrons. Whether this field reduction is necessary for completely excised tumours is the subject of a current UK study (VORTEX – Volume of Radiotherapy for Extremity Sarcomas).

Where there is macroscopic residual disease, the volume cannot be reduced in the same way as when the excision margins are clear. In this situation, a 5 cm margin around the tumour is sustained throughout treatment.

Three-dimensional treatment planning where available can assist in the delivery of a homogeneous dose throughout the treatment volume, while limiting the dose to normal tissues which may affect function and cosmesis. Intensity modulated radiotherapy (IMRT) may have a role in the irradiation of sites where minimization of dose to critical structures is particularly important, such as the skull base or the abdomen.

Technique

This will vary with the site of the tumour. For the limbs and retroperitoneum, a parallel-opposed pair of fields, often wedged, will provide a satisfactory dose distribution in most cases. In the shoulder region, tangential fields may be needed to reduce the volume of lung irradiated. Tangential fields are also appropriate for superficial trunk lesions to spare the bowel. For tumours in the buttock, a direct posterior field and two wedged lateral fields will reduce the dose to the rectum. In the head and neck, the principles of planning and respect for the tolerance of critical structures, such as the spinal cord, are the same as for squamous carcinoma of the head and neck. Target volumes tend to be smaller than below the clavicles and so higher doses can often be delivered with acceptable morbidity. Computer planning is essential to obtain a homogeneous distribution of dose within the target volume.

Stability of the limb is best assisted by a shell and appropriately positioned bolus bags. Bolus can be applied to the scar to ensure it receives the maximum dose to minimize the risk of scar recurrence but this is not the practice of all oncologists. The application of bolus to the scar is not recommended in the current UK VORTEX trial. Sagittal lasers are especially useful in lining up the limbs.

Care is taken to avoid irradiating the whole circumference of a limb to reduce the likelihood of lymphedema as a late complication. This is achieved by adjusting the width of the field to leave a longitudinal strip of unirradiated tissue outside the target volume. In the proximal part of the limb, especially in the thigh, this strip occupies a large proportion of the limb (Figures *evolve* 32.9–32.11).

When the retroperitoneum is irradiated, part or the whole of one kidney may need to be included in the target volume. Shielding of the other kidney by lead blocks on the anterior and posterior fields may be necessary, depending upon the site of the tumour (Figure *evolve* 32.12).

Dose and fractionation

There is little information on total dose and response in sarcomas. Most centres tend to give 50 Gy to a wide volume, shrinking to a final boost of 10–16 Gy. There is limited information on the relationship between total dose and response. However, fraction sizes should be kept small (1.8–2 Gy) to minimize the risks of late damage to normal tissue. Hypofractionated and hyperfractionated schedules have shown no advantage over conventional fractionation.

Limbs

No gross residual disease

1. Large volume

50 Gy in 25 daily fractions over 5 weeks at megavoltage (6–10 MV photons).

2. Boost volume

10–16 Gy in 5–8 daily fractions over 1–1.5 weeks.

(1) and (2) deliver a total dose of 66 Gy in 33 fractions over 6.5 weeks to the tumour-bearing area.

Gross residual disease

66 Gy in 33 daily fractions over 6.5 weeks at megavoltage (6–10 MV photons)
or up to 70 Gy in 35 fractions over 7 weeks, if volume permits in the boosted area.

Implantation

Because of the low radiosensitivity of sarcomas, an implant may be used in appropriate circumstances to give a high dose to the boost volume, or to gross residual disease.

Retroperitoneum

Dosage is limited by small bowel tolerance.

45–50 Gy in 25 fractions over 5 weeks.

Head and neck

66 Gy in 33 daily fractions over 6 weeks.

Acute reactions

Skin reactions are often a problem. This is because very high doses are needed in the boost volume and are sometimes given to graft areas with surface bolus. Dry desquamation normally develops and is treated as for other skin reactions. Moist desquamation is more likely to occur in the axilla, groin and perineum and is treated with hydrocortisone cream or ointment. If there is secondary infection, flamazine (silver sulfadiazine) can promote healing.

Late reactions

Atrophy of the skin and subcutaneous tissues and fibrosis within the muscles are common. Stiffness of a limb may be partly due to fibrosis of the intermuscular septa and partly due to fibrosis in the joint capsule.

Osteoporosis of bone is common since bone is frequently included in the target volume. Occasionally, particularly if the bone is invaded by tumour, radionecrosis may occur. In the ribs, this may cause pathological fractures.

Palliative radiotherapy

Palliative doses of radiation only have a limited role in the management of advanced sarcomas. Little benefit is seen following irradiation of massive, locally advanced primary tumours with doses such as 30 Gy in 10 fractions. Bleeding fungating masses, not amenable to toilet surgery, are best treated by a large single fraction of 8–10 Gy. This usually stops bleeding and occasionally there is shrinkage of the tumour.

Chemotherapy

In the past 30 years, improvements in both surgery and radiotherapy have led to marked improvements in local control and a subsequent decrease in the incidence of amputation. However, there has been less progress in the eradication of micrometastases which, ultimately, lead to the death of many patients. Doxorubicin and ifosfamide are the only chemotherapeutic agents that consistently have a greater than 20% response rate against soft tissue sarcomas. A meta-analysis of 13 randomized trials of adjuvant chemotherapy versus control in soft tissue sarcomas demonstrated that doxorubicin- (Adriamycin) based chemotherapy has increased overall recurrence-free survival of 10% (from 45 to 55% $P = 0.001$). The effect on overall survival was more modest. This increased from 50 to 54% ($P = 0.12$). The results of an EORTC trial randomizing between six cycles of adjuvant doxorubicin/ifosfamide compared with no chemotherapy are awaited. There is no clear evidence to show that preoperative chemotherapy offers a significant survival advantage, but this may be used in patients who are thought to be initially inoperable.

Chemotherapy should be reserved for patients with metastatic disease as the survival advantages are relatively small. Single agent doxorubicin is the treatment of choice, although there is a steep dose response curve. The highest rate of responses (37%) have been seen with doses of 75 mg/m^2 three weekly. However, complete responses are uncommon and the average duration of response is only 8 months. Somewhat higher response rates are seen with combination regimens but toxicity was increased with little or no survival advantage. One current EORTC trial is comparing doxorubicin with ifosfamide/doxorubicin in the younger (<60 years) fitter (PSO,1) patient, and another trial randomizes the older (>60 years) patient between single agent doxorubicin or brostacillin.

Results of treatment

In the best hands, conservative surgery and radiotherapy can achieve over 90% local control and 5-year survival in stage I disease. For stage II disease, local control is 85–90% and survival 90% (IIa) and 65% (IIb). For stage III, local control is similar to stage II but survival is lower, 85% (IIIa) and 45% (IIIb).

If there is only microscopic residual disease following surgery, overall survival is 65%, falling to 30% when there is gross residual disease.

BONE TUMOURS

Benign and malignant tumours may arise in bone. The pathological classification is shown in Table 32.4. Bone tumours represent 0.4% of all cancers. Primary bone tumours are rare and account for only 1% of bone neoplasia. The vast majority of bone lesions are secondary deposits. The main malignant tumour that forms bone is osteosarcoma; that forming cartilage is chondrosarcoma. Malignant tumours arising from the bone marrow are myeloma (see Chapter 29), Ewing's sarcoma and lymphoma (see Chapter 29).

Osteosarcoma (osteogenic sarcoma)

This is the commonest and most malignant primary bone tumour. It arises in bone-forming cells (osteoblasts) and is commonest between the ages of 10 and 20 years. There is a second peak incidence in the elderly, as a complication of Paget's disease of bone. The male to female ratio is 1.6:1.

The cause of the usual adolescent's tumour is unknown. There is an increased incidence (400-fold) of osteosarcoma in patients with bilateral retinoblastomas, presumably because of the same genetic abnormality or mutation of the Rb tumour suppressor gene developing outside the irradiated areas.

Pathology

Osteosarcoma is commonest near the knee in the metaphysis of the distal femur or proximal tibia. In the elderly, its distribution matches Paget's disease.

Macroscopically, the tumour is usually haemorrhagic. It expands the bone, destroying both the cortex and the medulla. The periosteum is frequently raised giving rise to the radiological features of Codman's triangle where the raised periosteum meets the cortex. Extension into the soft tissue follows.

Blood-borne metastases to the lungs occur early. Bone metastases, though less frequent, also occur. Microscopically, there are malignant osteoblasts laying down small pieces of irregular osteoid tissue. There is a variety of histological

appearances. The two main varieties are osteoblastic and telangiectatic (containing irregular blood vessels). The third variety is parosteal sarcoma. It arises from the surface of the bone and does not involve the medullary cavity.

Clinical features

The commonest presenting feature is pain, usually with swelling and a limp. Sometimes pathological fracture may follow minor trauma. Rarely, cough, dysponea and pneumothoraces may indicate lung involvement.

Diagnosis and staging investigations

Plain radiographs and CT scan (Figures *evolve* 32.13 🖱 and 32.14) of the affected part may show the typical features of bone destruction and soft tissue extension. The cortex may be raised with a 'sunburst' appearance. Full blood count,

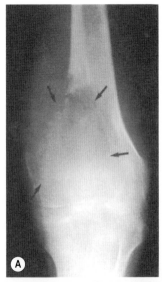

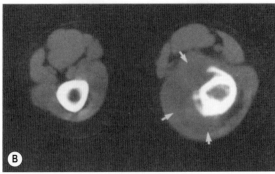

Figure 32.14 (A) Plain radiograph and (B) CT scan of the femur showing bone destruction from an osteogenic sarcoma (arrows). Compare normal CT appearance on opposite side. *(Courtesy of Dr R Nakielny, Sheffield.)*

Table 32.4 Classification of bone tumours
A. *Tumours forming bone*
1. Benign – e.g. osteoma
2. Malignant – osteosarcoma
B. *Tumours forming cartilage*
1. Benign – e.g. enchondroma
2. Malignant – chondrosarcoma
C. *Giant cell tumour (generally benign)*
D. *Tumours of the bone marrow – myeloma, lymphoma and Ewing's sarcoma*
E. *Other tumours*

liver function tests and chest radiograph (for lung metastases) are required.

A CT or MRI scan is necessary if surgery is contemplated, to assess the involvement of the medullary cavity and the extent of soft tissue involvement. CT is also helpful in assessing whether the capsule of a limb joint has been breached. An isotope bone scan may show increased uptake at the site of the tumour, in the adjacent bone (due to increased vascularity), in bone metastases and in bone-forming metastases in soft tissues. A biopsy should be carried out to confirm the diagnosis. It is important that the position of the biopsy is chosen so that the whole biopsy scar can be excised with the tumour to include potentially surgically-contaminated tissue along the track of the biopsy. The initial biopsy for histological confirmation and, in cases of high clinical and radiological suspicion, so-called 'clearance' biopsies to assess the distance of spread along the bone shaft, should be performed as the first procedure with a view to subsequent limb-sparing surgery. Ideally, both biopsy and definitive surgery should be performed by the same surgical team. The endoprosthesis has to be planned several weeks ahead of limb-sparing surgery.

Osteogenic sarcoma is often fatal owing to spread to the lungs, therefore, patients should have a CT scan of lungs prior to any local therapy.

Treatment

The management of osteosarcoma requires a multidisciplinary approach including orthopaedic surgeon, oncologist, pathologist and physiotherapist.

Chemotherapy

Adjuvant and neoadjuvant chemotherapy are an important part of the treatment of osteogenic sarcoma. Initial chemotherapy allows treatment to be instituted early, can shrink the primary tumour, any obvious metastases as well as obliterating micrometastases. Undoubtedly, neoadjuvant chemotherapy has reduced the rate of amputation in this disease. Moreover, chemotherapy has reduced the frequency of pulmonary metastases which used to occur in 80% of cases. Although only about 10% of inoperable tumours are rendered operable by neoadjuvant chemotherapy, in many more cases, surgery is much easier owing to the reduction of the tumour allowing for the insertion of an endoprosthesis and sparing of the limb. The effective agents are doxorubicin (Adriamycin) and cisplatin and methotrexate. A good response to neoadjuvant chemotherapy is an independent good prognostic factor and the degree of viable tumour at surgery is related to ultimate survival. In the current EURAMOS1 Trial, patients are randomized after two cycles of cisplatin, doxorubicin, methotrexate or surgery to four further cycles depending on the amount of tumour cell kill defined histologically.

Surgery

There has been an increasing trend since the early 1980s to conserve limb function as far as possible and avoid amputation. Limb preservation involves removing the tumour and replacing the bone defect with a custom-made artificial prosthesis (Figure 32.15). Careful preoperative assessment

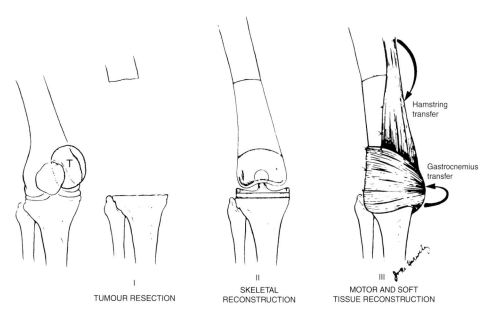

Figure 32.15 Schematic diagram of the three phases of a limb-sparing procedure.
(Reproduced with permission from DeVita VT, Hellman S, Rosenberg SA (2000) Cancer: Principles and Practice of Oncology, 6th end. Lippincott, Williams and Wilkins, Philadelphia.)

is necessary and referral to a specialist centre (Birmingham and London in the UK) is essential. To obtain adequate margins, the prosthesis incorporates an artificial joint as well as femoral and tibial components. Resections of pelvic primaries and replacing the bony defects with bone allograft or autografts are a major challenge.

Contraindications to limb conservation are:

1. extensive soft tissue infiltration
2. invasion of neurovascular bundles
3. involvement of the ankle joint.

Similar principles apply to the upper limb.

Resection of lung metastases

Lung metastases are occasionally isolated and, in the absence of metastases elsewhere, surgical resection should be considered. Results are best if lung metastases develop after a long disease-free interval. Surgery is contraindicated if there is pleural involvement. A 5-year survival of up to 30% has been reported following resection of pulmonary metastasis.

Radiotherapy

The indications for radiotherapy are:

1. use postoperatively where surgical margins are involved
2. palliation of pain from the primary tumour in the presence of metastatic disease or of bony metastases
3. radical treatment of inoperable sites (e.g. skull, vertebrae, ilium and sacrum). However, proximity of critical structures, such as the spinal cord, often limits the dose that can be delivered.

Palliative radiotherapy of primary tumour

Technique

A parallel-opposed pair of fields is suitable for limb primaries.

Dose and energy

30 Gy in 10 daily fractions over 2 weeks (4–6 MV photons or cobalt-60).

Radical radiotherapy

Technique

This will vary with the site of the primary. For tumours arising in a vertebra, a posterior oblique wedged pair (Figure 32.16) with or without an unwedged direct posterior field provides a satisfactory dose distribution. For the ilium, parallel-opposed fields suffice.

Dose and energy

Megavoltage is required. The choice of dose will be determined by critical organ tolerance. In the spine above L2, it will be limited by spinal cord tolerance to 47.5 Gy in 25 daily fractions over 5 weeks. In the iliac bone, the dose delivered is limited by small bowel tolerance to a central tumour dose of 45 Gy in 25 daily fractions over 5 weeks.

Results of treatment

The survival of osteosarcoma has improved with the development of more effective adjuvant chemotherapy. Average survival is 60% at 3 years. Osteoblastic and telangiectatic

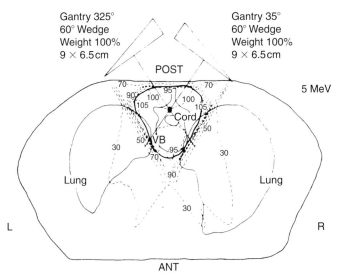

Gantry 325°
60° Wedge
Weight 100%
9 × 6.5 cm

Gantry 35°
60° Wedge
Weight 100%
9 × 6.5 cm

5 MeV

Figure 32.16 Posterior oblique wedged pair of fields to treat tumour of vertebral body (VB). *(Reproduced with permission of Arnold from Jane Dobbs, Ann Barrett, Daniel Ash, Practical Radiotherapy Planning, 3/e Arnold, 1999)*

tumours have a similar prognosis. Parosteal sarcomas have a better prognosis and may be cured by surgery alone.

Ewing's sarcoma

Ewing's sarcoma is the second most common primary bone tumour. In the UK, its incidence is 0.6 per million. The peak age is between 10 and 15 years. It is slightly commoner in males.

Pathology

Ewing's sarcoma probably arises from connective tissue within the bone marrow. The commonest sites in order of frequency are the pelvis, femur, tibia, fibula, rib, scapula, vertebra and humerus. In contrast to osteogenic sarcoma, a higher proportion of these tumours occur in the flat bones of the trunk. About 40% occur in the axial skeleton. Microscopically, there are sheets of uniform undifferentiated, small, deeply-staining round cells. The tumour needs to be distinguished from other small-round-cell tumours, including non-Hodgkin's lymphoma, Hodgkin's disease, neuroblastoma and metastatic carcinoma. Ninety percent of tumours have 11:22 chromosome translation.

There is local spread along the marrow cavity causing bone destruction. However, the epiphyseal plates are rarely breached. Blood-borne spread is early and common. About 50% will have lung metastases and 40% bone metastases and/or widespread bone marrow infiltration at presentation. Lymph node metastases are uncommon (less than 10%). Spread to the CNS may occur, usually late in the course of the disease.

Diagnosis and staging

Full blood count may show anaemia (leukoerythroblastic, if there is bone marrow infiltration) and a mildly raised white cell count. ESR is often moderately elevated. Liver function tests may be abnormal (raised lactate dehydrogenase (LDH) or alkaline phosphatase).

A biopsy of the tumour is required. As in osteogenic sarcoma, care is taken to ensure that the biopsy lies within the incision for any later proposed definitive surgical procedure. Plain radiographs of the primary are taken in two planes (usually anteroposterior and lateral). In long bones, this may show the typical multilayered 'onion-skin' (Figure 32.17) appearance of the periosteal reaction and often a large adjacent soft tissue mass. Pathological fracture occurs in 5% (less frequently than osteogenic sarcoma). CT scanning gives more detail of the local extent of the tumour and is useful in planning the site for a biopsy and subsequent surgery. MRI is superior to CT in assessment of the extent of infiltration within the medullary canal. A bone scan is necessary to screen for bone metastases.

As pulmonary metastases are common, a CT scan of chest is mandatory. A bone marrow and trephine are needed to exclude marrow infiltration.

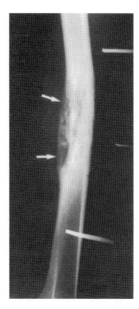

Figure 32.17 Plain radiograph of the femur showing typical appearance of Ewing's sarcoma of bone.
(Courtesy of Dr R Nakielny, Sheffield.)

Clinical features

Presentation is usually with a rapidly developing and painful swelling. Neurological symptoms may accompany this if there is nerve compression. Fever occurs in about 30% of patients.

Treatment

The choice of treatment will depend largely upon the site of the primary. Close liaison is required between orthopedic surgeon and oncologist. Treatment should, as with osteogenic sarcomas, only be carried out by an experienced team.

Chemotherapy

Ewing's sarcoma is a chemosensitive tumour and chemotherapy prior to surgery or radiotherapy has been shown to improve local control and reduce the incidence of distant metastasis. The most effective drugs are vincristine, ifosfamide, doxorubicin, etoposide and actinomycin D. Typically, patients receive four to six cycles of induction chemotherapy. This is followed by treatment to the primary site which may be surgery or radiotherapy or both depending on the location of the tumour. This is usually followed by six cycles of further chemotherapy for a total of 9 months' treatment. It is noteworthy that improvement in prognosis in Ewing's sarcoma has been because many patients were entered into clinical trials and, ideally, all patients should be considered for clinical trials. Owing to the rarity of Ewing's sarcoma, these trials are often international, multicentre studies. Very intensive chemo-therapy regimens, sometimes combined with peripheral blood stem cell rescue are required.

Radical radiotherapy

Target volume

Unlike osteogenic sarcomas, Ewing's sarcomas are radio-sensitive. Radiotherapy is indicated if the surgical excision margins are narrow.

It is not usually possible to deliver a radical dose uniformly to the whole bone unless it is very small, because of toxicity to normal tissue. For this reason, a 'shrinking field' approach is adopted with two consecutive phases based on the pretreatment volume. The initial volume is the tumour and a 5 cm margin of adjacent tissue. In long bones, an unirradiated strip of normal tissue containing lymphatics outside the tumour-bearing area is left, if possible, to reduce the risk of lymphedema as a late complication. In the second phase, the volume is reduced to encompass the primary tumour with a 2 cm margin of normal tissue.

Technique

The choice of technique will vary with the site of the primary. For the limbs, a parallel-opposed wedged pair of fields usually suffices. A 'shrinking field' technique is used for limb tumours. For pelvic primaries, it may be possible surgically to displace the bowel out of the radiation field, by inserting an absorbable mesh or a spacer. For rib primaries, electrons of appropriate energy may be used to diminish the dose to the underlying lung.

Dose and energy

A high local dose (of the order of 50–60 Gy conventionally fractionated) to the bulk of the tumour must be delivered at megavoltage, using photons or electrons as appropriate. Patients should be included in nationally agreed protocols. The following regimen is illustrative:

Phase 1: 39.6 Gy in 22 daily fractions over 30 days (4–6 MV photons).
Phase 2: 13.6 Gy in 8 daily fractions of 1.8 Gy over 10 days (4–6MV photons).

Acute and late reactions

These are the same as for soft tissue sarcoma.

Palliative radiotherapy

Whole lung irradiation is useful in relieving cough and dysponea from lung metastases.

Technique

A parallel-opposed pair of fields encompassing both lung fields is used.

Dose and energy

15 Gy in 10 fractions with lung correction for younger patients (<14 years).
A higher dose of 18 Gy in 10 fractions can be given to patients 15 or older.

Surgery

Surgery should be as radical as possible, hopefully with limb preservation but, occasionally, mandating amputation as the definitive operation. The same surgical principles as described in the section for osteosarcoma apply equally to Ewing's tumours. The likelihood of local tumour control is less if the primary tumour is large (9 cm or more). In these circumstances, unless the soft tissue component is very substantial, radical surgical removal of the whole bone (e.g. rib or fibula) is advised.

Where radical surgery to a limb would cause major functional impairment, a conservative approach, as in osteogenic sarcoma, can be adopted. A customized artificial prosthesis can be inserted at the end of the resected long bone. However, amputation may be preferable for proximal tibial or distal femoral tumours in growing children because of reduced bone growth in the affected limb following local radiotherapy. The latter may give rise to limbs of unequal length and therefore a permanent handicap.

Results of treatment

The outcome is better for patients with tumours of the peripheral rather than central skeleton. Up to 90% disease-free survival for peripheral tumours and 65% for central (axial) tumours has been achieved. Overall 5-year survival (and probably cure) is about 50%. Local recurrence occurs in about 10–15% of long bone primaries and 25–30% of pelvic tumours. The higher recurrence rate in the pelvis is probably due to the larger tumour size and the difficulty of irradiating the tumour homogeneously without damaging surrounding normal tissues.

Chondrosarcoma

Chondrosarcomas are malignant tumours of cartilage. They may arise in benign enchondromas or be malignant from the start. Adults aged 30–50 are affected. The commonest sites in order of frequency are the pelvis (50%), femur, humerus and scapula.

Macroscopically, the tumour is bulky, lobulated and semitranslucent. Microscopically, it is a sarcoma containing cartilage. Differentiation is variable. Poorly-differentiated tumours (mesenchymal chondrosarcomas) behave more aggressively. In the well-differentiated form, spread is slow locally. Blood-borne metastases occur late to the lungs.

Clinical features

Presentation is usually with a slowly progressive painless swelling which eventually becomes painful.

Diagnosis and investigation

A biopsy is required. Plain radiography shows bone destruction and commonly abnormal flecks of calcification. MRI scanning (Figure 32.18) helps define the local extent.

Treatment

Radical surgery is the treatment of choice. Limb preservation may be possible. It is a very radioresistant tumour. An exception is chondrosarcomas of the facial bones and the base of skull, where a combination of surgery and radiotherapy offer long-term control. Radiotherapy has only a palliative role for the relief of local symptoms, such as pain, and relatively high doses are required even for palliative effect.

Radiotherapy

Technique

A parallel-opposed wedged pair of fields is suitable for the long bones. A three-field technique for pelvic tumours using anterior and posterior wedged fields with an open lateral field may limit the dose to the bowel.

Dose and energy
60 Gy in 30 daily fractions over 6 weeks at megavoltage (4–6 MV photons).

Chemotherapy

By and large, chondrosarcomas are chemoresistant, although there has been a renewal of interest in chemotherapy recently using the same agents that have been

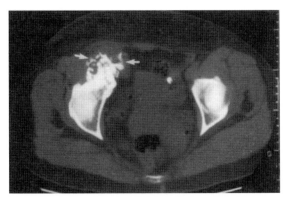

Figure 32.18 CT scan of the pelvis showing a chondrosarcoma of the ileum (arrows). Note the flecks of calcification.
(Courtesy of Dr R Nakielny, Sheffield.)

very useful in osteogenic sarcoma, particularly for the mesenchymal subtypes. However, the increase in overall survival following chemotherapy is small.

Results of treatment

Five-year survival is about 50% over the age of 21 years but falls to 35% under that age. Younger patients tend to have tumours in the pelvis, where radical surgery is more difficult than in long bones. They also have more poorly-differentiated tumours which metastasize more frequently.

Spindle cell sarcomas

These include malignant fibrous histiocytoma (MFH), angiosarcoma and sarcomas NOS (not otherwise stated). They occur later (30–60 years of age) than osteosarcoma. Origin is both in the diaphysis and the metaphysis from the periosteum or the medullary cavity. Any bone may be affected. Microscopically, there is variable collagen formation. Spread from the periosteum is to the soft tissues more than bone, and within the medullary cavity for endosteal tumours.

Clinical features

Pain and swelling are the main features.

Diagnosis and investigations

Plain radiography may show an area of bone similar in appearance to a bone infarct. A bone biopsy is necessary.

Treatment

Local excision is the treatment of choice with limb preservation if possible. Amputation may be necessary. Radiotherapy is only of palliative value. Adjuvant chemotherapy similar to that for osteogenic sarcoma is being evaluated.

Results of treatment

The prognosis is poor, with 5-year survival about 25%.

Secondary tumours in bone

The great majority of bone tumours are not primary but are of metastatic origin. They represent 15–20% of the workload of a radiotherapy department. The most common primary sites are breast, lung, prostate, myeloma and kidney. The prognosis of bone metastases is generally poor, though the course of the disease may be relatively slow over a period of years, for example, in some patients with breast cancer. Patients presenting with bone metastases from prostate or breast cancer may live for years while this tumour is hormone sensitive. Good symptomatic relief by a combination of analgesics and local radiotherapy can be achieved in most cases.

Clinical features and investigation

The usual presentation is with pain due to pressure on the periosteum or on nerve roots as they emerge from the spinal canal (Figure 32.19). Early diagnosis is important before bone destruction has advanced so far as to cause pathological fracture (Figure 32.20) or spinal cord compression.

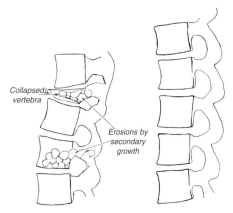

Figure 32.19 Diagrammatic radiological appearances of normal vertebral column and secondary deposits from cancer (e.g. breast).

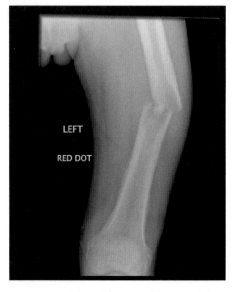

Figure 32.20 A pathological fracture of the mid-left femur. The patient had metastatic non-small cell lung cancer. A femoral pin was inserted and the femur irradiated.

Plain radiographs of the symptomatic area may show the deposits (osteolytic or osteosclerotic or both) or a pathological fracture. However, a metastasis in a vertebral body has to have reached a size of about 2 cm before it will be visible on a radiograph.

A radioisotope bone scan is helpful in detecting bone metastases too small to be visible on plain radiographs and to detect deposits elsewhere in the skeleton. Multiple bone metastases are common, predominantly in the spine, ribs, pelvis and upper femur. CT scanning of areas of the spine and sacrum where plain radiographs and bone scan are equivocal or normal may show bone destruction. If there is no known primary site, a CT-guided biopsy may be necessary.

Treatment

The treatment of bone metastases includes analgesics, radiotherapy, bisphosphonates and, occasionally, surgery. Treatment is aimed at relieving pain as simply and quickly as possible. Patients should always be given adequate analgesia escalating from paracetamol through non-steroidals, mild and then stronger opiates. The choice of treatment will depend on the site of the pain, its severity, complications, such as spinal cord compression or pathological fracture, the presence of hypercalcaemia, the underlying tumour and the general condition of the patient.

Numerous randomized clinical trials have shown that a single fraction of 8–10 Gy is as effective for relieving pain as a regimen of 30 Gy in 10 fractions when analgesic effect is measured at 6 weeks after treatment. The duration of pain relief after a single fraction is not known, but it is very easy to repeat the treatment. Depending on the site of the tumour, up to 80% of patients have a marked diminution of pain following a single radiation fraction and up to 50% have complete pain relief (Figure 32.21). There is an argument for giving higher doses (up to 40 Gy in 15 fractions) to a select group of patients. This may include young women

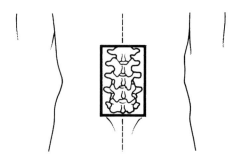

Figure 32.21 Palliative single field (16 × 8 cm) to the lumbar spine (4–6 MV photons).

with a solitary bone metastasis from breast cancer, especially when there has been a long disease-free interval. Similarly, patients with a solitary metastasis from a renal or thyroid carcinoma may gain durable palliation from a higher dose. Single fields are usually adequate for vertebral, sacral and rib deposits. Obese patients with lumbar metastasis should be treated with parallel-opposed fields. Kilovoltage radiation offers practical treatment advantages in the treatment of cervical spine lesions. Patients can be treated sitting in a chair, which is very useful if the neck is painful or the patient is wearing a supportive collar. As the absorbtion of kilovoltage x-rays in bone is greater than megavoltage, the exit dose is small with less mucositis. Similarly, rib lesions can easily be treated using 300 kV x-rays. Parallel-opposed fields are usually used for tumours in the pelvis, long bones and the base of skull. Usually, field sizes are generous, particularly in the spine. Fields usually include the uninvolved vertebra above and below the target lesions. In the treatment of long bone metastases, margins of 3–5 cm are added beyond visible lesions to deal with occult disease.

Pathological fracture

If there is a pathological fracture of a long bone, an orthopaedic opinion should be sought on the feasibility of reducing and stabilizing the fracture. Pinning a fracture usually provides prompt pain relief and a return to mobility.

If there is evidence of spinal cord compression, surgical decompression of the cord may be necessary prior to fractionated radiotherapy. Steroids should be given to patients with pain from nerve root infiltration and spinal cord compression.

Some patients are too unwell for even single fractions of radiotherapy. Their pain should be controlled medically.

Hemibody irradiation

If there are widespread painful bone metastases and the tumour is relatively radiosensitive (e.g. myeloma and prostate cancer), hemibody irradiation in a single fraction can be considered. Typically, single doses of 6 Gy are given to the upper and 8 Gy to the lower body. Doses greater than 6 Gy can induce an acute pulmonary reaction and pulmonary oedema. Radiation-induced nausea and vomiting can be suppressed by steroids such as dexamethasone and 5HT3 antagonists (granisetron and ondansetron).

Bisphosphonates

These drugs, usually given intravenously every 3 weeks, are effective by preventing further osteoclastic resorption of bone. Pain relief is durable. The main side effect is hypocalcaemia. They are licensed for use long-term in multiple myeloma and breast cancer. Studies are ongoing into their role in metastatic prostate cancer.

FURTHER READING

Suit H, Spiro I. Radiation as a therapeutic modality in sarcomas of the soft tissue. Hematol Oncol Clin North Am 1995;9:733–6.

Tierney JF, Stewart LA, Parmar MK. Adjuvant chemotherapy for localised resectable soft tissue sarcoma of adults: meta-analysis of individual patients data. Lancet 1997;350:1647–54.

Van Geel AN, Pastorino U, Jauch KW, et al. Surgical treatment of lung metastases: the EORTC soft tissue and bone sarcoma group study of 255 patients. Cancer 1996;77:675–82.

O'Sullivan B, Ward I, Haycock T, et al. Techniques to modulate radiotherapy toxicity and outcome in soft tissue sarcoma. Curr Opin Oncol 2003;4:453–64.

Price P, Hoskin PJ, Easton D. Prospective randomised trial of single and multifraction radiotherapy in the treatment of painful bone metastases. Radiother Oncol 1986;6:247–55.

La TH, Meyers PA, Wexler LH, et al. Radiation therapy for Ewing's sarcoma: results from Memorial Sloan-Kettering in the modern era. Int J Radiat Oncol Biol Phys 2006;64:544–50.

European Society for Medical Oncology. ESMO minimum clinical recommendations for diagnosis, treatment and follow-up of Ewing's sarcoma of bone. Ann Oncol 2005; 16(Suppl. 1):173–4.

Krasin MJ, Rodriguez-Galindo C, Billups CA, et al. Definitive irradiation in multidisciplinary management of localized Ewing sarcoma family of tumours in pediatric patients: outcome and prognostic factors. Int J Radiat Oncol Biol Phys 2004;60:830–8.

Aksnes LH, Hall KS, Folleraas S, et al. Management of high grade bone sarcoma over two decades: the Norwegian Radium Hospital experience. Acta Oncol 2006;45:38–46.

DeLaney TF, Trofimov AV, Engelsman M, Suit HD. Advanced-technology radiation therapy in the management of bone and soft tissue sarcomas. Cancer Control 2005;12:27–35.

Souhami RL, Craft AW, van der Eijken JW, et al. Randomised trial of two regimens of chemotherapy in operable osteosarcoma: a study of the European Osteosarcoma intergroup. Lancet 1997;350:911–7.

EVOLVE CONTENTS (available online at: http://evolve.elsevier.com/Symonds/radiotherapy/)

Chapter | 33 |

Paediatric oncology

Roger E. Taylor

INTRODUCTION

Cancer in childhood is uncommon. In the UK, approximately 1500 children below the age of 15 develop cancer each year. Approximately one individual child in 500 will develop cancer before the age of 15. The range of childhood cancers is very different from that seen in the adult population. Table 33.1 summarizes data on relative incidence of the various tumour types from the US Surveillance, Epidemiology and End Results (SEER) programme.

Table 33.1 Surveillance, epidemiology and end results (SEER) programme registrations 1975–2001, annual incidence rate per 1 000 000 and proportion of children aged 0–14 with cancer

DISEASE GROUP	ANNUAL INCIDENCE RATE PER 1 000 000	PERCENTAGE OF TOTAL
Acute lymphoblastic leukaemia (ALL)	32.8	23.6
Acute non-lymphoblastic leukaemia (ANNL)	6.4	4.6
Other leukaemias	3.0	2.2
All leukaemias	**42.2**	**30.3**
Astrocytoma	14.5	10.4
Medulloblastoma/PNET	6.6	4.7
Ependymoma	2.7	1.9
Intracranial germ cell tumours	1.1	0.8
Other CNS tumours	5.7	4.1
All CNS tumours	**29.4**	**21.1**
Hodgkin's disease	6.0	4.3
Non-Hodgkin's lymphoma	7.8	5.6
Osteosarcoma	3.5	2.5
Ewing's sarcoma/ peripheral PNET	2.4	1.7
Rhabdomyosarcoma	4.8	3.5
Other sarcoma	5.3	3.8
Neuroblastoma	10.3	7.4
Wilms' tumour	8.3	6.0
Total	**139.1**	

The evolution of the multidisciplinary care of children with cancer has been one of the success stories of modern oncology. Paediatric oncology collaborative groups have been very successful at entering a high proportion of children into clinical trials. In North America, clinical research has been coordinated via the Paediatric Oncology Group (POG), Children's Cancer Group (CCG), Intergroup Rhabdomyosarcoma Study Group (IRSG) and National Wilms' Tumour Study Group (NWTS). In 1999, these were amalgamated to form the Children's Oncology Group (COG), the largest paediatric oncology collaborative group in the world.

In the UK, treatment is coordinated by the network of twenty-two Children's Cancer and Leukaemia Group (CCLG) (formerly UKCCSG) paediatric oncology centres. Increasingly, collaboration is across European boundaries, with clinical trials coordinated via the International Society of Paediatric Oncology (SIOP).

Currently, approximately two-thirds of children treated for cancer can expect to be long-term survivors. For most diseases, this has been brought about largely as a result of the incorporation of chemotherapy as part of a multimodality approach, including surgery and radiotherapy. Since the introduction of chemotherapy into treatment programmes in the 1960s and 1970s, the proportion of children surviving cancer has shown a gratifying increase.

Approximately 40–50% of children with cancer receive radiotherapy as part of their initial treatment. Radiotherapy is an important modality of therapy in local tumour control and the majority of paediatric tumours are radiosensitive. Cure, however, often comes 'with a cost' as a result of the long-term sequelae of treatment. Long-term effects of radiotherapy include impaired bone and soft tissue growth, impaired neuropsychological development as a result of irradiation of the central nervous system (CNS) and radiation-induced malignancy. Increasing awareness of long-term effects in the 1970s and 1980s led to a general decline in the use of radiotherapy. However, more recently, it has become evident that chemotherapy is also associated with long-term side effects, including late myocardial damage due to anthracyclines, nephrotoxicity due to cisplatin or ifosfamide, and secondary leukaemia related to a number of chemotherapeutic agents including alkylating agents. The overall aim of paediatric oncology programmes is to maximize the chance of cure with the minimum impact of likely long-term effects of treatment. Continued vigilance for long-term effects of treatment is essential. This is ideally performed in the setting of dedicated long-term follow-up clinics and employing national treatment-related guidelines for long-term follow up, such as those produced by the CCLG and the Scottish Intercollegiate Group.

It is very important that the administration of chemotherapy and radiotherapy for children should be undertaken only in specialized oncology centres treating relatively large numbers of children. In the UK, these centres are usually affiliated to the CCLG. The multiprofessional paediatric radiotherapy team should include a specialist paediatric therapy radiographer, specialist nurse and play specialist. Young children, particularly those under the age of three to four, find it very difficult to lie still for radiotherapy planning and delivery, especially when a Perspex head shell is required. Sedation sufficient to ensure immobilization is difficult to achieve without it persisting for several hours and it is not feasible for this to be administered daily. Because of the importance of immobilization, short-acting general anaesthesia, such as DiprivanÒ (propofol), is sometimes needed. The daily fasting for this results in surprisingly little disruption to nutrition. An experienced play therapist can be very helpful in preparing the child for radiotherapy and may avoid the need for daily anaesthesia for some children.

TOXICITY OF RADIOTHERAPY FOR CHILDREN

Acute morbidity

The side effects of erythema, mucositis, nausea, diarrhoea etc. occur in children as in adults, and are generally managed by similar means.

Subacute effects

Liver

A large proportion of the liver may need to be irradiated when treating Wilms' tumour. Radiation hepatopathy may occur 1–3 months following radiotherapy, and consists of hepatomegaly, jaundice, ascites, thrombocytopenia and elevated transaminases. A risk factor is the administration of actinomycin-D following hepatic irradiation. Long-term dysfunction is rare and the risk is dose related.

Lung

The whole lungs may receive radiotherapy as part of total body irradiation, or in the treatment of pulmonary metastases from Wilms' tumour or Ewing's sarcoma. Mild radiation pneumonitis consists of a dry cough and mild dyspnoea. The risk of pneumonitis is dose and radiation volume related. Radiation pneumonitis is the dose limiting toxicity for total body irradiation. It is essential to consider potential interactions between chemotherapeutic drugs and lung irradiation and, in particular, to avoid lung irradiation in association with busulfan.

Central nervous system

The 'somnolence syndrome' occurs in at least 50% of children approximately 6 weeks after cranial irradiation and is probably related to temporary demyelination. Lhermitte's sign consists of an electric shock-like symptom radiating down the spine and into the limbs. It may follow radiation to the upper spinal cord, e.g. following mediastinal radiotherapy for lymphoma. Within the first 2 months following radiotherapy for brain tumours, children may experience a transient deterioration of neurological symptoms and signs.

Long-term effects

Bone growth

Impairment of bone growth and associated soft tissue hypoplasia can be one of the most obvious and distressing long-term effects, particularly when treating the head and neck region. Abnormalities of craniofacial growth can cause significant cosmetic and functional deformity, including micrognathia leading to problems with dentition. The epiphysial growth plates are very sensitive to radiation, and are excluded from the radiotherapy field whenever possible. Age at time of treatment, radiation dose and volume are factors which have an impact on the severity of these orthopaedic long-term effects. There is evidence of a dose response effect, with a greater effect seen for doses of >33 Gy compared with <33 Gy. Slipped femoral epiphysis and avascular necrosis have also been reported following irradiation of the hip. Laboratory evidence suggests a dose response effect between 5 Gy and 35–40 Gy, and an effect of dose per fraction. Careful consideration of the late orthopaedic effects of radiation is extremely important whenever planning radiotherapy for children. Epiphyses should be excluded from the irradiated volume where possible and, when irradiating the spine, an important principle of paediatric radiotherapy is that the full width of the vertebra should receive homogeneous irradiation in order to minimize long-term kyphoscoliosis.

Central nervous system

Paediatric radiation oncology involves a significant amount of time devoted to the treatment of children with brain tumours, and consideration needs to be given to the toxicity of therapy.

Radionecrosis is rare below 60 Gy, and generally occurs with a latency of 6 months to 2 years. It results from a direct effect on glial tissue. It is very unusual to have to deliver a dose of 60 Gy to any part of the CNS for a child and, for the radical treatment of children with brain tumours, it is very uncommon to exceed a dose of 50–54 Gy. It occurs in approximately 50% of patients treated by interstitial implantation for recurrent brain tumours following prior radical external beam radiotherapy. The clinical effects of radionecrosis vary according to the site within the CNS and are most devastating in the spinal cord. Radionecrosis of the spinal cord in children has been seen as a consequence of the interaction between radiation and cytosine arabinoside given intrathecally for metastatic rhabdomyosarcoma.

Necrotizing leukoencephalopathy may be seen when cranial irradiation is followed by high dose methotrexate for the treatment of leukaemia. The clinical features include ataxia, lethargy, epilepsy, spasticity and paresis.

Neuropsychological effects. The effects of cranial radiotherapy are now well established. Data from children treated with prophylactic radiotherapy for leukaemia have demonstrated that when compared with siblings, children given

24 Gy prophylactic cranial irradiation show an approximate fall in IQ of 12 points. Following higher radiation doses given for brain tumours, an increased risk of learning and behaviour difficulties is seen. An important risk factor for the incidence and severity of neuropsychological long-term effects is the age at diagnosis. Other factors include the impact of direct and indirect tumour-related parameters, treatment parameters with neuropsychological long-term effects worse for whole brain compared with partial brain irradiation, concomitant use of some chemotherapeutic agents, premorbid patient characteristics, such as intelligence, and the quality of 'catch up' education.

Kidney

Long-term effects on renal function are usually seen 2–3 years following a course of radiotherapy. The risk increases following a dose of greater than 15 Gy to both kidneys. The severity is related to the dose received, and when mild consists of hypertension. When more severe, following a higher dose, renal failure may ensue.

Endocrine

Endocrine deficiencies following radiotherapy are common. Of particular concern are the risk of growth hormone and other pituitary hormone deficiencies following pituitary irradiation for tumours of the CNS.

Following radiotherapy to the thyroid, the incidence of elevated TSH is 75% after 25–40 Gy.

Reproductive

In boys, the germinal epithelium is very sensitive to the effects of low dose irradiation. In adult males, transient oligospermia is seen after 2 Gy, but slow recovery can occur after 2–5 Gy.

In girls, the oocytes are also sensitive. Subsequent pregnancy is rare after 12 Gy whole body irradiation but anecdotal cases of pregnancy after bone marrow transplantation including whole body irradiation have been reported.

TOLERANCE OF CRITICAL ORGANS TO RADIOTHERAPY

The tolerance of critical organs frequently limits the dose of radiation that can be given. The critical organs and their 'tolerance doses' are listed in Table 33.2.

CHEMOTHERAPY/RADIOTHERAPY INTERACTIONS

Interactions between radiation and chemotherapy are complex and poorly understood. Interactions can be exploited in order to attempt to improve disease-free survival. The

Table 33.2 Normal tissue tolerance doses

TISSUE/ORGAN	TOLERANCE DOSE (Gy)
Whole lung	15–18
Both kidneys	12–15
Whole liver	20
Spinal cord	50

most frequently employed mechanism in paediatric oncology is 'spatial cooperation' whereby chemotherapy and radiotherapy are combined to exploit their differing roles in different anatomical sites. Examples are the use of radiation for local control of a primary, with chemotherapy for subclinical metastatic disease such as in the treatment of Ewing's sarcoma.

Chemotherapy and radiotherapy may be combined with the aim of increasing tumour cell kill without excess toxicity. An example is the use of combined chemotherapy and radiotherapy for children with Hodgkin's disease. It may be possible to reduce the intensity of both treatment modalities and hopefully reduce long-term morbidity. When using combined modality therapy the aim is to improve the therapeutic ratio. Many protocols for children involve the use of concurrent chemotherapy and radiotherapy. It is essential to be vigilant for additional early or long-term morbidity. Clinically important chemotherapy/radiotherapy interactions are often unpredictable and their mechanisms poorly understood. Actinomycin-D and cisplatin increase the slope of the radiation dose–response curve and actinomycin-D inhibits the repair of sublethal damage (SLD). Clinical interactions include enhanced skin and mucosal toxicity when radiation is followed by actinomycin-D (the 'recall phenomenon'), enhanced bladder toxicity when chemotherapy is combined with cyclophosphamide, enhanced CNS toxicity from combined radiation and methotrexate, cytosine arabinoside or busulfan, and the enhanced marrow toxicity from wide field irradiation and many myelotoxic chemotherapeutic agents. In the case of the effect of combined radiation and anthracyclines, such as doxorubicin on the heart, doxorubicin has its effects on the myocytes and radiation on the vasculature.

RADIOTHERAPY QUALITY ASSURANCE (QA)

Because of the high cure rate for most childhood cancers, it is important to achieve local tumour control and avoid a 'geographical miss'. It is also important to avoid unnecessarily large field sizes, in order to minimize long-term effects.

It is essential for all radiotherapy departments to deliver the highest possible standard of radiotherapy for all patients including children. Many radiotherapy departments have adopted quality systems.

In a number of studies, particularly those employing craniospinal radiotherapy for medulloblastoma, the accuracy of delivery of radiotherapy has impacted upon tumour control and patient survival. In many North American paediatric multicentre studies, radiotherapy quality, including beam data, dose prescription, planning and verification films are reviewed centrally in the Quality Assurance Review Centre (QARC) situated in Providence, Rhode Island. In the majority of European studies, QA is not as well organized. Ideally, review of radiotherapy simulator or verification films by study coordinators should be sufficiently fast to provide feedback early in the course of radiotherapy so that the treatment plan can be modified if necessary. The electronic transmission of planning films and associated clinical data can facilitate this process. This is logistically difficult but has been achieved in the USA for radiotherapy administered to children treated within POG, CCG and more recently COG trials. In Europe, where funding for these activities is more problematic, this has been achieved in Germany for radiotherapy for Ewing's sarcoma.

LEUKAEMIA

The improvement in survival of children with acute lymphoblastic leukaemia (ALL) was one of the early successes of paediatric oncology. Currently, more than 70% are long-term survivors. The leukaemias account for the most frequent group of paediatric malignancies. Approximately 80% have ALL and 20% acute non-lymphoblastic leukaemia (ANLL), usually acute myeloid leukaemia (AML) or rarely chronic myeloid leukaemia (CML).

Current treatment for ALL is stratified according to risk status based on presenting white count and cytogenetic profile. The four phases of treatment are:

1. remission induction, usually with vincristine, corticosteroids and asparaginase
2. intensification with multidrug combinations. The number of intensification modules is dependent upon risk status at presentation
3. CNS prophylaxis with intrathecal methotrexate. Cranial radiotherapy is no longer employed except for patients presenting with CNS involvement by leukaemia
4. maintenance, usually based on a continuous low dose antimetabolite drug such as 6-thioguanine, with a total duration of therapy of approximately 2 years.

During the 1960s and 1970s, the routine use of prophylactic whole brain radiotherapy and intrathecal methotrexate reduced the risk of CNS relapse to less than 10%. Whole brain radiotherapy may be employed for patients who present with CNS involvement (Figure *evolve* 33.1 🖱). Patients are immobilized in a head shell and treated with lateral-opposed 4–6 MV megavoltage fields which may be centred on outer canthus to minimize divergence into the contra-lateral lens. Shielding will cover the face, dentition, nasal structures and lenses. The clinical target volume (CTV) includes the intracranial meninges extending inferiorly to the lower border of the second or third cervical vertebra. Great care is taken to include the cribriform fossa, temporal lobe and base of skull. Although the lens is shielded, as much of the posterior orbit as possible is included as ocular relapses occasionally occur. The CTV is localized with lateral simulator radiographs or, more recently, computed tomography (CT) simulation. The prescribed dose in current UK protocols is 24 Gy in 15 fractions of 1.6 Gy daily.

Boys who suffer a testicular relapse are treated with testicular radiotherapy (Figure 33.2). The technique employed is an anterior field, generally electrons or orthovoltage (200–300 kV). The CTV includes both testes, scrotum and inguinal canal superlaterally as far as the deep inguinal ring with shielding of non-target skin and perineum. The prescribed dose is 24 Gy in 12 fractions of 2.0 Gy daily.

As for adults, children with ANNL are treated with intensive multidrug chemotherapy, which can achieve a survival rate of 60%. Bone marrow transplantation (BMT) is frequently employed for children who have an HLA-matched sibling. A survival rate of 65% can be achieved for children in first complete remission treated with BMT as consolidation therapy for acute myeloid leukaemia.

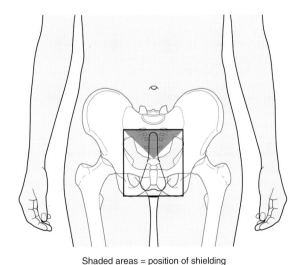

Shaded areas = position of shielding

Figure 33.2 Diagram of field for testicular radiotherapy.

Total body irradiation (TBI)

TBI is an important technique used together usually with high dose cyclophosphamide (Cyclo-TBI) as the conditioning regimen prior to BMT for adults and children. Bone marrow donors for BMT are generally HLA-matched siblings. However, increasingly, volunteer unrelated donors from donor panels donate marrow, resulting in a significant increase in the number of patients for whom BMT can be considered.

Techniques for TBI have evolved in different departments, generally depending on availability of treatment facilities. Modern linear accelerator design and field sizes allow the use of large anterior and posterior fields. TBI dosimetry is usually based on in vivo measurements.

As an example of a TBI technique, the Leeds technique is described. The patient lies in the lateral position in an evacuated polystyrene immobilization bag. Hands are placed under chin to provide 'lung compensation' (Figure *evolve* 33.3 🖰). Dosimetry is determined using in-vivo measurements performed at a 'test dose' of 0.2 Gy for each field. For such a large and complex target volume, it is not feasible to adhere to the ICRU 50 guidelines of a range of −5% to +7%, and a range of −10% to +10% is more realistic. The standard TBI dose for children in the UK is 14.4 Gy in eight fractions of 1.8 Gy twice daily with a minimum interfraction interval of 6 hours.

For children with ALL, many centres advise a cranial boost in addition to the TBI with the aim of reducing the risk of CNS relapse. Planning for the cranial boost is the same as for prophylactic cranial irradiation. Unlike the use of the standard TBI dose, policies for the cranial boost vary between individual centres. A typical regimen for the cranial boost would be 5.4 Gy in three daily fractions.

Indications for BMT/TBI in children

In the current UK Medical Research Council (MRC) Study, children with AML are selected for BMT and TBI based on risk status at presentation. Those with an HLA-matched sibling are selected for BMT if they fall into the intermediate or high-risk category, whereas those with low-risk disease, i.e. those with chromosome mutations t(8;21), t(15;17) or Inv 16 do well with standard chemotherapy. Children with ALL selected for BMT and TBI include relapsed patients and those presenting with features indicating a high risk of failure with standard chemotherapy. Other conditions considered for BMT where TBI is sometimes employed include severe aplastic anaemia, thalassaemia and immunodeficiency syndromes.

Morbidity of TBI

Acute effects include nausea and lethargy during TBI, mucositis, diarrhea, erythema and parotitis in the first few weeks following treatment and somnolence approximately 6 weeks after TBI. Long-term effects of TBI include impaired growth due to a direct effect from irradiation of epiphyses and also as a growth hormone deficiency. There is also a risk of cataract, hypothyroidism and, in some studies, the possibility of renal impairment. TBI is generally not considered for children under the age of 2 and, instead, a conditioning regimen with two drugs, busulfan and cyclophosphamide (Bu-Cy), is generally employed.

HODGKIN'S DISEASE

Hodgkin's disease spans the 'older' paediatric age range, through the adolescent and young adult age ranges. The overall survival rate for children with Hodgkin's disease is approximately 90% and an important aim is to maintain this good overall survival rate while reducing long-term treatment effects. These include orthopaedic long-term effects of radiotherapy, such as impaired bone growth resulting from direct irradiation of the epiphyses, and also infertility from alkylating agents and procarbazine. Wide field radiotherapy, such as the 'mantle' technique, has been avoided in children for several decades. In the UK, single modality therapy has been generally used. Children aged 10 or older with disease high in the neck will generally receive involved field radiotherapy. The dose prescribed is 35 Gy in 20 fractions. Both sides of the neck are irradiated to avoid asymmetric cervical spine growth, and the clavicles are shielded (Figure *evolve* 33.4 🖰). With this approach, approximately 70% of children with stage I disease will remain disease free. However, approximately 30% relapse, generally with disease outside the irradiated area, and require chemotherapy. For children aged less than 10 and for those with more extensive disease including all stages II–IV and children with stage I disease low in the neck, chemotherapy is used. The current CCLG regimen employs alternating cycles of chlorambucil, vinblastine, procarbazine and prednisolone (ChlVPP) with Adriamycin, bleomycin, vincristine and dacarbazine (ABVD).

Many North American and European protocols employ low intensity chemotherapy and low-dose involved field radiotherapy with the aim of avoiding infertility and serious orthopaedic effect. In the UK, the question of adopting more widespread use of combined modality therapy is under discussion. Also, positron emission tomography (PET) scanning following chemotherapy may have the potential for selecting patients who require consolidation radiotherapy. Those who are PET positive may require radiotherapy, whereas those who are PET negative may not require radiotherapy following chemotherapy. The role of PET scanning in this setting requires further evaluation.

The management of adolescents with Hodgkin's disease is an example of where local and national collaboration with adult oncology groups is important in order to provide age-related treatment protocols.

NON-HODGKIN'S LYMPHOMA (NHL)

A different spectrum of NHL is seen in children compared with adults. Follicle centre cell lymphoma and diffuse large B-cell lymphoma, which are common in adults, are uncommon in childhood. The majority of children have T-cell lymphoblastic lymphoma, Burkitt's, Burkitt-like, or anaplastic large cell lymphoma. Survival rates have improved in recent years and, currently, more than 80% survive long term. Patients are treated by intensive multiagent chemotherapy including CNS prophylaxis with intrathecal chemotherapy and there is no routine role for radiotherapy in their management. However, children with T-cell lymphoblastic lymphoma, which is managed according to the same principles as ALL, may be considered for BMT with TBI.

NEUROBLASTOMA

Neuroblastoma (NB) is the commonest solid tumour of childhood. NB is generally a disease of very young children. Approximately one-third are less than one year of age at presentation. NB arises in neural crest tissue in the autonomic nervous system, usually in the adrenal area, but can arise anywhere from the neck to the pelvis. The majority of children present with widespread metastases including bones, marrow, lungs and liver. Overall, current survival rates are generally poor, approximately 45% taking all stages and prognostic groups into account. Prognosis for individual clinical groups varies considerably and is related to a number of prognostic factors. Prognosis is better for young children aged less than one at presentation, and is worse for children whose tumours have amplification of the oncogene Myc-n. Deletion of the short arm of chromosome 1 has emerged as an important prognostic factor with a worse prognosis for those with 1p deletion. Tumours that are hyperdiploid have a better prognosis. Management is now stratified according to risk grouping. Patients in the best risk group with localized disease have a survival rate of greater than 90% following surgery alone. The majority are treated with intensive chemotherapy using drugs such as vincristine, cisplatin, carboplatin, etoposide, and cyclophosphamide.

For 'good-risk' patients, radiotherapy is unnecessary and for high-risk patients, the predominant relapse pattern is metastatic rather than local. The role of external beam radiotherapy for patients with high-risk disease (e.g. aged greater than one year with stage 4 disease at presentation) is to maximize the probability of local tumour control following surgical resection of the primary tumour. With current intensive chemotherapy, some patients with metastases at presentation can hopefully be 'cured' of their

metastatic disease, in which case local tumour control becomes important, employing a combination of surgical resection and postoperative radiotherapy. In the current European High-Risk NB protocol, the dose for postoperative radiotherapy to the tumour bed is 21 Gy in 14 fractions. In planning postoperative radiotherapy for NB, care has to be taken to consider dose limits to organs at risk (OARs), particularly liver and kidneys, the function of which may have been compromised by high-dose chemotherapy.

MIBG therapy for neuroblastoma

The majority of NBs take up the guanethidine analogue meta-iodobenzyl guanidine (MIBG). MIBG can be conjugated with iodine radionuclides for imaging and 'targeted' radiotherapy. Generally, ^{123}I-MIBG is the radionuclide used for diagnostic imaging. High-activity ^{131}I-MIBG (typically 3.7–7.4 GBq) can be used for targeted therapy. In a UK multicentre study, a response rate of 30% has been achieved for children with residual NB following first-line chemotherapy. After enthusiasm in the 1980s and early 1990s, interest in the potential role for therapeutic MIBG has diminished. However, in some European centres, 'up-front' MIBG is still employed and its role in the initial management of high-risk NB, together with chemotherapy, warrants further exploration. Logistic difficulties include radiation protection for very young children, who may not yet be continent of urine and the risk of radiation exposure to staff who may need to care for an ill child. Many UK radiotherapy departments are geographically separated in different hospitals from paediatric support. This is one of the main reasons why currently MIBG therapy is available in only a limited number of paediatric oncology centres in the UK.

WILMS' TUMOUR (NEPHROBLASTOMA)

Wilms' tumour is an embryonic renal tumour which generally presents as a large abdominal mass, sometimes with pain or hematuria. Wilms' tumour may be genetically associated with aniridia (congenital absence of the iris) and other inherited syndromes, such as the Beckwith-Wiedemann syndrome (variable features including macrosomia or hemihypertrophy, macroglossia, omphalocele). The WT1 gene is located on chromosome 11, and is a tumour suppressor gene. If both copies of the gene are lost by mutation, then Wilms' tumour may arise.

Median age at diagnosis is between 3 and 3.5 years. Patients are staged according to histopathological findings following nephrectomy. Table 33.3 shows the National Wilms' Tumour Study Group (NWTS) staging system for Wilms' tumour. In 4–8% of cases tumours are bilateral (stage V).

The current long-term survival rate for Wilms' tumour is in excess of 80%. Treatment is aimed at maintaining this

Table 33.3 National Wilms' Tumour Study Group (NWTS) staging system

STAGE	CLINICOPATHOLOGICAL FEATURES
I	Tumour confined to within renal capsule, completely excised
II	Tumour invading outside renal capsule, completely excised
III	Residual abdominal tumour – positive margins, tumour rupture, involved nodes
IV	Haematogenous metastases
V	Bilateral disease

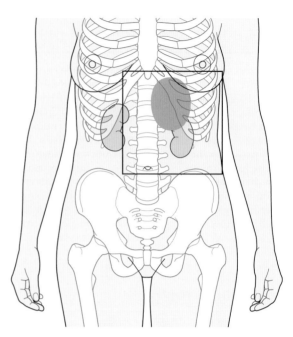

Figure 33.5 Diagram of flank radiotherapy field for Wilms' tumour.

high survival rate while attempting to reduce the long-term side effects of therapy. There is a major disparity between approaches adopted in Europe and North America. The North American series of NWTS, now COG protocols, employ immediate nephrectomy with staging and post-surgical adjuvant therapy based on histological examination of the primary tumour. Wilms' tumour histology is referred to as either favourable (FH) or unfavourable (UH) because of the presence of anaplasia.

Postoperative chemotherapy is given using the drugs vincristine, actinomycin-D and doxorubicin, the number of drugs and duration depending upon the staging.

In Europe, the series of International Society of Paediatric Oncology (SIOP) studies have been based on preoperative chemotherapy to 'downstage' the primary, reducing the surgical morbidity, particularly the number who have tumour rupture at surgery, and the number who require flank radiotherapy. The most recent study is the SIOP 2001 study into which patients from the UK are entered. All patients receive preoperative chemotherapy with actinomycin-D and vincristine, with delayed nephrectomy after 6 weeks of preoperative chemotherapy. Postoperative adjuvant therapy is based on subsequent pathological staging and allocation of risk status (good-risk versus intermediate-risk versus poor-risk histology). For intermediate-risk patients, there is a randomization to receive or not receive doxorubicin. The purpose of this is to determine whether doxorubicin can be omitted, thus reducing the risk of late cardiac sequelae.

Postoperative flank radiotherapy is employed for stage III patients, i.e. those with incompletely resected primary tumours, pre- or perioperative tumour rupture, or histologically involved lymph nodes. The technique employs anterior and posterior opposed fields. The CTV includes the preoperative extent of tumour and kidney, following preoperative chemotherapy with a margin of 1.0 cm. Fields extend across the midline in order to irradiate homogeneously the full width of the vertebral body in order to

minimize the risk of kyphoscoliosis (Figure 33.5 and Figure *evolve* 33.6 🖰). For patients with intermediate-risk histology, the dose is 14.4 Gy in eight fractions of 1.8 Gy daily, and for high-risk histology, 25.2 Gy in 14 fractions of 1.8 Gy. There is a boost to macroscopic disease or involved nodes: 10.8 Gy in six fractions of 1.8 Gy.

Whole abdominal radiotherapy has considerable acute and long-term morbidity and should be reserved for those who present with extensive intra-abdominal tumour spread or generalized preoperative or perioperative tumour rupture. The dose for this is 21 Gy in 1.5 Gy fractions with shielding to limit the dose to the remaining kidney to 12 Gy.

For children presenting with pulmonary metastases which do not resolve completely after the initial 6 weeks of preoperative chemotherapy, whole lung radiotherapy (Figure 33.7 and Figure *evolve* 33.8 🖰) is given. The fields have to include the costophrenic recess and the lower border generally extends to the lower border of the 12th thoracic vertebra. The humeral heads are shielded. In the current SIOP 2001 study, the lung dose is 15 Gy in 10 fractions with a lung density correction.

RHABDOMYOSARCOMA

Rhabdomyosarcoma (RMS) may arise at any site, although they tend to have a predilection for sites in the head and neck region. These include sites such as the orbit, nasopharynx and middle ear. Other relatively frequent sites

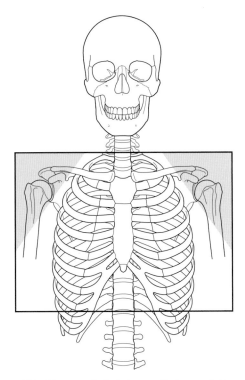

Figure 33.7 Diagram of whole lung radiotherapy field.

include those arising in the urogenital tract such as bladder, prostate and vagina. Tumours that arise in sites such as the nasopharynx and middle ear have the propensity for base of skull and intracranial invasion and are referred to as parameningeal RMS.

Although there are risks of both local and metastatic recurrence, local tumour control is an important consideration in the management of RMS and radiotherapy is an important modality for many patients. The sequelae following radiotherapy, particularly to the head and neck in young children, may be considerable. In Europe in the 1990s, these considerations limited its use, but there is now an increasing recognition of the importance of radiotherapy, not only on local tumour control, but also of its impact on overall survival. Currently, the long-term survival rate for RMS is approximately 65–70%. The challenges are to continue to increase the survival rate, but also to try to do this with acceptable long-term morbidity.

In many European countries including the UK, children have been treated according to the International Society of Paediatric Oncology (SIOP) MMT series of studies. The basis of these has been the use of intensive chemotherapy, with the aim of improving the survival and reducing the use of local therapy with surgery and/or radiotherapy and thus minimizing long-term effects. The strategy for this series of studies includes stratifying patients within risk groups based on histological subtype (embryonal versus alveolar histology), stage of disease and primary tumour site. Patients in the 'low-risk' category, i.e. those with localized tumours which are microscopically completely resected are treated with chemotherapy using actinomycin-D and vincristine for a duration of 9 weeks. Standard-risk tumours are those which are locally more extensive but at selected favourable sites, the vagina, uterus or paratestis and are treated with ifosfamide, vincristine and actinomycin-D. Poor responders switch to a six-drug combination. High-risk tumours include other incompletely resected tumours, including all those arising in parameningeal sites (nasopharynx, middle ear) and those with involved lymph nodes. These are treated with chemotherapy involving a randomization between three drugs (ifosfamide, vincristine, actinomycin-D) and six drugs (carboplatin, epirubicin, vincristine, ifosfamide, etoposide, and actinomycin-D).

In the recently closed MMT 95 study, radiotherapy was used for patients who failed to achieve a complete response following chemotherapy and surgery and, in effect, was used to convert a partial into a complete response. The standard radiotherapy dose in European trials has been 45 Gy in 25 daily fractions with a 'boost' of 5–10 Gy to sites of residual macroscopic disease evident at the start of radiotherapy. For high-risk parameningeal disease (skull base erosion or cranial nerve palsy), the target volume has been based on the pre-chemotherapy extent of disease. For those who require radiotherapy following relapse after initial treatment with chemotherapy alone, the target volume has been based on the tumour extent at the time of relapse and before second-line chemotherapy. For children with initially involved nodes, these are included in the target volume if they require radiotherapy. It is now recognized that patients presenting with primary tumours in the orbit (Figure 33.9) or limbs

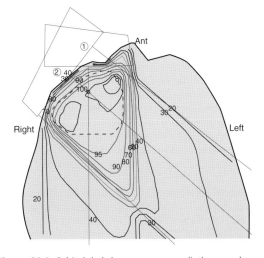

Figure 33.9 Orbital rhabdomyosarcoma radiotherapy plan.

have a high risk of recurrence and now routinely receive radiotherapy in recent European protocols.

Planning of radiotherapy requires meticulous attention to detail, avoiding excessive field sizes, particularly in the head and neck region.

Brachytherapy may be considered for a few highly selected children with RMS, usually with limited tumours arising in the head and neck, vagina, bladder or prostate. However, in the UK, the main area where brachytherapy has been successfully employed has been for the treatment of primary RMS arising in the vaginal vault. Brachytherapy can provide a means of local tumour control with reduced morbidity compared with external beam RT. However, for a child to be suitable for brachytherapy, the tumour must be sufficiently localized in order to achieve local control with a small planning target volume (PTV) suitable for brachytherapy rather than a larger volume suitable for only external beam radiotherapy (typically 2–3 cm). If brachytherapy is being considered for a genitourinary tract primary, discussion between oncologists and surgeons at an early stage is essential followed by a joint examination under anaesthetic (EUA). Both low dose rate and high dose rate afterloading brachytherapy techniques have been used with equal success. Most young children require sedation or general anaesthetic during treatment.

EWING'S SARCOMA/PERIPHERAL PRIMITIVE NEUROECTODERMAL TUMOUR (PPNET)

Ewing's sarcoma of bone is predominantly a disease of adolescents, having its peak incidence in the early teenage years. Survival rates of between 55 and 65% are reported. Approximately 60% of primary tumours occur in the long bones of the limbs, and 40% in the flat bones of the ribs, vertebrae or spine. Significant soft tissue extension is common. Peripheral primitive neuroectodermal tumour (PPNET), previously referred to as 'soft tissue Ewing's sarcoma' has become increasingly recognized in the last two decades. One of the first subtypes of PPNET to be described was the 'Askin tumour' of the chest wall. The majority of Ewing's sarcomas of bone share with PPNET a chromosomal translocation, t(11;22) (q24;q12). In recent years, Ewing's sarcoma and PPNET have generally been treated according to common protocols.

Managing children with Ewing's sarcoma and PPNET requires a multidisciplinary team approach. Initial treatment is with systemic chemotherapy which treats macroscopic tumour and any subclinical metastases. Appropriate use of local therapy, either surgical resection, radiotherapy, or a combination of both modalities is also necessary. Patients in the UK are currently entered into the European Ewing's Tumour Working Initiative of National Groups (Euro-EWING 99) study. Chemotherapy is commenced with VIDE (vincristine, ifosfamide, doxorubicin and etoposide). Patients are then stratified according to primary tumour volume. For patients with small tumours (<200 ml), and those with a good histological response to VIDE chemotherapy, treatment continues with doxorubicin and vincristine and a randomization to either cyclophosphamide or ifosfamide. For those with a poor histological response, there is a randomization between conventional chemotherapy or high dose chemotherapy with busulfan and melphalan.

Local tumour control is important and the decision as to whether surgery, radiotherapy or a combination of both should be employed demands careful multidisciplinary discussion. In previous series of patients treated in Europe, survival has been better following local treatment with surgery (with or without preoperative or postoperative radiotherapy), compared with radiotherapy alone. However, these series are confounded by selection bias with patients with smaller tumours selected for surgery and many patients with very large or inoperable pelvic tumours selected for radiotherapy alone.

Planning of radiotherapy for Ewing's sarcoma or PPNET is technically challenging. 'Multidisciplinary radiotherapy planning' involving radiologists, physicists, specialist therapy radiographers and mould room technicians is important at the outset. Three-dimensional planning may be employed in order to achieve a uniform dose within the target volume, which is frequently large and adjacent to critical organs.

Radiotherapy technique will depend upon the tumour site and anatomy. Individualized, generally multiple fields are used in order to deliver homogeneous irradiation to the PTV and to minimize dose to non-target tissues and organs at risk (Figure 33.10).

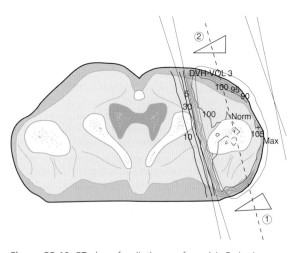

Figure 33.10 CT plan of radiotherapy for pelvic Ewing's sarcoma.

When planning the CTV, phase 1 includes the gross tumour volume (GTV) prior to chemotherapy and/or surgery if feasible with a minimum margin of 3–5 cm for extremity primaries and 2 cm for trunk or head and neck primaries. For a second phase, a margin of 2 cm is employed. Immobilization is dependent upon primary tumour site and anatomy. For limbs, an immobilization device, such as an evacuated polystyrene bag, may be useful. The CTV and PTV are localized on a planning CT scan. The prescribed doses are, for phase 1 and postoperative volume: 44.8 Gy in fractions of 1.8–2.0 Gy and, for phase 2, for macroscopic disease: 9.6 Gy in fractions of 1.8–2.0 Gy.

Selected patients may benefit from a higher dose, up to 64 Gy if this can be delivered without undue toxicity. However, patients selected for definitive radiotherapy frequently have large tumours, and dose may be limited by organ toxicity, and thus a dose of 64 Gy is generally difficult to achieve. For postoperative radiotherapy, the prescribed dose depends on the extent of surgery and histological response of the primary to initial chemotherapy. Following 'intralesional surgery' or 'marginal surgery' with poor histological response to chemotherapy (>10% residual tumour cells), 54.4 Gy is prescribed. For 'marginal surgery' with good histological response (<10% residual tumour cells) or 'wide surgery' with poor histological response, 44.8 Gy is prescribed. For patients who present with pulmonary metastases, whole lung RT is employed, 15 Gy for patients aged less than 14 and 18 Gy for those aged over 14. These doses are subject to homogeneity correction for reduced attenuation in lung.

Care has to be taken when combining chemotherapy and radiotherapy to avoid excessive morbidity from enhanced radiation reactions. Actinomycin-D is not given during radiotherapy and anthracyclines, such as doxorubicin and epirubicin, are omitted if there is a significant amount of bowel or mucosa in the treated volume. Patients requiring radical radiotherapy involving the spinal cord or significant radiotherapy to the lungs should not receive busulfan.

OSTEOSARCOMA

Osteosarcoma is the most frequent bone tumour of childhood, with the majority arising in teenagers. The lower femur and upper tibia are the most frequent primary sites, with approximately 65% developing around the knee. Less frequent sites include the humerus, fibula, sacrum, spine, mandible and pelvis. Prior to the advent of effective chemotherapy, approximately 80% of patients died because of progression of lung metastases. Currently, a survival rate of approximately 55% can be achieved with the use of intensive adjuvant chemotherapy. The majority of primary tumours can be resected and the affected bone replaced by a titanium endoprosthesis, thus avoiding the need for an amputation. The most frequently employed chemotherapy regimen is the combination of cisplatin and doxorubicin, although there is evidence that high dose methotrexate may further improve outcome. The European Osteosarcoma Intergroup (EOI) randomized study comparing six cycles of cisplatin and doxorubicin given either every 3 weeks or every 2 weeks using granulocyte colony stimulating factor (GCSF) to accelerate recovery of the blood count has recently closed. Early results suggest no significant difference in outcome.

Radiotherapy has only a minor role in the management of osteosarcoma. However, it is probably not as radioresistant as previously thought. In selected patients, after insertion of an endoprosthesis, postoperative radiotherapy may be employed for those felt to be at a high risk of local recurrence, i.e. those with tumour at a resection margin. Radiotherapy is sometimes employed for the treatment of an unresectable tumour, such as a spinal vertebral or extensive pelvic primary tumour. In these cases, the dose has to be as high as normal tissues will tolerate, i.e. 60 Gy if possible. Radiotherapy can be employed for the local palliation of metastases, using a relatively high dose, e.g. 40 Gy in 15 fractions.

CENTRAL NERVOUS SYSTEM TUMOURS

Tumours of the central nervous system (CNS) account for approximately 20–25% of malignant childhood tumours. Approximately 350 children develop CNS tumours each year in the UK. However, individual tumour types are uncommon and experience in the management of each type is limited. In contrast to most other paediatric malignancies, the use of chemotherapy has not yet resulted in significant improvements in survival for the majority of children with CNS tumours. The overall 5-year survival rate is approximately 50%, inferior to that reported for many other children's tumours. The 'burdens of survivorship' are high and the majority of survivors experience sequelae from either the tumour or therapy or, very frequently, a combination of both.

Children with CNS tumours and their families are managed by specialized paediatric neuro-oncology multidisciplinary teams. The UK intercollegiate publication 'Guidance for Services for Children and Young People with Brain and Spinal Tumours' describes the elements of a comprehensive multidisciplinary service.

Radiotherapy for children with CNS tumours is technically challenging. Many children require craniospinal radiotherapy, which is one of the most complex techniques employed in most oncology departments.

Long-term effects of radiotherapy for CNS tumours

Of greatest concern are the long-term neuropsychological effects of radiotherapy to the CNS, particularly for very young children. Other factors include direct and indirect effects of the tumour itself and also the effects of surgery. One of the most important factors which increases the risk and severity of long-term neuropsychological sequelae is young age at diagnosis. For children aged less than 3 years at diagnosis, radiotherapy is delayed if possible by the use of chemotherapy.

Children receiving craniospinal radiotherapy will experience spinal shortening as a direct effect of irradiation of the spine.

For many children, the hypothalamic/pituitary axis has to be included in the irradiated volume. This often results in growth hormone deficiency, but other endocrine deficiencies such as thyrotrophin-releasing hormone (TRH) or adrenocorticotrophic hormone (ACTH) deficiency may occur. TRH deficiency is relatively easily managed by thyroid hormone replacement, but ACTH deficiency may require life-long steroid replacement therapy, which may be problematic.

Chemotherapy for CNS tumours

Chemotherapy does not yet have an established role for the majority of paediatric CNS tumours. Secreting intracranial germ cell tumours are routinely treated with chemotherapy. Adjuvant chemotherapy improves the outcome for standard risk medulloblastoma compared with radiotherapy alone. The use of chemotherapy can delay the need for radiotherapy for very young children, particularly those with low-grade astrocytoma and probably ependymoma. However, in most cases, the use of chemotherapy is evaluated within the context of a clinical trial.

Low-grade astrocytoma

Low-grade astrocytomas (LGG) comprise the most frequent group of children's CNS tumours (see Table 31.1). The most frequent histological types are WHO grade I (pilocytic) or grade II (usually fibrillary), with other varieties, such as ganglioglioma and oligodendroglioma, much less frequent. The presence of neurofibromatosis type I (NF1) predisposes to the development of these tumours. It is now clear that LGG may undergo long periods of 'quiescence' even when not completely resected. It is now also clear that low-grade gliomas are more chemosensitive than previously thought. Following treatment of LGG, the 5-year survival rate is relatively high at approximately 80–85%, but late relapse is not uncommon.

Initial treatment is usually with surgical resection, which should be as complete as is considered safe. This is usually more straightforward for tumours arising in the cerebellum, where complete resection is usually feasible, compared with those arising from the optic tract or optic chiasm. Because of the considerable risk of surgery in this area, tumours with typical features on magnetic resonance imaging (MRI) scanning of a hypothalamic/optic tract astrocytoma are not necessarily biopsied, as many consider

the risk of the procedure (i.e. visual deterioration) outweighs the risk of an incorrect diagnosis.

During the last 10 years, North American and European collaborative group studies have attempted to standardize the management of children with LGG. The International Society of Paediatric Oncology (SIOP) series of studies has defined a strategy for managing these tumours. Following initial maximal surgical resection, patients undergo a period of observation. Patients with clinical or radiological evidence of progression, those with severe symptoms or threat to vision receive non-surgical treatment.

In the recently opened European SIOP study, those over the age of 7 years are treated by radiotherapy. Those aged 7 or under receive chemotherapy with the aim of delaying radiotherapy. It is hoped that by employing this strategy for younger children the long-term neuropsychological effects of radiotherapy may be lessened by the delay. Using the drug combination of carboplatin and vincristine, the majority of children with LGG can achieve either a response, or stabilization of previously progressive tumour. In the current SIOP study, patients are randomized to receive initial chemotherapy with either carboplatin and vincristine, or this drug combination with the addition of etoposide. The aim of this study will be to assess whether the addition of etoposide can reduce the risk of tumour progression within the first few months of chemotherapy, which was a significant problem in the previous SIOP LGG study. The total duration of chemotherapy is 18 months. Patients who are treated initially with chemotherapy and who experience progression will receive radiotherapy, and vice versa. For patients who present with spinal cord primary low-grade glioma, the management policy will be similar.

Radiotherapy for low-grade gliomas is based on a careful imaging for target volume definition (Figure *evolve* 33.11 🔊). The technique will depend upon tumour site and anatomy. Individualized multiple fields in order to deliver homogeneous RT to the PTV and to minimize dose to non-target tissues and OARs. The CTV includes the GTV and, in the case of surgical resection, any brain tissue previously surrounding the tumour with a margin in potential areas of spread of 0.5 cm. Patients are immobilized supine or prone depending upon anatomy, generally in a Perspex head shell. The extent of GTV is localized using T2 or 'flair' images on the MRI scan. Ideally, CT/MRI fusion should be employed. The radiotherapy dose is specified to the ICRU reference point. In international studies, the prescribed dose is 54 Gy in 30 fractions of 1.8 Gy daily. For patients with a spinal cord primary requiring radiotherapy, the dose is 50.4 Gy in 28 fractions of 1.8 Gy.

Three-dimensional conformal planning can reduce the amount of normal brain within the irradiated volume, and has the potential for reducing long-term effects, an important priority for this group of patients who have a high chance of long-term survival. In future, it is planned to assess the impact of radiotherapy parameters on long-term intellectual and functional outcome.

High-grade astrocytoma (HGG)

Unlike adults, where HGGS comprise the most frequent group of primary CNS tumours, HGGs are uncommon in childhood. As with HGGs arising in adults, the outlook is generally very poor, and survival rates are currently approximately 20% at 5 years. Treatment is based on surgical resection and postoperative radiotherapy, generally 54 Gy in 30 fractions. There is no definite routine role for chemotherapy and, in recent studies, chemotherapeutic agents have been examined, given prior to radiotherapy in the form of a 'window' phase II study. An example of this is the recently opened UK/French phase II study of cisplatin and temozolamide (CISTEM). In this study, patients receive up to four cycles of chemotherapy prior to radiotherapy, in order to assess response and identify potentially useful chemotherapeutic agents.

Brainstem glioma

This group of brain tumours comprises a heterogeneous mix of tumours arising in the midbrain, pons and medulla. They are classified as focal (5–10%), dorsal exophytic (10–20%), cervico-medullary (5–10%) and diffuse intrinsic tumours (75–85%). Focal, dorsal exophytic and cervico-medullary tumours are generally low-grade astrocytomas. Surgical excision is the treatment of choice with radiotherapy reserved for inoperable tumours.

The majority of children with brainstem gliomas have diffuse intrinsic pontine gliomas which, when subject to biopsy, have generally been shown to be high-grade astrocytomas. They can be diagnosed by their typical MRI appearance (Figure *evolve* 33.12 🎵). A biopsy procedure, such as a stereotactic biopsy, is often considered to be risky and many consider this to be contraindicated. The prognosis for diffuse intrinsic pontine gliomas is very poor. Because of the frequent relatively short history of these tumours, radiotherapy often needs to be commenced quickly. Although radiotherapy results in improvement of neurological symptoms for approximately 70% of children, median survival is about 9 months and there are very few long-term survivors. The management of these children remains a major challenge, and domiciliary palliative care usually has to be introduced at a relatively early stage.

Patients are treated with a relatively straightforward technique with lateral opposed fields (Figure *evolve* 33.13 🎵). The CTV includes the GTV as defined on diagnostic MRI scan with a margin of 2 cm along potential areas of spread superiorly, inferiorly and posteriorly along brainstem. Patients are generally treated supine in a Perspex shell or thermoplastic shell (e.g. 'orfit') with conventional or CT simulation. The dose is specified to the ICRU reference point and the prescribed dose is 54 Gy in 30 fractions of 1.8 Gy daily.

Conventional radiotherapy provides useful palliation for approximately 70% of children with diffuse intrinsic pontine glioma. However, the progression-free survival is short, usually less than 6 months. Neither hyperfractionated nor accelerated radiotherapy has improved outcome for these patients. Current protocols are evaluating novel drug therapy approaches.

Ependymoma

Ependymomas arise from the intracranial or spinal ependyma. Historically, management was with surgical excision, followed by radiotherapy, which was generally craniospinal for those with posterior fossa primaries or high-grade histology. However, it is now generally recognized that, although there is a risk of leptomeningeal metastases at relapse, this risk does not appear to be modified by the use of craniospinal radiotherapy. The overall 5-year survival rate is approximately 50–60%. In the majority of studies, prognostic factors include the extent of resection and tumour grade. The predominant site of relapse is within the surgical bed, and current research efforts are aimed at improving the prospect of local tumour control. It is important to try to achieve a complete or near complete resection. The current European SIOP ependymoma study recommends that, for completely resected tumours, postoperative focal radiotherapy (54 Gy in 30 fractions) should be given and, for incompletely resected tumours, a trial of chemotherapy using vincristine, cyclophosphamide and etoposide. In North America, patients are treated with a higher dose, (59.4 Gy with conformal planning). In this study, the margin for CTV around the GTV, and/or resection cavity is 1.0 cm.

Medulloblastoma/PNET

Medulloblastoma is a primitive neuronal tumour which arises in the cerebellum, usually from the vermis. It is characterized by its propensity for metastatic spread via the CSF (leptomeningeal), its radiosensitivity and chemosensitivity. Primitive neuroectodermal tumour (PNET) arises elsewhere in the CNS, usually the supratentorial cerebral cortex but sometimes the pineal area (pineoblastoma). Although histologically identical to medulloblastoma, supratentorial PNET has a significantly worse prognosis (approximately 40–50% 5-year survival compared with 60–70% for medulloblastoma).

Medulloblastoma and other PNETs are managed by initial surgical resection followed by craniospinal radiotherapy and a 'boost' to the primary site. Until recently in the UK, the 'standard' approach was craniospinal radiotherapy, 35 Gy with a 20 Gy 'boost' to the primary site. Between 1992 and 2000, the European SIOP/UKCCSG PNET-3 study employed craniospinal RT 35 Gy in 21 daily fractions of 1.67 Gy with a primary tumour boost of 20 Gy in 12 daily fractions of 1.67 Gy. There was a randomization to this radiotherapy alone or preceded by four cycles of chemotherapy (vincristine and etoposide with alternating

Table 33.4 Medulloblastoma and PNET risk status

STANDARD RISK	HIGH RISK
Medulloblastoma with no evidence of leptomeningeal metastases on MRI scan and Less than 1.5 cm^2 residual tumour on postoperative MRI scan and No evidence of cells in CSF from lumbar puncture	Medulloblastoma with evidence of leptomeningeal metastases on MRI scan or cells in CSF from lumbar puncture or Supratentorial primary, any stage

cyclophosphamide and carboplatin). This study demonstrated a significant advantage for chemotherapy, and has also demonstrated the importance of avoiding gaps in the radiotherapy schedule.

Current treatment strategies for medulloblastoma are based on the allocation of risk status (Table 33.4). Since the 1990s, in North America, it has been standard practice to employ adjuvant chemotherapy (vincristine, CCNU, and cisplatin) following radiotherapy and this has now become standard practice in European studies. Using initial radiotherapy, it has been possible to reduce the dose of craniospinal radiotherapy for patients with standard-risk medulloblastoma in North American studies to 23.4 Gy, with 55.8 Gy to the posterior fossa. Because of the poor survival of patients with CSF metastases, all these children receive chemotherapy and 'standard dose' radiotherapy.

Studies of altered fractionation for medulloblastoma/PNET

Hyperfractionated radiotherapy (HFRT) involves the use of a larger number of small fractions usually delivered twice daily. Long-term normal tissue effects are related to fraction size and the aim of HFRT is to improve the therapeutic ratio by increasing the anti-tumour effect or reducing long-term effects on the CNS or a combination of both.

Promising results have been reported from small North American studies of HFRT employing craniospinal radiotherapy 36 Gy in 36 fractions of 1 Gy twice daily, and a total dose of 72 Gy in 72 fractions of 1 Gy twice daily to the posterior fossa. A multicentre French study, employing a craniospinal radiotherapy (CSRT) dose of 36 Gy and a primary tumour dose of 68 Gy has also produced encouraging early results. The use of HFRT is being evaluated further in the European PNET-4 randomized study. The aim of the PNET-4 study is to assess whether survival can be improved by the use of HFRT without an increase in long-term effects. 'Conventionally' fractionated radiotherapy, employing a craniospinal dose of 23.4 Gy followed by 30.6 Gy to the posterior fossa is compared with an HFRT regimen. The HFRT dose per fraction is 1 Gy given twice daily with a minimum interval of 8 hours. The craniospinal dose is 36 Gy, with a second phase of 24 Gy to the whole posterior fossa and a final phase of 8 Gy to the tumour bed.

Craniospinal radiotherapy (CSRT)

CSRT is one of the most complex radiotherapy techniques delivered in oncology departments. The shape of the clinical target volume is complex, including the entire cranial and spinal meninges. The technique employs lateral-opposed cranial fields, with one or more posterior spinal fields carefully matched onto the lower border of the cranial fields. Fields may be centred on outer canthus to minimize divergence into the contralateral lens. Shielding of face, dentition, nasal structures and lenses is necessary. Moving junctions between fields minimize the risk of overlap or underdose.

The CTV includes the intracranial and spinal meninges extending inferiorly to the lower border of thecal sac. Great care is taken to include the cribriform fossa, temporal lobe and base of skull. In children, the cribriform fossa frequently lies between the lenses (Figure *evolve* 33.14 🖱). In many series of patients treated for medulloblastoma, the cribriform fossa has been the site for isolated recurrence in a significant minority of patients. It may not always be possible to treat the CTV and adequately shield the lenses, in which case, priority is given to treating the CTV.

The lower border of the spinal field has generally been placed at the lower border of the second sacral vertebra. However, there is evidence that the lower border of the thecal sac varies and planning of the lower border of the spinal field should be based on MRI scanning. The spinal field should be wide enough to encompass the extensions of the meninges along the nerve roots, and therefore wide enough to encompass the intervertebral foramina in the lumbar region. The spinal field will typically be 5–7 cm wide. Patients are usually treated prone in a Perspex head shell, although craniospinal RT in the supine position is feasible. The body may also be immobilized, e.g. in an evacuated polystyrene bag. For cranial fields, the dose is specified to the mid-point of central axis. For spinal fields, the dose is specified to the anterior spinal cord. The prescribed dose depends upon clinical scenario. Currently, 23.4 Gy in 13 fractions of 1.8 Gy daily is employed for standard risk medulloblastoma in the European PNET-4 study.

CSRT techniques employed in individual departments will vary in details but are generally based on these standard principles. Meticulous attention to detail in the planning and delivery of CSRT is essential and accuracy contributes to the chances of cure of medullo-blastoma and other PNETs. It is essential to avoid areas of underdose at field junctions and partially shielding of any part of the intracranial or spinal meninges. The 'moving junction' between abutting fields is a 'safety measure', which reduces the risk of underdose or overdose in the cervical spinal cord if a systematic error develops during CSRT.

When planning the posterior fossa 'boost' for medulloblastoma, it is generally accepted that the CTV should encompass the meninges of the entire posterior fossa, because of the risk of infiltration of the meninges adjacent to the primary tumour. It has been standard to employ a standard field arrangement, with a parallel-opposed pair of fields. However, to avoid a higher dose in the neck, it is usually necessary to employ wedges as tissue compensators. In many centres, the posterior fossa 'boost' volume is planned using a posterior oblique field arrangement which can reduce the radiation dose to the inner ears.

CSRT techniques are continuing to evolve, and need to incorporate technical developments in radiotherapy immobilization, planning and treatment delivery. For the posterior fossa 'boost', it is possible to employ three-dimensional conformal planning to reduce the radiation dose to non-target structures, such as the hypothalamus and middle ear. 'Virtual simulation' has been used to define the target volume for CSRT in critical areas such as the cribriform fossa (see Figure *evolve* 33.14 🖱).

Intracranial germ cell tumours

Intracranial germ cell tumours (GCT) account for approximately 30% of paediatric GCTs and arise in the suprasellar or pineal regions. Germinomas are the histological counterpart of testicular seminoma and may arise in either the suprasellar or pineal regions. Non-germinomatous germ cell tumours, also known as secreting germ cell tumours, are the histological equivalent of testicular non-seminomatous germ cell tumours. They generally arise in the pineal region and may secrete alpha-fetoprotein (AFP) and/or human chorionic gonadotrophin (HCG).

Management of germinoma

In common with testicular seminoma, germinomas are very radiosensitive. The traditional view has been that CSRT should be employed because of the risk of leptomeningeal metastases and, with this approach, more than 90% of germinomas are cured. However, as with testicular seminoma, there has been a gradual reduction in both the CSRT dose and the dose used for the 'boost' to the primary tumour in an attempt to minimize long-term effects. In the current SIOP protocol, the CSRT dose is 24 Gy in 15 fractions of 1.6 Gy and the boost dose to the primary is a further 16 Gy in 10 daily fractions of 1.6 Gy. Germinomas

have a tendency for subependymal spread, which has to be taken into account when planning the boost volume. A margin of 2 cm around the gross tumour volume should be employed. For non-germinomatous tumours, the prognosis is worse. Initial treatment is with platinum-containing chemotherapy followed by radiotherapy, either focal for localized non-metastatic tumours or CSRT for those with leptomeningeal meningeal metastases. For secreting GCT, the total radiotherapy dose is 54 Gy to the primary tumour, with 30 Gy CSRT for patients with leptomeningeal metastases.

Craniopharyngioma

These account for approximately 5–10% of intracranial tumours in childhood. These are predominantly cystic tumours which arise in the suprasellar area from remnants of Rathke's pouch. Although considered histologically 'benign', they are often associated with considerable morbidity. They are associated with pituitary deficiencies, including diabetes insipidus and disturbances of hypothalamic function such as obesity. They are frequently adherent to adjacent structures within the CNS. There is a significant risk of involvement of the optic chiasm with a risk of visual impairment or blindness. Small cranipharyngiomas may be amenable to complete surgical excision if this can be achieved without a risk of damage to the optic chiasm. An alternative approach is to consider partial or subtotal excision of the tumour with postoperative radiotherapy. The margin for CTV around the GTV is generally approximately 0.5 cm, with a dose of 50–55 Gy in a fraction size of 1.67–1.8 Gy. With either complete resection or partial resection and postoperative radiotherapy, long-term local control rates of approximately 80% can be achieved.

Proton therapy for paediatric tumours

Proton therapy has been available for several decades in selected centres, mainly in North America. There is now increasing interest in developing centres in Europe. However, in the UK, there is no proton facility of sufficient energy to deliver therapy for deep-seated tumours such as those of the CNS or skull base. In recent years, there has been increasing interest in the potential role for proton therapy in the management of paediatric tumours. The modulated Bragg peak can deliver homogeneous irradiation to the target volume while reducing the magnitude and/or extent of the low dose area beyond. This may be clinically relevant for long-term effects in children. For several decades, proton therapy has had an established role in the treatment of adults with skull base chordomas and chondrosarcomas. This role has now been extended to the treatment of children. In addition, planning studies have demonstrated the potential for improving the therapeutic ratio for radiotherapy for tumours either within or adjacent to the CNS and by achieving a uniform dose within the target volume, while potentially minimizing the severity of neuropsychological sequelae. In several North American proton therapy centres, the role of proton therapy for craniospinal radiotherapy is under investigation.

CONCLUSIONS

Paediatric oncology management continues to present many challenges and radiotherapy plays an important role in the treatment of many of these children. They require the highest standard of radiotherapy planning and delivery, incorporating modern technical developments. Children present with a wide variety of malignancies which pose many different problems for patients themselves and their families. Thus, management needs to be family-centred as well as patient-centred. Although cure rates for the majority of childhood cancers have continued to improve over the last decade, this has frequently been achieved with increased intensity of chemotherapy. Compared with adult radiation oncology practice, when planning radiotherapy for children, consideration of the long-term effects of treatment is always of paramount importance. With the increasing use of concurrent combined modality therapy, including intensive chemotherapy, constant vigilance for interactions between chemotherapy and radiotherapy is required. Therapeutic developments initially investigated in adults, such as hyperfractionation, also require investigation for childhood cancers.

FURTHER READING

Malpas J, editor. Cancer in children. Br Med Bull 1996;52(4):671–81.

Pizzo PA, Poplack DG. Principles and practice of pediatric oncology. 4th ed. Lippincott, Williams and Wilkins; 2002.

Pinkerton CR, Plowman PN. Paediatric oncology – clinical practice and controversies. 2nd ed. Chapman & Hall; 1997.

Halperin EC, Constine LS, Tarbell NJ, Kun LE. Pediatric radiation oncology. 3rd ed. Raven Press; 1999.

Royal College of Paediatrics and Child Health. Guidance for services for children and young people with brain and spinal tumours. Royal College of Paediatrics and Child Health; 1997.

Walker DA, Perilongo G, Punt JAG, Taylor RE. Brain and spinal tumours of childhood. Arnold; 2004.

Wallace H, Green D. Late effects of childhood cancer. Arnold; 2004.

EVOLVE CONTENTS (available online at: http://evolve.elsevier.com/Symonds/radiotherapy/)

Chapter 34

Care of patients during radiotherapy

Cathy Meredith, Lorraine Webster

When patients are referred for radiotherapy, they will expect that their treatment is planned and delivered in an optimal way and, indeed, previous chapters have addressed the scientific and medical knowledge that underpins this process.

However, everyone involved in this provision is well aware that patients have a right to expect that they will be well cared for and supported during this time. The quality of this care is dependent on a multiplicity of factors and the aim should be that it is all encompassing; addressing both the physical and emotional needs of patients and this should be our aspiration whether the treatment intent is to cure or to palliate. The most simplistic method of exploring supportive care in radiotherapy is to consider any aspect of care that may be experienced by the patient within the physical, psychosocial and spiritual realm and this chapter will introduce some of the key themes within supportive care of all radiotherapy patients. The physical aspects of supportive care in relation to the management of site-specific conditions are addressed in related chapters throughout this text. In addition, these and the other aspects of care can be explored further in specialist texts which deal with issues relating to palliative care, symptom control and psychosocial interventions [1, 2].

The responsibility of assessing how patients are as they progress through treatment and how they are coping with their treatment belongs to all. As is an acknowledgement of where individual's skills/expertise start and stop and when patients should be cared for by more appropriate members of the team. It is to be recommended that radiotherapy centres adopt a culture which encourages both the philosophy and the mechanisms to facilitate such a team approach and this team approach should reach out to the interface between primary and secondary care. Coordination of care therefore needs patients and their carers to remain the focus of the process and this means that they should be kept informed and involved and that their autonomy and rights to be included in the treatment decision-making process is respected at all times.

ASSESSMENT OF INDIVIDUAL PATIENT AND CARER NEEDS

To provide care appropriate to patient need requires first assessing and establishing what that need is. Inadequate assessment of the patient's physical symptoms and psychosocial needs may lead to a failure to recognize their need, with the result that necessary services may be denied to them. However, one of the challenges for today's cancer care is that effective assessment is dependent on providing appropriate training and education for healthcare professionals to allow them to appreciate the complexity of support needs. This presents another challenge for cancer and radiotherapy services because, in many instances, there is a lack of available supportive care services for the healthcare professional to call on.

So what aspects of the patient's well being should be assessed? While it is vital that the needs of the patient, in respect of their medical and physical condition, are addressed, it is important that all healthcare professionals acknowledge that central to this process should be asking patients how they are feeling and coping from an emotional and psychological level. In doing this, consideration should be given to patients' and carers' needs in relation to:

- control and management of physical effects of treatment and disease and associated side effects
- evidence-based quality assured patient information materials, including written, DVD, and utilizing digital and web based technologies
- good communication and involvement in decision making
- psychological, social and spiritual support
- family and carer support
- complementary therapies
- bereavement support services.

Physical and psychological symptoms do not sit in isolation from each other and can, indeed, be synergistic. Patients have varying coping mechanisms and family support available to them and this is something that must be considered when supportive care is being addressed.

Patients' quality of life is affected not only by the physical and emotional impact of their cancer but also the treatments prescribed to treat their condition. Since radiotherapy causes a degree of damage to the normal tissues of the body and can cause local and systemic side effects, this aspect of their management should be considered of pivotal importance. These side effects can be acute or delayed, with acute (early effects) occurring during radiation treatment and continuing after treatment or in the weeks and months following. Although side effects of radiotherapy are to an extent unavoidable, they can be kept to a minimum if patients are well supported and appropriate advice is given as they progress through treatment. Such support and education should be an essential component of the management process for all patients receiving radiotherapy.

SKIN REACTIONS

One such side effect is the reaction of skin to radiotherapy. Although there have been recent advances in the technical delivery of radiotherapy which have resulted in the use of higher energy beams, customised treatment shapes and escalated dose, skin toxicity still remains a challenge. Indeed the situation may also be further enhanced with the increasing trend of combined adjuvent therapies. All patients receiving external beam therapy are at some risk of skin damage [3] and as such, in most departments this is addressed by offering suitable advice and support by monitoring and recording the severity of these reactions during treatment.

Skin reactions range from mild erythema to moist desquamation and occur more frequently in the head and neck area, breast and chest wall and areas with skin folds. The most widely used assessment tool is the Radiation Therapy Oncology Group grading (Table 34.1).

The severity of skin reactions has been attributed to a number of extrinsic (treatment related) and intrinsic (how people react to radiotherapy) factors [4] and these may well have a genetic basis. However, the goal of good management is to have a system in place which facilitates the identification of risk and delays the onset of skin reactions. This can be facilitated by having a patient review process that includes the assessment grading and recording of skin reactions.

Patients should be provided with information explaining:

- how and why skin reactions occur
- when they are likely to appear
- what they will look and feel like
- how they will be treated
- where the reaction is likely to occur
- self-care strategies
- risk factors.

Involving patients in the prevention/care of skin reactions is an important element of the management process and reducing irritants to irradiated skin is a part of this self-care strategy. Skin can be exposed to a number of irritants which, if avoided, can lessen the likelihood of a troublesome reaction (Table 34.2) [5, 6].

How to care for radiation skin reactions once they have occurred and what products to recommend in this

Table 34.1 Radiation Therapy Oncology Group grading of acute skin reactions				
RTOG 0	**RTOG 1**	**RTOG 2A**	**RTOG 2B**	**RTOG 3**
No visible change	Faint or dull erythema	Tender or bright erythema with/without dry desquamation	Patchy moist desquamation; moderate oedema	Confluent moist desquamation; pitting oedema

Table 34.2 Recommendations for reducing irritants to irradiated skin during a course of radiotherapy

Sun exposure	Protect from direct sun exposure: cover with clothing or shade area. Stress that risk from sun exposure is lifelong and following radiotherapy a sun block should always be used if exposure unavoidable
Mechanical irritants	Minimize friction: wash or shower gently; avoid using a washcloth; pat dry with a soft, clean towel; wear loose fitting, soft clothing Avoid shaving or shave causing as little trauma to skin as possible- suggest electric shaver Avoid scratching Avoid rubbing vigorously and massaging Avoid use of adhesive tape in treatment field
Chemical irritants	Use mild soap (un-perfumed) and rinse thoroughly Apply only recommended products- check with treatment centre. Any topical cream or lotion to be used at room temperature Avoid perfume, aftershave, deodorant Use mild detergent to wash clothing
Thermal irritants	Use tepid water Avoid exposure to temperature extremes Avoid application of ice packs or heat (e.g. heating pad, hot water bottles, sun lamp)

Table 34.3 Characteristics of skin-care products for each stage of radiation skin reactions

No change in skin (RTOG0)	No intervention required. Aqueous cream if desired (n.b. this will not prevent or delay skin reaction
Faint or dull erythema (RTOG 1)	Aqueous cream applied to skin within the treatment field - may soothe and moisturise skin
Tender or bright erythema (RTOG 2a)	Aqueous cream – may soothe and moisturise skin, relieve itching Hydrocortisone cream – can be used sparingly for up to one week, skin to be reviewed and documented daily
Patchy moist desquamation (RTOG 2b)	Dressings should be non adhesive Hydrogel and non adhesive dressings, soft polymer dressings, hydrocolloid dressings
Moist desquamation (Pitting oedema) (RTOG 3)	Dressings should be non adhesive Hydrogel dressings, hydrocolloid dressings, anti microbial dressings, polyurethane foam dressings

event requires a knowledge of the more general wound care literature. It is important that advice and treatment given to patients is evidence based and that advice such as 'no washing' is now seen as inappropriate. Sadly this remains an area which lacks robust evidence from the literature, which in turn, creates challenges when making recommendations, Table 34.3 provides some small detail of skin-care products which can be utilized.

Other sources which may be useful include published national skin-care guidelines [7]. When moist desquamation becomes infected or infection is suspected, use of a silver or iodine based antimicrobial dressing may be used. Care should be taken to ensure the dressing is designed to prevent silver being absorbed by the wound (check manufacturer's information) and the dressing should be removed daily before treatment.

NUTRITION

Guidance on nutritional status and diet for patients undergoing radiotherapy can impact positively on patients if it is undertaken in a routine and evidence-based manner.

The nutritional status of patients may be adversely affected by not only their disease but by the impact of their radiotherapy. Treatment-induced toxicities such as dry mouth, mucositis, dysphagia, nausea, vomiting, diarrhoea and tenesmus can all impact negatively on nutritional status and, ultimately, upon the quality of life of patients. In addition, when patients are referred for radiotherapy they may already have undergone surgical intervention, chemotherapy or both and they may also be receiving concomitant treatment that could exacerbate further their nutritional status. These factors and the possibility that food intake may be modified during radiotherapy makes it essential that sound nutritional advice and support is available.

Although radiotherapy will not have a significant adverse impact on the nutritional status of all patients, they still require sufficient nutrition to support tissue repair. Patients often have coexisting medical and social conditions that can affect nutritional status and it is important that these are recognized and their impact incorporated into nutritional planning.

There are particular areas where side effects of treatment commonly jeopardize nutritional status, e.g. head and neck, oesophagus, colorectal and pelvis/abdomen. It has been suggested that these patients and others require to be screened to identify those who need a more in depth nutritional assessment. A study by Ravasco et al [8] has demonstrated the benefits that can be gained when early intervention and proper assessment of nutritional status and requirements is undertaken alongside early nutritional counselling and monitoring of diet.

Advice to patients should, wherever possible, have an evidence base and will be dependent upon the area being treated, the regimen employed and a myriad of other factors. Treatment and advice to patients should therefore be tailored to suit their needs. However, it is essential that initial assessment of all patients is carried out, in order that appropriate action can be taken at a time when any condition can be more easily dealt with. Identifying the reason for the impaired nutrition is pivotal to its adequate treatment and, although dieticians are the key professionals, this is the responsibility of the multidisciplinary team. Patients should be sign posted to existing good quality sources of information.

NAUSEA, VOMITING AND DIARRHOEA

There is little doubt that the above can cause a significant threat to the comfort and well being of patients and thus affect quality of life. It is important that patients are monitored for the development of such side effects, that their severity is assessed and appropriate treatment instigated.

Side effects such as dehydration and weight loss as a consequence of diarrhoea are to be avoided and, although some patients may find it difficult to discuss, a comprehensive assessment of the condition is essential in order that the appropriate pharmacological therapy can be made available. Loperamide (Imodium) is a frequently used standby in the treatment of diarrhoea. Codeine phosphate is especially useful if diarrhoea is associated with colicky abdominal pain.

In relation to the prevention of nausea and vomiting, granisetron 2 mg orally an hour before radiotherapy can be a very good prophylaxis even for wide field radiotherapy and is much more effective than old antiemetics such as metoclopramide.

FATIGUE

One of the most common symptoms experienced by cancer patients is fatigue although, not until recently, has it begun to be given the attention it deserves. It is a multidimensional phenomenon which makes it difficult to describe. It has been attributed to both the illness, 'cancer-related fatigue' and, as it develops, the term 'radiotherapy-related fatigue' is used. The evidence to support a relationship between radiotherapy and fatigue is difficult to isolate but what is known is that it can and does adversely affect patients' quality of life. Patients can describe fatigue in many ways, describing feelings of tiredness, exhaustion,

lethargy and being overwhelmed by events. Patients should be advised that, although their treatment may cause tiredness, they should try to get enough rest and sleep and try to continue some of their daily activities. This and even some gentle exercise can help to achieve a healthy balance and can prevent patients ending up in a fatigue/lethargy cycle. Macmillan Cancer Support have recently been proactive in disseminating information, underpinned by research, promoting the advantages of exercise in helping alleviate side effects, fatigue and depression as well as overall health benefits.

PSYCHOSOCIAL ISSUES

It is crucial to remember that patients do not exist with a particular illness in isolation and that the dynamics of family and social relationships that may or may not exist within their own supportive networks may influence the content, context and ability to offer the desired or needed care. In short, the patient should rarely be considered in isolation and due thought and support should also be given to the needs of close family and carers, as they will also experience many similar feelings to those of our patients. The family is an extended agent of patient care and a cancer illness can have a profound effect not only on patients but on their relatives and, indeed, the process of a patient informing relatives of their illness can be traumatic for all concerned.

Many patients and carers experience a range of psychological and emotional challenges as a result of their diagnosis and subsequent treatment effects. Research suggests that the prevalence of long-term psychological distress in cancer patients ranges from 20 to 66% [9]. In addition, there are also the practical implications of illness, and a patient and their family may have difficulties in terms of their financial and employment status, as well as disruption caused by changes in their role and the family dynamics.

For the patient coming to terms with a cancer diagnosis, it has become helpful to think of their emotional adjustment as a series of different emotional stages. Barraclough [10] describes patients initially experiencing shock, numbness or disbelief, often with the bad news seeming 'too much to take in'. This usually short-term denial is then followed by distress as the reality of the situation becomes clear and is often associated with anger, anxiety, protest and bargaining. This phase often lasts a number of weeks and can be followed by sadness and depression again taking several weeks before gradual movement to adjustment and acceptance, taking weeks and even months.

Although this is a useful guide to apply to many situations associated with 'loss' of any kind, it is important to caution against using it as a simple sequential model of what every patient (and their carers) will experience.

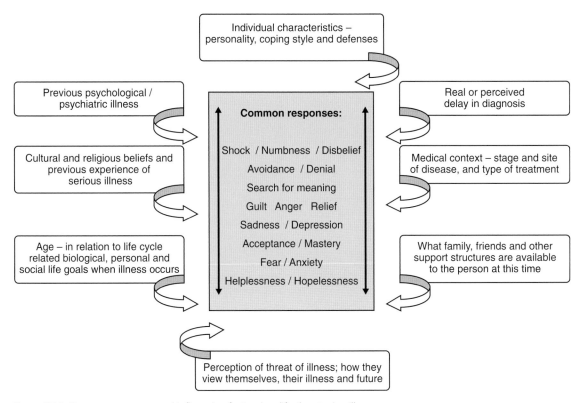

Figure 34.1 Common responses and influencing factors in a life-threatening illness.

Although many will react with some of the above emotions, we should not expect all to be initially shocked by a diagnosis and then work through all the stages to a final acceptance. Often there are more individual emotions and they may not occur in any clear order, or may overlap or may be gone through more than once, particularly in an illness that has remissions and relapses or a series of progressive deteriorations. Heightened anxiety and intensity of these emotions will occur most strongly at diagnosis, during treatment episodes and at times of recurrence and in terminal phase.

A summary of some of the common responses and influencing factors is illustrated in Figure 34.1, which aims to illustrate the dynamic that emotional adjustment changes through time, and is affected by many different factors which will be highly individualized for each patient. These reactions do not occur in any particular order and are particular to the individual who may move in and out of the different responses as the stimuli change.

COMMUNICATION

There is compelling evidence demonstrating that good, patient-centred communication is associated with important and meaningful health outcomes. The benefits of effective communication between healthcare professionals and patients include improvements in treatment compliance and satisfaction with their care and decision making as well as overall improvement in their psychosocial adjustment. In addition, it is important to highlight that a major effect of poor communication is dissatisfaction. When patients are dissatisfied and feel unable to speak freely, it has a negative effect on the likelihood that they will offer and seek the information necessary for a good informative exchange. The resultant effect of this is that the accurate exchange of information will be limited.

It must therefore be acknowledged that good communication is essential to allow patients and their carers to be involved with decisions about their care. Patients and carers place a lot of importance on face-to face communication with healthcare professionals and is the usual way information is given at crucial points in the patient's illness and treatment pathway. Indeed, the NHS cancer plan [11] cites that a 'willingness to listen and explain' is considered by patients to be one of the essential attributes of a health professional.

In addition, effective communication is central to the identification of an individual's specific needs and the provision of appropriate information and psychosocial support. Healthcare professionals also need to be sensitive to particular needs of each person in terms of awareness of issues of age, gender, culture and socioeconomic status.

Good communication also involves more than just being able to use the right words for a particular situation. It also requires an ability to listen and hear the person, and engage with them both emotionally and psychologically.

While all professionals involved in cancer care are increasingly aware of the need to interact effectively with patients, many feel inadequately trained in the various aspects of communication. There is also growing expectation from patients and their families that good communication is an essential component of their cancer treatment and care and it therefore becomes an important focus for all health professionals to judge whether they have addressed an individual patient or carers' communication and indeed information needs within any consultation or interaction.

INFORMATION

It is now widely accepted that seeking information is one strategy that many people use to help them cope with the challenges that a cancer diagnosis brings. The consensus would appear to be that the provision of appropriate, timely and honest information can make them feel more in control of their situation and can therefore be a key element for many people in managing the experience of cancer. In addition, there is evidence that the psychological distress in patients with serious illness is less when they think that they have received adequate information.

It is therefore important that any healthcare professional working with cancer patients should be attuned to the fact that patients are unlikely to have retained all the relevant information, particularly after one consultation. Hence, there is a need to assess this accurately and consistently repeat and reinforce this at subsequent consultations and visits for treatments.

Regardless of the amount of information retained, because patients tend to remember what they have been told first, rather than subsequent information, it can be difficult to undo any wrong perception and understanding of the patient and their carers in relation to this. It is therefore vital that there is consistency in explaining diagnosis, prognosis, treatment and effects. Consequently, it is exceptionally important that this is given accurately and not contradicted at a later date, by the same person or another member of the team.

However, it should be acknowledged that this remains an area of many challenges and tensions for all involved in working with patients with cancer for several reasons. While research has demonstrated that a majority of people want to be informed about all aspects of their disease and treatment, there is a responsibility also to be sensitive to the minority who do not. It is also important to acknowledge that patients' information needs will change through

time and that this needs to be judged at the level of the individual patient and carer need and should be assessed on an ongoing basis throughout the patient pathway. For example, a person's desire for information at the time of diagnosis may be very different at a time of relapse. Thus, the challenge is that it is vital that any information given is appropriate to an individual's personal needs and circumstances, therefore, when and how we communicate this information is crucial.

CONSENT

The NHS Plan [12] pledges that consent must be sought from all NHS patients. Both English and Scottish law state that before you examine, treat or care for competent adult patients you must obtain their consent. The Department of Health's Reference Guide to the consent process offers a comprehensive summary of the law on consent and offers help on frequently asked questions for both health professionals and patients (available at www.doh.gov.uk/consent). This provides a comprehensive guide and is usually well supplemented by individual health providers producing their own guidelines for use at a local level.

With respect to the issue of competence, as a general guide, the professional seeking consent should consider the question of whether a patient can understand and weigh up the information needed to make the required decision. It is also important to bear in mind that, if a patient reaches a decision that appears unexpected, it may not indicate incompetence, but rather a need for further information or explanation.

Thus, information giving is pivotal to underpinning a morally and ethically sound consent process. In essence, informed consent requires that patients have had their treatment options and procedures explained in a way that they can understand and, as patients are increasingly involved in their own healthcare, they need possession of the facts, including risks and benefits, to enable them to make decisions about their own treatment and care. This is important at all stages in the process but, particularly, at times when stages of illness and treatment options change. Indeed, the law regards giving and obtaining consent to be a process, not a one-off event and, therefore, must be valued as crucial in the treatment of cancer where different treatment options, such as further chemotherapy and radiotherapy, are required in the disease trajectory. It is also important to be aware that any patient may change their mind and withdraw consent at any time and this is applicable not only to those in clinical trials. As a general guidance point, if in any doubt, always check that the patient still consents to treatment.

With respect to explaining particular benefits and risks associated with treatment to patients, these will relate specifically to site and stage of disease as well as treatment intent and planned rationale. For example, whether radiotherapy is being combined with chemotherapy will affect not only outcome but early and late effects of treatment, as will whether the patient has had previous surgery. While the current Department of Health Guidelines state that patients should be advised on substantial or unusual risks of treatment, the detail of these for site-specific conditions are beyond the remit of this chapter. However, it is worth noting that many cancer centres now include specific details of both acute and late effects of treatment for specific cancers as an essential element in the consent process and this level of written detail can aid the professional seeking consent. In addition, it allows the patient to have time to reflect on many of the effects discussed and to give due consideration prior to actually consenting to treatment. The important message to get across to patients is one that should be balanced. That yes, indeed, radiotherapy does carry risks (and these should be explained individually for each patient and their related cancer) but must always be weighed up against the risks of not having any treatment at all. It should also be emphasized that, generally, the long-term risks tend to be rare and affect a very small number of people and that, generally, the benefits of radiotherapy treatment far outweigh the possibilities of involved risks.

In answer to the question of who should seek consent, it is advised that it is always best for the actual person who is in charge of treating the patient. However, it is deemed acceptable that consent may be sought on behalf of colleagues if the healthcare professional involved is capable of performing the procedure and can explain fully what the procedure involves or has been trained to seek consent for that procedure.

SPIRITUAL NEEDS

Over the last 20 years, the emphasis on spiritual care has become more acute, as has recognition that the spiritual dimension is important when patients and their carers face a life-threatening condition. Defining spirituality is challenging, to a degree it is intangible, but can be said to encompass those facets of an individual which give a sense of purpose and meaning to life. In essence, an awareness of the existential aspects of life and its meaning may be awakened. Contemporary medical literature supports the importance of spirituality for patients and proposes that strong spiritual beliefs can aid individuals fighting illness. It has been suggested that spiritual well being can have a positive effect on a patient's coping skills and their quality of life and can promote feelings of peace and acceptance, although there are those who identify the dangers of the spiritual challenge when patient's are asking 'Why me?'

Patients need to be supported to find coping mechanisms during their illness and the spiritual dimension may help in this process. There is a recognition that meeting spiritual need is important and policies to develop and implement spiritual care in our centres are now being advised. A study by Murray et al [13] concluded that 'spiritual issues were significant for many patients in their last year of life and their carers and that many health professionals lack the necessary time and skills to uncover and address such issues'.

Addressing patient's spirituality can be a challenge but communicating at this level can be a positive experience for healthcare professionals as well as patients.

COMPLEMENTARY THERAPIES

Complementary therapies do not offer patients an alternative approach to established treatments such as surgery, chemotherapy and radiotherapy but, as the name suggests, are designed to complement existing treatments. These therapies are diverse and varied and include self-help approaches, such as relaxation, meditation, visual therapies and touch therapies, such as aromatherapy, massage and reflexology, as well as more established practices of homeopathy and acupuncture.

While debate continues about the efficacy of many therapies, it has to be acknowledged that increasingly patients express an interest in their use and reports have indicated that up to one-third of patients with cancer have used complementary therapies [2]. While this debate is ongoing, and as demands for conventional reliable evidence for efficacy increases and research continues, the aim must be an acknowledgement among health professionals that patients will continue to search these therapies out. This means that we must be informed and open to dialogue with patients and their families. This is of particular importance, as some therapies patients may engage in may be viewed as more 'alternative' treatments which could possibly result in a tension with orthodox treatment and, indeed, there is growing concern among clinicians that sometimes their use can interfere with conventional treatments, such as chemotherapy or, indeed, produce harmful effects.

It should be recognized that the reasons given by patients for seeking out complementary therapies are varied and often relate to the perception that they are 'natural' and holistic, and that they will improve quality of life and help relieve the symptoms of both disease and the effects of treatment. They offer the patient a sense of personal involvement in their own care and often the feeling that they are taking some control of their disease. In addition, this form of treatment tends to a feeling of psychological empowerment as patients feel it allows them to cope better with their illness. So, while the reasons for seeking out complementary therapies are highly individual and may not be based on the same philosophical approach shared by many clinicians, they surely have to be regarded as personally valid for patients. Thus, the aims for heath professionals should first be to encourage disclosure by patients if they are using complementary therapies, and then to try to provide high quality information and opportunity for discussion that empowers patients to make their own decisions.

THE IMPACT ON STAFF

In cancer care, the main focus is justifiably on the needs of the patient and their families and friends. However, it is important to bear in mind that such care does not exist in a vacuum and can pose particular burdens for the health professionals involved. How we react to the pressures of caring is dependent on a multiplicity of factors but mainly our interpersonal resources, skills and life experiences. Indeed, many of the influencing factors that patients bring to coping with a diagnosis of a life-threatening illness (see Figure 34.1) also hold true for all of us in terms of our attitudes and beliefs and coping mechanisms as individuals, as well as our training, skills, knowledge and experience as healthcare professionals.

While this has historically been a rather neglected area, the issue of supporting the needs of those working with cancer patients is becoming more widely acknowledged within medicine and psycho-oncology and the levels and types of stress experienced by oncologists and other health professionals is becoming a growing area of interest and research.

There are particular different types of strategies for coping which can be aimed at dealing with preparing staff for many of the intense emotions they will be faced with.

Emotions such as anger, resentment, frustration and grief are often displayed by patients and their families, and communication skills training is particularly helpful and, indeed, desirable to help improve the situation for all concerned. It is also important to challenge unrealistic expectations of professional achievability. Often health professionals believe their task is to help people get better, however, in cancer care, it has to be accepted that this is not always possible. The juxtaposition between benefits and toxicities of treatment and concerns on the impact of quality of life for the patient and their close families can be issues of great concern and stress for staff which can result in significant emotional costs to those who feel unsupported in trying to meet these clinical demands.

Recognition and understanding of the emotional issues of health professionals working in cancer care is therefore important to help reduce the likelihood of stress. Attention must be paid to providing appropriate training in communication and coping strategies. In addition, multiprofessional team working should also aim to provide a supportive atmosphere and opportunity to allow staff to share their feelings and perceived difficulties in dealing with particular patient cases or situations which may present them with complex situations. This would allow them to draw on the expertise and support of others and negate any feelings of isolation and despondency.

Finally, it must be acknowledged that if health professionals are to work effectively with patients and families in cancer care, the emotional costs to them must be recognized, and not simply dismissed under the umbrella term of 'staff stress". Appropriate support mechanisms must be established to allow individuals to continue to offer high quality supportive care without this coming at the cost of staff stress and burn-out. In short, if we are to be able to care for our patients, we must also and perhaps first, be able to care for ourselves.

REFERENCES

[1] Faithfull S, Wells M. Supportive care in radiotherapy. Churchill Livingstone; 2003.

[2] National Institute for Clinical Excellence. Guidance on cancer services improving supportive and palliative care for adults with cancer: the manual. NICE; 2004.

[3] Maddocks Jennings W, Wilkinson JM, Shillington D. Novel approaches to radiotherapy-induced skin reactions: a literature review. Complement Therapy

Clinical Practice 2005;11 (4):224–31.

[4] Porock D, Kristjanson L, Nikoletti S, et al. Predicting the severity of radiation skin reactions in women with breast cancer. Oncol Nurs Forum 1998;25:1019–29.

[5] College of Radiographers. Summary of interventions for acute radiotherapy induced skin reactions in cancer patients: a clinical guideline. College of Radiographers; 2001.

[6] Glean E, Edwards S, et al. Interventions for acute radiotherapy induced skin reactions in cancer patients; the development of a clinical guideline recommended for use by the College of Radiographers. Journal of Radiotherapy in Practice 2001;2:75–84.

[7] Best Practice Statement NHS Quality Improvement Scotland (2010) www.nhshealthquality.org.

[8] Ravesco P, Monteiro-Grillo I, et al. Does nutrition influence quality of

life in cancer patients undergoing radiotherapy. Radiother Oncol 2003;67:213–20.

[9] Zabora J, BrintzenhofeSzock K, Curbow B, et al. The prevalence of psychological distress by cancer site. Psychooncology 2001;10:19–28.

[10] Barraclough J. Cancer and emotion. A practical guide to psycho-oncology. 3rd ed. John Wiley & Sons; 1999.

[11] Department of Health. The NHS cancer plan. HMSO; 2000.

[12] Department of Health. The NHS plan. HMSO; 2000.

[13] Murray SA, Kendall M, Boyd K, Worth A, Benton TF. Exploring the spiritual needs of people dying of lung cancer or heart failure: a prospective qualitative interview study of patients and their carers. Palliat Med 2004;18:39–45.

Chapter | 35 |

Medical complications of malignant disease

Robert Coleman

Cancer can cause a wide variety of medical and metabolic problems. These can be due to the physical presence of the tumour causing obstruction of, for example, the bile duct or a ureter, secretion of fluid into a body cavity, such as the pleura (an effusion), or local invasion of adjacent structures. Cancer and its treatment frequently predispose the patient to infection. In addition, cancer may cause constitutional disturbances which are not due to the local effect of the tumour but the consequence of secreted tumour products resulting in paraneoplastic syndromes. The problems of invasion into neighbouring structures are discussed in Chapter 15. In this chapter, we discuss the problems caused by effusions, infection and paraneoplastic syndromes (Table 35.1) in malignancy.

EFFUSIONS SECONDARY TO MALIGNANT DISEASE

Normally, the pleural, pericardial and peritoneal spaces contain only a few millilitres of fluid to lubricate the inner and outer surfaces of these membranous coverings. However, in cancer, the normal capillary and lymphatic vessels can become damaged and the hydrostatic pressures which regulate the transfer of fluid from one compartment of the body to another disturbed. A build-up of fluid at any of these three sites can cause unpleasant symptoms which may require treatment. Although effusions are usually a sign of advanced malignancy and treatment is only palliative, intervention is usually indicated as it can provide useful clinical benefit and improvement in quality of life.

Pleural effusions

The commonest malignancy to cause a pleural effusion is carcinoma of the bronchus. In addition, metastasis from carcinoma of the breast, other adenocarcinomas and lymphoma may also be implicated. Clinical detection is not possible until at least 500 ml has accumulated and, typically, a symptomatic effusion comprises 1000–4000 ml of fluid. This is usually straw coloured but may be blood stained and will cause increasing shortness of breath, a dry cough and sometimes pain as it increases in size. Diagnosis is usually made clinically and confirmed by chest x-ray. Ultrasound may occasionally be required to distinguish pleural fluid from a solid pleural mass.

Table 35.1 Endocrine and paraneoplastic manifestations of malignancy

SYSTEM	MANIFESTATION
Endocrine	Hypercalcaemia due to parathyroid hormone related peptide Water retention due to inappropriate ADH secretion Cushing's syndrome due to ACTH Hypoglycaemia due to insulin-like proteins/somatomedins Gynaecomastia due to human chorionic gonadotrophin Thyrotoxicosis due to human chorionic gonadotrophin
Neurological	Peripheral neuropathy Cerebellar ataxia Dementia Transverse myelitis Myasthenia gravis Eaton–Lambert syndrome
Haematological/vascular	Anaemia Thrombophlebitis Thromboembolism Disseminated intravascular coagulation Polycythemia Non-bacterial endocarditis Red cell aplasia
Musculoskeletal	Polymyalgia rheumatica Arthralgia Clubbing Hypertrophic pulmonary osteoarthropathy
Dermatological	Pruritus Various skin rashes
Renal	Nephrotic syndrome

Drainage of the fluid is required for relief of symptoms. This can be performed through a needle inserted into the pleural space, which provides good emergency management but, to prevent recurrence of the effusion, either effective treatment of the underlying cancer is required or the effusion should be drained to dryness and a pleurodesis performed. To achieve this, a flexible drainage tube needs to be inserted into the pleural space and the fluid allowed to drain via a sealed drainage system which prevents air from replacing the fluid. Increasingly often this is now performed with ultrasound guidance to reduce the risk of damage to underlying organs, and is particularly useful to identify the optimum site for drainage when the effusion is loculated. Drainage should be relatively slow as sudden removal of large volumes of fluid causes distress to the patient due to shift of the mediastinal structures, and this may precipitate acute pulmonary oedema. After 24–48 hours, when the effusion has drained to dryness, it is usual to inject a drug or chemical into the pleural space to effect a pleurodesis. This will inflame the pleural surfaces to encourage sticking together of the two layers and the development of fibrosis.

Tetracycline and bleomycin were the most commonly used agents for ward-based pleurodesis and will prevent recurrence of the effusion in 50–75% of patients. However, today, there is a much lower threshold for referral to a thoracic surgeon for drainage of the pleural fluid under general anaesthetic, breaking down of any adhesions causing loculation and insufflation of talcum powder. Overall, this more radical approach is more effective and probably both safer and more comfortable for the patient than traditional ward-based pleurodesis.

Pericardial effusions

These are much less common than pleural effusions. Again, the same tumour types are usually responsible, but probably less than 1% of cancer patients will develop a symptomatic collection of pericardial fluid. When this does occur, the build-up of fluid restricts normal cardiac function and produces symptoms and signs of cardiac failure, first affecting the right ventricle, which as it worsens subsequently impairs left ventricular function, resulting in a clinical syndrome referred to as cardiac tamponade.

Patients with tamponade are unable to lie flat, have chest discomfort, oedema and breathlessness. The diagnosis is made on the basis of clinical signs and confirmed by cardiac echocardiography. When cardiac tamponade develops, urgent drainage of the pericardial fluid can be life saving and generally indicated unless the patient is in the very terminal phases of the disease process. Pericardial drainage is technically more difficult than pleural drainage and is best performed by a cardiologist with ultrasound control to ensure safe placement of the drainage catheter. Ward-based pericardial drainage with electrocardiographic monitoring to identify contact between the drainage needle and myocardium is no longer recommended. Treatment of the underlying malignancy will usually prevent recurrence but, if this is not possible, injection of sclerosants into the pericardial space is occasionally advised, although the evidence base for this approach is limited. To prevent recurrent pericardial effusions, the formation of a pericardial window by a thoracic surgeon is preferred if the general condition of the patient makes this a realistic option.

Peritoneal effusions (ascites)

In cancer, ascites is usually caused by widespread peritoneal seedling metastases which exude protein-rich fluid. Liver metastases may contribute to the problem through hypoalbuminaemia or portal hypertension. Ascites is most commonly caused by advanced carcinomas of the ovary, gastrointestinal tract, breast and pancreas. Patients present with abdominal distension which becomes progressively uncomfortable, limits food intake and splints the diaphragm, making breathing difficult. Diagnosis is by clinical examination and is confirmed by ultrasound and aspiration cytology.

Treatment by tube drainage (paracentesis) and ultrasound-guided catheter insertion, or at least marking of a safe and appropriate position to insert the drain, is generally recommended to reduce the risk of bowel perforation. Drainage of the fluid should be performed relatively slowly, generally not exceeding a rate of 500 ml/hour. Drainage to dryness of ascites is not realistic and therefore sclerosants are much less effective for ascites than for pleural effusions. Diuretics are commonly prescribed to prevent reaccumulation, but are rarely effective in relieving established ascites. Intraperitoneal radioactive colloids or chemotherapy are sometimes of benefit and agents such as thiotepa, mitoxantrone (mitozantrone) and carboplatin have all been used with some success. For recurrent ascites, surgical procedures should be considered if medical treatments have failed to control the underlying disease. A peritoneovenous shunt can be inserted, which drains the fluid through a one-way valve into the venous system. Interestingly, despite drainage of large numbers of malignant cells into the circulation, metastatic disease in the lungs and other sites do not appear to be more common.

The most effective method of controlling ascites though is treatment of the underlying malignancy. Ascites can be abolished often in ovarian cancer as response rates are high but may be more difficult to control in gastrointestinal tumours as response rates to chemotherapy are comparatively low.

METABOLIC AND ENDOCRINE MANIFESTATIONS OF MALIGNANCY

Hypercalcaemia

Hypercalcaemia is a complication in around 5% of patients with advanced malignancy, and is particularly common in patients with carcinomas of the breast, lung and multiple myeloma. Three mechanisms are involved. First, metastatic cancer cells in bone stimulate osteoclasts, the normal bone cells which resorb (break down) bone, to destroy bone faster than the osteoblasts, the normal bone cells which build bone, can repair the damage. Secondly, the tumour may secrete proteins, such as parathyroid hormone related protein (PTHrP) into the circulation, which have similar destructive effects on bone but also promote the kidney to reabsorb more calcium from the urine than is appropriate. Finally, dehydration, which occurs due to the diuretic effect of an increased calcium load on the kidney, makes the situation worse, and tubular damage to the kidney, as commonly occurs in multiple myeloma, may also be important.

Hypercalcaemia causes many symptoms, including lethargy, nausea, thirst, constipation and drowsiness. Because the symptoms are non-specific and commonly encountered in many patients with advanced cancer, the diagnosis can be easily missed. As a result, a high index of suspicion is required. Often, however, the diagnosis is identified by routine biochemical testing which usually includes measurement of serum calcium. The level of serum calcium that causes symptoms varies from one patient to another and according to the speed of onset. Patients are better able to tolerate slowly developing hypercalcaemia than a sudden rise. However, most patients will have symptoms when the serum calcium exceeds 3.0 mmol/L.

Appropriate treatment will rapidly improve the patient's condition and relieve the unpleasant symptoms. This can be reliably achieved without side effects by rehydration of the patient and inhibition of bone breakdown by one of the class of drugs called bisphosphonates. Rehydration should be with normal saline and will typically require 3–6 litres over 24–48 hours. Rehydration reduces the serum calcium somewhat and relieves many of the symptoms, but is rarely sufficient treatment and the benefits are usually short lived over a matter of a few days. A single, short infusion of one of the potent bisphosphonates that are now available will restore the serum calcium to normal in around 90% of patients with a duration of action of around 3–4 weeks. Zoledronic acid is the most commonly used agent and has the highest probability of success, but pamidronate, ibandronate and clodronate are also effective in the majority of cases. Repeated infusions are usually required every 3–4 weeks unless successful systemic therapy can be instituted. For this reason, patients should be closely monitored every few weeks following a diagnosis of hypercalcaemia. Recurrent hypercalcaemia despite regular bisphosphonates has a very poor prognosis and may be a terminal event.

Inappropriate secretion of antidiuretic hormone (ADH)

This syndrome results in retention of fluid by the kidney and is characterized by a low serum sodium. This causes weakness and confusion, occurring most commonly in patients with small cell lung cancer. Treatment is by fluid restriction, drugs such as demeclocycline which inhibit the action of ADH, and chemotherapy for the underlying malignancy.

Other endocrine manifestations of malignancy

Many cancers produce hormones and peptides with biological activity. These include adrenocorticotrophic hormone (ACTH), which may result in the features of

Cushing's syndrome, hypoglycaemia from production of insulin-like substances and gynaecomastia from tumour production of human chorionic gonadotrophin (HCG).

Hyperuricaemia and tumour lysis syndrome

An acute metabolic disturbance may result from the rapid destruction of a tumour following chemotherapy. This is particularly likely to occur in childhood leukaemia and rapidly growing lymphomas or germ cell malignancies. As chemotherapy destroys the cancer, the cells release products of nitrogen metabolism, especially urea and urate, plus large amounts of potassium and phosphate into the circulation. The high urate concentration may result in urate crystal formation in the kidneys and lead to acute renal failure. A high potassium level is the most dangerous component of tumour lysis syndrome and may cause cardiac dysrhythmias and even sudden death. An increased phosphate level may complex with calcium and result in tetany. The syndrome can be prevented by prescribing allopurinol (or an intravenous equivalent) to prevent the production of large amounts of urate and intravenous fluids to encourage the kidneys to excrete the products of cell breakdown. Ideally, these interventions should be commenced a day or two before chemotherapy.

INFECTION

Infections are a major cause of death in cancer. Not only do they occur frequently, but they are often more severe than in other patients, less responsive to therapy and often related to organisms which, in normal health, would not cause any problem. The susceptibility of cancer patients to infection results from suppression of host defence mechanisms produced by the disease and its treatment. Infections are particularly frequent when the neutrophil count is suppressed by chemotherapy.

Advanced cancer and the treatments prescribed are associated with impaired neutrophil and lymphocyte function, depressed cell-mediated and humoral immunity, and damage to skin and mucous membranes, which allows organisms to enter the bloodstream more easily. *Escherischia coli*, pseudomonas, staphylococci and streptococci are the most frequent bacterial pathogens. Viruses, such as herpes simplex and herpes zoster (shingles), fungi, particularly *Candida*, and protozoal infection of the lungs with pneumocystis are important non-bacterial causes of infection requiring specific treatment. Most of the infecting organisms come from within the patient, for example gut bacteria and, providing sensible precautions are taken with regards to personal hygiene, infections transmitted from family or healthcare staff are of relatively minor importance.

If patients are infected while neutropenic, urgent admission to hospital is usually required, blood and urine cultures taken and, where clinically indicated, sputum, throat or wound swabs sent for culture. Treatment with broad-spectrum intravenous antibiotics should be commenced immediately after taking the necessary cultures, as untreated septicaemia can be rapidly fatal. The choice of antibiotics varies according to the clinical situation and individual hospital policy and may change from year to year as directed by the type of local pathogens and patterns of resistance. In some patients, intravenous fluids, inotropic support and high dependency care may be required. Occasionally, even in specialist cancer centres and despite efficient and aggressive treatment of infection, patients still die from overwhelming infection following chemotherapy.

PARANEOPLASTIC SYNDROMES

Neurological

Cancers, particularly of the bronchus, are associated with a number of neurological syndromes which are unrelated to direct compression or infiltration of neural tissue. The mechanisms that give rise to these problems are poorly understood. They are uncommon, and usually are possible to diagnose only by excluding the presence of malignant disease in the central nervous system or around nerve roots. The syndromes include numbness and weakness due to sensory and motor peripheral neuropathies respectively, paralysis from spinal cord damage, unsteadiness from cerebellar degeneration, dementia from cerebral damage and a form of muscle weakness which resembles myasthenia gravis. These neurological conditions may be the first manifestation of cancer. Sadly, treatment for the underlying cancer frequently fails to produce much neurological improvement.

Hypertrophic pulmonary osteoarthropathy

Lung cancer is the principal cause of this condition in which the bones of the forearms and shins become inflamed and painful. Plain radiographs show characteristic appearances and usually the patient has a deformity of the nails known as clubbing. Anti-inflammatory drugs relieve many of the symptoms and the condition may improve if the underlying tumour can be removed or destroyed.

Other paraneoplastic syndromes

A variety of general effects of cancer are sometimes described as paraneoplastic phenomena, and almost every organ in the body can be affected by one of these syndromes. Fever, cachexia, anaemia, thrombophlebitis and clotting disorders are all relatively common and may be the presenting symptoms of malignancy. In addition, arthritis, skin rashes, itching, muscle inflammation and renal impairment are uncommon but well-recognized complications of malignant disease. Each should be treated symptomatically while the increased risk of thromboembolism may warrant prophylactic anticoagulation.

FURTHER READING

Gushchin V, Demmy TL, Kane 3rd JM. Surgical management of metastatic peritonael or pleural disease. Semin Oncol 2007;34:215–25.

Luh SP, Chen CY, Tzao CY. Malignant pleural effusion treatment outcomes: pleurodesis via video-assisted thoracic surgery (VATS) versus tube thoracostomy. J Thorac Cardiovasc Surg 2006;54:332–6.

Tsang TS, Enriquez-Sarano M, Freeman WK, et al. Consecutive 1127 therapeutic echocardiographically guided pericardiocenteses: clinical profile, practice patterns, and outcomes spanning 21 years. Mayo Clin Proc 2002;77:429–36.

Becker G. Medical and palliative management of malignant ascites. Cancer Treat Res 2007;134:459–67.

Percherstorfer M, Brenner K, Zojer N. Current management strategies for hypercalcemia. Treat Endocrinol 2003;2:273–92.

Picazo JJ. Management of the febrile neutropenic patient: a consensus conference. Clin Infect Dis 2004;39 (Suppl. 1):S1–6.

Gemici C. Tumour lysis syndrome in solid tumours. Clin Oncol 2006;18:773–80.

Storstein A, Vedeler CA. Paraneoplastic neurological syndromes and onconeural antibodies: clinical and immunological aspects. Adv Clin Chem 2007;44:143–85.

Ellison DH, Berl T. Clinical practice. The syndrome of inappropriate antidiureses. N Engl J Med 2007;356:2064–72.

Index

Note: Page numbers followed by *b* indicate boxes, *f* indicate figures and *t* indicate tables.